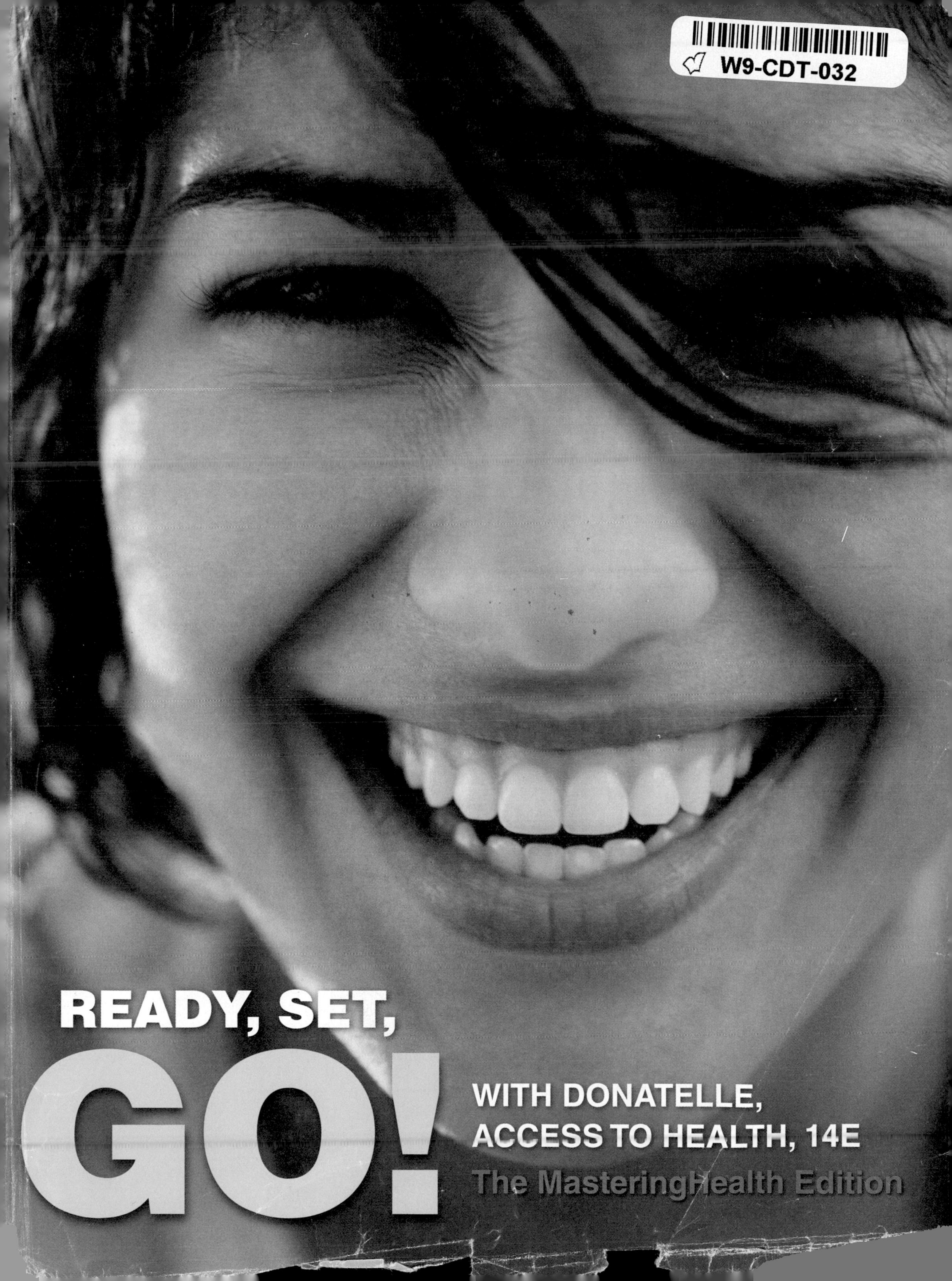

READY, SET, GO!

WITH DONATELLE, ACCESS TO HEALTH, 14E

The MasteringHealth Edition

GET YOUR **STUDENTS READY!**

Today's students expect their course materials to integrate text and media and to support interactive ways of learning that bring health concepts to life and make clear why those issues matter. With the MasteringHealth Edition of *Access to Health*, YOU have the the tools to help your students to effectively learn and master health concepts, both in the text and through online practice, and to apply those concepts to their daily lives.

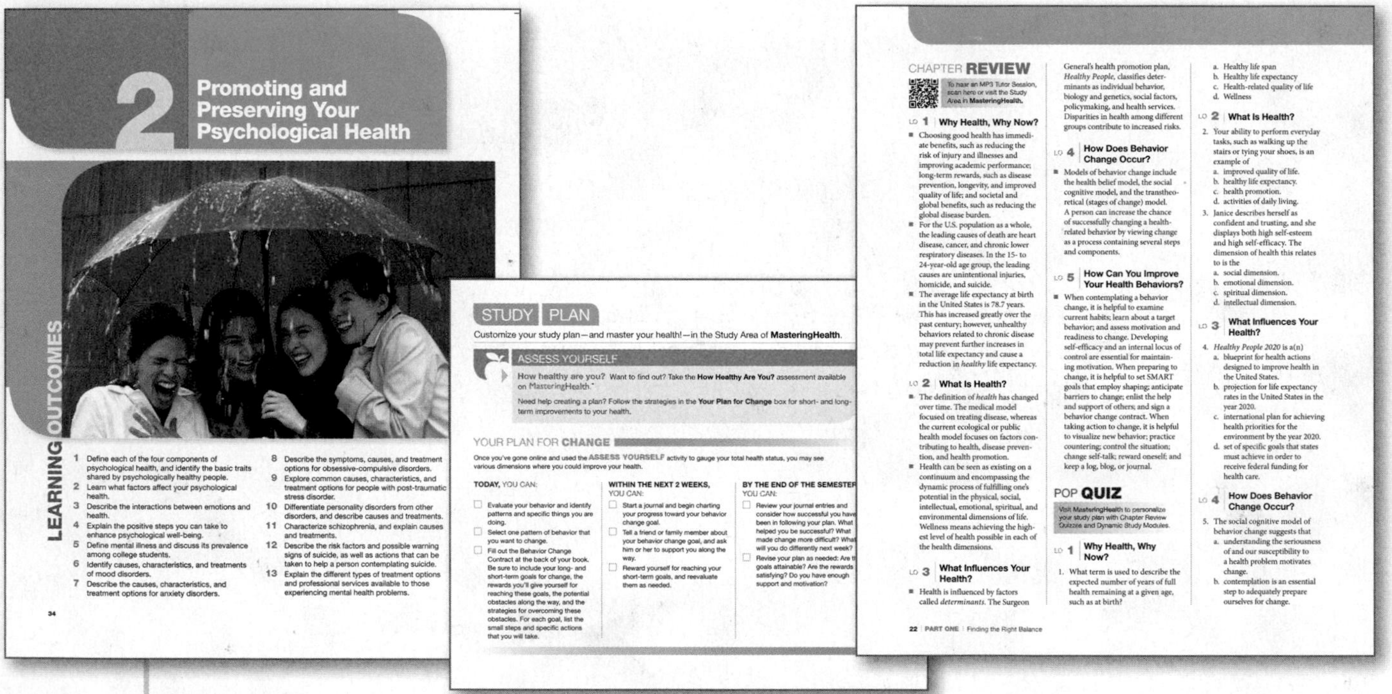

NEW! **Learning Outcomes and Study Plan**

Numbered learning outcomes (LOs) now introduce every chapter, giving students a roadmap for their reading. Each chapter concludes with a Study Plan, which summarizes key points of the chapter and provides review questions and critical thinking questions to check understanding, all tied to the chapter's learning outcomes and assignable in MasteringHealth.

Barbara Lamagna
Personal & Community Health

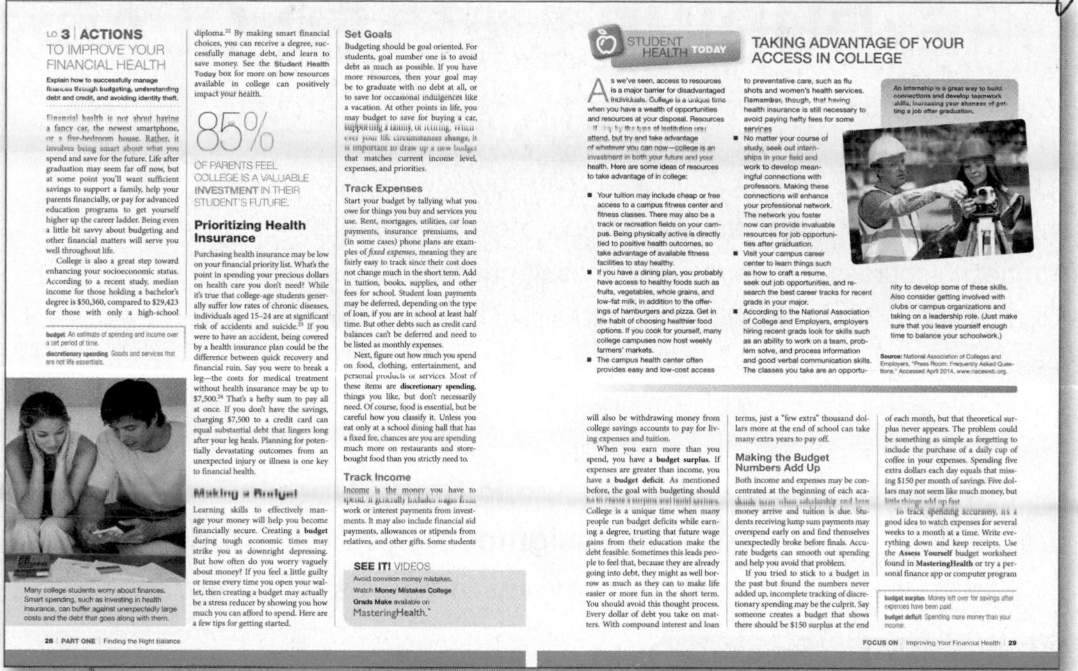

NEW! **Focus On: Improving Your Financial Health**

A new mini-chapter addresses the practical skills that students need to improve their financial health, from building a budget to understanding student loans. The mini-chapter also examines the connection between finances and health, including stress, nutrition, and more.

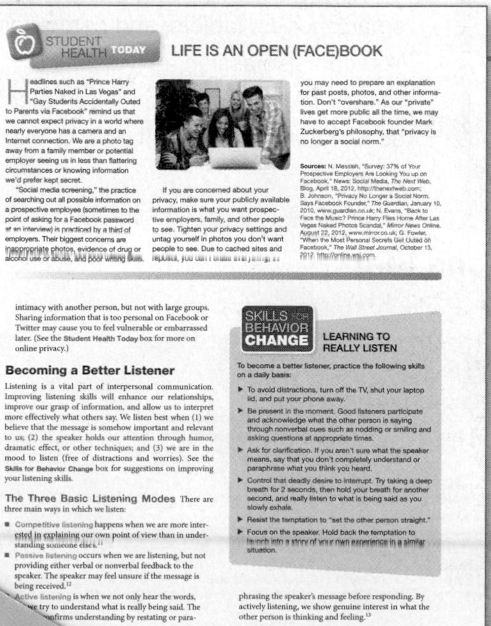

UPDATED!

Cutting-edge coverage of hot topics

Current health issues are covered throughout the new edition, speaking to students' questions and concerns. New and updated material covers such areas as the Affordable Care Act, gender differences in responses to stress, technology and sleep, learning disabilities, social media, "empty calorie" foods, apps to help smokers quit, marijuana legalization, new diabetes treatment options, rates of HPV vaccination, probiotics, "hook-up" culture, the relationship between violence and the media, and more.

GET YOUR **STUDENTS GOING** WITH MasteringHealth™ BEFORE, DURING & AFTER CLASS

Mastering is the most effective and widely used online homework, tutorial, and assessment system for the sciences and now includes content specifically for health courses. Mastering delivers self-paced tutorials that focus on your course objectives, provides individualized coaching, and responds to each student's progress.

BEFORE CLASS

Dynamic Study Modules and Pre-Class Assignments provide students with a preview of what's to come.

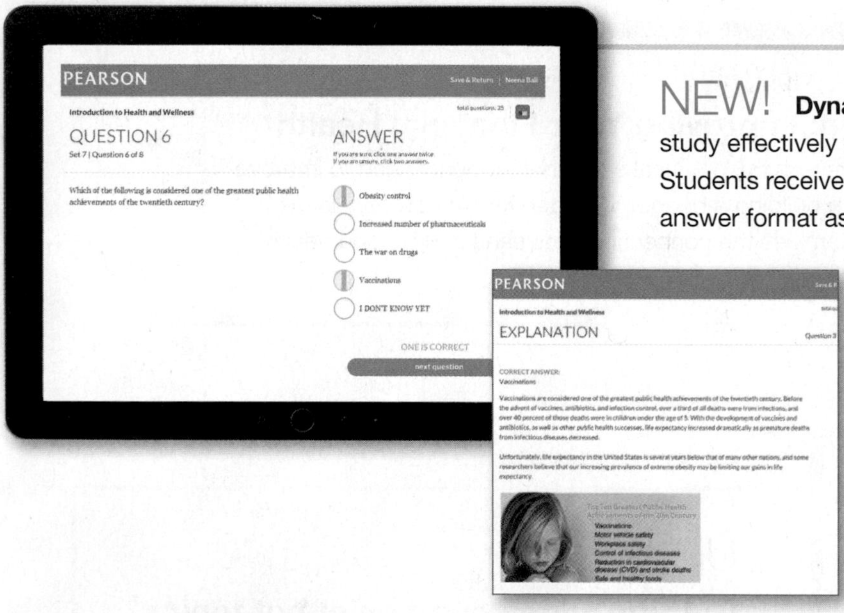
PEARSON
Introduction to Health and Wellness
QUESTION 6
Set 7 | Question 6 of 8
ANSWER
Which of the following is considered one of the greatest public health achievements of the twentieth century?
Obesity control
Increased number of pharmaceuticals
The war on drugs
Vaccinations
I DON'T KNOW YET
ONE IS CORRECT
next question
PEARSON
Introduction to Health and Wellness
EXPLANATION

NEW! **Dynamic Study Modules** enable students to study effectively on their own in an adaptive format. Students receive an initial set of questions with a unique answer format asking them to indicate their confidence level.

Once completed, Dynamic Study Modules include explanations using materials taken directly from the text. These modules can be accessed on smartphones, tablets, and computers. You can also assign an individual Dynamic Study Module for completion as a graded assignment prior to class.

MasteringHealth offers Pre-Lecture Quiz Questions that are easy to customize and assign.

NEW! **Reading Questions** ensure that students complete the assigned reading before class and understand the reading material. Reading Questions are 100% mobile ready to give students extra flexibility for study time.

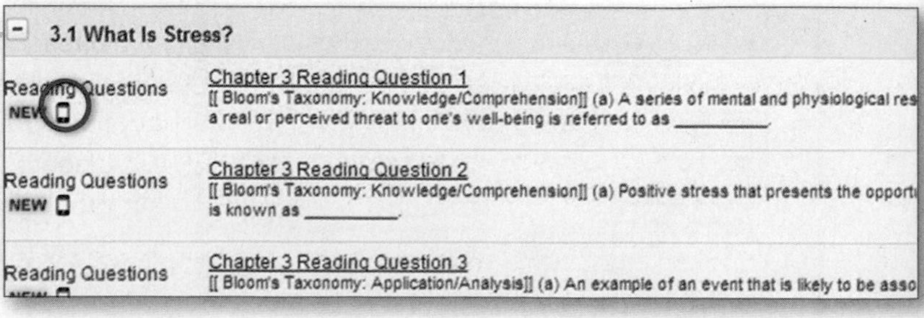
3.1 What Is Stress?
Reading Questions
Chapter 3 Reading Question 1
[[Bloom's Taxonomy: Knowledge/Comprehension]] (a) A series of mental and physiological res
a real or perceived threat to one's well-being is referred to as ________.
Reading Questions
NEW
Chapter 3 Reading Question 2
[[Bloom's Taxonomy: Knowledge/Comprehension]] (a) Positive stress that presents the opport
is known as ________.
Reading Questions
Chapter 3 Reading Question 3
[[Bloom's Taxonomy: Application/Analysis]] (a) An example of an event that is likely to be asso

DURING CLASS

Learning Catalytics™ and Engaging Media

What has professors and students so excited? Learning Catalytics, a "bring your own device" student engagement, assessment, and classroom intelligence system, allows students to use their smartphones, tablets, or laptops to respond to questions in class. With Learning Catalytics, you can:

- Assess students in real-time using open-ended question formats to uncover student misconceptions and adjust lectures accordingly.
- Automatically create groups for peer instruction based on student response patterns, to optimize discussion productivity.

> "My students are so busy and engaged answering Learning Catalytics questions during lecture that they don't have time for Facebook."
>
> Declan De Paor
> *Old Dominion University*

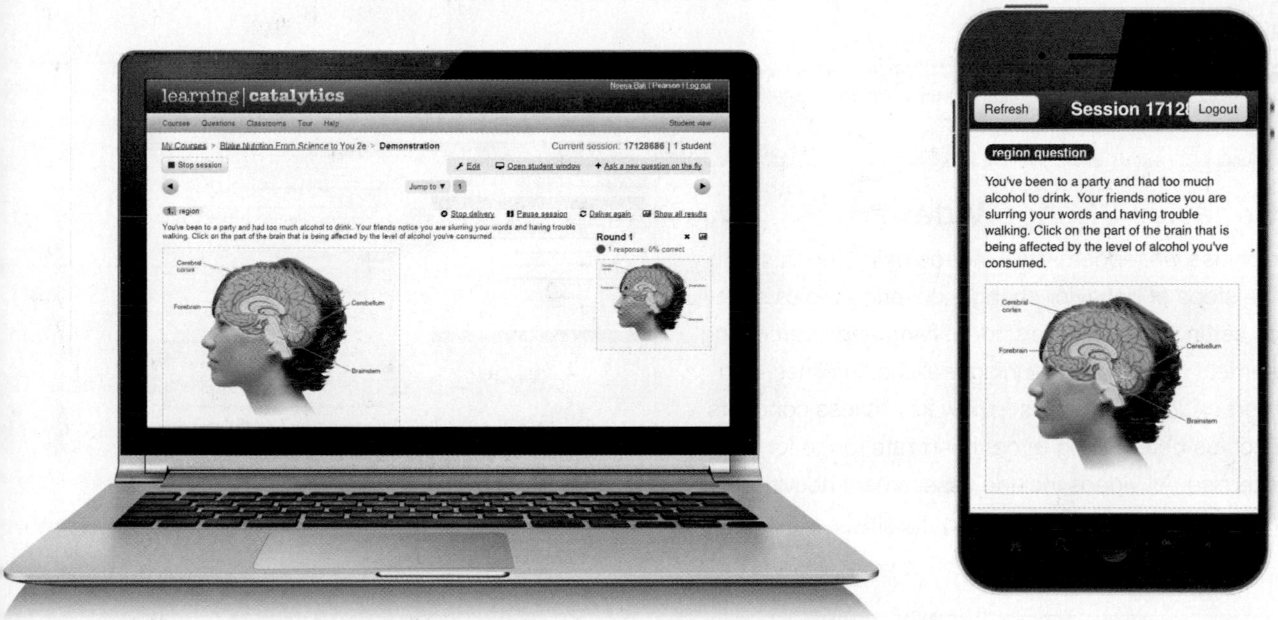

Engaging In-Class Media

Instructors can also incorporate dynamic media from the **Teaching Toolkit DVD** into lecture and build class discussions and activities around *ABC News* Lecture Launchers, Video Tutors, and more. For more information, please see the last page of this walkthrough.

MasteringHealth™

AFTER CLASS

Easy-to-Assign, Customizable, and Automatically Graded Assignments

The breadth and depth of content available to you to assign in MasteringHealth is unparalleled, allowing you to quickly and easily assign homework to reinforce key concepts.

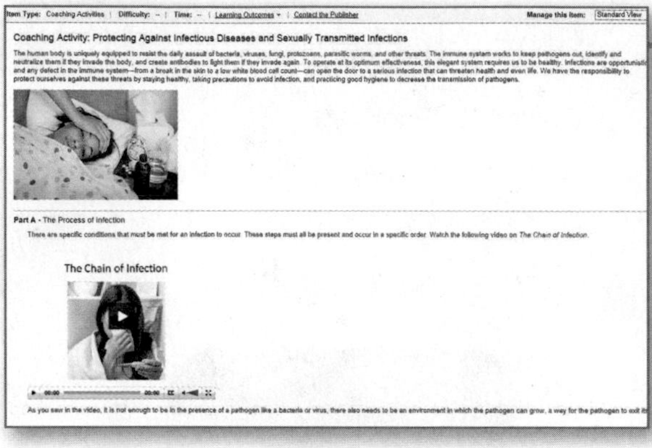

Health and Fitness Coaching Activities

Coaching activities guide students through key health and fitness concepts with interactive mini-lessons that provide hints and feedback.

Behavior Change Videos

Concise whiteboard-style videos help students with the steps of behavior change, covering topics such as setting SMART goals, identifying and overcoming barriers to change, planning realistic timelines, and more. Additional videos review key fitness concepts such as determining target heart rate range for exercise. All videos include assessment activities and are assignable in MasteringHealth.

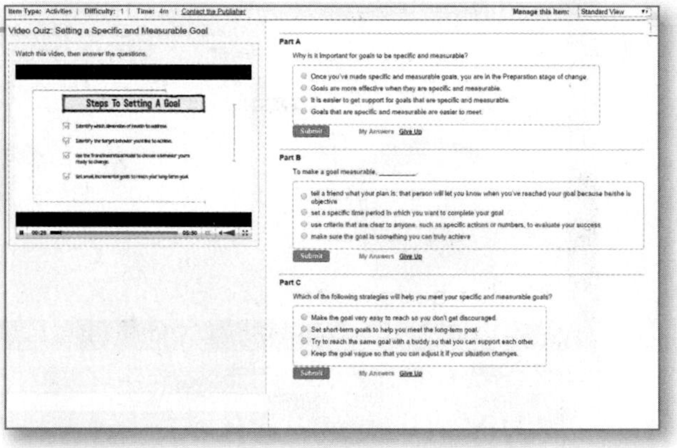

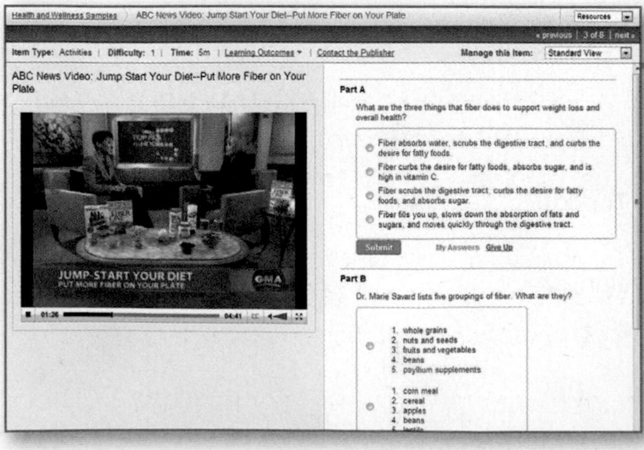

ABC News Videos

51 *ABC News* videos with assessment and feedback help health come to life and show how it's related to the real world.

Other automatically graded health and fitness activities include

Health Video Tutors
Chapter Reading Quizzes
MP3 Tutor Sessions

Self-Assessments from the Text

Do you want your students to write a self-reflection piece on their self-assessment? Or would you like them to complete the self-assessment and have it automatically speak to the gradebook so that students will get credit for these activities? Self assessments are assignable within MasteringHealth both in PDF format with a self-reflection section and as a multi-part activity.

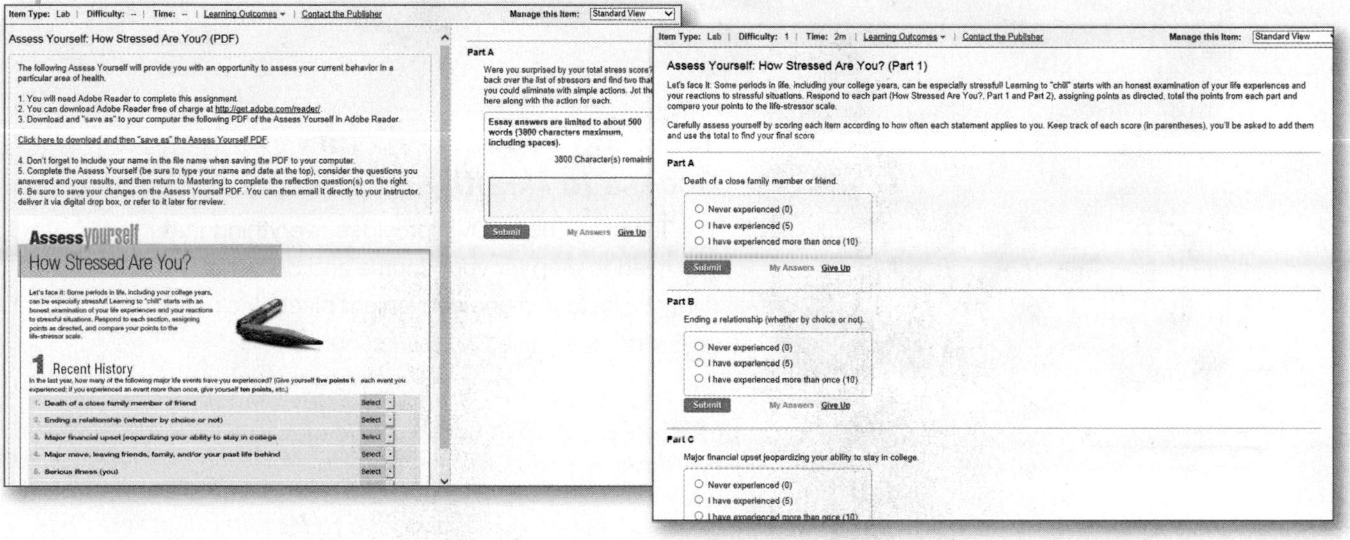

NutriTool Build-A-Meal Activities

These unique activities allow students to combine and experiment with different food options and learn first-hand how to build healthier meals.

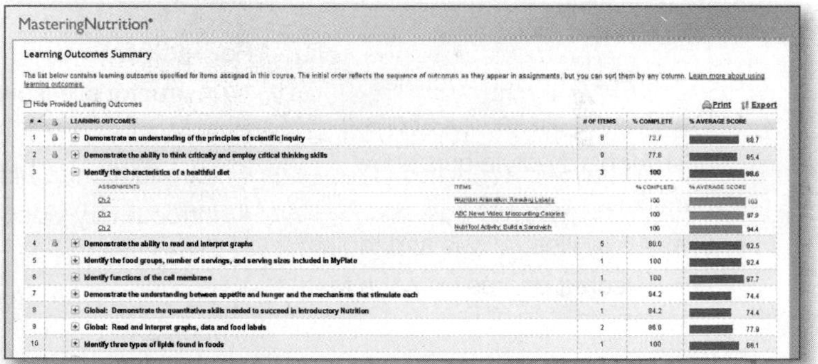

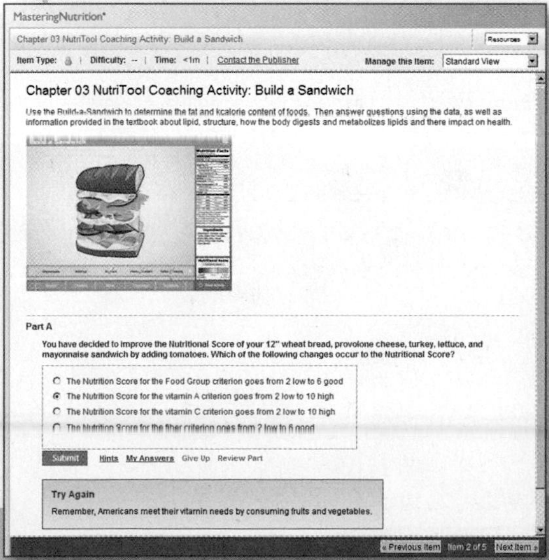

Learning Outcomes

All of the MasteringHealth assignable content is tagged to book content and to Bloom's Taxonomy. You also have the ability to add your own outcomes, helping you track student performance against your learning outcomes. You can view class performance against the specified learning outcomes and share those results quickly and easily by exporting to a spreadsheet.

EVERYTHING YOU NEED TO TEACH **IN ONE PLACE**

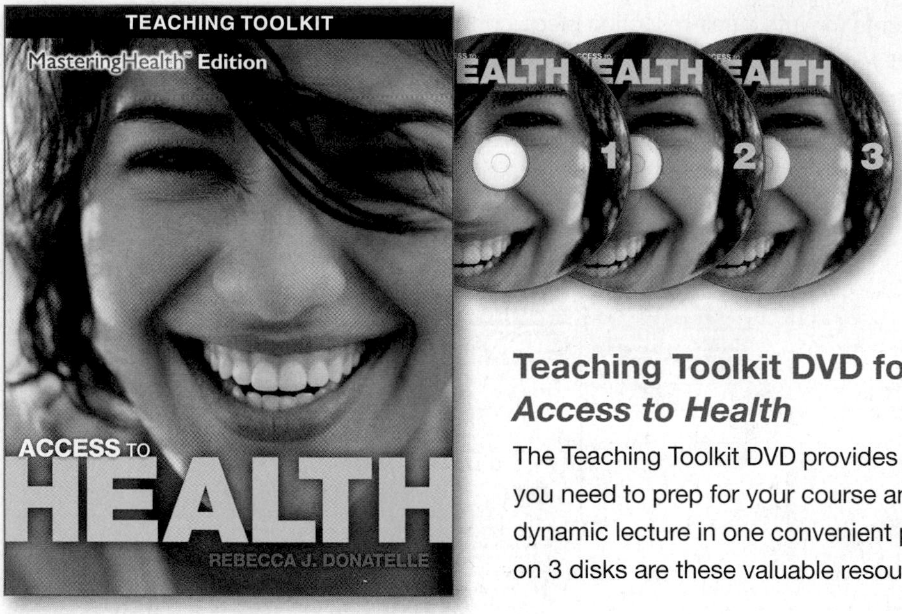

Teaching Toolkit DVD for *Access to Health*

The Teaching Toolkit DVD provides everything that you need to prep for your course and deliver a dynamic lecture in one convenient place. Included on 3 disks are these valuable resources:

DISK 1

Robust Media Assets for Each Chapter

- *51 ABC News* Lecture Launcher videos
- PowerPoint Lecture Outlines
- PowerPoint clicker questions and Jeopardy-style quiz show questions
- Files for all illustrations and tables and selected photos from the text

DISK 2

Comprehensive Test Bank

- Test Bank in Word and RTF formats
- Computerized Test Bank, which includes all of the questions from the test bank in a format that allows you to easily and intuitively build exams and quizzes

DISK 3

Additional Innovative Supplements for Instructors and Students

For Instructors

- Instructor's Resource Support Manual
- Introduction to MasteringHealth
- Introductory video for Learning Catalytics
- *Teaching with Student Learning Outcomes*
- *Teaching with Web 2.0*

For Students

- Take Charge of Your Health worksheets
- Assess Yourself worksheets
- Behavior Change Log Book and Wellness Journal
- *Live Right! Beating Stress in College and Beyond*
- *Eat Right! Healthy Eating in College and Beyond*
- Food Composition Table

User's Quick Guide for *Access to Health*

This easy-to-use printed supplement accompanies the Teaching Toolkit and offers easy instructions for both experienced and new faculty members to get started with rich Toolkit content, how to access assignments within MasteringHealth, and how to "flip" the classroom with Learning Catalytics.

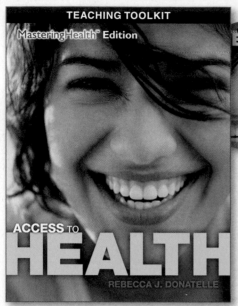

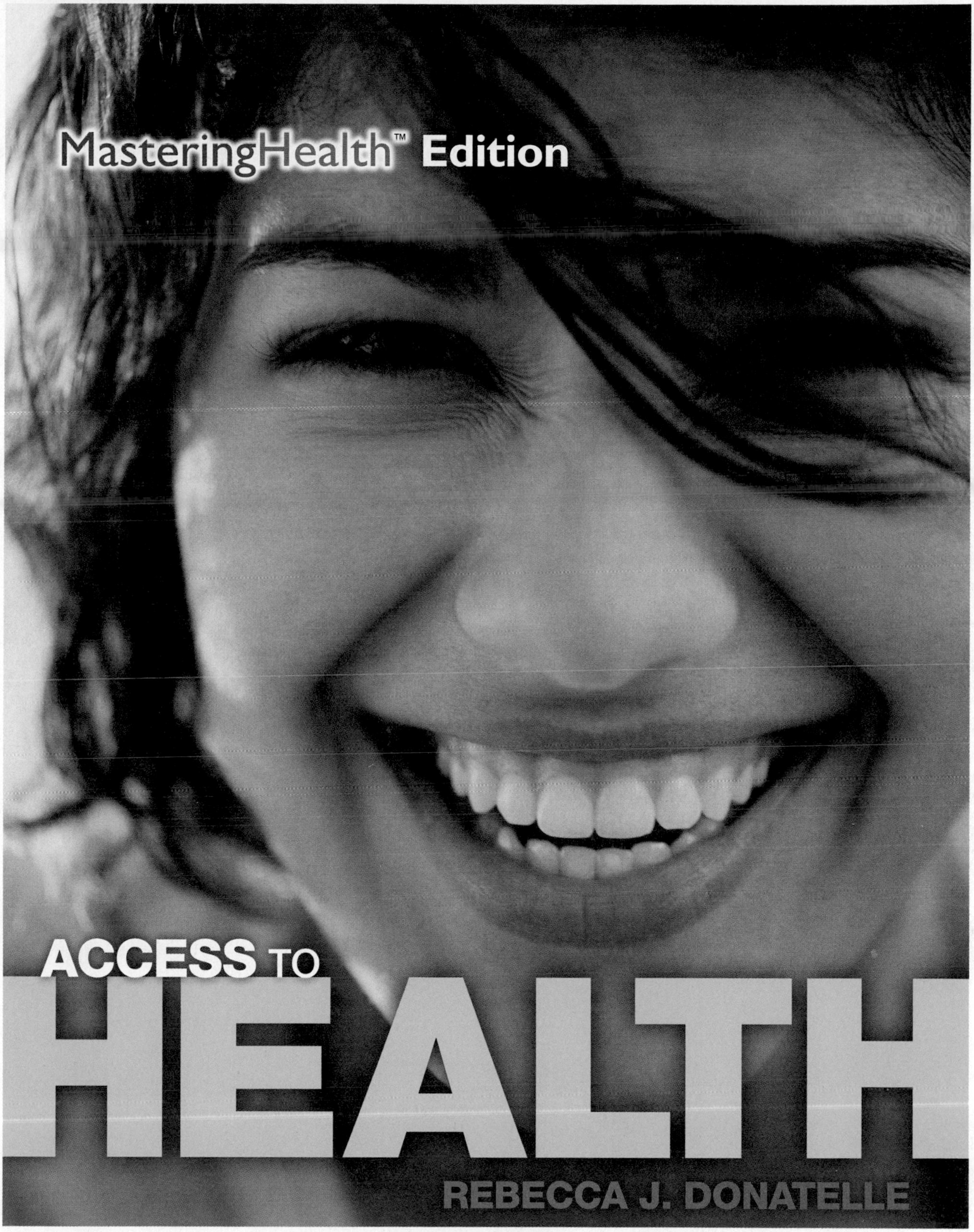
MasteringHealth™ Edition
ACCESS TO
HEALTH
REBECCA J. DONATELLE

PEARSON

Executive Editor: Sandra Lindelof
Senior Acquisitions Editor: Michelle Cadden
Project Manager: Lauren Beebe
Program Manager: Susan Malloy
Development Editors: Erin Schnair, Nic Albert
Editorial Assistant: Leah Sherwood
Text Permissions Project Manager: William Opaluch
Text Permissions Specialist: Liz Kincaid
Director of Development: Barbara Yien
Program Management Team Lead: Mike Early
Project Management Team Lead: Nancy Tabor
Production Management: Thistle Hill Publishing Services
Copy Editor: Jane Loftus
Compositor: Cenveo® Publisher Services
Art House: Precision Graphics
Design Manager: Derek Bacchus
Interior and Exterior Designer: Elise Lansdon
Photo Permissions Management: Eric Schrader, Maya Melenchuk
Photo Researcher: Stephen Merland, Jamey O'Quinn
Senior Procurement Specialist: Stacey Weinberger
Executive Marketing Manager: Neena Bali
Cover Photo Credit: Getty Images/Blend Images—JGI/Jamie Grill

Library of Congress Cataloging-in-Publication Data

Donatelle, Rebecca J., 1950–
Access to health/Rebecca J. Donatelle, Oregon State University. — Fourteenth edition.
pages cm
Includes bibliographical references and index.
ISBN 978-0-321-99548-3 — ISBN 0-321-99548-1
1. Health. I. Title.
RA776.D66 2016
613—dc23
2014041649

ISBN 10: 0-321-99548-1 (Student edition)
ISBN 13: 978-0-321-99548-3 (Student edition)
ISBN 10: 0-13-390387-7 (Instructor's Review Copy)
ISBN 13: 978-0-13-390387-4 (Instructor's Review Copy)

PEARSON

www.pearsonhighered.com

2 3 4 5 6 7 8 9 10—V303—16 15

BRIEF CONTENTS

CONTENTS

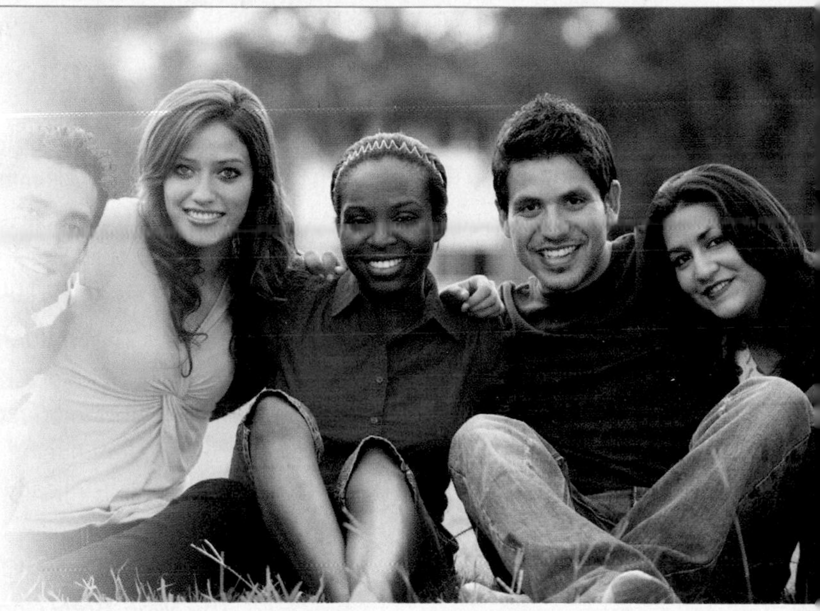

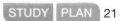

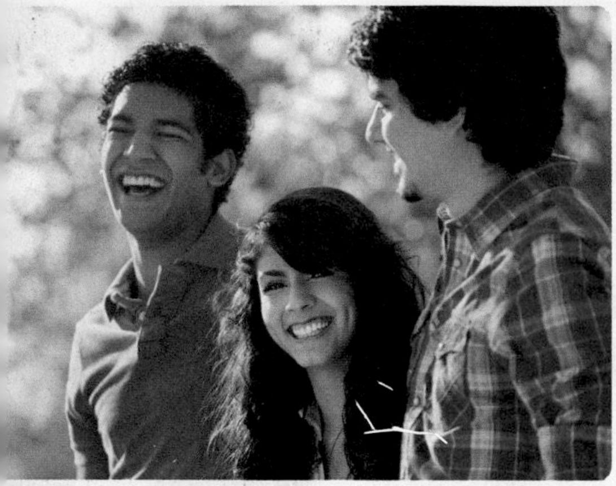

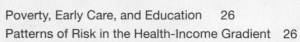

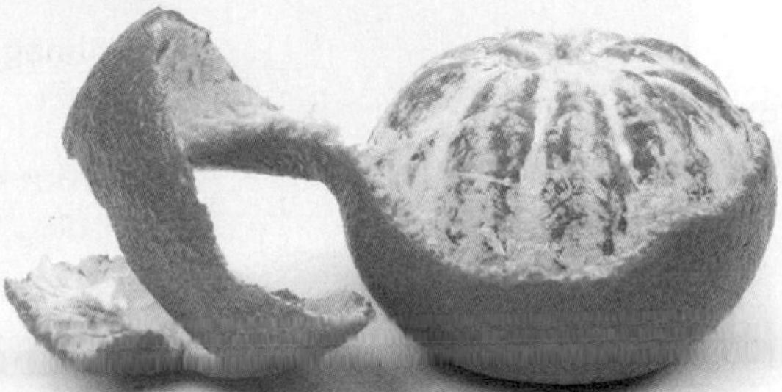

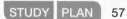

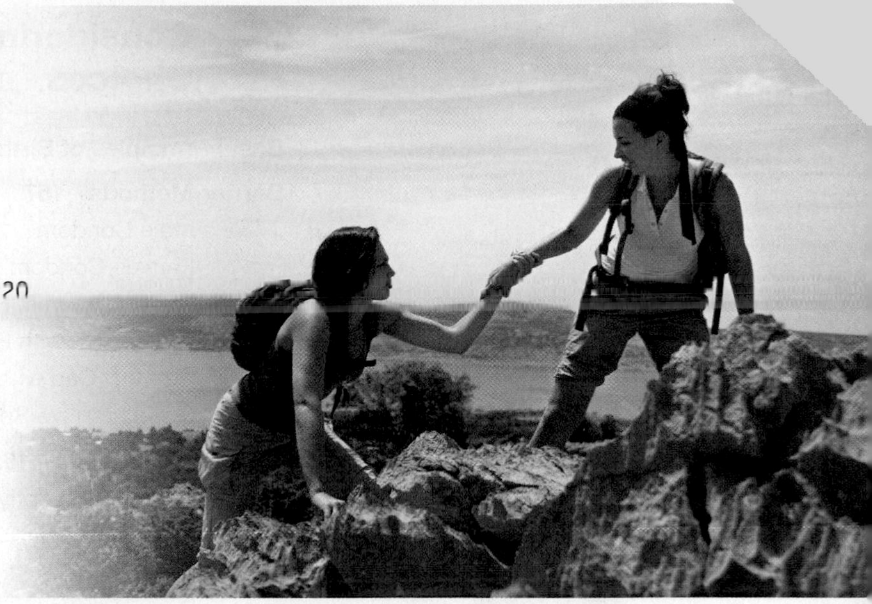

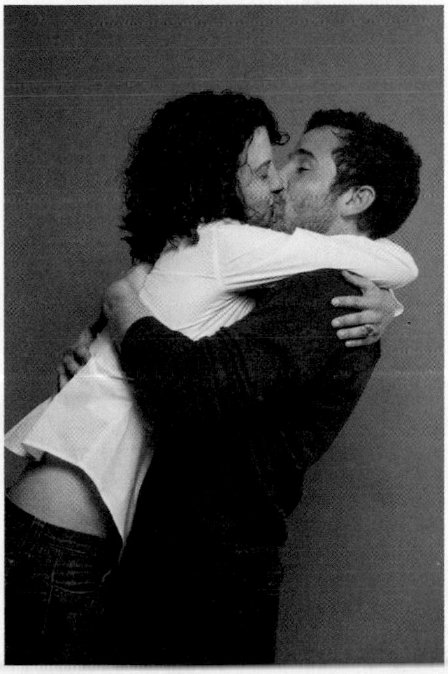

6 Considering Your Reproductive Choices 155

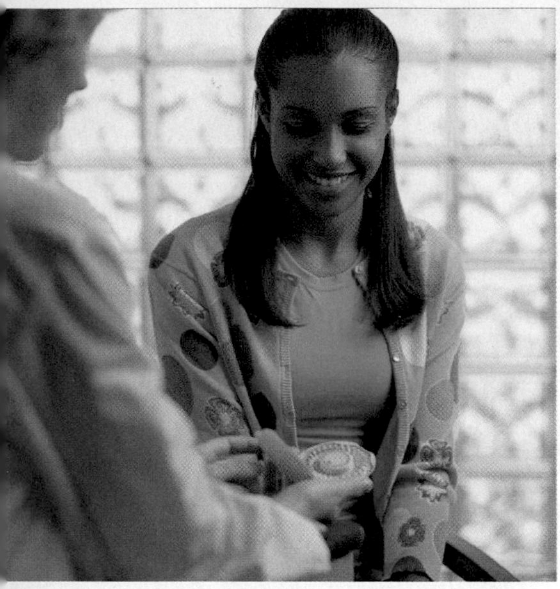

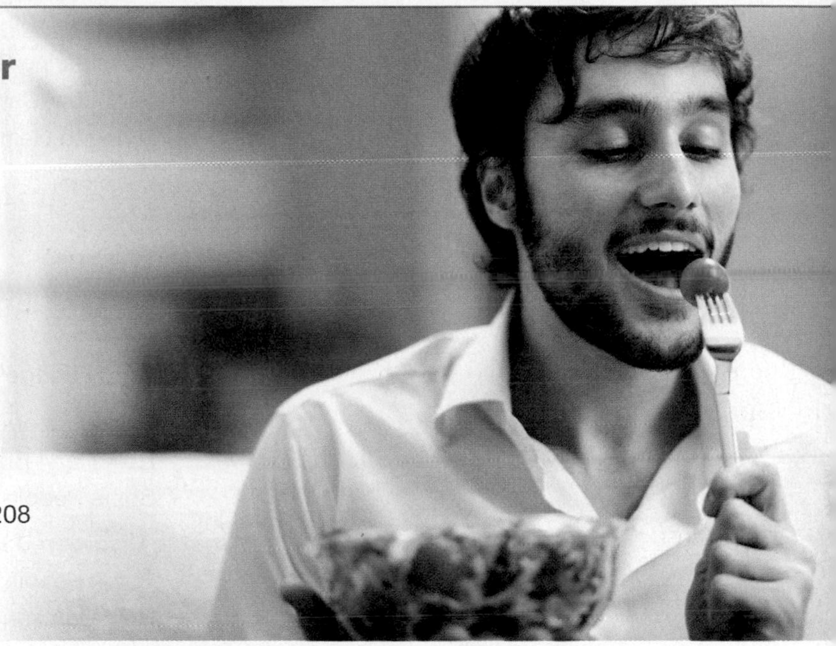

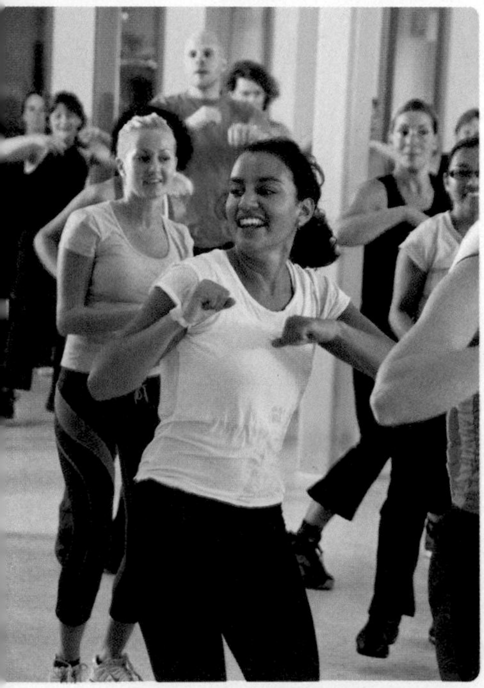

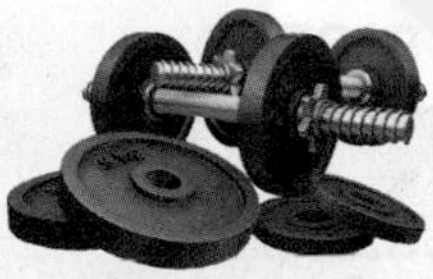

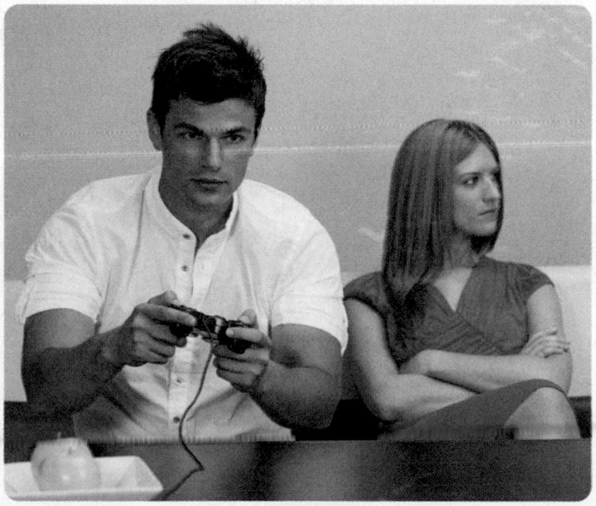

FOUR | Avoiding Risks from Harmful Habits

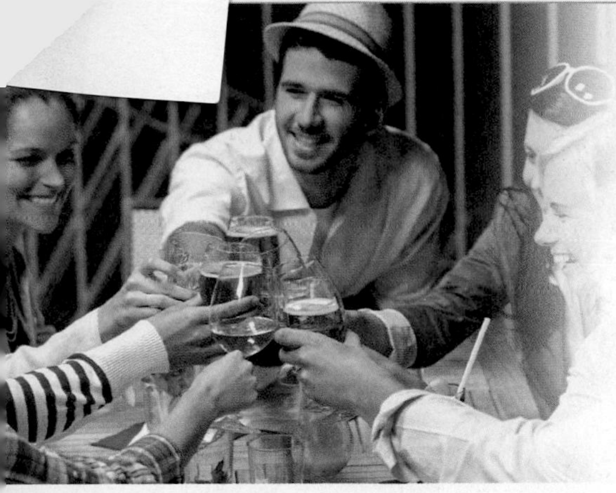

10 Drinking Alcohol Responsibly 301

11 Ending Tobacco Use 324

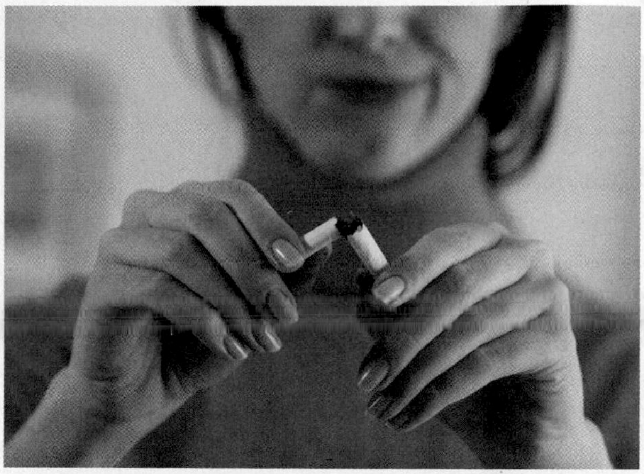

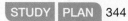

FIVE | Preventing and Fighting Disease

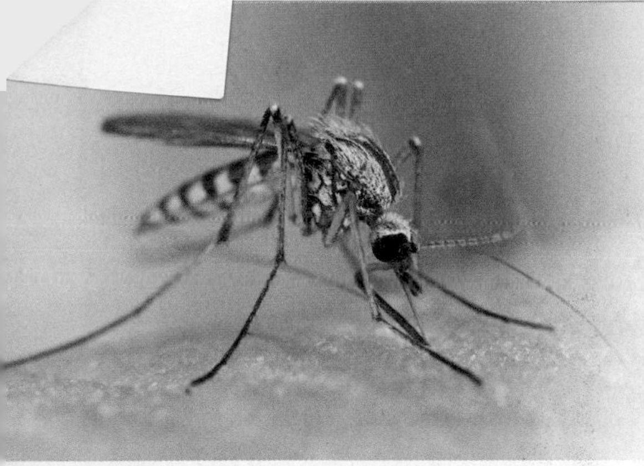

13 Protecting against Infectious Diseases 374

14 Protecting against Sexually Transmitted Infections 395

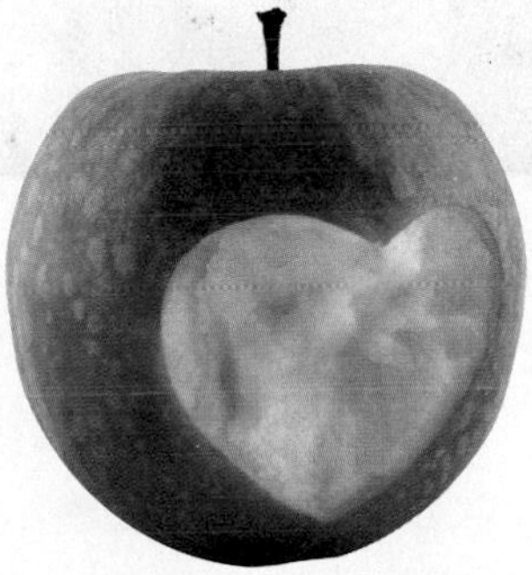

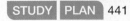

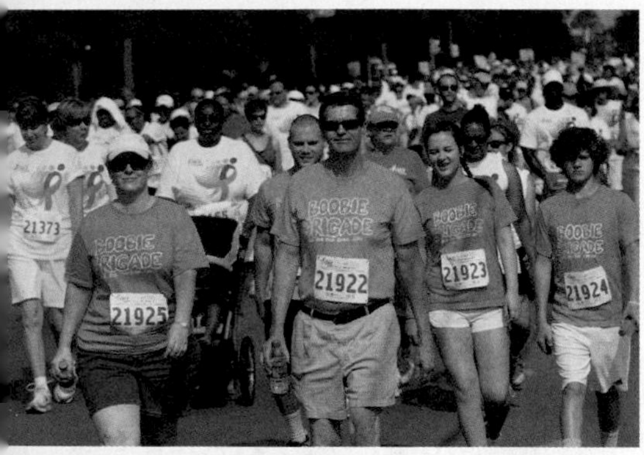

21373
BOOBIE BRIGADE
21925
21922
21923
21924

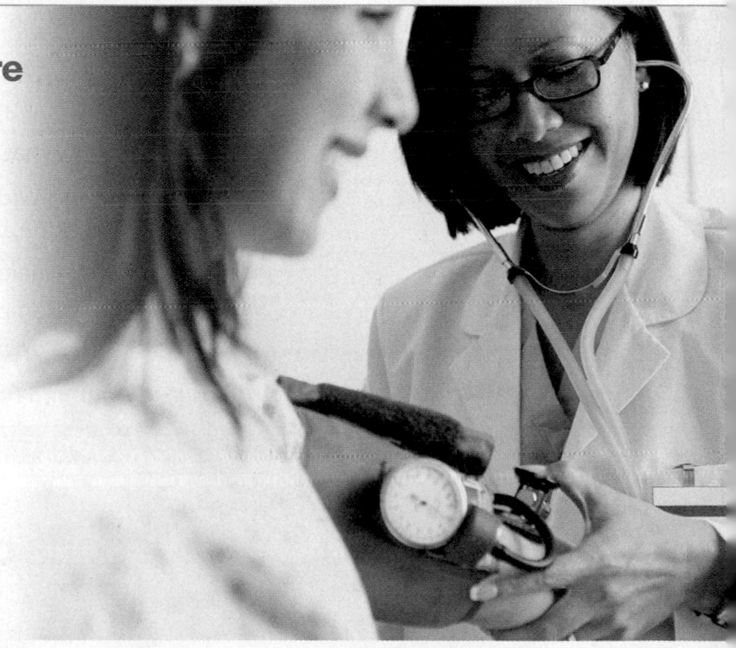

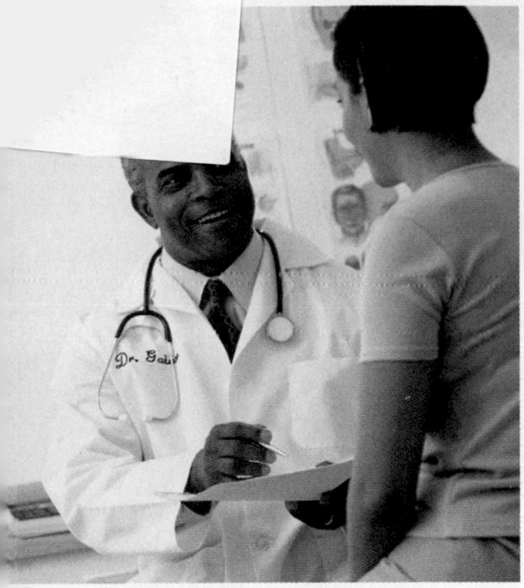

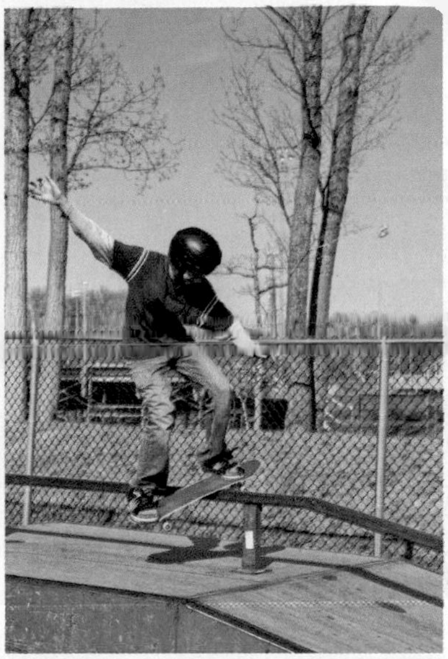

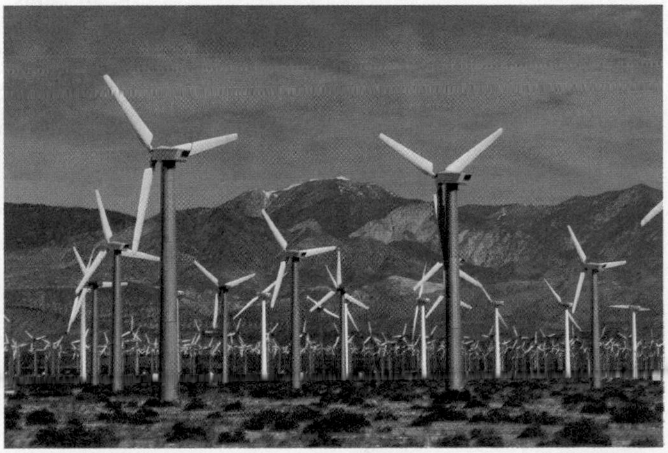

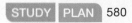

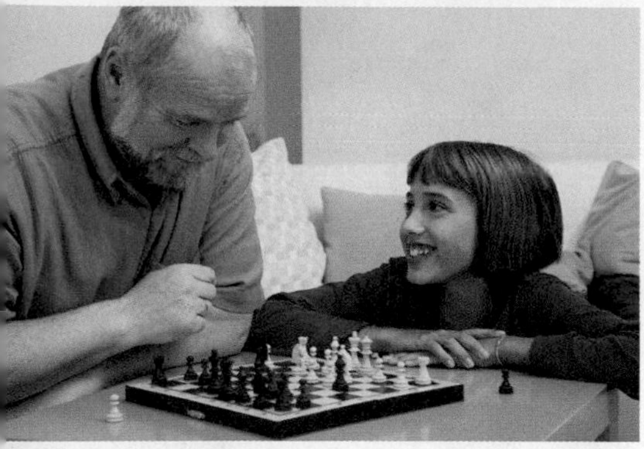

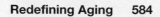

21 Preparing for Aging, Death, and Dying 583

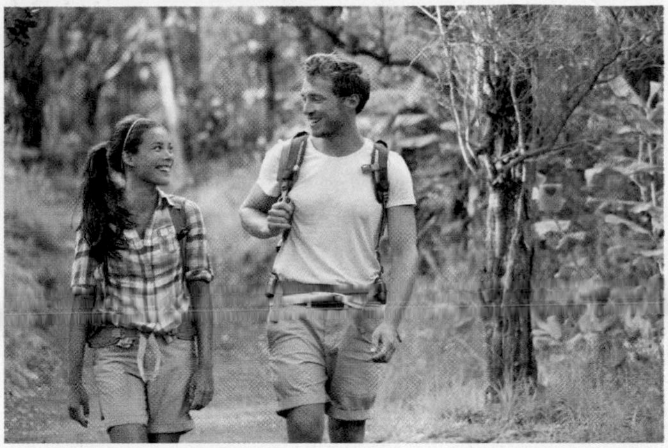

FEATURE BOXES

TECH & HEALTH

MONEY & HEALTH

SKILLS FOR BEHAVIOR CHANGE

STUDENT HEALTH TODAY

@ HEALTH HEADLINES

HEALTH IN A DIVERSE WORLD

ASSESS YOURSELF

The Assess Yourself activities are available online at MasteringHealth. Go to the MasteringHealth Study Area to find the chapter you want in the drop-down menu, and there you will see the Assess Yourself activities. Print them or save the PDF to your computer.

Chapter 1 How Healthy Are You?

Focus On Budgeting for College Students

Chapter 2 How Psychologically Healthy Are You?

Focus On What's Your Spiritual IQ?

Chapter 3 How Stressed Are You?

Focus On Are You Sleeping Well?

Chapter 4 How Well Do You Communicate?

Chapter 5 What Are Your Sexual Attitudes?

Chapter 6 Are You Comfortable with Your Contraception?

Chapter 7 How Healthy Are Your Eating Habits?

Chapter 8 Are You Ready to Start a Weight-Loss Program?

Focus On Are Your Efforts to Be Thin Sensible—or Spinning Out of Control?

Chapter 9 How Physically Fit Are You?

Focus On Are You Addicted?

Chapter 10 What's Your Risk of Alcohol Abuse?

Chapter 11 Tobacco: Are Your Habits Placing You at Risk?

Chapter 12 Learn to Recognize Drug Use and Potential Abuse

Chapter 13 Myth or Fact? Test Your Infectious Disease IQ

Chapter 14 STIs: Do You Really Know What You Think You Know?

Focus On What's Your Family Health History?

Chapter 15 What's Your Personal CVD Risk?

Focus On Are You at Risk for Diabetes?

Chapter 16 What's Your Personal Risk for Cancer?

Chapter 17 Are You at Risk for Chronic Illness?

Chapter 18 Are You a Smart Health Care Consumer?

Chapter 19 Are You at Risk for Violence?

Focus On Are You at Risk for a Motor Vehicle Accident?

Chapter 20 Are You Doing All You Can to Protect the Environment?

Chapter 21 Are You Afraid of Death?

PREFACE

In today's world, health is headline news. The issues and information seem so complex and contradictory that you may wonder how to make sense of it all. What can you do to ensure a life that is healthy and long and to help improve the health of the people around you? Getting healthy and staying healthy can be a challenge, but it is a worthwhile goal and one that is well within reach for most of us. No matter where your health is now, you can make positive changes for a healthier future, you can help others maintain health, and you can become an agent for healthy change in your community.

My goal in writing the MasteringHealth Edition of *Access to Health* is to provide students with just what that title says: access to health information and to their own health potential. This book provides the most scientifically valid information available to help students be smarter in their health decision making, more positively involved in their personal health, and more active as advocates for healthy changes in their communities. Change isn't something that just happens. Let's face it—if it were easy to lose weight, maintain a healthy diet, manage stress, and exercise regularly, we wouldn't have one of the fattest nations on Earth and one of the most costly, overburdened health care systems. However, the good news is that governmental agencies, communities, schools, and increasing numbers of individuals are taking steps (both small and large) to enhance, preserve, and protect our health. The key is to know where to look for accurate information, which information you can trust, and how to use the information to make the best choices for you and others. In short, it takes knowledge, preparation, and effort; therefore, this book places emphasis on empowering students to identify their health risks, create plans for reducing those risks, and make healthy lifestyle changes part of their daily routines.

Access to Health is designed to help students quickly grasp the information presented and understand its relevance to their own lives and the lives of others. Exciting revisions have been made to the art and design of the book in this new edition, with the purpose of capturing students' interest, engaging them in the subject matter, helping them find the most reliable resources available, and assisting them in weighing their options as they face health challenges today and in the future. In addition, there are eight Focus On chapters that delve into areas of health that are of practical importance to college students but are not always given sufficient coverage in typical personal health texts. These Focus On chapters spotlight financial health, spiritual health, sleep, body image, addiction, health inheritance, diabetes, and unintentional injury.

Looking back to the time when I taught my first Personal Health course as a teaching assistant in graduate school and remembering the years of teaching countless numbers of students in classes like this, I complete this, the MasteringHealth Edition of *Access to Health*, with overwhelming gratitude for the success that this text has enjoyed through its many revisions and changes. With each edition of the text, I have listened to the thoughtful suggestions of instructors and students using the book, as well as to the feedback from my own students in keeping the book relevant, interesting, and accessible. I hope that this edition's rich foundation of scientifically valid information, its wealth of technological tools and resources, and its thought-provoking features will stimulate you to share my enthusiasm for personal health and to become actively engaged in behaviors that will lead to better health for all.

NEW TO THIS EDITION

Access to Health, the MasteringHealth Edition, maintains many features that the text has become known for, while incorporating several major revisions and exciting new features. The most noteworthy changes to the text as a whole include the following:

- **New Learning Outcomes approach** In the new design of the book, numbered learning outcomes at the beginning of each chapter and Focus On are tied to each major chapter section, helping students navigate each chapter and measure their progress against specific learning goals and helping instructors assess the key information and skills students are meant to take away from each chapter.
- **Study Plan** Each chapter concludes with a Study Plan, which summarizes key points of the chapter and provides review questions and critical thinking questions to check understanding, all tied to the chapter's learning outcomes.
- **New Financial Health Focus On** This new Focus On helps students successfully manage finances through budgeting, understanding debt and credit, and avoiding identity theft, as well as helping students to understand the interrelationship between health and financial circumstances.
- **Separate chapter on Sexually Transmitted Infections (STIs)** Formerly part of the infectious diseases chapter, the topic of STIs now has a distinct chapter with specific learning outcomes, assessment materials, and a new video tutor.

- **Revised Tech & Health** These feature boxes have been updated to make the information even more applicable and to give the best apps and websites for additional learning and behavior change.
- **MasteringHealth** This online homework, tutorial, and assessment product is designed to improve results by helping students to quickly master concepts. Students benefit from self-paced tutorials that feature immediate wrong-answer feedback and hints that emulate the office-hour experience to help students stay on track. With a wide range of interactive, engaging, and assignable activities, students are encouraged to actively learn and retain tough course concepts. Specific features include:
  - **Health & Fitness Coaching Activities** that guide students through key health topics with engaging mini-lessons that provide hints and feedback.
  - **Behavior Change Videos** that offer concise whiteboard-style videos to help students with the steps of behavior change, covering topics such as setting SMART goals, identifying and overcoming barriers to change, planning realistic timelines, and more. Additional videos review key fitness concepts such as determining target heart rate range for exercise. All videos include assessment activities and are assignable in MasteringHealth.
  - **Dynamic Study Modules** that enable students to study effectively on their own in an adaptive format. Students receive an initial set of questions with a unique answer format asking them to indicate their confidence level.
  - **NutriTools Coaching Activities** for the nutrition chapter that allow students to combine and experiment with different food options and learn firsthand how to build healthier meals.
  - **MP3s linked with QR codes:** QR codes within the text lead to MP3s within MasteringHealth that recap key chapter content and include multiple-choice questions that provide wrong-answer feedback.
  - **51 *ABC News* Videos** bring health to life and spark discussion with hot topics. They also include multiple-choice questions that provide wrong-answer feedback to redirect students to the correct answer.
  - **Learning Catalytics™** provides open-ended questions students can answer in real time. Through targeted assessments, Learning Catalytics helps students develop the critical thinking skills they need for lasting behavior change.
  - **The Study Area** is broken down into learning areas and includes videos, MP3s, practice quizzing, and much more.

Chapter-by-Chapter Revisions

Access to Health, the MasteringHealth Edition, has been updated line by line to provide students with the most current information and references for further exploration. Portions of chapters have been reorganized to improve the flow of topics, while figures, tables, feature boxes, and photos have all been added, improved on, and updated. The following is a chapter-by-chapter listing of some of the most noteworthy changes, updates, and additions.

Chapter 1: Accessing Your Health

- Expanded coverage of the social cognitive model of behavior change
- New **Student Health Today** box on optimal wellness and chronic illness
- Updated research on health disparities
- New information on the Affordable Care Act

Focus On: Improving Your Financial Health

- New chapter on financial health covers:
  - Links between health and wealth
  - Financial struggles in college
  - Actions to take to improve financial health

Chapter 2: Promoting and Preserving Your Psychological Health

- New coverage of defense mechanisms
- Updated material on personality
- Updated research on PTSD
- New **Health Headlines** box on happiness
- New **Health Headlines** box on college success for those with learning disabilities and neurodevelopmental disorders

Focus On: Cultivating Your Spiritual Health

- New **Health Headlines** box on environmental mindfulness
- Updated research on the spiritual tendencies of undergraduates
- Updated figure on the qualities of mindfulness
- New coverage of the impact of mindfulness and meditation on overall health

Chapter 3: Managing Stress and Coping with Life's Challenges

- New **Student Health Today** box on *feng shui* and stress
- New coverage of the gender differences in responses to stress
- Updated research on the lifetime effects of stress

Focus On: Improving Your Sleep

- Updated research on students and sleep
- New section on technology's toll on sleep
- New section on sleepy workers

Chapter 4: Building Healthy Relationships and Communicating Effectively

- Updated statistics on cohabitation
- Updated information on same sex marriage
- New material on behaviors that signal trouble in relationships

- New **Student Health Today** box on privacy and social media
- New **Student Health Today** box on hooking up

Chapter 5: Understanding Your Sexuality

- Updated research on the relationship between birth control use and health problems
- Updated information on abstinence rates among college students
- New data on the sex trade in the United States
- New **Health in a Diverse World** box on living between genders
- New **Tech & Health** box on apps that can improve your sexual knowledge and confidence

Chapter 6: Considering Your Reproductive Choices

- Updated statistics on contraception use and unintended pregnancy
- Updated information on IUDs
- Updated information on emergency contraceptive pill availability
- Updated information on recent laws passed to restrict abortion rights

Chapter 7: Eating for a Healthier You

- Updated data on calcium supplements
- Updated research on beneficial, non-nutrient components of foods
- New coverage of empty calorie foods
- Expanded tips for eating healthy in college
- Updated research on impacts of genetically modified foods
- New **Student Health Today** box on nutrition rating systems

Chapter 8: Reaching and Maintaining a Healthy Weight

- Updated research on obesity rates and their impacts
- New research on the role of genetics in obesity
- Updated information on dietary supplement fraud and food fraud
- Updated information on the FDA and weight loss supplements
- Updated information on weight loss surgeries
- New **Money & Health** box on the economic impact of obesity

Focus On: Enhancing Your Body Image

- Updated information on the correlation between negative body image and traditional media
- Updated information on negative body image and social media
- New information on other unspecified feeding or eating disorders
- Additional resources on getting help with an eating disorder

Chapter 9: Improving Your Physical Fitness

- Updated data on the role of inactivity in heart disease, diabetes, and cancer
- Updated research on physical activity and increased academic performance
- Updated information on calculating target heart rate
- Updated information on progressive fitness programs

Focus On: Recognizing and Avoiding Addiction

- Updated information on the physiology of addiction
- Updated research on gambling disorder
- Updated research on compulsive buying

Chapter 10: Drinking Alcohol Responsibly

- New information on hangovers
- Updated research on alcohol use and injuries
- Updated information on alcohol, rape, sexual assault, and dating violence
- Updated information on alcohol and weight gain
- Updated information on alcohol and sleep
- New coverage of alcohol recovery programs for students

Chapter 11: Ending Tobacco Use

- Updated data on U.S. tobacco use
- Updated data on the financial costs of tobacco use
- Updated **Health in a Diverse World** box on the unique health risks for women who smoke
- New **Tech & Health** box on apps to help you quit smoking

Chapter 12: Avoiding Drug Misuse and Abuse

- Updated research on the prevalence of illicit drug use in the United States
- New research on the relationship between marijuana use and mental health issues
- New coverage of the legalization of marijuana for medical and recreational use
- Updated information on MDMA
- New data on the economic costs of illicit drug use

Chapter 13: Protecting against Infectious Diseases

- Updated information on recent infectious diseases and potential epidemics, including the Ebola virus
- Updated data on antibiotic resistance and antibiotic-resistant "superbugs"
- New coverage of urgent bacterial threats
- Updated commonsense strategies for preventing colds
- Updated information on recent measles cases in the United States

Chapter 14: Protecting against Sexually Transmitted Infections

- Updated information on reported rates of unprotected sex among college students
- Updated research on the prevalence of HPV
- Updated information on the prevalence of HIV/AIDS
- Updated research on HIV testing and treatment
- New **Student Health Today** box on safe oral sex

Focus On: Understanding Your Health Inheritance

- Updated information on sickle cell disease
- Updated coverage of epigenetics
- Updated information on the role of genetics in psychiatric disorders
- Updated material on the role of genetics in addiction

Chapter 15: Preventing Cardiovascular Disease

- Updated research on CVD death rates
- Updated information on the direct and indirect economic costs of CVD
- Updated information on ideal blood pressure and hypertension
- Updated research on the roles of smoking and cholesterol in CVD
- New information on ideal LDL and HDL levels

Focus On: Minimizing Your Risk for Diabetes

- Updated research on the global prevalence of diabetes
- New research on the prevalence of diabetes among youth
- Updated information on the impact of diabetes on pregnancy
- New coverage of most recent diabetes treatment options
- Updated information on the economic costs of diabetes

Chapter 16: Reducing Your Cancer Risk

- Updated data on cancer diagnoses and relative survival rates
- Updated data on prevalence of smoking worldwide
- Updated section on the relationship between inflammation and cancer
- New information on rates of HPV vaccinations

Chapter 17: Reducing Risks and Coping with Chronic Conditions

- Updated research on COPD prevalence and causes
- Updated coverage of allergies
- Updated coverage of coping with digestion-related disorders and diseases
- Updated research on arthritis and related conditions
- Updated **Health Headlines** box on treating chronic pain

Chapter 18: Becoming a Responsible Health Care Consumer

- Updated coverage of complementary and alternative medicine
- Updated information on massage therapy
- New information on probiotics
- Updated data on insurance coverage
- Updated research on the placebo effect

Chapter 19: Preventing Violence and Abuse

- Updated research on rates of violent crime in the United States
- Updated research on violence and relationship violence on U.S. college campuses
- New information on the relationship between media violence and actual violence
- Updated research on the prevalence of sexual assault
- Updated **Health Headlines** box on speaking up about sexual assault

Focus On: Reducing Your Risk of Unintentional Injury

- Updated information on distracted driving and motor vehicle safety
- Updated information on the unique risks motorcyclists face
- New research on poisoning rates and prevention

Chapter 20: Preserving and Protecting Your Environment

- Updated coverage of the impact of overpopulation on the environment
- New research on the amount of air pollution produced by vehicles with two-stroke engines
- Updated research on climate change and global warming
- New coverage of promising trends in sustainable development
- New **Money & Health** box on reducing food waste
- Updated **Health Headlines** box on e-waste

Chapter 21: Preparing for Aging, Death, and Dying

- Updated research on the economic impacts associated with an aging population
- Updated coverage of age-related hearing loss
- Updated research on rates of sexual activity among older adults
- Updated coverage of binge drinking and prescription drug abuse among older adults
- New section on financial planning for retirement
- New **Skills for Behavior Change** on aging well

TEXT FEATURES AND LEARNING AIDS

Access to Health, the MasteringHealth Edition, includes the following special features, all of which have been revised and improved upon for this edition:

- **Chapter learning outcomes** summarize the main competencies that students will gain from each chapter and alert students to the key concepts.
- **What Do You Think?** critical thinking questions within the chapter prompt students to reflect on personal and societal issues relating to the material they have just learned.
- **Why Should I Care?** features lead students to recognize the relevance of health issues to their own lives in the here and now.
- **Did You Know?** figures call attention to statistics that are relevant to the lives of college students in a fun format.
- **Assess Yourself and Your Plan for Change** boxes are combined in each chapter. Students assess their current health behaviors and are given specific ideas for setting goals and following through on behavior change.
- **Skills for Behavior Change** boxes give students specific strategies for making lasting changes to their health behaviors.
- **Tech & Health** boxes cover the new technology innovations, from medical tests to calorie-counting smartphone apps, that can help students stay healthy.
- **Student Health Today** boxes offer current data and information about health trends specific to college students, including potential risks and safety issues that affect students' lives.
- **Health Headlines** boxes highlight new discoveries and research, as well as interesting trends in the fields of public and personal health.
- **Health in a Diverse World** boxes expand discussion of health topics to diverse groups within the United States and around the world.
- **Money & Health** boxes cover health topics from the financial perspective, discussing everything from how to lessen money stress during school to how something like a plastic bag tax at the grocery store might impact behavior.
- A **running glossary** in the margins defines terms where students first encounter them, emphasizing and supporting understanding of material.
- **QR codes and media callout boxes** indicate when podcasts, videos, and assessments are available online for use with the book.
- The end-of-chapter **Study Plans** focus on student application: The **Summary** wraps up chapter content, **Pop Quiz** multiple-choice questions and **Think About It!** discussion questions encourage students to evaluate and apply new information, and **Accessing Your Health on the Internet** sections offer more opportunities to explore areas of interest.
- The **appendices** at the end of the book include practical information on providing emergency care and a table of nutritive values for selected foods and fast foods.
- A **Behavior Change Contract** for students to fill out is included in the back of the book.

SUPPLEMENTARY MATERIALS

Available with *Access to Health,* The MasteringHealth Edition, is a comprehensive set of ancillary materials designed to enhance learning and to facilitate teaching.

Instructor Supplements

- **MasteringHealth.** MasteringHealth coaches students through the toughest health topics. Instructors can assign engaging tools to help students visualize, practice, and understand crucial content, from the basics of health to the fundamentals of behavior change. **Coaching Activities** guide students through key health concepts with interactive mini-lessons, complete with hints and wrong-answer feedback. **Reading Quizzes** (20 questions per chapter) ensure students have completed the assigned reading before class. ***ABC News* Videos** stimulate classroom discussions and include multiple-choice questions with feedback for students. **NutriTools Coaching Activities** in the nutrition chapter allow students to combine and experiment with different food options and learn firsthand how to build healthier meals. MP3s relate to chapter content and come with multiple-choice questions that provide wrong-answer feedback. **Learning Catalytics** provides open-ended questions students can answer in real time. Through targeted assessments, Learning Catalytics helps students develop the critical-thinking skills they need for lasting behavior change.
- **Teaching Toolkit DVD.** The Teaching Toolkit DVD includes everything instructors need to prepare for their course and deliver a dynamic lecture in one convenient place. Resources include the following: *ABC News* videos, Video Tutor videos, clicker questions, Quiz Show questions, PowerPoint lecture outlines, all figures and tables from the text, PDFs and Microsoft Word files of the *Instructor Resource and Support Manual* and the Test Bank, the Computerized Test Bank, the User's Quick Guide, *Teaching with Student Learning Outcomes, Teaching with Web 2.0, Behavior Change Log Book and Wellness Journal, Eat Right!, Live Right!,* and *Take Charge of Your Health* worksheets.
- ***ABC News* Videos** and **Video Tutors.** Fifty-one new *ABC News* videos, each 5 to 10 minutes long, and 22 brand-new brief videos accessible via QR codes in the text help instructors stimulate critical discussion in the classroom. Videos are provided already linked within PowerPoint lectures and are also available separately

in large-screen format with optional closed captioning on the Teaching Toolkit DVD and through Mastering-Health.

- ***Instructor Resource and Support Manual.*** This teaching tool provides chapter summaries and outlines of each chapter. It includes information on available PowerPoint lectures, integrated ABC News video discussion questions, tips and strategies for managing large classrooms, ideas for in-class activities, and suggestions for integrating MasteringHealth and MyDietAnalysis into your classroom activities and homework assignments.
- **Test Bank.** The Test Bank incorporates Bloom's Taxonomy, or the higher order of learning, to help instructors create exams that encourage students to think analytically and critically, rather than simply to regurgitate information. Test Bank questions are tagged to global and book-specific student learning outcomes.
- **User's Quick Guide.** Newly redesigned to be even more useful, this valuable supplement acts as your road map to the Teaching Toolkit DVD.
- ***Teaching with Student Learning Outcomes.*** This publication contains essays from 11 instructors who are teaching using student learning outcomes. They share their goals in using outcomes and the processes that they follow to develop and refine them, and they provide many useful suggestions and examples for successfully incorporating outcomes into a personal health course.
- ***Teaching with Web 2.0.*** From Facebook to Twitter to blogs, students are using and interacting with Web 2.0 technologies. This handbook provides an introduction to these popular online tools and offers ideas for incorporating them into your personal health course. Written by personal health and health education instructors, each chapter examines the basics about each technology and ways to make it work for you and your students.
- ***Behavior Change Log Book and Wellness Journal.*** This assessment tool helps students track daily exercise and nutritional intake and create a long-term nutritional and fitness prescription plan. It also includes a Behavior Change Contract and topics for journal-based activities.

Student Supplements

- **The Study Area of MasteringHealth** is organized by learning areas. *Read It* houses the Pearson eText 2.0, with which users can create notes, highlight text in different colors, create bookmarks, zoom, click hyperlinked words for definitions, and change page view. Pearson eText 2.0 also links to associated media files. *See It* includes 51 *ABC News* videos on important health topics and the key concepts of each chapter. *Hear It* contains MP3 Study Tutor files and audio case studies. *Do It* contains critical-thinking questions and Web links. *Review It* contains study quizzes for each chapter. *Live It* helps jump-start students' behavior-change projects with assessments and resources to plan change; students can fill out a Behavior Change Contract, journal and log behaviors, and prepare a reflection piece.
- ***Behavior Change Log Book and Wellness Journal.*** This assessment tool helps students track daily exercise and nutritional intake and create a long-term nutrition and fitness prescription plan. It includes Behavior Change Contracts and topics for journal-based activities.
- ***Eat Right! Healthy Eating in College and Beyond.*** This booklet provides students with practical nutrition guidelines, shopper's guides, and recipes.
- ***Live Right! Beating Stress in College and Beyond.*** This booklet gives students useful tips for coping with stressful life challenges both during college and for the rest of their lives.
- **Digital 5-Step Pedometer** Take strides to better health with this pedometer, which measures steps, distance (miles), activity time, and calories, and provides a time clock.
- **MyDietAnalysis** (www.mydietanalysis.com). Powered by ESHA Research, Inc., MyDietAnalysis features a database of nearly 20,000 foods and multiple reports. It allows students to track their diet and activity using up to three profiles and to generate and submit reports electronically.

ACKNOWLEDGMENTS

It is hard for me to believe that *Access to Health* is in its fourteenth edition and that this one may be the best one yet! Since its inception, the personal health textbook market has undergone remarkable changes. Whereas the text remains the foundation of information, the ability to communicate with students through the Internet and a wide range of other media and devices such as smartphones and tablets provides textbook authors and publishers entirely new and exciting ways of teaching, sharing information, motivating students to become actively engaged in the learning experience, and covering up-to-the-minute health topics in every class. Today's text offers opportunities for student engagement and thought-provoking exercises that help students understand complex issues surrounding health so they can make better decisions related to health care and behaviors. To maximize student learning, we sought input from faculty members and experts in technology and e-learning—those who work with students daily and who understand how to engage today's learners with written and visual content. We also interviewed students and asked them about how they used technology in their learning and incorporated their recommendations in our student-centered approach. Producing a text that students actually want to pick up and read—one that they find interesting and that encourages critical thinking and learning—is no small task. In fact, in addition to having an author and contributors with the professional training and expertise in the scientific foundations of the health field, it takes a small army of publishing professionals and media specialists who take the basic information and make it come alive for the reader. Each step in planning, developing, and marketing a high-quality textbook and supplemental materials requires a tremendous amount of work from many skilled and dedicated professionals. I often think how fortunate I have been to work with the many gifted and talented professionals who make up the Pearson family. Upon reflection, there have been so many names and faces along the way—from people who have carried a tremendous amount of responsibility from beginning to end to those who have quietly worked behind the scenes on special tasks, in many cases, to make *Access to Health* a resounding success from the first edition to this one. I owe each of them tremendous gratitude, for without their efforts, this book may have languished on the shelves along the way. From this author's perspective, Pearson personnel personify key aspects of what it takes to be successful in the publishing world: (1) skill and competence; (2) drive and motivation; (3) creativity and commitment to excellence; (4) a vibrant, youthful, and enthusiastic approach; and (5) personalities that motivate an author to continually strive to produce market-leading texts.

In particular, I am indebted to my new project manager, Lauren Beebe, who took over the reins with this edition of *Access to Health* and never missed a beat in ensuring that the project kept on schedule and continued to reflect excellent editorial skills. Lauren was able to juggle numerous responsibilities, provide thoughtful recommendations, and problem-solve along the way to keep the team on task and working to provide a final manuscript on a tight schedule—all the while gently nudging the author, who has a slight tendency to want to add more and more in a limited space! In short, Lauren did a fantastic job in making this edition continue as a leading text in the field. In addition to Lauren, I am thankful to Erin Schnair, previous project editor, who agreed to continue working with us to refine and develop a newer, cutting-edge edition. Her history with the project allowed her to make excellent recommendations for revisions and incorporate new information seamlessly into each chapter. Her creative suggestions helped maintain continuity and excellence in the final product. A gifted writer herself and a knowledgeable health editor, she was able to refine and improve sections of the manuscript with a deft stroke of the keyboard—skills that are invaluable in the editorial process. Consistent with Pearson's team approach to publishing, so many people work with these projects over the years, and their collective memory, edition to edition, makes for a fantastic author/editor interaction. In short, Lauren and Erin were part of the "dream team" that allowed the author and contributors to focus on the task at hand—using their knowledge to provide scientifically valid information about health. Thank you, Erin and Lauren.

I would also like to thank Nic Albert for his behind-the-scenes work as developmental editor on our chapters as we submitted our revisions, and the copy editor, Jane Loftus, who played a key role in refining material, synthesizing my long narratives, and keeping the text clean and concise for students.

I also wish to give profound thanks to Susan Malloy, Program Manager, for her continued oversight, careful management, and wise decision making. Without Susan's dedicated support behind the scenes, this project would not have been possible.

Although many executive editors play a more detached role in project management and development, I was fortunate in being able to work with a hands-on and enthusiastic editor over the last several editions of the book. Much appreciation and many thanks go to executive editor Sandra Lindelof. Whether traveling to assist with adoptions, negotiating contracts, dealing with issues that inevitably arise in a changing health marketplace, or securing necessary resources to stay on top of a competitive field, Sandy has been key to the success of my books and the health list at the Pearson publishing enterprise. A tireless worker, an enthusiastic advocate for authors and her staff, Sandy has been a driving force in moving the *Access to Health* series into the twenty-first century of technologically savvy textbooks. Clearly, she "gets it" when it comes to keeping a steady hand on the pulse of the personal health market and what instructors are looking for and what students need. Thank you, Sandy, for your consistent and outstanding work as my executive editor over the last several editions and for all you've done to put together an outstanding team of publishing professionals, one that any author would be proud to work with!

Although these women were key contributors to the finished work, there were many other people who worked on this revision of *Access to Health.* In particular, I would like to thank Angela Williams Urquhart and Andrea Archer at Thistle Hill Publishing Services, who put everything together to make a polished finished product. Elise Lansdon worked wonders in giving the book an exciting and fresh new look, both inside and out. Editorial Assistant Leah Sherwood gets major kudos for skillfully overseeing the supplements package, as does Liz Winer, Executive Content Producer, who developed a comprehensive MasteringHealth program. Additional thanks go to the rest of the team at Pearson, especially Design Manager Derek Bacchus, Rights and Permissions Project Manager Eric Schrader, and Director of Development Barbara Yien.

The editorial and production teams are critical to a book's success, but I would be remiss if I didn't thank another key group who ultimately help determine a book's success: the textbook representative and sales group and their leader, Product Marketing Manager Neena Bali. Over the years, Neena has traveled extensively, visiting with hundreds of Personal Health instructors and explaining why *Access to Health* is uniquely suited to provide a compelling and interesting learning experience for students. Neena's long history with the Pearson group is a testament to how fantastic she is and the superb job that she does in marketing health texts. From providing training for representatives to meeting with professors and explaining product nuances and available resources, Neena does a terrific job of getting texts into instructors' hands and maximizing their use of available technology and materials. Once a book is adopted, she provides the kind of support and service that customers deserve. In keeping with my overall experiences with Pearson, the members of the marketing and sales staff are among the best of the best. I am very lucky to have them working with me on this project and want to extend a special thanks to all of them!

CONTRIBUTORS TO THE FOURTEENTH EDITION

Many colleagues, students, and staff members have provided the feedback, reviews, extra time, assistance, and encouragement that have helped me meet the rigorous demands of publishing this book over the years. Whether acting as reviewers, generating new ideas, providing expert commentary, or revising chapters, each of these professionals has added his or her skills to our collective endeavor.

I would like to thank other key contributors to chapters in this edition. As always, I would like to give particular thanks to Dr. Patricia Ketcham, who has helped with the *Access to Health* series since its beginnings. As associate director of health promotion in Student Health Services at Oregon State University, as president of the American College Health Association, and with her high level of involvement in national groups focused on college student issues, Dr. Ketcham has provided a current and unique perspective on key campus challenges and the innovative ways in which campuses are responding to a wide range of student health issues. Although she has been instrumental in the development and updating of several different chapters over the years, for this edition she used her skills in careful revisions of "Focus On: Recognizing and Avoiding Addiction"; Chapter 10, "Drinking Alcohol Responsibly"; Chapter 11, "Ending Tobacco Use"; Chapter 12, "Avoiding Drug Misuse and Abuse"; and Chapter 21, "Preparing for Aging, Death, and Dying."

Dr. Erica Jackson, associate professor in the Department of Public and Allied Health Sciences at Delaware State University, used her extensive background in exercise science and kinesiology to prepare an excellent update and revision for the chapter on physical fitness.

Dr. Karen Elliot, senior instructor in the Department of Social and Behavioral Health, College of Public Health, at Oregon State University, has assisted with several outstanding chapter revisions in *Access to Health* over the last editions. In this edition, she used her expertise in the health promotion and health behavior areas (with a specialty in disordered eating) to update "Focus On: Cultivating Your Spiritual Health"; "Focus On: Enhancing Your Body Image"; and Chapter 14, "Protecting against Sexually Transmitted Infections." In each edition Karen has provided detailed, cutting-edge information to improve the content and quality of each chapter and help students find appropriate strategies for coping with related issues.

Laura Bonazzoli, development editor and author, provided a thorough and timely revision of Chapter 1, "Accessing Your Health"; Chapter 7, "Eating for a Healthier You"; "Focus On: Understanding Your Health Inheritance"; Chapter 18, "Becoming a Responsible Health Care Consumer"; and "Focus On: Reducing Your Risk of Unintentional Injury." Laura has done an outstanding job in creating an innovative chapter on health inheritance, and breathing new life into chapters that have high interest for students.

The new "Focus On: Improving Your Financial Health" was contributed by Erin Schnair, Development Editor and skilled writer and researcher. Thank you for crafting this new and timely addition to *Access to Health.*

Finally, a special thank you to Dr. Susan Dobie, associate professor in the Department of Health, Physical Education and Leisure Sciences at the University of Northern Iowa, for her outstanding work in revising Chapter 2, "Promoting and

Preserving Your Psychological Health"; Chapter 4, "Building Healthy Relationships and Communicating Effectively"; Chapter 5, "Understanding Your Sexuality"; and Chapter 6, "Considering Your Reproductive Choices." Her attention to detail, expertise in these content areas, and excellent writing style combined to provide a top-notch revision of these important chapters. As an educator, mentor, and researcher, Dr. Dobie has a superb grasp of what today's students need in a health text.

The above contributors were brought on because of their history of working with college students and their vital, enthusiastic approach to student learning. Importantly, they are all experts in subject matter content and have proven academic training and research background in related fields. Thank you to each of you for your help in making this edition of *Access to Health* one of the best yet!

REVIEWERS FOR THE FOURTEENTH EDITION

With each new edition of *Access to Health*, we have built on the combined expertise of many colleagues throughout the country who are dedicated to the education and healthy behavioral changes of students. I thank the many reviewers of the past 13 editions of *Access to Health* who have made such valuable contributions. I want you, the instructors who have used and reviewed the book over the years, to know that I am grateful for your support and guidance. You are an essential resource for knowing how to best stimulate students to learn, grow, and tackle the health challenges that lie ahead of them.

For the MasteringHealth Edition, reviewers who have helped us continue this tradition of excellence include the following:

Elizabeth Ash (Morehead State University)
Marshina Baker (Bowie State University)
Vanessa Byrd (Tallahassee Community College)
Jessica Casey (Merced College)
Leslie Crocker (Virginia State University)
Terry Dibble (Oakland University)
Ping Johnston (Kennesaw State University)
Jonathan T. Moss (Montclair State University)
Priscilla Rice (Bucks County Community College)
Todd Sabato (University of North Dakota)
Teresa K. Snow (Georgia Institute of Technology)

Many thanks to all,
Rebecca J. Donatelle, PhD

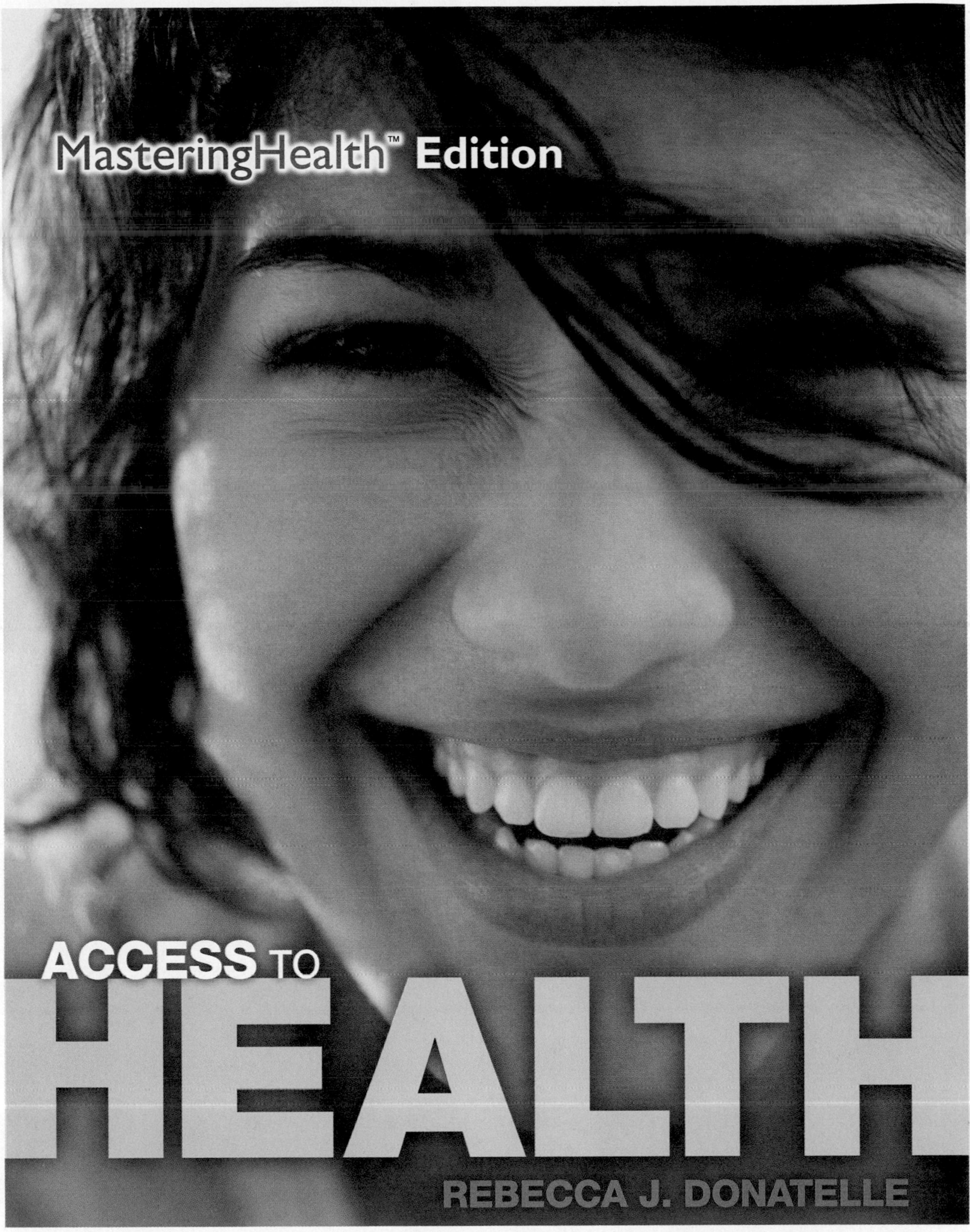
MasteringHealth™ Edition
ACCESS TO
HEALTH
REBECCA J. DONATELLE

1 Accessing Your Health

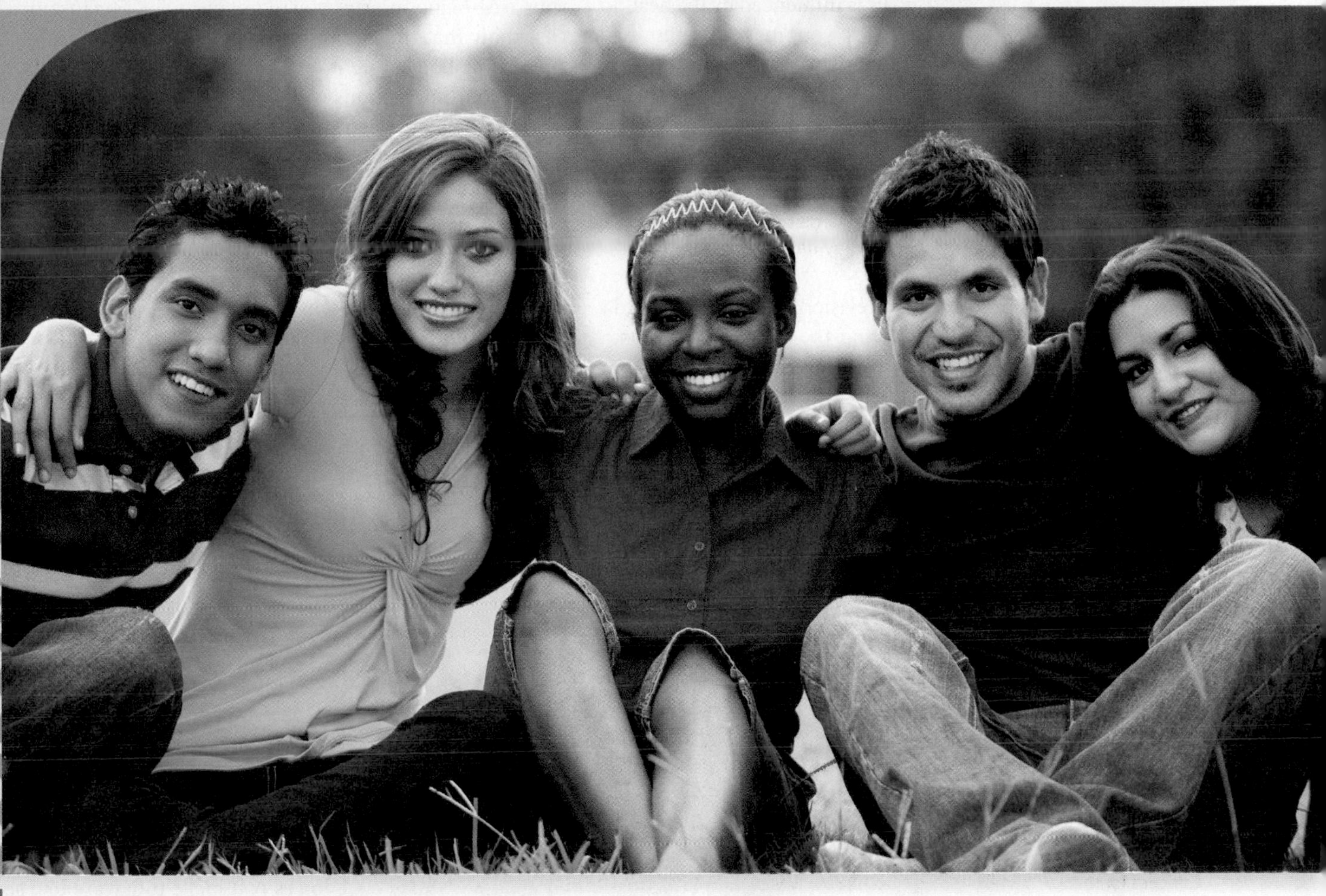

LEARNING OUTCOMES

1. Describe the immediate and long-term rewards of healthy behaviors and the effects that your health choices may have on others.
2. Compare and contrast the medical model of health and the public health model, and discuss the six dimensions of health.
3. Identify modifiable and nonmodifiable personal and social factors that influence your health; discuss the importance of a global perspective on health; and explain how gender, racial, economic, and cultural factors influence health disparities.
4. Compare and contrast the health belief model, the social cognitive model, and the transtheoretical model of behavior change, and explain how you might use them in making a specific behavior change.
5. Identify your own current risk behaviors, the factors that influence those behaviors, and the strategies you can use to change them.

Got health? That may sound like a simple question, but it isn't. Health is a process, not something we just "get." People who are healthy in their forties, fifties, sixties, and beyond aren't just lucky or the beneficiaries of hardy genes. In most cases, those who are healthy and thriving in later years set the stage for good health by making it a priority in their early years. You've probably heard from your parents and grandparents that your college years are some of the best of your life. Whether the coming decades are filled with good health, productive careers, special relationships, and fulfillment of life goals is influenced by the health choices you make—beginning right now.

mortality The proportion of deaths to population.

life expectancy Expected number of years of life remaining at a given age, such as at birth.

LO 1 | WHY HEALTH, WHY NOW?

Describe the immediate and long-term rewards of healthy behaviors and the effects that your health choices may have on others.

Every day, you're reminded via television, the Internet, and magazines of health challenges facing the world, the nation, your community—maybe even your campus. You might want to ignore these issues, but you can't. In the twenty-first century, your health is connected to the health of people with whom you directly interact, as well as to people you've never met, and to the well-being of your local environment, as well as the entire planet. Let's take a look at how.

Choose Health Now for Immediate Benefits

Almost everyone knows that overeating leads to weight gain, or that drinking and driving increases the risk of motor vehicle accidents. But other choices you make every day may influence your well-being in ways you're not aware of. For instance, did you know that the amount of sleep you get each night could affect your body weight, your ability to ward off colds, your mood, your interactions with others, and your driving? What's more, inadequate sleep is one of the most commonly reported impediments to academic success (**FIGURE 1.1**). Similarly, drinking alcohol reduces your immediate health and your academic performance. It also sharply increases your risk of unintentional injuries—not only motor vehicle accidents, but also falls, drownings, and other harm or damage. This is especially significant because for people between the ages of 15 and 44, unintentional injury—whether related to alcohol use or any other factor—is the leading cause of death (**TABLE 1.1**).

It isn't an exaggeration to say that healthy choices have immediate benefits. When you're well nourished, fit, rested, and free from the influence of nicotine, alcohol, and other drugs, you're more likely to avoid illness, succeed in school, maintain supportive relationships, participate in meaningful work and community activities, and enjoy your leisure time.

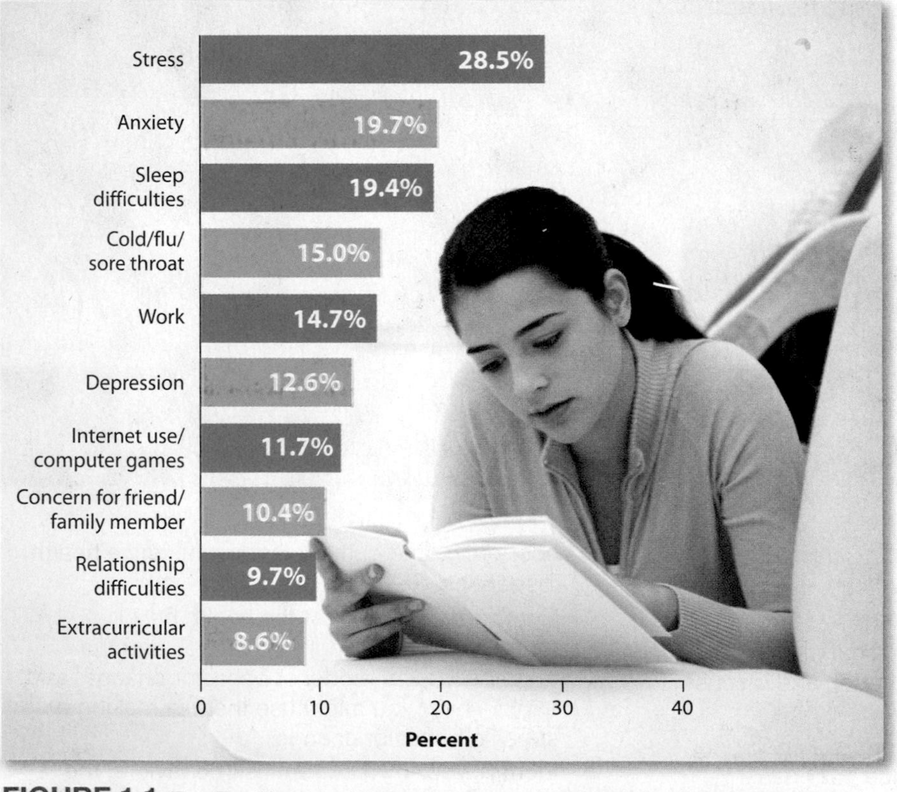

FIGURE 1.1 **Top Ten Reported Impediments to Academic Performance—Past 12 Months** In a recent survey by the National College Health Association, students indicated that stress, anxiety, poor sleep, and recurrent minor illnesses, among other things, had prevented them from performing at their academic best.

Source: Data are from American College Health Association, *American College Health Association—National College Health Assessment II (ACHA-NCHA II) Reference Group Data Report, Spring 2013* (Baltimore: ACHA, 2013).

Choose Health Now for Long-Term Rewards

Successful aging starts now. The choices you make today are like seeds: Planting good seeds means you're more likely to enjoy the fruits of a longer and healthier life. In contrast, poor choices increase the likelihood of a shorter life, as well as persistent illness, addiction, and other limitations on quality and quantity of life.

Personal Choices Influence Your Life Expectancy According to current **mortality** rates and death statistics—which reflect the proportion of deaths within a population—the average **life expectancy** at birth in the United States is projected to be 78.7 years for a

TABLE **1.1** | **Leading Causes of Death in the United States, 2010, Overall and by Age Group (15 and older)**

All Ages	Number of Deaths
Diseases of the heart	597,680
Malignant neoplasms (cancer)	574,743
Chronic lower respiratory diseases	138,080
Cerebrovascular diseases	128,476
Accidents (unintentional injuries)	120,859
Aged 15–24	
Accidents (unintentional injuries)	12,341
Assault (homicide)	4,678
Suicide	4,600
Malignant neoplasms (cancer)	1,604
Diseases of the heart	1,028
Aged 25–44	
Accidents (unintentional injuries)	29,365
Malignant neoplasms (cancer)	15,428
Diseases of the heart	13,816
Suicide	12,306
Assault (homicide)	6,731
Aged 45–64	
Malignant neoplasms (cancer)	159,712
Diseases of the heart	104,806
Accidents (unintentional injuries)	33,690
Chronic lower respiratory diseases	18,694
Chronic liver disease and cirrhosis	18,415
Aged 65+	
Diseases of the heart	477,338
Malignant neoplasms (cancer)	396,670
Chronic lower respiratory diseases	118,031
Cerebrovascular diseases	109,990
Alzheimer's disease	82,616

Source: Data from M. Heron, "Deaths: Leading Causes for 2010, Table 1," *National Vital Statistics Reports* 62, no. 6 (2013):17–18, www.cdc.gov/nchs/data/nvsr/nvsr62/nvsr62_06.pdf.

child born in 2011.[1] In other words, we can expect that American infants born today will live to an average age of over 78 years, much longer than the 47-year life expectancy for people born in the early 1900s. That's because life expectancy a century ago was largely determined by our susceptibility to infectious disease. In 1900, over 30 percent of all deaths occurred among children younger than 5 years old, and the leading cause of death was infection.[2] Even among adults, infectious diseases such as tuberculosis and pneumonia were the leading causes of death, and widespread epidemics of infectious diseases such as influenza crossed national boundaries to kill millions.

With the development of vaccines and antibiotics, life expectancy increased dramatically as premature deaths from infectious diseases decreased. As a result, the leading cause of death shifted to **chronic diseases** such as heart disease, cerebrovascular disease (which leads to strokes), cancer, and chronic lower respiratory diseases. At the same time, advances in diagnostic technologies, heart and brain surgery, and radiation and other cancer treatments, as well as new medications, continued the trend of increasing life expectancy into the twenty-first century.

Unfortunately, life expectancy in the United States is several years below that of many other nations, and some researchers believe that our increasing prevalence of extreme obesity may be limiting our gains.[3] Others cite more complex issues, including poor access to health care, poor health behaviors, social inequality, and poverty.[4]

WHY SHOULD I CARE?

Just as health problems can create challenges for success, improving your health can lead to better academics, career success, increased relationship satisfaction, and more joy in living overall.

chronic disease A disease that typically begins slowly, progresses, and persists, with a variety of signs and symptoms that can be treated but not cured by medication.

healthy life expectancy Expected number of years of full health remaining at a given age, such as at birth.

health-related quality of life Assessment of impact of health status—including elements of physical, mental, emotional, and social function—on overall quality of life.

65 & 67

ARE THE HEALTHY **LIFE EXPECTANCY** AGES OF MEN AND WOMEN, RESPECTIVELY, IN THE UNITED STATES, WHILE THE AVERAGE TOTAL LIFE EXPECTANCY AGES ARE 76.3 AND 81.1.

Personal Choices Influence Your *Healthy* Life Expectancy Another benefit of healthful choices is that they increase your **healthy life expectancy**, that is, the number of years remaining at a given age without disability, chronic pain, or significant illness. One dimension of healthy life expectancy is **health-related quality of life** (HRQoL), a concept that goes beyond mortality rates and life expectancy and focuses on the impact health status has on physical, mental, emotional, and social

HEAR IT! PODCASTS

Want a study podcast for this chapter? Download **Promoting Healthy Behavior Change** on MasteringHealth.™

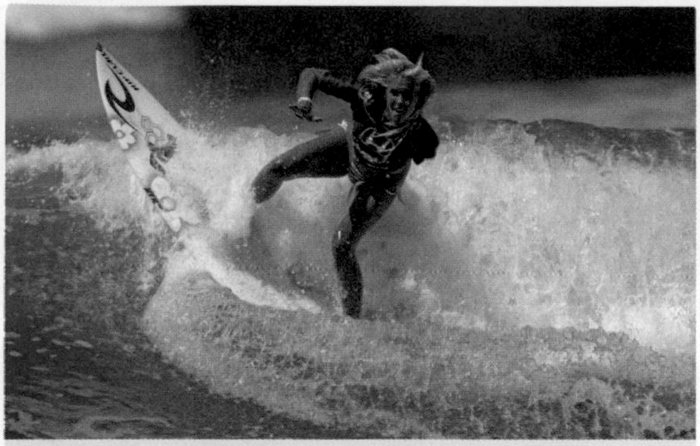

What is meant by *quality of life*? Hawaiian surfer Bethany Hamilton lost her arm in a shark attack while surfing at age 13, but that hasn't prevented her from achieving her goals as a professional surfer.

function. Closely related to this is *well-being*, which assesses the positive aspects of a person's life, such as positive emotions and life satisfaction.[5]

Choose Health Now to Benefit Others

Our personal health choices affect the lives of others in addition to our own because they contribute to global health or the global burden of disease. For example, we've said that overeating and inadequate physical activity contribute to obesity. But obesity isn't a problem only for the individual. Along with its associated health problems, obesity burdens the U.S. health care system and the U.S. economy overall. According to a report from the Brookings Institution, nearly 21 percent of current medical spending in the United States is due to obesity. Without obesity, Medicaid spending would drop by roughly 12 percent, according to one analysis.[6] In addition, obesity costs the public *indirectly*. These indirect costs include reduced tax revenues because of income lost from absenteeism and premature death, increased disability payments because of an inability to remain in the workforce, and increased health insurance rates as claims rise for treatment of obesity itself as well as its associated diseases.

health The ever-changing process of achieving individual potential in the physical, social, emotional, mental, spiritual, and environmental dimensions.

medical model A view of health in which health status focuses primarily on the individual and a biological or diseased organ perspective.

Smoking, excessive alcohol consumption, and illegal drug use also place an economic burden on our communities and society. Moreover, these behaviors have social and emotional consequences. The burden on caregivers who make personal sacrifices to take care of those disabled by diseases is another part of this problem.

SEE IT! VIDEOS

Why are women experiencing a decline in life expectancy? Watch **Women's Life Expectancy in Decline** available on MasteringHealth.™

At the root of the concern that individual health choices cost society is an ethical question causing considerable debate: To what extent should the public be held accountable for an individual's unhealthy choices? Should we require individuals to somehow pay for their poor choices? Of course, in some cases, we already do. We tax cigarettes and alcohol, and 34 states tax sweetened soft drinks, which have been blamed for rising obesity rates.[7] On the other side of the debate are those who argue that smoking and drinking are addictions that require treatment, not punishment, and that obesity is either an addiction or a product of a society of excess. Should individuals be punished for choices that society influenced and the media promoted? Are seemingly personal choices that influence health always entirely within our control? Before we explore these questions further, it's essential to understand what health actually is.

LO 2 | WHAT IS HEALTH?

Compare and contrast the medical model of health and the public health model, and discuss the six dimensions of health.

For some, the word **health** simply means the antithesis of sickness. To others, it means fitness, wellness, or well-being—an increasingly enlightened way of viewing health that has taken shape over time. As our collective understanding of illness has improved, so has our ability to understand the many nuances of health.

Models of Health

Over the centuries, different ideals—or models—of human health have dominated. Our current model of health has broadened from a focus on the individual physical body to an understanding of health as a reflection not only of ourselves, but also of our communities.

Medical Model Prior to the twentieth century, if you made it to your fiftieth birthday, you were regarded as lucky. Survivors were believed to be of hearty, healthy stock—having what we might refer to today as "good genes." We didn't have the means to delve into factors influencing risks, and as such, cleanliness, good behavior, and a bit of luck were part of the good health formula.

Throughout these years, perceptions of health were dominated by the **medical model**, in which health status focused primarily on the individual and his or her tissues and organs. The surest way to improve health was to cure the individual's disease, either with medication to treat the disease-causing

WHAT DO YOU THINK?

Is obesity always a matter of lacking willpower or discipline?

- Since we tax cigarettes, is it reasonable to tax high-calorie sugary drinks?
- What about taxing prepackaged, high-fat foods?
- Who should decide?

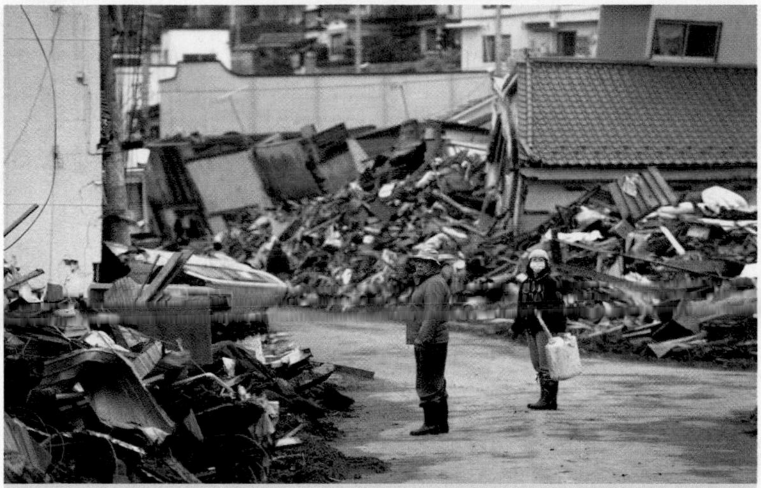

Conditions and events in one location can have far-reaching impacts. A 2011 earthquake and tsunami caused devastation in Japan and damaged the Fukushima Daiichi nuclear power plant, releasing radiation and spreading fear of widespread nuclear fallout.

agent or through surgery to remove the diseased body part. Thus, government resources focused on initiatives that led to treatment, rather than prevention, of disease.

Public Health Model Not until the early decades of the 1900s did researchers begin to recognize that entire populations of poor people, particularly those living in certain locations, were victims of environmental factors over which they had little control: polluted water and air, a low-quality diet, poor housing, and unsafe work settings. As a result, researchers began to focus on an **ecological** or **public health model**, which views diseases and other negative health events as a result of an individual's interaction with his or her social and physical environment.

Recognition of the public health model enabled health officials to move to control contaminants in water, for example, by building adequate sewers, and to control burning and other forms of air pollution. In the early 1900s, colleges began offering courses in health and hygiene. Over time, public health officials began to recognize and address many other forces affecting human health, including hazardous work conditions; air, soil, and water pollution; negative influences in the home and social environment; abuse of drugs and alcohol; stress; unsafe behavior; diet; sedentary lifestyle; and cost, quality, and access to health care.

By the 1940s progressive thinkers began calling for policies, programs, and services to improve individual health and that of the population as a whole—shifting focus from treatment of individual illness to **disease prevention**. For example, childhood vaccination programs reduced the incidence and severity of infectious disease; installation of safety features such as seatbelts and airbags in motor vehicles reduced traffic injuries and fatalities; and laws governing occupational safety reduced injuries to and deaths of American workers. In 1947 at an international conference focusing on global health issues, the World Health Organization (WHO), proposed a new definition of health: "Health is the state of complete physical, mental, and social well-being, not just the absence of disease or infirmity."[8] This new definition definitively rejected the old medical model.

Alongside prevention, the public health model began to emphasize **health promotion**—policies and programs that promote behaviors known to support good health. Health-promotion programs identify people who are engaging in **risk behaviors** (those that increase susceptibility to negative health outcomes) and motivate them to change their actions by improving their knowledge, attitudes, and skills. Numerous public policies and services, technological advances, and individual actions have worked to improve our overall health status greatly in the past 100 years. **FIGURE 1.2** lists the ten greatest public health achievements of the twentieth century.

ecological or public health model A view of health in which diseases and other negative health events are seen as a result of an individual's interaction with his or her social and physical environment.

disease prevention Actions or behaviors designed to keep people from getting sick.

health promotion The combined educational, organizational, procedural, environmental, social, and financial supports that help individuals and groups reduce negative health behaviors and promote positive change.

risk behaviors Actions that increase susceptibility to negative health outcomes.

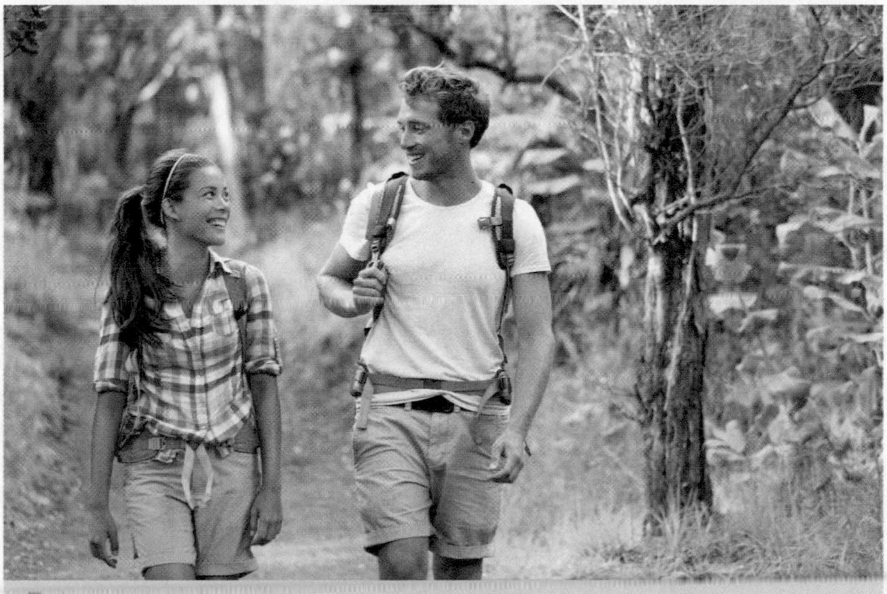

Today, health and wellness mean taking a positive, proactive attitude toward life and living it to the fullest.

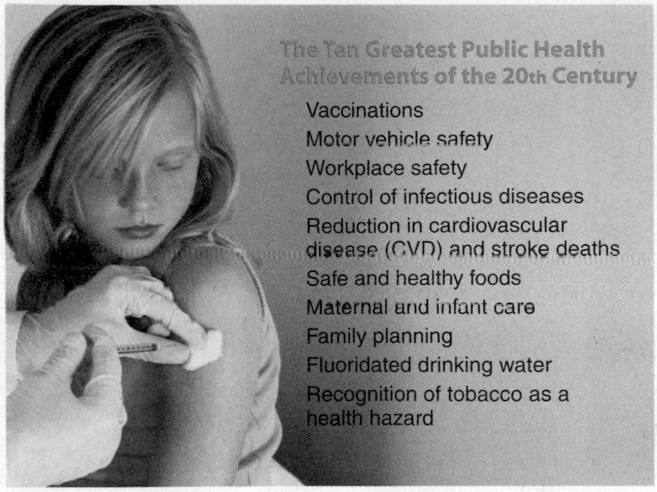
The Ten Greatest Public Health Achievements of the 20th Century
Vaccinations
Motor vehicle safety
Workplace safety
Control of infectious diseases
Reduction in cardiovascular disease (CVD) and stroke deaths
Safe and healthy foods
Maternal and infant care
Family planning
Fluoridated drinking water
Recognition of tobacco as a health hazard

FIGURE 1.2 The Ten Greatest Public Health Achievements of the Twentieth Century

Source: Adapted from Centers for Disease Control and Prevention, "Ten Great Public Health Achievements—United States, 1900–1999," *Morbidity and Mortality Weekly Report* 48, no. 12 (April 1999): 241–43.

Wellness and the Dimensions of Health

In 1968, biologist, environmentalist, and philosopher René Dubos proposed an even broader definition of health. In his Pulitzer Prize–winning book, *So Human an Animal,* Dubos defined health as "a quality of life, involving social, emotional, mental, spiritual, and biological fitness on the part of the individual, which results from adaptations to the environment."[9] This concept of adaptability, or the ability to cope successfully with life's ups and downs, became a key element in our overall understanding of health.

wellness The achievement of the highest level of health possible in each of several dimensions.

Eventually, the concept of **wellness** emerged. This concept enlarged Dubos's definition of health by recognizing levels—or gradations—of health (**FIGURE 1.3**). To achieve *high-level wellness,* a person must move progressively higher on a continuum of positive health indicators. Those who fail to achieve these levels may slip into illness, premature disability, or death.

Today, the words *health* and *wellness* are often used interchangeably to mean the dynamic, ever-changing process of trying to achieve one's potential in each of six interrelated dimensions (**FIGURE 1.4**):

- **Physical health.** Physical health includes features like the shape and size of your body, how responsive and acute your senses are, and how susceptible you are to disease and disorders, as well as general body functioning, overall physical fitness, and your body's ability to heal. More recent definitions of physical health encompass a person's ability to perform *activities of daily living* (*ADLs*), or those activities that are essential to function normally in society—including things like getting up out of a chair, bending over to tie your shoes, or writing a check.
- **Social health.** The ability to have a broad social network and maintain satisfying interpersonal relationships with friends, family members, and partners is a key part of overall wellness. This implies being able to give and receive love and to be nurturing and supportive in social interactions. Successfully interacting and communicating with others, adapting to various social situations, and other daily behaviors are all part of social health.
- **Intellectual health.** The ability to think clearly, reason objectively, analyze critically, and use brainpower effectively to meet life's challenges are all part of this dimension. This includes learning from successes and mistakes and making sound, responsible decisions. It also includes having a healthy curiosity about life and an interest in learning new things.
- **Emotional health.** This is the feeling component—being able to express emotions when appropriate, and to control them when not. Self-esteem, self-confidence, trust, love, and many other emotional reactions and responses are all part of emotional health.
- **Spiritual health.** This dimension involves having a sense of meaning and purpose in your life. This may include believing in a supreme being or following a particular religion's rules and customs. It also may involve the ability to understand and express one's purpose in life; to feel a part of a greater spectrum of existence; to experience peace, contentment, and wonder over life's experiences; and to care about and respect all living things.
- **Environmental health.** This dimension entails understanding how the health of the environments in which you live, work, and play can positively or negatively affect you; protecting yourself from hazards in your own environment; and working to preserve, protect, and improve environmental conditions for everyone.

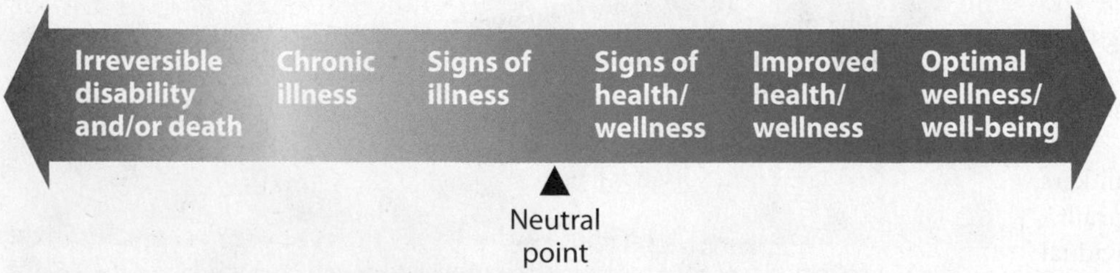
Irreversible disability and/or death
Chronic illness
Signs of illness
Signs of health/ wellness
Improved health/ wellness
Optimal wellness/ well-being
Neutral point

FIGURE 1.3 The Wellness Continuum

Achieving wellness means attaining the optimal level of well-being for your unique limitations and strengths. For example, a physically disabled person may function at his or her optimal level of performance; enjoy satisfying interpersonal relationships; work to maintain emotional, spiritual, and

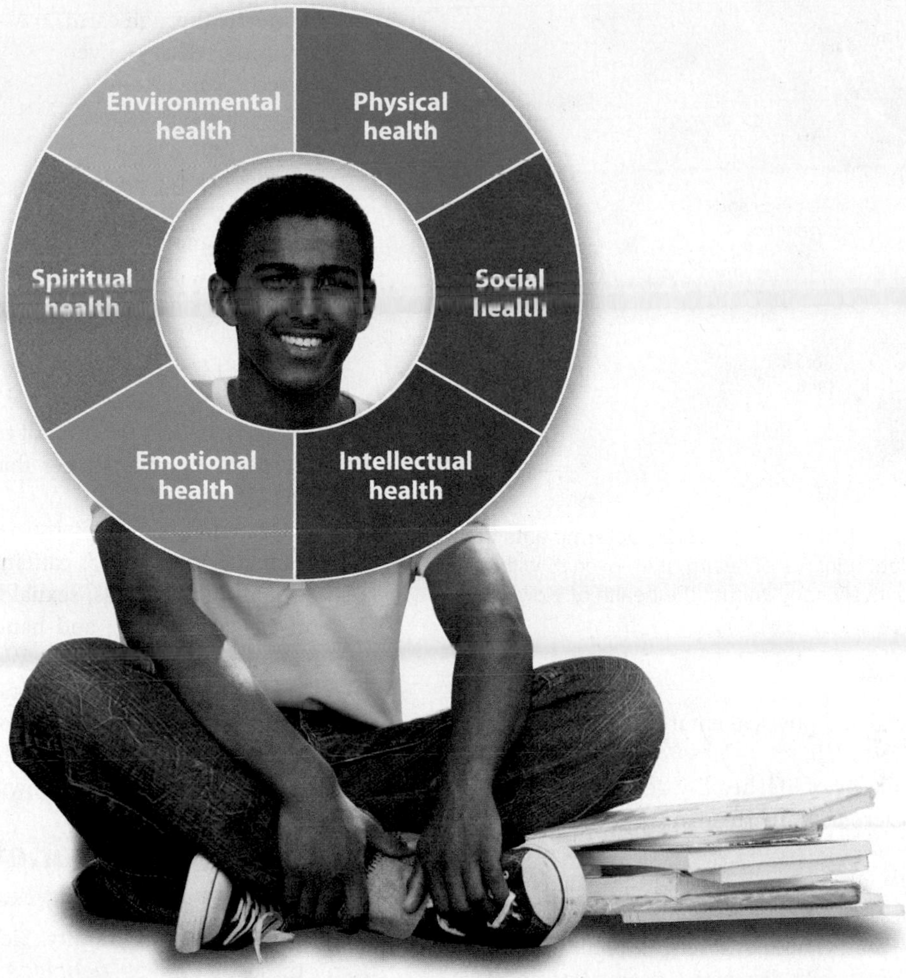

FIGURE 1.4 **The Dimensions of Health** When all dimensions are balanced and well developed, they support your active, thriving lifestyle.

VIDEO TUTOR Dimensions of Health

intellectual health; and have a strong interest in environmental concerns. In contrast, those who spend hours lifting weights to perfect the size and shape of each muscle but pay little attention to their social or emotional health may look healthy but may not maintain a good balance in all dimensions. The perspective we need is *holistic,* emphasizing the balanced integration of mind, body, and spirit.

LO 3 | WHAT INFLUENCES YOUR HEALTH?

Identify modifiable and nonmodifiable personal and social factors that influence your health; discuss the importance of a global perspective on health; and explain how gender, racial, economic, and cultural factors influence health disparities.

If you're lucky, aspects of your world conspire to promote your health: Everyone in your family is slender and fit; there are fresh apples on sale at the neighborhood farmer's market; and a new bike trail opens along the river (and you have a bike!). If you're not so lucky, aspects of your world discourage health: Everyone in your family is overweight; your peers urge you to keep up with their drinking; there are only cigarettes, alcohol, and junk food for sale at the corner market; and you wouldn't dare walk or ride alongside the river for fear of being mugged. In short, seemingly personal choices aren't always totally within an individual's control.

Public health experts refer to the factors that influence health as **determinants of health**, a term the U.S. Surgeon General defines as "the range of personal, social, economic, and environmental factors that influence health status."[10] The Surgeon General's health promotion plan, called *Healthy People,* has been published every 10 years since 1990 with the goal of improving the quality and increasing the years of life for all Americans. The overarching goals set out by the newest version, *Healthy People 2020,* are as follows:

determinants of health The range of personal, social, economic, and environmental factors that influence health status.

- Attain high-quality, longer lives free of preventable diseases.
- Achieve health equity, eliminate disparities, and improve health of all groups.

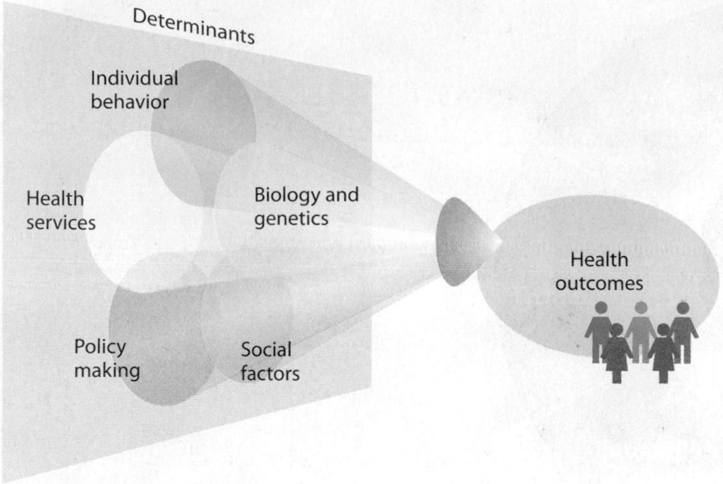

FIGURE 1.5 Healthy People 2020 Determinants of Health The determinants of health often overlap with one another. Collectively, they impact the health of individuals and communities.

- Create social and physical environments that promote good health for all.
- Promote quality of life, healthy development, and healthy behaviors across all life stages.

Healthy People 2020 classifies health determinants into five categories: individual behavior, biology and genetics, social factors, policymaking, and health services (**FIGURE 1.5**). A sixth category, health disparities, is equally important.

Individual Behavior

Individual behaviors can help you attain, maintain, or regain good health, or they can deteriorate your health and promote disease. Because most behaviors are within your power to change, health experts refer to them as *modifiable determinants*. Modifiable determinants significantly influence your risk for chronic disease—responsible for 7 out of 10 deaths.[11] Incredibly, just four modifiable determinants are responsible for most chronic disease (**FIGURE 1.6**). These are the following:[12]

- **Poor nutrition.** Diets low in whole foods like fruits, vegetables, nuts, and seeds, but high in sodium, processed meats, and *trans* fats are associated with the greatest burden of disease.[13]
- **Lack of physical activity.** Low levels of physical activity contribute to over 200,000 deaths in the United States annually.[14]
- **Excessive alcohol consumption.** Alcohol causes 88,000 deaths in adults annually through cardiovascular disease, liver disease, cancer, and other diseases, as well as motor vehicle accidents and violence.[15]
- **Tobacco use.** Tobacco smoking and the cancer, high blood pressure, and respiratory disease it causes are responsible for about 1 in 5 deaths in American adults.[16]

SEE IT! VIDEOS
How can a community's cafe help fight hunger? Watch **Hunger at Home** available on MasteringHealth.™

On the flip side, studies show people who drink only in moderation, do not smoke, exercise 2 or more hours per week, and eat three servings of fruits and vegetables daily live, on average, 12 years longer than those who do not choose these behaviors.[17]

Other modifiable determinants include use of vitamins and other supplements, caffeine, over-the-counter medications, and illegal drugs; sexual behaviors and use of contraceptives; sleep habits; and hand washing and other simple infection-control measures. We'll explore these and many other behaviors in later chapters.

For more on how today's choices affect how long you live, and how long you live *well*, check out the nearby **Student Health Today** box on the following page.

Biology and Genetics

Biological and genetic determinants are things you can't typically change or modify. Health experts frequently refer to these factors as *nonmodifiable determinants*. Genetically inherited traits are important nonmodifiable determinants. They include genetic disorders such as sickle cell disease, hemophilia, and cystic fibrosis, as well as inherited

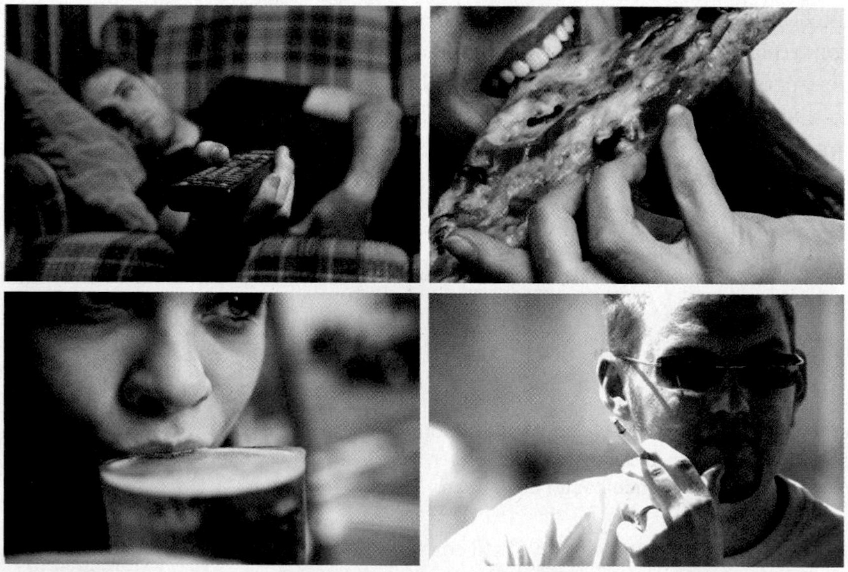

FIGURE 1.6 Four Leading Causes of Chronic Disease in the United States Lack of physical activity, poor nutrition, excessive alcohol consumption, and tobacco use—all modifiable health determinants—are the four most significant factors leading to chronic disease among Americans today.

STUDENT HEALTH TODAY

OPTIMAL WELLNESS OR CHRONIC ILLNESS *What Will Your Future Bring?*

Every 2 years, American athletes gather to compete in the Senior Games. In the summer of 2013, gold medalists Saundra Rue won the 200-meter dash in 33 seconds—at age 67 and Delwin Cobb ran the 400-meter dash in a minute and 29 seconds—at age 85! How do these athletes stay so fit when the majority of older Americans struggle with overweight and chronic disease? And what will your future bring?

Although imprecise, research into healthy aging has identified five modifiable factors that appear to most strongly influence your chances of living a longer and healthier life:

- **Diet.** Next time you're debating between the hot dog and the veggie burrito, bear this in mind: A landmark report by the U.S. Burden of Disease Collaborators found that dietary factors—such as high intake of processed meats and sodium and low intake of fruits and vegetables—contribute to 26 percent of all deaths in the United States. In fact, since smoking rates have declined, dietary factors now cause the greatest reductions in life expectancy and healthy life expectancy. To increase your chances of healthy living in your senior years, one of the smartest things you can do is eat a healthful diet. (See Chapter 7.)
- **Smoking.** Smokers have an average life expectancy more than 10 years shorter than people who don't smoke. Smoking directly causes or contributes to the four diseases responsible for the greatest number of years of life lost: heart disease, lung cancer, stroke, and chronic obstructive pulmonary disease. Moreover, smoking can make your life miserable, causing shortness of breath, coughing, frequent respiratory infections, dulled senses of taste and smell, premature wrinkling of the skin, vision loss, erectile dysfunction, and many other disorders. (See Chapter 12.)
- **Physical activity.** An overwhelming number of studies indicate that an active life is a longer life. A recent population study involving more than 600,000 people found that even very modest physical activity, such as a brisk 15-minute walk 5 days a week, was associated with a gain of 1.8 years in life expectancy over sedentary people. Extend that walk to 30 minutes 5 days a week and gain an average of 3.4 to 4.5 years! While you do, you'll be improving your quality of life by strengthening your bones, heart, and lungs; increasing your breathing capacity and your muscle strength and endurance; boosting your immune system; and lifting your spirits. Moreover, exercise helps you maintain a healthful weight, both by burning calories directly and by speeding up the rate at which your body uses calories over time. (See Chapter 9.)
- **Body weight.** The role of body weight as an independent factor in life expectancy is the subject of a great deal of controversy. What we do know is that your risk of premature death increases modestly if you're either underweight or overweight and increases substantially if your weight reaches the level associated with moderate to severe obesity. Researchers also agree that obesity significantly reduces your disability-free years of life. It's associated with an increased risk for heart disease, stroke, type 2 diabetes, certain cancers, arthritis, sleep disorders, and many other health problems. (See Chapter 8.)
- **Alcohol consumption.** Alcohol abuse is involved in 40 percent of fatal motor vehicle crashes, which themselves cause the fifth-greatest loss of years of life. Alcohol is also a factor in 60 percent of fatal burns, drownings, and homicides, and 40 percent of suicides. Alcohol abuse is a risk factor for several cancers, heart disease, and liver disease. So to preserve your life—as well as your life span—drink moderately if at all. (See Chapter 11.)

Sources: U.S. Burden of Disease Collaborators, "The State of U.S. Health, 1990–2010: Burden of Diseases, Injuries, and Risk Factors," *Journal of the American Medical Association* 310, no. 6 (2013): 591–606, doi:10.1001/jama.2013.13805; P. Jha et al. "21st Century Hazards of Smoking and Benefits of Cessation in the United States," *New England Journal of Medicine* 368 (2013): 341–50; E. G. Wilmot et al. "Sedentary Time in Adults and the Association with Diabetes, Cardiovascular Disease and Death: Systematic Review and Meta-Analysis," *Diabetologia* 55, no. 11 (2012): 2895; P. T. Katzmarzyk, I-M Lee, "Sedentary Behaviour and Life Expectancy in the USA: A Cause-Deleted Life Table Analysis," *British Medical Journal Open* 2 (2012): e000828, doi:10.1136/bmjopen-2012-000828; S. C. Moore et al. "Leisure Time Physical Activity of Moderate to Vigorous Intensity and Mortality: A Large Pooled Cohort Analysis," *PLoS Medicine* 9, no. 11 (2012): e1001335, doi:10.1371/ journal.pmed.1001335; H. L. Walls et al., "Obesity and Trends in Life Expectancy," *Journal of Obesity* (2012): 107989, www.ncbi.nlm.nih.gov/pmc/articles/PMC3359718/; National Institute on Alcohol Abuse and Alcoholism. "Rethinking Drinking: Alcohol and Your Health: What Are the Risks?" (no date), http://rethinkingdrinking.niaaa.nih.gov/WhatsTheHarm/WhatAreTheRisks.asp.

predispositions to conditions such as allergies and asthma, cardiovascular disease, diabetes, and certain cancers. Nonmodifiable determinants also refer to certain innate characteristics, such as your age, race, ethnicity, metabolic rate, and body structure. Your sex is a key biological determinant: As compared to men, women have an increased risk for low bone density and autoimmune diseases (in which the body attacks its own cells), whereas men have an increased risk for heart disease compared to women. Your own history of illness and injury also classifies as biology; for instance, if you had a serious knee injury in high school, it may cause pain with walking and exercise, which in turn may predispose you to weight gain.

Social Factors

Social factors include both the social and physical conditions in the environment in which people are born or live. Exposure to crime, violence, mass media, technology, and poverty, as well as availability of healthful foods, transportation, living wages, social support, and educational or job opportunities, are all examples. Physical conditions include the natural environment; good lighting, trees, or benches; the state of buildings, such as homes, schools, or workplaces; exposure to toxic substances; and the presence of physical barriers, which can present problems, particularly for people with disabilities.

Economic Factors Even in affluent nations such as the United States, people who are in lower socioeconomic brackets on average have substantially shorter life expectancies and more illnesses than do people who are wealthy.[18] Economic disadvantages exert their effects on human health within nearly all domains of life, including the following:

- Lacking access to quality education from early childhood through adulthood
- Living in poor housing with potential exposure to asbestos, lead, dust mites, rodents and other pests, inadequate sanitation, unsafe drinking water, and high levels of crime
- Being unable to pay for nourishing food, warm clothes, and sturdy shoes; heat and other utilities; medications and medical supplies; transportation; and counseling services, fitness classes, and other wellness measures
- Having insecure employment or being stuck in a low-paying job with few benefits
- Having few assets to fall back on in case of illness or injury

As a student, you're likely to face economic challenges. In a recent survey, over 34 percent of college students reported that in the past year their finances had been "very difficult to handle."[19] When you're injured or sick and the money is tight, what can you do to get the best care for the lowest price? Read the **Money & Health** box on page 522 for ideas on maximizing care while minimizing costs.

The Built Environment One part of the physical environment that is getting a fair amount of attention from public health officials is the *built environment*. As the name implies, the built environment includes anything created or modified by human beings, from buildings to roads that serve recreation areas and transportation systems to electric transmission lines and communications cables.

Researchers in public health have increasingly been promoting changes to the built environment that can improve the health of community members.[20] These include, for example, increased construction of sidewalks, "open streets" free of motor traffic, and bike paths, as well as public transit systems to which commuters typically walk or bike.[21] Some communities are enticing supermarkets to open in inner-city neighborhoods to increase residents' access to fresh fruits and vegetables.[22]

Pollutants and Infectious Agents Physical conditions also include the quality of the air we breathe, our land, our water, and our foods. When individuals and communities are exposed to toxins, radiation, irritants, and infectious agents via their environment, they can suffer significant harm.

With the rise of global travel and commerce, the health status of people in one region can affect the health of people around the world. These environmental determinants are a grim reminder of the need for a proactive international response for disease prevention and climate change.

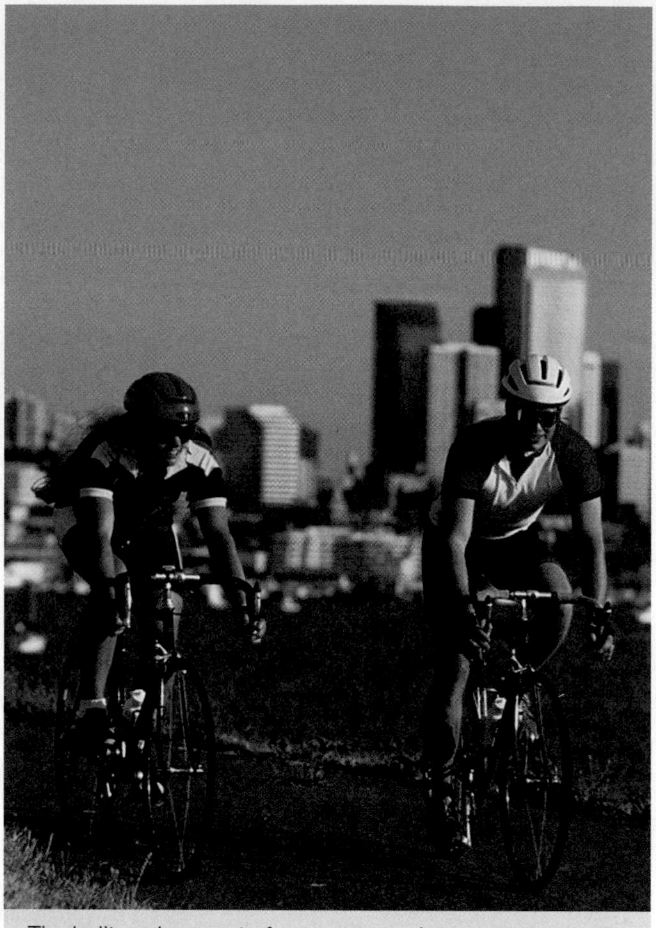

The built environment of your community can promote positive health behaviors. Wide bike paths and major thoroughfares closed to automobile traffic encourage residents to incorporate healthy physical activity into their daily lives.

Access to Quality Health Services

The health of individuals and communities is also determined by access to quality health care, including not only services for physical and mental health, but also accurate and relevant health information and products such as eyeglasses, medical supplies, and medications. By May of 2014, nearly 20 percent of young adults aged 18 to 25 lacked health insurance. Americans aged 26 to 34 are the most likely to be uninsured.[23] Individuals without health insurance may delay going to the doctor for regular preventative care. If they are sick, their disease may not be diagnosed until it is advanced, reducing the chance of recovery and leading to higher rates of hospitalization, longer stays, and more costly health care

HEALTH HEADLINES

NATIONAL HEALTH CARE REFORM

The United States saw four major political movements supporting national health insurance during the past century, but none succeeded. The Obama administration put health care reform at the top of its domestic agenda, and on March 23, 2010, the Patient Protection and Affordable Care Act (ACA) became law. The main goal of the ACA is to provide access to health insurance for more than 30 million previously uninsured Americans and also to reform some insurance practices and policies deemed unfair or counter to the public good. The legislation is structured to achieve its goals by expanding Medicaid eligibility to include an additional 17 million people. This expansion is largely funded by federal dollars, and as of early 2014, 25 states and the District of Columbia had begun implementation. The law also provides tax credits to small businesses to help them pay for coverage for their employees.

One of the most contentious aspects of the ACA is the so-called individual mandate: All Americans are required to carry health insurance or face an annual (and progressively increasing) fine if they fail to do so. The individual mandate is necessary to push young, healthy Americans into the insurance pool and thereby dilute the cost of care overall. Incidentally, coverage under your college's student health plan typically qualifies under the health care law.

Opponents have argued that compelling individuals to purchase an expensive product such as health insurance is an overreaching by the federal government; however, in June 2012 the U.S. Supreme Court ruled that Congress could enact the ACA under its authority to raise and collect taxes.

Significant reforms of the ACA include a provision allowing young adults to stay on their parents' health insurance plan up to age 26 if they do not have access to coverage through an employer. In addition, most employer-based and individual plans are required to cover preventive services with no co-payment or deductible.

Other provisions ban or place restrictions on certain insurance industry practices such as the following:

- Insurers are no longer allowed to deny coverage to people with preexisting conditions.
- Insurers are not allowed to cancel coverage because the insured made an honest mistake on his or her application.
- Insurers have to publicly justify rate hikes of 10 percent or more and must spend at least 80 percent of premiums on health care as opposed to administration, marketing, etc.
- New health insurance plans cannot impose annual or lifetime coverage limits.

To find the most affordable plan for their needs, most Americans can shop for and compare plans in state-based Affordable Insurance Exchanges, which opened in October 2013. You can find more information and updates on health care reform at www.healthcare.gov.

Sources: Kaiser Family Foundation, "Status of State Action on the Medicaid Expansion Decision, 2014" (January 28, 2014), http://kff.org/health-reform/state-indicator/state-activity-around-expanding-medicaid-under-the-affordable-care-act/; U.S. Centers for Medicare & Medicaid Services, "If I'm a College Student, What Do I Need to Know About the Marketplace?" www.healthcare.gov/if-i-m-a-college-student-what-do-i-need-to-know-about-the-marketplace.

than for those who have insurance and get preventive screenings and prompt treatment.

In addition to the uninsured is the problem of the millions of "underinsured"—those who have some coverage, but not enough. These individuals cannot afford to pay the difference between what their insurance covers and what their providers and medications cost. Therefore, like the uninsured, they tend to delay care or try other cost-saving measures such as taking only half of the prescribed dose of their medications.

Policymaking

Public policies and interventions can have a powerful and positive effect on the health of individuals and communities. Examples include policies banning smoking in public places, laws mandating seatbelt use in motor vehicles and helmets for bikes and motorcycles, policies that require you be vaccinated before enrolling in classes, and laws that ban cell phone use while driving. Health policies serve a key role in protecting public health and motivating individuals and communities to change.

Access to health services is also affected by policymaking—including health insurance legislation. Early in 2010, President Obama signed into law the Affordable Care Act (ACA), a set of reforms intended to reduce the nation's health care costs while increasing Americans' access to quality care. In the first 4 months of open enrollment, nearly 3.3 million Americans signed up for coverage under the ACA, and about one-fourth of them were young adults.[24] The ACA is discussed in the **Health Headlines** box.

Health Disparities

In recognition of the changing demographics of the U.S. population and the vast differences in health status based on

13.4%

OF AMERICANS DO NOT HAVE HEALTH **INSURANCE.**

HEALTH IN A DIVERSE WORLD

THE CHALLENGE OF HEALTH DISPARITIES

The following factors can affect an individual's ability to attain optimal health:

- **Race and ethnicity.** Research indicates dramatic health disparities among people of certain racial and ethnic backgrounds. For example, African Americans have the highest rates of heart disease, colorectal cancer, and infant mortality of any ethnic group. Socioeconomic differences, stigma based on "minority status," poor access to health care, lower quality health insurance, cultural barriers and beliefs, discrimination, and limited education and employment opportunities can all affect health status.
- **Sex and gender.** At all ages and stages of life, men and women experience major differences in rates of disease and disability. For instance, men smoke more than women, but women who smoke have higher rates of lung disease. Also, women with asthma are more likely than men to experience an acute exacerbation (asthma attack). In contrast, men have much higher rates of drug-induced deaths, as well as deaths from suicide and homicide. This contributes to their lower life expectancy overall. Males also have a lower healthy life expectancy than females.

Remote Area Medical (RAM) clinics attempt to address the problem of health disparities caused by location, poverty, and lack of insurance. At RAM clinics, rural families wait in line for hours to receive free health care from hundreds of professional doctors, nurses, dentists, and other health workers.

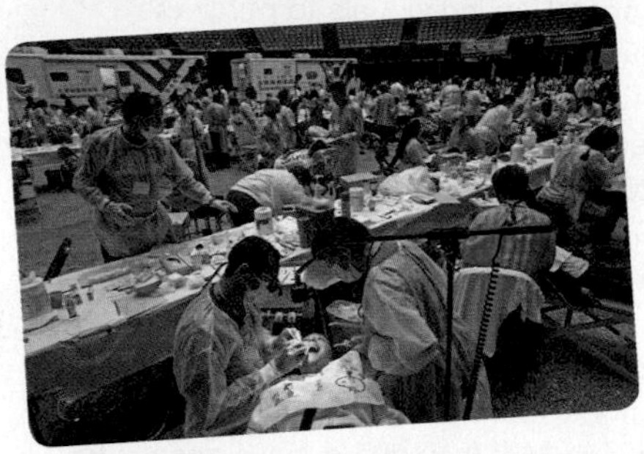

- **Economics and education.** Income and education provide resources that protect against health problems throughout life. Poor Americans with a low level of education experience increased rates of illness, premature death, and risk-taking behaviors such as smoking and binge drinking. Moreover, persistent poverty may make it difficult to buy healthy food, medications, quality housing, and access to safe, affordable exercise options.
- **Inadequate health insurance.** People who are uninsured or underinsured may face unaffordable payments or copayments, high deductibles, or limited care in their area.
- **Geographic location.** Whether you live in an urban or rural area and have access to public transportation or your own vehicle can have a huge impact on what you eat, the amount of physical activity you get, and your ability to visit the doctor or dentist. Moreover, healthy life expectancy is lowest throughout the Southeastern United States, with the exception of Florida.
- **Sexual orientation.** Gay, lesbian, bisexual, or transgender individuals may lack social support, may be denied health benefits due to unrecognized marital status, and may experience unusually high stress levels and stigmatization by other groups.
- **Disability.** Disproportionate numbers of disabled individuals lack access to health care services, social support, and community resources that would enhance their quality of life.

Source: Data from Centers for Disease Control and Prevention, "CDC Health Disparities and Inequalities Report—United States, 2013," *Morbidity and Mortality Weekly Report* 62, Supplement 3 (November 22, 2013): 1–187, Available at www.cdc.gov/mmwr/preview/ind2013_su.html#HealthDisparities2013; Centers for Disease Control and Prevention, "State-Specific Healthy Life Expectancy at Age 65 Years—United States, 2007–2009," *Morbidity and Mortality Weekly Report* 62, no. 28 (July 19, 2013): 561–66.

health disparities Differences in the incidence, prevalence, mortality, and burden of diseases and other health conditions among specific population groups.

belief Appraisal of the relationship between some object, action, or idea and some attribute of that object, action, or idea.

racial or ethnic background, *Healthy People 2020* includes strong language about the importance of reducing these **health disparities.**[25] See the **Health in a Diverse World** box for examples of groups that often experience health disparities.

LO 4 | HOW DOES BEHAVIOR CHANGE OCCUR?

Compare and contrast the health belief model, the social cognitive model, and the transtheoretical model of behavior change, and explain how you might use them in making a specific behavior change.

While many factors influence your health status, you have the most control over factors in just one category: your individual behaviors. Over the years, social scientists and public health researchers have developed a variety of models to illustrate how individual behavior change occurs. We explore three of those here.

Health Belief Model

We often assume that when rational people realize their behaviors put them at risk, they will change those behaviors and reduce that risk. However, it doesn't work that way for many of us. Consider the number of health professionals who smoke, consume junk food, and act in other unhealthy ways. They surely know better, but their "knowing" is disconnected from their "doing." One classic model of behavior change proposes that our beliefs may help to explain why this occurs.

A **belief** is an appraisal of the relationship between some object, action, or idea (e.g., smoking) and some attribute of that object, action, or idea (e.g., "Smoking is expensive, dirty, and causes cancer" or "Smoking is sociable and relaxing"). Psychologists studying the relationship between beliefs and health behaviors have determined that although beliefs may subtly influence behavior, they may or may not cause people to behave differently. In 1966, psychologist I. Rosenstock developed a classic theory, the **health belief model (HBM)**, to show when beliefs affect behavior change.[26] The HBM holds that several factors must support a belief before change is likely:

- **Perceived seriousness of the health problem.** The more serious the perceived effects are, the more likely it is that action will be taken.
- **Perceived susceptibility to the health problem.** People who perceive themselves at high risk are more likely to take preventive action.
- **Perceived benefits.** People are more likely to take action if they believe that this action will benefit them.
- **Perceived barriers.** Even if a recommended action is perceived to be effective, the individual may believe it is too expensive, difficult, inconvenient, or time-consuming. These perceived barriers must be overcome or acknowledged as less important than the perceived benefits.
- **Cues to action.** A person who is reminded or alerted about a potential health problem—by anything from early symptoms to an e-mail from a health care provider—is more likely to take action.

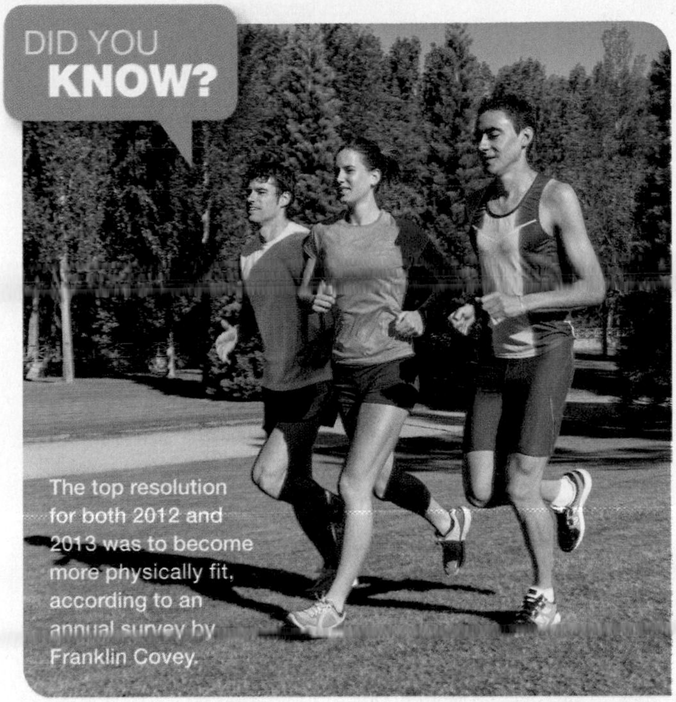
DID YOU
KNOW?
The top resolution for both 2012 and 2013 was to become more physically fit, according to an annual survey by Franklin Covey.

People follow the HBM many times every day. Take, for example, smokers. Older smokers are likely to know other smokers who have developed serious heart or lung problems. They are thus more likely to perceive tobacco as a threat to their health than are teenagers who have just begun smoking. The greater the perceived threat of health problems caused by smoking, the greater the chance a person will quit.

However, many chronic smokers know the risks yet continue to smoke. Why? According to Rosenstock, some people do not believe they are susceptible to a severe problem—they act as though they are immune to it—and are unlikely to change their behavior. They also may feel that the immediate pleasure outweighs the long-range cost.

Social Cognitive Model

The **social cognitive model (SCM)** developed from the work of several researchers over decades, but it is most closely associated with the work of psychologist Albert Bandura.[27] Fundamentally, the model proposes that three factors interact in a reciprocal fashion to promote and motivate change. These are the social environment in which we live, our thoughts or cognition (including our values, perceptions, beliefs, expectations, and sense of self-efficacy), and our behaviors. We change our behavior in part by observing models in our environments—from childhood to the present moment—reflecting on our observations, and regulating ourselves accordingly.

For instance, if we observe a family member successfully quitting smoking, we are more apt to believe we can do it, too. In addition, when we succeed in changing ourselves, we change our thoughts about ourselves, and this in turn may promote further behavior change. For instance, after we've successfully quit smoking, we may feel empowered to increase our level of physical activity. Moreover, as we change ourselves, we become a model for others to observe. Thus, we are not just products of our environments, but producers.

health belief model (HBM) Model for explaining how beliefs may influence behaviors.

social cognitive model (SCM) Model of behavior change emphasizing the role of social factors and thought processes (cognition) in behavior change.

transtheoretical model Model of behavior change that identifies six distinct stages people go through in altering behavior patterns; also called the *stages of change model*.

The SCM is often used to design health promotion programs. For example, one public health program engaged overweight fathers to influence the eating and activity patterns of their children. The families were supported with health care, nutrition counseling, fitness instruction, access to a gym, and other community resources. As they lost weight, the fathers modeled healthful eating and regular physical activity, changing their home environments in ways that encouraged similar behavior change in their children.[28]

Correspondingly, positive change is less likely when role models are inadequate or absent. Poor family functioning, for example, is a risk factor for youth violence; thus, public health efforts that follow the SCM to reduce youth violence typically include mentoring programs that pair at-risk children with adults and youth who model nonviolent methods of conflict resolution.[29]

Transtheoretical Model

Why do so many New Year's resolutions fail before Valentine's Day? According to Drs. James Prochaska and Carlos DiClemente, it's because most of us aren't really prepared to take action. Their research indicates that behavior changes usually do not succeed if they start with the change itself. Instead, we must go through a series of stages to adequately prepare ourselves for that eventual change.[30] According to Prochaska and DiClemente's **transtheoretical model** of behavior change

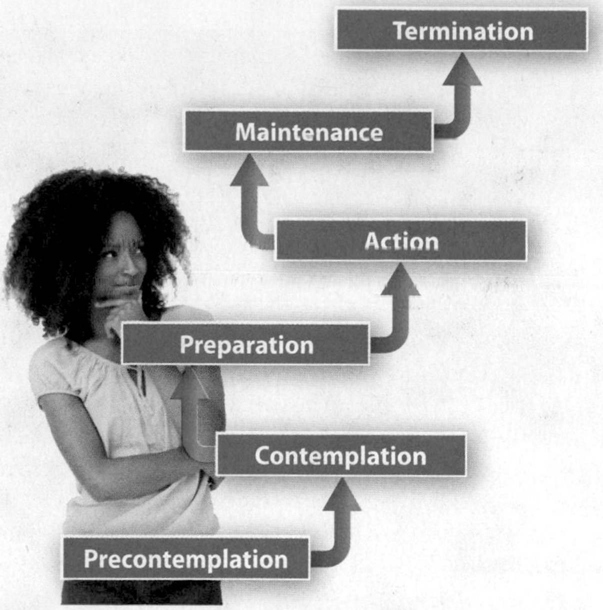

FIGURE 1.7 **Transtheoretical Model** People don't move through the transtheoretical model stages in sequence. We may make progress in more than one stage at one time, or we may shuttle back and forth from one to another—say, contemplation to preparation, then back to contemplation—before we succeed in making a change.

(also called the *stages of change model*), our chances of keeping those New Year's resolutions will be greatly enhanced if we have proper reinforcement and help during each of the following stages:

1. **Precontemplation.** People in the precontemplation stage have no current intention of changing. They may have tried to change a behavior before and given up, or they may be in denial and unaware of any problem.
2. **Contemplation.** In this phase, people recognize that they have a problem and begin to contemplate the need to change. Despite this acknowledgment, people can languish in this stage for years, realizing that they have a problem but lacking the time or energy to make the change.
3. **Preparation.** Most people at this point are close to taking action. They've thought about what they might do and may even have come up with a plan.
4. **Action.** In this stage, people begin to follow their action plans. Those who have prepared for change appropriately and made a plan of action are more ready for action than are those who have given it little thought.
5. **Maintenance.** During the maintenance stage, a person continues the actions begun in the action stage and works toward making these changes a permanent part of his or her life. In this stage, it is important to be aware of the potential for relapses and to develop strategies for dealing with such challenges.
6. **Termination.** By this point, the behavior is so ingrained that constant vigilance may be unnecessary. The new behavior has become an essential part of daily living.

SEE IT! VIDEOS

How can you change your habits and stick with it? Watch **New Year's Resolutions** available on MasteringHealth.™

We don't necessarily go through these stages sequentially. They may overlap, or we may shuttle back and forth from one to another—say, contemplation to preparation, then back to contemplation—for a while before we become truly committed to making the change (**FIGURE 1.7**). Still, it's useful to recognize "where we are" with a change, so that we can consider the appropriate strategies to move us forward.

LO 5 | HOW CAN YOU IMPROVE YOUR HEALTH BEHAVIORS?

Identify your own current risk behaviors, the factors that influence those behaviors, and the strategies you can use to change them.

Clearly, change is not always easy. To successfully change a behavior, you need to see change not as a singular *event* but instead as a *process* by which you substitute positive patterns for new ones—a process that requires preparation, has several stages, and takes time to occur. The following four-step plan integrates ideas from each of the above behavior change models into a simple guide to help you move forward.

Step One: Increase Your Awareness

Before you can decide what you might want to change, you need to learn what researchers know about the behaviors that contribute to and detract from your health. Each chapter in this book provides a foundation of information focused on these factors. Check out the Table of Contents at the front of the book to locate chapters with the information you're looking for.

This is also a good time to take stock of the health determinants in your life: What aspects of your biology and behavior support your health, and which are obstacles to overcome? What elements of your social and physical environment could you tap into to help you change, and what elements might hold you back? Making a list of all of the health determinants that affect you—both positively and negatively—should greatly increase your understanding of what you might want to change and what you might need to do to make that change happen.

Step Two: Contemplate Change

Now that you've increased your awareness of the behaviors that contribute to wellness in populations and the specific health determinants that affect you, you may find yourself contemplating change. In this stage, the following strategies may be helpful.

Examine Your Current Health Habits and Patterns Do you routinely stop at Dunkin' Donuts for breakfast? Smoke when you're feeling stressed? Party too much on the weekends? Get to bed way past 2 A.M.? When considering behavior you may want to change, ask yourself the following:

- How long has this behavior existed, and how frequently do I do it?
- How serious are the long- and short-term consequences of the habit or pattern?
- What are some of your reasons for continuing this problematic behavior?
- What kinds of situations trigger the behavior?
- Are other people involved in this behavior? If so, how?

Health behaviors involve elements of personal choice, but they are also influenced by other determinants. Some are *predisposing factors*—for instance, if your parents smoke, you're more likely to start smoking than someone whose parents don't smoke. Some are *enabling factors*—for example, peers who smoke enable one another's smoking. Identifying the factors that encourage or discourage a habit is part of contemplating behavior change.

Various *reinforcing factors* can support or undermine your effort to change. If you decide to stop smoking, but your family and friends all smoke, then you may lose your resolve. In such cases, it can be helpful to employ the social cognitive model and deliberately change aspects of your social environment. For instance, you could spend more time with nonsmoking friends to give yourself a chance to observe people modeling the positive behavior you want to emulate.

Identify a Target Behavior To clarify your thinking about the various behaviors you might like to target, ask yourself these questions:

- **What do I want?** Is your ultimate goal to lose weight? To exercise more? To reduce stress? To have a lasting relationship? You need a clear picture of your target outcome.
- **Which change is the greatest priority at this time?** Rather than saying, "I need to eat less *and* start exercising," identify one specific behavior that contributes significantly to your greatest problem, and tackle that first.
- **Why is this important to me?** Think through why you want to change. Are you doing it because of your health? To improve your academic performance? To look better? To win someone else's approval? It's best to target a behavior because it's right for you rather than because you think it will help you win others' approval.

Learn More about the Target Behavior Once you've clarified exactly what behavior you'd like to change, you're ready to learn more about that behavior. This textbook will help, and this is a great time to learn how to gain access to accurate and reliable health information on the Internet (see the **Tech & Health** box on page 16).

As you conduct your research, don't limit your focus to the behavior and its effects. Learn all you can about aspects of your world that might pose obstacles to your success. For instance, let's say you decide you want to meditate for 15 minutes a day. You face a big ramp-up just in learning what meditation is, how it's practiced, and what benefits you might expect from it. But in addition, what might pose an obstacle to meditation? Do you think of yourself as hyper? Do you live in a super-noisy dorm? Are you afraid your friends might think meditating is weird? In short, learn everything you can—positive and negative—about your target behavior now, and you'll be better prepared for change.

Assess Your Motivation and Your Readiness to Change Wanting to change is an essential prerequisite of the change process, but to achieve change, you need more than desire. You need real **motivation**, which isn't just a feeling, but a social and cognitive force that directs your behavior. To understand what goes into motivation, let's return for a moment to two models of change discussed earlier: the health belief model and the social cognitive model.

motivation A social, cognitive, and emotional force that directs human behavior.

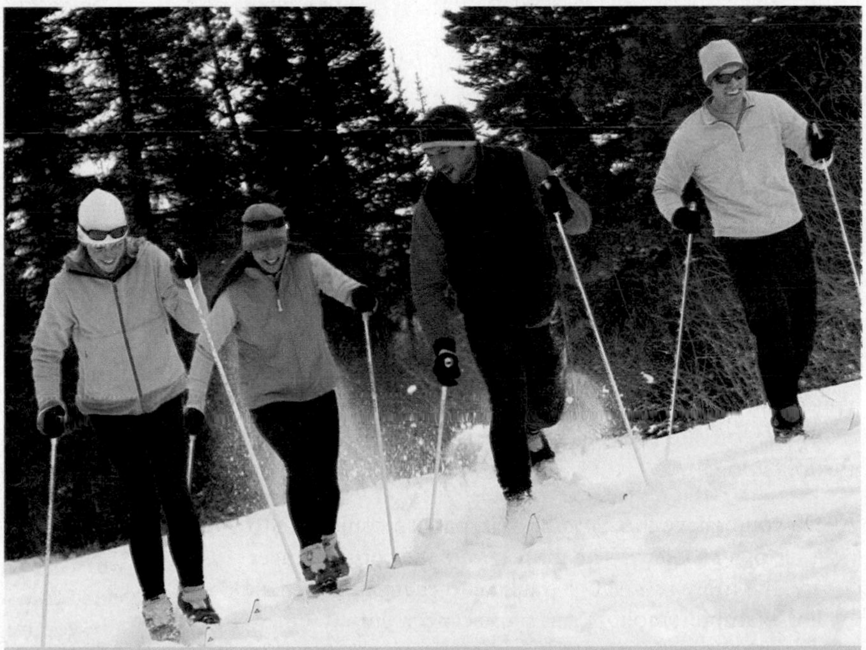

Many people find it easiest to stay motivated by planning small incremental changes, working toward a goal, and rewarding themselves along the way. Friends can also help you stay motivated by modeling healthy behaviors, offering support, joining you in your change efforts, and providing reinforcement.

TECH & HEALTH | SURFING FOR THE LATEST IN HEALTH

The Internet can be a wonderful resource for quickly finding answers to your questions, but it can also be a source of much *misinformation*. To ensure that the sites you visit are reliable and trustworthy, follow these tips.

- Look for websites sponsored by an official government agency, a university or college, or a hospital/medical center. Government sites are easily identified by their *.gov* extensions, college and university sites typically have *.edu* extensions, and many hospitals have a *.org* extension (e.g., the Mayo Clinic's website is www.mayoclinic.org). Major philanthropic foundations, such as the Robert Wood Johnson Foundation, the Kellogg Foundation, and others, often provide information about selected health topics. In addition, national nonprofit organizations, such as the American Heart Association and the American Cancer Society, are often good, authoritative sources of information. Foundations and nonprofits usually have URLs ending with a *.org* extension.
- Search for well-established, professionally peer-reviewed journals such as the *New England Journal of Medicine* (**http://content.nejm.org**) or the *Journal of the American Medical Association (JAMA,* **http://jama.ama-assn.org**). Although some of these sites require a fee for access, you can often locate concise abstracts and information that can help you conduct a search. Your college may make these journals available to students for no cost.
- Consult the Centers for Disease Control and Prevention (www.cdc.gov) for consumer news, updates, and alerts.
- For a global perspective on health issues, visit the World Health Organization (www.who.int/en).

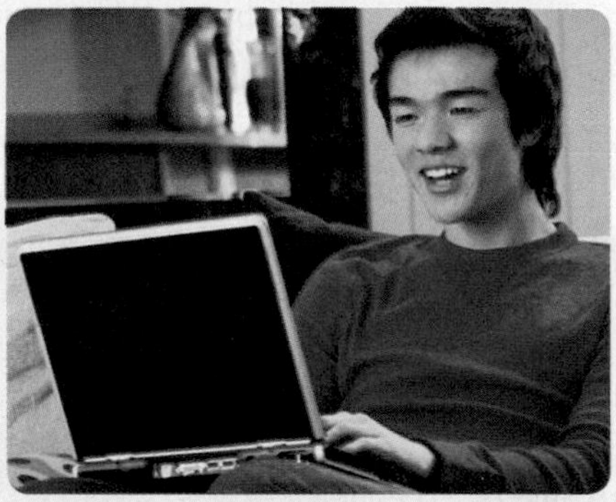

Find reliable health information at your fingertips!

- There are many government- and education-based sites that are independently sponsored and reliable. Some of these include:
  1. Aetna Intelihealth: www.intelihealth.com
  2. FamilyDoctor.org: familydoctor.org
  3. MedlinePlus: www.nlm.nih.gov/medlineplus
  4. Go Ask Alice!: www.goaskalice.columbia.edu
  5. WebMD Health: webmd.com
- The nonprofit health care accrediting organization Utilization Accreditation Review Commission (URAC; www.urac.org) has devised more than 50 criteria that health sites must satisfy to display its seal. Look for the "URAC Accredited Health Web Site" seal on websites you visit.
- Finally, gather information from two or more reliable sources to see whether facts and figures are consistent. Avoid websites that try to sell you something, whether products like dietary supplements or services such as medical testing. When in doubt, check with your own health care provider, health education professor, or state health division website.

Remember that, according to the HBM, your beliefs affect your ability to change. For example, when reaching for another cigarette, smokers sometimes tell themselves, "I'll stop tomorrow," or "They'll have a cure for lung cancer before I get it." These beliefs allow them to continue what they're doing. To put it another way, they dampen motivation. As you contemplate change, consider whether your beliefs are likely to motivate you to achieve lasting change. Ask yourself the following:

- Do you believe that your current pattern could lead to a serious problem? The more severe the consequences are, the more motivated you'll be to change the behavior. For example, smoking can cause cancer, emphysema, and other deadly diseases. The fear of developing those diseases can help you stop smoking. But what if cancer and emphysema were just words to you? In that case, you could study up on these disorders and the tissue destruction, pain, loss of function, and emotional suffering they cause. Doing so might increase your motivation: In Canada, a law requires that graphic images of gangrenous limbs, diseased organs, and chests sawed open for autopsy cover at least half of cigarette packages. Researchers estimate that this graphic labeling has reduced smoking rates in Canada by 2.9 to 4.7 percent, cutting the total number of smokers by at least one-eighth.[31]
- Do you believe that you are personally likely to experience the consequences of your behavior? For example, losing a loved one to lung cancer could motivate you to work harder to stop smoking. If you really couldn't convince yourself that your behavior will affect you personally, you might ask your health care provider to give you an honest assessment of your risk.

Let's say you're still struggling to perceive the behavior as serious or the consequences as personal. Try employing the

SCM to help change those beliefs. For instance, you could interview people struggling with the consequences of the behavior you want to change. Ask them what their life is like, and if, when they were engaging in the behavior, they believed that it would harm them. Your health care provider may be able to put you in touch with patients who would be happy to support your behavior change plan in this way. And don't ignore the motivating potential of positive role models. Do you know people who have successfully lost weight, stopped drinking, or quit smoking? Hang out with them! Finding ways to stay motivated is behind many of the behavior change steps and processes we have been describing throughout this section.

Even though motivation is powerful, by itself it's not enough to achieve change. Motivation has to be combined with common sense, commitment, and a realistic understanding of how best to move from point A to point B. *Readiness* is the state of being that precedes behavior change. People who are ready to change possess the knowledge, skills, and external and internal resources that make change possible.

Develop Self-Efficacy One of the most important factors influencing health status is **self-efficacy**, an individual's belief that he or she is capable of achieving certain goals or of performing at a level that may influence events in life. In general, people who exhibit high self-efficacy approach challenges with a positive attitude and are confident that they can succeed. In turn, they may be more motivated to change and more likely to succeed. Prior success will lead to expectations of success in the future.

Conversely, someone with low self-efficacy or with self-doubts may give up easily or never even try to change a behavior. These people tend to shy away from difficult challenges. They may have failed before, and when the going gets tough, they are more likely to give up or revert to old patterns of behavior.

If you suspect you have low self-efficacy, the contemplation stage is a great time to get to work developing it! A technique called *cognitive restructuring* can help. (See **Chapter 3** for information on cognitive restructuring.) Find out more by visiting your campus student counseling services.

Cultivate an Internal Locus of Control The conviction that you have the power and ability to change is a powerful motivator. People who have a strong *internal* **locus of control** believe that they have power over their own actions. They are more driven by their own thoughts and are more likely to state their opinions and be true to their own beliefs. In contrast, people who believe that they have no control over a situation or that others control what they do have an *external* locus of control. They may easily succumb to feelings of anxiety and disempowerment and give up. For example, a recent review study found that, compared to people with an internal locus of control, people with an external locus of control are likely to suffer more significant symptoms of psychiatric illness following a natural disaster, military service, or other traumatic experience.[32]

Having an internal or external locus of control can vary according to circumstance. For instance, someone who learns that diabetes runs in his family may resign himself to facing the disease one day instead of taking an active role in modifying his lifestyle to minimize his risk of developing diabetes. On this front, he would be demonstrating an external locus of control. However, the same individual might exhibit an internal locus of control when resisting a friend's pressure to smoke.

WHAT DO YOU THINK?

Do you have an internal or an external locus of control?

- Can you think of some friends whom you would describe as more internally or externally controlled?
- How do people with the different views deal with similar situations?

Step Three: Prepare for Change

You've contemplated change for long enough! Now it's time to set a realistic goal, anticipate barriers, reach out to others, and commit. Here's how.

Set a SMART Goal Unsuccessful goals are vague and open-ended: for instance, "Get into shape by exercising more." In contrast, SMART goals are:

- **Specific.** "Attend a Tuesday/Thursday aerobics class at the YMCA."
- **Measurable.** "Reduce my alcohol intake on Saturday nights from three drinks to two."
- **Action oriented.** "Volunteer at the animal shelter on Friday afternoons."
- **Realistic.** "Increase my daily walk from 15 to 20 minutes."
- **Time oriented.** "Stay in my strength-training class for the full 10-week session, then reassess."

Knowing that your SMART goal is attainable—that you can achieve it within the current circumstances of your life—increases your motivation. This, in turn, leads to a better chance of success and to a greater sense of self-efficacy—which can motivate you to succeed even more.

Use Shaping A stepwise process of making a series of small changes known as **shaping** can help you achieve your goal. Suppose you want to start jogging 3 miles every other day, but right now you get tired and winded after half a mile. Shaping would dictate a process of slow, progressive steps, such as walking 1 hour every other day at a

self-efficacy Belief in one's ability to perform a task successfully.

locus of control The location, *external* (outside oneself) or *internal* (within oneself), that an individual perceives as the source and underlying cause of events in his or her life.

shaping Using a series of small steps to gradually achieve a particular goal.

modeling Learning specific behaviors by watching others perform them.

slow, relaxed pace for the first week; walking for an hour every other day, but at a faster pace that covers more distance the second week; and speeding up to a slow run the third week.

Regardless of the change you plan, remember that current habits didn't develop overnight, and they won't change overnight, either. Start changes slowly to avoid hurting yourself or causing undue stress. Keep the steps of your program small, and master one step before moving on to the next. Be flexible and willing to change the original plan if it proves too uncomfortable.

Anticipate Barriers to Change

Recognizing possible stumbling blocks in advance will help you prepare fully for change. Various social determinants, aspects of the built environment, or lack of adequate health care can inhibit change. In addition to negative determinants, a few general barriers to change include the following:

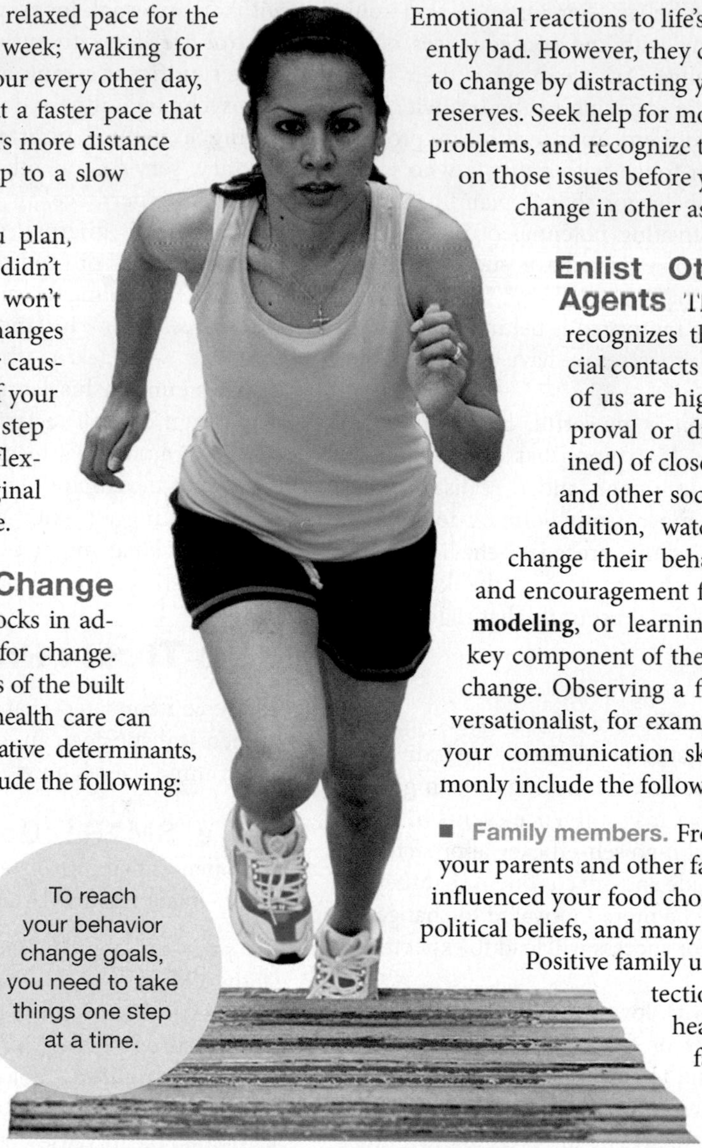

To reach your behavior change goals, you need to take things one step at a time.

- **Overambitious goals.** Remember the advice to set realistic goals? Even with the strongest motivation, overambitious goals can derail change. Habits are best changed one small step at a time.
- **Self-defeating beliefs and attitudes.** As the health belief model explains, believing you're too young, fit, or lucky to worry about the consequences of your behavior can keep you from making a solid commitment to change. Likewise, thinking you are helpless to change your habits can also undermine efforts.
- **Failure to accurately assess your current state of wellness.** You might assume that you will be able to walk 2 miles to campus each morning, for example, only to discover that you're aching and winded after 1 mile. Failing to make sure that the planned change is realistic for *you* can be a barrier that leaves you with weakened motivation and commitment.
- **Lack of support and guidance.** If you want to cut down on your drinking, socializing with peers who drink heavily may be a powerful barrier to that change. To succeed, you need to recognize and limit interactions with people in your life who might oppose your decision to change.
- **Emotions that sabotage your efforts and sap your will.** Sometimes the best-laid plans go awry because you're having a bad day or are fighting with someone. Emotional reactions to life's challenges aren't inherently bad. However, they can sabotage your efforts to change by distracting you and draining your reserves. Seek help for more severe psychological problems, and recognize that you may need to focus on those issues before you can effect significant change in other aspects of your health.

Enlist Others as Change Agents

The social cognitive model recognizes the importance of our social contacts in successful change. Most of us are highly influenced by the approval or disapproval (real or imagined) of close friends, family members, and other social and cultural groups. In addition, watching others successfully change their behavior can give you ideas and encouragement for your own change. This **modeling**, or learning from role models, is a key component of the social cognitive model of change. Observing a friend who is a good conversationalist, for example, can help you improve your communication skills. Change agents commonly include the following:

- **Family members.** From the time of your birth, your parents and other family members have influenced your food choices, activity patterns, political beliefs, and many other actions and values. Positive family units provide care and protection, are dedicated to the healthful development of all family members, and work together to solve problems. When the loving family unit does not exist or when it does not provide for basic human needs, many young people have great difficulties.
- **Friends.** As you leave childhood behind, your friends increasingly influence your behaviors. If your friends offer encouragement, or even express interest in joining with you in the behavior change, you are more likely to remain motivated. Thus, friends who share your personal values can greatly support your behavior change.
- **Professionals.** Consider enlisting support from professionals such as your health or PE instructor, coach, health care provider, or other adviser. As appropriate, consider the counseling services offered on campus, as well as community services such as smoking cessation programs, Alcoholics Anonymous support groups, and your local YMCA.

Sign a Contract

It's time to get it in writing! A formal *behavior change contract* serves many powerful purposes. It functions as a promise to yourself, as a public declaration of intent, as an organized plan that lays out start and end dates and daily actions, as a listing of barriers you may encounter,

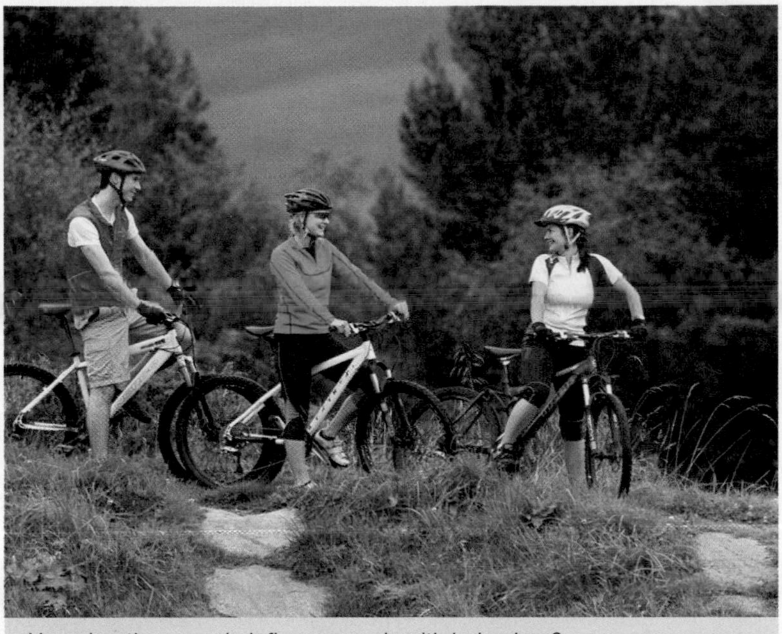

How do other people influence my health behaviors?

as a place to brainstorm strategies to overcome barriers, as a list of sources of support, and as a reminder of the benefits of sticking with the program. Writing a behavior change contract will help you clarify your goals and make a commitment to change. Fill out the **Behavior Change Contract** at the back of this book to help you set a goal, anticipate obstacles, and create strategies to overcome obstacles. **FIGURE 1.8** shows an example of a completed contract.

Step Four: Take Action to Change

It's time to put your plan into action! Behavior change strategies include visualization, countering, controlling the situation, changing your self-talk, rewarding yourself, and journaling. The options don't stop here, but these are a good place to start.

Visualize New Behavior Mental practice can transform unhealthy behaviors into healthy ones. Athletes and others often use a technique known as **imagined rehearsal** to reach their goals. Careful mental and verbal rehearsal of how you intend to act will help you anticipate problems and greatly improve the likelihood of success.

Learn to "Counter" **Countering** means substituting a desired behavior for an undesirable one. If you want to stop eating junk food, for example, compile a list of substitute foods and places to get them and have this ready before your mouth starts to water at the smell of a burger and fries.

Control the Situation Sometimes, the right setting or the right group of people will positively influence your behaviors. Any behavior has both antecedents and consequences. *Antecedents* are the aspects of the situation that come beforehand; these cue or stimulate a person to act in certain ways. *Consequences*—the results of behavior—affect whether a person will repeat that action. Both antecedents and consequences can be physical events, thoughts, emotions, or the actions of other people.

A diary noting your undesirable behaviors and identifying the settings in which they occur can be useful in helping you determine antecedents and consequences involved. Once you have recognized the antecedents of a given behavior, you can employ **situational inducement** to modify those that are working against you—you can seek settings, people, and circumstances that support your efforts to change, as well as avoid those likely to derail your change. Similarly, identifying substitute antecedents that can

imagined rehearsal Practicing, through mental imagery, to become better able to perform a task in actuality.

countering Substituting a desired behavior for an undesirable one.

situational inducement Attempts to influence a behavior through situations and occasions that are structured to exert control over that behavior.

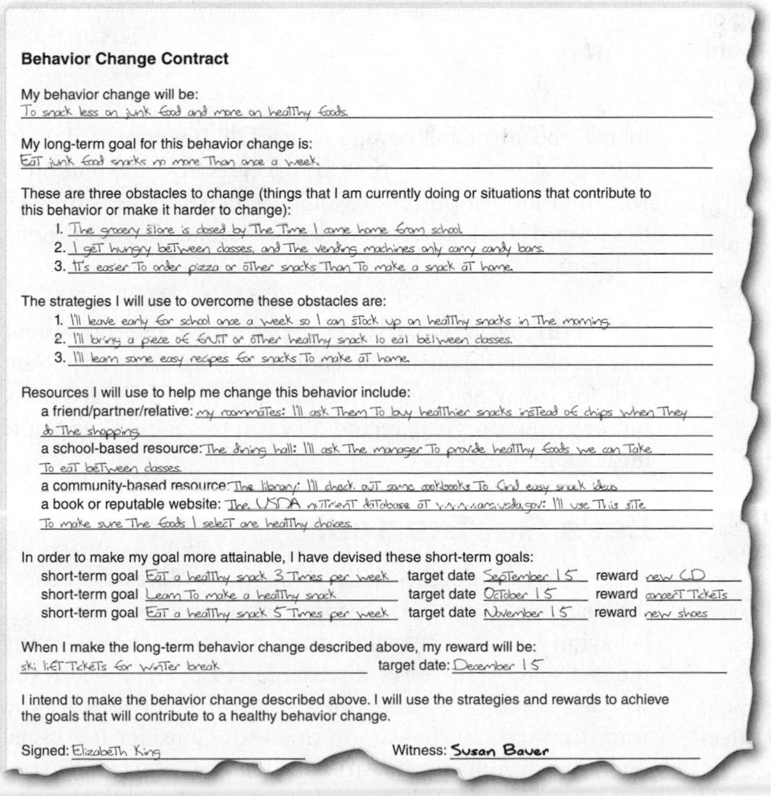

Behavior Change Contract

My behavior change will be:
To snack less on junk food and more on healthy foods.

My long-term goal for this behavior change is:
Eat junk food snacks no more than once a week.

These are three obstacles to change (things that I am currently doing or situations that contribute to this behavior or make it harder to change):
1. The grocery store is closed by the time I come home from school.
2. I get hungry between classes, and the vending machines only carry candy bars.
3. It's easier to order pizza or other snacks than to make a snack at home.

The strategies I will use to overcome these obstacles are:
1. I'll leave early for school once a week so I can stock up on healthy snacks in the morning.
2. I'll bring a piece of fruit or other healthy snack to eat between classes.
3. I'll learn some easy recipes for snacks to make at home.

Resources I will use to help me change this behavior include:
a friend/partner/relative: my roommates: I'll ask them to buy healthier snacks instead of chips when they do the shopping.
a school-based resource: The dining hall: I'll ask the manager to provide healthy foods we can take to eat between classes.
a community-based resource: The library: I'll check out some cookbooks to find easy snack ideas
a book or reputable website: The USDA nutrient database at www.ars.usda.gov: I'll use this site to make sure the foods I select are healthy choices.

In order to make my goal more attainable, I have devised these short-term goals:
short-term goal Eat a healthy snack 3 times per week target date September 15 reward new CD
short-term goal Learn to make a healthy snack target date October 15 reward concert tickets
short-term goal Eat a healthy snack 5 times per week target date November 15 reward new shoes

When I make the long-term behavior change described above, my reward will be:
ski lift tickets for winter break target date: December 15

I intend to make the behavior change described above. I will use the strategies and rewards to achieve the goals that will contribute to a healthy behavior change.

Signed: Elizabeth King Witness: Susan Bauer

FIGURE 1.8 Example of a Completed Behavior Change Contract
A blank version is included in the back of the book for you to fill out.

…nary manner …g to yourself, …r self-image.

…nt Presenting …llowing a behavior that is being reinforced.

support a more positive result gives you a strategy for controlling the situation.

Change Your Self-Talk There is a close connection between what people say to themselves, known as **self-talk**, and how they feel. According to psychologist Albert Ellis, most emotional problems and related behaviors stem from irrational statements that people make to themselves when events in their lives are different from what they would like them to be.[33]

> **WHAT DO YOU THINK?**
>
> **What type of reinforcers would most likely get you to change a behavior: money, praise, or recognition from someone?**
>
> - Why would it motivate you?
> - Can you think of options to reinforce behavior changes?

For example, suppose that after doing poorly on a test you say to yourself, "I can't believe I flunked that easy exam. I'm so stupid." Now change this irrational, negative self-talk into rational, positive statements about what is really going on: "I really didn't study enough for that exam. I'm certainly not stupid; I just need to prepare better for the next test." Such self-talk will help you recover quickly from disappointment and take positive steps to correct the situation.

Another technique for changing self-talk is to practice blocking and stopping. For example, suppose you are preoccupied with thoughts of your ex-partner, who has recently left you for someone else. You can block those thoughts by focusing on the actions you're taking right now to help you move forward. The **Skills for Behavior Change** box offers more strategies for changing self-talk.

Reward Yourself Another way to promote positive behavior change is to reward yourself for it. This is called **positive reinforcement**. Each of us is motivated by different reinforcers, which can be classified as follows:

- *Consumable reinforcers* are edible items, such as your favorite fruit or snack mix.
- *Activity reinforcers* are opportunities to do something enjoyable, such as going on a hike or taking a trip.
- *Manipulative reinforcers* are incentives such as getting a lower rent in exchange for mowing the lawn or the promise of a better grade for doing an extra-credit project.
- *Possessional reinforcers* are tangible rewards, such as a new electronic gadget or sports car.
- *Social reinforcers* are signs of appreciation, approval, or love, such as loving looks, affectionate hugs, and praise.

The difficulty with employing positive reinforcement often lies in determining which incentive will be most effective. Your reinforcers may initially come from others (*extrinsic* rewards), but as you see positive changes in yourself, you will begin to reward and reinforce yourself (*intrinsic* rewards). Keep in mind that reinforcers should immediately follow a behavior, but beware of overkill. If you reward yourself with a movie every time you go jogging, this reinforcer will soon lose its power. It would be better to give yourself this reward after, say, a full week of adherence to your jogging program.

> **SKILLS FOR BEHAVIOR CHANGE**
>
> **CHALLENGE THE THOUGHTS THAT SABOTAGE CHANGE**
>
> **Are any of the following thought patterns and beliefs holding you back? Try these strategies to combat self-sabotage:**
>
> - **"I don't have enough time!"** Chart your hourly activities for 1 day. What are your highest priorities and what can you eliminate? Plan to make time for a healthy change next week.
> - **"I'm too stressed!"** Assess your major stressors right now. List those you can control and those you can change or avoid. Then identify two things you enjoy that can help you reduce stress now.
> - **"I'm worried about what others may think."** Ask yourself how much others influence your decisions about drinking, sex, eating habits, and the like. What is most important to you? What actions can you take to act in line with these values?
> - **"I don't think I can do it."** Just because you haven't done something before doesn't mean you can't do it now. To develop some confidence, take baby steps and break tasks into small segments of time.
> - **"I can't break this habit!"** Habits are difficult to break, but not impossible. What triggers your behavior? List ways you can avoid these triggers. Ask for support from friends and family.

Journal Writing personal experiences, interpretations, and results in a journal, notebook, or blog is an important skill for behavior change. You can log your daily activities, monitor your progress, record how you feel about it, and note ideas for improvement.

Let's Get Started!

After you acquire the skills to support successful behavior change, you're ready to apply those skills to your target behavior. Create a behavior change contract incorporating the goals and skills we've discussed, and place it where you will see it every day and where you can refer to it as you work through the chapters in this text. Consider it a visual reminder that change doesn't "just happen." Reviewing your contract helps you to stay alert to potential problems, to be aware of your alternatives, to maintain a firm sense of your values, and to stick to your goals under pressure.

STUDY PLAN

Customize your study plan—and master your health!—in the Study Area of **MasteringHealth**.

ASSESS YOURSELF

How healthy are you? Want to find out? Take the **How Healthy Are You?** assessment available on MasteringHealth.™

Need help creating a plan? Follow the strategies in the **Your Plan for Change** box for short- and long-term improvements to your health.

YOUR PLAN FOR **CHANGE**

Once you've gone online and used the **ASSESS YOURSELF** activity to gauge your total health status, you may see various dimensions where you could improve your health.

TODAY, YOU CAN:

- ☐ Evaluate your behavior and identify patterns and specific things you are doing.
- ☐ Select one pattern of behavior that you want to change.
- ☐ Fill out the Behavior Change Contract at the back of your book. Be sure to include your long- and short-term goals for change, the rewards you'll give yourself for reaching these goals, the potential obstacles along the way, and the strategies for overcoming these obstacles. For each goal, list the small steps and specific actions that you will take.

WITHIN THE NEXT 2 WEEKS, YOU CAN:

- ☐ Start a journal and begin charting your progress toward your behavior change goal.
- ☐ Tell a friend or family member about your behavior change goal, and ask him or her to support you along the way.
- ☐ Reward yourself for reaching your short-term goals, and reevaluate them as needed.

BY THE END OF THE SEMESTER, YOU CAN:

- ☐ Review your journal entries and consider how successful you have been in following your plan. What helped you be successful? What made change more difficult? What will you do differently next week?
- ☐ Revise your plan as needed: Are the goals attainable? Are the rewards satisfying? Do you have enough support and motivation?

R REVIEW

hear an MP3 Tutor Session, scan here or visit the Study Area in **MasteringHealth.**

LO 1 Why Health, Why Now?

- Choosing good health has immediate benefits, such as reducing the risk of injury and illnesses and improving academic performance; long-term rewards, such as disease prevention, longevity, and improved quality of life; and societal and global benefits, such as reducing the global disease burden.
- For the U.S. population as a whole, the leading causes of death are heart disease, cancer, and chronic lower respiratory diseases. In the 15- to 24-year-old age group, the leading causes are unintentional injuries, homicide, and suicide.
- The average life expectancy at birth in the United States is 78.7 years. This has increased greatly over the past century; however, unhealthy behaviors related to chronic disease may prevent further increases in total life expectancy and cause a reduction in *healthy* life expectancy.

LO 2 What Is Health?

- The definition of *health* has changed over time. The medical model focused on treating disease, whereas the current ecological or public health model focuses on factors contributing to health, disease prevention, and health promotion.
- Health can be seen as existing on a continuum and encompassing the dynamic process of fulfilling one's potential in the physical, social, intellectual, emotional, spiritual, and environmental dimensions of life. Wellness means achieving the highest level of health possible in each of the health dimensions.

LO 3 What Influences Your Health?

- Health is influenced by factors called *determinants*. The Surgeon General's health promotion plan, *Healthy People,* classifies determinants as individual behavior, biology and genetics, social factors, policymaking, and health services. Disparities in health among different groups contribute to increased risks.

LO 4 How Does Behavior Change Occur?

- Models of behavior change include the health belief model, the social cognitive model, and the transtheoretical (stages of change) model. A person can increase the chance of successfully changing a health-related behavior by viewing change as a process containing several steps and components.

LO 5 How Can You Improve Your Health Behaviors?

- When contemplating a behavior change, it is helpful to examine current habits; learn about a target behavior; and assess motivation and readiness to change. Developing self-efficacy and an internal locus of control are essential for maintaining motivation. When preparing to change, it is helpful to set SMART goals that employ shaping; anticipate barriers to change; enlist the help and support of others; and sign a behavior change contract. When taking action to change, it is helpful to visualize new behavior; practice countering; control the situation; change self-talk; reward oneself; and keep a log, blog, or journal.

POP QUIZ

Visit **MasteringHealth** to personalize your study plan with Chapter Review Quizzes and Dynamic Study Modules.

LO 1 Why Health, Why Now?

1. What term is used to describe the expected number of years of full health remaining at a given age, such as at birth?
   a. Healthy life span
   b. Healthy life expectancy
   c. Health-related quality of life
   d. Wellness

LO 2 What Is Health?

2. Your ability to perform everyday tasks, such as walking up the stairs or tying your shoes, is an example of
   a. improved quality of life.
   b. healthy life expectancy.
   c. health promotion.
   d. activities of daily living.
3. Janice describes herself as confident and trusting, and she displays both high self-esteem and high self-efficacy. The dimension of health this relates to is the
   a. social dimension.
   b. emotional dimension.
   c. spiritual dimension.
   d. intellectual dimension.

LO 3 What Influences Your Health?

4. *Healthy People 2020* is a(n)
   a. blueprint for health actions designed to improve health in the United States.
   b. projection for life expectancy rates in the United States in the year 2020.
   c. international plan for achieving health priorities for the environment by the year 2020.
   d. set of specific goals that states must achieve in order to receive federal funding for health care.

LO 4 How Does Behavior Change Occur?

5. The social cognitive model of behavior change suggests that
   a. understanding the seriousness of and our susceptibility to a health problem motivates change.
   b. contemplation is an essential step to adequately prepare ourselves for change.

c. behavior change usually does not succeed if it begins with action.
d. the environment in which we live—from childhood to the present—influences change.

LO 5 How Can You Improve Your Health Behaviors?

6. Suppose you want to lose 20 pounds. To reach your goal, you take small steps. You start by joining a support group and counting calories. After 2 weeks, you begin an exercise program and gradually build up to your desired fitness level. What behavior change strategy are you using?
   a. Shaping
   b. Visualization
   c. Modeling
   d. Reinforcement
7. After Kirk and Tammy pay their bills, they reward themselves by watching TV together. The type of positive reinforcement that motivates them to pay their bills is a(n)
   a. activity reinforcer.
   b. consumable reinforcer.
   c. manipulative reinforcer.
   d. possessional reinforcer.
8. Jake is exhibiting *self-efficacy* when he
   a. believes that he can and will be able to bench-press 125 pounds in his specified time frame.
   b. is doubtful that his bad shoulder will heal enough to bench-press the weight he is hoping for.
   c. claims he is not good enough to do any physical exercise that will ever allow him to bench-press 125 pounds.
   d. believes that he does not possess personal control over this situation.
9. The setting events for a behavior that cue or stimulate a person to act in certain ways are called
   a. antecedents.
   b. frequency of events.
   c. consequences.
   d. cues to action.
10. Which of the following strategies is most important during the preparation step in behavior change?
    a. Identifying behaviors that support or undermine health
    b. Recognizing that a health problem exists
    c. Setting a SMART goal
    d. Rewarding progress toward a goal

Answers to the Pop Quiz can be found on page A-1. If you answered a question incorrectly, review the section identified by the Learning Outcome. For even more study tools, visit MasteringHealth.

THINK ABOUT IT!

LO 1 Why Health, Why Now?

1. How healthy is the U.S. population today? What factors influence today's disparities in health?

LO 2 What Is Health?

2. How are the words *health* and *wellness* similar? What, if any, are important distinctions between these terms? What is health promotion? Disease prevention?

LO 3 What Influences Your Health?

3. What are some of the health disparities existing in the United States today? Why do you think these differences exist? What policies do you think would most effectively address or eliminate health disparities?

LO 4 How Does Behavior Change Occur?

4. What is the health belief model? How may this model be working when a young woman decides to smoke her first cigarette? Her last cigarette?

LO 5 How Can You Improve Your Health Behaviors?

5. Using our four-step plan for behavior change, discuss how you might act as a change agent to help a friend stop smoking. Why is it important that your friend be ready to change before trying to change?

ACCESS YOUR HEALTH ON THE INTERNET

Visit **MasteringHealth** for links to the websites and RSS feeds.

The following websites explore further topics and issues related to personal health.

CDC Wonder. This is a clearinghouse for comprehensive information from the Centers for Disease Control and Prevention (CDC), including special reports, guidelines, and access to national health data. **http://wonder.cdc.gov**

MayoClinic.com. This reputable resource for specific information about health topics, diseases, and treatment options is provided by the staff of the Mayo Clinic. It is easy to navigate and is consumer friendly. **www.mayoclinic.com**

National Center for Health Statistics. This resource contains links to key reports; national survey information; information on mortality by age, race, gender, and geographic location; and other important information about health status in the United States. **www.cdc.gov/nchs**

National Health Information Center. This is an excellent resource for consumer information about health. **www.health.gov/nhic**

World Health Organization. This resource for global health information provides information on the current state of health around the world, such as illness and disease statistics, trends, and illness outbreak alerts. **www.who.int/en**

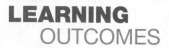

FOCUS ON Improving Your Financial Health

The ability to budget and manage personal finance plays a key role in psychological and physical health—both in college and beyond.

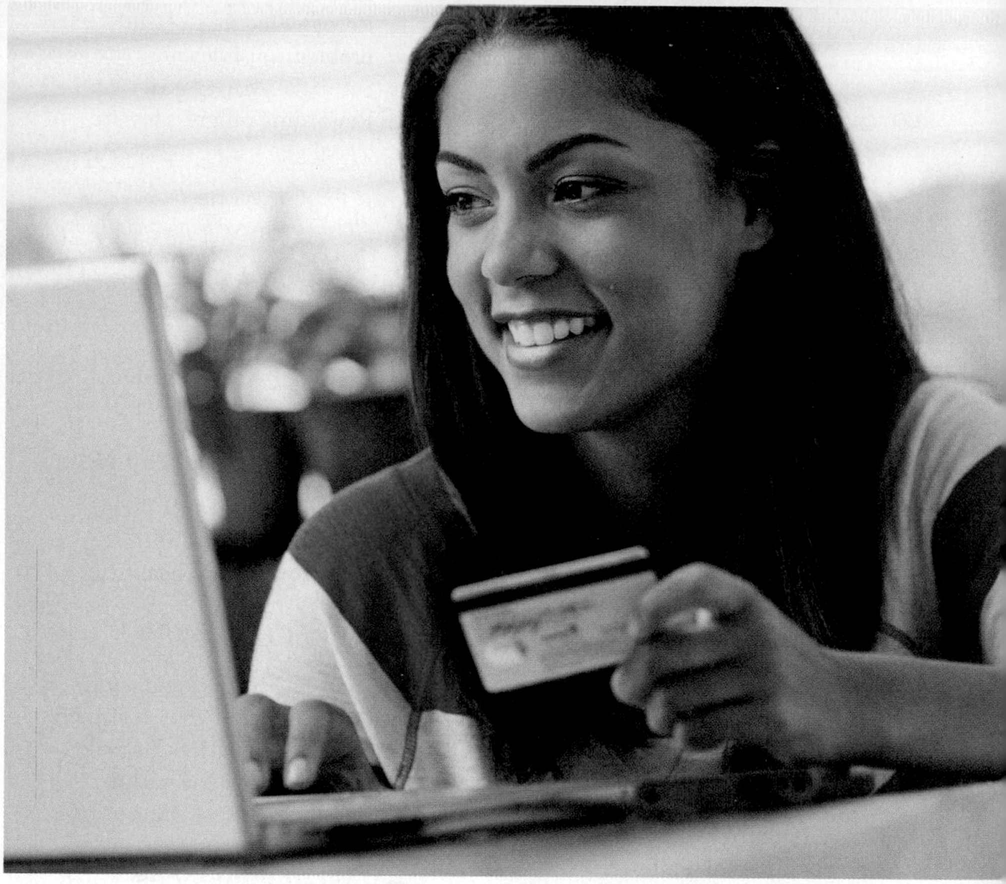

LEARNING OUTCOMES

1. List and explain factors that influence the health-income gradient.
2. Describe common financial struggles students face in college and the impact these may have on their health and well-being
3. Explain how to successfully manage finances through budgeting, understanding debt and credit, and avoiding identity theft.

They say money can't buy happiness or love—but can it buy health? We do know that individuals of a greater **socioeconomic status (SES)** tend to live healthier and longer lives than those living in poverty. This phenomenon is known as the **health-income gradient** (**FIGURE 1**). Based on the health-income gradient, a lower income individual has more to gain, health-wise, with a smaller increase in income. But a higher income doesn't necessarily guarantee greater health benefits.[1]

The gradient between poverty and health can be demonstrated worldwide, whether it's based on individual income, the wealth of the community, or the overall gross national product of the country.[2] People living in wealthy, developed countries have much longer life expectancies than do those in poor countries (**FIGURE 2**). There also tends to be an inverse relationship between SES and overweight (body mass index); that is, the lower someone's income, the greater her odds for being overweight or obese. Carrying extra weight is a major risk factor for developing heart disease, stroke, and diabetes, so the relationship between body mass and overall health is important.

Now, a person doesn't have to be rich to attain wellness. There are some notable exceptions to these patterns. For example, U.S. men have similar obesity rates at all income levels, with the highest rates stacked at the top income tiers.[3]

socioeconomic status (SES) An individual or family's social and economic position in relation to others with regards to education, income, and occupation.

health-income gradient The relationship between the health of individuals or communities and income, where health outcomes increase as income increases.

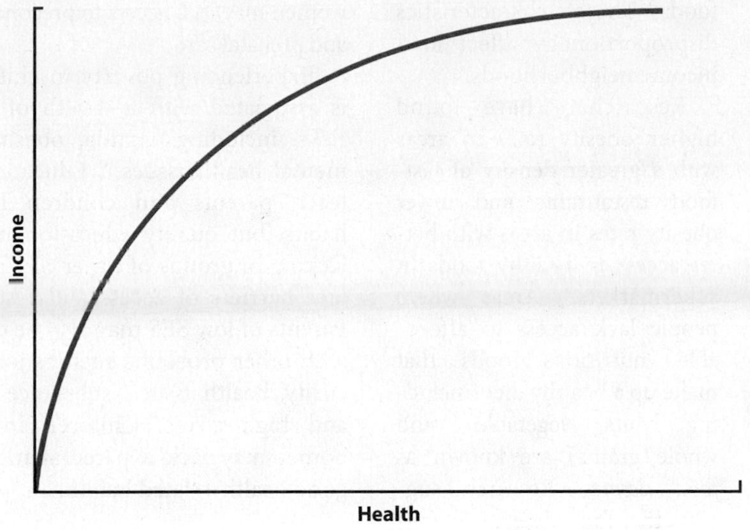

FIGURE 1 **The Health-Income Gradient** The health-income gradient shows a steeper curve in the lower income levels and flattens out toward higher income levels. Individuals at the lower end of the gradient typically have poorer health outcomes.

Source: W. Evans, B. Wolfe, and N. Adler, "The Income-Health Gradient," *Institute for Research on Poverty: Focus* 30, no. 1 (2013), Available at www.irp.wisc.edu /publications/focus/pdfs/foc301b.pdf.

Researchers continue to debate the exact relationship between income and health, with some arguing that the issues are less clear-cut than graphs such as those in Figures 1 and 2 depict.[4] Still, it's safe to say that, while money may not exactly buy good health, it makes attaining it much easier. This chapter will address some of the factors that influence health and wealth and what you can do now to increase your financial health.

LO 1 | WHAT INFLUENCES THE LINK BETWEEN HEALTH AND WEALTH?

List and explain factors that influence the health-income gradient.

The relationship between health and wealth is based on a complex interplay of many interconnected factors, including what the U.S. Surgeon General defines as *determinants of health*: individual behavior, the physical environment, and access to health services. (See **Chapter 1** for more on the determinants of health.) For example, research has associated higher rates of smoking with lower socioeconomic groups.[5] We also know that tobacco ads frequently target low-income neighborhoods. Along with the influence of advertisements, low-income individuals may smoke for many reasons: They may lack education regarding the risk factors involved with smoking, they may turn to smoking to reduce stress, or they may have become addicted at an early age after witnessing family members smoking. Smoking is associated with a wide range of negative health effects, including cancer, cardiovascular disease, and respiratory disorders. It's an increasingly expensive habit, too, and it places a huge economic burden on society with health-related economic losses. (See **Chapter 11** for more on the impacts of smoking.)

relative deprivation The inability of lower in. groups to sustain the same lifestyle as higher income groups in their same community, often resulting in feelings of anxiety and inferiority.

Let's take a closer look at additional risks low-income individuals face and factors that influence the health-income gradient.

Money and Stress

We've all experienced some degree of financial anxiety. Have you ever been embarrassed to admit to your friends that you can't afford a concert ticket, when everyone else is going to the show? Or have you been jealous of your roommate's new smartphone when you're stuck with an aging older model? While these feelings may quickly pass, on the whole we do have a tendency to compare ourselves to others. Because we value money as an indicator of status and success, those with long-term financial insecurity may experience increased feelings of inferiority, low self-esteem, and self-doubt. These feelings are in part due to **relative deprivation**—the inability of lower income groups to sustain the same lifestyle as higher income groups in their same community. For low-income individuals, experiencing constant feelings of inferiority

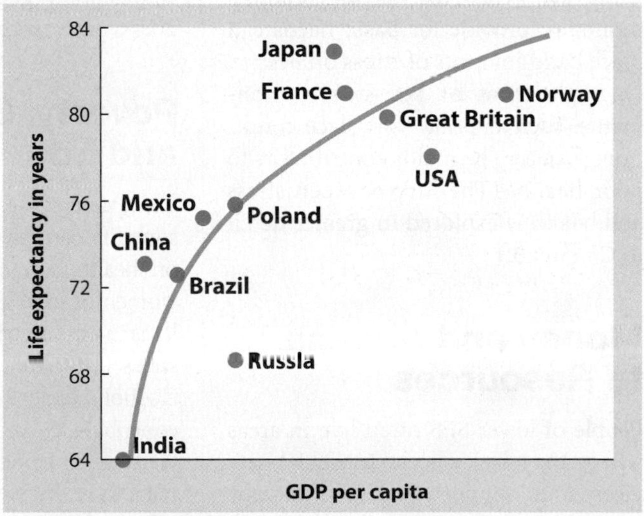

FIGURE 2 Life Expectancy at Birth and GDP per Capita, 2009 (or nearest year)

Source: Based on Figure 1.1.2, "Health at a Glance 2011: OECD Indicators," The Organisation for Economic Co-operation and Development (OECD), November 2011, Available at www .oecd-ilibrary.org.

VIDEO TUTOR
Financial Health

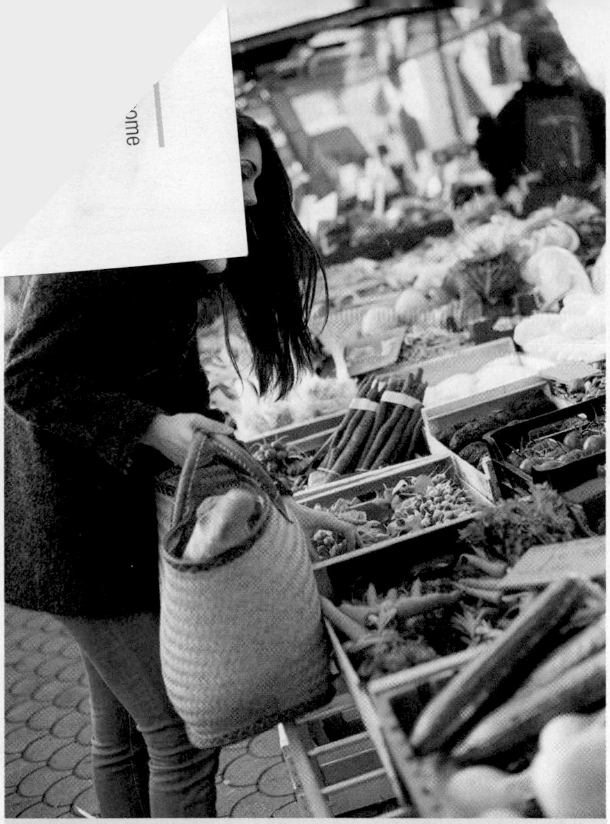

Living in an area with more farmers' markets than liquor stores provides ample access to healthy foods.

and anxiety in a money-driven society can progress into chronic stress. Chronic stress, and in particular financial stress, is associated with a plethora of negative health outcomes, such as cardiovascular disease or infectious diseases.[6]

Financial stress manifests in other ways as well. Not having enough money to provide for basic needs can place large amounts of stress on people. Unemployment or stressful environments, such as poor workplace conditions, can also be major contributors to poor health. (The link between stress and health is explored in greater detail in **Chapter 3**.)

Money and Access to Resources

People of lower SES often live in areas where they lack access to social services and support, such as nearby medical facilities, educational opportunities, safe housing, or clean water. Take the following example: A high-crime neighborhood filled with fast-food restaurants but few supermarkets presents huge barriers to safety, ability to exercise, and access to nutritious food. These characteristics disproportionally affect low-income neighborhoods.

Researchers have found higher obesity rates in areas with a greater density of fast-food restaurants and lower obesity rates in areas with better access to healthy foods in supermarkets.[7] Areas where people lack access to affordable, nutritious foods that make up a healthy diet (including fruits, vegetables, and whole grains) are known as *food deserts*. Research suggests that food deserts do exist in the United States, where some people lack access to supermarkets.[8] The difference between living in a fast-food dense neighborhood lacking supermarkets and a place that promotes good health—a safe, walkable neighborhood with a weekend farmer's market, for instance—usually comes down to money.

Researchers also link some lower income counties in the United States with lower government spending on social services, safety, affordable housing, and education.[9] While living in a high-income area with ample access to resources won't automatically guarantee good health, it does reduce certain risk factors.

Poverty, Early Care, and Education

Disadvantages early on in a person's life can have a lasting impact on health. For example, pregnant women of low SES may face problems with nutrition inadequacy, stress, smoking, and drug or alcohol abuse—all of which can contribute to an unhealthy fetus. Getting preconception and prenatal care includes regular medical checkups as well as stopping unhealthy habits—both of which have a major impact on the growth and development of a healthy child. (You'll learn more about preconception care and prenatal care in **Chapter 6**.) Low-income pregnant women may lack access to preconception and prenatal care.

Experiencing poverty in childhood is associated with a wealth of health risks, including asthma, obesity, and mental health issues.[10] Education can teach parents and children healthy habits, but quality education may be lacking in groups of lower SES as they face barriers of access and resources. Parents of low SES may also be dealing with other problems such as job insecurity, health issues, substance abuse, and high stress. Children in these homes may lack a parental model of good health-related habits.

Patterns of Risk in the Health-Income Gradient

Social capital (the social and institutional connections that provide support and assistance) at both the individual and community/institutional levels is tied to the risk for poor health faced by those of lower SES. A recent study compared premature mortality among low-, mid-, and high-income counties in the United States (where low-income meant the median annual household income was \$29,631; mid-income was \$29,631–\$39,401; and high-income was \$39,401 or more).[11] As expected, overall premature mortality was higher in low-income counties. However, patterns of risk varied by county. For example, the percentage of adults who smoked was the greatest predictor of premature mortality in low-income counties. On

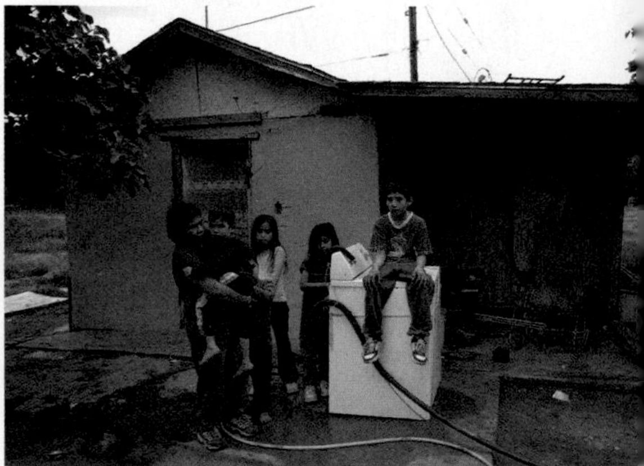

Experiencing poverty in childhood makes people susceptible to a variety of health problems, including asthma, obesity, and mental health issues.

the other hand, **income inequality** (the gap in income between the wealthy and the poor) didn't affect premature mortality in low-income counties. In high-income counties, income inequality *was* associated with greater rates of premature morality. Why this discrepancy in the effects of income inequality between low and high-income counties? While access to resources may be better in high-income counties, lower socioeconomic groups may actually fare worse due to relative deprivation and other reasons.[12] In other words, simply living in a higher income area doesn't buffer all the risks for poor health from low SES. To improve health outcomes for groups of lower SES, it's necessary to consider the entire social, economic, and physical context in which risk factors exist.

LO 2 | FINANCIAL STRUGGLES IN COLLEGE

Describe common financial struggles students face in college and the impact these may have on their health and well-being.

Many first feel the burden of financial struggles in college. Students have it particularly rough these days: A recession followed by a period of sluggish economic growth reduced many family incomes and savings. A government budget crisis then led to tuition and fee hikes at most state and city colleges. The average college tuition at public 4-year colleges and universities increased by a staggering 27 percent between 2008–2009 and 2013–2014.[13] Along with tuition, other costs such as course materials, housing, food, and travel expenses can all add up.

It's not surprising that a recent survey of 15,000 college students found that 60 percent worried often or very often about meeting regular expenses, and over half also worried frequently about paying for school.[14] Over one third of undergraduate students queried in a different survey said that finances have been "traumatic or very difficult to handle" in the past year.[15] The financial burden students face can have a debilitating effect on their mental health and likelihood of graduating.

Making College More Affordable

In a recent survey of incoming college first-year students, almost half indicated that financial aid is a major determining factor in the college they chose to attend.[16] Among students who were admitted to their top choice school but decided not to attend, 62 percent received financial aid from the school they chose. Another recent study found about 27 percent of students and parents borrowed money to pay for college.[17]

In 2013, President Obama announced a controversial set of plans aimed at making college more affordable. Some notable reforms included a new rating system tying financial aid to college performance; holding students receiving financial aid responsible for receiving a degree; and matching student loan repayment plans to income.[18] Currently, schools receive financial aid from the federal government based on enrollment. Under the proposed education plan, schools would receive funding based on factors such as how many students from disadvantaged backgrounds attend and how many scholarships are awarded. The idea of a federal rating system based on these factors created a major backlash from many higher education groups.[19] But what's clear is that as college tuition is rising, financial aid is becoming increasingly important.

Families are also taking steps to make college more affordable. These steps include having students reduce spending, increase their workload, or take on another roommate (**FIGURE 3**).[20] While these solutions can help, there are some drawbacks. For example, having a job in college certainly has perks and looks good on a resume. But the difficulty of balancing work and school can cause students to spend less time on coursework or drop out altogether. In the United States, only about half of students who enter a college degree program finish.[21] Common reasons why students drop out include growing debt; inability to cope with work, school, and life; and not believing that college is a valuable investment for the payoff.

income inequality The discrepancy in income between the wealthy and the poor.

WHAT DO YOU THINK?

Do you think the federal government should provide financial aid to colleges based on how well they serve low- and middle-income students?

- Should such funding be reduced if colleges don't perform well?
- What constitutes a valuable education?

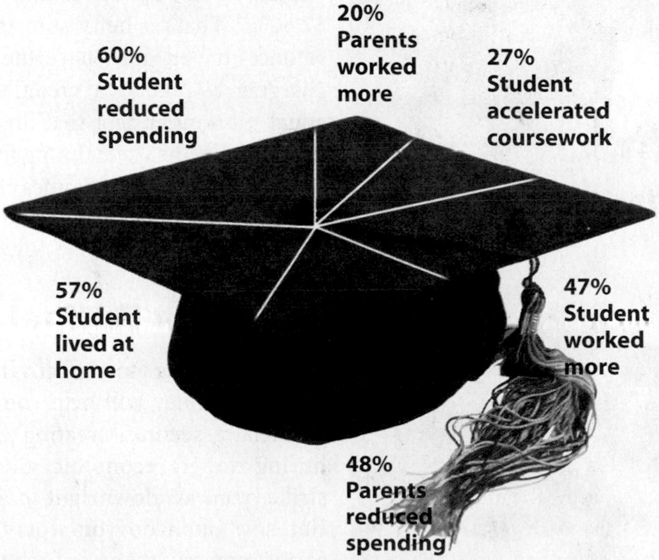

FIGURE 3 How Families Cut Costs to Make College More Affordable

Source: Data are from Sallie Mae, "A Snapshot of How America Pays for College 2013," 2013, www1.salliemae.com

LO 3 | ACTIONS TO IMPROVE YOUR FINANCIAL HEALTH

Explain how to successfully manage finances through budgeting, understanding debt and credit, and avoiding identity theft.

Financial health is not about having a fancy car, the newest smartphone, or a five-bedroom house. Rather, it involves being smart about what you spend and save for the future. Life after graduation may seem far off now, but at some point you'll want sufficient savings to support a family, help your parents financially, or pay for advanced education programs to get yourself higher up the career ladder. Being even a little bit savvy about budgeting and other financial matters will serve you well throughout life.

College is also a great step toward enhancing your socioeconomic status. According to a recent study, median income for those holding a bachelor's degree is $50,360, compared to $29,423 for those with only a high-school diploma.[22] By making smart financial choices, you can receive a degree, successfully manage debt, and learn to save money. See the **Student Health Today** box for more on how resources available in college can positively impact your health.

budget An estimate of spending and income over a set period of time.

discretionary spending Goods and services that are not life essentials.

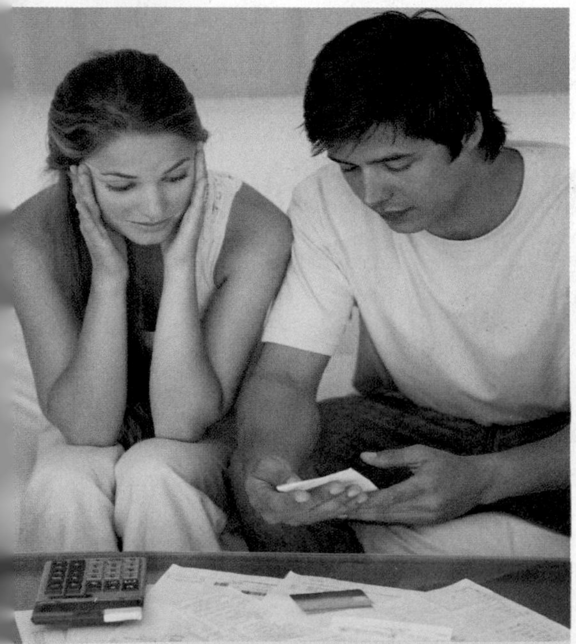

Many college students worry about finances. Smart spending, such as investing in health insurance, can buffer against unexpectedly large costs and the debt that goes along with them.

85%

OF PARENTS FEEL COLLEGE IS A VALUABLE **INVESTMENT** IN THEIR STUDENT'S FUTURE.

Prioritizing Health Insurance

Purchasing health insurance may be low on your financial priority list. What's the point in spending your precious dollars on health care you don't need? While it's true that college-age students generally suffer low rates of chronic diseases, individuals aged 15–24 are at significant risk of accidents and suicide.[23] If you were to have an accident, being covered by a health insurance plan could be the difference between quick recovery and financial ruin. Say you were to break a leg—the costs for medical treatment without health insurance may be up to $7,500.[24] That's a hefty sum to pay all at once. If you don't have the savings, charging $7,500 to a credit card can equal substantial debt that lingers long after your leg heals. Planning for potentially devastating outcomes from an unexpected injury or illness is one key to financial health.

Making a Budget

Learning skills to effectively manage your money will help you become financially secure. Creating a **budget** during tough economic times may strike you as downright depressing. But how often do you worry vaguely about money? If you feel a little guilty or tense every time you open your wallet, then creating a budget may actually be a stress reducer by showing you how much you can afford to spend. Here are a few tips for getting started.

Set Goals

Budgeting should be goal oriented. For students, goal number one is to avoid debt as much as possible. If you have more resources, then your goal may be to graduate with no debt at all, or to save for occasional indulgences like a vacation. At other points in life, you may budget to save for buying a car, supporting a family, or retiring. Whenever your life circumstances change, it is important to draw up a new budget that matches current income level, expenses, and priorities.

Track Expenses

Start your budget by tallying what you owe for things you buy and services you use. Rent, mortgages, utilities, car loan payments, insurance premiums, and (in some cases) phone plans are examples of *fixed expenses*, meaning they are fairly easy to track since their cost does not change much in the short term. Add in tuition, books, supplies, and other fees for school. Student loan payments may be deferred, depending on the type of loan, if you are in school at least half time. But other debts such as credit card balances can't be deferred and need to be listed as monthly expenses.

Next, figure out how much you spend on food, clothing, entertainment, and personal products or services. Most of these items are **discretionary spending**, things you like, but don't necessarily need. Of course, food is essential, but be careful how you classify it. Unless you eat only at a school dining hall that has a fixed fee, chances are you are spending much more on restaurants and store-bought food than you strictly need to.

Track Income

Income is the money you have to spend. It generally includes wages from work or interest payments from investments. It may also include financial aid payments, allowances or stipends from relatives, and other gifts. Some students

SEE IT! VIDEOS

Avoid common money mistakes. Watch **Money Mistakes College Grads Make** available on MasteringHealth.™

STUDENT HEALTH TODAY

TAKING ADVANTAGE OF YOUR ACCESS IN COLLEGE

As we've seen, access to resources is a major barrier for disadvantaged individuals. College is a unique time when you have a wealth of opportunities and resources at your disposal. Resources will vary by the type of institution you attend, but try and take advantage of whatever you can now—college is an investment in both your future and your health. Here are some ideas of resources to take advantage of in college:

- Your tuition may include cheap or free access to a campus fitness center and fitness classes. There may also be a track or recreation fields on your campus. Being physically active is directly tied to positive health outcomes, so take advantage of available fitness facilities to stay healthy.
- If you have a dining plan, you probably have access to healthy foods such as fruits, vegetables, whole grains, and low-fat milk, in addition to the offerings of hamburgers and pizza. Get in the habit of choosing healthier food options. If you cook for yourself, many college campuses now host weekly farmers' markets.
- The campus health center often provides easy and low-cost access to preventative care, such as flu shots and women's health services. Remember, though, that having health insurance is still necessary to avoid paying hefty fees for some services.
- No matter your course of study, seek out internships in your field and work to develop meaningful connections with professors. Making these connections will enhance your professional network. The network you foster now can provide invaluable resources for job opportunities after graduation.
- Visit your campus career center to learn things such as how to craft a resume, seek out job opportunities, and research the best career tracks for recent grads in your major.
- According to the National Association of College and Employers, employers hiring recent grads look for skills such as an ability to work on a team, problem solve, and process information and good verbal communication skills. The classes you take are an opportunity to develop some of these skills. Also consider getting involved with clubs or campus organizations and taking on a leadership role. (Just make sure that you leave yourself enough time to balance your schoolwork.)

An internship is a great way to build connections and develop teamwork skills, increasing your chances of getting a job after graduation.

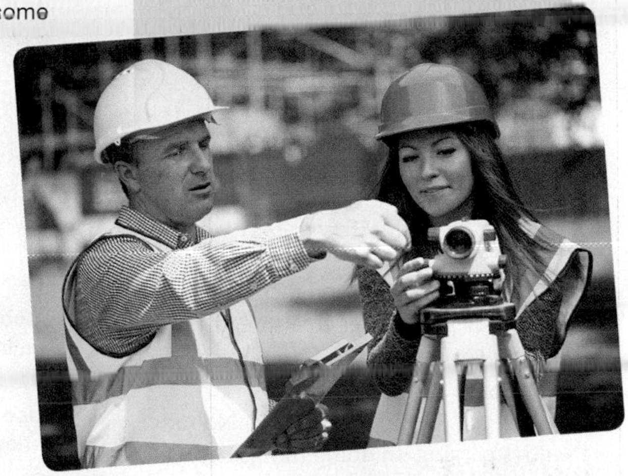

Source: National Association of Colleges and Employers, "Press Room: Frequently Asked Questions," Accessed April 2014, www.naceweb.org.

will also be withdrawing money from college savings accounts to pay for living expenses and tuition.

When you earn more than you spend, you have a **budget surplus**. If expenses are greater than income, you have a **budget deficit**. As mentioned before, the goal with budgeting should be to create a surplus and build savings. College is a unique time when many people run budget deficits while earning a degree, trusting that future wage gains from their education make the debt feasible. Sometimes this leads people to feel that, because they are already going into debt, they might as well borrow as much as they can to make life easier or more fun in the short term. You should avoid this thought process. Every dollar of debt you take on matters. With compound interest and loan terms, just a "few extra" thousand dollars more at the end of school can take many extra years to pay off.

Making the Budget Numbers Add Up

Both income and expenses may be concentrated at the beginning of each academic term when scholarship and loan money arrive and tuition is due. Students receiving lump sum payments may overspend early on and find themselves unexpectedly broke before finals. Accurate budgets can smooth out spending and help you avoid that problem.

If you tried to stick to a budget in the past but found the numbers never added up, incomplete tracking of discretionary spending may be the culprit. Say someone creates a budget that shows there should be $150 surplus at the end of each month, but that theoretical surplus never appears. The problem could be something as simple as forgetting to include the purchase of a daily cup of coffee in your expenses. Spending five extra dollars each day equals that missing $150 per month of savings. Five dollars may not seem like much money, but little things add up fast.

To track spending accurately, it's a good idea to watch expenses for several weeks to a month at a time. Write everything down and keep receipts. Use the **Assess Yourself** budget worksheet found in **MasteringHealth** or try a personal finance app or computer program

budget surplus Money left over for savings after expenses have been paid.

budget deficit Spending more money than your income.

debt Money owed for goods and services that have been purchased.

credit The ability to buy goods and services in advance of paying for them.

loan Giving money to someone today with an agreement that it will be paid off under certain terms in the future.

principal Either the original loan amount or the amount left outstanding on a loan, excluding interest.

interest A fee paid by the borrower of a loan.

student loans Financial student aid that must be repaid in the future.

grant Financial student aid that does not need to be repaid.

federal work study A type of financial aid in which part-time jobs for students are arranged to help them pay for school.

that tracks spending and income. Many universities also offer free spreadsheets for student budgeting. Check your own school's website for options.

Budget cutting is hard. Nobody enjoys passing on doing things because of money woes. To be happier while reducing spending, try to focus on what you gain: self-discipline, control, and more money in your future. Also remind yourself that there are many ways to socialize and be entertained that are inexpensive. Make lower-cost options part of your regular routine and reserve higher-cost things for rare treats. Once the period of adjustment is over, you will likely find that your "new financial normal" feels just fine. The **Skills for Behavior Change** box gives some examples of little things you can do to help trim spending.

SKILLS FOR BEHAVIOR CHANGE

CREATIVE WAYS TO CUT SPENDING

Little changes in behavior can add up to big savings. Consider some of the following:

- **Cut back on the cappuccinos.** A large espresso drink from a coffee shop can cost $4 or $5. Making coffee at home or switching your order to less costly drip varieties saves money.
- **Add 2 more weeks between haircuts.** Book hair appointments every 6 weeks instead of 4. You'll end up paying for three to four fewer haircuts per year than if you scheduled monthly.
- **Drive less.** Carpooling saves on gas and bridge tolls. If you live in an area where car sharing or good public transportation exists, getting rid of your car entirely could save thousands of dollars. You can avoid insurance, gas, maintenance, parking fees, and car payments.
- **Cook more.** Cooking meals from scratch is often cheaper (and healthier) than eating out. If you live on campus and cannot cook, consider the lower-cost dining plan options available.
- **Use your phone on WiFi.** If you don't have an unlimited data plan for your smart phone, then texting and downloading on a cellular network gets expensive fast. Avoid charges by using the phone on WiFi networks whenever possible.
- **Carry cash instead of credit cards.** Withdraw a set amount of cash each week for daily expenses and reserve the credit cards for less frequent, big-ticket buying.

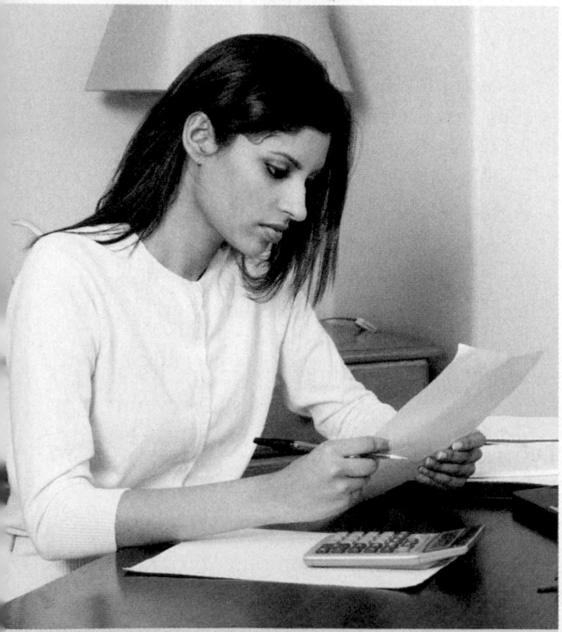

A budget helps you put limits on spending and save for your goals. No matter the income level, a budget is important.

Understanding Debt and Credit Basics

It would be nearly impossible for governments, businesses, and individuals to function in the modern world without credit and debt. These tools allow huge projects such as highway systems and airports to be built all at once and then paid for gradually. Families can buy homes and cars or fund college educations, too. Used wisely, credit and debt are incredibly helpful. But overuse of credit and debt are also major contributors to recessions, job losses, and other turmoil.

Debt is the condition of owing money for something that was purchased. **Credit** is the ability to purchase things in advance of paying for them: Put another way, credit is a **loan**, or the ability to incur debt. The original amount borrowed is referred to as the loan **principal**. Loans also include **interest** charges. Interest is sometimes described as "rent" for using someone else's money. *Fixed interest rate loans* have payments that will not fluctuate for the life of the loan. *Variable interest rate loans* have interest rates that fluctuate over time.

Types of Student Aid

The first experience many young adults have with loans comes when reviewing student aid packages. Financial aid options may come from the university itself, the government, or through private banks or firms. Government aid is often awarded according to financial need, whereas other aid may be awarded based on achievements in sports or academics.

Student Loans

Some people think "aid" and "loans" are exactly the same, but **student loans** refer just to aid options that require repayment. A **grant** is another aid type—money you don't repay. Most scholarships are grants. You also may have heard of Pell grants, which are issued by the federal government to some undergraduate students. **Federal work study** is another type of aid in which part-time jobs are arranged either on or off campus to help pay for education.

If you take out student loans, it is crucial to understand the details regarding repayment, deferrals (situations where you can put off repaying), interest rates, and loan length. The stakes are high. In past decades, someone who got into financial trouble could declare bankruptcy, which nullified all current debts. But bankruptcy laws have since changed to exclude education loans, meaning debt you incur in college will stick with you for a very long time.[25]

The two main categories of student loans are private and federal loans. **Private student loans** are issued by banks, credit unions, state agencies, or schools. **Federal student loans** are funded by the federal government. If you have a choice, pick a federal loan. They are almost always more consumer friendly than private loans when it comes to interest rates, deferral options, penalties, tax breaks, and fees. **TABLE 1** compares how both types of loans stack up.

TABLE 1 | Differences in Federal and Private Student Loans

Loan Issue	Federal Student Loans	Private Student Loans
Repayment timeline	You don't start repaying federal student loans until you graduate, leave school, or enroll less than half-time.	Many private student loans require payments while you are still in school.
Interest rate	Fixed interest rates won't change and are often lower than private loans—much lower than credit card interest rates.	May have variable interest rates, some greater than 18%. Variable rates may substantially increase the total amount you repay.
Subsidies	Undergraduates with financial need may qualify for *subsidized loans* in which the government pays the interest if you are in school at least half-time.	Private student loans are not subsidized. No one pays the interest on your loan but you.
Credit checks	You don't need to get a credit check or have a credit history for most federal student loans.	May require a credit record, and the loan cost depends on credit score and other factors.
Interest tax deduction	Interest may be tax deductible.	Interest may not be tax deductible.
Deferrals	If you have trouble repaying your loan, you may be able to temporarily postpone or lower payments.	Private student loans may not offer *forbearance* or *deferment* options.
Repayment plans	There are several repayment plans, including an option to tie your monthly payment to your income.	Some, but not all, private loans offer repayment plans.
Loan forgiveness	You may be eligible to have some portion of your loans forgiven (removed) if you work in public service.	It is unlikely that your lender will offer a loan forgiveness program.

Source: Table adapted from "What Types of Aid Can I Get?," Federal Student Aid, an Office of the U.S. Department of Education, http://studentaid.ed.gov, Accessed May 2014.

Credit Cards

There are 382 million open credit card accounts in the United States today, which averages to more than one card for every man, woman, and child.[26] Credit cards are *unsecured loans*, meaning the only thing guaranteeing their repayment is your promise. This differs from *secured loans* such as home mortgages, where the loan giver is allowed to seize an asset (for home mortgages, the house itself) if payments are not made on time.

Getting your first credit card is an important, but also potentially dangerous rite of passage. On the positive side, there are some things such as renting a car or booking a hotel that are almost impossible to do without a credit card. Likewise, many high-end cards ("gold" or "platinum" varieties) provide purchase protection programs, so if your new phone falls into the bathtub, your card may actually compensate for the loss. On the other hand, the danger of credit cards is that they can make shopping too easy and pain free. Once spending is out of control, extra fees and compounding interest can make your debt balloon fast.

$15,159

IS THE AVERAGE AMOUNT OF U.S. CREDIT CARD **DEBT**.

Interest and Fees

Because credit cards are loans, the banks and firms that issue them make money by charging interest on what you owe (your *account balance*) as well as other fees. Common fee types include *cash advance fees,* charged when you withdraw money from a credit card at an ATM; *annual fees,* charged once every 12 months; and *late fees,* charged when you pay your monthly bill late.

Credit card interest is calculated in a variety of ways. Some cards have variable rates; others have fixed rates. (Fixed rates can change; lenders just need to inform you in writing before they alter anything.) Add in a dizzying array of fees, and you get widespread confusion about which card is a good deal. A good rule of thumb is to find the card with the fewest fees and lowest interest rate possible.

A good starting point for comparison shopping is the **annual percentage rate (APR)**, which is the officially quoted interest rate you pay over a year-long period. The Truth in Lending Act makes

private student loans Student financial aid loans that are financed by private banks or other institutions.

federal student loans Student financial aid loans that are financed by the government.

annual percentage rate (APR) The yearly cost of a credit card account, including interest and certain fees, expressed as a percentage.

all credit cards clearly state the APR. Card APRs vary greatly: One person may have a card featuring a 10 percent rate and another a card charging 22 or 23 percent. Think about it: A person with a 10 percent APR is charged less than *half* the interest than is someone with the higher APR. It almost literally pays to get the best credit card deal possible.

What counts as your official "first credit card" is one created in your name only, with no cosigner who is guaranteeing that charges will be covered. The first card you have independently likely has a small **credit limit**. This is good. It allows you to build credit history without getting far into debt. Start with a single account. Most people get into trouble when they run up balances on multiple cards.

Although your first credit card may have a low credit limit, it will almost certainly have a high APR. Since you don't have any credit history yet, it is hard for companies to judge how much of a risk it is to loan to you. To compensate for this, credit cards charge you high interest.

Another important issue is whether a card has an interest rate *grace period*. Many cards do not charge interest if you pay the balance off in full each month. Knowing what day of the month your payment is due (it's not always the first) as well as your grace period can allow you to avoid most interest charges and other fees.

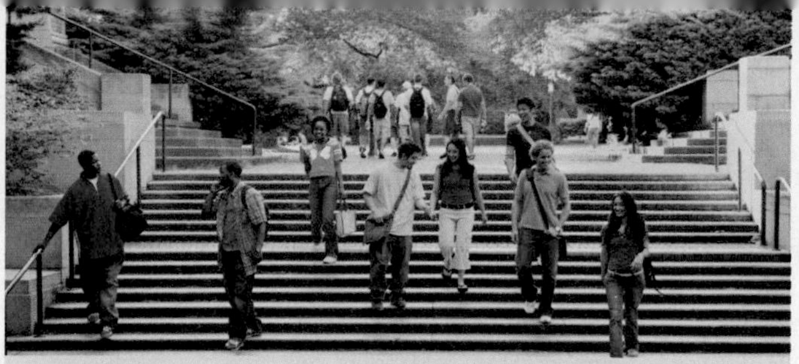

Usually, government-sponsored loans are a better deal in the long haul than private loans. Be sure you do research before you take on any loans for school.

Know Your Consumer Credit Rights

If your credit card application is rejected, you have the right to find out why. Being rejected should be investigated, since it may indicate identity theft or a credit report mistake. After rejection, you can always apply for a credit card somewhere else. A "no" at one company doesn't automatically mean "no" elsewhere.

For many years, credit card companies were criticized for unfair practices related to young adults. Firms paid universities for easy access to students on campus. Students received mugs, T-shirts, and other items in exchange for filling out brief applications. People of limited financial means could rapidly get multiple cards. Interest rates and fees were high, and penalties for missed payments extreme. In 2009, the Credit Card Accountability Responsibility and Disclosure (CARD) Act was enacted. It included rules to prevent predatory practices aimed at young consumers, including the following:[27]

- Credit card issuers who set up on or near campus can't give students gifts in exchange for applying for cards.
- Colleges must publicly disclose marketing contracts with credit card companies.
- Those under age 21 must provide proof of ability to repay charges by themselves in card applications. Otherwise, the card must be cosigned by someone over age 21 who has financial means to cover potential debts.
- If a card is cosigned, then credit limits cannot be raised without written permission of the cosigner.

The CARD Act also banned retroactive rate increases, limited fees, removed certain limits on store gift cards (like expiration dates), and required "plain language" disclosure of fees and rates.

The Consumer Financial Protection Bureau (CFPB) is a new government agency whose goal is to educate, conduct research, and enforce federal laws that protect consumers. The CFPB is the place to look for recent developments in credit card rules and other financial information. You can find their website at www.consumerfinance.gov.

Protecting against Fraud and Identity Theft

Identity theft occurs when someone steals personal information (name, address, social security number, credit card, or bank account numbers) and uses it without permission. Identity crimes have always existed, but they really exploded when credit cards, computers, and online banking became widespread. In 2013, identity theft cost Americans about $18 billion and impacted 13.1 million people.[28] Technology makes people particularly vulnerable to identity theft. Non–credit card fraud tripled in 2013, including compromised Internet accounts (e.g., eBay, Amazon) and e-mail accounts associated with commerce sites such as PayPal.[29]

44%

OF IDENTITY **FRAUD** INVOLVES INTERNET TRANSACTIONS.

Credit Card Theft

If you see unfamiliar charges on your statement, call the fraud number on the back of your card immediately. You will not be held responsible for charges if they happen after you report the card theft. After the first few days, you may be liable for up to $50 in charges.

Bank (Debit) Card Theft

As with credit cards, if you report theft of ATM or debit cards before any charges have occurred, you won't be liable for any charges. Reporting a theft within 2 business days will only cost you $50. But reporting bank card fraud 2 to 60 days after a crime leaves you liable for up to $500 of losses, and if you discover the problem after 60 days, you will be unable to recover *any* lost money.[30] Watch those bank cards and balances carefully!

credit limit The maximum amount a person can charge on a credit card account.

identity theft Stealing personal information and using it without permission.

Protecting Personal Information and Avoiding Scams

Sometimes accounts are compromised through data breaches from hacker attacks at credit card and banking facilities. The companies in question should notify you of the problem and, if necessary, close the compromised accounts and transfer your balances to new accounts. Monitor your credit card statements for signs of identity theft.

You don't have control over identity breaches, but there are other types of fraud you can help prevent. Here are some tips:

- **Steer clear of phishers.** Phishing is an e-mail scam where someone impersonates a bank, credit card company, or other entity in an attempt to trick you into divulging account numbers or passwords. Most financial institutions will not contact you via e-mail asking for personal information. Never supply personal information without verifying the request is genuine—and verifying is not clicking on a link or calling a number listed in the suspicious e-mail. Look up contact information independently to check the requester out.
- **Update your smartphone operating system and computer software regularly.** When security vulnerabilities are discovered, programmers "bug patch" them quickly to resolve threats. But you remain open to attack if you don't update to newer versions.
- **Remove key information from social media accounts.** Sharing birth dates and other life details commonly used for passwords, such as names of pets and hometowns, on social media sites makes you vulnerable to fraud. Passwords should not contain words a stranger can easily look up.

Get a Smart Card

Traditional credit and debit cards have magnetic strip technology that is fairly easy to steal from. New smart cards contain microchips that make it harder to hijack account information. Merchants and banks in the United States have been slow to adopt smart cards, but increased fraud means they are likely to become more widely available soon.

Password Lock Your Smartphone and PC

If you don't put a password on the home screen of your PC or other devices, they become a goldmine of names, numbers, and other information for identity thieves when stolen.

Shred Anything with Your Credit Card Number on It

Don't throw away old card statements or communications unless the account numbers have been rendered unreadable.

Cleaning Up Identity Theft Messes

Once you discover identity theft, place a fraud alert on your credit reports and ask for report copies to review for problems. Close any accounts that were misused or set up fraudulently. Fill out dispute forms so related debts won't be held against you. Visit the Federal Trade Commission website at www.ftc.gov to learn more about complaint forms and how to correct credit reports. You should also file a police report to document the crime.

ASSESS YOURSELF

Want to improve your budgeting skills? Complete the **Budgeting for College Students** worksheet available on MasteringHealth.™

Need help creating a plan? Follow the strategies in the **Your Plan for Change** box for short- and long-term improvements to your health.

YOUR PLAN FOR CHANGE

The **ASSESS YOURSELF** activity allowed you to begin tracking spending, income, and saving. If you face a budget deficit, then consider some of the following steps to fix it:

TODAY, YOU CAN:

- ☐ Calculate a dollar amount you need to reduce spending to eliminate your budget shortfall.
- ☐ Reduce purchases of new clothing, switch to less expensive brands for food or personal products, and go to the movies and restaurants less often.
- ☐ Unless something is broken, postpone purchases of phones, cars, or computers.

WITHIN THE NEXT 2 WEEKS, YOU CAN:

- ☐ Research lower cost options for Internet service providers, and consider downgrading or eliminating cable TV service.
- ☐ Look up your phone plan details. See if it is possible to switch to a lower-cost option without incurring penalties or fees.

BY THE END OF THE SEMESTER, YOU CAN:

- ☐ Ditch car loans. Sell the vehicle, pay off the loan, and buy a car you can afford outright. If you live on campus you might sell the car and not replace it.
- ☐ Reduce housing expenses. If you rent a residence near family, consider moving home. If that's not possible, find a cheaper apartment or roommates to reduce costs.

2 Promoting and Preserving Your Psychological Health

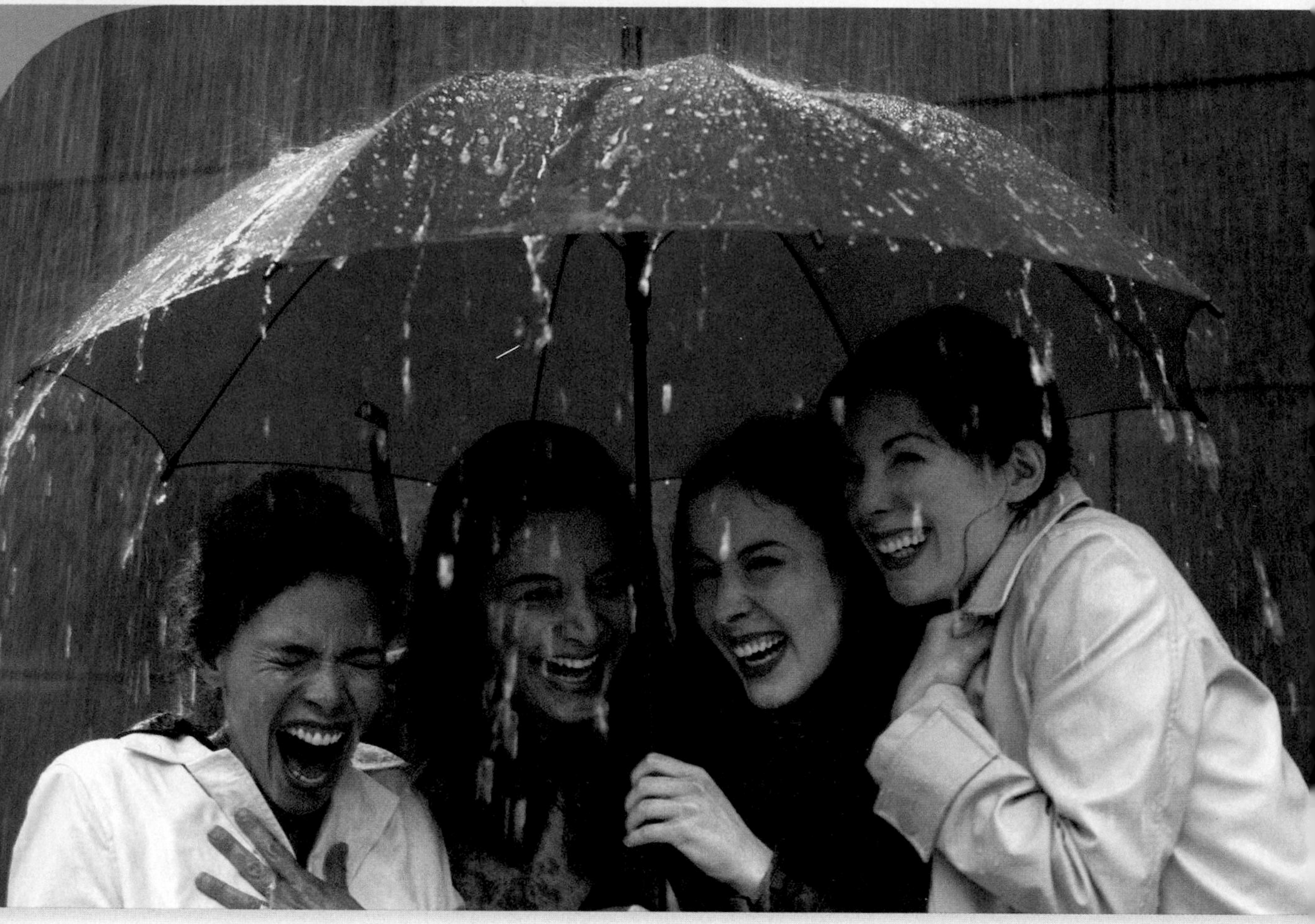

LEARNING OUTCOMES

1 Define each of the four components of psychological health, and identify the basic traits shared by psychologically healthy people.
2 Learn what factors affect your psychological health.
3 Describe the interactions between emotions and health.
4 Explain the positive steps you can take to enhance psychological well-being.
5 Define mental illness and discuss its prevalence among college students.
6 Identify causes, characteristics, and treatments of mood disorders.
7 Describe the causes, characteristics, and treatment options for anxiety disorders.
8 Describe the symptoms, causes, and treatment options for obsessive-compulsive disorders.
9 Explore common causes, characteristics, and treatment options for people with post-traumatic stress disorder.
10 Differentiate personality disorders from other disorders, and describe causes and treatments.
11 Characterize schizophrenia, and explain causes and treatments.
12 Describe the risk factors and possible warning signs of suicide, as well as actions that can be taken to help a person contemplating suicide.
13 Explain the different types of treatment options and professional services available to those experiencing mental health problems.

Most students describe their college years as among the best of their lives, but they may also find the pressure of grades, finances, and relationships, along with the struggle to find themselves, to be extraordinarily difficult. Psychological distress caused by relationship issues, family concerns, academic competition, and adjusting to college life is common. Experts believe that the anxiety-inducing campus environment is a major contributor to poor health decisions such as high levels of alcohol consumption and overeating. These, in turn, can affect academic success and overall health.

Fortunately, humans possess **resiliency,** a trait that enables us to cope, adapt, and thrive, regardless of life's challenges. How we feel and think about ourselves, those around us, and our environment can tell us a lot about our psychological health.

LO 1 | WHAT IS PSYCHOLOGICAL HEALTH?

Define each of the four components of psychological health, and identify the basic traits shared by psychologically healthy people.

Psychological health is the sum of how we think, feel, relate, and exist in our day-to-day lives. Our thoughts, perceptions, emotions, motivations, interpersonal relationships, and behaviors are a product of our experiences and the skills we have developed to meet life's challenges. **Psychological health** includes mental, emotional, social, and spiritual dimensions (**FIGURE 2.1**).

Most experts identify several basic elements psychologically healthy people regularly display:

- **They feel good about themselves.** They are not typically overwhelmed by fear, love, anger, jealousy, guilt, or worry. They know who they are, have a realistic sense of their capabilities, and respect themselves even though they realize they aren't perfect.
- **They feel comfortable with other people, respect others, and have compassion.** They enjoy satisfying and lasting personal relationships and do not take advantage of others or allow others to take advantage of them. They accept that there are others whose needs are greater than their own and take responsibility for fellow human beings. They can give love, consider others' interests, take time to help others, and respect personal differences.
- **They control tension and anxiety.** They recognize the underlying causes and symptoms of stress and anxiety in their lives and consciously avoid irrational thoughts, hostility, excessive excuse making, and blaming others for their problems. They use resources and learn skills to control reactions to stressful situations.
- **They meet the demands of life.** They try to solve problems as they arise, accept responsibility, and plan ahead. They set realistic goals, think for themselves, and make independent decisions. Acknowledging that change is inevitable, they welcome new experiences.

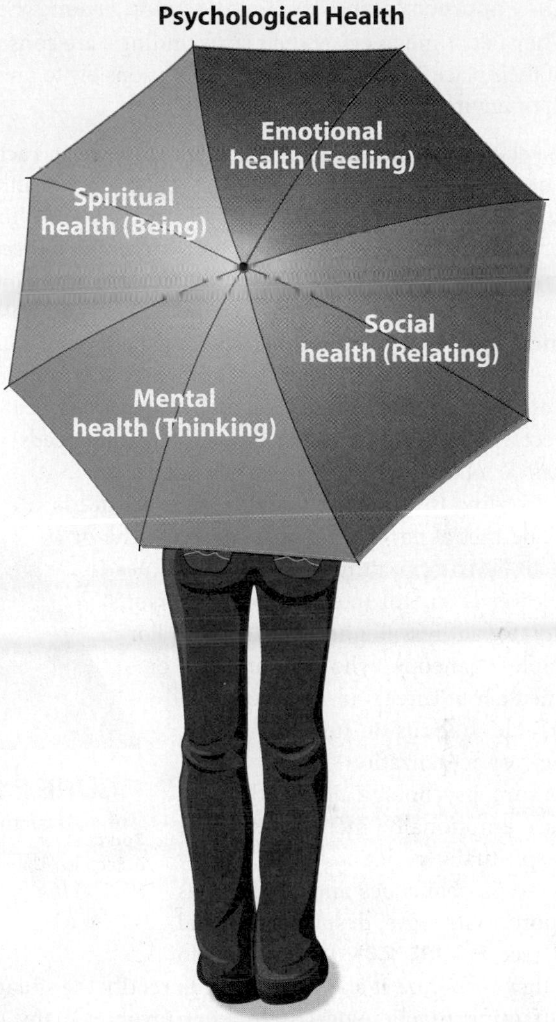

FIGURE 2.1 **Psychological Health** Psychological health is a complex interaction of the mental, emotional, social, and spiritual dimensions of health. Possessing strength and resiliency in these dimensions can maintain your overall well-being and help you weather the storms of life.

- **They curb hate and guilt.** They acknowledge and combat tendencies to respond with anger, thoughtlessness, selfishness, vengefulness, or feelings of inadequacy. They do not try to knock others aside to get ahead, but rather reach out to help others.
- **They maintain a positive outlook.** They approach each day with a presumption that things will go well. They look to the future with enthusiasm rather than dread. Having fun and making time for themselves are integral parts of their lives.
- **They value diversity.** They do not feel threatened by those of a different gender, religion, sexual orientation, race, ethnicity, age, or political party. They are nonjudgmental and do not force their beliefs and values on others.

resiliency The ability to adapt to change and stressful events in healthy and flexible ways.

psychological health The mental, emotional, social, and spiritual dimensions of health.

- **They appreciate and respect the world around them.** They take time to enjoy their surroundings, are conscious of their place in the universe, and act responsibly to preserve their environment.

Psychologists have long argued that before we can achieve any of the above characteristics of psychological health, we must meet certain basic human needs. In the 1960s, human theorist Abraham Maslow developed a *hierarchy of needs* to describe this idea (**FIGURE 2.2**): At the bottom of his hierarchy are basic *survival needs,* such as food, sleep, and water; at the next level are *security needs,* such as shelter and safety; at the third level—*social needs*—is a sense of belonging and affection; at the fourth level are *esteem needs,* self-respect and respect for others; and at the top are needs for *self-actualization* and self-transcendence.

According to Maslow's theory, a person's needs must be met at each of these levels before he or she can be truly healthy. Failure to meet needs at a lower level will interfere with a person's ability to address higher-level needs. For example, someone who is homeless or worried about threats from violence will be unable to focus on fulfilling social, esteem, or actualization needs.[1]

In sum, psychologically healthy people are emotionally, mentally, socially, and spiritually resilient. They usually respond to challenges and frustrations in appropriate ways, despite occasional slips (see **FIGURE 2.3**). When they do slip, they recognize it and take action to rectify the situation.

Attaining psychological well-being involves many complex processes. Learning how to assess your own health and take action to help yourself are important aspects of psychological health.

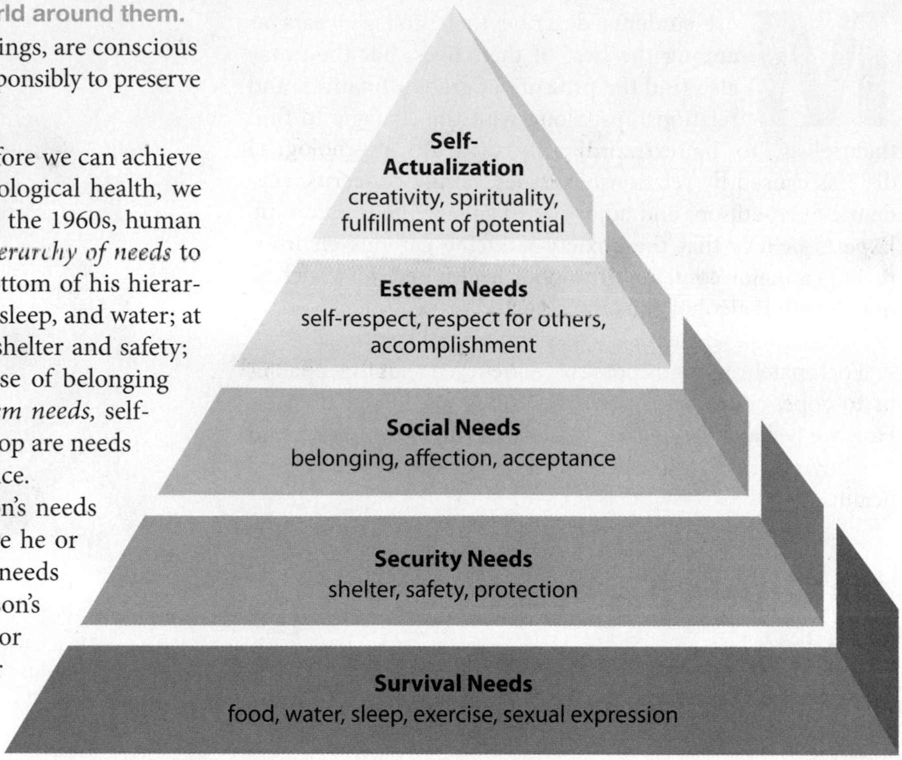

FIGURE 2.2 Maslow's Hierarchy of Needs

Source: From A. H. Maslow, *Motivation and Personality*, 3rd ed., eds. R. D. Frager and J. Fadiman (Upper Saddle River, NJ: Pearson Education, Inc., 1987). Reprinted with permission.

VIDEO TUTOR
Maslow's Hierarchy of Needs

mental health The thinking part of psychological health; includes your values, attitudes, and beliefs.

emotional health The feeling part of psychological health; includes your emotional reactions to life.

emotions Intensified feelings or complex patterns of feelings.

emotional intelligence (EI) A person's ability to identify, understand, use, and manage emotional states in positive and constructive ways.

Mental Health

The term **mental health** is used to describe the "thinking" or "rational" dimension of our health. A mentally healthy person perceives life in realistic ways, can adapt to change, can develop rational strategies to solve problems, and can carry out personal and professional responsibilities. In addition, a mentally healthy person has the intellectual ability to learn and use information effectively and strive for continued growth. This is often referred to as *intellectual health,* a subset of mental health.[2]

HEAR IT! PODCASTS

Want a study podcast for this chapter? Download the podcast **Psychological Health: Being Mentally, Emotionally, and Spiritually Well** on MasteringHealth.™

Emotional Health

The term **emotional health** refers to the feeling, or subjective, side of psychological health. **Emotions** are intensified feelings or complex patterns of feelings that we experience on a regular basis, including love, hate, frustration, anxiety, and joy, just to name a few. Typically, emotions are described as the interplay of four components: physiological arousal, feelings, cognitive (thought) processes, and behavioral reactions. As rational beings, we are responsible for evaluating our individual emotional responses, their causes, and the appropriateness of our actions.

Emotionally healthy people usually respond appropriately to upsetting events. Rather than reacting in an extreme fashion or behaving inconsistently or offensively, they can express their feelings, communicate with others, and show emotions in appropriate ways. In contrast, emotionally unhealthy people are much more likely to let their feelings overpower them. They may be highly volatile and prone to unpredictable emotional responses, which may be followed by inappropriate communication or actions. **Emotional intelligence (EI)** is the ability to identify, use, understand, and manage one's emotions in positive and constructive ways. It is about recognizing your own emotional state and the emotional states of others and using that information to maintain good relationships. Emotional intelligence consists of four core abilities: self-awareness, self-management, relationship management, and social awareness.

Psychologically unhealthy			Psychologically healthy
No zest for life; pessimistic/cynical most of the time; spiritually down	Shows poorer coping than most, often overwhelmed by circumstances	Works to improve in all areas, recognizes strengths and weaknesses	Possesses zest for life; spiritually healthy and intellectually thriving
Laughs, but usually at others, has little fun	Has regular relationship problems, finds that others often disappoint	Healthy relationships with family and friends, capable of giving and receiving love and affection	High energy, resilient, enjoys challenges, focused
Has serious bouts of depression, "down" and tired much of time; has suicidal thoughts	Tends to be cynical/critical of others; tends to have negative/critical friends	Has strong social support, may need to work on improving social skills but usually no major problems	Realistic sense of self and others, sound coping skills, open-minded
A "challenge" to be around, socially isolated	Lacks focus much of the time, hard to keep intellectual acuity sharp	Has occasional emotional "dips," but overall good mental/emotional adaptors	Adapts to change easily, sensitive to others and environment
Experiences many illnesses, headaches, aches/pains, gets colds/infections easily	Quick to anger, sense of humor and fun evident less often		Has strong social support and healthy relationships with family and friends

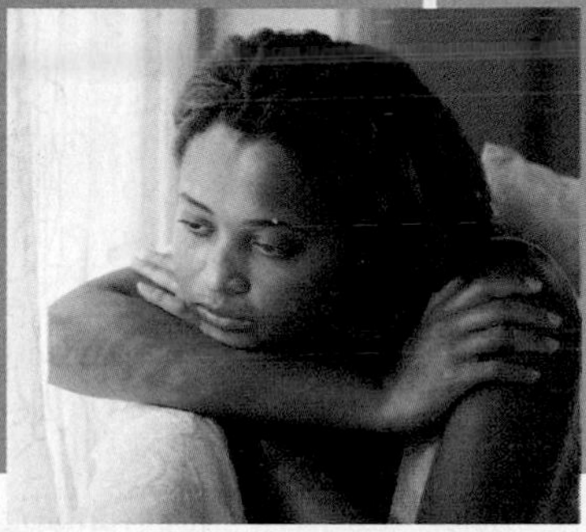

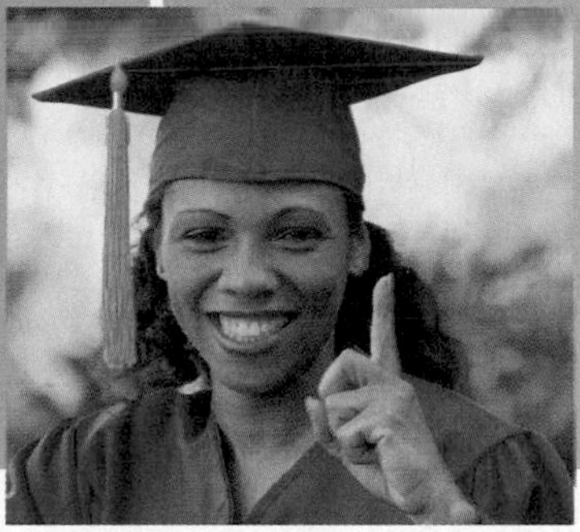

FIGURE 2.3 Characteristics of Psychologically Healthy and Unhealthy People
Where do you fall on this continuum?

Proponents of EI suggest that developing or increasing your emotional intelligence can help you build strong relationships, succeed at work, and achieve your goals.[3]

Emotional health also affects social and intellectual health. People who feel hostile, withdrawn, or moody may become socially isolated. Because they are not much fun to be around, people may avoid them at the very time they are most in need of emotional support. For students, a more immediate concern is the impact of emotional upset on academic performance. Have you ever tried to study for an exam after a fight with a friend or family member? Emotional turmoil can seriously affect your ability to think, reason, and act rationally.

Social Health

Social health includes your interactions with others on an individual and group basis, your ability to use social resources and support in times of need, and your ability to adapt to a variety of social situations. Socially healthy individuals enjoy a wide range of interactions with family, friends, and acquaintances and are able to have healthy interactions with an intimate partner. Typically, socially healthy individuals can listen, express themselves, form healthy attachments, act in socially acceptable and responsible ways, and find the best fit for themselves in society. Numerous studies have documented the importance of positive relationships with family members, friends, and significant others to overall well-being and longevity.[4]

Social bonds reflect the level of closeness and attachment that we develop with individuals and are the very foundation of human life. They provide intimacy, feelings of belonging, opportunities for giving and receiving nurturance, reassurance of one's worth, assistance and guidance, and advice. Social bonds take multiple forms, the most common of which are social support and community involvement.

social health Aspect of psychological health that includes interactions with others, ability to use social supports, and ability to adapt to various situations.

social bonds The level of closeness and attachment with other individuals.

social support Network of people and services with whom you share ties and from whom you get support.

The concept of **social support** is more complex than many people realize. In general, it refers to the people and services with whom we interact and share social connections. These ties can provide *tangible support,* such as babysitting services or money to help pay the bills, or *intangible support,* such as encouraging you to share your concerns. Sometimes, support can just be the knowledge that someone would be there for you in a crisis. Generally, the closer and the higher the quality of the social bond, the more likely a person is to ask for and receive social support. For example, if your car broke down late at night, who could you call for help and know that the person would do everything humanly possible to help you? Common descriptions of strong social support include the following:[5]

- Being cared for and loved, with shared understanding
- Being esteemed and valued
- Sharing companionship, communication, and mutual obligations with others; having a sense of belonging
- Having "informational" support—access to information, advice, community services, and guidance from others

Social health also reflects the way we react to others. (Look for more information about interpersonal relationships in **Chapter 4**.)

Spiritual Health

It is possible to be mentally, emotionally, and socially healthy and still not achieve optimal psychological well-being. For many people, the difficult-to-describe element that gives life purpose is the spiritual dimension.

The term *spirituality* is broader in meaning than religion and is defined as an individual's sense of purpose and meaning in life; it involves a sense of peace and connection to others.[6] Spirituality may be practiced in many ways, including through religion; however, religion does not have to be part of a spiritual person's life. **Spiritual health** refers to the sense of belonging to something greater than the purely physical or personal dimensions of existence. For some, this unifying force is nature; for others, it is a feeling of connection to other people; for still others, the unifying force is a god or other higher power. (**Focus On: Cultivating Your Spiritual Health,** which begins on page 61, explores spiritual health and the role spirituality plays in your overall psychological health in more detail.)

spiritual health Aspect of psychological health that relates to having a sense of meaning and purpose to one's life, as well as a feeling of connection with others and with nature.

dysfunctional families Families in which there is violence; physical, emotional, or sexual abuse; significant parental discord; or other negative family interactions.

LO 2 | FACTORS THAT INFLUENCE PSYCHOLOGICAL HEALTH

Learn what factors affect your psychological health.

Psychological health is the product of many influences throughout our lives, including family, social supports, and the community in which you live. Your psychological health is also shaped by your sense of self-efficacy and self-esteem, your personality, and your maturity.

Your family members play an important role in your psychological health. As you were growing up, they modeled behaviors and skills that helped you develop cognitively and socially. Their love and support can give you a sense of self worth and encourage you to treat others with compassion and care.

The Family

Families have a significant influence on psychological development. Healthy families model and help develop the cognitive and social skills necessary to solve problems, express emotions in socially acceptable ways, manage stress, and develop a sense of self-worth and purpose. Children raised in healthy, nurturing homes are more likely to become well-adjusted, productive adults. In adulthood, family support is one of the best predictors of health and happiness.[7] Children brought up in **dysfunctional families**—in which there is violence; distrust; anger; dietary deprivation; drug abuse; significant parental discord; or sexual, physical, or emotional abuse—may have a harder time adapting to life and may run an increased risk of psychological problems. In dysfunctional families, love, security, and unconditional trust may be so lacking that children become psychologically damaged. Yet not all people raised in dysfunctional families become psychologically unhealthy, and not all people from healthy environments become well adjusted. The difference may lie in their support system, community, self-esteem, and personality.

Support System

Our initial social support may be provided by family members, but as we grow and develop, the support of peers and friends becomes more and more important. We rely on friends to help us figure out who we are and what we want to do with our lives. We often bounce ideas off friends to see if they think we are being logical, smart, or fair. Research shows that college students with adequate social support have improved overall

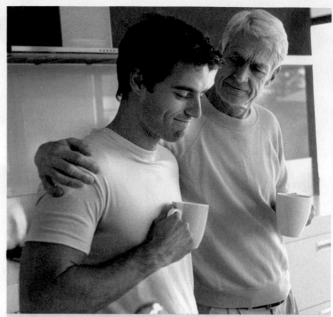

SEE IT! VIDEOS

How can we help veterans who suffer from PTSD? Watch **Battling Post Traumatic Stress** available on MasteringHealth.™

well-being, including higher GPAs, higher perceived ability in math and science courses, less peer pressure for binge drinking, lower rates of suicide, and higher overall life satisfaction.[8] Having people in our lives who provide positive support and who we can rely on is important to our psychological health at every stage of our lives.

Community

The communities we live in can have a positive impact on our psychological health through collective actions. For example, neighbors may join together to get rid of trash on the street, participate in a neighborhood watch to keep children and our homes safe, help each other with home repairs, or organize community social events. Religious institutions, schools, clinics, and local businesses can also engage in efforts that demonstrate support and caring for community members. Likewise, you are a part of a campus community. That community can support and care for your psychological health by creating a safe environment to explore and develop your mental, emotional, social, and spiritual dimensions.

WHAT DO YOU THINK?

What are some ways in which people in your community work together toward a common goal?

- What type of groundwork must be established before this type of working together can occur?
- What factors can get in the way of collaboration and cooperation?

64 MILLION

AMERICANS **VOLUNTEER** AT LEAST ONCE A YEAR.

Self-Efficacy and Self-Esteem

During our formative years, successes and failures in school, athletics, friendships, intimate relationships, jobs, and every other aspect of life subtly shape our beliefs about our personal worth and abilities. These beliefs in turn become internal influences on our psychological health.

Self-efficacy describes a person's belief about whether he or she can successfully engage in and execute a specific behavior. **Self-esteem** refers to one's realistic sense of self-respect or self-worth. People with high levels of self-efficacy and self-esteem tend to express a positive outlook on life.

Self-esteem results from the relationships we have with our parents and family growing up; with friends as we grow older; with our significant others as we form intimate relationships; and with our teachers, coworkers, and others throughout our lives. While we tend to think of self-esteem as a positive thing, the **Health Headlines** box on the following page discusses the possible downside of having too much self-esteem.

Learned Helplessness versus Learned Optimism Psychologist Martin Seligman proposed that people who continually experience failure may develop a pattern of response known as **learned helplessness** in which they give up and fail to take action to help themselves. Seligman ascribes this response in part to society's tendency toward *victimology*—blaming one's problems on other people and circumstances.[9] Although viewing ourselves as victims may make us feel better temporarily, it does not address the underlying causes of a problem. Ultimately, it can erode self-efficacy by making us feel that we cannot do anything to improve the situation.

Today, many self-help programs use elements of Seligman's principle of **learned optimism**. The basis for these programs is the idea that we can teach ourselves to be optimistic. By changing our self-talk, examining our reactions, and blocking negative thoughts, we can "unlearn" negative thought processes that have become habitual. Some programs practice positive affirmations with clients, teaching them the habit of acknowledging positive things about themselves. Often we are our own worst critics, and learning to be kinder to ourselves can be difficult.

self-efficacy Describes a person's belief about whether he or she can successfully engage in and execute a specific behavior.

self-esteem One's realistic sense of self-respect or self-worth.

learned helplessness Pattern of responding to situations by giving up because of repeated failure in the past.

learned optimism Teaching oneself to think positively.

Defense Mechanisms Famed psychoanalyst Sigmund Freud proposed that, in order to deflect negative emotions and stress, we develop defense mechanisms, strategies we unconsciously use to distort our present reality to help avoid anxiety. While defense mechanisms can be pathological if taken to an extreme, fantasizing about a vacation to cope with work stress or rationalizing why you weren't selected for the lead role in a play can help to relieve stress and disappointment.[10]

Personality

Your personality is the unique mix of characteristics that distinguishes you from others. Heredity, environment, culture, and experience influence how each person develops. Personality determines how we react to the challenges of life, interpret our feelings, and resolve conflicts. A leading personality theory called the five-factor model distills personality into five traits, often called the "big five":[11]

- **Agreeableness.** People who score high are trusting, likable, and demonstrate friendly compliance and love, while low scorers are critical and suspicious.

HEALTH HEADLINES

OVERDOSING ON SELF-ESTEEM?

Fostering self-esteem in children has been seen as key to keeping them away from drugs and violence and to ensuring well-adjusted lives. While it's true people tend to thrive when praised for hard work and accomplishments, society is now seeing a possible downside to handing out trophies just for showing up. There is a fine line between healthy self-esteem and vanity or narcissism, leading some to have an exaggerated self-image, a need for constant compliments, and a sense of feeling entitled to special treatment. A friend who posts selfies all day on Facebook or Snapchat so everyone knows what he's doing/eating/wearing may have crossed that line!

The self-esteem generation's need for positive feedback is strong. Although the sample size was small, a University of Michigan study showed students reported liking and wanting moments that boost their self-esteem more than having sex, eating a favorite food, drinking, or nearly all other pleasurable events!

Call it the "soccer trophy effect" if you will, but it appears to have serious downsides. First, preliminary research indicates people who have been protected from failure (perhaps by well-meaning parents and teachers) and have extremely high levels of self-esteem might be more prone to anger, aggression, and other negative behaviors when others don't praise them or meet their needs for instant gratification. Second, learning to lose may teach us valuable lessons. Carol Dweck, a psychology professor at Stanford University, found that after a steady diet of praise, kids collapsed at the first experience of difficulty. Failure can teach us to keep trying—and that just showing up is not enough to excel in college or the subsequent work world; in real life, there are no participation ribbons.

Psychologists continue to support the idea that self-esteem is important for positive growth and development. More research is needed to examine potential risks of too much self-esteem and the best ways to deal with it once it occurs.

Sources: Aspen Educational Group, "Narcissistic and Entitled to Everything—Does Gen Y Have Too Much Self-Esteem?," Accessed February 11, 2012, www.aspeneducation.com/article-entitlement.html; M. Wei, K. Yu-Hsin Liao, T. Ku, and P. Shaffer, "Attachment, Self Compassion, Empathy, and Subjective Well-Being among College Students and Community Adults," *Journal of Personality*, 79, no. 1 (2011): 191–221; B. J. Bushman, S. J. Moeller, and J. Crocker, "Sweets, Sex, or Self-Esteem? Comparing the Value of Self-Esteem Boosts with Other Pleasant Rewards," *Journal of Personality* (2011), DOI: 10.1111/j.1467-6494.2011.00712; A. Merryman, "Losing Is Good for You," *New York Times* (September 24, 2013), http://www.nytimes.com/2013/09/25/opinion/losing-is-good-for-you.html?_r=0.

- **Openness.** People who score high demonstrate curiosity, independence, and imagination, while low scorers are more conventional and down-to-earth.
- **Neuroticism.** People who score high in neuroticism are anxious and insecure, while those who score low show the ability to maintain emotional control.
- **Conscientiousness.** People who score high are dependable and demonstrate self-control, discipline, and a need to achieve, while low scorers are disorganized and impulsive.
- **Extroversion.** People who score high adapt well to social situations, demonstrate assertiveness, and draw enjoyment from the company of others, while low scorers are more reserved and passive.

One way to examine personality is to consider which traits are associated with psychological health. Scoring high on agreeableness, openness, conscientiousness, and extroversion, while scoring low on neuroticism, is often related to psychological well-being. The link between these traits and well-being may lie in the social connections people who display these personality traits often form.[12]

The good news is that most recent schools of psychological theory indicate that we have the power to understand our behavior and change it, thus molding our own personalities, even as adults.[13] Although inhospitable social environments make it more difficult, there are opportunities for making changes and improving our long-term psychological well-being.

Life Span and Maturity

Although our temperaments are largely determined by genetics, as we age we learn to control the volatile emotions of youth and channel our feelings in more acceptable ways. For example, as children we might have screamed, thrown things, or hit people when upset, but as we mature we learn to control angry outbursts. People who have not completed early developmental tasks may find it impacts their life in later stages. For example, if you did not learn to trust others in childhood, you may have difficulty establishing intimate relationships as an adult.

The college years mark a critical transition period as young adults move away from families and establish themselves as independent adults. This transition is easier for those who have successfully accomplished earlier developmental tasks such as learning how to solve problems, make and evaluate decisions, define and adhere to personal values, and establish both casual and intimate relationships. Graduating from college can also be another transition for many into adulthood and further independence. Anticipating an adjustment period and exploring campus resources for new graduates can help in developing autonomy after graduation.

LO 3 | THE MIND-BODY CONNECTION

Describe the interactions between emotions and health.

Can negative emotions make us physically ill? Can positive emotions help us stay well? Researchers are exploring the interaction between emotions and health, especially in conditions of uncontrolled, persistent stress. In fact, the National Center for Complementary and Alternative Medicine (NCCAM) and other organizations are investing more and more dollars in large research projects designed to explore the link between mind and body. At the core of the mind-body connection is **psychoneuroimmunology (PNI)**, the study of the interactions of behavioral, neural, and endocrine functions and the functioning of the body's immune system.

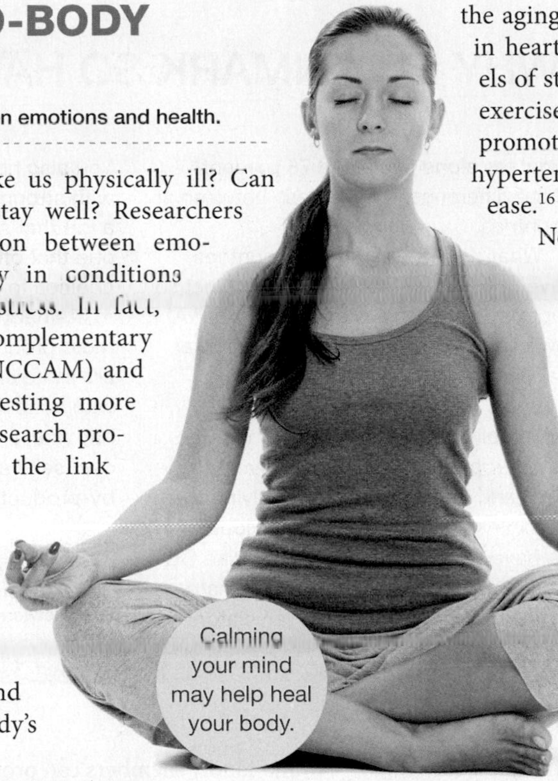

Calming your mind may help heal your body.

One area of study that appears to be particularly promising in enhancing physical health is *happiness*—a collective term for several positive states in which individuals actively embrace the world around them.[14] In examining the characteristics of happy people, scientists have found that this emotion can have a profound impact on the body. Happiness, or related mental states such as hopefulness, optimism, and contentment, appears to reduce the risk or limit the severity of cardiovascular disease, pulmonary disease, diabetes, hypertension, colds, and other infections, and even slow down the aging process.[15] Laughter can promote increases in heart and respiration rates and can reduce levels of stress hormones in much the same way light exercise can. For this reason, laughter has been promoted as a possible risk reducer for people with hypertension and other forms of cardiovascular disease.[16] Not all happiness is created equal though. New research indicates that happiness derived from doing kind deeds or working towards your life's purpose improves health more than happiness found in pleasure-seeking activities like watching TV.[17] For more information on happiness, see the **Health Headlines** box on the following page.

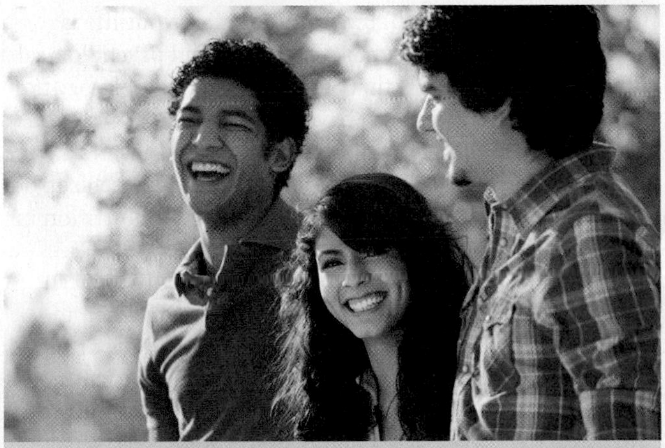

Research suggests that laughter can increase blood flow, boost the immune response, lower blood sugar levels, and facilitate better sleep. Additionally, sharing laughter and fun with others can strengthen social ties and bring joy to your everyday life.

Subjective well-being is that uplifting feeling of inner peace or an overall "feel-good" state, which includes happiness. Subjective well-being is defined by three central components: satisfaction with present life, relative presence of positive emotions, and relative absence of negative emotions.[18] You do not have to be happy all the time to achieve overall subjective well-being. Everyone experiences disappointments, unhappiness, and times when life seems unfair. However, people with a high level of subjective well-being are typically resilient, are able to look on the positive side and get back on track fairly quickly, and are less likely to fall into despair over setbacks.

Scientists suggest that some people may be biologically predisposed to happiness. One study of 2,574 Americans showed that variants of a gene actually influenced how satisfied or dissatisfied people were with their lives and their overall levels of happiness. This marks an advance toward explaining why some people seem naturally happier than others. However, researchers are careful to point out that happiness is only partly influenced by genetics.[19] Other psychologists, most notably Martin Seligman, suggest that we can develop well-being by practicing positive psychological actions. Seligman describes five elements of well-being (represented by the acronym PERMA) that help humans flourish:[20]

- **Positive emotion.** How happy and satisfied are you?
- **Engagement.** Can you get completely absorbed in a task?
- **Relationships.** Are there people in life who really care about you?

psychoneuroimmunology (PNI) The study of the interactions of behavioral, neural, and endocrine functions and the functioning of the body's immune system.

subjective well-being An uplifting feeling of inner peace.

@ HEALTH HEADLINES

WHY IS DENMARK SO HAPPY?

Denmark, a small country in northern Europe that only has a few hours of light per day in winter, scored highest on the World Happiness Survey, followed by Norway, Switzerland, The Netherlands, and Sweden.

So, what makes people in Denmark so happy? According to the United Nations Sustainable Development Solutions Network, the measures that best predicted happiness were real gross domestic product (GDP) per capita, having people to count on, healthy life expectancy, the perception of freedom to make life choices, absence of government corruption, and generosity. Those six variables alone explained 75 percent of the difference in happiness between countries.

What do the top-ranking countries have in common that makes them feel so supported and free to make choices? A few things, including generous parental leave for new parents, high-quality available child care, gender equality, and a collective sense of responsibility for other people. Instead of moving to Denmark, we can consider applying these principles in our own lives. Individually, we have little control over issues like GDP, but we do have the ability to advocate for these supports from our legislators. You also have the power to build a life with strong social ties. You can choose a job that allows you more flexibility over one that offers less, and we can all make choices to be more generous.

As happy people live longer lives, are more productive at work, earn more, and are more engaged in their community with actions like voting and volunteering, happiness should be nurtured for its own sake and also for the sake of its by-products.

Source: J. F. Helliwell, R. Layard, and J. D. Sachs, eds. *World Happiness Report 2013* (New York: United Nations Sustainable Development Solutions Network, 2013).

- **Meaning.** Are you working toward something bigger than yourself?
- **Accomplishment.** How hard will you work for something?

The **Skills for Behavior Change** box provides some suggestions for things you can do to incorporate PERMA principles in your own life.

LO 4 | STRATEGIES TO ENHANCE PSYCHOLOGICAL HEALTH

Explain the positive steps you can take to enhance psychological well-being.

As we have seen, psychological health involves four dimensions. Attaining self-fulfillment is a lifelong, conscious process that involves enhancing each of these components. Strategies include building self-efficacy and self-esteem, understanding and controlling emotions, maintaining support networks, and employing a positive outlook. Here are some tips on managing stress and other tools for enhancing your psychological health. (See **Chapter 3** for more tips for managing stress.)

- **Develop a support system.** One of the best ways to promote self-esteem is through a support system of peers and others who share your values. Members of your support system can help you feel good about yourself and force you to take an honest look at your actions and choices. Keeping in contact with old friends and family members can provide a foundation of unconditional love that will help you through life's transitions.
- **Complete required tasks to the best of your ability.** A good way to boost your sense of self-efficacy is to learn new skills and develop a history of success. Most college campuses provide study groups and learning centers that can help you manage time, improve study and writing skills, and prepare for tests.
- **Form realistic expectations.** If you expect perfect grades, a steady stream of Saturday-night dates, and the perfect job, you may be setting yourself up for failure. Assess your current resources and the direction in which you are heading. Set small, incremental goals that you can likely meet.
- **Make time for you.** Taking time to enjoy your life is another way to boost your self-esteem and psychological health. View a new activity as something to look forward to and an opportunity to have fun.
- **Maintain physical health.** Regular exercise fosters a sense of well-being. More and more research supports the role of exercise and good nutrition in improved mental health.
- **Examine problems and seek help when necessary.** Knowing when to seek help from friends, family, or professionals is an important factor in boosting self-esteem. Sometimes you can handle life's problems alone; at other times, you need assistance.
- **Get adequate sleep.** Getting enough sleep on a daily basis is a key factor in physical and psychological health. Not only do our bodies need to rest to conserve energy for daily activities, but we also need to restore supplies of many of the

WHY SHOULD I CARE?

Mental health problems can have a huge impact on the kind of life you lead—including your success in academics, career, and relationships, as well as your general ability to function and enjoy life. Also, mental health concerns are so prevalent among college students that it is possible your roommate or a friend could have a problem and may need your help and support.

SKILLS FOR BEHAVIOR CHANGE

USING PERMA TO ENHANCE YOUR HAPPINESS

Implement the following strategies to enhance well-being and employ a more positive outlook:

"P"—POSITIVE EMOTIONS

- Consider what brings you the most happiness and engage in that behavior often.
- Be open to new experiences, be curious, and be kind.

"E"—ENGAGEMENT

- Adopt mindfulness and appreciation for being in the present moment.
- Consider what activities completely absorb you and invest more time in those activities.

"R"—RELATIONSHIPS

- Open yourself to building new relationships and deepen existing ones.
- Offer others social support and accept support that is offered to you.

"M"—MEANING

- Consider, what is your legacy?
- Invest time in activities that bring you peace: pray, meditate, or care for others.

"A"—ACHIEVEMENT

- Set realistic goals and pursue them.
- If achievement equals skills plus effort, put forth the effort to build strong skills.

Adapted from: E. Terantin-O'Brien, IDEA Health and Fitness Association, "Applying the PERMA Model," June 2013, Available at: www.ideafit.com/fitness-library/applying-the-perma-model; M. Seligman, *Flourish: A Visionary New Understanding of Happiness and Well-Being* (New York: Free Press, 2011).

neurotransmitters that we use up during our waking hours. (For more information on the importance of sleep, see **Focus On: Improving Your Sleep** beginning on page 98.)

LO 5 | WHEN PSYCHOLOGICAL HEALTH DETERIORATES

Define mental illness and discuss its prevalence among college students.

Sometimes circumstances overwhelm us to such a degree that we need help to get back on track to healthful living. Stress, abusive relationships, anxiety, loneliness, financial upheavals, and other traumatic events can derail our coping resources. Chemical imbalances, drug interactions, trauma, neurological disruptions, and other physical problems also may contribute to mental health problems.

Mental illnesses are disorders that disrupt thinking, feeling, moods, and behaviors and cause varying degrees of impaired functioning in daily living. They are believed to be caused by a variety of biochemical, genetic, and environmental factors.[21] Risk factors for developing or triggering mental illness include the following: having other biological relatives with a mental illness; malnutrition or exposure to viruses while in the womb; stressful life situations, such as financial problems, a loved one's death, or a divorce; chronic medical conditions, such as cancer; combat; taking psychoactive drugs during adolescence; childhood abuse or neglect; and lack of friendships or healthy relationships.[22] As with physical disease, mental illnesses can range from mild to severe and can exact a heavy toll on quality of life, both for people with the illnesses and for those who interact with them.

neurotransmitters Chemicals that relay messages between nerve cells or from nerve cells to other body cells.

mental illnesses Disorders that disrupt thinking, feeling, moods, and behaviors and that impair daily functioning.

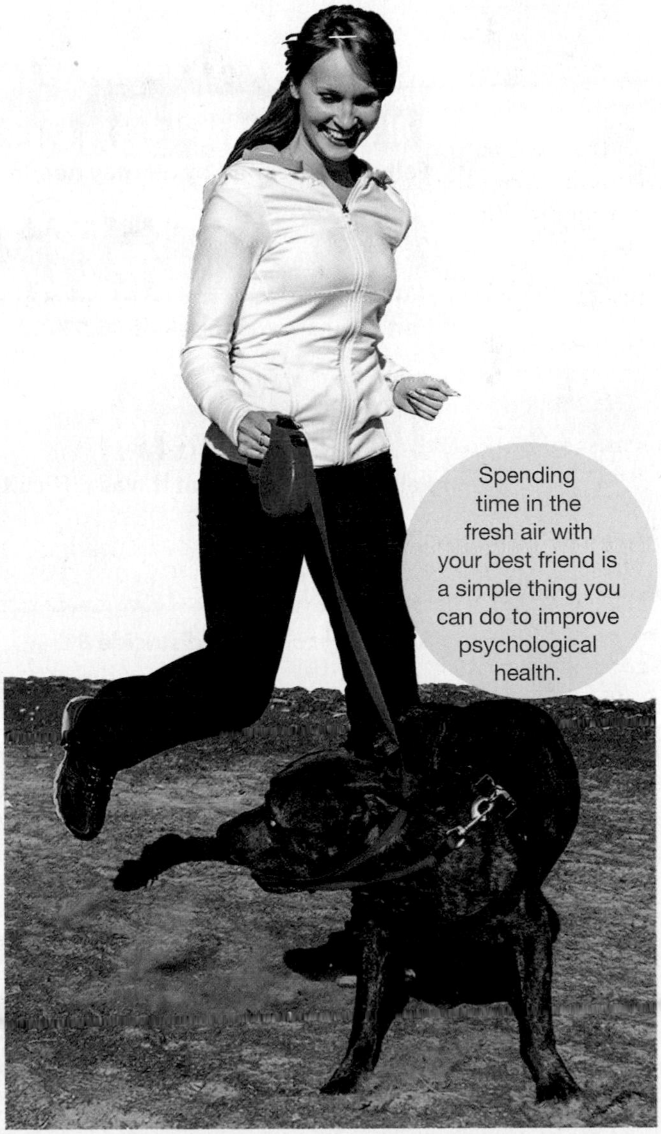

Spending time in the fresh air with your best friend is a simple thing you can do to improve psychological health.

43 MILLION

NUMBER OF ADULTS IN THE UNITED STATES WHO HAD A DIAGNOSABLE **MENTAL ILLNESS** OVER THE PAST 12 MONTHS.

Mental disorders are common in the United States and worldwide. The basis for diagnosing mental disorders in the United States is the *Diagnostic and Statistical Manual of Mental Disorders,* Fifth Edition (*DSM-5*). An estimated 20 percent of Americans aged 18 and older—about 1 in 5 adults—suffer from a diagnosable mental disorder in a given year, and nearly half of them have more than one mental illness at the same time. About 5 percent, or 1 in 20, suffer from a serious mental illness requiring close monitoring, residential care in many instances, and medication.[23] Mental disorders are the leading cause of disability worldwide for people aged 15 to 44, costing more than $100 billion annually in the United States alone.[24]

Mental Health Threats to College Students

Mental health problems are increasingly common among college students, growing in both number and severity.[25] The most recent National College Health Assessment survey found that approximately 1 in 3 undergraduates reported "feeling so depressed it was difficult to function" at least once in the past year, and 8 percent of students reported "seriously considering attempting suicide" in the past year.[26] In all, more than 1 in 4 college students experience a mental health issue each year.[27] Although these data may appear alarming, it is important to note that increases in help-seeking behavior, in addition to actual increases in overall prevalence of disorders, may contribute to these trends. **FIGURE 2.4** shows the mental health concerns reported by American college students.

Although there are many types of mental illnesses, we will focus here on those disorders that are most common among college students: mood disorders, anxiety disorders, obsessive-compulsive disorder (OCD), post-traumatic stress disorder (PTSD), personality disorders, and schizophrenia. See the **Health Headlines** box on the following page for

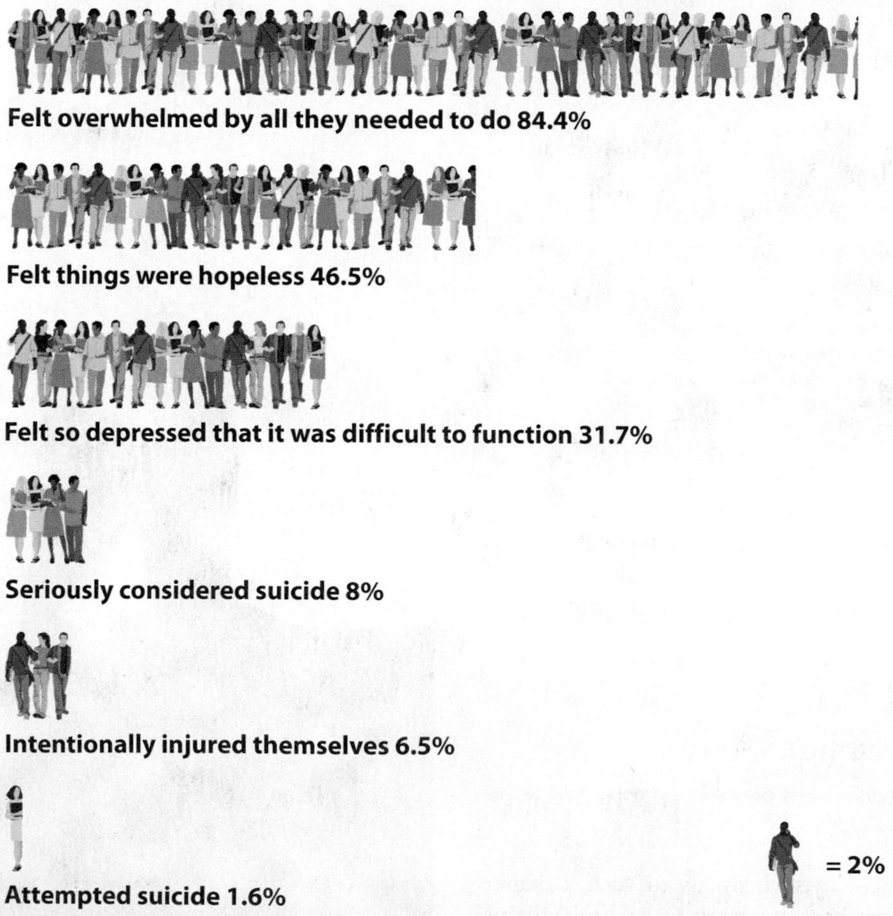

FIGURE 2.4 Mental Health Concerns of American College Students, Past 12 Months

Source: Data from American College Health Association, *American College Health Association—National College Health Assessment II (ACHA-NCHA II): Undergraduate Students, Reference Group Data Report, Spring 2013* (Baltimore, MD: American College Health Association, 2013).

@ HEALTH HEADLINES

COLLEGE SUCCESS WITH LEARNING DISABILITIES & NEURODEVELOPMENTAL DISORDERS

The mental illnesses discussed in this chapter are all based in the brain, but there are other brain-based disorders that are not mental illnesses. Just as people living with mental illness can be successful in college with appropriate counseling, medication, and/or accommodations, people living with learning disabilities (LDs) and neurodevelopmental disorders can also be successful in college when the proper supports are in place.

Attention-deficit (hyperactive) disorder (ADD/ADHD) is a learning disability usually associated with school-aged children, but for many people, symptoms persist into adulthood. People with ADD/ADHD are distracted much of the time. Even when they try to concentrate, they find it hard to pay attention. Organizing things, listening to instructions, and remembering details are especially difficult.

Dyslexia is a language-based learning disorder that can pose problems for reading, writing, and spelling. Lesser known, but equally challenging, are **dyscalculia** (a learning disability involving math) and **dysgraphia** (a learning disability involving writing). People with dysgraphia may have difficulty putting letters, numbers, and words on a page into order.

Autism spectrum disorder (ASD) is not a learning disability, but a neurodevelopmental disorder (an impairment in brain development).

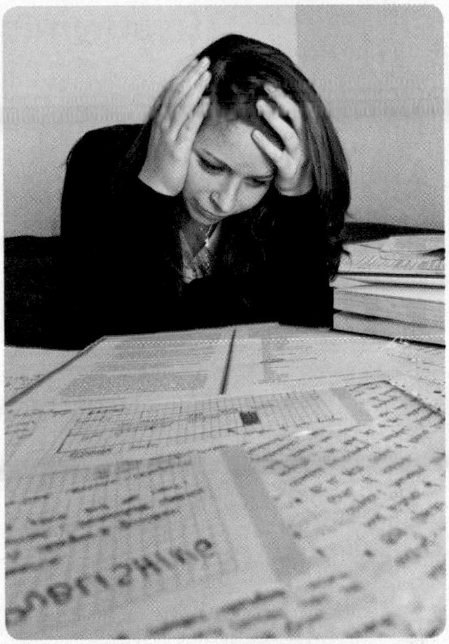

Disorder and chaos can be headaches for us all, but ADHD sufferers may find them insurmountable obstacles.

People with an ASD will continue to learn and grow intellectually throughout their lives, but struggle to master communication and social behavior skills, which impacts their performance in school and work. Some adults with an ASD (especially those with high-functioning autism or **Asperger syndrome**) will attend college and go on to succeed in the workforce.

Universities regularly offer a variety of support services to help students with learning disabilities. These may include testing and diagnosis for LDs, including prescribing medication for ADD/ADHD; reading and writing supports; exam accommodations, such as extra time or a quiet location; and classes on study skills and test anxiety. These supports are generally offered at no cost through an office of disability services or health center. Universities are newly considering what supports can be offered to allow more students on the ASD spectrum to attend and be successful in college. A small number of campuses have developed programs specifically targeted toward students on the ASD spectrum. ASD students will usually need a significant amount of support to be successful in college. In addition to the free services offered to students with LDs, some schools offer additional fee-based assistance including tutoring, help with financial management, and support groups for social interaction and leisure activities.

Sources: S. Shapiro, "Are We Afraid of Treating Adult ADHD?," March 31, 2013, www.psychologytoday.com/blog/the-best-strategies-managing-adult-adhd/201303/are-we-afraid-treating-adult-adhd; National Center for Learning Disabilities, "Types of LD," Accessed February 2014, www.ncld.org/types-learning-disabilities; Autism Speaks, "Preparing for Post-Secondary Education," 2013, www.autismspeaks.org/sites/default/files/docs/preparing_for_postsecondary_education.pdf.

information on other brain-based disorders in young adults. (For coverage of addiction, which is classified as a mental disorder, see **Focus On: Recognizing and Avoiding Addiction** beginning on page 289.) For information about other disorders, consult the websites listed at the end of this chapter or ask your instructor for local resources.

LO 6 | MOOD DISORDERS

Identify causes, characteristics, and treatments of mood disorders.

Chronic mood disorders are disorders that affect how you feel, such as persistent sadness or feelings of euphoria. They include major depression, dysthymic disorder, bipolar disorder, and seasonal affective disorder. In any given year, approximately 10 percent of Americans aged 18 or older suffer from a mood disorder.[28]

chronic mood disorder Experience of persistent emotional states, such as sadness, despair, hopelessness, or euphoria.

major depression Severe depressive disorder with physical effects such as sleep disturbance and exhaustion, and mental effects such as the inability to concentrate; also called *clinical depression.*

Major Depression

Sometimes life throws us a curveball. We experience loss, pain, disappointment, or frustration, and we can be left feeling beaten and bruised. How do we know if these emotions are really signs of **major depression**? Major or clinical depression is not the same as having a bad day or feeling down after a negative experience. It is also not something that can be willed or wished away,

dysthymic disorder (dysthymia) Type of depression that is milder and harder to recognize than major depression; chronic; and often characterized by fatigue, pessimism, or a short temper.

bipolar disorder Form of mood disorder characterized by alternating mania and depression; also called *manic depression.*

seasonal affective disorder (SAD) Type of depression that occurs in the winter months, when sunlight levels are low.

nor can a person just "cheer up." Major depression is the most common mood disorder, affecting approximately 8 percent of the U.S. population in a given year.[29] This number, however, does not reflect all those who suffer from depression because many are misdiagnosed or undiagnosed.

Major depression is characterized by a combination of symptoms that interfere with work, study, sleep, appetite, relationships, and enjoyment of life. Symptoms can last for weeks, months, or years and vary in intensity.[30] Sadness and despair are the main symptoms of depression.[31] Other common signs include:

- Loss of motivation or interest in pleasurable activities
- Preoccupation with failures and inadequacies; concern over what others are thinking
- Difficulty concentrating; indecisiveness; memory lapses
- Loss of sex drive or interest in close interactions with others
- Fatigue and loss of energy; slow reactions
- Sleeping too much or too little; insomnia
- Feeling agitated, worthless, or hopeless
- Withdrawal from friends and family
- Diminished or increased appetite
- Significant weight loss or weight gain
- Recurring thoughts that life isn't worth living; thoughts of death or suicide

Depression in College Students Mental health problems, particularly depression, have gained increased recognition as major obstacles to healthy adjustment and success in college. Students who have weak communication skills, who find that college isn't what they expected, or who lack motivation often have difficulties. Stressors such as anxiety over relationships, pressure to get good grades and win social acceptance, abuse of alcohol and other drugs, poor diet, and lack of sleep can create a toxic cocktail that can overwhelm even the most resilient students. In a recent survey by the American College Health Association, 10.7 percent of college students reported having been diagnosed with or treated for depression in the past 12 months.[32]

Being far from home without the security of family and friends can exacerbate problems. International students are particularly vulnerable to depression and other mental health concerns. Most campuses have counseling centers and other services available; however, many students do not use them because of persistent stigma about seeing a counselor. The **Health in a Diverse World** box on the following page discusses the differences in depression prevalence across different ages, genders, and ethnicities.

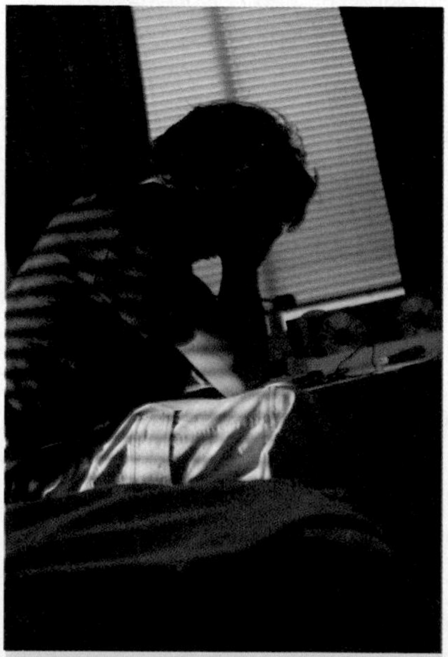

There is more to depression than simply feeling blue. When a person is clinically depressed, he or she finds it difficult to function, sometimes struggling just to get out of bed in the morning or to follow a conversation.

Dysthymic Disorder

Dysthymic disorder (dysthymia), a less severe syndrome of chronic mild depression, can be harder to recognize than major depression. Dysthymic individuals may appear to function well, but they may lack energy or may fatigue easily; be short-tempered, overly pessimistic, and ornery; or just not feel quite up to par but not have any significant, overt symptoms. People with dysthymia may cycle into major depression over time. For a diagnosis, symptoms must persist for at least 2 years in adults (1 year in children). This disorder affects approximately 5 percent of the adult population in the United States in a given year.[33]

Bipolar Disorder

People with **bipolar disorder** (also called *manic depression*) often have severe mood swings, ranging from extreme highs (mania) to extreme lows (depression). Sometimes these swings are dramatic and rapid; other times they are slow and gradual. When in the manic phase, people may be overactive, talkative, and have tons of energy; in the depressed phase, they may experience some or all of the symptoms of major depression.

Although the cause of bipolar disorder is unknown, biological, genetic, and environmental factors, such as drug abuse and stressful or psychologically traumatic events, seem to be involved in triggering episodes. Once diagnosed, persons with bipolar disorder have several counseling and pharmaceutical options, and most will be able to live a healthy, functional life while being treated. Bipolar disorder affects approximately 2 percent of the adult population in the United States.[34]

Seasonal Affective Disorder

Another form of depression, **seasonal affective disorder (SAD)**, strikes during the winter months and is associated with reduced exposure to sunlight. People with SAD suffer from irritability, apathy, carbohydrate craving and weight gain, increased sleep time, and general sadness. Several factors are implicated in SAD development, including disruption in the body's circadian rhythms and changes in levels of the hormone melatonin and the brain chemical serotonin.[35]

HEALTH IN A DIVERSE WORLD

DEPRESSION ACROSS GENDER, AGE, AND ETHNICITY

Although depression may affect persons of every age, gender, and ethnicity, it does not always manifest itself in the same way across all populations.

Depression and Gender

Women are almost twice as likely as men to experience depression. Hormonal changes may be one factor. Women also face various stressors related to multiple responsibilities—work, child rearing, single parenthood, household work, and caring for elderly parents—at rates that are higher than those of men. Researchers have observed gender differences in coping strategies (responses to negative events) and suggest that some women's strategies make them more vulnerable to depression. For example, men may try to distract themselves from a depressed mood, whereas women may focus on it. If focusing on negative feelings intensifies these feelings, women who do this may predispose themselves to depression.

Depression in men is often masked by alcohol or drug abuse, or by the socially acceptable habit of working excessively long hours. Typically, depressed men present not as hopeless and helpless, but as irritable, angry, and discouraged—often personifying a "tough guy" image. Men are less likely to admit they are depressed, and doctors are less likely to suspect it, based on what men report during doctor's visits.

Depression can affect men's physical health differently than it can women's health. Although depression is associated with an increased risk of coronary heart disease in both men and women, it is associated with a higher risk of death in men.

Depression and Age

Today, depression in children is increasingly reported, with 1 in 10 children between ages 6 and 12 experiencing persistent feelings of sadness, the hallmark of depression. Depressed children may pretend to be sick, refuse to go to school or have a sudden drop in school performance, sleep excessively, engage in self-injury, abuse drugs or alcohol, feel misunderstood, or attempt suicide.

Before adolescence, girls and boys experience depression at about the same rate, but by adolescence and young adulthood, girls experience depression more than boys do. This may be due to biological and hormonal changes; girls' struggles with self-esteem and perceptions of success and approval; and an increase in girls' exposure to traumas, such as childhood sexual abuse, that may contribute to depression.

As adults reach their middle and older years, most are emotionally stable and lead active and satisfying lives. With aging, though, comes higher rates of depression; in fact, depression is considered the most common mental disorder of people aged 65 and older. Rates are likely even higher than reported, as the symptoms of depression can be mistaken for dementia and thus be misdiagnosed.

Depression and Race/Ethnicity

The Centers for Disease Control and Prevention (CDC) reports that rates of depression are higher among African Americans and Latinos than among whites; however, true rates of depression among minority populations are difficult to determine, as members of these groups may have difficulty accessing mental health services because of economic barriers, social and cultural differences, language barriers, and lack of culturally competent providers. African American males specifically may avoid professional help owing to stigma attached to mental illness in the African American community as well as greater distrust of physicians and poor patient-physician communication. Unfortunately, when African Americans do report depression symptoms to a health care provider, they are significantly less likely to receive a depression diagnosis from a health care provider than are non-Hispanic whites, and those who are diagnosed are less likely to be treated for depression.

There is no simple fix for this type of health disparity, but including universal depression screening in all primary care visits would be a good first step to ensure every patient's symptoms were equally considered for a depression diagnosis and treatment.

Regardless of gender, age, or ethnicity, no one is immune to depression.

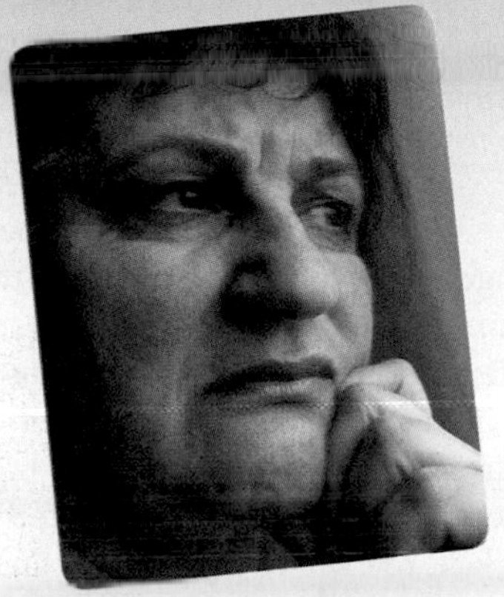

Sources: Mayo Clinic, MayoClinic.com, "Depression in Women: Understanding the Gender Gap," January 2013, www.mayoclinic.org/diseases-conditions/depression/in-depth/depression/art-20047725; HelpGuide.org, "Depression in Men," 2014, www.helpguide.org/mental/depression_men_male.htm; American Psychiatric Association (APA), Mental Health, "Children," Accessed February 2014, www.psychiatry.org/mental-health/people/children; APA, Mental Health, "Seniors," Accessed February 2014, www.psychiatry.org/mental-health/people/seniors; CDC, "An Estimated 1 in 10 U.S. Adults Report Depression," March 31, 2011, www.cdc.gov/features/dsdepression/; A. Akincigil, "Racial and Ethnic Disparities in Depression Care in Community-Dwelling Elderly in the United States," *American Journal of Public Health* 102, no. 2 (2012): 319–28.

The most beneficial treatment for SAD is light therapy, which exposes patients to lamps that simulate sunlight. Other treatments for SAD include diet change (such as eating more complex carbohydrates), increased exercise, stress-management techniques, sleep restriction (limiting the number of hours slept in a 24-hour period), psychotherapy, and prescription medications.

What Causes Mood Disorders?

Mood disorders are caused by the interaction between multiple factors, including biological differences, hormones, inherited traits, life events, and early childhood trauma.[36] The biology of mood disorders is related to individual levels of brain chemicals called *neurotransmitters.* Several

anxiety disorders Mental illness characterized by persistent feelings of threat and worry in coping with everyday problems.

generalized anxiety disorder (GAD) A constant sense of worry that may cause restlessness, difficulty in concentrating, tension, and other symptoms.

panic attack Severe anxiety reaction in which a particular situation, often for unknown reasons, causes terror.

types of depression, including bipolar disorder, appear to have a genetic component. Depression can also be triggered by a serious loss, difficult relationships, financial problems, and pressure to succeed. Early childhood trauma, such as loss of a parent, may cause permanent changes in the brain, making one more prone to depression. Changes in the body's physical health can be accompanied by mental changes, particularly depression. Stroke, heart attack, cancer, Parkinson's disease, chronic pain, type 2 diabetes, certain medications, alcohol, hormonal disorders, and a wide range of other afflictions can cause a person to become depressed, frustrated, or angry. When this happens, recovery is often more difficult, as a person who feels exhausted and defeated may lack the will to fight illness and do what is necessary to optimize recovery.

LO 7 | ANXIETY DISORDERS

Describe the causes, characteristics, and treatment options for anxiety disorders.

Anxiety disorders include generalized anxiety disorder, panic disorders, and phobic disorders. They are characterized by persistent feelings of threat and worry. Consider John Madden, former head coach of the Oakland Raiders, who outfitted his own bus and, for many years, drove every weekend across the country to serve as commentator for NFL games. Why the exhausting driving schedule? Madden was terrified of getting on a plane.

DID YOU KNOW?

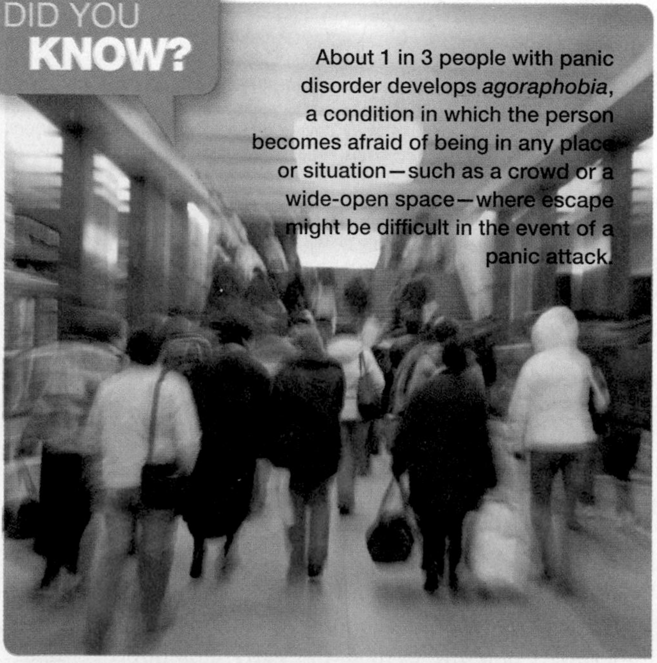

About 1 in 3 people with panic disorder develops *agoraphobia*, a condition in which the person becomes afraid of being in any place or situation—such as a crowd or a wide-open space—where escape might be difficult in the event of a panic attack.

Source: Anxiety and Depression Association of America, "Panic Disorder and Agoraphobia, https://www.adaa.org/understanding-anxiety/panic-disorder-agoraphobia.

SEE IT! VIDEOS

Why are women more likely than men to take antidepressants? Watch **Antidepressant Use Increases Among Women** available on MasteringHealth.™

Anxiety disorders are the number one mental health problem in the United States, affecting more than 21 percent of all adults ages 18–64.[37] Anxiety is also a leading mental health problem among adolescents, affecting 25 percent of Americans aged 13 to 17.[38] About 12 percent of U.S. undergraduates report being diagnosed with or treated for anxiety in the past year.[39]

Generalized Anxiety Disorder

One common form of anxiety disorder, **generalized anxiety disorder (GAD)**, is severe enough to interfere significantly with daily life. Generally, a person with GAD is a consummate worrier who develops a debilitating level of anxiety. To be diagnosed with GAD, one must exhibit at least three of the following symptoms for more days than not during a 6-month period: restlessness or feeling keyed up or on edge, being easily fatigued, difficulty concentrating or mind going blank, irritability, muscle tension, and/or sleep disturbances.[40] Generalized anxiety disorder often runs in families, but it is readily treatable.

Panic Disorder

Panic disorder is characterized by the occurrence of **panic attacks**, an acute anxiety reaction that brings on an intense physical reaction. You may dismiss the feelings as the jitters from too much stress, or the reaction may be so severe that you fear you will have a heart attack and die. Approximately 3 percent of Americans aged 18 and older experience panic attacks, usually in early adulthood.[41] Panic attacks and disorders are increasing in incidence, particularly among young women.

Although highly treatable, panic attacks may become debilitating and destructive, particularly if they happen often and cause the person to avoid going out in public or interacting with others. A panic attack typically starts abruptly, peaks within 10 minutes, lasts about 30 minutes, and leaves the person tired and drained. Symptoms include increased respiration, chills, hot flashes, shortness of breath, stomach cramps, chest pain, difficulty swallowing, and a sense of doom or impending death.[42]

Although researchers aren't sure what causes panic attacks, heredity, stress, and certain biochemical factors may play a role. Your chances of having a panic attack increase if a close relative has them. Some researchers believe that people who suffer panic attacks are experiencing an overreactive fight-or-flight physical response. (See **Chapter 3** for more on the fight-or-flight response.)

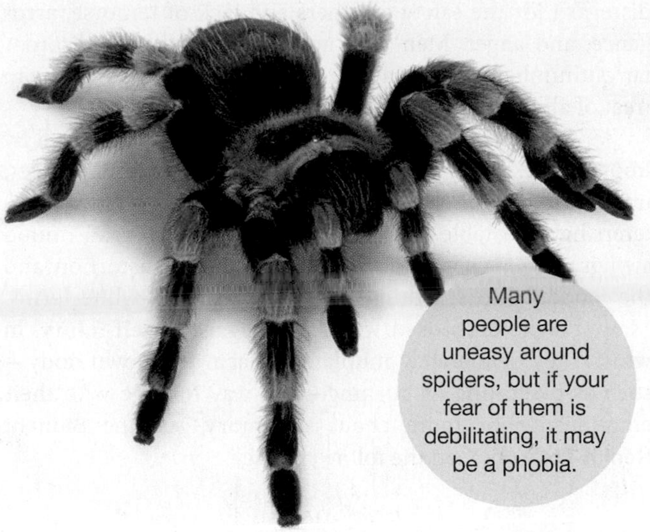

Many people are uneasy around spiders, but if your fear of them is debilitating, it may be a phobia.

Phobic Disorders

Phobias, or phobic disorders, involve a persistent and irrational fear of a specific object, activity, or situation, often out of proportion to the circumstances. Phobias result in a compelling desire to avoid the source of the fear. About 10 percent of American adults suffer from specific phobias, such as fear of spiders or snakes or riding in elevators.[43]

Another 8 percent of American adults suffer from **social anxiety disorder**, also called *social phobia*.[44] Social phobia is an anxiety disorder characterized by the persistent fear and avoidance of social situations. Essentially, the person dreads these situations for fear of being humiliated, embarrassed, or even looked at. These disorders vary in scope. Some cause difficulty only in specific situations, such as getting up in front of the class to give a presentation, while in extreme cases, a person avoids all contact with others.[45]

What Causes Anxiety Disorders?

Because anxiety disorders vary in complexity and degree, scientists have yet to find clear reasons why one person develops them and another doesn't. The following factors are often cited as possible causes:[46]

- **Biology.** Some scientists trace the origin of anxiety to the brain and its functioning. Using sophisticated positron-emission tomography (PET) scans, scientists can analyze areas of the brain that react during anxiety-producing events. Families appear to display similar brain and physiological reactivity, so we may inherit tendencies toward anxiety disorders.
- **Environment.** Anxiety can be a learned response. Although genetic tendencies may exist, experiencing a repeated pattern of reaction to certain situations programs the brain to respond in a certain way. For example, if your sibling screamed whenever a large spider crept into view or if other anxiety-raising events occurred frequently, you might be predisposed to react with anxiety to similar events later in life.
- **Social and cultural roles.** Cultural and social roles also may be a factor in risks for anxiety. Because men and women are taught to assume different roles, women may find it more acceptable to scream, tremble, or otherwise express extreme anxiety. Men, in contrast, may have learned to repress anxious feelings rather than act on them.

LO 8 | OBSESSIVE-COMPULSIVE DISORDER

Describe the symptoms, causes, and treatment options for obsessive-compulsive disorders.

People who feel compelled to perform rituals over and over again; who are fearful of dirt or contamination; who have an unnatural concern about order, symmetry, and exactness; or who have persistent intrusive thoughts that they can't shake may be suffering from **obsessive-compulsive disorder (OCD)**. Approximately 1 percent of Americans aged 18 and over have OCD.[47] Not to be confused with being a perfectionist, a person with OCD often knows the behaviors are irrational, yet is powerless to stop them. According to the *DSM-5*, for a person to be diagnosed with OCD, the obsessions must consume more than 1 hour per day and interfere with normal social or life activities. Although the exact cause is unknown, genetics, biological abnormalities, learned behaviors, and environmental factors have all been considered. Obsessive-compulsive disorder usually begins in childhood or the teen years; most people are diagnosed before age 20.[48]

phobia Deep and persistent fear of a specific object, activity, or situation that results in a compelling desire to avoid the source of the fear.

social anxiety disorder Phobia characterized by fear and avoidance of social situations; also called *social phobia*.

obsessive-compulsive disorder (OCD) Form of anxiety disorder characterized by recurrent, unwanted thoughts and repetitive behaviors.

post-traumatic stress disorder (PTSD) Collection of symptoms that may occur as a delayed response to a traumatic event or series of events.

LO 9 | POST-TRAUMATIC STRESS DISORDER

Explore common causes, characteristics, and treatment options for people with post-traumatic stress disorder.

People who have experienced or witnessed a traumatic event may develop **post-traumatic stress disorder (PTSD)**. While only about 4 percent of Americans suffer from PTSD each year, about 8 percent will experience PTSD in their lifetimes, with women experiencing rates twice as high as men.[49] Fourteen percent of U.S. combat veterans who fought in Iraq and Afghanistan have experienced PTSD, and their stories frequent the national news. However, the "worst stressful experiences" reported most frequently by those with PTSD are not war-related, but rather the unexpected death, serious illness, or injury of someone close, and sexual assault. Others report experiences such as a natural disaster, serious accident, violent assault, or terrorism. It is important to understand that PTSD is not rooted in weakness or an inability to cope; traumatic events can actually cause chemical changes in the brain, leading to PTSD.[50]

Symptoms of PTSD include:

- Dissociation, or perceived detachment of the mind from the emotional state or even the body
- Intrusive recollections of the traumatic event, such as flashbacks, nightmares, and recurrent thoughts or images
- Acute anxiety or nervousness, in which the person is hyperaroused, may cry easily, or experiences mood swings
- Insomnia and difficulty concentrating
- Intense physiological reactions, such as shaking or nausea, when something reminds the person of the traumatic event

Although these symptoms may be appropriate as initial responses to traumatic events, PTSD may be diagnosed if a person experiences them for at least 1 month following the traumatic event. However, in some cases, symptoms don't appear until months or even years later.

LO 10 | PERSONALITY DISORDERS

Differentiate personality disorders from other disorders, and describe causes and treatments.

According to the *DSM-5*, a **personality disorder** is an "enduring pattern of inner experience and behavior that deviates markedly from the expectation of the individual's culture and is pervasive and inflexible."[51] It is estimated that at least 10 percent of adults in the United States have some form of personality disorder as defined by the *DSM-5*.[52] People who live, work, or are in relationships with individuals suffering from personality disorders often find interactions with them to be challenging and destructive.

One common type of personality disorder is *paranoid personality disorder,* which involves pervasive, unfounded suspicion and mistrust of other people, irrational jealousy, and secretiveness. Persons with this illness have delusions of being persecuted by everyone, from family members and loved ones to the government.

Narcissistic personality disorders involve an exaggerated sense of self-importance and self-absorption. Persons with narcissistic personalities are preoccupied with fantasies of how wonderful they are. Typically, they are overly needy and demanding and believe that they are "entitled" to nothing but the best.

Persons with *antisocial personality disorders* display a long-term pattern of manipulation and taking advantage of others, often in a criminal manner. Symptoms include disregard for the safety of others and lack of remorse, arrogance, and anger. Men with antisocial personality disorder far outnumber women, and it remains one of the hardest to treat of all personality disorders.[53]

Borderline personality disorder (BPD) is characterized by impulsiveness and risky behaviors such as gambling sprees, unsafe sex, use of illicit drugs, and daredevil driving.[54] Sufferers have unstable moods and can experience erratic mood swings. Other characteristics include reality distortion and the tendency to see things in only black-and-white terms. Many people diagnosed with BPD engage in **self-injury**, in which they deliberately mutilate or harm their own body—such as by cutting or burning—as a way to cope with their emotions.[55] For more about self-injury, see the **Student Health Today** box on the following page.

personality disorder Mental disorder characterized by inflexible patterns of thought and beliefs that lead to socially distressing behavior.

self-injury Intentionally causing injury to one's own body in an attempt to cope with overwhelming negative emotions; also called *self-mutilation, self-harm,* or *nonsuicidal self-injury* (NSSI).

schizophrenia Mental illness with biological origins characterized by irrational behavior, severe alterations of the senses, and often an inability to function in society.

LO 11 | SCHIZOPHRENIA

Characterize schizophrenia, and explain causes and treatments.

Schizophrenia is a severe psychological disorder that affects about 1 percent of the U.S. population.[56] Schizophrenia is characterized by alterations of the senses (including auditory and visual hallucinations); the inability to sort and process incoming stimuli and make appropriate responses; an altered sense of self; and radical changes in emotions, movements, and behaviors. Typical symptoms of schizophrenia include fluctuating courses of delusional behavior, hallucinations, incoherent and rambling speech, inability to think logically, erratic movement, odd gesturing, and difficulty with normal activities of daily living.[57] Such individuals are often regarded as odd or dangerous, and viewed that way, they have difficulties in social interactions and may withdraw.

For decades, scientists believed that schizophrenia was a form of madness provoked by the environment in which a child lived. They blamed abnormal family interactions or early childhood traumas. In the mid-1980s, magnetic resonance imaging (MRI) and positron emission tomography (PET) scans

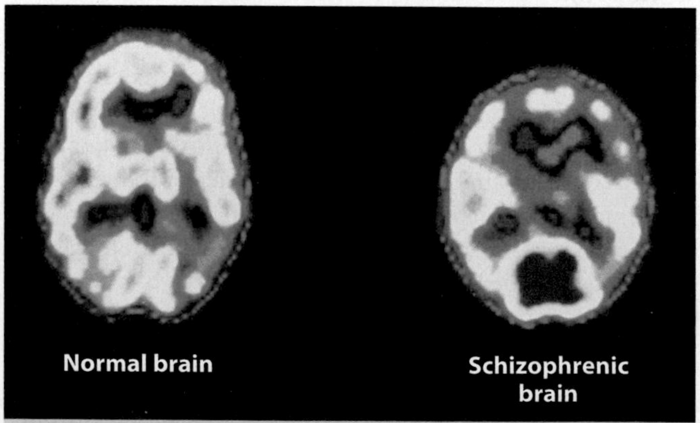

These brain images reveal the difference in brain activity in persons with and without schizophrenia. The yellow and red correspond to areas with greatest activity, and blue signifies reduced activity.

STUDENT HEALTH TODAY

CUTTING THROUGH THE PAIN

When some people are unable to deal with the pain, pressure, or stress they experience in everyday life, they may resort to self-harm in an effort to cope. Self injury, also termed self mutilation, self-harm, or nonsuicidal self-injury (NSSI), is the act of deliberately harming one's body in an attempt to cope with overwhelming negative emotions. Self-injury is an attempt at coping; it is not an attempt at suicide.

The most common method of self-harm is cutting (with razors, glass, knives, or other sharp objects). Other methods include burning, bruising, excessive nail biting, breaking bones, pulling out hair, and embedding sharp objects under the skin.

Reports on prevalence of NSSI in college students vary, ranging from 7 percent to 15 percent. Estimates are higher in the high school population, with the majority of studies reporting about 20 percent of adolescents engaging in self-injury at least once in their lifetime. Many people who harm themselves suffer from other mental health conditions and have experienced sexual, physical, or emotional abuse as children or adults. Self-harm is also commonly associated with mental illnesses such as borderline personality disorder, depression, anxiety disorders, substance abuse disorders, post-traumatic stress disorder, and eating disorders.

Signs of self-injury include multiple scars, current cuts and abrasions, and implausible explanations for wounds and ongoing injuries. A self-injurer may attempt to conceal scars and injuries by wearing long sleeves and pants. Other symptoms can include difficulty handling anger, social withdrawal, sensitivity to rejection, or body alienation. If you or someone you know is engaging in self-injury, seek professional help. Treatment is challenging; not only must the self-injurious behavior be stopped, but the sufferer must also learn to recognize and manage the feelings that triggered the behavior.

If you are a recovering self-injurer, some of the following steps may be part of your treatment:

1. Start by being aware of feelings and situations that trigger your urge to hurt yourself.
2. Identify a plan of what you can do instead when you feel the urge.
3. Create a list of alternatives, including:
   - Things that might distract you
   - Things that might soothe and calm you
   - Things that might help you express the pain and deep emotion
   - Things that might help release physical tension and distress
   - Things that might help you feel supported and connected
   - Things that might substitute for the cutting sensation

For more information, visit these resources: S.A.F.E. Alternatives, **www.selfinjury.com**, and Help Guide, **www.helpguide.org/mental/self_injury.htm.**

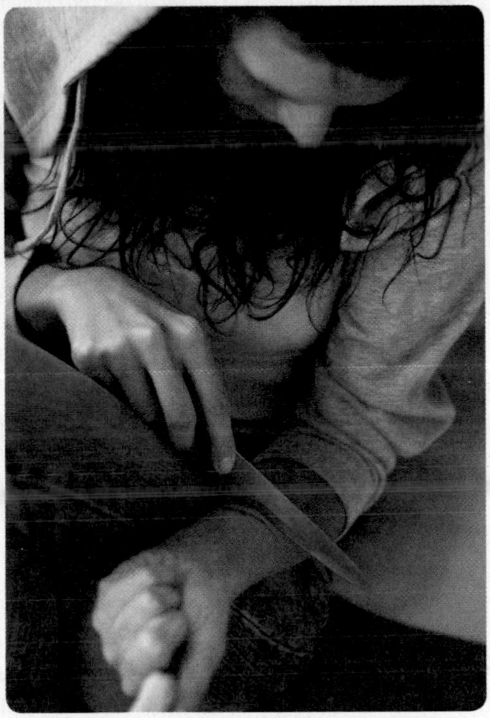

Cutting and scratching behaviors are more common in females, while burning and hitting behaviors are more common in males.

Sources: American College Health Association, *ACHA–NCHA II: Reference Group Data Report, Spring 2013,* (Baltimore, MD: American College Health Association, 2013); M. J. Sornberger et al., "Nonsuicidal Self-Injury and Gender: Patterns of Prevalence, Methods, and Locations among Adolescents," *Suicide and Life-Threatening Behavior* 42, no. 3 (2012): 266–78; J. Whitlock et al., "Nonsuicidal Self-Injury in a College Population: General Trends and Sex Differences," *Journal of American College Health* 59, no. 8 (2011): 691–98; M. Smith and J. Segal, HelpGuide.org, "Cutting and Self-Harm," updated February 2014, www.helpguide.org/mental/self_injury.htm.

began allowing scientists to study brain function more closely; based on that knowledge, schizophrenia was found to be a biological disease of the brain. The brain damage occurs early in life, possibly as early as the second trimester of fetal development. Fetal exposure to toxic substances, infections, and medications have been studied as a possible risk, and hereditary links are being explored. Symptoms usually appear in men in their late teens and twenties and in women in their late twenties and early thirties.[58]

Even though theories that blame abnormal family life or childhood trauma for schizophrenia have been discarded in favor of biological theories, a stigma remains attached to the disease. Families of people with schizophrenia frequently experience anger and guilt. They often need information, family counseling, and advice on how to meet the schizophrenic person's needs for shelter, medical care, vocational training, and social interaction.

At present, schizophrenia is treatable but not curable. Treatments usually include some combination of hospitalization, medication, and psychotherapy. Supportive psychotherapy, as opposed to psychoanalysis, can help the patient acquire skills for living in society. With proper medication, public understanding, support of loved ones, and access to therapy, many schizophrenics lead normal lives. Without these forms of assistance and treatment, they often have great difficulty.

LO 12 | SUICIDE: GIVING UP ON LIFE

Describe the risk factors and possible warning signs of suicide, as well as actions that can be taken to help a person contemplating suicide.

Suicide is the third leading cause of death for 15- to 19-year-olds and the second leading cause of death for 19- to 24-year-olds in the United States.[59] The pressures, disappointments, challenges, and changes of the college years are believed to be partially responsible for the emotional turmoil that can lead a young person to contemplate suicide. However, young adults who do not attend college but who are searching for direction in careers, relationships, and other areas are also at risk; in fact, suicide rates for young adults are higher in the general population than among college students.[60] Risk factors include a family history of suicide, previous suicide attempts, excessive drug and alcohol use, prolonged depression, financial difficulties, serious illness in oneself or a loved one, and loss of a loved one through death or rejection.

Whether they are more likely to attempt suicide or are more often successful, nearly four times as many men die by suicide as women.[61] Firearms, suffocation, and poison are the most common methods of suicide. Males are almost twice as likely as females to commit suicide with firearms, whereas younger females (age 10 to 24 years) are more likely to commit suicide by suffocation and older females (25 years and older) are more likely to commit suicide by poisoning.[62]

Warning Signs of Suicide

People who commit suicide usually indicate their intentions, although others do not always recognize their warnings.[63] Anyone who expresses a desire to kill himself or herself or who has made an attempt is at risk. Common signs that a person may be contemplating suicide include:[64]

- Recent loss and a seeming inability to let go of grief
- History of depression
- Change in personality, such as sadness, withdrawal, irritability, anxiety, tiredness, indecisiveness, apathy
- Change in behavior, such as inability to concentrate, loss of interest in classes or work, unexplained demonstration of happiness following a period of depression, or risk-taking behavior
- Change in sexual interest
- Change in sleep patterns and/or eating habits
- A direct statement (including statements posted on social media) about committing suicide, such as "I might as well end it all"
- An indirect statement (including statements posted on social media), such as "You won't have to worry about me anymore"
- Final preparations such as writing a will, giving away prized possessions, or writing revealing letters or social media posts
- Preoccupation with themes of death
- Marked changes in personal appearance

Preventing Suicide

Most people who attempt suicide really want to live but see death as the only way out of an intolerable situation. Crisis counselors and suicide hotlines may help temporarily, but the best way to prevent suicide is to get rid of conditions and substances that may precipitate attempts, including alcohol, drugs, loneliness, isolation, and access to guns.

If someone you know threatens suicide or displays warning signs, get involved—ask questions and seek help. Specific actions you can take include:[65]

- **Monitor the warning signals.** Keep an eye on the person or see that someone else is present. Don't leave the person alone.
- **Take threats seriously.** Don't brush them off as "cries for attention." Act now.
- **Let the person know how much you care.** State that you are there to help.
- **Ask directly,** "Are you thinking of hurting or killing yourself?"
- **Take action.** Remove any firearms or objects that could be used for suicide from the area.
- **Help the person think about alternatives to suicide.** Offer to go for help along with the person. Call your local suicide hotline, and use all available community and campus resources.
- **Tell the person's spouse, partner, parents, siblings, or counselor.** Do not keep your suspicions to yourself. Don't let a suicidal friend talk you into keeping your discussions confidential. If your friend succeeds in a suicide attempt, you may blame yourself.

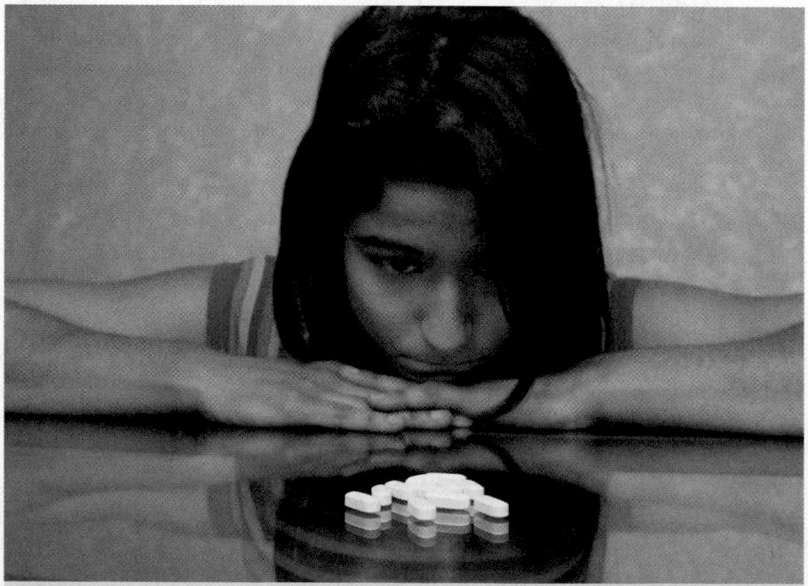

If you notice warning signs of suicide in someone, you must take action. Suicidal people urgently need professional assistance. Always take thoughts of or plans for suicide seriously—a life may depend on it.

MONEY & HEALTH | LOW-COST TREATMENT OPTIONS FOR MENTAL HEALTH CONDITIONS

Mental health disorders are treatable, yet people don't always seek help. Often the cost of therapy and prescription drugs is a major barrier, since insurance plans may provide only limited coverage of mental health services. If you are on a tight budget and struggle with depression, anxiety, or other mental health issues, it's a good idea to speak with your family physician about low-cost treatment resources in your region and state. Here is a roundup of possible treatment options one can pursue, along with tips on easing the expense.

Therapy

Cognitive behavioral therapy (CBT) can cost $100 or more per hour. However, some therapists or clinics offer therapy on a sliding scale, which means the fee fluctuates based on income. Ask about a sliding scale or other payment options when you call or visit for a consultation. Federally funded health centers can also be a good resource for those with a limited budget. Many of these centers include mental health services, and they also have sliding scales for payment. Finally, some colleges and universities offer low-cost therapy for mental health problems through the health center. You can also call the psychology, psychiatry, or behavioral health department and inquire about sessions with graduate students, who are supervised and can provide services at a lower cost as they gain counseling experience.

Prescription Drugs

Medication can help reduce symptoms of certain mental health disorders, including anxiety and depression, but for many people drugs can be expensive. Most pharmaceutical companies offer patient-assistance programs for low-income patients. These programs provide prescribed medication at little to no cost. It's also a good idea to ask your doctor if a generic (non-brand-name) drug might work as well for you as a brand-name drug. The cost difference between generic and brand-name drugs can be substantial. You can also see if your doctor might have medication samples he or she could give you for free.

Note that if you are considering medication, it must be prescribed and monitored by your physician. Do not adjust the dosage or frequency or stop taking it abruptly, even if cost is a factor, without first discussing it with your doctor.

Sources: ADAA, "Low Cost Treatment," Accessed February 2014, www.adaa.org/finding-help/treatment/low-cost-treatment; Partnership for Prescription Assistance, Accessed February 2014, "Patient Frequently Asked Questions," www.pparx.org/en/patient_faqs; J. Grohol, 2011, "Finding Low-Cost Psychotherapy," PsychCentral, Accessed February 10, 2014, http://psychcentral.com/lib/2007/finding-low-cost-psychotherapy; Psych Central Staff, "Mental Health Care Benefits Under Affordable Care Act," July 2, 2012, http://psychcentral.com/news/2012/06/30/mental-health-care-benefits-under-affordable-care-act-obamacare/41052.html.

LO 13 | SEEKING PROFESSIONAL HELP

Explain the different types of treatment options and professional services available to those experiencing mental health problems.

A physical ailment will readily send most of us to the nearest health professional, but many people view seeking professional help for psychological problems as an admission of personal failure. Although estimates show that 20 percent of adults have some kind of mental disorder, only 6 to 7 percent of adults use mental health counseling services.[66]

Researchers view breakdowns in support systems, high societal expectations, and dysfunctional families as three major reasons why people need more assistance than ever before. Consider seeking help if:

- You feel that you need help or feel out of control.
- You experience wild mood swings or inappropriate emotional responses to normal stimuli.
- Your fears or feelings of guilt frequently distract your attention.
- You begin to withdraw from others.
- You have hallucinations.
- You feel inadequate or worthless or that life is not worth living.
- Your daily life seems to be nothing but a series of repeated crises.
- You are considering suicide.
- You turn to drugs or alcohol to escape your problems.

stigma Negative perception about a group of people or a certain situation or condition.

Low-cost or free counseling sessions or support groups are often available on college campuses to help students deal with all types of issues, including mental illness; recovery from eating disorders, substance abuse, and other addictions; dealing with health conditions such as diabetes or cancer; and addressing other challenges, such as managing stress, overcoming fear of public speaking, becoming more physically fit, or changing eating habits. See the **Money & Health** box for tips on how to get good mental health care on a tight budget. You may find certain websites or phone apps useful as well, but be cautious in your selection.

Mental Illness Stigma

Stigmas are negative perceptions about groups of people or about a certain situation or condition. Common stigmas about people with mental illness are that they are dangerous, irresponsible, require constant care, or that they "just need to get over it." Derogatory terms such as *nut job, whacko, crazy, insane, madman,* *bonkers,* and *demented* are still commonly used to describe persons with mental illness. In truth, a small percentage of people with a mental illness are dangerous. Most people with a mental illness live independently, go to school, hold jobs, and are productive members of society. A mental illness is like any other chronic disease. You can't just decide to "get over it."

WHAT DO **YOU** THINK?

Do you notice a stigma associated with mental illness in your community?

- How often do you hear terms like "crazy" or "whacko" used to describe people who appear to have a mental health problem? Why are those words harmful?
- What could you do to combat the stigma of mental illness?

The stigma of mental illness often leads to feelings of shame, guilt, loss of self-esteem, and a sense of isolation and hopelessness. Many people who have successfully managed their mental illness report that the stigma they faced was more disabling at times than the illness itself.[67] This stigma may cause people who are struggling with a mental illness to delay seeking treatment or avoid care that could dramatically improve their symptoms and quality of life.

1 IN 3

COLLEGE STUDENTS WITH A MENTAL ILLNESS IDENTIFY **STIGMA** AS THE BIGGEST BARRIER TO RECEIVING TREATMENT.

Getting Evaluated for Treatment

If you are considering treatment for a psychological problem, schedule a complete evaluation first. Consult a credentialed health professional for a thorough examination, which should include three parts:

1. *A physical checkup,* which will rule out thyroid disorders, viral infections, and anemia—all of which can result in depression-like symptoms—and a neurological check of coordination, reflexes, and balance to rule out brain disorders.
2. *A psychiatric history,* which will trace the course of the apparent disorder, genetic or family factors, and any past treatments.
3. *A mental status examination,* which will assess thoughts, speaking processes, and memory, and will include an in-depth interview with tests for other psychiatric symptoms.

Once physical factors have been ruled out, you may decide to consult a professional who specializes in psychological health.

Mental Health Professionals

Several types of mental health professionals are available; **TABLE 2.1** provides information on the most common types of practitioners. When choosing a therapist, it is important to verify that he or she has the appropriate training and certification. But the most important factor is whether you feel you can work with him or her. A qualified mental health professional should be willing to answer all your questions during an initial consultation. Questions to ask the therapist or yourself include:

- **Can you interview the therapist before starting treatment?** An initial meeting will help you determine whether this person will be a good fit for you.
- **Do you like the therapist as a person?** Can you talk to him or her comfortably?
- **Is the therapist watching the clock or easily distracted?** You should be the main focus of the session.
- **Does the therapist demonstrate professionalism?** Be concerned if your therapist is frequently late or breaks appointments, suggests social interactions outside therapy sessions, talks inappropriately about himself or herself, has questionable billing practices, or resists releasing you from therapy.
- **Will the therapist help you set your own goals and timetables?** A good professional should evaluate your general situation and help you set small goals to work on between sessions.

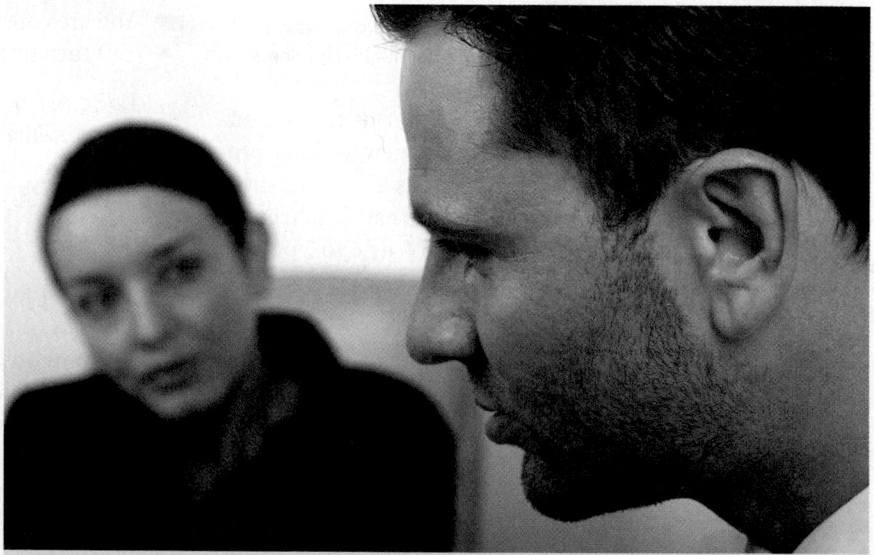

When you begin seeing a mental health professional, you enter into a relationship with that person, and just as with any person, you will connect better with some therapists than others. If one doesn't "feel right," trust your instincts and look for someone else.

TABLE 2.1 | Mental Health Professionals

What Are They Called?	What Kind of Training Do They Have?	What Kind of Therapy Do They Do?	Professional Association
Psychiatrist	Medical doctor degree (MD), followed by 4 years of mental health training	Can prescribe medications and may have admitting privileges at a local hospital.	American Psychiatric Association **www.psych.org**
Psychologist	Doctoral degree in counseling or clinical psychology (PhD), plus several years of supervised practice to earn license	Various types, such as cognitive-behavioral therapy and specialties including family or sexual counseling	American Psychological Association **www.apa.org**
Clinical/psychiatric social worker	Master's degree in social work (MSW), followed by 2 years of experience in a clinical setting to earn license	May be trained in certain specialties, such as substance abuse counseling or child counseling	National Association of Social Workers **www.socialworkers.org**
Counselor	Master's degree in counseling, psychology, educational psychology, or related human service; generally must complete at least 2 years of supervised practice to obtain a license	Many are trained to provide individual and group therapy; may specialize in one type of counseling, such as family, marital, relationship, children, or substance abuse	American Counseling Association **www.counseling.org**
Psychoanalyst	Postgraduate degree in psychology or psychiatry (PhD or MD), followed by 8 to 10 years of training in psychoanalysis, which includes undergoing analysis themselves	Based on the theories of Freud and others, focuses on patterns of thinking and behavior and recalling early traumas that block personal growth. Treatment lasts 5 to 10 years, with three to four sessions per week.	American Psychoanalytic Association **www.apsa.org**
Licensed marriage and family therapist (LMFT)	Master's or doctoral degree in psychology, social work, or counseling, specializing in family and interpersonal dynamics; generally must complete at least 2 years of supervised practice to obtain a license	Treats individuals or families who want relationship counseling. Treatment is often brief and focused on finding solutions to specific relational problems.	American Association for Marriage and Family Therapy **www.aamft.org**

Note that the use of the title *therapist* or *counselor* is not nationally regulated. Check credentials and make your choice carefully.

What to Expect in Therapy

Before making an appointment, call for information and to briefly explain your needs. Ask about office hours, policies and procedures, fees, and insurance participation. The first trip to a therapist can be unsettling. Most of us have misconceptions about what therapy is and what it can do. The first visit serves as a sizing-up between you and the therapist. If you decide that this professional is not for you, you will at least have learned how to present your problem and what qualities you need in a therapist.

Dress however you feel most comfortable, arrive on time, and expect your visit to last about an hour. The therapist will record your history and details about the problem that has brought you to therapy. Answer honestly and do not be embarrassed to acknowledge your feelings. It is critical to the success of your treatment that you trust the therapist enough to be open and honest.

Do not expect the therapist to tell you what to do or how to behave. The responsibility for improved behavior lies with you. If after your first visit (or even after several visits), you feel you cannot work with this person, say so. You have the right to find a therapist with whom you feel comfortable.

Treatment Models Many different types of counseling exist, including psychodynamic therapy, interpersonal therapy, and cognitive-behavioral therapy.

Psychodynamic therapy focuses on the psychological roots of emotional suffering. This type of therapy has roots in Freud's theories and involves self-reflection, self-examination, and the use of the relationship between therapist and patient as a window into problematic relationship patterns in the patient's life. Its goal is not only to alleviate the most obvious symptoms, but also to help people lead healthier lives.[68]

Interpersonal therapy is a variation of psychodynamic therapy and focuses on social roles and relationships. The patient works with a therapist to evaluate specific problem areas in the patient's life, such as conflicts with family and friends or significant life changes or transition. While past experiences help inform the process, interpersonal therapy focuses mainly on improving relationships in the present.[69]

Treatment for mental disorders can include various cognitive-behavioral therapies. *Cognitive therapy* focuses on the impact of thoughts and ideas on feelings and behavior. It helps a person to look at life rationally and correct habitually pessimistic or faulty thinking patterns. *Behavioral therapy,* as the name implies, focuses on what we do. Behavioral therapy uses the concepts of stimulus, response, and reinforcement to alter behavior patterns. With cognitive-behavioral therapy, you work with a mental health professional in a structured way, attending a limited number of sessions to become aware of inaccurate or negative thinking. Cognitive-behavioral therapy enables you to view challenging situations more clearly and respond to them in a more effective and positive way. This therapy can be a very helpful tool in treating mental anxiety or depression.[70]

Pharmacological Treatment

Treatment for some conditions combines cognitive-behavioral therapies with psychoactive medication prescribed by the patient's physician or by a psychiatrist. **TABLE 2.2** includes information about the major classes of medications used to treat the most common mental illnesses. Psychoactive drugs require a doctor's prescription and carry approval from the U.S. Food and Drug Administration (FDA). Side effects of psychoactive drugs commonly include dry mouth, headaches, nausea, sexual dysfunction, and weight gain, among others. Additionally, the FDA requires warnings for antidepressant medications, including labeling that warns of increased risks of suicidal thinking and behavior during initial treatment in young adults aged 18 to 24.[71]

Potency, dosage, and side effects of drugs can vary greatly. It is vital to talk to your health care provider and completely

TABLE **2.2** | Types of Medications Used to Treat Mental Illness

Antidepressants	**Used to Treat Depression, Panic Disorders, Anxiety Disorders**	
Selective serotonin-reuptake inhibitors (SSRIs)	*Examples:* fluoxetine (Prozac), paroxetine (Paxil), escitalopram (Lexapro, Esipram), citalopram (Celexa)	The current standard drug treatment for depression; also frequently prescribed for anxiety disorders
Noradrenergic and specific serotonergic antidepressants (NaSSAs)	*Examples:* mirtazapine (Remeron)	Reportedly has fewer sexual dysfunction side effects than do SSRIs
Serotonin-norepinephrine reuptake inhibitors (SNRIs)	*Examples:* venlafaxine (Effexor), duloxetine (Cymbalta)	Also sometimes prescribed for ADHD
Norepinephrine-dopamine reuptake inhibitors (NDRIs)	*Examples:* bupropion (Wellbutrin)	Also used in smoking cessation; fewer weight gain or sexual dysfunction side effects than SSRIs
Tricyclic antidepressants (TCAs)	*Examples:* imipramine (Tofranil), amitriptyline, nortriptyline (Aventyl), and desipramine (Norpramin)	Negative side effects; usually used as a 2nd or 3rd line of treatment when other medications prove ineffective
Monoamine oxidase inhibitors (MAOIs)	*Examples:* phenelzine (Nardil), tranylcypromine (Parnate), and isocarboxazid (Marplan)	Dangerous interactions with many other drugs and substances in food; generally no longer prescribed
Anxiolytics (antianxiety drugs)	**Used to Treat Anxiety Disorders, GAD, Panic Disorders, Phobias, OCD, PTSD**	
Benzodiazepines	*Examples:* lorazepam (Ativan), clonazepam (Klonopin), alprazolam (Xanax), diazepam (Valium)	Short-term relief, sometimes taken on an as-needed basis; dangerous interactions with alcohol; possible to develop tolerance or dependence
Serotonin 1A agonists	*Examples:* buspirone (BuSpar)	Longer-term relief; must be taken for at least 2 weeks to achieve antianxiety effects
Mood Stabilizers	**Used to Treat Bipolar Disorder, Schizophrenia**	
Lithium	*Examples:* lithium carbonate (Eskalith)	Drug most commonly used to treat bipolar disorder; blood levels must be closely monitored to determine proper dosage and avoid toxic effects
Anticonvulsants	*Examples:* valproic acid/divalproex sodium (Depakote)	Used more frequently for acute mania than for long-term maintenance of bipolar disorder
Antipsychotics (neuroleptics)	**Used to Treat Schizophrenia, Mania, Bipolar Disorder**	
Atypical antipsychotics	*Examples:* clozapine (Clozaril), risperidone (Risperdal)	First line of treatment for schizophrenia; fewer adverse effects than earlier antipsychotics
First-generation antipsychotics	*Examples:* haloperidol (Haldol), chlorpromazine (Thorazine)	Earliest forms of antipsychotics; unpleasant side effects such as tremor and muscle stiffness
Stimulants	**Used to Treat ADHD, Narcolepsy**	
Methylphenidate	*Examples:* Ritalin, Metadate CD, Concerta	Can lead to tolerance and dependence; frequently abused for both performance enhancement and recreational use
Amphetamines	*Examples:* amphetamine (Adderall), dextroamphetamine (Dexedrine, Dextrostat)	Can lead to tolerance and dependence; frequently abused for both performance enhancement and recreational use

Source: Data from National Institute of Mental Health, Mental Health Medications, "Alphabetical List of Medications," 2012, www.nimh.nih.gov/health/publications/mental-health-medications/nimh-mental-health-medications.pdf.

understand the risks and benefits of any prescribed medication. Likewise, your doctor needs to be notified as soon as possible of any adverse effects you may experience. With some drug therapies, such as antidepressants, you may not feel the therapeutic effects for several weeks, so patience is important. Finally, be sure to follow your doctor's recommendations for beginning or ending a course of any medication.

To avoid the side effects of psychoactive drugs, some patients choose complementary or alternative therapies such as St. John's Wort or omega-3 fatty acids for depression and kava or acupuncture for anxiety.

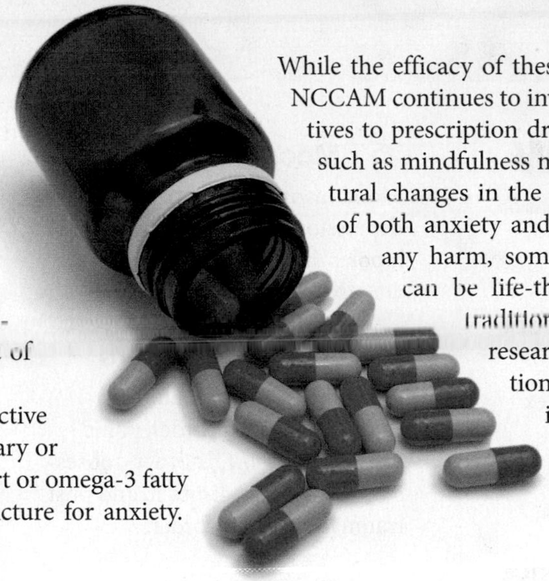

While the efficacy of these therapies is not yet conclusive, NCCAM continues to invest in research to explore alternatives to prescription drugs. While some CAM therapies, such as mindfulness meditation—associated with structural changes in the brain that may reduce symptoms of both anxiety and depression—is unlikely to cause any harm, some therapies, like St. John's Wort, can be life-threatening when combined with traditional depression medications. Much research is still needed on both traditional and CAM therapies for mental illness, making it essential to talk to a medical professional when considering any new treatment or change in treatment.[72]

STUDY PLAN

Customize your study plan—and master your health!—in the Study Area of **MasteringHealth.**

ASSESS **YOURSELF**

How is your psychological health? Want to find out? Take the **How Psychologically Healthy Are You?** assessment available on MasteringHealth.™

Need help creating a plan? Follow the strategies in the **Your Plan for Change** box for short- and long-term improvements to your health.

YOUR PLAN FOR **CHANGE**

The **ASSESS YOURSELF** activity "How Psychologically Healthy Are You?" gives you the chance to look at various aspects of your psychological health and compare your self-assessment with a friend's perceptions. After considering these results, you can take steps to change behaviors that may be harmful.

TODAY, YOU CAN:

- ☐ Evaluate your behavior and identify patterns and specific things you are doing that negatively affect your psychological health. What can you change now? What can you change in the near future?
- ☐ Start a journal and list people you can rely on and trust in life. Describe what you are really engaged in and what gives your life meaning.
- ☐ List the things that bring you joy—friends, family, activities, entertainment, nature. Commit yourself to making more room for these joy-givers in your life.

WITHIN THE NEXT 2 WEEKS, YOU CAN:

- ☐ Visit your campus health center's website and find out about counseling services they offer. If you are feeling overwhelmed, depressed, or anxious, make an appointment with a counselor.
- ☐ Pay attention to negative thoughts that pop up throughout the day. Note times when you find yourself undermining your abilities and notice when you project negative attitudes. Bringing your awareness to these thoughts gives you an opportunity to stop and reevaluate them.

BY THE END OF THE SEMESTER, YOU CAN:

- ☐ Make a commitment to an ongoing practice aimed at improving your psychological health. Depending on your current situation, this could mean anything from seeing a counselor or joining a support group to practicing meditation or attending religious services.
- ☐ Volunteer regularly with a local organization you care about. Focus your energy and gain meaning by helping to improve others' lives or the environment.

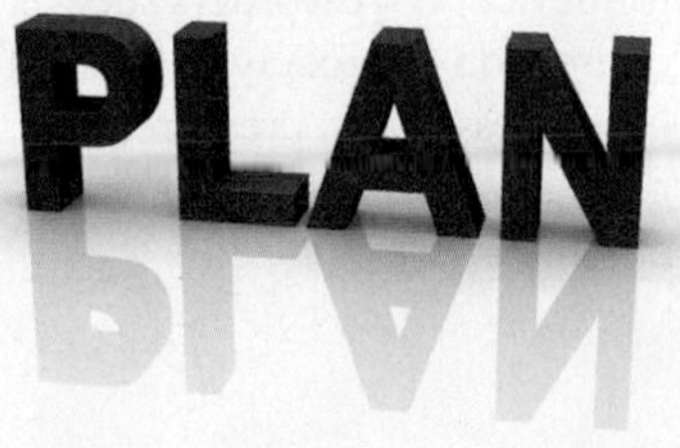

CHAPTER REVIEW

To hear an MP3 Tutor Session, scan here or visit the Study Area in **MasteringHealth.**

LO 1 What Is Psychological Health?

- Psychological health is a complex phenomenon involving mental, emotional, social, and spiritual dimensions.

LO 2 Factors That Influence Psychological Health

- Many factors influence psychological health, including life experiences, family, the environment, other people, self-esteem, self-efficacy, and personality.

LO 3 The Mind-Body Connection

- The mind-body connection is an important link in overall health and well-being. Positive psychology emphasizes well-being as a key factor in determining overall reactions to life's challenges. Psychoneuroimmunology indicates that mental health and physical health are linked.

LO 4 Strategies to Enhance Psychological Health

- Developing self-esteem and self-efficacy, making healthy connections, having a positive outlook on life, and maintaining physical health are key to enhancing psychological health.

LO 5 Mental Illness on Campus

- College life is a high-risk time for developing disorders such as depression or anxiety because of high stress levels, pressures for grades, and financial problems, among others.

LO 6 Mood Disorders

- Mood disorders include major depression, dysthymic disorder, bipolar disorder, and seasonal affective disorder.

LO 7 Anxiety Disorders

- Anxiety disorders include generalized anxiety disorder, panic disorders, phobic disorders, obsessive-compulsive disorder, and post-traumatic stress disorder.

LO 8 Obsessive-Compulsive Disorders

- People with OCD often have irrational concern about order, symmetry, or exactness, or have persistent intrusive thoughts.

LO 9 Post-Traumatic Stress Disorders

- PTSD is caused by experiencing or witnessing a traumatic event, such as those that occur in war, natural disasters, or the loss of a loved one.

LO 10 Personality Disorders

- Personality disorders include paranoid, narcissistic, antisocial, and borderline personality disorders.

LO 11 Schizophrenia

- Schizophrenia is often characterized by visual and auditory hallucinations, an altered sense of self, and radical changes in emotions, among others.

LO 12 Suicide: Giving Up on Life

- Suicide is a result of negative psychological reactions to life. People intending to commit suicide often give warning signs of their intentions and can often be helped. Suicide prevention involves eliminating the conditions that may lead to attempts.

LO 13 Seeking Professional Help

- Mental health professionals include psychiatrists, psychoanalysts, psychologists, social workers, and counselors/therapists. Many therapy methods exist, including psychodynamic, interpersonal, and cognitive-behavioral therapy.
- Treatment of mental disorders can combine talk therapy and drug therapy using psychoactive drugs, such as antidepressants or anxiolytics.

POP QUIZ

Visit **MasteringHealth** to personalize your study plan with Chapter Review Quizzes and Dynamic Study Modules.

LO 1 What Is Psychological Health?

1. All of the following traits have been identified as characterizing psychologically healthy people *except*
   a. conscientiousness.
   b. understanding.
   c. openness.
   d. agreeableness.

LO 2 Factors That Influence Psychological Health

2. A person with high self-esteem
   a. possesses feelings of self-respect and self-worth.
   b. believes he or she can successfully engage in a specific behavior.
   c. believes external influences shape one's psychological health.
   d. has a high altruistic capacity.

LO 3 The Mind-Body Connection

3. Subjective well-being includes all of the following components *except*
   a. psychological hardiness.
   b. satisfaction with present life.

c. relative presence of positive emotions.
d. relative absence of negative emotions.

LO 4 Strategies to Enhance Psychological Health

4. Which of the following is *not* part of a good strategy for building self-esteem?
   a. Develop a support system
   b. Concentrate more on mental health than physical health
   c. Make time for you
   d. Form realistic expectations

LO 5 Mental Illness on Campus

5. Which statement below is *false*?
   a. One in five adults in the United States suffers from a diagnosable mental disorder in a given year.
   b. Mental disorders are the leading cause of disability in the United States.
   c. Dysthymia is an example of an anxiety disorder.
   d. Bipolar disorder can also be referred to as manic depression.

LO 6 Mood Disorders

6. Every winter, Stan suffers from irritability, apathy, weight gain, and sadness. He most likely has
   a. seasonal depression.
   b. generalized anxiety disorder.
   c. seasonal affective disorder.
   d. chronic mood disorder

LO 7 Anxiety Disorders

7. Sarah has a compulsion to wash her hands over and over again and she's extremely fearful of dirt. She most likely has
   a. generalized anxiety disorder
   b. panic disorder
   c. obsessive-compulsive disorder
   d. dysthymic disorder

LO 8 Obsessive-Compulsive Disorders

8. This disorder is characterized by a need to perform rituals over and over again; fear of dirt or contamination; or an unnatural concern with order, symmetry, and exactness.
   a. Personality disorder
   b. Obsessive-compulsive disorder
   c. Phobic disorder
   d. Post-traumatic stress disorder

LO 9 Post-Traumatic Stress Disorder

9. How many Americans will experience post-traumatic stress disorder in their lifetime?
   a. 1%
   b. 8%
   c. 16%
   d. 32%

LO 10 Personality Disorders

10. This type of disorder is characterized by an exaggerated sense of self-importance and self-absorption.
    a. borderline personality disorder
    b. narcissistic personality disorder
    c. antisocial personality disorder
    d. paranoid personality disorder

LO 11 Schizophrenia

11. What percentage of the United States population has schizophrenia?
    a. 1 percent
    b. 5 percent
    c. 10 percent
    d. 20 percent

LO 12 Suicide

12. For 15- to 24-year-olds in the United States, suicide is the ____ leading cause of death.
    a. first
    b. second
    c. third
    d. fourth

LO 13 Seeking Professional Help

13. A person with a Ph.D. in counseling psychology and training in various types of therapy is a
    a. psychiatrist.
    b. psychologist.
    c. social worker.
    d. psychoanalyst.

Answers to the Pop Quiz can be found on page A-1. If you answered a question incorrectly, review the section identified by the Learning Outcome. For even more study tools, visit MasteringHealth.

THINK ABOUT IT!

LO 1 What Is Psychological Health?

1. What is psychological health? What indicates that you are or are not psychologically healthy? Why might the college environment provide a challenge to psychological health?

LO 2 Factors That Influence Psychological Health

2. Consider the factors that influence your overall level of psychological health. Which factors can you change? Which ones may be more difficult to change?

LO 3 The Mind-Body Connection

3. What connections can you make between physical and psychological health?

LO 4 Strategies to Enhance Psychological Health

4. Which psychological dimensions do you need to work on? Which are most important to you, and why? What actions can you take today?

LO 5 Mental Illness on Campus

5. What proportion of the student population suffers from some type of mental illness? What types of support network exist on your campus?

LO 6 Mood Disorders

6. What are the symptoms of major depression? How is major depression different from other mood disorders?

LO 7 Anxiety Disorders

7. What are the symptoms of an anxiety disorder? How is feeling anxious different from having an anxiety disorder or having a panic attack?

LO 8 Obsessive-Compulsive Disorders

8. How common is obsessive-compulsive disorder? How is having OCD different from being a perfectionist?

LO 9 Post-Traumatic Stress Disorders

9. What are the causes of post-traumatic stress disorder? Why do some go less reported than others?

LO 10 Personality Disorders

10. What are the characteristics of borderline personality disorder? How is it different from other personality disorders?

LO 11 Personality Disorders

11. How has our understanding of schizophrenia evolved? What is responsible for this shift in understanding? Why might it be difficult for people with schizophrenia to lead normal lives without support and other treatment?

LO 12 Suicide: Giving Up on Life

12. What are the warning signs of suicide? Why are some people more vulnerable to suicide than others? What could you do if you heard a classmate say to no one in particular that he was going to "do the world a favor and end it all"?

LO 13 Seeking Professional Help

13. Describe the various types of mental health professionals and types of therapies. If you felt depressed about breaking off a long-term relationship, which professional and which therapy do you think would be most beneficial to you?

ACCESS YOUR HEALTH ON THE INTERNET

Visit **MasteringHealth** for links to the websites and RSS feeds.

The following websites explore further topics related to psychological health.

American Foundation for Suicide Prevention. Provides resources for suicide prevention and support for family and friends of those who have committed suicide. Includes info on the National Suicide Prevention Hotline, 1-800-273-TALK (8255). www.afsp.org

American Psychological Association Help Center. Includes information on psychology at work, the mind body connection, understanding depression, psychological responses to war, and other topics. www.apa.org/helpcenter/wellness

National Alliance on Mental Illness. Support and advocacy organization of families and friends of people with severe mental illnesses. www.nami.org

National Institute of Mental Health (NIMH). Provides an overview of mental health information and new research. www.nimh.nih.gov

Helpguide. Resources for improving mental and emotional health as well as specific information on topics such as self-injury, sleep, depressive disorders, and anxiety disorders. www.helpguide.org

Active Minds. Campus education and advocacy organization formed to combat the stigma of mental illness, encourage students who need help to seek it early, and prevent tragedies related to untreated mental illness. www.activeminds.org

Jed Foundation. Works to promote emotional health and prevent suicide among college students. Provides information for parents, students, campus professionals, and friends. www.jedfoundation.org

FOCUS ON Cultivating Your Spiritual Health

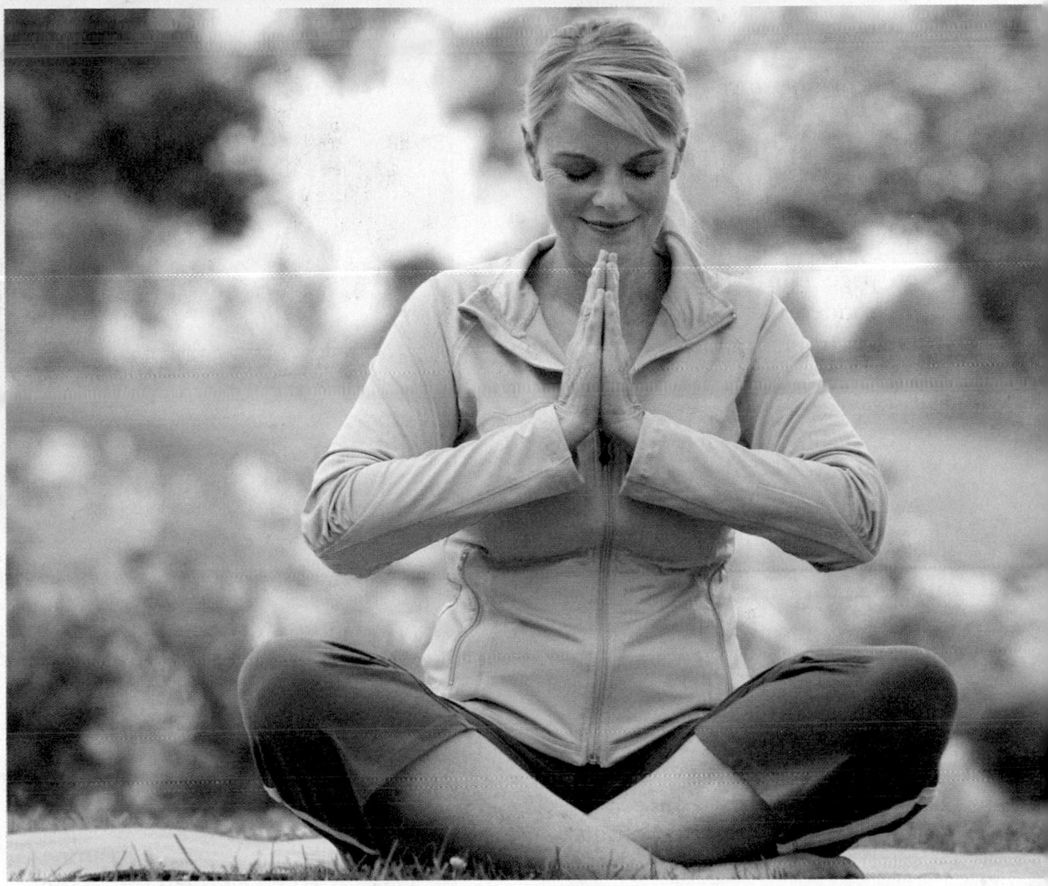

A secluded garden can be an ideal spot for quiet contemplation and spiritual renewal.

LEARNING OUTCOMES

1 Define spirituality, describe its three facets, and distinguish between religion and spirituality.
2 List and explain the accumulated evidence that spiritual health has physical benefits, has psychological benefits, and lowers stress.
3 Describe three ways you can develop your spiritual health.

Lia's favorite spot on campus is the secluded Japanese garden on the south side of the library. Whether she's feeling stressed about exams or is mulling over an important decision, a few minutes alone in the garden always seem to help. Sometimes she sits quietly and watches the birds come and go. Sometimes she gets out her camera and photographs particularly brilliant blossoms. Often she simply rests, eyes closed, feeling the sun's warmth on her face, and lets her thoughts turn to gratitude for her health, her loving family, and her opportunity to study. However she spends it, her "garden break" leaves Lia feeling refreshed and refocused, with greater confidence in her ability to tackle the challenges of her day.

Lia's desire to find a sense of purpose, meaning, and harmony in her life is shared by a majority of American college students. According to UCLA's Higher Education Research Institute (HERI), incoming undergraduate students have a wide spectrum of spiritual and ethical considerations.[1] More than 165,743 students at 243 colleges and universities were surveyed as they entered college in the fall of 2013. The data showed that, compared to their peers, 37.9 percent of incoming first-year students rated themselves above average in spirituality, 53 percent in emotional health, and 83.4 percent in being able to work with a diverse population.[2] Of the students surveyed, 88.5 percent also reported volunteering in

HEAR IT! PODCASTS

Want a study podcast for this chapter? Download the podcast **Psychological Health: Being Mentally, Emotionally, and Spiritually Well** available on MasteringHealth.™

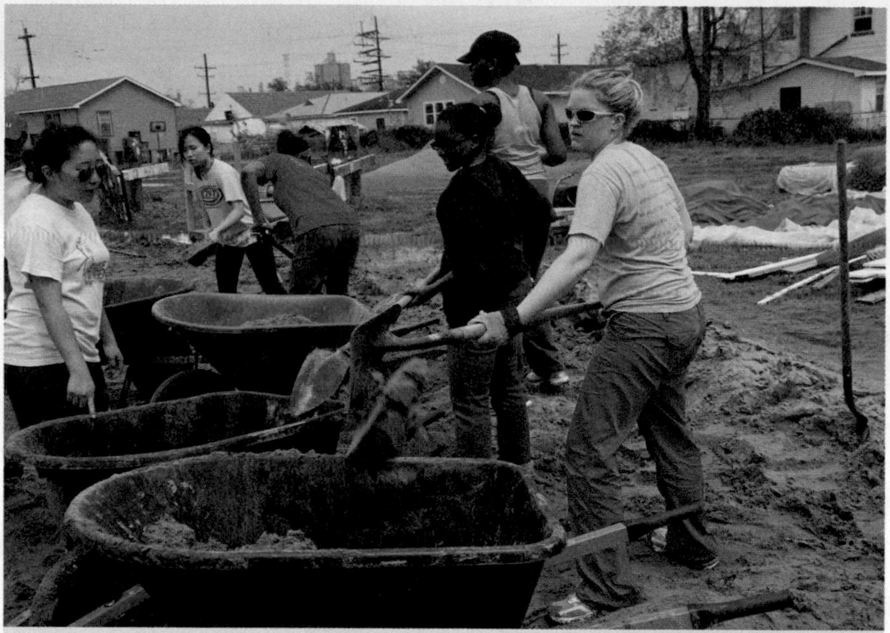

Spiritual and ethical concerns are important to most American college students. One of the ways students express their spirituality is by working to reduce suffering in the world; many contribute their time and skills to volunteer organizations, as these students are doing by working to build homes for Habitat for Humanity.

the past year, and 57.3 percent reported participating in community service as part of a class. Lastly, 80.5 percent of students reported high levels of being tolerant of diverse beliefs.[3]

Spiritual health is one of six key dimensions of health (see **Figure 1.4** on page 7 in **Chapter 1**). Lia's sense of wonder and respect for the natural world, her gratitude for the good things in her life, and her belief in a "universal spirit" suggest that spiritual health is an important focus of her daily life, bringing her greater awareness and serenity. If you're feeling as if you could use a little more of these qualities in your own life, read on: This chapter will help you explore ways to enhance your spiritual focus.

LO 1 | WHAT IS SPIRITUALITY?

Define spirituality, describe its three facets, and distinguish between religion and spirituality.

From one day to the next, many of us attempt to satisfy our needs for belonging and self-esteem by acquiring material possessions. At some point, many come to realize that new gadgets, clothes, or concert tickets don't necessarily bring happiness or improve our sense of self-worth. That's when many of us begin to contemplate another side of ourselves: our spirituality.

But what is spirituality? It isn't easy to define. Although part of the universal human experience, it's highly personal and involves feelings and senses that are often intangible. As such, it tends to defy the boundaries that strict definitions would impose. Let's begin by exploring its root, *spirit,* which in many cultures refers to *breath,* or the force that animates life. When you're "inspired," your energy flows. You're not held back by doubts about the purpose or meaning of your work and life. Indeed, many definitions of spirituality incorporate this sense of transcendence, focused on an internal experience. Harold G. Koenig, MD, one of the foremost researchers of spirituality and health, defines **spirituality** as the personal quest for understanding answers to ultimate questions about life, about meaning, and about our relationship with the sacred or transcendent.[4] The sacred or transcendent could be a higher power, or it could refer to our relationship with nature or forces we cannot explain.

spirituality An individual's sense of peace, purpose, and connection to others and beliefs about the meaning of life.

religion System of beliefs, practices, rituals, and symbols designed to facilitate closeness to the sacred or transcendent.

Religion and Spirituality Are Distinct Concepts

Spirituality may or may not lead to participation in organized **religion**, that is, a system of beliefs, practices, rituals, and symbols designed to facilitate closeness to the sacred or transcendent.[5] Although spirituality and religion share some common elements, they are not the same thing. Most individuals consider spirituality to be important in their lives, but not necessarily in the form of religion or through affiliation with a particular religion: A global survey revealed that 1 in 6 people worldwide (1.1 billion, or 16%) are religiously unaffiliated.[6] Even though they might not ascribe to a particular religion or faith, many people without religious affiliation still have certain religious or spiritual beliefs.[7] Thus, it's clear that religion does not have to be part of a spiritual

31.8% OF COLLEGE STUDENTS IDENTIFY THEIR **WORLDVIEW** AS RELIGIOUS, 32.4% AS SPIRITUAL, AND 28.2% AS SECULAR (NON-RELIGIOUS).

TABLE 1 | Characteristics Distinguishing Religion and Spirituality

Religion	Spirituality
Observable, measurable, objective	Less measurable, more subjective
Formal, orthodox, organized	Less formal, less orthodox, less systematic
Behavior-oriented, outward practices	Emotionally oriented, inwardly directed
Authoritarian in terms of behaviors	Not authoritarian, little accountability
Doctrine separating good from evil	Unifying, not doctrine oriented

Source: National Center for Complementary and Alternative Medicine (NCCAM), "Prayer and Spirituality in Health: Ancient Practices, Modern Science," *CAM at the NIH* 12 no. 1 (2005): 1–4.

values Principles that influence our thoughts and emotions and guide the choices we make in our lives.

spiritual intelligence (SI) The ability to access higher meanings, values, abiding purposes, and unconscious aspects of the self, a characteristic that helps us find a moral and ethical path to guide us through life.

person's life. **TABLE 1** identifies some characteristics that can help you distinguish religion and spirituality.

Spirituality Integrates Three Facets

Brian Luke Seaward, a professor at the University of Northern Colorado and author of several books on spirituality and mind-body healing, identifies three facets of human existence that together constitute the core of human spirituality: relationships, values, and purpose in life (**FIGURE 1**).[8] Questions arising in these three domains prompt many of us to look for spiritual answers. At the same time, spiritual well-being is characterized by healthy relationships, strong personal values, and a sense that we have a meaningful purpose in life.

Relationships

Have you ever wondered if someone you were attracted to is really right for you? Or, conversely, wondered if you should break off a long-term relationship? Have you ever wished you had more friends, or that you were a better friend to yourself? For many people, such questions and yearnings are natural triggers for spiritual growth: As we contemplate who we should choose as a life partner or how to mend a quarrel with a friend, we begin to foster our own inner wisdom. At the same time, healthy relationships are a sign of spiritual well-being. When we treat ourselves and others with respect, honesty, integrity, and love, we are manifesting our spiritual health.

Values

Our personal **values** are our principles—not only the things we say we care about, but also the things that cause us to behave the way we do. For instance, if you value honesty, then you are not likely to call in sick for work when you intend to spend the day at the beach. In other words, our value system is the set of fundamental rules by which we conduct our lives. It's what we stand for. When we attempt to clarify our values, and then to live according to those values, we're engaging in spiritual work. Spiritual health is characterized by a strong personal value system.

Meaningful Purpose in Life

What career do you plan to pursue? Do you hope to marry? Do you plan to have or adopt children? What things will make you feel happy and "complete"? How do these choices reflect what you hold as your purpose in life? At the end of your days, what would you want people to say about how you've lived your life and what your life has meant to others? Contemplating these questions fosters spiritual growth. People who are spiritually healthy are able to articulate their purpose and to make choices that manifest that purpose. In thinking about your own purpose, avoid the temptation to get too ambitious, as in, "I'm here to eradicate world hunger!" Instead, try to articulate what you see as your unique contribution to the world—something you can actually do, starting now.

Spiritual Intelligence Is an Inner Wisdom

Our relationships, values, and sense of purpose together contribute to our overall **spiritual intelligence (SI)**. This term was introduced by physicist and philosopher Danah Zohar, who defined it as "an ability to access higher meanings, values, abiding purposes, and unconscious aspects of the self."[9] Zohar includes qualities such as the ability to think outside the box, humility, and an access to energies that come from a source

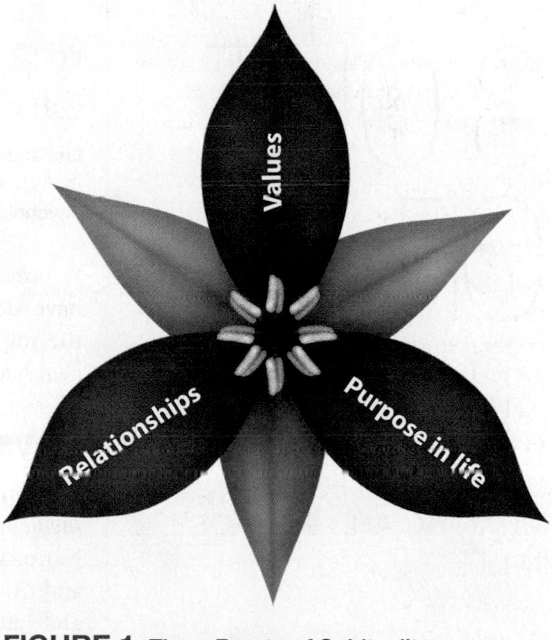

FIGURE 1 Three Facets of Spirituality
Most of us are prompted to explore our spirituality because of questions relating to our relationships, values, and purpose in life. At the same time, these three facets together constitute spiritual well-being.

VIDEO TUTOR
Facets of Spirituality

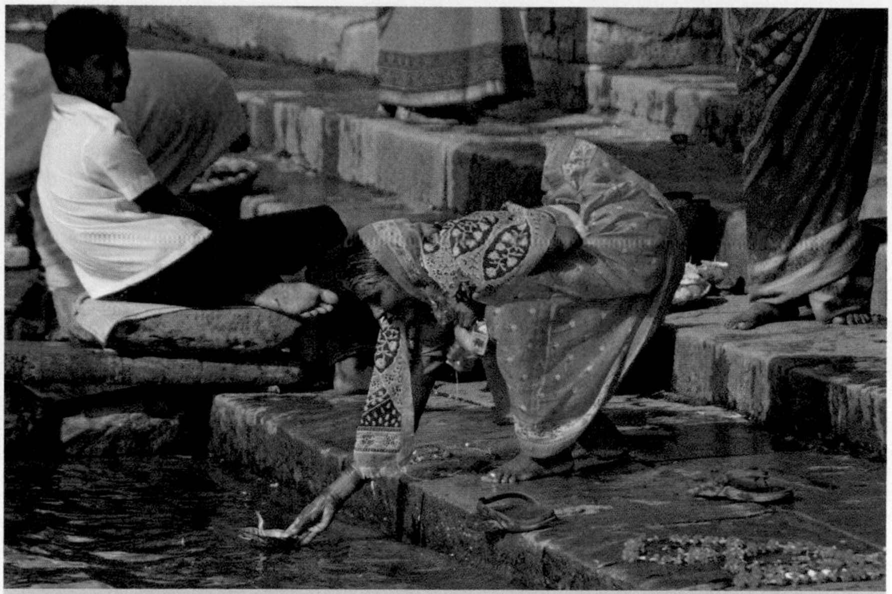

Spirituality and religion are not the same. Many people find that religious practices, for example, attending services or making offerings—such as the flowers these Hindus are preparing to place in the sacred Ganges River—help them to focus on their spirituality. However, religion does not have to be part of a spiritual person's life.

beyond the ego in her definition of *spiritual intelligence*, explaining that SI helps us use meanings, values, and purposes to live richer and more creative lives.

3 OUT OF 4

FIRST-YEAR COLLEGE STUDENTS REPORT THAT THEY ARE ACTIVELY "SEARCHING FOR **MEANING** AND **PURPOSE** IN LIFE."

Since Zohar's introduction of SI, dozens of clerics, psychologists, and even business consultants have expanded on the definition. For example, spiritual intelligence expert Cindy Wigglesworth explains that SI helps us find compassion and wisdom to help guide us through life.[10] SI also helps us maintain our peaceful center. Would you like to find out your own spiritual IQ? See the Assess Yourself activity in Mastering-Health.

LO 2 | THE BENEFITS OF SPIRITUAL HEALTH

List and explain the accumulated evidence that spiritual health has physical benefits, has psychological benefits, and lowers stress.

A broad range of large-scale surveys have documented the importance of the mind-body connection to human health and wellness.[11]

Physical Benefits

The emerging science of *mind-body medicine* is a research focus of the National Center for Complementary and Alternative Medicine (NCCAM) and an important objective of the organization's 2011–2015 Strategic Plan. One area under study is the association between spiritual health and general health. The NCCAM cites evidence that spirituality can have a positive influence on health and suggests that the connection may be due to improved immune function, cardiovascular function, or a combination of physiological changes.[12] Increasing numbers of studies are examining the role that certain spiritual practices, such as yoga, deep meditation, and prayer, have on the mind, body, and behavior and how these practices may improve health and promote healthy behaviors.[13]

Some researchers believe that a key to understanding the improved health and longer life of spiritually healthy people is mindfulness training. In a recent study, participants who practiced mindfulness meditation showed notable changes in regions of the brain associated with stress and memory. These changes indicate that they may be more likely to cope better with stress on a daily basis.[14]

Other research has shown positive results in the use of mindfulness to reduce smoking behavior[15] and in controlling binge eating and obesity.[16]

The National Cancer Institute (NCI) contends that when we get sick, spiritual or religious well-being may help restore health and improve quality of life as follows:

- Decreasing anxiety, depression, anger, discomfort, and feelings of isolation
- Decreasing alcohol and drug abuse
- Decreasing blood pressure and the risk of heart disease
- Increasing the person's ability to cope with the effects of illness and with medical treatments
- Increasing feelings of hope and optimism, freedom from regret, satisfaction with life, and inner peace[17]

Several studies show an association between spiritual health and a person's ability to cope with a variety of physical illnesses, including cancer.[18] For example, a study of cardiac patients showed a benefit related to spiritual health and mind-body techniques.[19] Researchers have also looked into the overall association between spiritual practices and mortality, and a review of over a decade of research studies indicated that individuals who incorporate spiritual practices regularly have a significant reduction in mortality and risk of cardiovascular events.[20]

Psychological Benefits

Current research also suggests that spiritual health contributes to psychological health. For instance, the NCI and independent studies have found that spirituality reduces levels of anxiety and depression.[21]

People who have found a spiritual community also benefit from increased social support. For instance, participation in religious services, charitable organizations, and social gatherings can help members avoid isolation. At such gatherings, clerics and others may offer spiritual support in regard to challenges that members may be facing. A community may include retired members who offer child care for working parents, meals for those with disabilities, or transportation to medical appointments. All such measures can contribute to members' overall feelings of security and belonging.

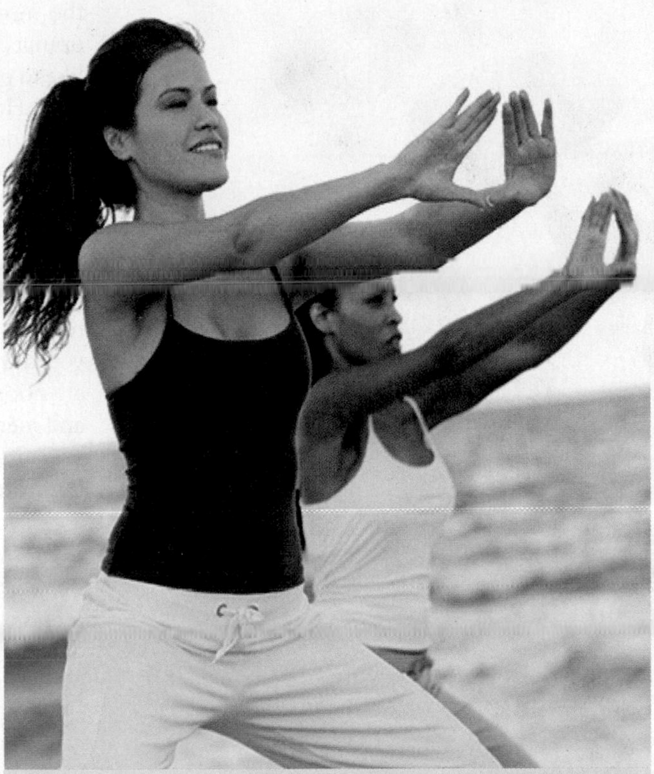

Spirituality is widely acknowledged to have a positive impact on health and wellness, from reductions in overall morbidity and mortality to improved abilities to cope with illness and stress. These students are using the movement techniques of tai chi to improve their spiritual health.

Stress Reduction Benefits

The NCI cites stress reduction as one probable mechanism among spiritually healthy people for improved health and longevity and for better coping with illness.[22] In addition, several small studies support the contention that positive religious practices aid effective stress management.[23] Studies also suggest that increasing mindfulness through meditation reduces stress levels not only in people with physical and mental disorders, but in healthy people as well.[24]

LO 3 | WHAT CAN YOU DO TO FOCUS ON YOUR SPIRITUAL HEALTH?

Describe three ways you can develop your spiritual health.

Cultivating your spiritual side takes just as much work as becoming physically fit or improving your diet. Ways to develop your spiritual health include tuning in, training your body, expanding your mind, and reaching out.

Tune in to Yourself and Your Surroundings

Focusing on your spiritual health has been likened to tuning in on a radio: Inner wisdom is perpetually available to us, but if we fail to tune our "receiver," we won't be able to hear it through all the "static" of daily life. Fortunately, four ancient practices still in use today can help you tune in. These are *contemplation* (studying), *mindfulness* (observing), *meditation* (quieting), and *prayer* (communing with the Divine).

Contemplation

In a dictionary, the word *contemplation* means a study of something—whether a candle flame or a theory of quantum mechanics. In the domain of spirituality, **contemplation** refers to concentrating the mind on a spiritual or ethical question or subject, a view of the natural world, or an icon or other image representative of divinity. For instance, a Zen Buddhist might contemplate a riddle, called a *koan,* such as "What is the sound of one hand clapping?" A Sufi might contemplate the 99 names of God. A Roman Catholic might contemplate an image of the Virgin Mary. Spiritual people with no religious affiliation might contemplate the natural world, a favorite poem, or an ethical question such as "What is the origin of evil?" Most religious and spiritual traditions advocate engaging in the contemplation of gratitude, forgiveness, and unconditional love.

When practicing contemplation, it can be helpful to keep a journal to record any insights that arise, and journaling itself can be a form of contemplation. For example, you might want to make a list of 20 things in your life you are grateful for or write a poem of forgiveness for yourself or a loved one. You might also use your journal to record inspirational quotations that you encounter in your readings. Journaling can fill a larger role in spiritual health and development by providing a sense of overall calmness.

contemplation Practice of concentrating the mind on a spiritual or ethical question or subject, a view of the natural world, or an icon or other image representative of divinity.

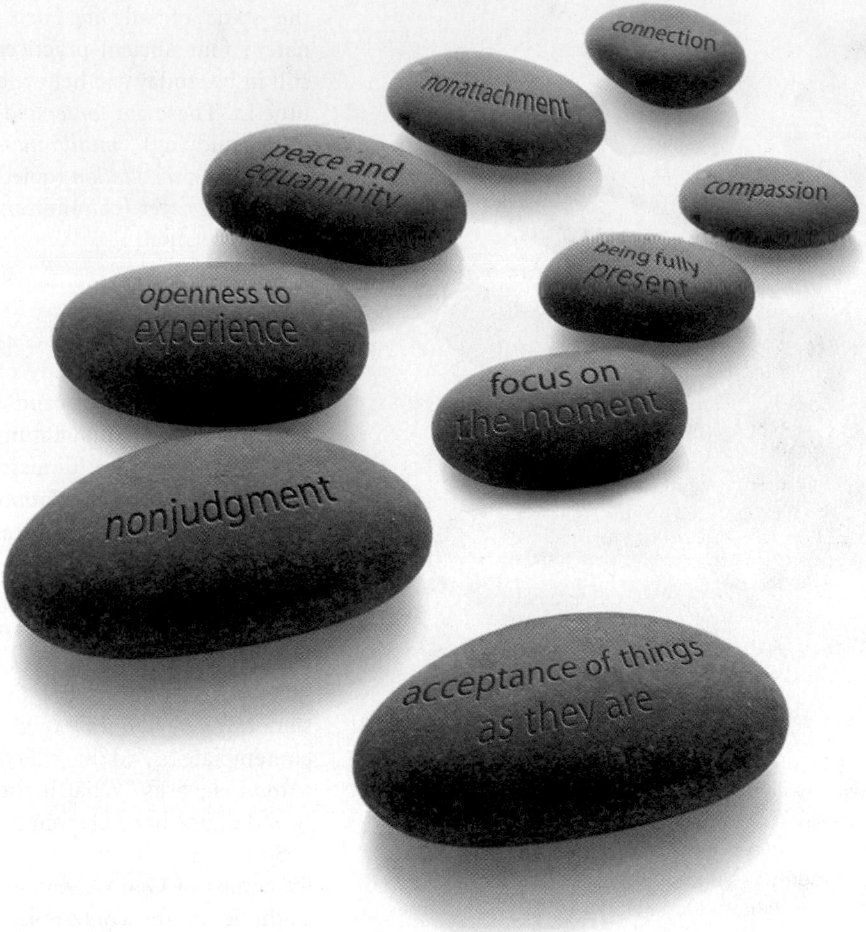

FIGURE 2 Qualities of Mindfulness

Source: M. Greenberg, "Nine Essential Qualities of Mindfulness," *Psychology Today*, February 22, 2012, www.psychologytoday.com/blog/the-mindful-self-express/201202/nine-essential-qualities-mindfulness.

Mindfulness

A practice of focused, nonjudgmental observation, **mindfulness** is the ability to be fully present in the moment (**FIGURE 2**). If you have ever been immersed in a moment, experiencing it completely with all your senses, this is mindfulness. You could be watching a sunset, listening to a great pianist, or even perfecting your golf swing. In any case, mindfulness is an awareness of present-moment reality—a holistic sensation of being totally involved in the moment rather than focused on some worry or being on "autopilot."[25]

So how do you practice mindfulness? The range of opportunities is as infinite as the moments of our lives. Living mindfully means allowing ourselves to become more deeply and completely aware of what we are sensing in each moment.[26] For instance, the next time you are going to eat an orange, pay attention! What does it feel like to pierce the skin with your thumbnail? How does it smell as you peel it? What does the rind really look like? Do the drops of juice splatter as you pull apart the segments? What does it taste like, and how does the taste change from the first bite to the last?

Pursuing almost any endeavor that requires close concentration can help you develop mindfulness. Think of the attention required to perform physical and mental challenges, such as the focus used by a competitive diver in leaping from the board, or the precision of a surgeon attempting a difficult operation. Or consider the close concentration needed for creative and performing arts such as sculpting, painting, writing, dancing, or playing a musical instrument. Even household activities such as cooking or cleaning can foster mindfulness—as long as you pay attention while you do them!

In this era of global environmental concerns, we can also cultivate mindfulness by paying attention to how our choices affect our world. Now, this doesn't just mean recycling soda cans and taking the subway instead of driving. Mindfulness of our environment calls on us to examine our values and behaviors as we share our Earth with the global population of humans, plants, animals and all living creatures every moment of each day. It includes having a shared sense of responsibility for improving the world for future generations. See the

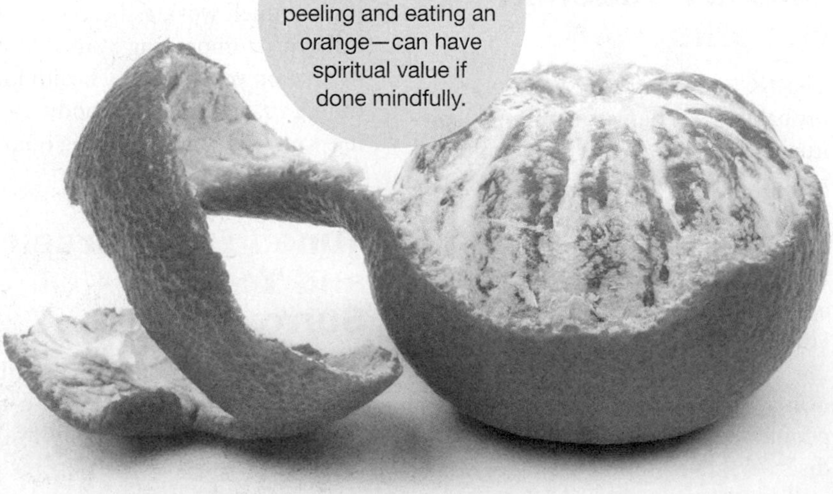

Even the most mundane activities—such as peeling and eating an orange—can have spiritual value if done mindfully.

mindfulness Practice of purposeful, nonjudgmental observation in which we are fully present in the moment.

@ HEALTH HEADLINES

DEVELOPING ENVIRONMENTAL MINDFULNESS

We know that the Earth's oil reserves won't last forever, yet in 2013 many U.S. automakers saw a continued increase in sales of large pickups and SUVs. General Motors reported their sales of pickups increased 15 percent and SUVs 29 percent. Chrysler and Ford Motor Company also reported significant increases in their heavy-duty pickups and large SUVs. We know that beef production releases gobs of greenhouse gases, yet Americans consume nearly 26 billion pounds of beef annually. Why do we make such choices? We want to "go green," so what's in our way?

If the environmental movement seems to be running out of steam, many activists say that it's due to an overemphasis on our external choices, whereas the real challenge is to change our state of mind. They argue that until we confront the mental habits and identities that fuel our consumption patterns, meaningful change won't happen. In short, they advocate mindfulness.

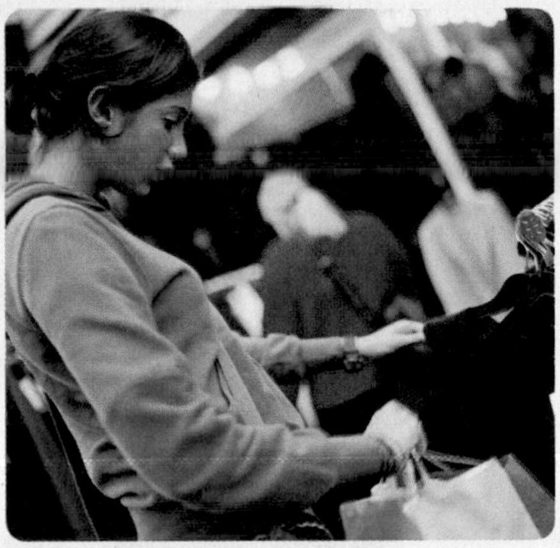

To be mindfully green requires us to ask ourselves some tough questions, such as What is my fair share? and How much do I really need?

When we pay attention to our thoughts as we make choices, we might notice guilt, insecurity, disparagement of ourselves or others, or even righteous claims to entitlement. Only by becoming aware of these "inner demons" can we begin to take action to expel them. So how do we cultivate environmental mindfulness? Environmentalist Stephanie Kaza explains that mindfulness requires us to stay present with our actions moment by moment, always asking, "What is the kind thing to do now?"

Sources: J. R. Healey, C. Woodyard, and F. Meier, "Detroit's August Sales Lead the Way, Pickups and SUVs Lead the Way," *USAToday*, September 4, 2013, www.usatoday.com/story/money/cars/2013/09/04/general-motors-gm-ford-chrysler-detroit-sales-august/2700795/; U.S. Department of Agriculture, Economics Research Service, "Statistics and Information," October 31, 2013, www.ers.usda.gov/topics/animal-products/cattle-beef/statistics-information.aspx; E. Nichtern, *Exploring the Internal Landscape of Consumption*, 2008 (Stockbridge, MA: Kripalu Center); S. Kaza, *Mindfully Green* (Boston, MA: Shambhala Publications, 2008).

Health Headlines box for more information about developing environmental mindfulness.

Meditation

Meditation is a practice of cultivating a still or quiet mind (you'll read more on meditation in **Chapter 3**). Although the precise details vary with different schools of meditation, the fundamental task is the same: to quiet the mind's noise (referred to as "chatter," "static," or "monkey mind").

Why would you want to cultivate stillness? For thousands of years, human beings of different cultures and traditions have found that achieving periods of meditative stillness each day enhances their spiritual health. Today, researchers are beginning to discover why. The NCCAM reports that researchers using brain-scanning techniques found experienced meditators to show a significantly increased level of *empathy*—the ability to understand and share another person's experience.[27] Similar research has shown that participants who practiced a specific form of meditation, known as *compassion-meditation*, further increased their levels of compassion toward others.[28] Studies also suggest that meditation improves the brain's ability to process information; reduces stress, anxiety, and depression; improves concentration; and decreases blood pressure.[29] The physiological processes that produce these effects are only partially understood. One theory suggests meditation works by reducing the body's stress response. By practicing deep, calm contemplation, people who meditate seem to promote activity in the body's systems, leading to slower breathing, lower blood pressure, and easier digestion, along with the spiritual benefits.[30]

So how do you meditate? Detailed instructions are beyond the scope of this text, but most teachers suggest beginning by sitting in a quiet place with low lighting where you won't be interrupted. Many advocate assuming a "full lotus" position, with legs bent fully at the knees, each ankle over the opposite knee. However, this position can be painful for beginners and those with poor flexibility or joint pain. Thus, you may want to assume a modified lotus position, with your legs simply crossed in front of you. Lying down is not recommended because you may fall asleep. Rest your hands on your knees, palms upward. Beginners usually find it easier to meditate with the eyes closed.

Once you're in position, it's time to start emptying your mind. The various schools of meditation teach different methods to achieve this.

WHY SHOULD I CARE?

Practicing meditation can improve concentration and your brain's ability to process information; it can also reduce stress, anxiety, and depression, all important factors when trying to manage your classes and handle daily demands.

- **Mantra meditation.** Focus on a *mantra,* a single word such as *Om, Amen, Love,* or *God,* and repeat this word silently. When a distracting thought arises, simply set it aside. It may help to imagine the thought as a leaf, and visualize placing it on a gently flowing stream that carries it away. Do not fault yourself for becoming distracted. Simply notice the thought, release it, and return to your mantra.
- **Breath meditation.** Count each breath: Pay attention to each inhalation, the brief pause that follows, and the exhalation. Together, these equal one breath. When you have counted ten breaths, return to one. As with mantra meditation, release distractions as they arise, and return to following the breath.

prayer Communication with a transcendent Presence.

yoga System of physical and mental training involving controlled breathing, physical postures (*asanas*), meditation, chanting, and other practices believed to cultivate unity with the *Atman,* or spiritual life principle of the universe

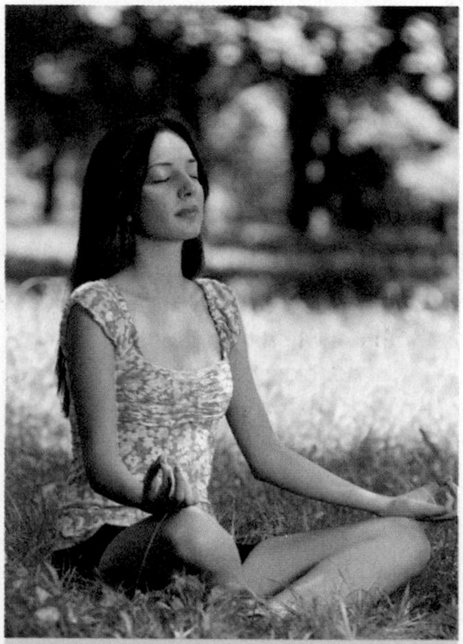

Professor Adam Burke, Director of San Francisco State's Institute for Holistic Health Studies, says that the key to sticking with meditation is choosing a technique that you like. He points out that there are a variety of different meditation techniques. It is important to try them and not settle for the most popular type, but rather to pick the one that works best for you.

DID YOU **KNOW?**

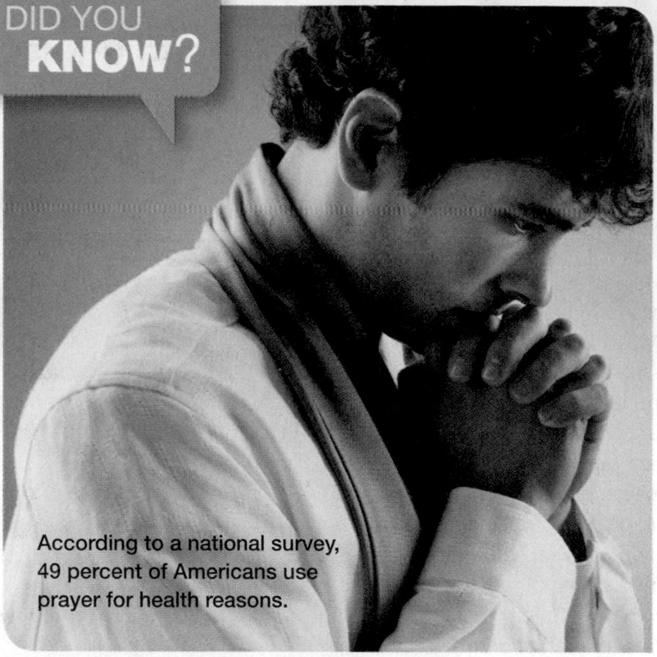

According to a national survey, 49 percent of Americans use prayer for health reasons.

Source: A. Wachholtz and U. Sambamoorthi, "National Trends in Prayer Use as a Coping Mechanism for Health Concerns: Changes from 2002 to 2007," *Psychology of Religion and Spirituality* 3, no. 2 (2011): 67, DOI 10.1037/a0021598.

- **Color meditation.** When your eyes are closed, you may perceive a field of color, such as a deep, restful blue. Focus on this color. Treat distractions as in other forms of meditation.
- **Candle meditation.** With your eyes open, focus on the flame of a candle. Allow your eyes to soften as you meditate on this object. Treat distractions as in the other forms of meditation.

After several minutes of meditation, and with practice, you may come to experience a sensation sometimes described as "dropping down," in which you feel yourself release into the meditation. In this state, which can be likened to a wakeful sleep, distracting thoughts are far less likely to arise, and yet you may receive surprising insights.

Initially, try meditating for just 10 to 20 minutes, once or twice a day. In time, you can increase your sessions to 30 minutes or more. As you meditate for longer periods, you will likely find yourself feeling more rested and less stressed, and you may begin to experience the increased levels of empathy recorded among expert meditators.

Prayer

In **prayer**, an individual focuses the mind in communication with a transcendent Presence. Spiritual traditions throughout the world distinguish several forms that this communication can take. For many, prayer offers a sense of comfort, a sense that we are not alone. It can be the means of expressing concern for others, for admission of transgressions, for seeking forgiveness, and for renewing hope and purpose. Focusing on the things we are grateful for can move people to look to the future with hope and give them the strength to get through the most challenging times. Research has shown that spiritual wellbeing, including the use of prayer, can increase the ability to cope and decrease stress.[31]

Train Your Body

For thousands of years, in regions throughout the world, spiritual seekers have cultivated transcendence through physical means. One of the foremost examples is the practice of various forms of **yoga**. Although in the West we think of yoga as involving controlled breathing and physical postures, traditional forms also emphasize meditation, chanting, and other practices that are believed to cultivate unity with the *Atman,* or spiritual life principle of the universe.

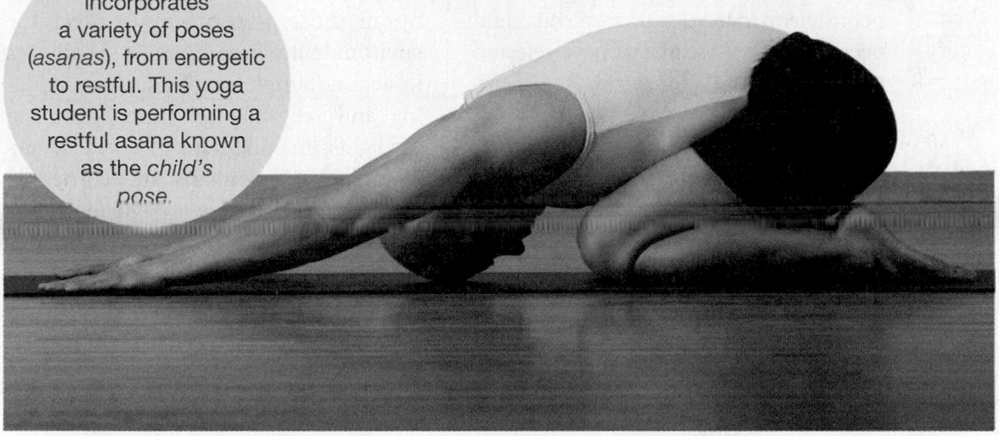

Yoga incorporates a variety of poses (*asanas*), from energetic to restful. This yoga student is performing a restful asana known as the *child's pose*.

20.4 MILLION

U.S. ADULTS PRACTICE **YOGA**, ACCORDING TO A RECENT SURVEY BY *YOGA JOURNAL*.

If you are interested in exploring yoga, sign up for a class on campus, at your local YMCA, or at a yoga center. Choose a form that seems right to you: Some, such as *hatha yoga,* focus on developing flexibility, deep breathing, and tranquility, whereas others, such as *ashtanga yoga,* are fast-paced and demanding and thus more focused on developing physical fitness than spiritual health. (See **Chapter 3** and **Chapter 9** for more on various styles of yoga.) For your first class, dress comfortably in fabrics that are somewhat close-fitting, but also allow movement. Be able to bend at the waist or lift your leg without feeling constricted or exposed. No shoes or socks are worn. Some facilities provide yoga mats, or you may need to bring your own. The instructor will likely begin the class with a series of gentle warm-up poses (*asanas*) and then add more challenging poses with coordinated breathing to align, stretch, and invigorate each body region. Classes usually conclude with several minutes of relaxation and deep breathing.

Training your body to improve your spiritual health doesn't necessarily require you to engage in a formal practice such as yoga. By energizing your body and sharpening your mental focus, jogging, biking, aerobics, dance, or any other exercise you do regularly can contribute to your spiritual health. The Eastern meditative movement practices of tai chi or qigong can also increase physical activity and mental focus. Both have been shown to have beneficial effects on bone health, stress, cardiopulmonary fitness, mood, balance, and quality of life.[32] To transform exercise into a spiritual workout, begin by acknowledging gratitude for your body and its abilities, and throughout the session, maintain mindfulness of your breathing. (We'll say more about mindful breathing later in the discussion on meditation.)

You can also cultivate spirituality through fully engaging your body's senses. In fact, you can think of vision, hearing, taste, smell, and touch as five portals to spiritual health. Viewing an engaging piece of art or listening to beautiful music can calm the mind and soothe the spirit. A key reason that Lia, in our opening story, finds sustenance in nature is because she fully engages her senses—smelling freshly cut grass, listening to the birds, and photographing the flowers.

The flip side of cultivating your senses is depriving them! Closing your eyes and sitting in silence removes the distraction of visual and auditory stimuli, helping you to focus within. To take advantage of silence, turn off your cell phone and take a long, solitary walk. You might even spend a weekend at one of the many retreat centers throughout the United States. To find one, see the listings at www.SpiritSite.com.

WHAT DO YOU THINK?

Why do you think mindfulness practices are gaining more recognition?

- What are the benefits of mindfulness?
- In today's fast-paced, multitasking world, do you think it is challenging to practice mindfulness on a regular basis?

Expand Your Mind

For many people, psychological counseling is a first step toward improving their spiritual health. Therapy helps you let go of past hurts, accept your limitations, manage stress and anger, reduce anxiety and depression, and take control of your life—all steps toward spiritual growth. If you've never engaged in therapy, making the first appointment can feel daunting. Your campus health department can usually help by providing a referral.

Another practical way to expand your mind is to study the sacred texts of the world's major religions and spiritual practices. Many find guidance in the writings of great spiritual teachers. Libraries and bookstores are filled with volumes that explore the diverse approaches humans take to achieving spiritual fulfillment.

Finally, you can expand your awareness of different spiritual practices by exploring on-campus meditation or service-oriented groups, taking classes in spiritual or religious subjects, attending religious meetings or services, attending public lectures, and checking out the websites of various spiritual and religious organizations. In each case, you can evaluate the messages and ideas you encounter and decide which practices or beliefs hold meaning for you.

altruism Giving of oneself out of genuine concern for others.

environmental stewardship Responsibility for environmental quality shared by all those whose actions affect the environment.

Reach Out to Others

Altruism, the giving of oneself out of genuine concern for others, is a key aspect of a spiritually healthy lifestyle. Volunteering to help others, working for a nonprofit organization, donating money or other resources to a food bank or other program—even spending an afternoon picking up litter in your neighborhood—are all ways to serve others and simultaneously enhance your own spiritual and overall health. Researchers have referred to the benefits of volunteering as a "helpers high," or a distinct physical sensation associated with helping. About half of participants in one study reported that they feel stronger and more energetic after helping others; many also reported feeling calmer and less depressed, with increased feelings of self-worth.[33]

Community service can also take the form of **environmental stewardship**, which the Environmental Protection Agency (EPA) defines as the responsibility for environmental quality shared by all those whose actions affect the environment. Responsibility manifests in action. Simple actions such as reducing and recycling packaging, turn-ing off lights, making sure the heat or air-conditioning maintains an ecofriendly temperature, using energy-efficient lightbulbs and appliances, and taking shorter showers can make a difference.

For more strategies to enhance your spiritual health by reaching out to others, refer to the **Skills for Behavior Change** box.

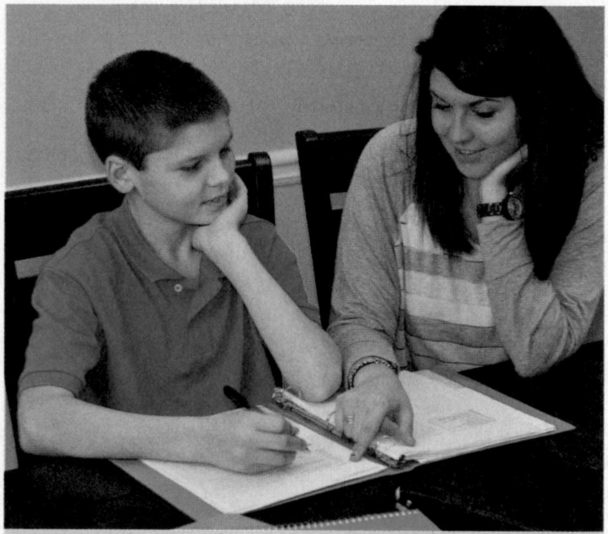

Volunteering can be a fun and fulfilling way to broaden your experience, connect with your community, and focus on your spiritual health.

SKILLS FOR BEHAVIOR CHANGE

FINDING YOUR SPIRITUAL SIDE THROUGH SERVICE

Recognizing that we are all part of a greater system with responsibilities to and for others is a key part of spiritual growth. Volunteering your time and energy is a great way to connect with others and help make the world a better place while improving your own health. Here are a few ideas:

- Offer to help elderly neighbors with lawn care or simple household repairs.
- Volunteer with Meals on Wheels, a local soup kitchen, a food bank, or another program that helps people obtain adequate food.
- Organize or participate in an after-school or summertime activity for neighborhood children.
- Participate in a highway, beach, or neighborhood cleanup; restoration of park trails and waterways; or other environmental preservation projects.
- Volunteer at the local humane society.
- Apply to become a Big Brother or Big Sister and mentor a child who may face significant challenges or have poor role models.
- Join an organization working on a cause such as global warming or hunger, or start one yourself. Check out these inspiring examples: Students Against Global Apathy (SAGA), Students for the Environment (S4E), The National Student Campaign Against Hunger and Homelessness.
- Volunteer in a neighborhood challenged by poverty, low literacy levels, or a natural disaster. Or volunteer with an organization such as Habitat for Humanity to build homes or provide other aid to developing communities.

To find out more information on service, the following are some online resources:

Ties community service to learning for K–12 through college: www.servicelearning.org

Locates service opportunities: www.volunteermatch.org

Lists overseas volunteer opportunities: www.projects-abroad.org

Oriented toward students: www.dosomething.org

Competition for money for service projects: www.truehero.org

ASSESS **YOURSELF**

Are you a spiritual person? Want to find out? Take the **What's Your Spiritual IQ?** assessment available on MasteringHealth.™

Need help creating a plan? Follow the strategies in the **Your Plan for Change** box for short- and long-term improvements to your health.

YOUR PLAN FOR **CHANGE**

The **ASSESS YOURSELF** activity gives you the chance to evaluate your spiritual intelligence, and the text introduced you to some practices used successfully by millions over many generations to enhance their spiritual health. If you are interested in further cultivating your spirituality, consider some of the small but significant steps listed below.

TODAY, YOU CAN:

- ☐ Find a quiet spot, turn off your cell phone, close your eyes, and contemplate, meditate, or pray for 10 minutes. Or spend 10 minutes in quiet mindfulness of your surroundings.
- ☐ In a journal or on your computer, compose a list of at least ten things you are grateful for. Include people, pets, talents and abilities, achievements, places, foods . . . whatever comes to mind!

WITHIN THE NEXT 2 WEEKS, YOU CAN:

- ☐ Explore the options on campus for beginning psychotherapy, joining a spiritual or religious group, or volunteering with an organization working for positive change.
- ☐ Think of a person in your life with whom you have experienced conflict. Spend a few minutes contemplating forgiveness toward this person and then write a letter or e-mail apologizing for any offense and offering your forgiveness in return. Wait a day or two before deciding whether you are truly ready to send the message.

BY THE END OF THE SEMESTER, YOU CAN:

- ☐ Develop a list of several spiritual texts you would like to read during your break.
- ☐ Begin exploring options for volunteer work that would serve others and have meaning for you.

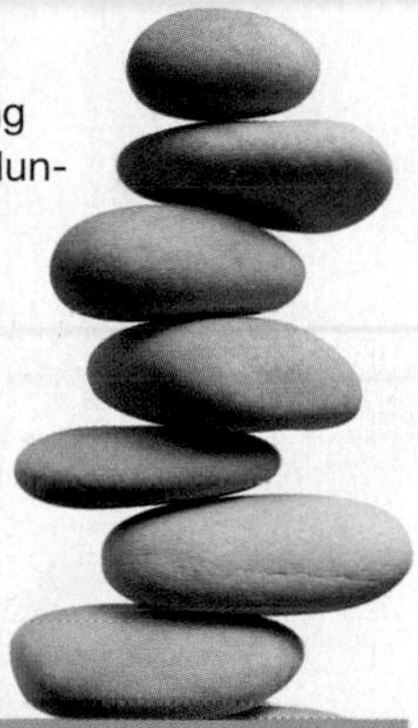

3 Managing Stress and Coping with Life's Challenges

LEARNING OUTCOMES

1 Define stress and examine its potential impact on health, relationships, and success in college.

2 Explain the phases of the general adaptation syndrome and the physiological changes that occur during them.

3 Examine the physical health risks that may occur with chronic stress.

4 Examine the intellectual and psychological effects of stress and their impacts on college students.

5 Discuss sources of stress and examine the unique stressors that affect college students.

6 Explore stress-management techniques and ways to enrich your life with positive experiences and attitudes.

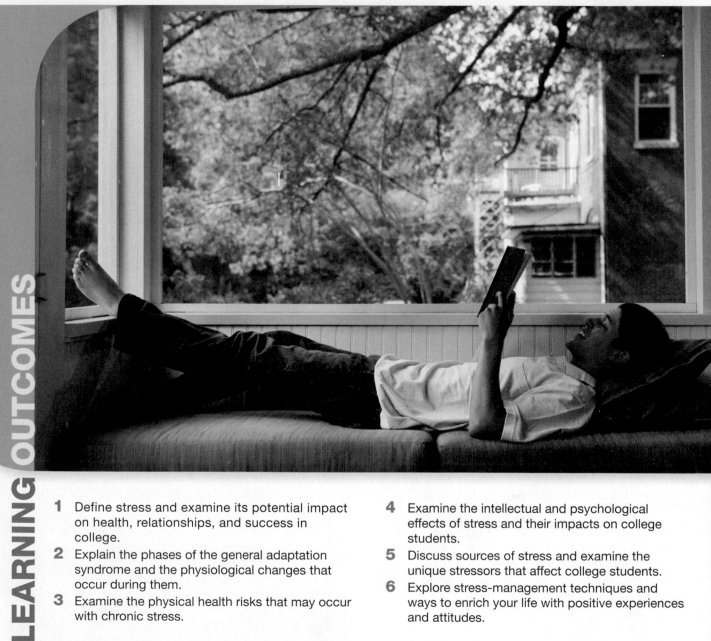

Skyrocketing tuition, roommates who bug you, dating anxiety, pressure about grades, finances, and worries about getting a job after graduation—they all lead up to STRESS! In today's fast-paced, 24/7 connected world, stress can be overwhelming. It can also bring excitement, push us to improve performance, and help us thrive. While we work, play, socialize, and sleep, stress affects us in myriad ways—some we may not even notice.

Chronic stress is stress that inhibits normal functioning for a length of time, and it is growing to be a public health crisis. According to a recent American Psychological Association poll, the health care system is not giving Americans the support they need to cope with stress and build healthy lifestyles. Key findings from the study indicate the following:[1]

- Although reported stress levels are down slightly in the last 5 years, Americans consistently report high stress levels (20% report extreme stress).
- Adults ages 18–46 report the highest levels of stress and the greatest increases in stress levels.
- The biggest sources of stress for adults ages 18–33 are work, money, and job stability. Individuals aged 67 and older are more likely to cite personal health concerns as a key source of stress.

While key sources of stress are similar for men and women (money, work, the economy), huge gender differences exist in how people experience, report, and cope with stress. Both men and women report above average levels of stress, but women are more likely to report stress levels that are on the rise and more extreme than those of their male counterparts. Additionally, although men may recognize and report stress, they are much less likely to take action to reduce it.[2]

The exact toll stress exerts on us during a lifetime of overload is unknown, but we know stress affects virtually every system of the body, causing problems for us at work, in the home, and in our interactions with others. Being "stressed out" can take a major toll on even the youngest among us, with some youth suffering from stress-related headaches, stomachaches, and difficulty sleeping. Stress seems to be a particular threat to youth who are overweight. Stress-related eating, lack of exercise, parental influences, and social stigma contribute to youth weight gain and higher levels of stress.[3]

39%

OF MILLENNIALS (AGES 18–33) SAY THEIR **STRESS** LEVELS HAVE INCREASED IN THE LAST YEAR, WITH 52% SAYING THEIR STRESS LEVELS KEEP THEM AWAKE AT NIGHT.

Is too much stress inevitably negative? Fortunately, the answer is no. How we react to real and perceived threats often is key to whether stressors are enabling or debilitating. Learning to assess our perceptions and to anticipate, avoid, and develop skills to reduce or better manage those stressors is crucial. The first step in controlling or reducing stress is to understand what stress is and how it affects the body.

LO 1 | WHAT IS STRESS?

Define stress and examine its potential impact on health, relationships, and success in college.

Stress seems to be the new norm for people of all races during all ages and stages of life. We blame our fights with loved ones on it; we attribute our sleep deficits, illnesses, anxieties, frustrations, successes, and failures to it. As much as we talk about being stressed, we each experience stressful events in different ways based on our past experiences, fears, and perceptions. While being in the backseat of a high-flying rollercoaster would send some of us into screaming fits, complete with white knuckles, nausea, and pure horror—an entire set of negative stress consequences—others in the same situation would be having an emotionally positive and fun experience, complete with wide-eyed laughter and excitement. While the latter group might pay for another ride, the first group would be running for the exits!

chronic stress An ongoing state of physiological arousal in response to ongoing or numerous perceived threats.

stress A series of mental and physiological responses and adaptations to a real or perceived threat to one's well-being.

stressor A physical, social, or psychological event or condition that upsets homeostasis and produces a stress response.

Although "stress" may be a common term, defining it isn't as easy as it might seem. Most current definitions state that **stress** is the mental and physical response and adaptation by our bodies to real or perceived changes and challenges. Things that get us revved up are **stressors**—real or perceived physical, social, environmental, or psychological events or stimuli that strain our abilities to cope. For some, extreme rollercoaster rides may not be enjoyable; for others, these rides may be just the stimulus needed to renew and energize.

Several factors influence whether one's response to stressors ends up being positive or negative, including *characteristics of the stressor* (e.g., How traumatic is it? Can you control it? Is it something you were mentally prepared for, or did it catch you by surprise? Has anything in your life experience prepared you for it?); *biological factors* (e.g., your age or gender, your current health status, whether you've had enough sleep recently); and *past experiences or fears* (e.g., things that have happened to you, their consequences, and how you felt or responded to the situation). Stressors may be *tangible*, such as a failing grade on a test, or *intangible*, such as the angst associated with meeting your significant other's parents for

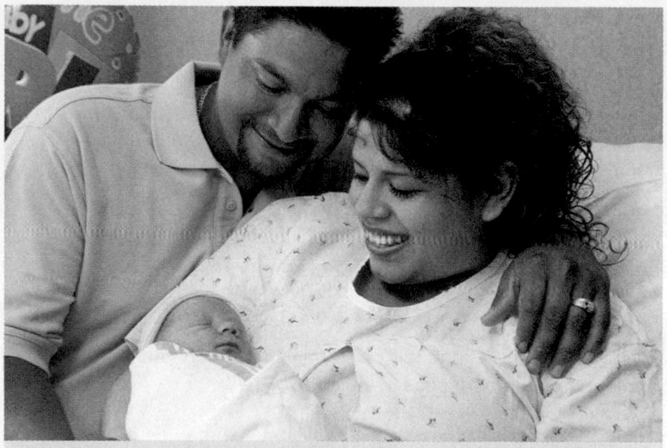

Not all stress is bad for you! Although events that cause prolonged *distress,* such as a natural disaster, can undermine your health, events that cause *eustress,* such as the birth of a child, can have positive effects on your growth and well-being. People usually live their lives to the fullest when they experience a moderate level of stress—just enough to keep them challenged and motivated—and deal with that stress in a productive manner. Just as too much stress can be detrimental to your health, too little stress leaves you stagnant and unfulfilled.

the first time. **Distress**, or negative stress, is more likely to occur when you are tired, under the influence of alcohol or other drugs, or coping with an illness, financial trouble, or relationship problems.

distress Stress that can have a detrimental effect on health; negative stress.

eustress Stress that presents opportunities for personal growth; positive stress.

acute stress The short-term physiological response to an immediate perceived threat.

episodic acute stress The state of regularly reacting with wild, acute stress about one thing or another.

traumatic stress A physiological and mental response that occurs for a prolonged period of time after a major accident, war, assault, natural disaster, or an event in which one may be seriously hurt, or killed, or witness horrible things.

homeostasis A balanced physiological state in which all the body's systems function smoothly.

Generally, positive stress is called **eustress.** Eustress presents the opportunity for personal growth and satisfaction and can actually improve health. It can energize you, motivate you, and raise you up when you are down. Getting married or winning a major competition can give rise to the pleasurable rush associated with eustress.

There are several types of stress. The most common type, **acute stress**, comes from demands and pressures of the recent past and anticipated demands and pressures of the near future.[4] Usually acute stress is intense, flares quickly, and disappears quickly without permanent damage to your health. Seeing someone you have a crush on could cause your heart to race and your muscles to tense while you appear cool, calm, and collected on the outside. The positive reaction to acute stress is that you rise to the occasion and put your most charming self forward. In contrast, anticipating a class presentation could cause shaking hands, nausea, headache, cramping, or diarrhea, along with a galloping heartbeat, stammering, and forgetfulness. **Episodic acute stress** is the state of *regularly* reacting with wild, acute stress to various situations. Individuals experiencing episodic acute stress may complain about all they have to do and focus on negative events that may or may not occur. These *"awfulizers"* are often reactive and anxious, but their thoughts and behaviors can be so habitual that to them they seem normal. Others may regularly react with episodic outbursts that are over-the-top "chirpy" or "happy, happy, happy," and may not recognize them as stress reactions.

Acute stress and episodic acute stress can both cause physical and emotional reactions, but they may or may not result in negative physical or emotional outcomes. In contrast, **chronic stress** can linger indefinitely and wreak silent havoc on your body systems. Caregivers are especially vulnerable to prolonged physiological stress as they watch a loved one struggle with cancer, heart disease, or other physical or mental disabilities. Upon a loved one's eventual death, survivors may struggle to balance the need to process emotions such as anger, grief, loneliness, and guilt with the need to stay caught up in classes, work, and everyday life. Sleep deprivation during times of emotional upset may result in more negative reactions to stressors. Another type of stress, **traumatic stress**, is often a result of witnessing or experiencing events like major accidents, war, shootings, assault, or natural disasters. Effects of traumatic stress may be felt for years after the event and cause significant disability, potentially leading to *post-traumatic stress disorder* or *PTSD* (see **Chapter 2** for a discussion of PTSD).[5]

LO 2 | YOUR BODY'S RESPONSES TO STRESS

Explain the phases of the general adaptation syndrome and the physiological changes that occur during them.

Our physiological responses evolved to protect humans from harm. Thousands of years ago, if your ancestors didn't respond by fighting or fleeing, they might have been eaten by a saber-toothed tiger or killed by a marauding enemy clan. Today, when we face real or perceived threats, these same physiological responses kick into gear, but our instinctual reactions to fight, scream, or flee the enemy must be held in check. Restraining these responses rather than allowing them to run their course can make us physiologically charged for longer periods—sometimes chronically. Over time, a simmering stress response can wreak havoc on the body.

The General Adaptation Syndrome

When stress levels are low, the body is often in a state of **homeostasis**—all body systems are operating smoothly to maintain equilibrium. Stressors trigger a "crisis mode" physiological response, after which the body attempts to

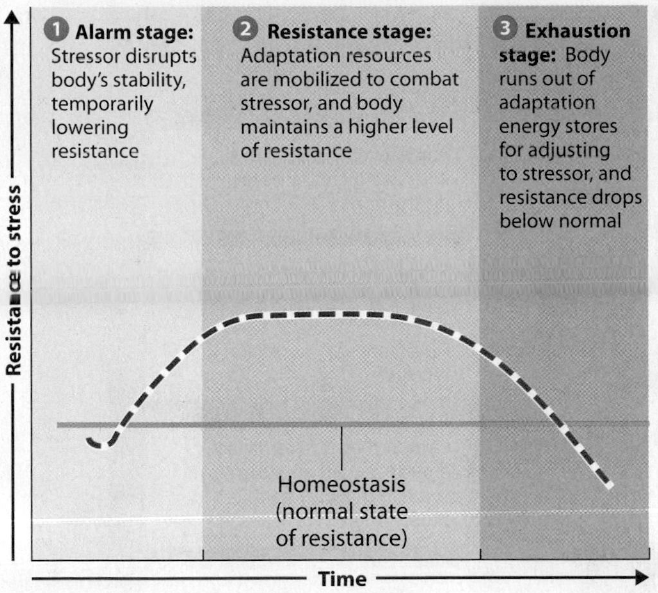

1 Alarm stage: Stressor disrupts body's stability, temporarily lowering resistance
2 Resistance stage: Adaptation resources are mobilized to combat stressor, and body maintains a higher level of resistance
3 Exhaustion stage: Body runs out of adaptation energy stores for adjusting to stressor, and resistance drops below normal
Resistance to stress
Homeostasis (normal state of resistance)
Time

FIGURE 3.1 The General Adaptation Syndrome (GAS) The GAS describes how we cope with prolonged stress.

return to homeostasis by means of an **adaptive response**. First characterized by Hans Selye in 1936, the internal fight to restore homeostasis in the face of a stressor is known as the **general adaptation syndrome (GAS)** (**FIGURE 3.1**). The GAS has three distinct phases: alarm, resistance, and exhaustion.[6]

Regardless of whether you are experiencing distress or eustress, similar physiological changes occur. The GAS can occur in varying degrees of intensity, last varying lengths of time, and be experienced differently by different individuals.

Alarm Phase Suppose you are walking home after a night class on a dimly lit campus. You hear someone cough behind you and sense them approaching rapidly. You walk faster, only to hear the other person's footsteps quicken. Your senses become increasingly alert, your breathing quickens, your heart races, and you begin to perspire. In desperation you stop, rip off your backpack, and prepare to fling it at your would-be attacker to defend yourself. You turn around, ready to rumble, and let out a blood-curdling yell. To your surprise, the would-be-attacker screeches back. It's not an attacker after all, but one of your classmates trying to stay close out of her own fear of being alone in the dark! You both gasp, and then laugh hysterically as you release built up tension. You have just experienced the *alarm* phase of the GAS. Also known as the **fight-or-flight response**, this physiological reaction is one of our most basic, innate survival instincts.[7] (See **FIGURE 3.2**.)

When the mind perceives a real or imaginary stressor, the cerebral cortex, the region of the brain that interprets the nature of an event, triggers an **autonomic nervous system (ANS)** response that prepares the body for action. The ANS is the portion of the central nervous system regulating body functions that we do not normally consciously control, such as heart and glandular functions and breathing.

The ANS has two branches: sympathetic and parasympathetic. The **sympathetic nervous system** energizes the body for fight or flight by signaling the release of several stress hormones. The **parasympathetic nervous system** slows systems stimulated by the stress response—in effect, it counteracts the actions of the sympathetic branch.

The responses of the sympathetic nervous system to stress involve a series of biochemical exchanges between different parts of the body. The brain's **hypothalamus** functions as the control center of the sympathetic nervous system and determines the overall reaction to stressors. When the hypothalamus perceives that extra energy is needed to fight a stressor, it stimulates the adrenal glands, located near the top of the kidneys, to release the hormone **epinephrine**, also called *adrenaline*. Epinephrine revs you for action, pumping more blood with each heartbeat, dilating the airways in the lungs to increase oxygen intake, increasing the breathing rate, stimulating the liver to release more glucose (which fuels muscular exertion), and dilating the pupils to improve visual sensitivity.

In addition to the fight-or-flight response, the alarm phase can trigger a longer-term reaction to stress. The hypothalamus uses chemical messages to trigger the pituitary gland within the brain to release a powerful hormone, *adrenocorticotropic hormone (ACTH)*. ACTH signals the adrenal glands to release **cortisol**, a hormone that makes stored nutrients more readily available to meet energy demands. Finally, other parts of the brain and body release *endorphins*, which relieve pain that a stressor may cause.

Resistance Phase In the resistance phase of the GAS, the body tries to return to homeostasis by resisting alarm responses. However, because some perceived stressor still exists, the body does not achieve complete calm or rest. Instead, the body remains at a level that causes a higher metabolic rate in some organ tissues.

HEAR IT! PODCASTS

Want a study podcast for this chapter? Download the podcast **Managing Stress: Coping with Life's Challenges** available on MasteringHealth.™

adaptive response The physiological adjustments the body makes in an attempt to restore homeostasis.

general adaptation syndrome (GAS) The pattern followed in the physiological response to stress, consisting of the alarm, resistance, and exhaustion phases.

fight-or-flight response Physiological arousal response in which the body prepares to combat or escape a real or perceived threat.

autonomic nervous system (ANS) The portion of the central nervous system regulating body functions that a person does not normally consciously control.

sympathetic nervous system Branch of the autonomic nervous system responsible for stress arousal.

parasympathetic nervous system Branch of the autonomic nervous system responsible for slowing systems stimulated by the stress response.

hypothalamus A structure in the brain that controls the sympathetic nervous system and directs the stress response.

epinephrine Also called *adrenaline*, a hormone that stimulates body systems in response to stress.

cortisol Hormone released by the adrenal glands that makes stored nutrients more readily available to meet energy demands.

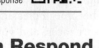

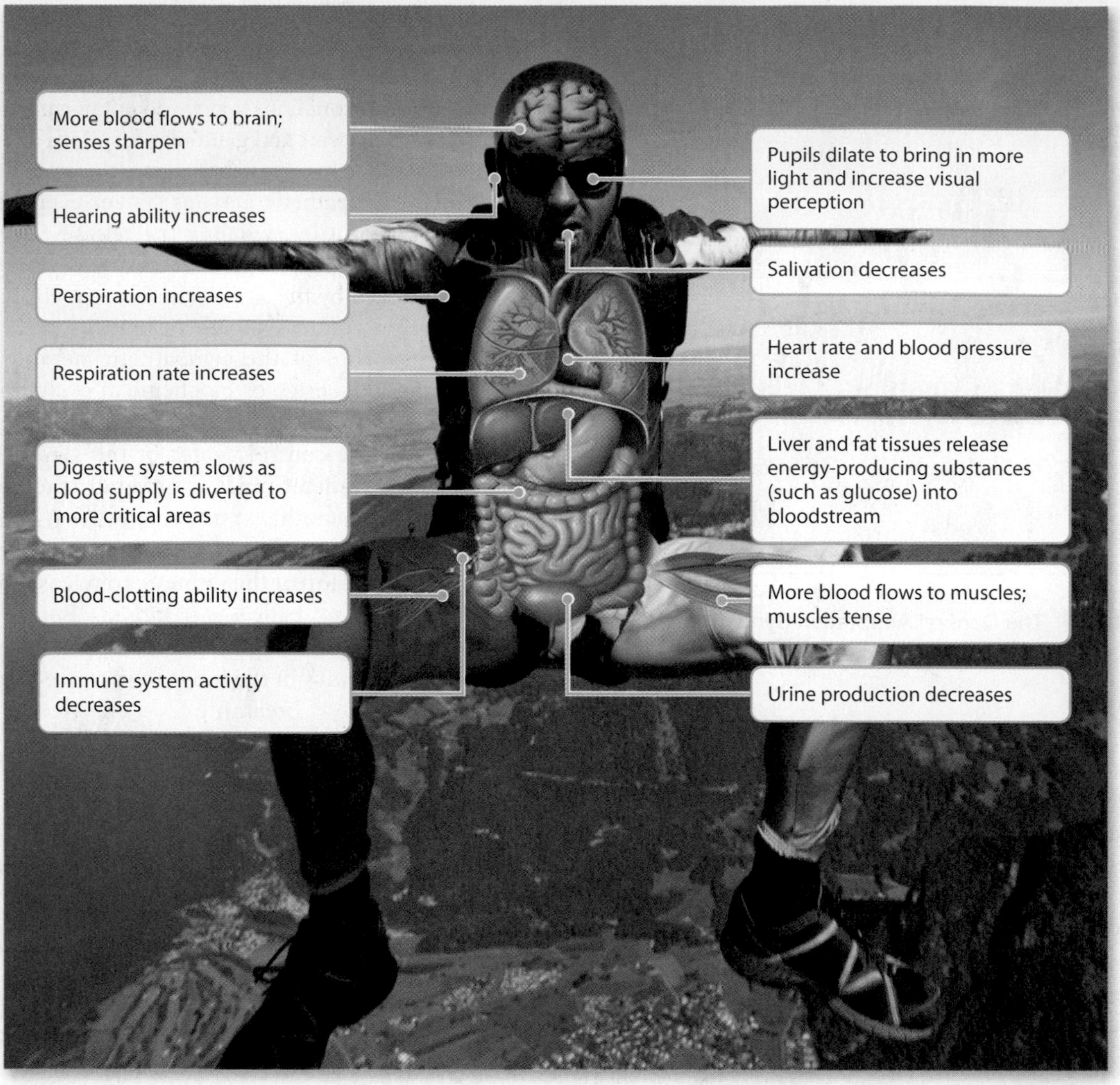
More blood flows to brain; senses sharpen
Hearing ability increases
Perspiration increases
Respiration rate increases
Digestive system slows as blood supply is diverted to more critical areas
Blood-clotting ability increases
Immune system activity decreases
Pupils dilate to bring in more light and increase visual perception
Salivation decreases
Heart rate and blood pressure increase
Liver and fat tissues release energy-producing substances (such as glucose) into bloodstream
More blood flows to muscles; muscles tense
Urine production decreases

FIGURE 3.2 The Body's Acute Stress Response Exposure to stress of any kind causes a complex series of involuntary physiological responses.

VIDEO TUTOR: Body's Stress Response

Exhaustion Phase In the exhaustion phase of the GAS, the hormones, chemicals, and systems that trigger and maintain the stress response are depleted, and the body returns to *allostasis,* or balance. You may feel tired or drained as your body returns to normal. In situations where stress is *chronic,* triggers may reverberate in the body, keeping body systems at a heightened arousal state. The prolonged effort to adapt to the stress response leads to **allostatic load**, or exhaustive wear and tear on the body. As the body adjusts to chronic unresolved stress, the adrenal glands continue to release cortisol, which remains in the bloodstream for longer periods of time as a result of slower metabolic responsiveness. Over time, cortisol can reduce **immunocompetence**—the ability of the immune system to respond to attack—as well as increase risk of diabetes, cardiovascular disease (CVD), and other chronic diseases.[8]

allostatic load Wear and tear on the body caused by prolonged or excessive stress responses.

immunocompetence The ability of the immune system to respond to attack.

Do Men and Women Respond Differently to Stress?

Ever since Walter Cannon's landmark studies in the 1930s, it's been thought that humans as well as many species of animals respond similarly to stressful events with the fight-or-flight response. However, several recent researchers believe that men and women may actually respond very differently to stressors. While men may be prone to fighting or fleeing, women may be more likely to "tend and befriend" by either trying to befriend the enemy or by obtaining social support from others to ease stress-related reactions.[9] According to a recent Australian study, a gene known as *SRY* may prime males to secrete more stress-related hormones and be more aggressive than women.[10] Other studies point to the fact that one's mind-set may influence stress responses and that males and females may differ in their in stress responses based on the way they perceive stressful events.[11]

34.8%

OF COLLEGE STUDENTS REPORT THAT THEIR **FINANCES** HAVE BEEN VERY DIFFICULT TO HANDLE DURING THE PAST 12 MONTHS.

LO 3 | LIFETIME EFFECTS OF STRESS

Examine the physical health risks that may occur with chronic stress.

Researchers have only recently begun to untangle the complex web of physiological and emotional responses that can take a toll on a person's physical, intellectual, and emotional well-being. Stress is often described as a "disease of prolonged arousal" that leads to a cascade of potentially devastating health effects. Some warning symptoms of prolonged stress are shown in **FIGURE 3.3**.

Physical Effects of Stress

The higher the levels of stress you experience and the longer that stress continues, the greater the likelihood of damage to your physical health.[12] A recent international study indicated a universal tendency toward negative health consequences among those with chronically high stress in their lives. Specifically, the more traumatic life events a person experiences, the greater the risk of a wide range of subsequent illnesses, including cardiovascular diseases, arthritis, gastrointestinal disorders, and others.[13] In addition to physical threats, increases in rates of suicide, mental illness, homicide, and domestic violence are symptoms of a nation that is chronically stressed.

Stress and Cardiovascular Disease Perhaps the most studied and documented health consequence of unresolved stress is CVD. A recent summary of accumulated knowledge indicates that chronic stress plays a significant role in heart rate problems, high blood pressure, and atherosclerosis, as well as increased risk for a wide range of cardiovascular diseases.[14]

Chronic stress has been linked to increased arterial plaque buildup due to elevated cholesterol, hardening of the arteries, increase in inflammatory responses in the body, alterations in heart rhythm, increased and fluctuating blood pressures, and other CVD risks.[15] In recent decades, a wide range of social conditions, such as job strain, job instability, social isolation, discrimination, housing and environmental threats, lack of access to quality health care, caregiving responsibilities, bereavement, and natural disasters have been linked to increased CVD risks.[16] (For more information about CVD, see **Chapter 15**.)

Stress and Weight Gain If you think that when you are extremely stressed, you tend to eat more and gain weight, you didn't imagine it. Higher stress levels may increase cortisol levels in the bloodstream, which contributes to increased hunger and seems to activate fat-storing enzymes. Animal and human studies, including those in which subjects suffer from post-traumatic stress, seem to support the theory that cortisol plays a role in laying down extra belly fat and increasing eating behaviors.[17]

FIGURE 3.3 **Common Physical Symptoms of Stress** Sometimes you may not even notice how stressed you are until your body starts sending you signals. Do you frequently experience any of these physical symptoms of stress?

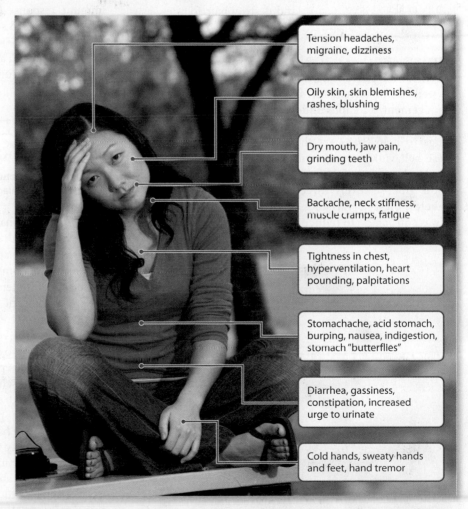

Stress and Alcohol Dependence New research has found a specific stress hormone, the *corticotropin-releasing factor* (CRF), is key to the development and maintenance of alcohol dependence in animals. CRF—a naturally occurring chemical—stimulates stress hormone secretion as part of the bodies stress response. It may play a similar role in humans, making it harder for stressed alcoholics to abstain from alcohol. If proven, options for dealing with stress-related alcohol abstinence difficulties may focus on substances that diminish CRF receptor activity. More research is necessary to fully understand potential options.[18]

Stress and Hair Loss Too much stress can lead to thinning hair, and even baldness, in men and women. The most common type of stress-induced hair loss is *telogen effluvium*. Often seen in individuals who have lost a loved one or experienced severe weight loss or other trauma, this condition pushes colonies of hair into a resting phase. Over time, hair may begin to fall out. A similar stress-related condition known as *alopecia areata* occurs when stress triggers white blood cells to attack and destroy hair follicles, usually in patches.[19]

psychoneuroimmunology (PNI) The study of the interrelationship between the mind and body on immune system functioning.

Stress and Diabetes Controlling stress levels is critical for preventing development of type 2 diabetes, as well as for successful short- and long-term diabetes management.[20] People under lots of stress often don't get enough sleep, don't eat well, and may drink or take other drugs to help them get through a stressful time. All of these behaviors can alter blood sugar levels and promote the development of diabetes. Stress hormones may affect blood glucose levels directly. (For full information on diabetes, lifestyle variables that may contribute to it, and things you can do to reduce your risks, see **Focus On: Minimizing Your Risk for Diabetes**.)

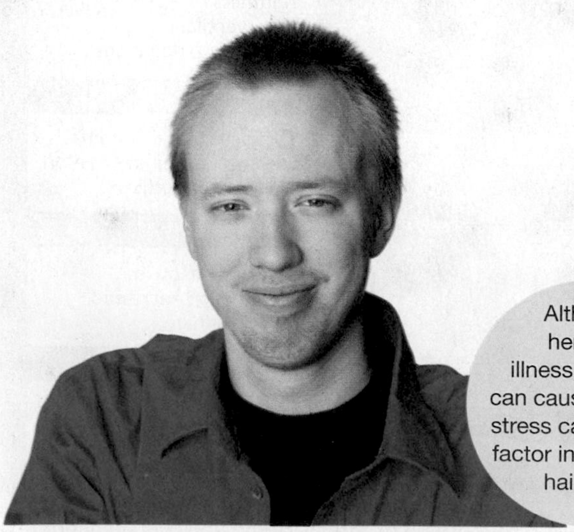

Although heredity, illness, and diet can cause hair loss, stress can be a key factor in premature hair loss.

Stress and Digestive Problems Millions of Americans suffer from one or more digestive diseases or disorders (see **Chapter 17** on chronic diseases). Although stress may not directly cause these symptoms, it is clearly related and may actually make your risk of having symptoms worse.[21] For example, people with depression or anxiety are more susceptible to dehydration, inflammation, and other digestive problems. Irritable bowel syndrome may be more likely, in part because stress stimulates colon spasms by means of the nervous system. Relaxation techniques and mindfulness training (found later in this chapter) may reduce the activity of the sympathetic nervous system, leading to decreases in heart rate, blood pressure, and other stress responses that trigger gastrointestinal (GI) tract flare-ups.[22]

Stress and Impaired Immunity A growing area of scientific investigation known as **psychoneuroimmunology (PNI)** analyzes the intricate relationship between the mind's response to stress and the immune system's ability to function effectively. (See more on PNI in **Chapter 2**.) Several recent reviews of research linking stress to adverse health consequences suggest that too much stress over a long period can negatively affect various aspects of the cellular immune response (see **Chapter 13** on infectious diseases). This increases risks for upper respiratory infections and certain chronic conditions, increases adverse birth outcomes and fetal development, and exacerbates problems for children and adults suffering from post-traumatic stress.[23]

LO 4 | INTELLECTUAL EFFECTS OF STRESS

Examine the intellectual and psychological effects of stress and their impacts on college students.

In a recent national survey of college students, nearly half (48.5 percent) of the respondents said that they had felt overwhelmed by all that they had to do within the past 2 weeks, with a similar number reporting they felt exhausted. Nearly 43 percent of students said they had experienced a larger than average amount of stress, and another 10 percent said they had experienced tremendous stress during the past year. Not surprisingly, these same students rated stress as their number one impediment to academic performance, followed by anxiety and lack of sleep.[24] Stress can play a huge role in whether students stay in school, get good grades, and succeed on their career path. It can also wreak havoc on students' ability to concentrate, affect memory, and decrease ability to understand and retain complex information.

SEE IT! VIDEOS

Can a test identify your risk for stress-related illnesses? Watch **Stress Can Damage Women's Health** available on MasteringHealth.™

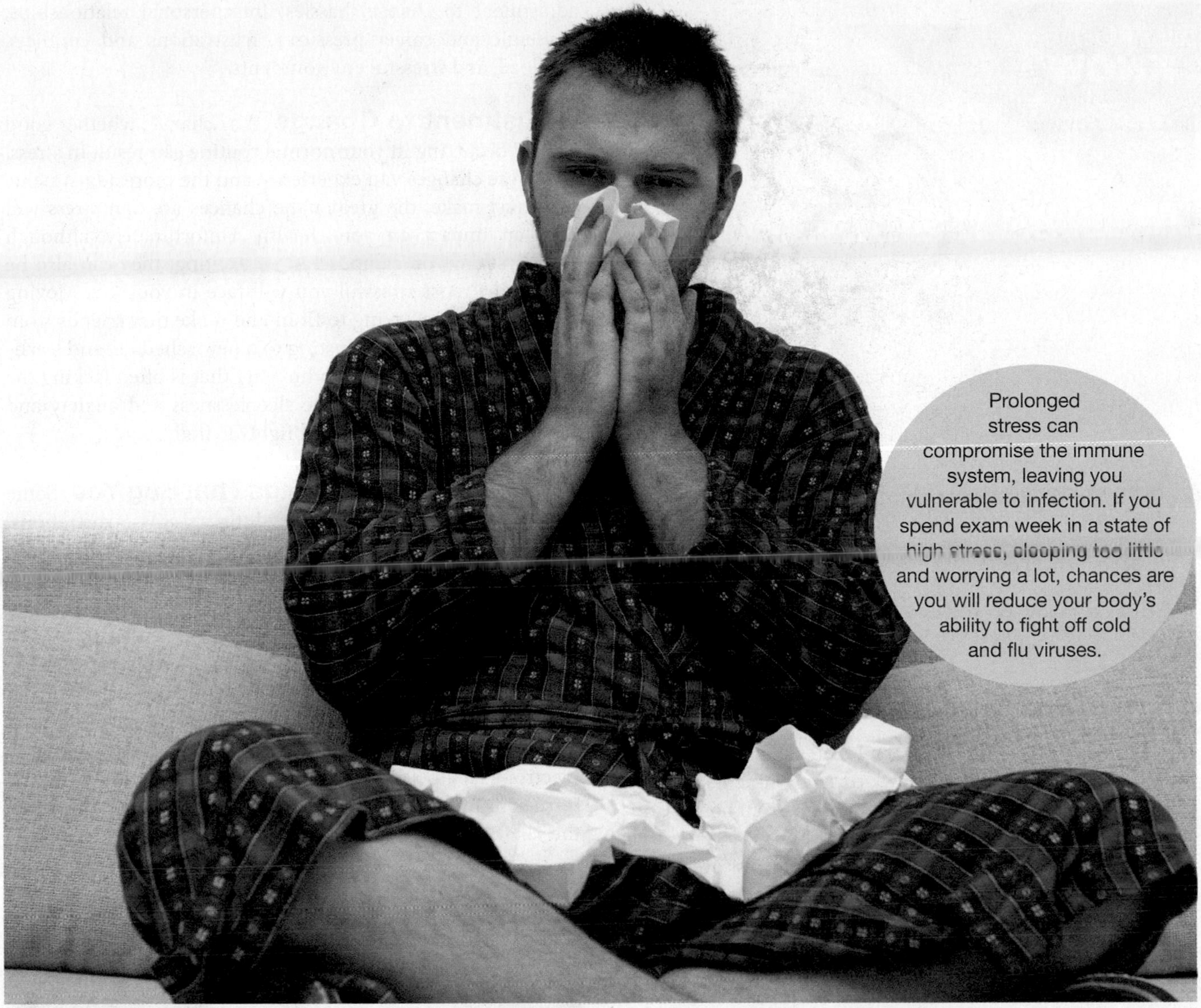

Prolonged stress can compromise the immune system, leaving you vulnerable to infection. If you spend exam week in a state of high stress, sleeping too little and worrying a lot, chances are you will reduce your body's ability to fight off cold and flu viruses.

Stress, Memory, and Concentration Although the exact reasons stress can affect grades are complex, new research has provided possible clues. Animal studies have provided compelling indicators of how chronic exposure to glucocorticoids—stress hormones released from the adrenal cortex—are believed to affect cognitive functioning and overall mental health. In humans, memory is impaired when acute stress bombards the brain with hormones and neurotransmitters—affecting the way we think, make decisions, and respond behaviorally in stressful situations.[25] Recent laboratory studies with rats have linked prolonged exposure to cortisol to actual shrinking of the hippocampus, the brain's major memory center.[26] Other research indicates that prolonged exposure to high levels of stress hormones may actually predispose women, in particular, to Alzheimer's disease. More research is necessary to determine the validity of these theories.[27]

Psychological Effects of Stress

Stress may be one of the single greatest contributors to mental disability and emotional dysfunction in industrialized nations. Studies have shown that the rates of mental disorders, particularly depression and anxiety, are associated with various environmental stressors from childhood through adulthood, including violence and abuse, marital and relationship conflict, poverty, and other stressful life events.[28]

Stress and the Transition to Adulthood

College students not only face the typical stressors of adulthood, they also face additional stressors stemming from housing searches, financial independence, career choices and

DID YOU **KNOW?**

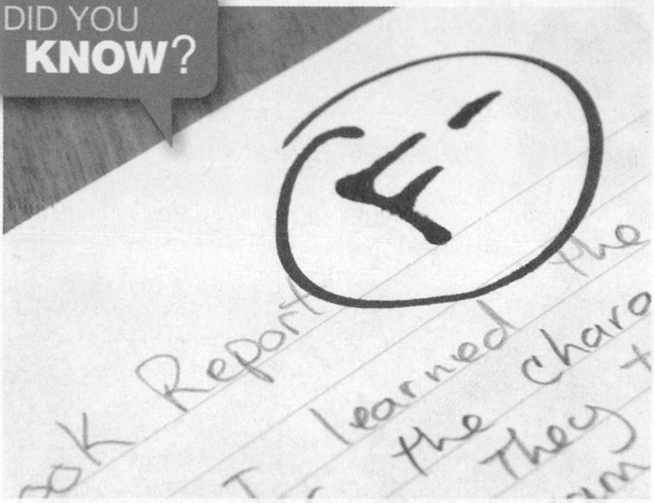

In the most recent National College Health Assessment, over 28.5 percent of college students reported that stress negatively impacted their grade on an exam or course, or caused them to drop a course.

Source: Data are from American College Health Association, *American College Health Association–National College Health Assessment II (ACHA-NCHA II): Reference Group Data Report Spring 2013* (Baltimore: American College Health Association, 2014).

employment (or the lack thereof), relationships, interactions with family and peers, and perceived environmental threats. Change is a huge part of their first year away from home. Coping skills and social support from family, friends, and community services can buffer the negative effects of stress overload.[29]

LO 5 | WHAT CAUSES STRESS?

Discuss sources of stress and examine the unique stressors that affect college students.

On any given day, everyone experiences eustress and distress from a wide range of sources, some more obvious than others. The American Psychological Association conducts one of the most comprehensive studies examining sources of stress among various populations annually. The 2012 survey found that concerns over money, work, the economy, family responsibilities, and relationships were major sources of stress among American adults (**FIGURE 3.4**).[30] College students, in particular, face stressors from internal sources, as well as external pressures to succeed in a competitive environment that is often geographically far from the support of family and lifelong friends. Awareness of the sources of stress can do much to help you develop a plan to avoid, prevent, or control the things that cause you stress.

Psychosocial Stressors

Psychosocial stressors refer to the factors in our daily routines and in our social and physical environments that cause us to experience stress. Key psychosocial stressors include adjustment to change, hassles, interpersonal relationships, academic and career pressures, frustrations and conflicts, overload, and stressful environments.

Adjustment to Change Any change, whether good or bad, occurring in your normal routine can result in stress. The more changes you experience and the more adjustments you must make, the greater the chances are that stress will have an impact on your health. Unfortunately, although your first days on campus can be exciting, they can also be among the most stressful you will face in your life. Moving away from home, trying to fit in and make new friends from diverse backgrounds, adjusting to a new schedule, and learning to live with strangers in housing that is often lacking the comforts of home can cause sleeplessness and anxiety and keep your body in a continual fight-or-flight mode.

Hassles: The Little Things That Bug You Some psychologists have proposed that little stressors, frustrations, and petty annoyances, known collectively as *hassles*, can eventually be just as stressful as major life changes.[31] Put another way, cumulative hassles add up, increasing allostatic load and resulting in wear and tear on body systems. Listening to others monopolize class time, not finding parking on campus, having people tweeting and texting while you are trying to study, and a host of other irritants can push your buttons and result in frustration, anger, and fight-or-flight responses.[32] Electronic devices we can't seem to live without can also cause intrusions into our lives, sap energy, and increase anxiety. See the **Tech & Health** box on page 82 for more on technostress.

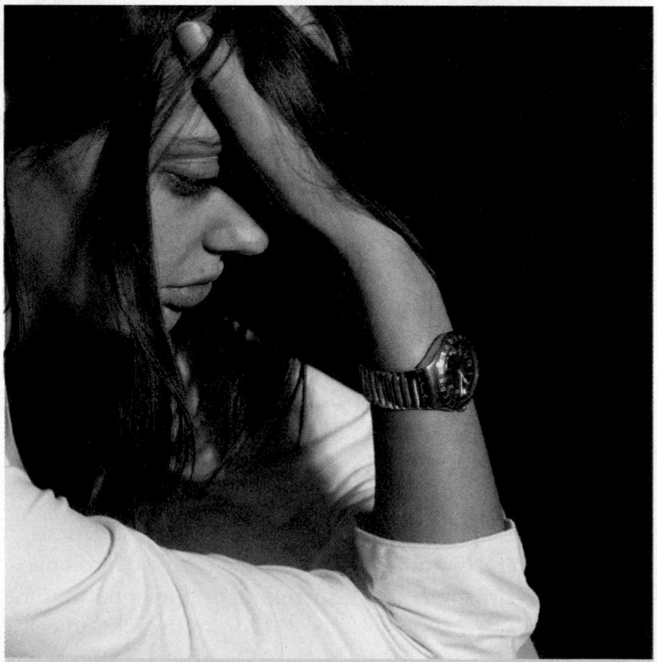

Stress and depression have complicated interconnections based on emotional, physiological, and biochemical processes. Prolonged stress can trigger depression in susceptible people, and prior periods of depression can leave individuals more susceptible to stress.

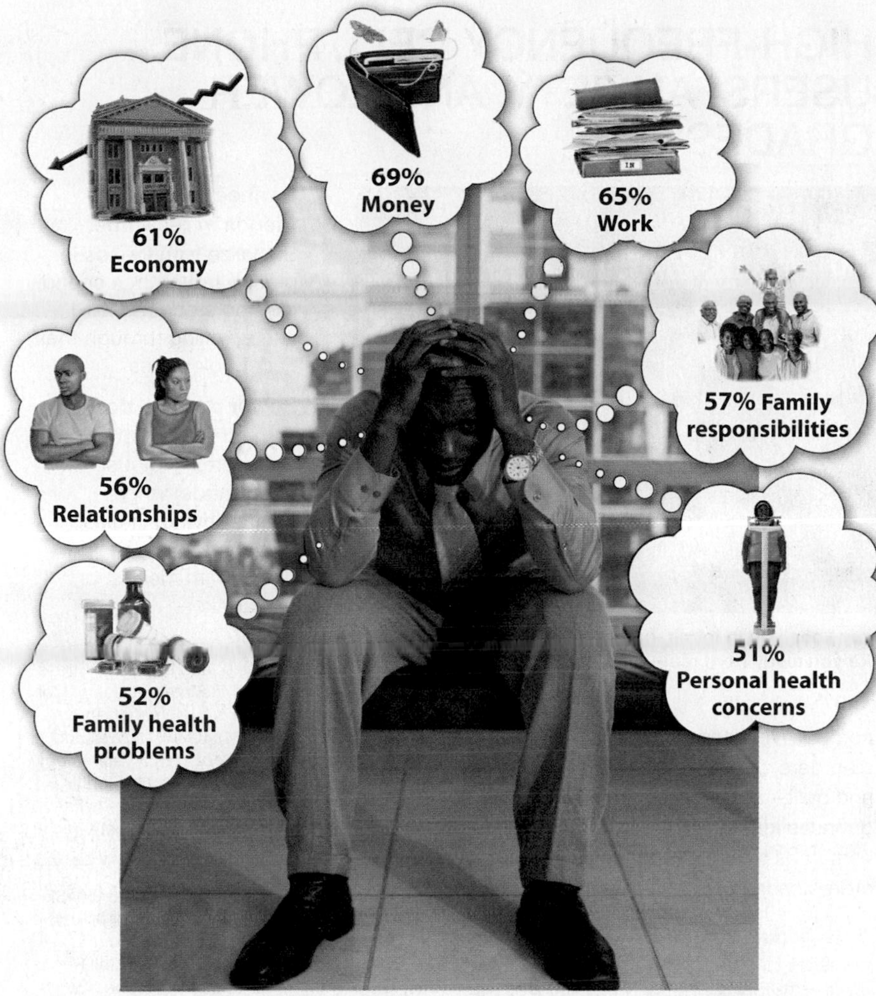

FIGURE 3.4 **What Do We Say Stresses Us?** The annual *Stress in America* survey indicates American adults are increasingly experiencing money, work, and housing concerns as major sources of stress in their lives.

Source: Data are from the American Psychological Association, *2012 Stress in America, Key Findings*, 2013, www.apa.org/news/press/releases/stress/2012/full-report.pdf.

The Toll of Relationships Let's face it, relationships can trigger some of the biggest fight-or-flight reactions of all time. Although love relationships are the ones we often think of first, relationships with friends, family members, and coworkers can be the sources of overwhelming struggles just as easily as they can be sources of strength and support. A recent comparison of nearly 80 studies of stress and work provides strong evidence that work situations with high demands, little control, and coworkers who are difficult to get along with increase the likelihood of employee complaints about gastrointestinal ailments and sleep difficulties. Competition for rewards and systems that favor certain classes of employees or pit workers against one another are among the most stressful job situations.[33] Healthy interactions with supportive others can not only reduce our stress levels, but keep us motivated and energized.

Academic and Financial Pressure It isn't surprising that today's college and university students face mind-boggling amounts of pressure competing for grades, athletic positions, internships, and jobs. Challenging classes can be tough enough, but many students must also juggle work in order to pay bills. When economic conditions become strained, the effects on people with limited resources (particularly students) can be significant. An economic downturn can even make student dreams seem unattainable. (For tips on how to head off some financial stressors before they start, see **Focus On: Improving Your Financial Health**.) Increasing reports of mental health problems on college campuses may be one of the results of too much stress.

Frustrations and Conflicts

Whenever there is a disparity between our goals (what we hope to obtain in life) and our behaviors (actions that may or may not lead to these goals), frustration can occur. For example, you realize that you must get good grades in college to enter graduate school, which is your ultimate goal. If your social life is cutting into your studying time, you may find your goals slipping away, leading to increased stress.

Conflicts occur when we are forced to decide among competing motives, impulses, desires, and behaviors (for example, to party or study) or when we are forced to face pressures of demands that are incompatible with our own values and sense of importance (for example, get good grades or compete in college athletics). College students who are away from their families for the first time may face a variety of conflicts among parental values, their own beliefs, and the beliefs of others who are very different from themselves.

Overload We've all experienced times in our lives when the demands of work, responsibilities, deadlines, and relationships all seem to be pulling us underwater. **Overload** occurs when we are overextended and, try as we might, there are not nearly enough hours in the day to do everything. Students suffering from overload may experience depression, sleeplessness, mood swings, frustration, anxiety, or a host of other symptoms. Binge drinking; high consumption of junk foods; and fighting with friends, family, and coworkers can all add fuel to the overload fire. Unrelenting stress and overload can lead to a state of physical and mental exhaustion known as *burnout*.

overload A condition in which a person feels overly pressured by demands.

TECH & HEALTH

HIGH-FREQUENCY CELL PHONE USERS, ANXIETY, AND LOWER GRADES?

Are you "tweeted out"? Is all that texting causing your thumbs to seize up in protest? Do you find yourself constantly checking your phone? If so, you're not alone. *High-frequency cell phone* use is on the rise, and with it come a variety of problems. According to a new study, college students who can't keep their hands off their mobile devices are reporting higher levels of anxiety, less satisfaction with life, and lower grades than peers who use their devices less often. The average student surveyed spent nearly 5 hours per day using their cell phones for everything from calling and texting (over 77 messages/day), to Facebook, e-mails, gaming, and more. Surprised?

Like millions of others, you may find that all of the pressure for contact is causing *technostress*—stress created by a dependence on technology and the constant state of connection, which can include a perceived obligation to respond, chat, or tweet. Research supports the concept that being wired 24/7 can lead to anxiety, obsessive compulsive disorder, narcissism, sleep disorders, frustration, time pressures, and guilt—some of the negative consequences known as iDisorders. Here are some tips to avoid technostress or iDisorders caused by technology overload:

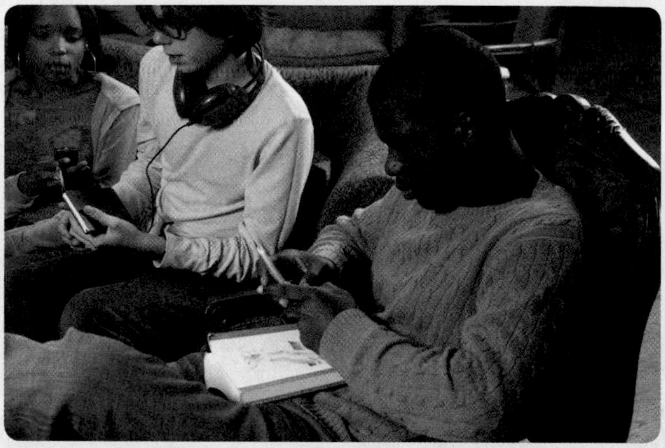

Technology may keep you in touch, but it can also add to your stress and take you away from real-world interactions.

- **Schedule screen time.** Set time aside to check e-mail, text messages, and Twitter feeds, such as once in the morning and once in the evening for no more than a half hour. Resist the urge to check if you're outside your set time frame. NO reading messages in the middle of the night!
- **Connect with your friends in real-time.** Socialize with friends in person rather than spending hours commenting and scrolling through their Facebook pages.
- **Power devices down.** Turn off all your devises completely (not just silent mode) when you're driving, in class, at work, in bed, having dinner with friends, or on vacation.

Sources: S. Deatherage, H. Servaty-Seib, and I. Aksoz. "Stress, Coping and the Internet Use of College Students." *Journal of American Health* 62, no. 1 (2014):40–46; M. Weil and L. Rosen, *Technostress: Coping with Technology @Work, @Home, @Play* (Hoboken, NJ: John Wiley & Sons, 1997); L. D. Rosen et al., "Is Facebook Creating "iDisorders"? The Link between Clinical Symptoms of Psychiatric Disorders and Technology Use, Attitudes and Anxiety," *Computers in Human Behavior* 29, no. 3 (2013): 1243–54, Available at http://dx.doi.org/10.1016/j.chb.2012.11.012; A. Lepp, T. Barkley, and A. Karpinski, "The Relationship Between Cell Phone Use, Academic Performance, Anxiety and Satisfaction with Life in College Students." *Computers in Human Behavior*. 2014. 31: 343–350; NIH Medline Plus, "Avid Cellphone Use by College Kids Tied to Anxiety, Lower Grades," December 2013, www.nlm.nih.gov/medlineplus/news/fullstory_143389.html

Stressful Environments For many students, where they live and the environment around them cause significant levels of stress. Perhaps you cannot afford safe, healthy housing, or a bad roommate constantly makes life uncomfortable, or loud neighbors keep you up at night. Noise, pressure of people in crowded living situations, and uncertainties over food and whether you have a place to sleep can keep even the most resilient person on edge.

Imagine waking up to find that your family is missing, your home is wiped out, you have no cell phone or communication methods, your city and university are in shambles, and all you have are the clothes on your back! This type of stress would make that little spat you had with your roommate seem pretty insignificant in comparison. Unexpected natural disasters can cause tremendous stress at the time and for years later. Typhoon Haiyan, Superstorm Sandy, and Hurricane Katrina; the Sumatra, Japan, and Haiti earthquakes; killer tornadoes in Oklahoma, Iowa, and Kansas; human disasters such as the Gulf Oil Spill, and have threatened millions, disrupted lives, and damaged ecosystems. Even after the initial images of suffering pass and the crisis has subsided, shortages of vital resources such as gasoline, clean water, food, housing, health care, sewage disposal and other necessities, as well as electricity outages and transportation problems, can wreak havoc in local communities and on campuses.

background distressors Environmental stressors of which people are often unaware.

While not as newsworthy as major disasters, **background distressors** in the environment, such as noise, air, and water pollution; allergy-aggravating pollen and dust; unsafe food; and environmental tobacco smoke can also be incredibly stressful. As with other challenges, our bodies respond to environmental distressors with the GAS. People who cannot escape background distressors may exist in a constant resistance phase.

Bias and Discrimination Racial and ethnic diversity of students, faculty members, and staff enriches everyone's

HEALTH IN A DIVERSE WORLD

INTERNATIONAL STUDENT STRESS

International students experience unique adjustment issues such as language barriers, financial issues, cultural barriers, and a lack of social support. Academic stress may pose a particular problem for the nearly 765,000 international students who left family and friends in their native countries to study in the United States in 2011–2012. Accumulating evidence suggests seeking emotional support from others is one effective way to cope with stressful and upsetting situations. Yet many international students feel ashamed to struggle and fear seeking support is a sign of weakness—calling inappropriate attention to both the individual and the individual's respective ethnic group. This reluctance, coupled with cultural conflicts and other stressors, can lead international students to suffer significantly more stress-related illnesses than their American counterparts.

Language barriers, cultural conflicts, racial prejudices, and a reluctance to seek social support all contribute to a significantly higher rate of stress-related illnesses among international students studying in the United States.

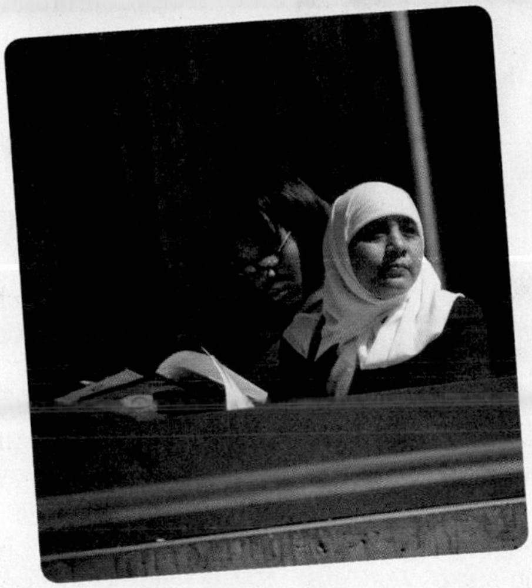

Even if we can't solve the many problems international students encounter, we can each share companionship, helping to offset loneliness, improve communication, and make each other's lives easier. To paraphrase a popular Hindu proverb: "Help thy neighbor's boat across and thine own boat will also reach the shore."

Sources: K. Cokley, et al. "An Examination of the Impact of Minority Status Stress and Imposter Feelings on the Mental Health of Diverse Ethnic Minority College Students." *Journal of Multicultural Counseling and Development* 41, no. 2 (2013): 82–93; P. Hoffman, *Examining Factors of Acculturative Stress on International Students as They Affect Utilization of Campus-Based Health and Counseling Services at Four-Year Public Universities in Ohio*, doctoral dissertation, Bowling Green University, https://etd.ohiolink.edu/rws_etd/document/get/bgsu1288203526/inline2010; S. Sumner, *Students' Psychological and Sociocultural Adaptation in the United States*, doctoral dissertation, Georgia State University, 2009, http://digitalarchive.gsu.edu/cps_diss/34; Institute of International Education, "Record Numbers of International Students in U.S. Higher Education," Fast Facts, OpenDoors, 2013, http://nces.ed.gov/fastfacts/display.asp?id=372.

educational experience on campus. It also challenges us to examine our personal attitudes, beliefs, and biases. As campuses become more internationalized, a diverse cultural base of vastly different life experiences, languages, and customs is emerging. Often, those perceived as dissimilar may become victims of subtle and not-so-subtle forms of bigotry, insensitivity, harassment, or hostility, or they may simply be ignored.

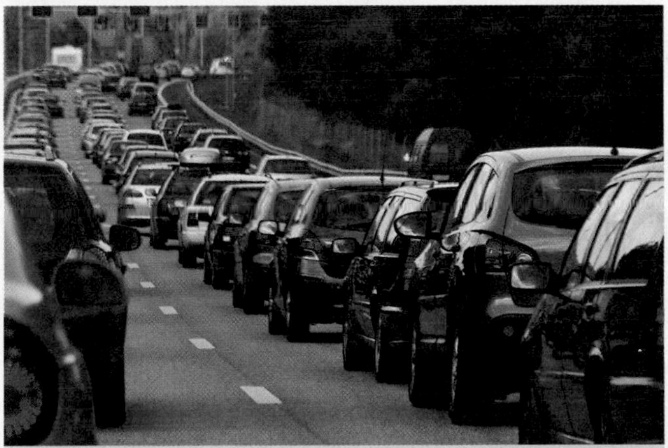

Traffic jams and noise pollution are examples of the daily hassles and frustrations that can add up and jeopardize our health.

Bias and discrimination based on race, ethnicity, religious affiliation, age, sexual orientation, or other "differences"—whether in viewpoints, appearance, behaviors, or backgrounds—may hang like a dark cloud over these students.[34] See the **Health in a Diverse World** box for more on stress and international students.

Evidence of the health effects of excessive stress in minority groups abounds. For example, African Americans suffer higher rates of hypertension, CVD, and most cancers than do whites.[35] Although poverty and socioeconomic status have been blamed for much of the spike in hypertension rates for African Americans and other marginalized groups, this chronic, physically debilitating stress may reflect real and perceived effects of institutional racism rather than individual/interpersonal poverty and perceived racism. More research is necessary to show direct associations between racism, stress, and hypertension; however, it is important to realize that all types of "isms" may influence stress-related hypertension and make it more difficult for those affected to engage in healthy lifestyle behaviors.[36]

WHAT DO YOU THINK?

Do you get stressed out by things in your home or school environment?

- Which environmental stressors bug you the most?
- When you encounter these environmental stressors, what actions do you take, if any?

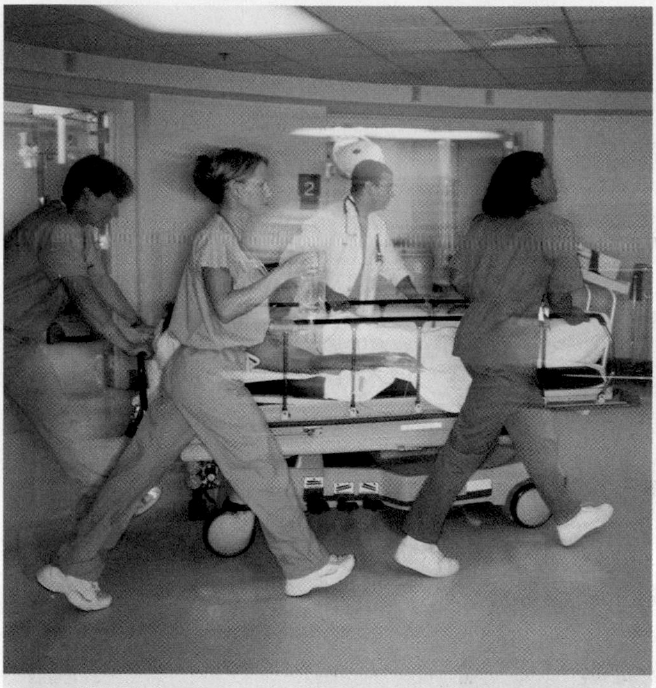

Certain jobs can be especially stressful, particularly those where the stakes are high and coworkers have little control over many outcomes. Individuals such as doctors and nurses face long work hours and a high-stakes work environment, making them especially prone to stress, overload, and burnout.

SKILLS FOR BEHAVIOR CHANGE
OVERCOMING TEST-TAKING ANXIETY

Testing well is a skill needed in college and beyond. Try these helpful hints on your next exam.

BEFORE THE EXAM

- Manage your study time. Keep up with reading during the term; don't wait until the last minute to cram. At least 1 week before your test, start studying for a set amount of time each day. Do a limited review the night before, get a good night's sleep, and arrive for the exam early.
- Eat a balanced meal before the exam. Avoid sugar and rich or heavy foods, as well as foods that might upset your stomach. You want to feel your best.
- Wear a watch to class on the day of the test, in case there is no clock.

DURING THE TEST

- Manage your time during the test. See how many questions there are and prioritize the high-point questions, allowing a certain amount of time for each. Make sure that you leave some time for the rest. Hold to this schedule.
- Slow down and pay attention. Focus on one question at a time. Check off each part of multipart questions to make sure your answers are complete.

Internal Stressors

Although stress can come from the environment and other external sources, it can result from internal factors as well. Internal stressors such as negative appraisal, low self-esteem, and low self-efficacy can cause unsettling thoughts or feelings, affect perceptions, and can ultimately affect your health. It is important to address and manage these internal stressors.

Appraisal, Perceptions, and Stress Throughout life, we encounter many different types of demands and potential stressors—some biological, some psychological, and others sociological. In any case, it is our appraisal of these demands, not the demands themselves, that results in our experiencing stress. **Appraisal** is defined as the interpretation and evaluation of information provided to the brain by the senses. As new information becomes available, appraisal helps us recognize stressors, evaluate them on the basis of past experiences and emotions, and decide whether or not we have the ability to cope. When you feel that the stressors of life are overwhelming and you lack control, you are more likely to feel strain and distress.

appraisal The interpretation and evaluation of information provided to the brain by the senses.

suicidal ideation A desire to die and thoughts about suicide.

Self-Esteem and Self-Efficacy Recall that *self-esteem* refers to how you feel about yourself. Self-esteem varies; it can and does continually change.[37] When you feel good about yourself, you are less likely to view certain events as stressful and more likely to be able to cope.[38] Of particular concern, research with high school and college students has found that low self-esteem and stressful life events significantly predict **suicidal ideation**, a desire to die and thoughts about suicide. On a more positive note, research has also indicated that it is possible to increase an individual's ability to cope with stress by increasing self-esteem.[39]

Self-efficacy, or confidence in one's skills and ability to cope with life's challenges, appears to be a key buffer in preventing negative stress effects. Research has shown that people with high levels of self-efficacy tend to feel more in control of stressful situations and, as such, report fewer stress effects.[40] Self-efficacy is considered one of the most important personality traits that influence psychological and physiological stress responses.[41] Developing self-efficacy is also vital to coping with and overcoming academic pressures and worries. For example, by learning to handle anxiety around testing situations, you improve your chances of performing well; the more you feel yourself capable of handle testing situations, the greater will be your sense of academic self-efficacy. For tips on how to deal with test-taking anxiety and build your testing self-efficacy, see the **Skills for Behavior Change** box.

Type A and Type B Personalities It should come as no surprise that personality can have an impact on whether you are happy and socially well-adjusted or sad and socially isolated. However, your personality may affect more than just your social interactions: It may be a critical factor in your stress level, as well as in your risk for CVD, cancer, and other chronic and infectious diseases.

In 1974, physicians Meyer Friedman and Ray Rosenman published a book indicating that Type A individuals had a greatly increased risk of heart disease.[42] *Type A* personalities are defined as hard-driving, competitive, time-driven perfectionists. In contrast, *Type B* personalities are described as being relaxed, noncompetitive, and more tolerant of others.

Today, most researchers recognize that none of us will be wholly Type A or Type B all of the time, and we may exhibit either type in selected situations. In addition, recent research indicates that not all Type A people experience negative health consequences; in fact, some hard-driving individuals seem to thrive on their supercharged lifestyles. Often those Type A individuals who exhibit a "toxic core," that is, have disproportionate amounts of anger; are distrustful of others; and have a cynical, glass-half-empty approach to life—a set of characteristics referred to as **hostility**—are at increased risk for heart disease. Relationships fraught with problems may not just be unpleasant happenings in life. In fact, a recent study has shown that couples who have marital discord—who are often in turmoil and are angry and hostile toward each other—have a significantly higher risk of early coronary heart disease.[43]

Type C and Type D Personalities In addition to CVD, personality types have been linked to increased risk for a variety of other illnesses, ranging from asthma to cancer, even though much of this research remains in question. A type in vogue today is the *Type C* personality, characterized as stoic with a tendency to stuff feelings down and conform to the wishes of others (or be "pleasers"). Preliminary research suggests that Type C individuals may be more susceptible to illnesses such as asthma, multiple sclerosis, autoimmune disorders, and cancer; however more research is necessary to support this relationship.[44]

A more recently identified personality type is *Type D* (distressed), which is characterized by a tendency toward excessive negative worry, irritability, gloom, and social inhibition. Several recent studies have indicated that Type D people may be up to eight times more likely to die of a heart attack or sudden cardiac death.[45]

Are Internal Stressors Inescapable?

For most people, most of the time, enough exposure to stressors will evoke the stress response. With the long list of stressors we've just reviewed, especially for people prone to Type A behavior, it might seem like stress is a given. But two factors seem to break the cycle and offer some protection from stress: psychological hardiness and resilience and the shift-and-persist strategy.

Psychological Hardiness and Resilience

According to psychologist Susanne Kobasa, **psychological hardiness** was the key to reducing self-imposed stress associated with Type A behavior. Psychologically hardy people were characterized by *control*, *commitment*, and willingness to embrace *challenge*.[46] People with a sense of *control* are able to accept responsibility for their behaviors and work to change situations they discover to be debilitating. People with a sense of *commitment* have healthy self-esteem and know their purpose in life. Those who embrace *challenge* see change as a stimulating opportunity for personal growth. Today, the concept of hardiness has evolved to include a person's overall ability to cope with stress and adversity.[47] In recent years, it has become common for people to think of this general hardiness concept in terms of **psychological resilience**. Essentially, resilience refers to our capacity to maintain or regain psychological well-being in the face of challenge.[48] Resilient individuals are often able to do well in the face of adversity because of "*protective factors*" such as strong support networks of family, friends, and healthy communities and their own coping skills. Resilience has been studied extensively and appears to be a key indicator of good psychological and social development.[49]

hostility The cognitive, affective, and behavioral tendencies toward anger and cynicism.

psychological hardiness A personality trait characterized by control, commitment, and the embrace of challenge.

psychological resilience The process of adapting well in the face of adversity, trauma, tragedy, threats, or significant sources of stress, such as family and relationship problems, serious health problems, or workplace and financial stressors.

Shift and Persist Some youth who face extreme poverty, abuse, and unspeakable living conditions as they grow up seem to thrive when their conditions are bleak. Why? An exciting, emerging body of sociological research proposes that in the midst of extreme, persistent adversity, youth—often with the help of positive role models in their lives—are able to reframe appraisals of current stressors more positively (*shifting*), while *persisting* in focusing on a future that has something to offer them. These youth are able to endure the present by adapting, holding on to meaningful things in

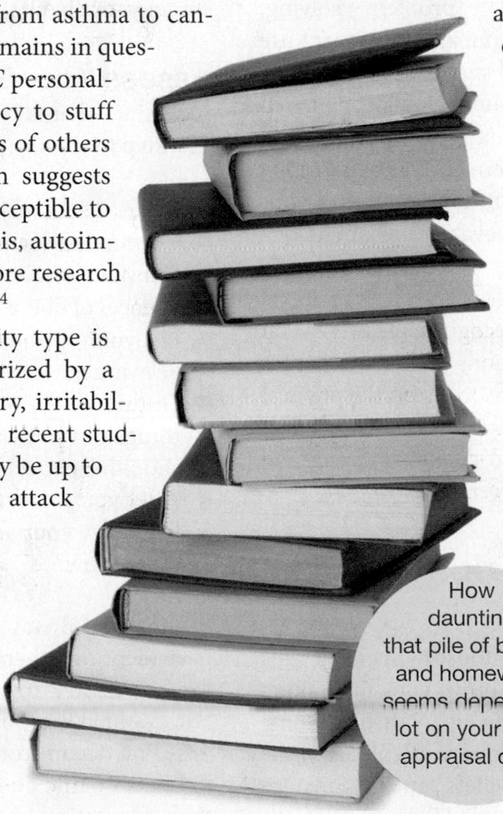

How daunting that pile of books and homework seems depends a lot on your own appraisal of it.

their lives, and staying optimistic and positive. These "**shift and persist**" strategies are among the most recently identified factors that protect against the negative effects of too much stress in our lives.[50]

LO 6 | MANAGING STRESS IN COLLEGE

Explore stress-management techniques and ways to enrich your life with positive experiences and attitudes.

College students thrive under a certain amount of stress; however, excessive stress can leave them overwhelmed and unable to cope. Recent studies of college students indicate that the emotional health self-rating of first-year college students is at an all-time low. At the same time, increased percentages (nearly 65%) report feeling overwhelmed during the last 2-week to 1-month period. These same students report more emotional reactivity in the form of anger, hostility, frustration, and a greater sense of being out of control.[51] Sophomores and juniors reported fewer problems with these issues, and seniors reported the fewest problems. This may indicate students' progressive emotional growth through experience, maturity, increased awareness of support services, and more social connections.[52]

Numerous researchers have found stress among young adults to be correlated to unhealthy behaviors such as substance abuse, lack of physical activity, poor psychological and physical health, lack of social problem solving, depression, and infrequent use of social support networks.[53]

shift and persist A strategy of reframing appraisals of current stressors and focusing on a meaningful future that protects a person from the negative effects of too much stress.

coping Managing events or conditions to lessen the physical or psychological effects of excess stress.

stress inoculation Stress-management technique in which a person consciously anticipates and prepares for potential stressors.

Newfound independence in college may pose challenges, but it also provides an opportunity for you to take control of your life, to evaluate your unique situation, and to take steps that fit your schedule and lifestyle to reduce negative stressors. Although you can't eliminate all life stressors, you can train yourself to recognize the events that cause stress and to anticipate your reactions to them. **Coping** is the act of managing events or conditions to lessen the physical or psychological effects of excess stress.[54] One of the most effective ways to combat stressors is to build coping strategies and skills, known collectively as *stress-management techniques*.

Practicing Mental Work to Reduce Stress

Stress management isn't something that just happens. It calls for getting a handle on what is going on in your life, taking a careful look at yourself, and coming up with a personal plan of action. Because your perceptions are often part of the problem, assessing your "self-talk," beliefs, and actions are good first steps. Why are you so stressed? How much of it is due to perception rather than reality? What's a realistic plan of action for you? Think about your situation and map out a strategy for change. The tools in this section will help you.

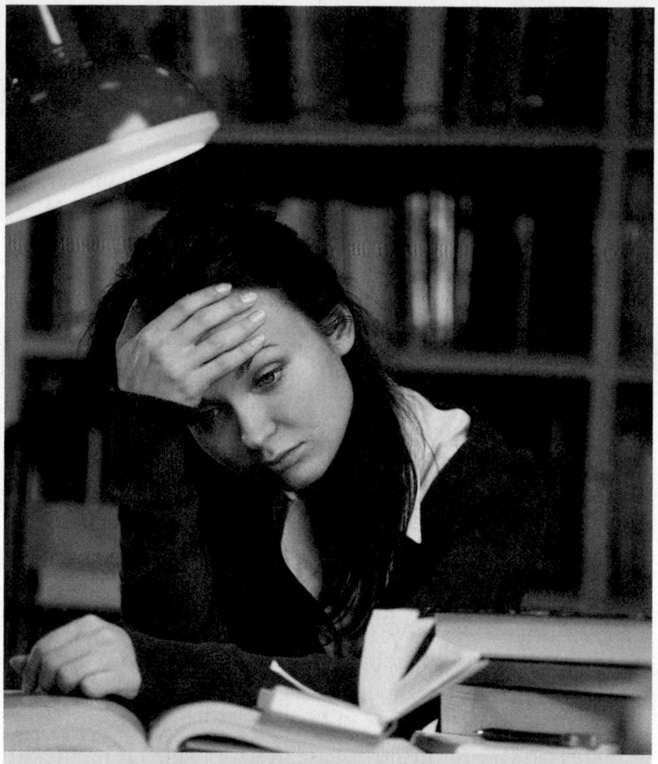

Studies suggest college students are more stressed out than other groups—the combination of new environment, peer and parent pressures, and juggling the demands of work, school, and a social life likely contribute to this phenomenon.

Assess Your Stressors and Solve Problems

Assessing what is really going on in your life is an important first step to solving problems and reducing stress. Here's how:

- Make a list of major things you are worried about right now.
- Examine the causes of the problems and worries.
- Consider how big each problem is. What are the consequences of doing nothing versus taking action?
- List your options, including ones that you may not like very much.
- Outline an action plan, and *act*. Remember that even little things can sometimes make a big difference and that you shouldn't expect immediate results.
- After you act, evaluate. How did you do? Do you need to change your actions to achieve a better outcome next time? How?

One useful way of coping with your stressors, once you have identified them, is to consciously anticipate and prepare for specific stressors, a technique known as **stress inoculation**. For example, suppose that speaking in front of a class scares you. Practice in front of friends or in front of a video camera to banish panic and prevent your freezing up on the day of the presentation.

Change How You Think and Talk to Yourself As noted earlier, our appraisal of people and situations and our own self-talk can increase stress in subtle ways. Several types of negative self-talk exist, but among the most common are *pessimism,* or focusing on the negative; *perfectionism,* or expecting superhuman standards; *"shoulding,"* or reprimanding yourself for items that you should have done; *blaming* yourself or others for circumstances and events; and *dichotomous thinking,* in which everything is either black or white (good or bad) instead of gradations. To combat negative self-talk, we must first become aware of it, then stop it, and finally replace the negative thoughts with positive ones—a process referred to as **cognitive restructuring**. Once you realize that some of your thoughts may be negative, irrational, or overreactive, interrupt this self-talk by saying "stop" (under your breath or out loud) and make a conscious effort to think positively.

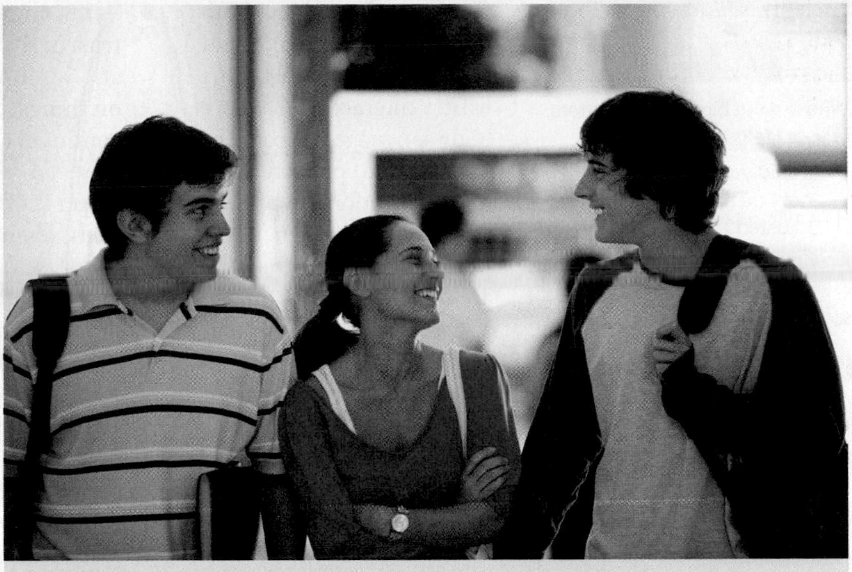

Spending time communicating and socializing can be an important part of building a support network and reducing your stress level

80%

OF ALL AMERICANS SAY THEIR STRESS LEVELS HAVE STAYED THE SAME OR INCREASED IN THE LAST YEAR, BUT ONLY 37% OF AMERICANS FEEL THEY ARE ACTUALLY DOING AN EXCELLENT OR VERY GOOD JOB OF **MANAGING** THEIR STRESS.

Developing a Support Network

As you plan a stress-management program, remember the importance of social networks and social bonds. Friendships are important for inoculating yourself against harmful stressors. Studies of college students have demonstrated the importance of social support in *buffering* individuals from the effects of stress.[55] It isn't necessary to have a large number of friends. However, different friends often serve different needs, so having more than one is usually beneficial.

Find Supportive People Family members and friends are often a steady base of support when the pressures of life seem overwhelming. But if friends or family are unavailable or if your friends tend to bring you down rather than build you up, most colleges and universities offer counseling services at no cost for short-term crises. Clergy, instructors, and residence hall supervisors also may be excellent resources, and most communities offer low-cost counseling through mental health clinics.

Invest in Your Loved Ones Imagine if you had absolutely no one you could call when you were in financial trouble or had a death in the family. Many people find that they've spent so much time pushing ahead in careers or self-improvement that they are alone at the worst times of their lives. As our lives get busy and obligations become overwhelming, we often don't make time for the very people who are most important to us: our friends, family, and other loved ones. To have a healthy social support network, we have to invest time and energy. Cultivate and nurture the relationships that matter: those built on trust, mutual acceptance and understanding, honesty, and genuine caring. If you want others to be there for you to help you cope with life's stressors, you need to be there for them.

cognitive restructuring The modification of thoughts, ideas, and beliefs that contribute to stress.

Cultivating Your Spiritual Side

One of the most important factors in reducing overall stress in your life is making the time and commitment to cultivate your spiritual side: finding your purpose in life and living your days more fully. Spiritual health and spiritual practices can be vital components of your support system, often linking you to a community of like-minded individuals and giving you perspective on the things that truly matter in your life. (For more information, see **Focus On: Cultivating Your Spiritual Health** beginning on page 61.)

Managing Emotional Responses

Have you ever gotten all worked up about something only to find that your perceptions were totally wrong? We often get upset not by realities, but rather by our faulty perceptions. Social networking sites and e-mails are often perfect places

WHAT DO YOU THINK?

Who are the biggest supporters in your life?

- Would you characterize them as stressed out or well-adjusted?
- Could you follow their lead if they are more relaxed?
- What tips would you give them if they're stressed?

for reading meaning into things that are said and perceiving issues that don't exist. Interactions where body language, voice intonation, and opportunities for clarification are present are much better for interpreting true meanings than are cryptic texts or e-mails.

Stress management requires that you learn to tell the difference between normal emotions and emotions based on irrational beliefs or expressed and interpreted in an over-the-top manner and requires you to either stop the emotion or express it in a healthy and appropriate way.

Fight the Anger Urge Anger usually results when we feel we have lost control of a situation or are frustrated by a situation that we can do little about. Major sources of anger include (1) perceived *threats* to self or others we care about; (2) *reactions to injustice* such as unfair actions, policies, or behaviors; (3) *fear,* which leads to negative responses; (4) *faulty emotional reasoning,* or misinterpretation of normal events; (5) *low frustration tolerance,* often fueled by stress, drugs, lack of sleep, and other factors; (6) *unreasonable expectations* about ourselves and others; and (7) *people rating,* or applying derogatory ratings to others.

There are three main approaches to dealing with anger: *expressing it, suppressing it,* or *calming it.* You may be surprised to find out that expressing anger is probably the healthiest thing to do in the long run, if you express anger in an assertive rather than an aggressive way. However, it's natural to react aggressively, and we must learn to keep that reaction at bay. There are several strategies you can use.[56]

- **Identify your anger style.** Do you express anger passively or actively? Do you hold anger in, or do you explode? Do you throw the phone, smash things, or scream at others?
- **Learn to recognize patterns in your anger responses and how to de-escalate them.** For 1 week, keep track of everything that angers you or keeps you stewing. What thoughts or feelings lead up to your boiling point? Keep a journal and listen to your anger. Try to change your self-talk. Explore ways to interrupt patterns of anger, such as counting to ten, getting a drink of water, or taking some deep breaths.
- **Find the right words to de-escalate conflict.** Communicate to de-escalate. When conflict arises, be respectful and state your needs or feelings rather than shooting zingers at the other person. Avoid "you always" or "you never" and instead say, "I feel___ when you____" or "I would really appreciate it if you could___." If you find you are continually revved up for a battle, consider taking a class or workshop on assertiveness training or anger management.
- **Plan ahead.** Explore options to minimize your exposure to anger-provoking situations such as traffic jams.
- **Vent to your friends.** Find a few close friends you trust and who can be honest with you about your situation. Allow them to listen and give their perspectives on things, but don't wear down your supporter with continual rants.
- **Develop realistic expectations of yourself and others.** Anger is often the result of unmet expectations, frustrations, resentments, and impatience. Are your expectations of yourself and others realistic? Pick your battles. When upset, don't send nasty texts or emails as a knee jerk reaction. Take time to chill, and then try communicating your feelings, calmly.
- **Turn complaints into requests.** When frustrated or angry with someone, try reworking the problem into a request. Instead of screaming and pounding on the wall because your neighbors are blaring music at 2 A.M., talk with them. Think about the words you will use, and try to reach an agreement that works for everyone.
- **Leave past anger in the past.** Learn to resolve issues and not bring them up over and over. If you can't, seek the counsel of a professional to learn how.

Learn to Laugh, Be Joyful, and Cry Have you ever noticed that you feel better after a belly laugh or a good cry? Adages such as "laughter is the best medicine" and "smile and the world smiles with you" didn't evolve out of the blue. Humans have long recognized that smiling, laughing, singing, dancing, and other actions can elevate our moods, relieve stress, and help us improve our relationships. Learning to laugh at your own silly actions and taking yourself less seriously is a good starting place. Crying can have similar positive physiological effects in relieving tension. Several studies have indicated that laughter and joy may increase endorphin levels, increase oxygen levels in the blood, decrease stress levels, relieve pain, enhance productivity, and reduce risks of chronic disease; the evidence for *long-term* effects on immune functioning and protective effects for chronic diseases is only just starting to be understood.[57] For ideas on how to find more joy in your daily life, see the **Health Headlines** box.

Taking Physical Action

Are you feeling sluggish and ready to nap too much of the time? Or are you feeling wired, restless, and ready to explode? Both reactions could be the result of too much stress.

Get Enough Exercise Remember that the human stress response is intended to end in physical activity. Exercise "burns off" existing stress hormones by directing them toward their intended metabolic function.[58] Exercise can also help combat stress by raising levels of endorphins—mood-elevating, painkilling hormones—in the bloodstream, increasing energy, reducing hostility, and improving mental alertness. Still, according to a recent meta-analysis of stress and exercise research, those who would benefit most—particularly sedentary, overweight individuals—are more likely to eat when they are stressed and less likely to

@ HEALTH HEADLINES

HAPPINESS AND FLOURISHING

New Strategies to Reduce Stress

For decades, noted psychologist Martin Seligman has conducted research focused on *positive psychology* and *authentic happiness*. His work has been the framework for a new way of looking at life with a more "glass half full" perspective. His theories have carried over into new movements to help us find happiness in the face of adversity, with research supporting the idea that people who are optimistic and happier have fewer mental and physical problems. Today, Seligman takes happiness a step further, focusing on the concept of "flourishing," which consists of *positive emotion, engagement, relationships, meaning, and accomplishments* (PERMA). With these elements in your life, positive psychologists believe that you will flourish in all aspects of life, avoid stress, and be healthier.

- **Positive Emotion:** Take time to get to know people's names. Share highs of the day rather than lows. Be active in complimenting others, verbalize their strengths, laugh, show appreciation, be kind. Be real with others. When you start to assess people in the negative, find something *good* about them. Ditch the negative thoughts!
- **Engagement:** Practice mindfulness. See, hear, touch, feel—experience your present. Live and notice the moments, rather than focusing on the past or the future. Make time for things that bring you joy, and remember to be good to others.
- **Relationships:** Listen and ask questions. Connect in *person*. Look people in the eyes. Empower others to see their strengths. Hug freely. Be honest and sincere. Check in to show that you care. Acknowledge that people matter.
- **Meaning:** Think about how you would like to be remembered. Show appreciation. Give to others, and show your emotions. Renew and refresh continually. Read and explore new things. Learn about different cultures and history. Work to help others. Bring happiness to them. Improve the world. Cherish the environment.
- **Achievement:** What are the steps to achieving your goals? Try new things; don't be afraid to fail. View change as opportunity. Celebrate accomplishments; both yours and those of others. Acknowledge the good things that others do. Remember the little things that are important in your day. Give praise, and be unselfish in your support to others.

While flourishing offers an expanded approach to individual and community well-being, another group has developed the Action for Happiness movement—a ten-step set of recommendations designed to provide momentum for actions that will lead to a more positive society. Among these ten keys to happier living are the following recommendations:

- Do things for others.
- Connect with people.
- Take care of your body.
- Notice the world around you.
- Keep learning new things.
- Have goals to look forward to.
- Find ways to bounce back.
- Take a positive approach.
- Be comfortable with who you are.
- Be part of something bigger.

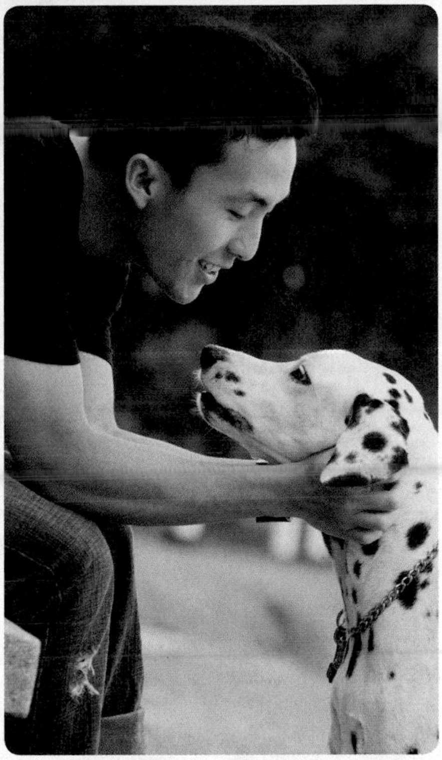

Four-legged friends can be great stress relievers as they allow you to focus on something besides yourself and can add laughter to your life.

Sources: M. E. Seligman, *Flourishing: A Visionary New Understanding of Happiness and Well-Being,* (New York, NY: Free Press/Simon and Schuster, 2011); M. E. P. Seligman, *Authentic Happiness: Using the New Positive Psychology to Realize Your Potential for Lasting Fulfillment* (New York, NY: Free Press/Simon & Schuster, 2002). Action for Happiness website: www.actionforhappiness.org/10-keys-to-happier-living.

exercise. Motivating people unready to exercise for health and stress relief is a major challenge that could reap huge rewards.[59] (For more information on the beneficial effects of exercise, see **Chapter 9**.)

Get Enough Sleep Adequate amounts of sleep allow you to refresh your vital energy, cope with multiple stressors more effectively, and be productive when you need to be. In fact, sleep is one of the biggest stress busters of them all. (These benefits and others are discussed in much more depth in **Focus On: Improving Your Sleep** beginning on page 98.)

Practice Self-Nurturing Find time each day for something fun—something that you enjoy and that calms you. Take a hot bath, get a massage, and allow yourself a set amount of guilt-free time texting or chatting with friends. Turn on your iPod or MP3 and listen to your favorite songs. Remember that taking time out for you should be a part of every day. Like exercise, relaxation can help you cope with

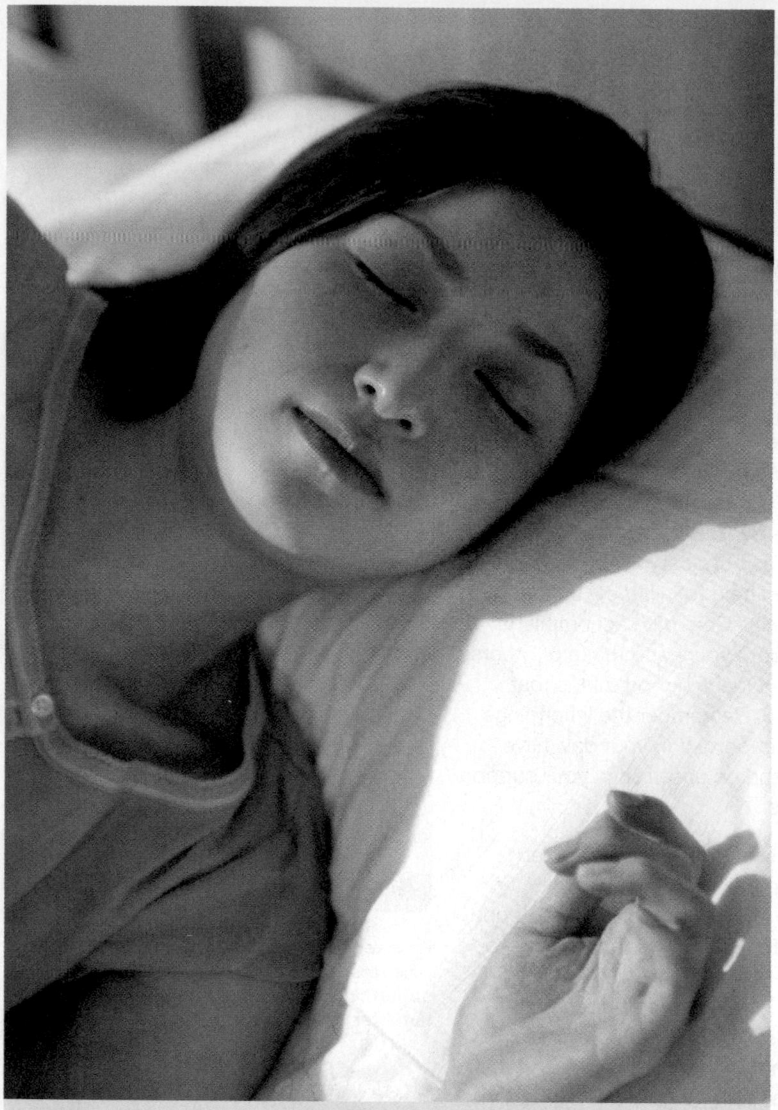

Taking care of your physical health—through quality sleep, sufficient exercise, and healthful nutrition—is a crucial component of stress management.

despite being worse off because of it. Procrastination results in academic difficulties, financial problems, relationship problems, and a multitude of stress-related ailments.

How can you avoid the procrastination bug? According to psychologist Peter Gollwitzer and colleagues, setting clear "implementation intentions," a series of goals to accomplish toward a specific end, is key.[60] Having a plan that includes specific deadlines (and rewards for meeting deadlines) can help you stay on task. Start with a simple plan and be flexible. Another strategy is to get started early and set a personal end date that is well ahead of the deadline.

Keep a journal for 2 days to become aware of how you spend your time. Write down your activities every day—everything from going to class to doing your laundry to texting your friends—and the amount of time you spend doing each. What can you do to make better use of your time? Use the following time-management tips in your stress-management program:

- **Do one thing at a time.** Don't try to watch television, wash clothes, and write your term paper all at once. Stay focused.
- **Clean off your desk.** Go through the things on your desk, toss unnecessary papers, and keep important documents in folders. Read your mail, recycle what you don't need, and file what you will need later. (For more on organizing to de-stress, see the **Student Health Today** box.)
- **Prioritize your tasks.** Make a daily "to do" list and stick to it. Categorize the things you must do today, the things that must eventually get done, and the things that it would be nice to do. Consider the "nice to do" items only if you finish the others (or if they include something fun).
- **Find a clean, comfortable place to work, and avoid interruptions.** When you have a project that requires total concentration, schedule uninterrupted time. Don't answer the phone, close your door and post a "Do Not Disturb" sign, or go to a quiet room in the library or student union.
- **Reward yourself for work completed.** When you finish a task, do something nice for yourself. Rest breaks give you time to yourself to help you recharge and refresh your energy levels.
- **Work when you're at your best.** If you're a morning person, study and write papers in the morning, and take breaks when you start to slow down.
- **Remember that time is precious.** Many people learn to value their time only when they face a terminal illness. Try to value each day. If you have trouble saying no to people and projects that steal your time, see the **Skills for Behavior Change** box for some suggestions.

sympathomimetics Food substances that can produce stresslike physiological responses.

procrastinate To intentionally put off doing something.

stressful feelings, as well as preserve and refocus your energies.

Eat Healthfully
It is clear that eating a balanced, healthy diet will help provide the stamina you need to get through problems and will stress-proof you in ways that are not fully understood. It is also known that undereating, overeating, and eating the wrong kinds of foods can create distress in the body. In particular, avoid **sympathomimetics**, foods that produce (or mimic) stresslike responses, such as caffeine. (For more information about the benefits of sound nutrition, see **Chapter 7**.)

Managing Your Time

Ever put off writing a paper until the night before it was due? We all **procrastinate**—voluntarily delay doing some task

STUDENT HEALTH TODAY

FENG SHUI FOR STRESS RELIEF

Today, many space designers are trying to create peaceful "me caves" for reducing the stress of harried lives. One strategy, known as *feng shui* (translation "wind and water"), is part of an ancient Chinese art designed to restore balance of *chi* and create peace and harmony with help from the built environment. There are several feng shui tips for reducing stress in your bedroom area:

1. **De-clutter.** Get rid of any extra "things" in your space. Pick up and put things away each day.
2. **Paint.** Use peaceful and welcoming colors. Coordinate linens and tapestry colors to enhance warmth.
3. **Relocate.** Your bed should never be in line with the door; nightstands should be balanced on either side of bed, and mirrors should *never* reflect the bed.
4. **Shut out the world.** Use shades that allow you to darken or dim the room.
5. **Beautify.** Include things that make you feel peaceful.
6. **Invest.** Get a set of soft sheets, duvet covers, and blankets. Plump and soften pillows.
7. **Refresh.** Open windows to remove stale odors. If needed, use relaxing fragrances such as lavender.
8. **Block.** If you can't get rid of a desk covered in work, use a curtain to keep things out of sight. Put your phone away, and *relax*.

How might you balance the *chi* in your environment?

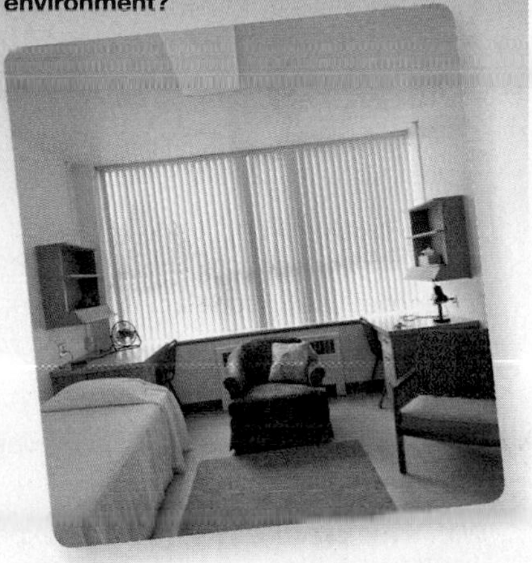

SKILLS FOR BEHAVIOR CHANGE

LEARN TO SAY NO AND MEAN IT!

Is your calendar always so full you barely have time to breathe? Are you unable to say no to other people? When you're asked to do something you don't really want to do, practice the following tips to avoid overcommitment:

- **Be sympathetic, but firm.** Explain that although you think it's a great cause or idea, you just can't take on one more project right now. Don't waver if they persist in pressuring you.
- **Don't say you want to think about it and will get back to them.** This only leads to more forceful requests later.
- **Don't give in to guilt.** Stick to your guns. Remember you don't owe anyone your time.
- **Even if something sounds good, avoid spontaneous "yes" responses to new projects.** Make a rule that you will take at least a day to think about committing your time.
- **Schedule time for yourself first.** If you don't have time for the things you love to do, stop and prioritize your activities. Don't let time get sucked up doing things you don't want to do.

Consider Downshifting

Today's lifestyles are hectic, and stress often comes from trying to keep up. Many people are questioning whether "having it all" is worth it and are taking a step back and simplifying their lives. This trend has been labeled **downshifting**, or *voluntary simplicity*. Moving from a large urban area to a smaller town, leaving a high-paying and high-stress job for one that makes you happy, de-cluttering your life, and making a host of other changes in lifestyle typify downshifting.

downshifting Taking a step back and simplifying a lifestyle that is hectic, packed with pressure and stress, and focused on trying to keep up; also known as *voluntary simplicity*.

Downshifting involves a fundamental alteration in values and honest introspection about what is important in life. It means cutting down on shopping habits, buying only what you need, and living within modest means. When you contemplate any form of downshift (or start your career this way), it's important to move slowly and consider the following:

- **Complete a financial inventory.** How much money will you need to do the things you want to do? Will you live alone or share costs with roommates? Do you need a car, or can you rely on public transportation? (See **Focus On: Improving Your Financial Health** for more on assessing your finances.)
- **Develop an expense plan.** Manage your budget and plan ahead for things like college tuition, book costs, rent, food, and entertainment expenses. It's also extremely

TECH & HEALTH | APPS FOR THE RELAXATION RESPONSE

Looking for a way to relax that you can carry with you? Check out the following apps to help you de-stress.

- **Stress Check** (Free: Android, iPhone, iPod), www.azumio.com/apps/stress-check

This nifty app has a stress gauge and heart monitor onboard. Just put your finger over your phone's camera hole; it will pick up your heart rate and give you readouts.

- **Pocket Yoga** (Modest cost: iPhone), http://pocket-sports.com

With three practices designed by experienced instructors, three levels of difficulty, and three session durations, you can tailor the app to your needs. Both visual and voice-over instructions are included.

- **Breathe2Relax** (Free: Android, iPhone, iPod, iPad), http://t2health.org/apps/breathe2relax

This relaxation tool uses guided information to help you learn and practice diaphragmatic breathing.

- **Ambiance** (Modest cost: Android, iPhone, iPod, iPad, Desktop), http://ambianceapp.com

This app is marketed as an "environmental enhancer" and includes over 2,500 downloadable sounds, from ocean waves to electronic sounds and music.

- **GPS for the Soul** (Free: iPhone), www.heartmath.org/free-services/solutions-for-stress/gps-for-the-soul.html

This app uses your device's camera to gauge stress levels by measuring your heart rate. It contains guided meditation, poetry, visuals, sound or music, and a breathing pacer to help you relax.

There is a broad array of stress management and relaxation apps. Remember, technology can be a stressor if you let it, but you can also use it to beat stress.

important to understand your health insurance plan so that you know what services are covered and what you have to cover.

- **Make both short- and long-term plans for simplifying your life.** Set up your plans in doable steps, and work slowly toward each step.
- **Select the right career.** Look for work that you enjoy and think about whether enjoyment and financial goals are compatible. Happiness isn't necessarily driven by salary. Can you be happy taking a lower-paying job if it is less stressful?
- **Consider options for saving money.** Downshifting doesn't mean you renounce money; it means you choose not to let money rule your life. Saving is still important. If you're just getting started, you need to prepare for emergencies and for future plans.

Relaxation Techniques for Stress Management

Relaxation techniques to reduce stress have been practiced for centuries and offer opportunities for calming your nervous energy and coping with life's challenges. Some common techniques include yoga, qigong, tai chi, deep breathing, meditation, visualization, progressive muscle relaxation, massage therapy, biofeedback, and hypnosis. Newer forms of relaxation may be found in the latest technology; see the **Tech & Health** box for more information.

Not enough money to cover all those monthly purchases can be a major stressor.

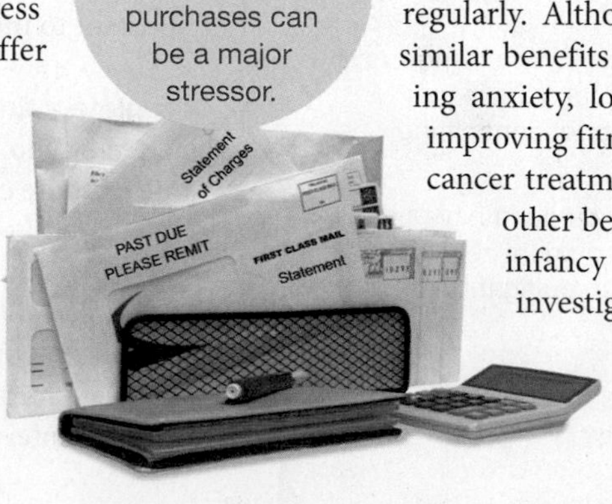

Yoga Yoga is an ancient practice that combines meditation, stretching, and breathing exercises designed to relax, refresh, and rejuvenate. It began about 5,000 years ago in India and has been evolving ever since. Although exact numbers are difficult to obtain, approximately 20.4 million Americans practice yoga, according to a recent study. The majority of these people are women between the ages of 18 and 44. The most common reasons reported were general conditioning, stress relief, fitness and flexibility, and improvements in overall health.[61]

Classical yoga is the ancestor of nearly all modern forms of yoga. Breathing, poses, and verbal mantras are often part of classical yoga. Of the many branches of classical yoga, *Hatha yoga* is best known because it is the most body focused. Hatha yoga involves the practice of breath control and *asanas*—held postures and choreographed movements that enhance strength and flexibility. (Several other, more athletic, forms of yoga are discussed in **Chapter 9**.) Recent research shows increased evidence of benefits of Hatha yoga in reducing inflammation, boosting mood, increasing relaxation, and reducing stress among those who practice regularly. Although studies have shown yoga to have similar benefits in treating insomnia and PTSD, reducing anxiety, lowering heart rate and blood pressure, improving fitness and flexibility, providing relief from cancer treatment pain, alleviating low back pain, and other benefits, much of this research is still in its infancy and could benefit from more rigorous investigation.[62]

Qigong *Qigong* (pronounced "chee-kong"), one of the fastest-growing and most widely accepted forms of mind-body health exercises, is used by some of the country's largest health care organizations, particularly for people suffering from chronic pain or stress. Qigong is an ancient Chinese practice that involves becoming aware of and learning to control *qi* (or *chi,* pronounced "chee")—vital energy in your body. According to Chinese medicine, a complex system of internal pathways called *meridians* carry *qi* throughout your body. If your *qi* becomes stagnant or blocked, you'll feel sluggish or powerless. Qigong incorporates a series of flowing movements, breathing techniques, mental visualization exercises, and vocalizations of healing sounds designed to restore balance and integrate and refresh the mind and body.

Tai Chi *Tai chi* (pronounced "ty-chee") is sometimes described as "meditation in motion." Originally developed in China as a form of self-defense, this graceful form of exercise has existed for about 2,000 years. Tai chi is noncompetitive and self-paced. To do tai chi, you perform a defined series of postures or movements in a slow, graceful manner. Each movement or posture flows into the next without pause. Tai chi has been widely practiced in China for centuries and is now becoming increasingly popular around the world, both as a basic exercise program and as a complement to other health care methods. Health benefits include stress reduction, greater balance, and increased flexibility.

Diaphragmatic or Deep Breathing Typically, we breathe using only the upper chest and thoracic region rather than involving the abdominal region. Simply stated, diaphragmatic breathing is deep breathing that maximally fills the lungs by involving the movement of the diaphragm and lower abdomen. This technique is commonly used in yoga exercises and in other meditative practices. (Try the diaphragmatic breathing exercise in **FIGURE 3.5** right now and see whether you feel more relaxed!)

Meditation There are many different forms of **meditation**. Most involve sitting quietly for 15 or 20 minutes, focusing on a particular word or symbol, and controlling breathing. Practiced by Eastern religions for centuries, meditation is believed to be an important form of introspection and personal renewal. In stress management, it can calm the body and quiet the mind, creating a sense of peace. A recent review of accumulated research found that one form of meditation, *transcendental meditation* (TM), results in adults reducing their blood pressure as well as need for blood pressure medications. Importantly, TM reduced symptoms of angina, CVD risks, and overall CVD mortality.[63] (Meditation and other aspects of spiritual health

meditation A relaxation technique that involves deep breathing and concentration.

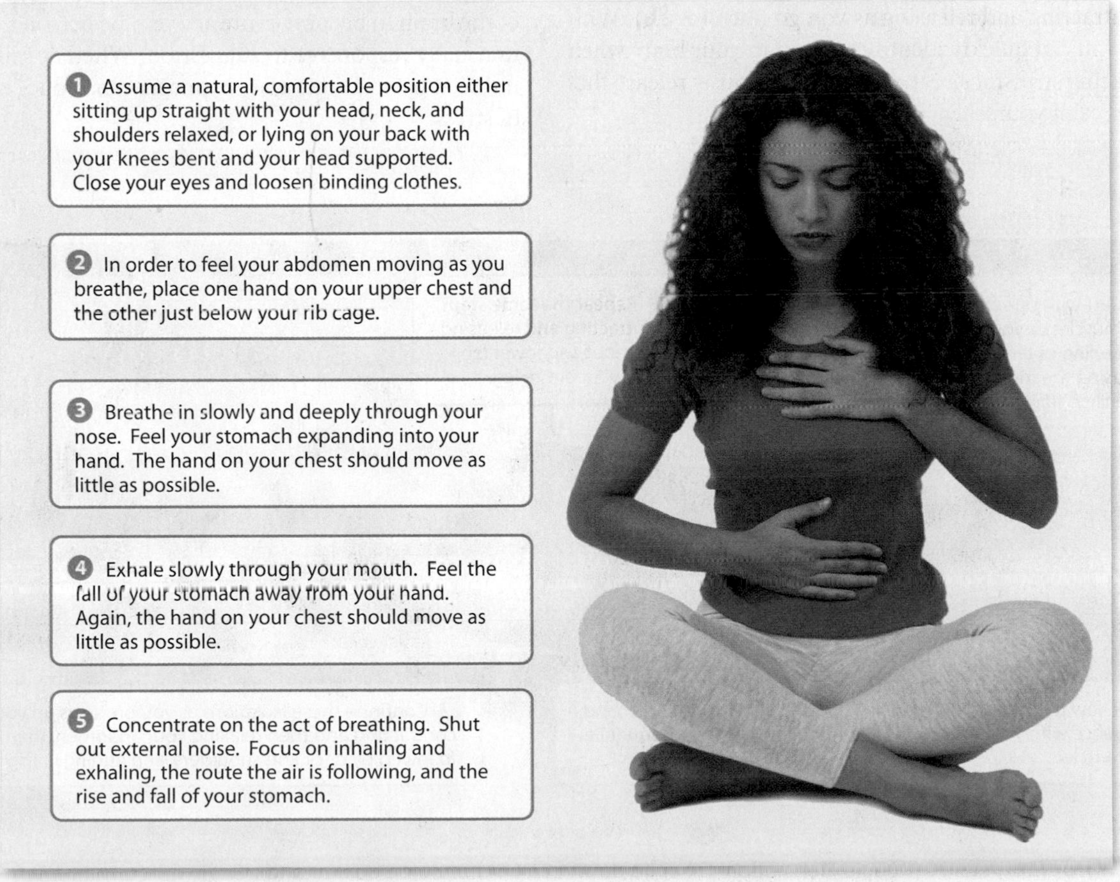

1 Assume a natural, comfortable position either sitting up straight with your head, neck, and shoulders relaxed, or lying on your back with your knees bent and your head supported. Close your eyes and loosen binding clothes.
2 In order to feel your abdomen moving as you breathe, place one hand on your upper chest and the other just below your rib cage.
3 Breathe in slowly and deeply through your nose. Feel your stomach expanding into your hand. The hand on your chest should move as little as possible.
4 Exhale slowly through your mouth. Feel the fall of your stomach away from your hand. Again, the hand on your chest should move as little as possible.
5 Concentrate on the act of breathing. Shut out external noise. Focus on inhaling and exhaling, the route the air is following, and the rise and fall of your stomach.

FIGURE 3.5 Diaphragmatic Breathing This exercise will help you learn to breathe deeply as a way to relieve stress. Practice this for 5 to 10 minutes several times a day, and soon diaphragmatic breathing will become natural for you.

visualization The creation of mental images to promote relaxation.

biofeedback A technique using a machine to self-monitor physical responses to stress.

hypnosis A trancelike state that allows people to become unusually responsive to suggestion.

are discussed in detail in **Focus On: Cultivating Your Spiritual Health** beginning on page 61.) Meditation can be performed alone or in a group. Many colleges and universities offer classes on how to meditate. Check with your campus wellness center.

Visualization Often, our thoughts and imagination provoke distress by conjuring up worst-case scenarios. Our imagination, however, can also be tapped to reduce stress. In **visualization**, you use your imagination to visualize calming scenes. The choice of mental images is unlimited, but natural settings such as ocean beaches and mountain lakes are often used to represent stress-free environments. Recalling physical sensations of sight, sound, smell, taste, and touch can replace stressful stimuli with peaceful or pleasurable thoughts. Try to make your visualization as real and detailed as possible.

Progressive Muscle Relaxation Progressive muscle relaxation involves teaching awareness of the feeling of tension and release by systematically contracting and relaxing different muscle groups in your body. The standard pattern is to begin with the feet and work your way up your body, contracting and releasing as you go (**FIGURE 3.6**). With practice, you can quickly identify tension in your body when you are facing stressful situations and consciously release that tension to calm yourself.

Massage Therapy If you have ever had someone massage your stiff neck, you know that massage not only feels great, it is also an excellent way to relax. Techniques vary from deep-tissue massage to the gentler acupressure. One study indicates that Swedish massage may have beneficial effects on hormones that regulate blood pressure and reduce inflammation, as well as invoke a general relaxation response in the body.[64] Though promising, research on the effectiveness of massage as a stress-reducer, pain reliever, and mood enhancer is in its infancy. (**Chapter 18** provides more information about the benefits of massage and other body-based methods.)

Biofeedback **Biofeedback** is a technique in which a person learns to use the mind to consciously control body functions like heart rate, body temperature, and breathing rate. Using machines from those as simple as stress dots that change color with body temperature variation to sophisticated electrical sensors, individuals learn to listen to their bodies and make necessary adjustments, such as relaxing certain muscles, changing breathing, or concentrating to slow heart rate and relax. Eventually, individuals develop the ability to recognize and lower stress responses without machines and can practice it anywhere.

Hypnosis **Hypnosis** requires a person to focus on one thought, object, or voice, thereby freeing the right hemisphere of the brain to become more active. The person then becomes unusually responsive to suggestion. Whether self-induced or induced by someone else, hypnosis can reduce certain types of stress.

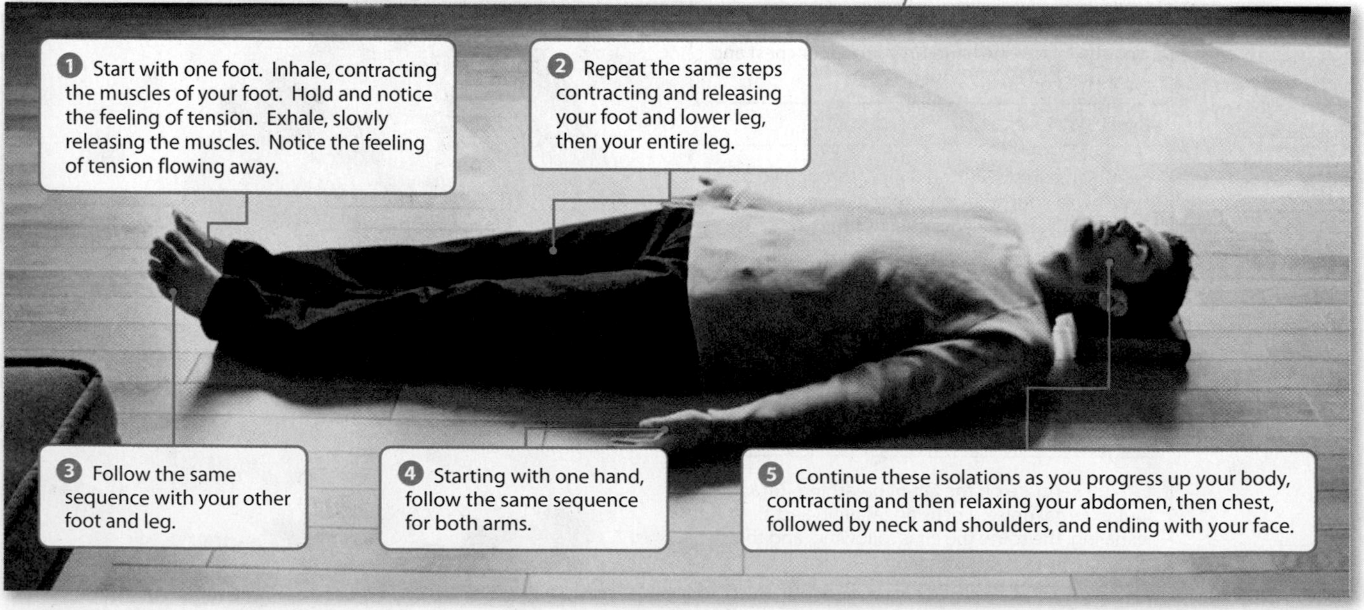

1 Start with one foot. Inhale, contracting the muscles of your foot. Hold and notice the feeling of tension. Exhale, slowly releasing the muscles. Notice the feeling of tension flowing away.
2 Repeat the same steps contracting and releasing your foot and lower leg, then your entire leg.
3 Follow the same sequence with your other foot and leg.
4 Starting with one hand, follow the same sequence for both arms.
5 Continue these isolations as you progress up your body, contracting and then relaxing your abdomen, then chest, followed by neck and shoulders, and ending with your face.

FIGURE 3.6 Progressive Muscle Relaxation Sit or lie down in a comfortable position and follow the steps described to increase your awareness of tension in your body.

STUDY PLAN

Customize your study plan—and master your health!—in the Study Area of **MasteringHealth.**

ASSESS YOURSELF

Is stress negatively affecting your life? Want to find out? Take the **How Stressed Are You?** assessment available on MasteringHealth.™

Need help creating a plan? Follow the strategies in the **Your Plan for Change** box for short- and long-term improvements to your health.

YOUR PLAN FOR CHANGE

Use the **ASSESS YOURSELF** activity "How Stressed Are You?" to rate your stress level. If it is higher than desired, use these tips to reduce stress.

TODAY, YOU CAN:

- ☐ Practice one new stress-management technique. For example, you could spend 10 minutes doing a deep-breathing exercise or find a good spot on campus to meditate.
- ☐ In a journal, write down stressful events or symptoms of stress that you experience. Try to focus on intense emotional experiences and explore how they affect you.

WITHIN THE NEXT 2 WEEKS, YOU CAN:

- ☐ Attend a class or workshop on a stress-relieving activity. Look for beginner classes offered on campus or in your community.
- ☐ Make a list of the papers, projects, and tests that you have over the coming semester and create a schedule for them. Break projects and term papers into small, manageable tasks with a plan for completing each. Try to be realistic about how much time you'll need to get these tasks done.

BY THE END OF THE SEMESTER, YOU CAN:

- ☐ Keep track of the money you spend and where it goes. Establish a budget, and follow it for at least a month.
- ☐ Find some form of exercise you can do regularly. You may consider joining a gym or just arranging regular "walk dates" or pickup basketball games with your friends. Try to exercise at least 30 minutes every day. (See **Chapter 9** for more information about physical fitness.)

CHAPTER REVIEW

To hear an MP3 Tutor Session, scan here or visit the Study Area in **MasteringHealth.**

LO 1 What Is Stress?

- Stress is always part of life. *Eustress* refers to stress associated with positive events; *distress* is stress associated with negative events.

LO 2 Body Responses to Stress

- The alarm, resistance, and exhaustion phases of the general adaptation syndrome (GAS) involve physiological responses to both real and imagined stressors and cause complex hormonal reactions.

LO 3 Lifetime Effects of Stress

- Undue stress for extended periods of time can compromise the immune system. Stress has been linked to numerous health problems, including cardiovascular disease (CVD), weight gain, hair loss, diabetes, digestive problems, and increased susceptibility to infectious diseases. *Psychoneuroimmunology* is the study of stress and the immune response.

LO 4 Intellectual Effects of Stress

- Stress can have negative impacts on your intellectual and psychological health, including impaired memory, poor concentration, depression, anxiety, and other disorders.

LO 5 What Causes Stress?

- Psychosocial factors that impact stress include change, hassles, relationships, pressure, conflict, overload, financial pressures, and environmental stressors. Discrimination or bias may cause unusually high stress. Some sources are internal and are related to appraisal, self-esteem, self-efficacy, personality, and psychological hardiness.

LO 6 Managing Stress in College

- College can be especially stressful. Managing stress begins with learning coping skills. Managing emotional responses, examining perceptions, adjusting to change, taking mental or physical action, downshifting, managing finances and time, setting goals, and/or learning relaxation techniques will help you cope in the long run.

POP QUIZ

Visit **MasteringHealth** to personalize your study plan with Chapter Review Quizzes and Dynamic Study Modules.

LO 1 What Is Stress?

1. Even though Andre experienced stress when he graduated from college and moved to a new city, he viewed these changes as an opportunity for growth. What is Andre's stress called?
   a. Strain
   b. Distress
   c. Eustress
   d. Adaptive response

LO 2 Body Responses to Stress

2. In which stage of the general adaptation syndrome does the fight-or-flight response occur?
   a. Exhaustion stage
   b. Alarm stage
   c. Resistance stage
   d. Response stage
3. The branch of the autonomic nervous system that is responsible for energizing the body for either fight or flight and for triggering many other stress responses is the
   a. central nervous system.
   b. parasympathetic nervous system.
   c. sympathetic nervous system.
   d. endocrine system.

LO 3 Lifetime Effects of Stress

4. The area of scientific investigation that analyzes the relationship between the mind's response to stress and the immune system's ability to function effectively is called
   a. psychoneuroimmunology.
   b. immunocompetence.
   c. psychoimmunology.
   d. psychology.

LO 4 Intellectual Effects of Stress

5. When Jesse encounters a stressful situation, he adapts well and tends to bounce back easily, even though the same situation may derail others. What protective factor is Jesse exhibiting to deal with stress?
   a. Cognitive restructuring
   b. Type A personality
   c. High self-esteem
   d. Psychological resilience

LO 5 What Causes Stress?

6. A state of physical and mental exhaustion caused by excessive stress is called
   a. conflict.
   b. overload.
   c. hassles.
   d. burnout.
7. Losing your keys is an example of what psychosocial source of stress?
   a. Pressure
   b. Inconsistent behaviors
   c. Hassles
   d. Conflict

LO 6 Managing Stress in College

8. After 5 years of 70-hour workweeks, Tom decided to leave his high-paying, high-stress law firm and lead a simpler lifestyle. What is this trend called?
   a. Adaptation
   b. Conflict resolution
   c. Burnout reduction
   d. Downshifting

9. Which of the following is the best strategy to avoid test-taking anxiety on an exam?
   a. Do the majority of your studying the night before the exam so it is fresh in your mind.
   b. Plan ahead and study over a period of time for the exam with a limited, yet thorough, review the night before.
   c. Drink a caffeinated beverage right before the exam because sympathomimetics are known to reduce stress.
   d. Go through the exam as quickly as possible so you don't dwell on potential mistakes.
10. Which of the following is an example of a chronic stressor?
   a. Giving a talk in public
   b. Meeting a big project deadline
   c. Having a permanent disability
   d. Finding out one of your parents just had a heart attack.

Answers to the Pop Quiz can be found on page A-1. If you answered a question incorrectly, review the section identified by the Learning Outcome. For even more study tools, visit MasteringHealth.

THINK ABOUT IT!

LO 1 | What Is Stress?

1. Define stress. What are some examples of scenarios where you might feel distress? Eustress?

LO 2 | Body Responses to Stress

2. Describe the general adaptation syndrome phases and the body's response to stress. Does stress lead to more irritability or emotionality, or does emotionality lead to stress? Provide examples.

LO 3 | Lifetime Effects of Stress

3. What are some of the health risks connected with chronic stress? How does the study of psychoneuroimmunology link stress and illness?

LO 4 | Intellectual Effects of Stress

4. Why might stress and the occurrence of mental disorders be correlated?

LO 5 | What Causes Stress?

5. Why are the college years often high stress? What factors increase stress risks? How stressed are you?

LO 6 | Managing Stress in College

6. What actions can you take to manage your stressors?
7. How does anger affect the body? How do you typically react when you get really angry? Discuss the steps you can take to prevent and/or control your anger reactions.
8. How much do you procrastinate? What sorts of situations make you the most likely to be a "procrastinator"? What could you do to reduce the likelihood of procrastinating in these situations?

ACCESS YOUR HEALTH ON THE INTERNET

Visit **MasteringHealth** for links to the websites and RSS feeds.

The following websites explore further topics and issues related to personal health.

American College Counseling Association. This organization for college counselors has useful links and articles. **www.collegecounseling.org**

American College Health Association. This site provides information and data from the National College Health Assessment survey, which covers stress, anxiety, and other health issues for students every year. **www.acha.org**

American Psychological Association. Here you can find current information and research on stress and stress-related conditions. **www.apa.org**

Higher Education Research Institute. This organization provides annual surveys of first-year and senior college students that cover academic, financial, and health-related issues and problems. **www.heri.ucla.edu**

National Institute of Mental Health. This comprehensive site from the National Institutes of Health is a resource for information on all aspects of mental health, including the effects of stress. **www.nimh.nih.gov**

FOCUS ON Improving Your Sleep

Overloaded with papers and exams, classes and caffeine, extracurricular events and social lives, today's college students are largely a sleep-deprived bunch—and their health may be in jeopardy as a result.

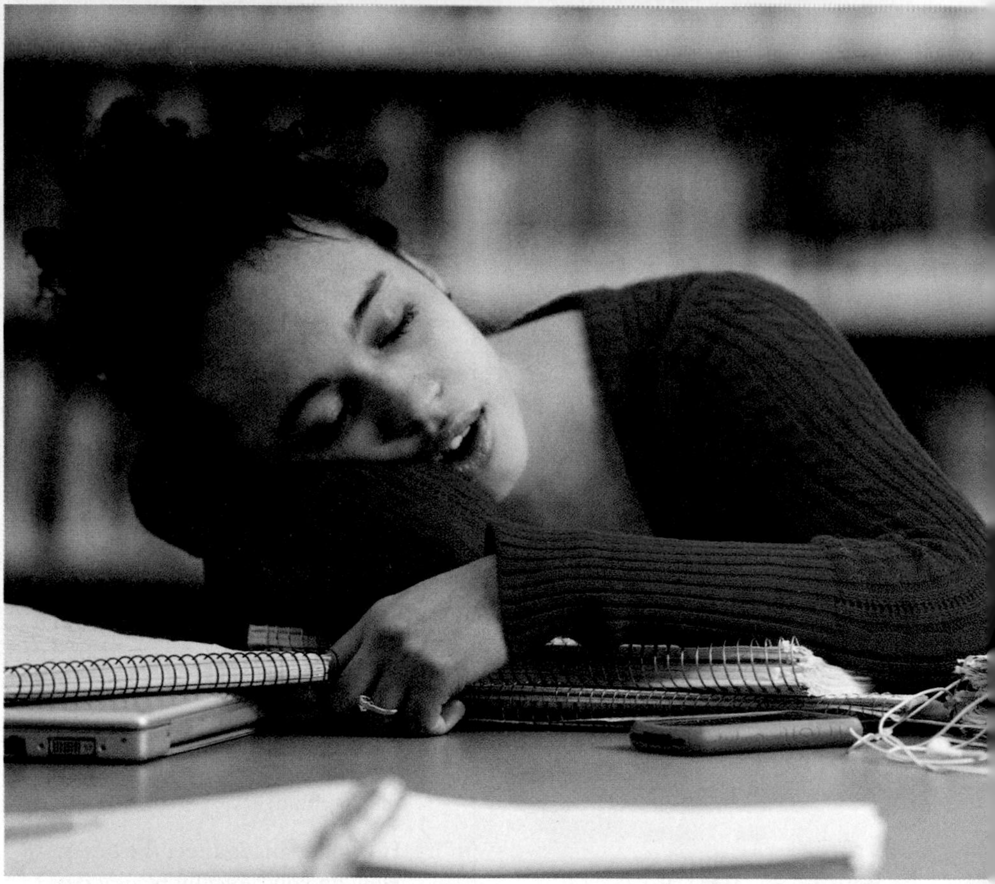

LEARNING OUTCOMES

1. Describe the problem of sleep deprivation both in the United States and globally.
2. Explain why we need sleep and what happens if we don't get enough, including potential physical, emotional, social, and safety threats to health.
3. Explain circadian rhythms and why they are important to daily functioning, and identify both how much sleep we need and how we can catch up on missed sleep.
4. Explore factors that contribute to sleep deficits and what you can do to make sure you get enough sleep.
5. Describe the common sleep disorders insomnia, sleep apnea, restless legs syndrome, and narcolepsy, and what, if anything, we can do to prevent or control them.

Josh knew he wasn't ready for tomorrow's physics exam, but he went to his roommate's basketball game anyway. It was past 11 P.M. when he finally hit the books. To keep himself awake he drank an energy drink and then a cup of coffee as he plowed through the text, his notes, and the online study guide. Just before 4 A.M., he fell into bed, exhausted. His mind raced. *Dynamics, inertia, action*, and *reaction* tumbled around with disjointed thoughts of recent stressful events: losing his cell phone, arguing with his parents, realizing he had three more papers due in the next week. He glanced at the clock: It was 5:30 A.M., and the exam was in 3 hours.

You can probably predict what happened—Josh bombed the test.

Nearly every night, we leave our waking world and slide into a series of sleep stages, punctuated by changes in heart rate, respiration rate, blood pressure, and other bodily processes. Like Josh, we all need sleep—the stages and changes that allow the body to repair, restore and refresh itself. Still, between 50 and 70 million adults in the United States don't get the sleep they need due to sleep or wakefulness disorders.[1]

New evidence links inadequate sleep with a variety of health problems, including obesity, high blood pressure, impaired insulin resistance, sexual problems, depression, lowered immunity, and other ailments. It's no wonder that 76 percent of Americans want to improve the quantity and quality of the sleep they get. Inadequate sleep isn't just an American problem. Sleep deprivation is believed to affect the quality of life of 45 percent of the world's population, and those numbers are on the increase.[2]

LO 1 | SLEEPLESS IN AMERICA

Describe the problem of sleep deprivation both in the United States and globally.

College students seem to be particularly vulnerable to sleep problems. In a recent survey from the American College Health Association (ACHA), only 11.9 percent of students reported getting enough sleep to feel well rested in the morning 6 or more days a week. Nearly 60 percent of students said they felt tired, dragged out, or sleepy for 3 or more days in the past week.[3] It's widely acknowledged that college students are among the most sleep-deprived age group in the United States, with nearly 60 percent of those in the 18- to 29-year-old age group describing themselves as night owls who are still awake in the wee hours of the morning, even though they must get up early—resulting in regular sleep deficiency.[4] These sleep deficiencies have been linked to a host of student issues, including poor academic performance, weight gain, increased alcohol abuse, accidents, daytime drowsiness, relationship issues, depression, and other problems.[5]

60%

OF STUDENTS SAY THEY FELT TIRED, DRAGGED OUT, OR **SLEEPY** FOR 3 OR MORE DAYS IN THE PAST WEEK.

College students are not alone. The sleepiest members of the U.S. population are people aged 13 to 29, with people aged 30 to 64 reporting they are less sleepy than their younger counterparts

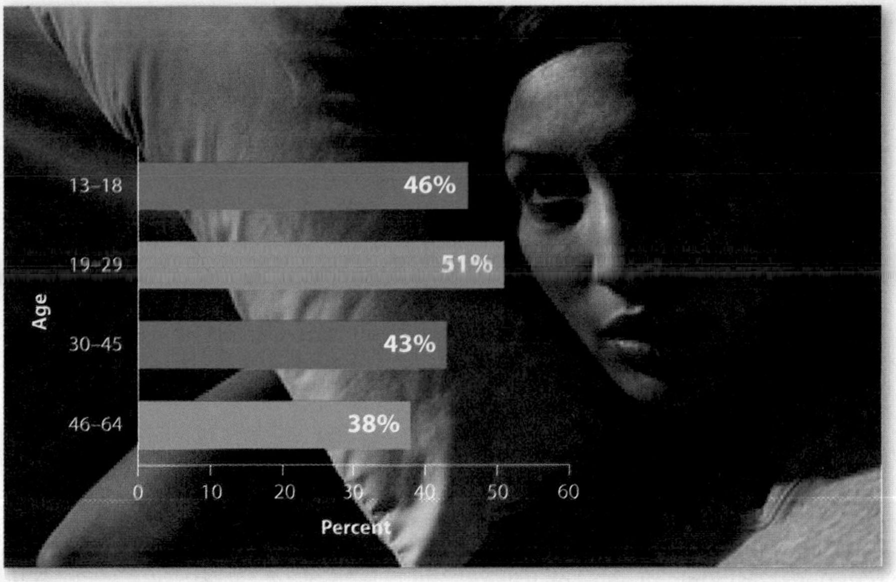

FIGURE 1 Percentage of the U.S. Population Who Rarely/Never Get a Good Night's Sleep on Weekdays

Source: Data from National Sleep Foundation, "2011 Sleep in America Poll: Communications Technology in the Bedroom, Summary of Findings," (Washington, DC: National Sleep Foundation, 2011). Available at www.nationalsleepfoundation.org.

(**FIGURE 1**).[6] Several major studies also indicate that Americans between the ages of 18 and 24 and those over the age of 65 are most likely to fall asleep unintentionally during the day, suffering from a condition known as **excessive daytime sleepiness**. In clinical terms, **primary idiopathic hypersomnia** refers to excessive daytime sleepiness without narcolepsy or the associated features of other sleep disorders.[7] People aged 25 to 35 are the most likely to have nodded off or fallen asleep while driving in the last month, while those 65 and over were the least likely.[8]

Wired and Tired: Technology's Toll on Our Sleep

Why are younger Americans so tired? According to some sources, the average 18- to 34-year-old college student has up to seven tech devices (including TVs) and may be using a smartphone from 1 to 4 hours each day![9] If you can't live without your interactive device or are compelled to constantly check your tweets and texts, you may be among the growing number of *wired and tired* Americans. In fact, according to a recent poll, technology invades the bedrooms of millions, with over 95 percent of respondents reporting using electronic devices before bed and during the night. Is it any wonder that sleep may suffer?

excessive daytime sleepiness A disorder characterized by unusual patterns of falling asleep during normal waking hours.

primary idiopathic hypersomnia Excessive daytime sleepiness without narcolepsy or the associated features of other sleep disorders.

melatonin A hormone that affects sleep cycles, increasing drowsiness.

Sleep experts indicate that increased exposure to interactive technology and "multiscreening" with several devices at a time may increase alertness compared to just watching television.[10] Artificial light exposure from multiple devices in the hours before we go to bed may suppress the release of **melatonin**, a hormone that helps regulate biological rhythms and promotes sleep, while increasing alertness and shifting circadian rhythms to a later hour, making it harder to fall asleep. Some experts believe that as children develop into their teenage years, their bodies may be biologically predisposed toward later bedtimes and shorter sleep times, causing morning wake-up problems.[11]

Sleepy Workers

Adult workers, particularly shift workers, also suffer from sleepiness in unprecedented numbers, and the costs are high. Drowsiness may contribute to poor work performance, off-task thinking, difficulties in concentrating, and irritability or edginess on the job. Tired workers are also more likely to have on-the-job accidents, be depressed, miss work, and have motor vehicle accidents when commuting. When drowsy driving results in vehicle crashes, the underlying contributors are usually sleep loss, driving patterns (long hours as in commercial driving or being up too late at night), taking sedative prescriptions, drinking alcohol, or having unrecognized or untreated sleep disorders, such as sleep apnea. Shift workers and males between the ages of 16 and 29 are at highest risk.[12]

When there just aren't enough hours in the day, sleep typically gets shortchanged. Because Americans are managing to function with less sleep, you might conclude that sufficient sleep isn't all that necessary. In fact, the evidence grows daily for the importance of adequate sleep to overall health and daily functioning. Let's look at the benefits of sleep and find out what happens when you don't get enough.

LO 2 | WHY DO YOU NEED TO SLEEP?

Explain why we need sleep and what happens if we don't get enough, including potential physical, emotional, social, and safety threats to health.

Sleep serves to maintain your physical health, affect your ability to function effectively, and enhance your psychological health. It achieves these results by serving at least two biological purposes:

- **It conserves body energy.** When you sleep, your core body temperature and the rate at which you burn calories drop. This leaves you with more energy to perform activities throughout your waking hours.
- **It restores you both physically and mentally.** For example, certain reparative chemicals are released while you sleep. And there is some evidence, discussed shortly, that during sleep the brain is cleared of daily minutiae, learning is synthesized, and memories are consolidated.

Sleep Maintains Your Physical Health

Sleep has beneficial effects on most body systems. That's why, when you consistently don't get a good night's rest, your body doesn't function as well, and you become more vulnerable to a wide variety of health problems.[13] Researchers are only just beginning to explore the physical benefits of sleep. Here is a brief summary of the physical benefits of sleep.

- **Sleep helps maintain your immune system.** The common cold, strep throat, flu, mononucleosis, cold sores, and a variety of other ailments are more common when your immune system is depressed. And that's more likely to happen if you're not getting enough sleep. Recent studies found that poor sleep quality and shorter sleep duration increased susceptibility to the common cold.[14] Another study reports that sleep disruption, particularly when circadian rhythms are disturbed repeatedly, disrupts overall immune function.[15]

20%

OF STUDENTS SAY THAT SLEEP IS A **PROBLEM** THAT HAS AFFECTED THEIR ACADEMIC PERFORMANCE.

- **Sleep helps reduce your risk for cardiovascular disease.** Several studies have indicated that high blood pressure is more common in people who get fewer than 7 hours of sleep a night.[16] Newer research points to a strong association between short-duration sleep and increased risk of developing and/or dying from cardiovascular disease.[17]
- **Sleep contributes to a healthy metabolism.** Chemical reactions in your body's cells break down food and synthesize compounds that the body needs. The sum of all these reactions is called *metabolism*. Several recent studies suggest that sleep contributes to healthy metabolism and possibly a healthy body weight. In fact, those who sleep less than 5 hours per night have a 40 percent higher risk of developing obesity than those sleeping 7 to 8 hours per night.[18] Sleeping less is associated with eating more—particularly high-fat, high-protein foods—and exercising less.[19] There is evidence that sleep deficiencies, particularly sleep disorders such as sleep apnea, can increase the risk of *type 2 diabetes*, a disorder of glucose metabolism.[20]
- **Sleep may be a factor in male reproductive health.** Although issues with sexual interest and sexual performance are common problems for tired people, new research suggests sleep deprivation may affect males more than they realize.

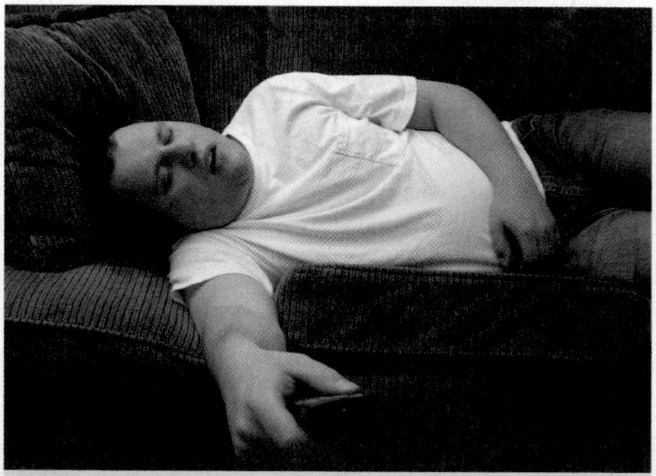

Being overweight can increase your risk of certain sleep disorders.

SEE IT! VIDEOS

What kind of sleep keeps your memory sharp? Watch **How Sleep Affects Your Memory** available on MasteringHealth.™

Young males who suffered from chronic sleep deficits were shown to have reduced semen quality, reduced sperm motility, and smaller testicular size than men with higher sleep levels. More research is necessary to determine the mechanisms contributing to these problems.[21]

- **Sleep contributes to neurological functioning.** Restricting sleep can cause a wide range of neurological problems, including lapses of attention, slowed or poor memory, reduced cognitive ability, difficulty in concentrating, and a tendency for your thinking to get "stuck in a rut."[22] Your ability not only to remember facts, but also to integrate them, make meaningful generalizations about them, and consolidate what you've learned into lasting memories requires adequate sleep time.[23] College students who pull all-nighters, as well as students who are short sleepers, have significantly lower overall grade-point averages compared with classmates who get adequate sleep.[24]
- **Sleep improves motor tasks.** Sleep also has a restorative effect on motor function, or the ability to perform tasks such as shooting a basket, playing a musical instrument, or driving a car. Motor function is affected by sleep throughout the life span among otherwise healthy individuals.[25] Some researchers contend that a night without sleep impairs your motor skills and reaction time as much as if you were driving drunk.[26] As Americans have become more and more sleep deprived, the incidence of drowsy driving and so-called fall-asleep crashes has become a national concern. A recent survey found that, in the last month, nearly one-third of drivers drove when they couldn't keep their eyes open.[27] Drivers 16 to 24 are the most likely of any age group to report falling asleep at the wheel within the last year, and men of all ages are more likely to fall asleep than are women. Data from the National Highway Traffic Safety Administration (NHTSA) indicate that sleepy drivers are involved in 2 percent of all fatal crashes; however, other sources estimate these figures may be considerably higher, ranging from 15 to 33 percent.[28]

Sleep Promotes Your Psychosocial Health

It is believed that certain brain regions, including the cerebral cortex (your "master mind"), get essential rest only during sleep. Metabolism may slow, but other brain functions may actually increase during sleep.[29]

In addition, you're more likely to be reactive, as well as feel stressed-out, worried, or sad, when you're sleep deprived. The relationship between sleep and

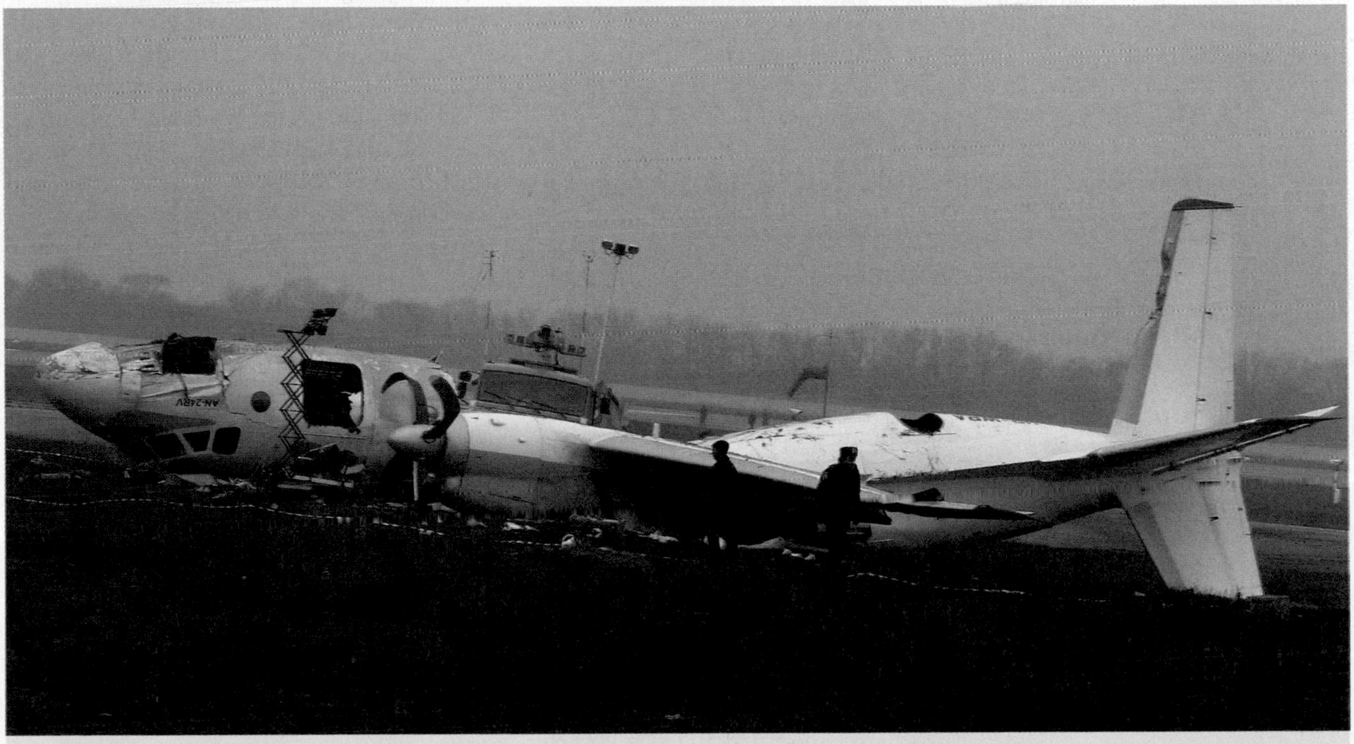

People we trust for transportation suffer from on-the-job sleepiness at alarming rates. Over 26 percent of train operators and 23 percent of pilots admit to sleepiness on the job in the last week. Twenty percent of pilots, 18 percent of train operators, and 14 percent of truck drivers report making a serious error or having a "near miss" while at work.

Source: Data from National Sleep Foundation, "Sleepy Pilots, Train Operators and Drivers," March 2012, www.sleepfoundation.org.

circadian rhythm The 24-hour cycle by which you are accustomed to going to sleep, waking up, and performing habitual behaviors.

REM sleep A period of sleep characterized by brain-wave activity similar to that seen in wakefulness; rapid eye movement and dreaming occur during REM sleep.

non-REM (NREM) sleep A period of restful sleep dominated by slow brain waves; during non-REM sleep, rapid eye movement is rare.

stress is highly complex: Stress can cause or contribute to sleep problems, and sleep problems can cause or increase your level of stress! The same is true of clinical psychiatric conditions such as depression and anxiety disorders: Reduced or poor-quality sleep can trigger these disorders, but it's also a common symptom resulting from them. Nondepressed individuals who suffer from chronic insomnia have over twice the risk of developing depression.[30]

LO 3 | WHAT GOES ON WHEN YOU SLEEP?

Explain circadian rhythms and why they are important to daily functioning, and identify both how much sleep we need and how we can catch up on missed sleep.

If you've ever taken a flight that crossed two or more time zones, you've probably experienced *jet lag,* a feeling that your body's "internal clock" is out of sync with the hours of daylight and darkness at your destination. Jet lag happens because the new day/night pattern disrupts the 24-hour biological clock by which you are accustomed to going to sleep, waking up, and performing habitual behaviors. This cycle, known as your **circadian rhythm**, is regulated by a master clock that coordinates the activity of nerve cells, protein, and genes. The hypothalamus and a tiny gland in your brain called the *pineal body*—responsible for the drowsiness-inducing hormone called melatonin—are key to these cyclical rhythms.[31]

You can fight the effects of melatonin for hours—even days!—especially if, like Josh in our opening story, you load up on caffeine. But all mammals will eventually succumb to sleep. Humans should spend roughly one-third of every day asleep. Sleep researchers generally distinguish between two primary sleep stages. During **REM sleep**, rapid eye movement and dreams occur, and brain-wave activity appears similar to that when you are awake. **Non-REM (NREM) sleep**, in contrast, is the period of restful sleep with slowed brain activity that does *not* include rapid eye movement. During the night, you alternate between periods of NREM and REM sleep, repeating one full cycle about once every 90 minutes.[32] Overall, you spend about 75 percent of each night in NREM sleep and 25 percent in REM (**FIGURE 2**).

Non-REM Sleep Is Restorative

During non-REM sleep, the body rests. Movement can occur, for instance, to shift your position in bed, but muscle tension is reduced. Both your body temperature and your energy use drop; sensation is dulled; and your brain waves, heart rate, and breathing slow. In contrast, digestive processes speed up, and your body stores nutrients. During NREM sleep—also called *slow-wave sleep*—you do not typically dream. Rather, the deepest part of sleep occurs, and your body begins organizing your day's memories. Four distinct stages of NREM sleep have been distinguished by their characteristic brainwave patterns.

Stage 1 is the lightest stage of sleep, lasts only a few minutes, and involves the transition between waking and sleep. Your brain begins to produce *theta waves* (slow brain waves), and you may experience sensations of falling with quick, jerky muscle reaction. During *Stage 2,* your eyes close, body movement slows, and you disengage from your environment. During *Stages 3* and *4,* a sleeper's brain generates slow, large-amplitude delta waves as shown on an electroencephalogram (EEG). Blood pressure drops, your heart rate and respiration slow considerably, and you enter deep sleep. Human growth hormone is released, signaling the body to repair worn tissues. Speech and movement are rare during the final stage (but

SEE IT! VIDEOs
How you can avoid nodding off behind the wheel? Watch **Dozing and Driving** available on MasteringHealth.™

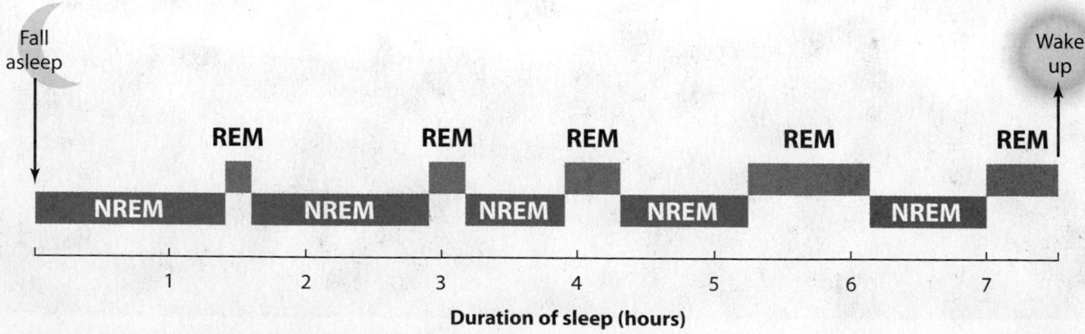

FIGURE 2 **The Nightly Sleep Cycle** As the number of hours you sleep increases, your brain spends more and more time in REM sleep. Thus, sleeping for too few hours could mean you're depriving yourself primarily of needed REM sleep.

VIDEO TUTOR Sleep Cycle

sometimes people sleepwalk, cook, clean, or drive during this stage!).

REM Sleep Energizes

Dreaming takes place primarily during REM sleep. On an EEG, a REM sleeper's brain-wave activity is almost indistinguishable from that of someone who is wide awake, and the brain's energy use is higher than that of a person who is performing a difficult math problem![33] Your muscles are paralyzed during REM sleep: You may dream that you're rock climbing, but your body is incapable of movement. Almost the only exceptions are your respiratory muscles, which allow you to breathe, and the tiny muscles of your eyes, which move your eyes rapidly as if you were following the scenario of your dream. This rapid eye movement gives REM sleep its name.

While REM sleep was once thought to be the key to memory retention, newer research indicates that the deep phases of slow-wave sleep consolidate and organize the day's information and that REM sleep stabilizes consolidated memory. Without adequate slow-wave sleep and REM sleep, your short-term memory may suffer.[34]

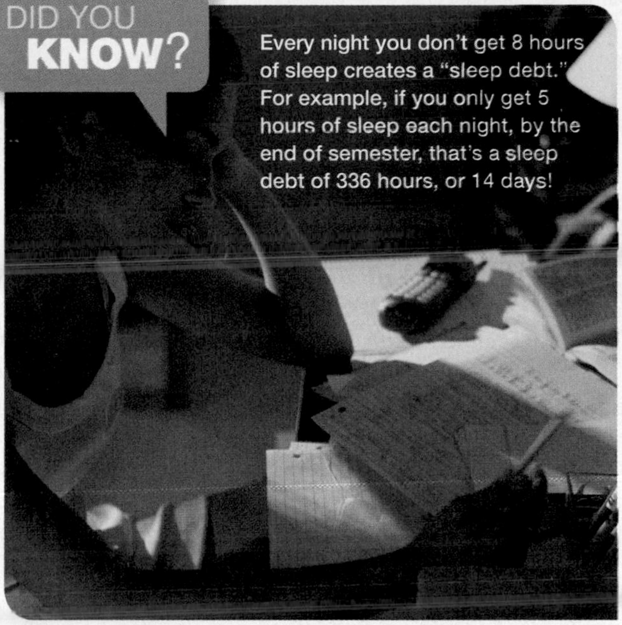

DID YOU KNOW?

Every night you don't get 8 hours of sleep creates a "sleep debt." For example, if you only get 5 hours of sleep each night, by the end of semester, that's a sleep debt of 336 hours, or 14 days!

How Much Sleep Do You Need?

Researchers find that most people need between 7 and 8 hours of sleep per day, on average.[35] But sleep needs vary from person to person, and your gender, health, and lifestyle will also affect how much rest your body demands. For example, women need more sleep than men overall.

It is worth noting that sleep patterns change over the life span. Newborns need 16 to 18 hours of sleep daily, and teens and younger adults need 8 to 9 hours per night, slightly more than the adult average. Older adults may experience sleep difficulties that result in fewer hours of rest per night owing to health conditions, pain, and the need to use the bathroom more frequently.[36]

Research has consistently shown that sleep deprivation and disorders contribute significantly to premature death and disability from a variety of conditions, including cardiovascular disease, cancer, depression, obesity, and diabetes. Many scientists believe that diabetes, obesity, and other metabolic disorders may be linked with biological clock activity.[37] In general, those who get adequate sleep live longer and enjoy more quality days than those who don't.[38]

WHAT DO YOU THINK?

Do you find it difficult to get 7 or 8 hours of sleep each night?

- Do you think you are able to catch up on sleep you miss?
- Have you noticed any negative consequences in your own life when you get too little sleep?

Sleep Need Includes Baseline Plus Debt

Pay attention to how you feel after different amounts of sleep, and aim for the duration that feels best for you.[39] In addition to your body's physiological need, consider your current **sleep debt**. That's the total number of hours of missed sleep you're carrying around with you, either because you got up before you were fully rested or because your sleep was interrupted. Let's say that last week you managed just 5 hours of sleep a night Monday through Thursday. Even if you get 7 to 8 hours a night Friday through Sunday, your unresolved sleep debt of 8 to 12 hours will leave you tired and groggy when you start the week again. That means you need *more than* 8 hours a night for the next several nights to "catch up."

The good news is that you *can* catch up if you go about it sensibly. Getting 5 hours of sleep a night all semester long, then sleeping 48 hours the first weekend you're home on break won't restore your functioning, and it's likely to disrupt your circadian rhythm. Instead, whittle away at that sleep debt by sleeping 9 hours a night throughout your break—then start the new term resolved to sleep 7 to 8 hours a night.

Do Naps Count?

Speaking of catching up, do naps count? Although naps can't entirely cancel out a significant sleep debt, they can improve your mood, alertness, and performance. Regular naps may also improve immune functioning and help ward off infections.[40] It's best to nap in the early to midafternoon, when the pineal body in your brain releases a small amount of melatonin and your body experiences a natural dip in its circadian rhythm. Never nap in the late afternoon, as it could interfere with your ability to fall asleep that night. Keep your naps short, because a nap of more than 30 minutes can leave you in a state of **sleep inertia**,

sleep debt The difference between the number of hours of sleep an individual needed in a given time period and the number of hours he or she actually slept.

sleep inertia A state characterized by cognitive impairment, grogginess, and disorientation that is experienced upon rising from short sleep or an overly long nap.

which is characterized by cognitive impairment, nausea, light-headedness, grogginess, and a disoriented feeling.

LO 4 | HOW TO GET A GOOD NIGHT'S SLEEP

Explore factors that contribute to sleep deficits and what you can do to make sure you get enough sleep.

Do you need a jolt of caffeine to get started in the morning? Do you find it hard to stay awake in class? Have you ever nodded off behind the wheel? These are all signs of inadequate or poor quality sleep. To find out whether you're sleep deprived, go online to www.pearsonhighered.com/donatelle and take the **Assess Yourself** questionnaire.

Do's and Don'ts for Restful Sleep

The following tips can help you get a more restful night's sleep.

- **Let there be light.** Throughout the day, stay in sync with your circadian rhythm by spending time in the sunlight. Exposure to natural light outdoors is most beneficial, but opening the shades indoors and, on overcast days, turning on room lights can also help keep you alert.
- **Stay active.** Exercisers are much more likely to feel rested than those who are sedentary—regardless of timing. According to recent polls, there was no significant difference in sleepiness or quality of sleep between those who exercised less than 4 hours before bedtime and those who exercised more than 4 hours before bedtime. However, those who engaged in vigorous exercises during the day appeared to sleep best overall.[41]
- **Sleep tight.** Don't let a lumpy or pancake pillow, scratchy or pilled sheets, or a threadbare blanket keep you from sleeping soundly. Keep pets off the bed. Invest in a good mattress. And make your bed in the morning and air out your room; cool sheets and bedding and a lavender-scented room have been shown to help you sleep better.
- **Create a sleep "cave."** Take a lesson from bats, bears, and burrowing animals! As bedtime approaches, keep your bedroom quiet, cool, dark, and *free of technology* during sleep hours. Start by turning off your TV and computer and don't leave your cell phone anywhere near your bed. Better yet, turn it off! If your living area is noisy from roommates or neighbors, wear earplugs or play "white noise," such as the sound of gentle rain. Turn down the thermostat or, on hot nights, run an electric fan. If you can't block out the light, wear an eye mask.
- **Condition yourself into better sleep.** Go to bed and get up at the same time each day. Establish a bedtime ritual that signals to your body that it's time for sleep. For instance, listen to a quiet song, take a warm shower, or read something that lets you quietly wind down. Practice relaxation strategies such as deep breathing.
- **Make your bedroom a mental escape.** Don't stew about things you can't fix right now. Clear your mind of worries and frustrations. Breathe deeply. Allow your body to unwind.
- **Avoid foods and drinks that keep you awake.** Large meals, nicotine, energy drinks, caffeine, and alcohol close to bedtime can affect your ability to fall asleep and stay asleep. Caffeine starts to work about 15 minutes after that first cup of coffee, and it takes over 6 hours to clear half of it from your system.[42]
- **Don't drink large amounts of any liquid before bed.** Drinking liquids may contribute to **nocturia**, or overactive bladder, meaning you have to get up several times during the night. A variety of conditions, including urinary tract infection or other ailments, can also cause nocturia. See your doctor if bathroom trips have begun to be a regular thing at night.
- **Don't get revved by emotional upheavals.** Avoid late-night phone calls, texts, or e-mails that can end up in arguments, disappointments, and other emotional stressors. If something does jazz you up before bed, journal about

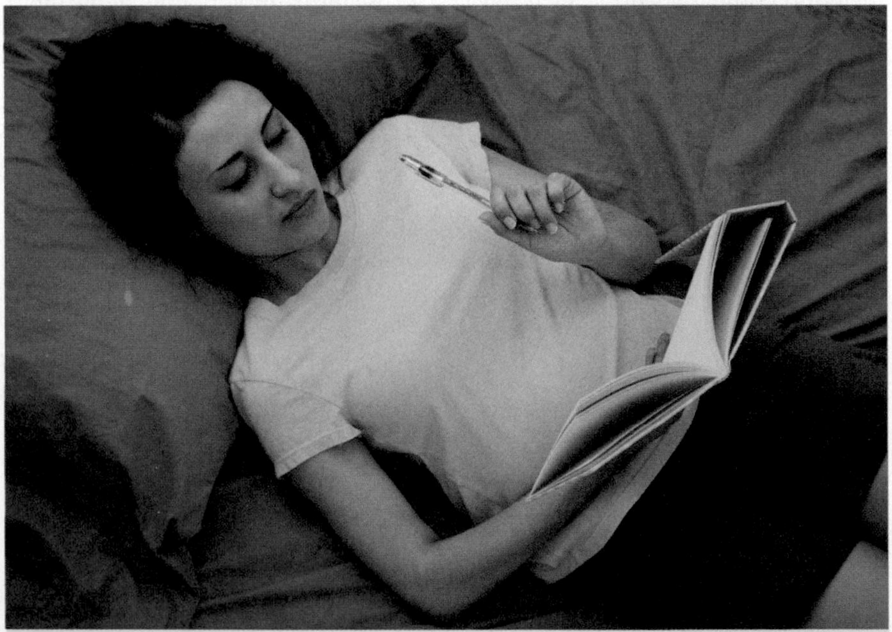

If a worry keeps you awake, jot it down in a journal. You'll be better prepared to handle it in the morning after a good night's sleep.

nocturia Frequent urination at night caused by an overactive bladder.

it briefly, then promise yourself that you'll make time the next day to explore your feelings more deeply.

- **Don't toss and turn.** If you're not asleep after 20 minutes, get up. Turn on a low light, read something relaxing, or listen to some gentle music. Once you feel sleepy, go back to bed.
- **Don't take nonprescribed sleeping pills or nighttime pain medications.** Casual use of over-the-counter sleeping aids can interfere with your brain's natural progression through the healthy stages of sleep.

LO 5 | WHAT DO YOU DO IF YOU'RE STILL NOT SLEEPING WELL?

Describe the common sleep disorders insomnia, sleep apnea, restless legs syndrome, and narcolepsy, and what, if anything, we can do to prevent or control them.

Sleep deprivation is becoming an increasing problem for the world's population. Although over 4 percent of college students report regularly suffering from insomnia and 2.2 percent have diagnosed sleep disorders, the exact number receiving treatment is unknown.[43] Nearly 27 percent of students say that they have had sleep difficulties in the last year that were traumatic or difficult to handle.[44] If you're following the advice in this chapter and you still aren't sleeping well, it's time to visit your health care provider. To aid in diagnosis, you will probably be asked to keep a sleep diary like the one in **FIGURE 3**. You may also be referred to a sleep disorders center for an overnight clinical **sleep study**. While

sleep study A clinical assessment of sleep in which the patient is monitored while spending the night in a sleep disorders center.

	Day 1	Day 2	Day 3
Fill out in morning			
Bedtime	11 pm	11:30 pm	
Wake time	7:30 am	8:30 am	
Time to fall asleep	45 min	30 min	
Awakenings (how many and how long?)	2 times 1 hour	1 time 45 min	
Total sleep time	6.75 hrs	7.75 hrs	
Feeling at waking (refreshed, groggy, etc.)	Still tired	Energized	
Fill out at bedtime			
Exercise (what, when, how long?)	Jog at 2 pm 30 min	Soccer practice at 4 pm; 2 hrs	
Naps (when, where, how long?)	4 pm, my bed 30 min	2 pm, library 1 hour	
Caffeine (what, when, how much?)	2 cups coffee at 8 am	1 latte at 10 am; 1 soda at 9 pm	
Alcohol (what, when, how much?)	1 beer at 8 pm	None	
Evening snacks (what, when, how much?)	Bag of popcorn at 10 pm	Chips and soda at 9 pm	
Medications (what, when, how much?)	None	None	
Feelings (happiness, anxiety, major cause, etc.)	Stressed about paper	Worried about sister	
Activities 1 hour before bed (what and how long?)	Wrote paper	Watched TV	

FIGURE 3 Sample Sleep Diary Using a sleep diary such as this one can help you and your health care provider discover behavioral factors that might be contributing to your sleep problem.

you are asleep in the sleep center, sensors and electrodes record data that will be reviewed by a sleep specialist who will work with your doctor to diagnose and treat your sleep problem.

The American Academy of Sleep Medicine identifies more than 80 sleep disorders. The most common disorders in adults are *insomnia, sleep apnea, restless legs syndrome,* and *narcolepsy.*

SKILLS FOR BEHAVIOR CHANGE

BEAT JET LAG

Insomnia, fatigue, stomachache, and headache: These are symptoms of jet lag and not a great way to spend a vacation. In general, the more time zones you cross, the worse the jet lag will be. Here's how to avoid or reduce jet lag:

- Begin the trip rested (preexisting sleep deprivation intensifies jet lag).
- Schedule a daytime flight.
- Reset your watch as soon as you depart.
- Avoid alcohol and caffeine while traveling.
- Eat small meals at the appropriate mealtime for your destination.
- A few days before going west, go to bed and wake up 1 hour later each day.
- Once in the west, seek morning light and avoid afternoon light.
- A few days before going east, go to bed and wake up 1 hour earlier each day.
- Once in the east, seek evening light and avoid morning light.
- If you take an overnight flight, avoid sleeping too much on the day of your arrival. You'll find it hard to fight the fatigue, but sleeping during the day will make it harder for you to adjust to your new time zone's schedule.

Insomnia

Insomnia—difficulty in falling asleep, frequent arousals during sleep, or early morning awakening—is the most common sleep complaint. Young adults aged 18 to 29 experience the most insomnia, with 68 percent of them reporting symptoms. Somewhat fewer adults (59%) aged 30 to 64 experience regular symptoms, and only 44 percent of those over age 65 have regular symptoms.[45] Adults with children in the household tend to report more insomnia symptoms than those without children.[46] Approximately 10 to 15 percent of Americans have chronic insomnia that lasts longer than a month.[47] About 4 percent of college students are being treated for insomnia.[48] Insomnia is more common among women than men, and its prevalence increases with age.

insomnia A disorder characterized by difficulty in falling asleep quickly, frequent arousals during sleep, or early morning awakening.

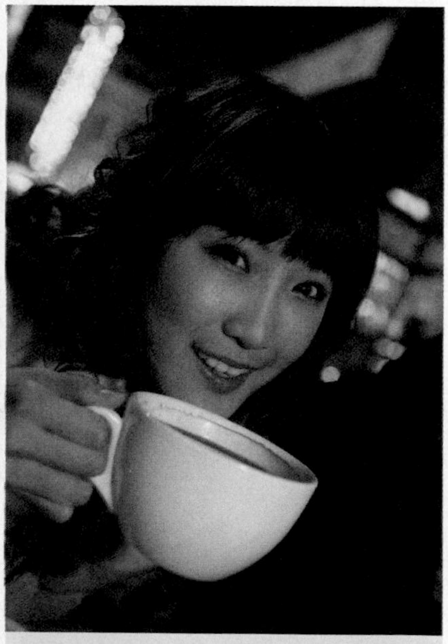

After-dinner coffee? Not unless it's decaf. Caffeine promotes alertness by blocking the neurotransmitter adenosine in your brain—a useful thing when you are studying, but a potential problem when you are trying to sleep.

Symptoms and Causes of Insomnia

Symptoms of insomnia include difficulty falling asleep, waking up frequently during the night, difficulty returning to sleep, waking up too early in the morning, unrefreshing sleep, daytime sleepiness, and irritability. Sometimes insomnia is related to stress and worry. In other cases it may be related to disrupted circadian rhythms, which may occur with travel across time zones, shift work, and other major schedule changes. Insomnia can also occur as a side effect from taking certain medications. Untreated insomnia can be associated with increased illness or morbidity. See the **Skills for Behavior Change** box on ways to beat travel-related insomnia.

Treatment for Insomnia

Because of the close connection between behavior and insomnia, cognitive behavioral therapy is often part of treatment. A cognitive behavioral therapist assists a patient in identifying thought and behavioral patterns that contribute to the inability to fall asleep. Sometimes, hormonal changes or issues with the gastrointestinal tract or bladder may be an underlying cause. Excess stress is also a key factor in insomnia, and strategies designed to treat or control the underlying contributors can be helpful in reducing insomnia.

In some cases of insomnia, *hypnotic* or *sedative* medications may be prescribed. Over 4 percent of adults aged 20 and over use prescription sleep aids.[49] These drugs induce sleep, and some may help relieve anxiety. However, some have undesirable side effects ranging from daytime sleepiness and hallucinations to sleepwalking and other strange nighttime behaviors. Some actually promote anxiety or depression. Many sedatives are also addictive and can lead to tolerance and dependence. Antidepressants are also commonly prescribed for insomnia.

Relaxation strategies, including yoga and meditation, can be helpful in inducing sleep, as can exercise. Talk to a health professional if insomnia is unresolved in spite of your best efforts to make changes.

Sleep Apnea

Sleep apnea is a disorder in which breathing is briefly and repeatedly interrupted during sleep.[50] *Apnea* refers to a breathing pause that lasts at least 10 seconds. Sleep apnea affects more than 18 million Americans, or 1 in every 15 people; it affects all age groups and both sexes.[51]

Symptoms and Causes of Sleep Apnea

There are two major types of sleep apnea: central and obstructive. *Central sleep apnea* occurs when the brain fails to tell the respiratory muscles to initiate breathing. Consumption of alcohol, certain illegal drugs, and certain medications can contribute to central sleep apnea.

Obstructive sleep apnea (OSA) is more common and occurs when air cannot move in and out of a person's nose or mouth, even though the body tries to breathe. Typically, OSA occurs when a person's throat muscles and tongue relax during sleep and block the airways, causing snorting, snoring, and gagging. These sounds occur because falling oxygen saturation levels in the blood stimulate the body's autonomic nervous system to trigger inhalation, often via a sudden gasp of breath. This response may wake the person, preventing deep sleep and causing the person to wake in the morning feeling like he or she hasn't slept.

People who are overweight often have sagging internal throat tissue, which puts them at higher risk for sleep apnea. In addition to overweight, other risk factors include smoking and alcohol use, being age 40 or older, and ethnicity—sleep apnea occurs at higher rates in African Americans, Pacific Islanders, and Hispanics.[52] Anatomical risk factors for OSA can include a small upper airway (or large tongue, tonsils or uvula), a recessed chin, small jaw or a large overbite, and a large neck size. Because OSA runs in some families, genetics may also play a role.[53] More serious risks of OSA include chronic high blood pressure, irregular heartbeats, heart damage and heart attack, and stroke. Apnea-associated sleeplessness may also increase the risk of type 2 diabetes, immune system deficiencies, and a host of other problems.[54]

Treatment for Sleep Apnea

The most commonly prescribed therapy for OSA is *continuous positive airway pressure (CPAP),* which consists of an airflow device, long tube, and mask (see **FIGURE 4**). People with sleep apnea wear this mask during sleep, and air is forced into the nose to keep the airway open.

Other methods for treating OSA include dental appliances, which reposition the lower jaw and tongue, and surgery to remove tissue in the upper airway. In general, these approaches are most helpful for mild disease or heavy snoring. Lifestyle changes, which may include losing weight, avoiding alcohol, and quitting smoking, are often effective ways of reducing symptoms of OSA.

sleep apnea A disorder in which breathing is briefly and repeatedly interrupted during sleep.

restless legs syndrome (RLS) A neurological disorder characterized by an overwhelming urge to move the legs when they are at rest.

Restless Legs Syndrome

Restless legs syndrome (RLS) is a neurological disorder characterized by unpleasant sensations in the legs when at rest combined with an uncontrollable urge to move in an effort to relieve these feelings. These sensations range in severity from uncomfortable to irritating to painful. Some researchers estimate that RLS affects over 10 percent of the U.S. population, with increasing diagnosis in all age groups. Many believe it is even more common, but that it is often underdiagnosed or misdiagnosed.[55]

Symptoms and Causes of RLS

Restless legs syndrome sensations are often described as burning, creeping, or tugging, or like insects crawling inside the legs. In general, the symptoms are more pronounced at night. Lying down

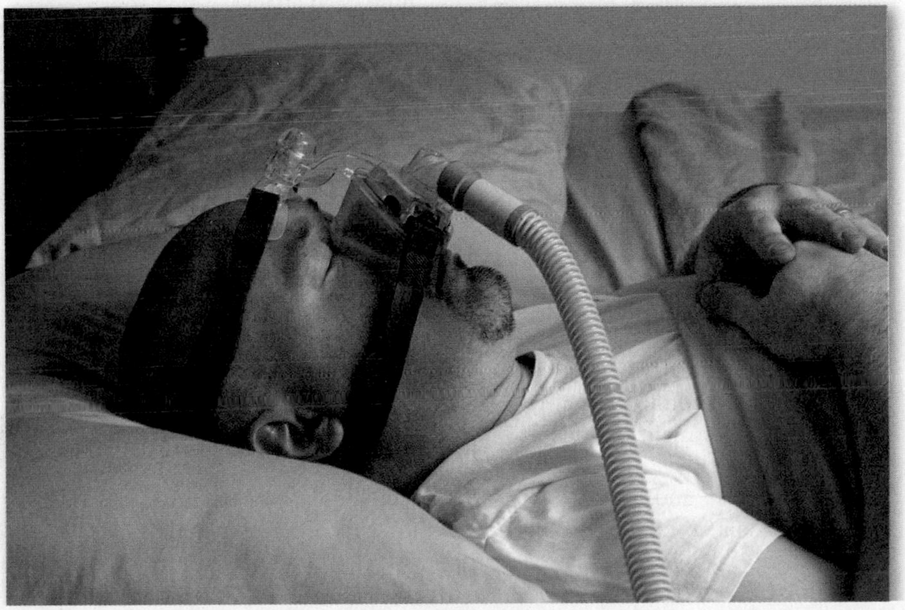

FIGURE 4 **Continuous Positive Airway Pressure (CPAP) Device** People with sleep apnea can get a better night's sleep by wearing a CPAP device. A gentle stream of air flows continuously into the nose through a tube connected to a mask. This steady stream of air helps keep the sleeper's airway open.

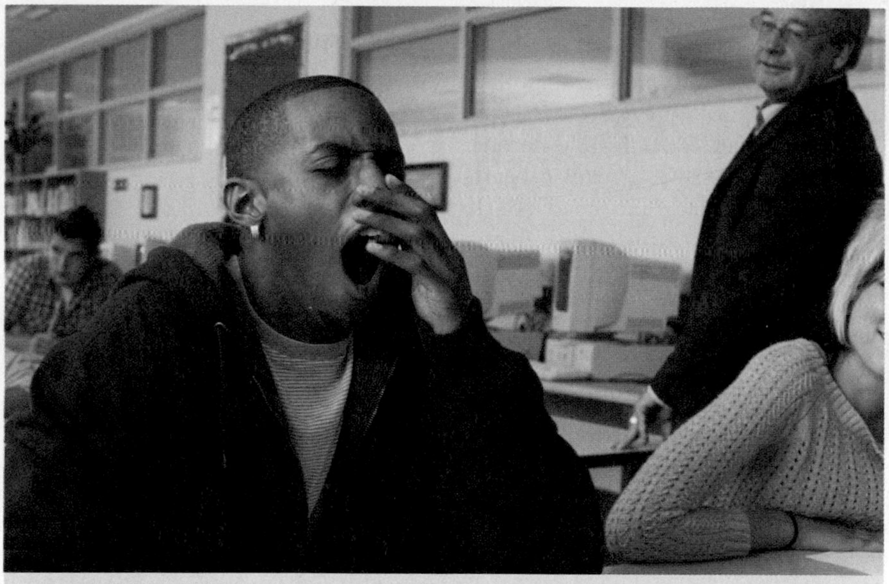

From insomnia to narcolepsy, sleep disorders are more common than you might think. There are more than 80 different clinical sleep disorders, and it is estimated that 50 to 70 million Americans—children and adults—suffer from one. Many aren't even aware of their disorder, and many others never seek treatment.

or trying to relax activates the symptoms, and moving the legs relieves the discomfort, so people with RLS often have difficulty falling and staying asleep.

In most cases, the cause of RLS is unknown. A family history of the condition is seen in approximately 50 percent of cases, suggesting some genetic link. People with familial RLS tend to be younger when symptoms start and have a slower progression of the condition. In other cases, RLS appears to be related to other conditions, including Parkinson's disease, kidney failure, diabetes, peripheral neuropathy, and anemia. Pregnancy or hormonal changes can worsen symptoms.[56]

Treatment of RLS

If there is an underlying condition, treatment of that condition may provide relief. Other treatment options include prescribed medications, decreasing tobacco and alcohol use, and applying heat to the legs. For some people, relaxation techniques or stretching exercises can alleviate symptoms.

narcolepsy A neurological disorder that causes people to fall asleep involuntarily during the day.

Narcolepsy

Narcolepsy is a neurological disorder caused by the brain's inability to properly regulate sleep-wake cycles. The result of this disorder is excessive, intrusive sleepiness and daytime sleep attacks. Narcolepsy occurs in about 1 of every 3,000 people and affects men and women equally. Narcolepsy is not rare, but it is an underrecognized and underdiagnosed condition.[57]

Symptoms and Causes of Narcolepsy

Narcolepsy is characterized by overwhelming and uncontrollable sleepiness during the day. Narcoleptics are prone to falling asleep at inappropriate times and places—in class, at work, while driving or eating, or even mid-conversation. These sleep attacks can last from a few seconds to several minutes. Other symptoms include *cataplexy* (the sudden loss of voluntary muscle tone, often triggered by emotional stimuli), hallucinations during sleep onset or upon awakening, and brief episodes of paralysis during sleep-wake transitions.

In most cases narcolepsy appears to be caused by a deficiency of chemicals in the brain that regulate sleep. Genetics may also play a role.[58] Other factors, including having another sleep disorder, using certain medications, or having a mental disorder or substance abuse disorder, may also be factors.

Treatment for Narcolepsy

Narcolepsy is commonly treated with medications that improve alertness, and antidepressants may be prescribed to treat cataplexy, hallucinations, and sleep paralysis. Behavioral therapy can also help narcoleptics cope with their condition. Some lifestyle changes, such as scheduling brief naps during the day or eating smaller meals on a regular schedule, may be helpful.

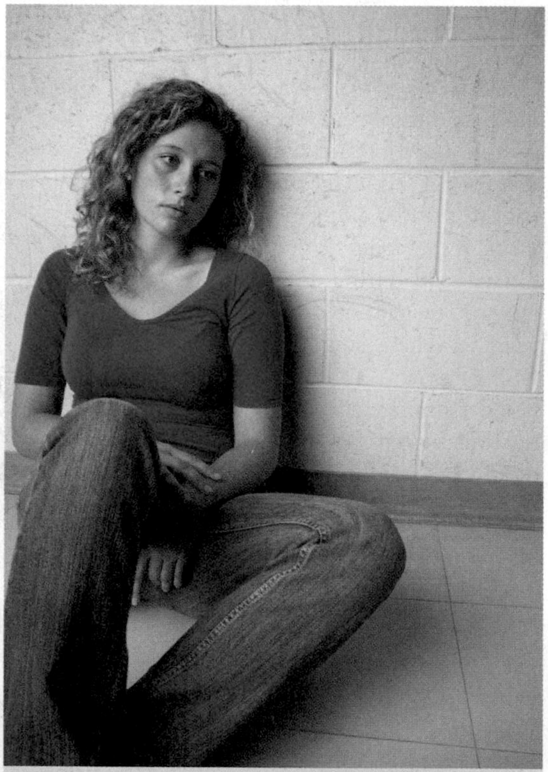

While grades, finances, and conflicts with others can cause worries that keep you from sleep, learning to block these thoughts through thought stopping, listening to relaxing music, reading, or other restful activities can help you change your focus and sleep.

ASSESS **YOURSELF**

Are you getting enough sleep? Want to find out? Take the **Are You Sleeping Well?** assessment available on MasteringHealth.™

Need help creating a plan? Follow the strategies in the **Your Plan for Change** box for short- and long-term improvements to your health.

YOUR PLAN FOR **CHANGE**

Now that you have considered how sleep deprived you may be by completing the **ASSESS YOURSELF** activity, you can take steps to improve your sleep, starting tonight.

TODAY, YOU CAN:

- ☐ Evaluate your behaviors and identify things in your life that may prevent you from getting a good night's sleep. Develop a plan. What can you do differently starting today?
- ☐ Write a list of personal Do's and Don'ts. For instance: Do turn off your cell phone after 11 P.M. Don't drink anything with caffeine after 3 P.M.

WITHIN THE NEXT 2 WEEKS, YOU CAN:

- ☐ Keep a sleep diary, noting not only how many hours of sleep you get each night, but also how you feel and how you function the next day
- ☐ Arrange your room to promote restful sleep. Remember the "cave": Keep it quiet, cool, dark, and comfortable.
- ☐ Visit your campus health center and ask for more information about getting a good night's sleep.

BY THE END OF THE SEMESTER, YOU CAN:

- ☐ Establish a regular sleep schedule. Get in the habit of going to bed and waking up at the same time, even on weekends.
- ☐ Create a ritual, such as stretching, meditation, reading something light, or listening to music, that you follow each night to help your body ease from the activity of the day into restful sleep.
- ☐ If you are still having difficulty sleeping and feel you may have a sleep disorder or an underlying health problem disrupting your sleep, contact your health care provider.

4 Building Healthy Relationships and Communicating Effectively

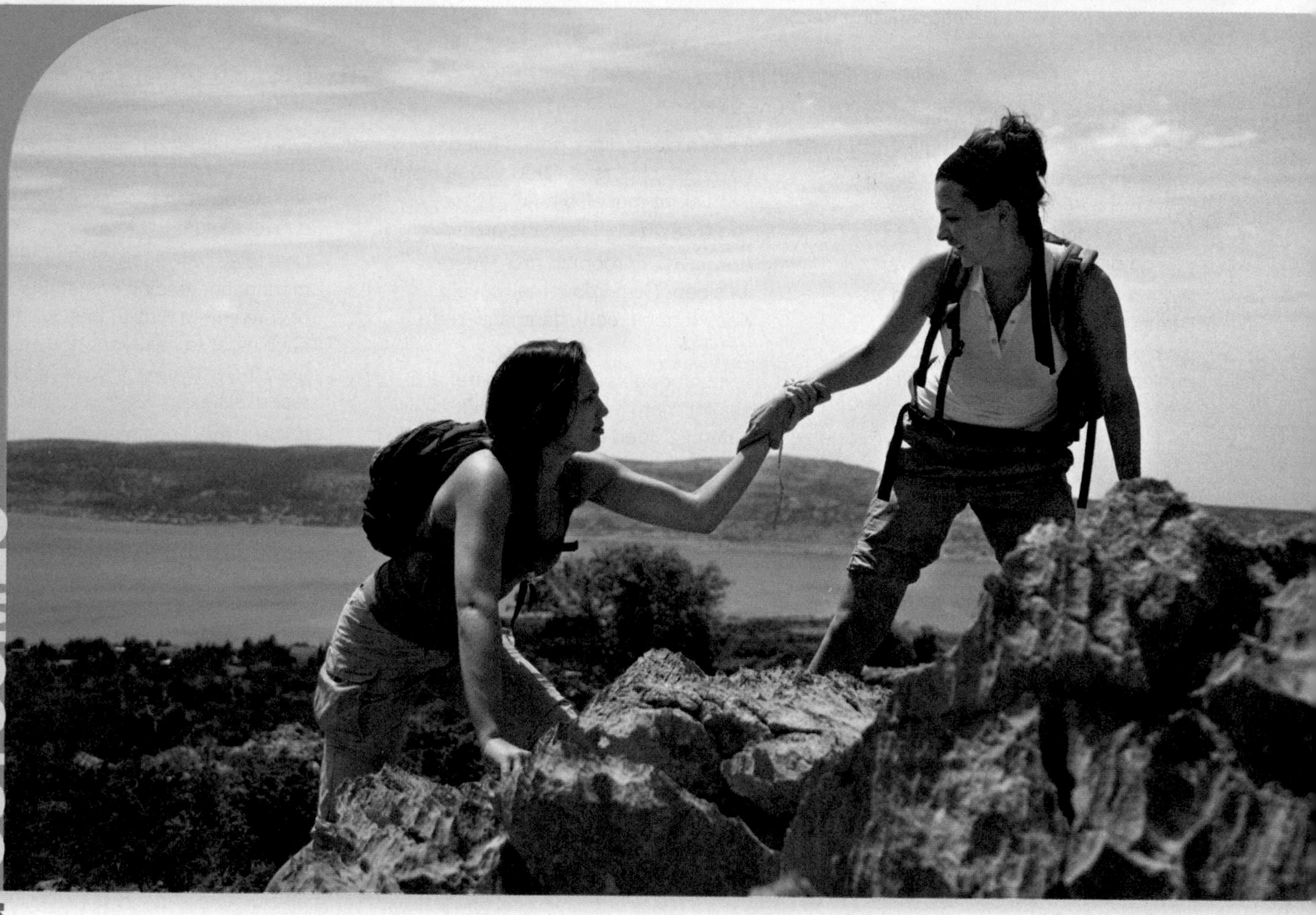

LEARNING OUTCOMES

1. Explain the purpose and common types of intimate relationships.
2. Identify the characteristics of successful relationships, including how to maintain them and overcome common barriers.
3. Describe ways to improve communication skills and interpersonal interactions.
4. Compare and contrast the different types of committed relationships.
5. Describe the demographic trends related to remaining single.
6. Examine the factors that affect decisions related to whether or when to have children.
7. Explain why relationships end and how to cope when they do.

Humans are social beings—we have a basic need to belong and to feel loved, accepted, and wanted. We can't live without interacting with others in some way. The ability to relate well and to give and receive love and support are essential components of a healthy and productive life.

We build networks of supportive friends, significant others, family members, and others who play important roles in helping us meet life's challenges. Numerous studies have shown that having supportive interpersonal relationships is beneficial to health.[1]

All relationships involve a degree of risk. However, only by taking these risks can we grow and truly experience all that life has to offer. In this chapter, we examine healthy relationships and the communication skills necessary to create and maintain them. Expressing ourselves well and knowing how to understand others are vitally important skills. These abilities lay the groundwork for healthy relationships, which are critical to overall health.

LO 1 | INTIMATE RELATIONSHIPS

Explain the purpose and common types of intimate relationships.

We can define **intimate relationships** in terms of four characteristics: *behavioral interdependence, need fulfillment, emotional attachment,* and *emotional availability.* Each of these characteristics may be related to interactions with family, close friends, and romantic partners.

Behavioral interdependence refers to the mutual impact that people have on each other as their lives intertwine. What one person does influences what the other person wants to do and can do. Behavioral interdependence may become stronger over time, to the point that each person would feel a void if the other were gone.

Intimate relationships are also a means of *need fulfillment.* Through relationships with others, we fulfill our needs for:

- **Intimacy**—someone with whom we can share our feelings freely.
- **Social integration**—someone with whom we can share worries and concerns.
- **Nurturance**—someone we can take care of and who will take care of us.
- **Assistance**—someone to help us in times of need.
- **Affirmation**—someone who will reassure us of our own worth and tell us that we matter.

In mutually rewarding intimate relationships, partners and friends meet each other's needs. They disclose feelings, share confidences, and provide support and reassurance. Each person comes away feeling better for the interaction and validated by the other person.

In addition to behavioral interdependence and need fulfillment, intimate relationships involve strong bonds of *emotional attachment,* or feelings of love. When we hear the word *intimacy,* we often think of a sexual relationship. Although sex can play an important role in emotional attachment, a relationship can be very intimate without being sexual; for example, two people can be emotionally intimate (share feelings) or spiritually intimate (share spiritual beliefs and meanings) without being sexually intimate.

intimate relationships Relationships with family members, friends, and romantic partners, characterized by behavioral interdependence, need fulfillment, emotional attachment, and emotional availability.

Emotional availability, the ability to give to and receive emotionally from others without fear of being hurt or rejected, is the fourth characteristic of intimate relationships. At times, all of us may limit our emotional availability. For example, after a painful breakup, we may decide not to jump into another relationship immediately, or we may decide to talk about it only with close friends. Holding back can offer time for introspection, healing, and considering lessons learned. Some people who have experienced intense trauma find it difficult to ever be fully available emotionally.[2] This limits their ability to experience intimate relationships.

Relating to Yourself

You have probably heard people say that you must love and care for yourself before you can love someone else. Ultimately, the most important relationship in your life is the one you have with yourself. But how do you learn to value and accept who you are? People with high self-esteem show respect for themselves by remaining true to their values and beliefs. They feel worthy of success in love, relationships, and life in general.

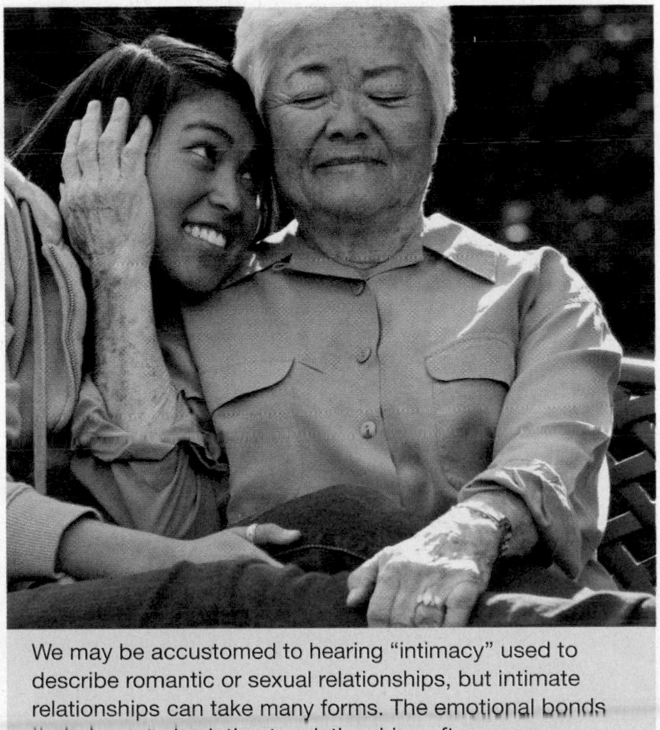

We may be accustomed to hearing "intimacy" used to describe romantic or sexual relationships, but intimate relationships can take many forms. The emotional bonds that characterize intimate relationships often span the generations and help individuals gain insight and understanding into each other's worlds.

HEAR IT! PODCASTS

Want a study podcast for this chapter text? Download the podcast **Healthy Relationships and Sexuality: Making Commitments** available on MasteringHealth.™

Two personal qualities that are especially important to any good relationship are *accountability* and *self-nurturance.* **Accountability** means that you recognize responsibility for your own decisions, choices, and actions. You don't hold others responsible for positive or negative experiences. **Self-nurturance,** which goes hand in hand with accountability, means developing individual potential through a balanced and realistic appreciation of self-worth and ability. To make good choices in life, a person must balance many physical and emotional needs, including sleeping, eating, exercising, working, relaxing, and socializing. When the balance is disrupted, as it will inevitably be at times, self-nurturing people are patient with themselves as they put things back on course. Learning to live in a balanced and healthy way is a lifelong process. Individuals who are on a path of accountability and self-nurturance have a much better chance of achieving this balance and maintaining satisfying relationships with others.

accountability Accepting responsibility for personal decisions, choices, and actions.

self-nurturance Developing individual potential through a balanced and realistic appreciation of self-worth and ability.

family of origin People present in the household during a child's first years of life—usually parents and siblings.

Self-Esteem and Self-Acceptance Important factors that affect your ability to nurture yourself and maintain healthy relationships with others include the way you define yourself (*self-concept*) and the way you evaluate yourself (*self-esteem*). Your self-concept is like a mental mirror that reflects how you view your physical features, emotional states, talents, likes and dislikes, values, and roles. A person might define herself as an activist, a mother, an honor student, an athlete, or a musician. In contrast, how you feel about yourself or evaluate yourself constitutes your self-esteem. You might consider yourself an excellent student, a horrible singer, a great lover, or a "10" in terms of appearance. Taken together, such judgments indicate your level of self-esteem or self-evaluation.

Your perception and acceptance of yourself influence your relationship choices. If you feel unattractive, insecure, or inferior to others, you may choose not to interact with other people or to avoid social events. You may even unconsciously seek out individuals who confirm your negative view of yourself by treating you poorly. Conversely, if you are secure about your unique characteristics and talents, that positive self-concept will make it easier to form relationships with people who support and nurture you and to interact with a variety of people in a healthy, balanced way.

WHAT DO YOU THINK?

What values about relationships did you learn from your family?

- Did your family foster open, caring communication?
- Were they demonstrative in showing their love and feelings for others?
- How do you think they influenced you in your relationships today?

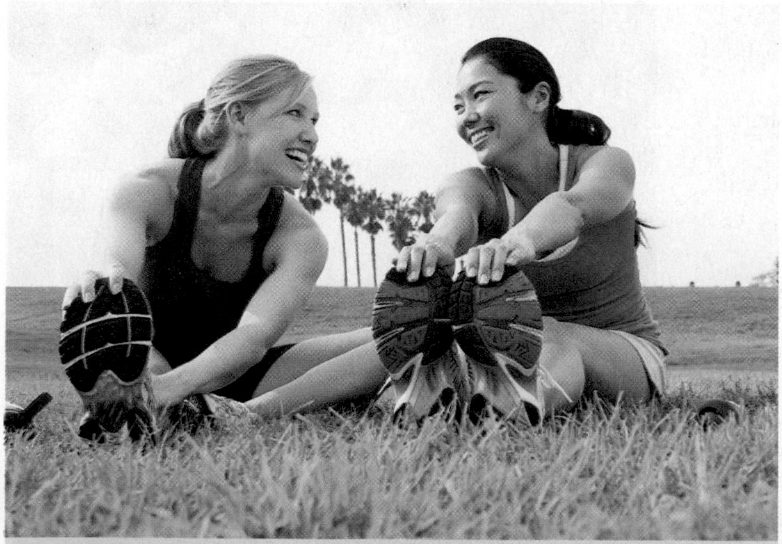

Good friends can add joy and meaning to your life. As Abraham Lincoln said, "The better part of one's life consists of his friendships."

Family Relationships

A family is a recognizable group of people with roles, tasks, boundaries, and personalities whose central focus is to protect, care for, love, and socialize with one another. Because the family is a dynamic institution that changes as society changes, the definition of *family* changes over time. Historically, most families have been made up of people related by blood, marriage or long-term committed relationships, or adoption. Yet today, many other groups of people are recognized and function as family units. Although there is no "best" family type, we do know that a healthy family's key roles and tasks are to nurture and support. Healthy families foster a sense of security and feelings of belonging that are central to growth and development.

During the childhood years, families provide our most significant relationships. It is from our **family of origin,** the people present in our household during our first years of life, that we initially learn about feelings, problem solving, love, intimacy, and gender roles. We learn to negotiate relationships and have opportunities to communicate effectively, develop attitudes and values, and explore spiritual belief systems. It is not uncommon when we establish relationships outside the family to rely on these initial experiences and on skills modeled by our family of origin.

Friendships

Friendships are often the first relationships we form outside of our immediate families, and they can be some of life's most stable and enduring relationships. Establishing and maintaining strong friendships may be a good predictor of your success in establishing loving relationships, as each requires shared interests and values, mutual acceptance, trust, understanding, respect, and levels of confidence.

WHAT DO YOU THINK?

What characteristics keep your friendships intact?

- What do you gain from your friendships?
- What do your friends gain in return?

Developing meaningful friendships is more than merely "friending" someone on Facebook. Getting to know someone well requires time, effort, and commitment. But the effort is worth it: A good friend can be a trustworthy companion, someone who respects your strengths as well as your weaknesses, someone who can share your joys and your sorrows, and someone you can count on for support.

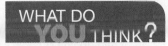

Romantic Relationships

At some point, most people choose to enter an intimate romantic and sexual relationship with another person. Romantic relationships typically include all the characteristics of friendship as well as the following characteristics related to passion and caring:

- **Fascination.** Lovers tend to pay attention to the other person even when they should be involved in other activities. They are preoccupied with the other and want to think about, talk to, and be with the other.
- **Exclusivity.** Lovers have a special relationship that usually precludes having the same kind of relationship with a third party. The love relationship often takes priority over all others.
- **Sexual desire.** Lovers desire physical intimacy and want to touch, hold, and engage in sexual activities with the other.
- **Giving the utmost.** Lovers care enough to give the utmost when the other is in need, sometimes to the point of extreme sacrifice.
- **Being a champion or advocate.** Lovers actively champion each other's interests and attempt to ensure that the other succeeds.

Theories of Love There is no single definition of *love*, and the word may mean different things to different people, depending on cultural values, age, gender, and situation. Although we may not know how to put our feelings into words, we know it when the "lightning bolt" of love strikes.

consummate love A relationship that combines intimacy, compassion, and commitment.

Several theories related to how and why love develops have been proposed. In his classic triangular theory of love, psychologist Robert Sternberg proposes the following three key components to loving relationships (**FIGURE 4.1**):[3]

- **Intimacy.** The emotional component, which involves closeness, sharing, and mutual support.
- **Passion.** The motivational component, which includes lust, attraction, and sexual arousal.
- **Commitment.** The cognitive component, which includes the decision to be open to love in the short term and the commitment to the relationship in the long term.

The quality of a love relationship is related to the level of intimacy, passion, and commitment each person brings to the relationship over time. Sternberg suggests that relationships that include two or more of these components are more likely to endure than those that include only one. He uses the term **consummate love** to describe a combination of intimacy, passion, and commitment—an ideal and deep form of love that is, unfortunately, rare.[4]

Quite different from Sternberg's approach are theories of love and attraction based on brain circuitry and chemistry. Anthropologist Helen Fisher, among others, hypothesizes that attraction and falling in love follow a fairly predictable pattern based on (1) *imprinting*, in which our evolutionary patterns, genetic predispositions, and past

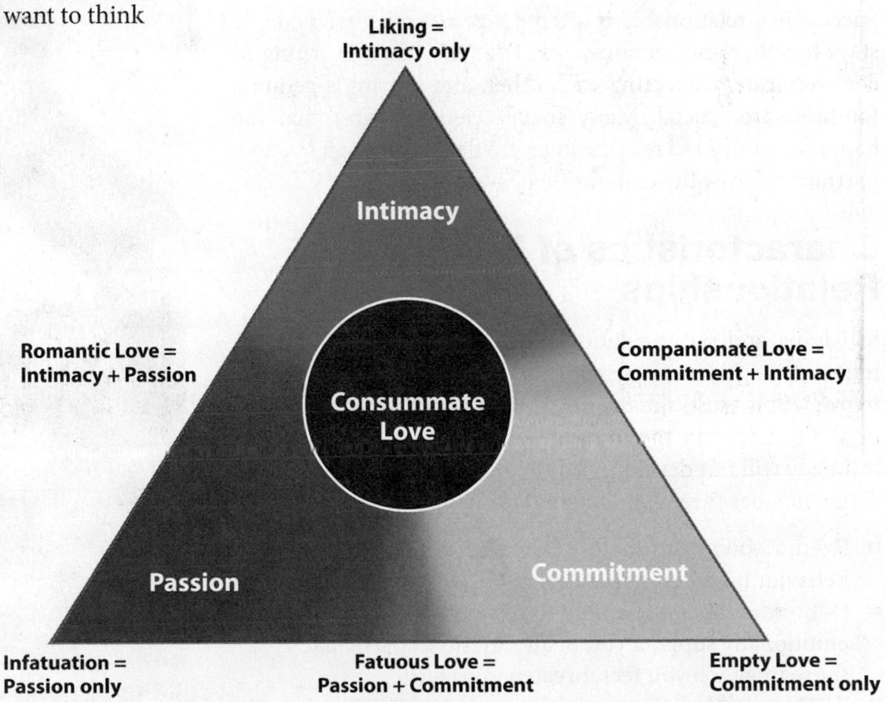

FIGURE 4.1 Sternberg's Triangular Theory of Love According to Sternberg's model, three elements—intimacy, passion, and commitment—existing alone or in combination, form different types of love. The most complete, ideal type of love in the model is consummate love, which combines balanced amounts of all three elements.

experiences trigger a romantic reaction; (2) *attraction,* in which neurochemicals produce feelings of euphoria and elation; (3) *attachment,* in which endorphins (natural opiates) cause lovers to feel peaceful, secure, and calm; and (4) *production of a cuddle chemical;* that is, the brain secretes the hormone oxytocin, which stimulates sensations during lovemaking and elicits feelings of satisfaction and attachment.[5]

According to Fisher's theory, lovers who claim to be swept away by passion may not be far from the truth. A love-smitten person's endocrine system secretes chemical substances such as dopamine, norepinephrine, and phenylethylamine (PEA), which are chemical cousins of amphetamines.[6] Attraction may in fact be a "natural high"; however, this passion "buzz" loses effectiveness over time as the body builds up a tolerance. Fisher speculates that some people become attraction junkies, seeking out the intoxication of new love much as a drug user seeks a chemical high. Fisher also suggests that the significant drop in PEA levels over a 3- to 4-year period leads to the "4-year itch" that manifests in the peaking fourth-year divorce rates present in more than 60 cultures. Romances that last beyond the 4-year mark are influenced by endorphins that give lovers a sense of security, peace, and calm.[7]

LO 2 | STRATEGIES FOR SUCCESSFUL RELATIONSHIPS

Identify the characteristics of successful relationships, including how to maintain them and overcome common barriers.

Success in a relationship is often defined as whether a couple stays together and remains close over the years. Learning to communicate, respecting each other, and sharing a genuine fondness are crucial. Many social scientists agree that the happiest committed relationships are flexible enough to allow partners to grow throughout their lives.

Characteristics of Healthy Relationships

Satisfying and stable relationships are based on good communication, intimacy, friendship, and other factors. A key ingredient is trust, the degree to which each partner feels he or she can rely on the integrity of the other. Without trust, intimacy will not develop, and the relationship will likely fail. Trust includes three fundamental elements:[8]

- **Predictability**—the ability to predict your partner's behavior based on past actions.
- **Dependability**—the ability to rely on your partner to emotionally support you in all situations, particularly those in which you feel threatened or hurt.
- **Faith**—your belief in your partner having positive intentions and behavior.

What does a healthy relationship look and feel like? Characteristics of healthy and unhealthy relationships are contrasted in **FIGURE 4.2**. Answering some basic questions can also help you determine if a relationship is working.

- Do you love and care for yourself to the same extent that you did before the relationship? Can you be yourself in the relationship?
- Is there genuine caring and goodwill? Do you share interests, values, and opinions? Is there mutual respect for differences?
- Is there mutual encouragement? Are you there for each other and do you support each other unconditionally?
- Do you trust each other? Are you honest with each other? Can you comfortably express your feelings, opinions, and needs?
- Is there room in your relationship for growth as you both evolve and mature?

Relationships are nurtured by consistent communication, actions, and self-reflection. Poor communication can weaken bonds and create mistrust. We all need to reflect periodically on how we typically relate to others through our words and actions. Have we been honest, direct, and fair in our conversations?

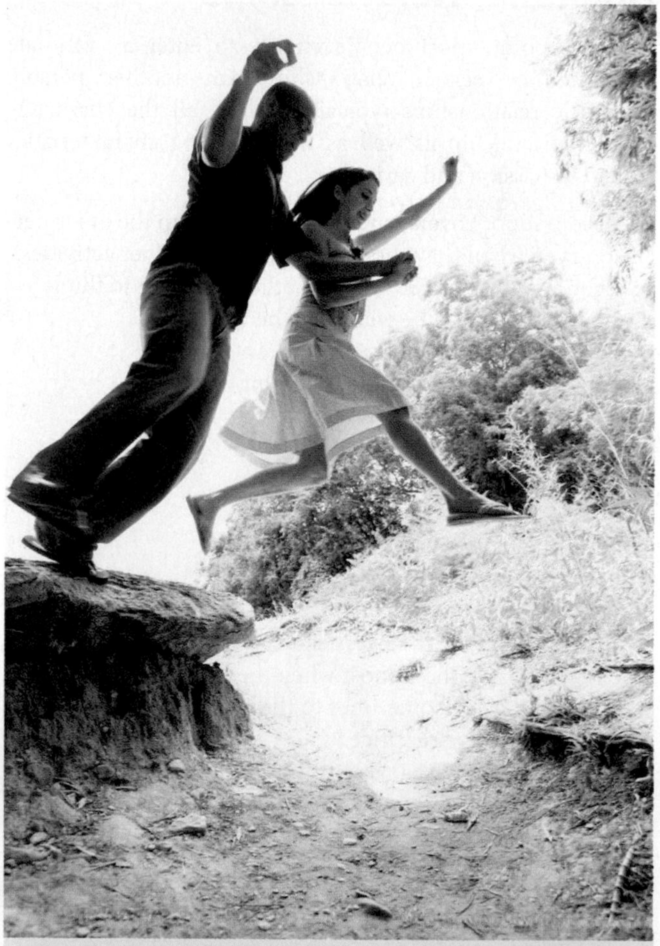

Healthy relationships can come in all shapes and sizes, but they do have some characteristics in common, including communication, caring, respect, and support. One of the most important components of a strong relationship is trust, which is made up of predictability, dependability, and faith.

In an unhealthy relationship . . .	In a healthy relationship . . .
You care for and focus on another person only and neglect yourself or you focus only on yourself and neglect the other person.	You both love and take care of yourselves before and while in a relationship.
One of you feels pressure to change to meet the other person's standards and is afraid to disagree or voice ideas.	You respect each other's individuality, embrace your differences, and allow each other to "be yourselves."
One of you has to justify what you do, where you go, and whom you see.	You both do things with friends and family and have activities independent of each other.
One of you makes all the decisions and controls everything without listening to the other's input.	You discuss things with each other, allow for differences of opinion, and compromise equally.
One of you feels unheard and is unable to communicate what you want.	You express and listen to each other's feelings, needs, and desires.
You lie to each other and find yourself making excuses for the other person.	You both trust and are honest with yourselves and with each other.
You don't have any personal space and have to share everything with the other person.	You respect each other's need for privacy.
Your partner keeps his or her sexual history a secret or hides a sexually transmitted infection from you, or you do not disclose your history to your partner.	You share sexual histories and information about sexual health with each other.
One of you is scared of asking the other to use protection or has refused the other's requests for safer sex.	You both practice safer sex methods.
One of you has forced or coerced the other to have sex.	You both respect sexual boundaries and are able to say no to sex.
One of you yells and hits, shoves, or throws things at the other in an argument.	You resolve conflicts in a rational, peaceful, and mutually agreed upon way.
You feel stifled, trapped, and stagnant. You are unable to escape the pressures of the relationship.	You both have room for positive growth, and you both learn more about each other as you develop and mature.

FIGURE 4.2 Healthy versus Unhealthy Relationships

Source: Advocates for Youth, Washington, DC, 2006, www.advocatesforyouth.org. Copyright © 2000. Used with permission.

Have we listened to others' thoughts, wants, and needs? Have we behaved in ways consistent with our words, values, and beliefs?

Choosing a Romantic Partner

Choosing a partner is influenced by more than just chemical and psychological processes. Another factor is *proximity*, or being in the same place at the same time. The more often you see a person at school, work, religious or social events, or as part of volunteer activities, the more likely it is that interaction will occur. However, with the growth of Internet dating sites, it has become easier to meet others outside your geographic proximity. (See the **Student Health Today** box on page 116 for guidelines on meeting people online.)

You also choose a partner based on *similarities* (in attitudes, values, intellect, interests, education, and socioeconomic status); the old adage that "opposites attract" usually isn't true. If your potential partner expresses interest or liking, you may react with mutual regard known as *reciprocity*. The more you express interest, the safer it is for someone else to do the same, and the cycle continues.

A final factor that plays a significant role in selecting a partner is *physical attraction*. Whether such attraction is caused by a chemical reaction or a learned behavior, men and women appear to have different attraction criteria. Men tend to be attracted by youth and beauty, while women tend to be attracted to older mates with good financial prospects who appear to be dependable and industrious.

WHAT DO YOU THINK?

What factors do you consider most important in a potential partner?

- Are any absolute musts?
- Does what you believe to be important in a relationship differ from what your parents feel is important?

STUDENT HEALTH TODAY

LOVE IN THE TIME OF TWITTER

Technology has revolutionized our access to information and the ways we communicate. Couples can meet on a site like Match.com, keep in constant contact via texting, and inform the world of their relationship highs and lows via Facebook and Twitter. With all these tools available, it can be easy to share TMI (too much information). Ilana Gershon, author of *The Breakup 2.0: Disconnecting over New Media*, suggests we lack standard etiquette for the use of new media in relationships. At its best, social media can bring people closer together; at its worst, it can be used intentionally or unintentionally to embarrass or hurt. Consider the following suggestions to safeguard yourself:

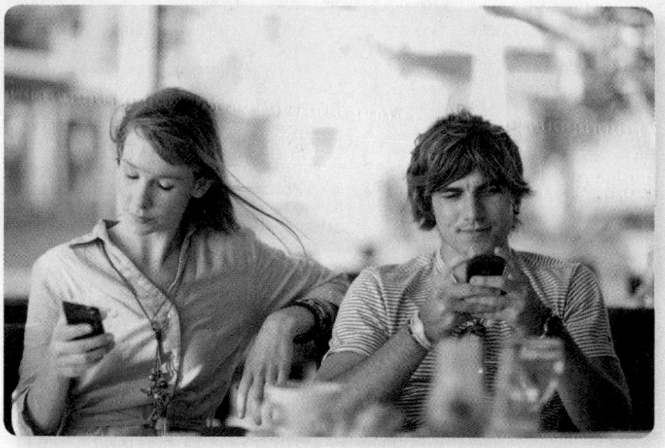

When meeting:

- If you join a dating site, be honest about yourself; state your own interests and characteristics fairly, including things that you think might be less attractive than stereotypes and cultural norms dictate.
- If you meet someone online and want to meet in person, put safety first! Plan something brief, preferably during daylight hours. Meet in a public place, like a coffee shop. Do not meet with anyone who wants to keep the time and location a secret. Tell a friend or family member the details of when and where you are meeting and any information you have on the person you are meeting.

While dating:

- Discuss limits with your partner on the type of information you each want shared online. Agree to share only within those limits.
- Recognize that constant electronic updates throughout the day can leave little to share when you are together. Save some information for face-to-face talks!
- Sober up before you click "submit." Things that seem funny under the influence may not seem funny the next morning.
- Remember that the Internet is forever. Once a picture or a post is sent, it can never be completely erased. Never post anything that would embarrass someone if it was seen by a family member or potential employer.
- Respect your partner's privacy. Logging onto his or her e-mail or Facebook account to look at private messages is a breach of trust.
- Know that the GPS in a phone can be used to track your location, and cell phone spyware can be installed that allows e-mail and texts to be read from another device. If you think you may be a victim of "cyberstalking" by a current (or former) partner, get a new phone or ask the phone company to reinstall the phone's operating system to wipe out the software.

If breaking up:

- Do not break up with someone via text/e-mail/tweet/Facebook/chat. People deserve the respect of a more personal breakup.
- Upon breaking up, be sure to change any passwords you may have confided in your partner. The temptation to use those for ill may be too strong to resist.

Source: I. Gershon, *The Breakup 2.0: Disconnecting over New Media:* Ithaca, NY: Cornell University Press, 2012.

Attraction is a complex notion, and influenced by social, biological, and cultural factors.[9] (See the **Student Health Today** box on the next page for a discussion of "hooking up.")

LO 3 | COMMUNICATING: A KEY TO GOOD RELATIONSHIPS

Describe ways to improve communication skills and interpersonal interactions.

From the moment of birth, we struggle to be understood. We flail our arms, cry, scream, smile, frown, and make sounds and gestures to attract attention or to communicate what we want or need. By adulthood, each of us has developed a unique way of communicating with others through gestures, words, expressions, and body language. No two people communicate exactly the same way or have the same need for connecting with others.

Different cultures have different ways of expressing feelings and using body language. Members of some cultures gesture broadly; others maintain a closed body posture. Some are offended by direct eye contact; others welcome a steady gaze. Men and women also tend to have different styles of communication that are largely dictated by culture and socialization (see the **Health in a Diverse World** box).

Although people differ in the way they communicate, this doesn't mean that one gender, culture, or group is better at communication than another. We have to be willing to accept differences and work to keep communication lines

STUDENT HEALTH TODAY

HOOKING UP

The New Norm or Nothing New?

Hooking up is a vague term often used to describe sexual encounters, from kissing to intercourse, without the expectation of commitment. While college students may feel that there is a new "hookup culture" on campus, research tells a different story. Longitudinal data tells us that young adults' sexual behavior hasn't changed much in the past few decades in terms of the number of sexual encounters or the number of partners. And while students are more likely to describe their sex partner as a friend than in the past, college students are twice as likely to have sex with a romantic partner than with a "hookup."

While hookup behavior may not be as pervasive as some think, college students should understand the risks involved:

1. **Recognize the role of emotions in sex.** Sternberg's "triangle of love" would place hooking up in the "infatuation" category, passion with no commitment or intimacy, far from Sternberg's picture of "ideal." Additionally, according to Fisher, attraction and sex create a chemical reaction in the brain that fosters an emotional response, even if we say "it's just about the sex."
2. **Recognize the role of alcohol in hooking up.** In a recent study of college hookups, students reported that they were more likely to hook up if they had been drinking alcohol. Among participants who consumed alcohol prior to their last hookup, 31 percent of females and 28 percent of males indicated that they would likely not have hooked up with their partners had alcohol not been involved.
3. **Recognize the risk of unintended pregnancy and sexually transmitted infections (STIs).** Reduced inhibitions due to alcohol plus a lack of communication with a new partner increases the risk of unprotected sex, and thus the risk for unintended pregnancy and STIs.

Sources: M. A. Monto and A. G. Carey, "A New Standard of Sexual Behavior? Are Claims Associated with the 'Hookup Culture' Supported by Nationally Representative Data?" *The Journal of Sex Research* (2014), DOI: 10.1080/00224499.2014.906031; R. L. Fielder, K. B. Carey, and M. P. Carey, "Are Hookups Replacing Romantic Relationships? A Longitudinal Study of First-Year Female College Students," *Journal of Adolescent Health* 52, no. 5 (2012): 657–59.

open and fluid. Remaining interested, actively engaged in interaction, and open and willing to exchange ideas and thoughts are all things that we can typically learn with practice. By understanding how to deliver and interpret information, we can enhance our relationships. Three aspects of strong communication skills are sharing information through self-disclosure, becoming a better listener, and understanding nonverbal communication.

Learning Appropriate Self-Disclosure

Sharing personal information with others is called **self-disclosure.** If you are willing to share personal information with others, they will likely share personal information with you. Likewise, if you want to learn more about someone, you have to be willing to share some of your personal background and interests with that person. Self-disclosure is not only storytelling or sharing secrets; it is also revealing how you are reacting to the present situation and giving any information about the past that is relevant to the other person's understanding of your current reactions.

Self-disclosure can be a double-edged sword because there is risk in divulging personal insights and feelings. If you sense that sharing feelings and personal thoughts will result in a closer relationship, you will likely take such a risk. But if you believe that the disclosure may result in rejection or alienation, you may not open up so easily. If the confidentiality of previously shared information has been violated, you may hesitate to be as open in the future. However, the risk in not disclosing yourself to others is that you will lack intimacy in relationships. Famed psychologist Carl Rogers, founder of the client-centered approach to therapy, stressed the importance of understanding yourself and others through self-disclosure. He believed that weak relationships were characterized by inhibited self-disclosure.[10]

self-disclosure Sharing feelings or personal information with others.

All couples have conflicts. Learning to handle them maturely is vital to relationship success.

If self-disclosure is a key element in creating healthy communication, but fear is a barrier to that process, what can we do? The following suggestions can help:

- **Get to know yourself.** Remember that your *self* includes your feelings, beliefs, thoughts, and concerns. The more you know about yourself, the more likely you will be able to share yourself with others.
- **Become more accepting of yourself.** No one is perfect or has to be.
- **Be willing to talk about sex.** The U.S. culture puts many taboos on

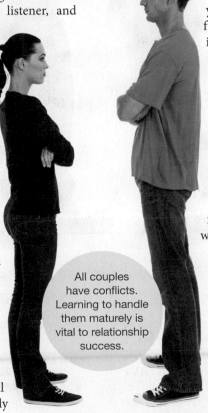

HEALTH IN A DIVERSE WORLD

HE SAYS/SHE SAYS

There are some gender-specific communication patterns and behaviors that are obvious to the casual observer (see graphic). However, according to Dr. Cynthia Burggraf Torppa at Ohio State University, the bigger difference is the way in which men and women interpret or process the same message. She indicates that women are more sensitive to interpersonal meanings "between the lines," and men are more sensitive to subtle messages about status. Recognizing these differences and how they make us unique is a good first step in avoiding unnecessary frustrations and miscommunications.

Sources: C. Burggraf Torppa, Family and Consumer Sciences, Ohio State University Extension, "Gender Issues: Communication Differences in Interpersonal Relationships," 2010, http://ohioline.osu.edu/flm02/pdf/fs04.pdf; J. Wood, *Gendered Lives: Communication, Gender, and Culture*, 10th ed. (Belmont, CA: Cengage, 2013).

VIDEO TUTOR Gender Differences in Communication

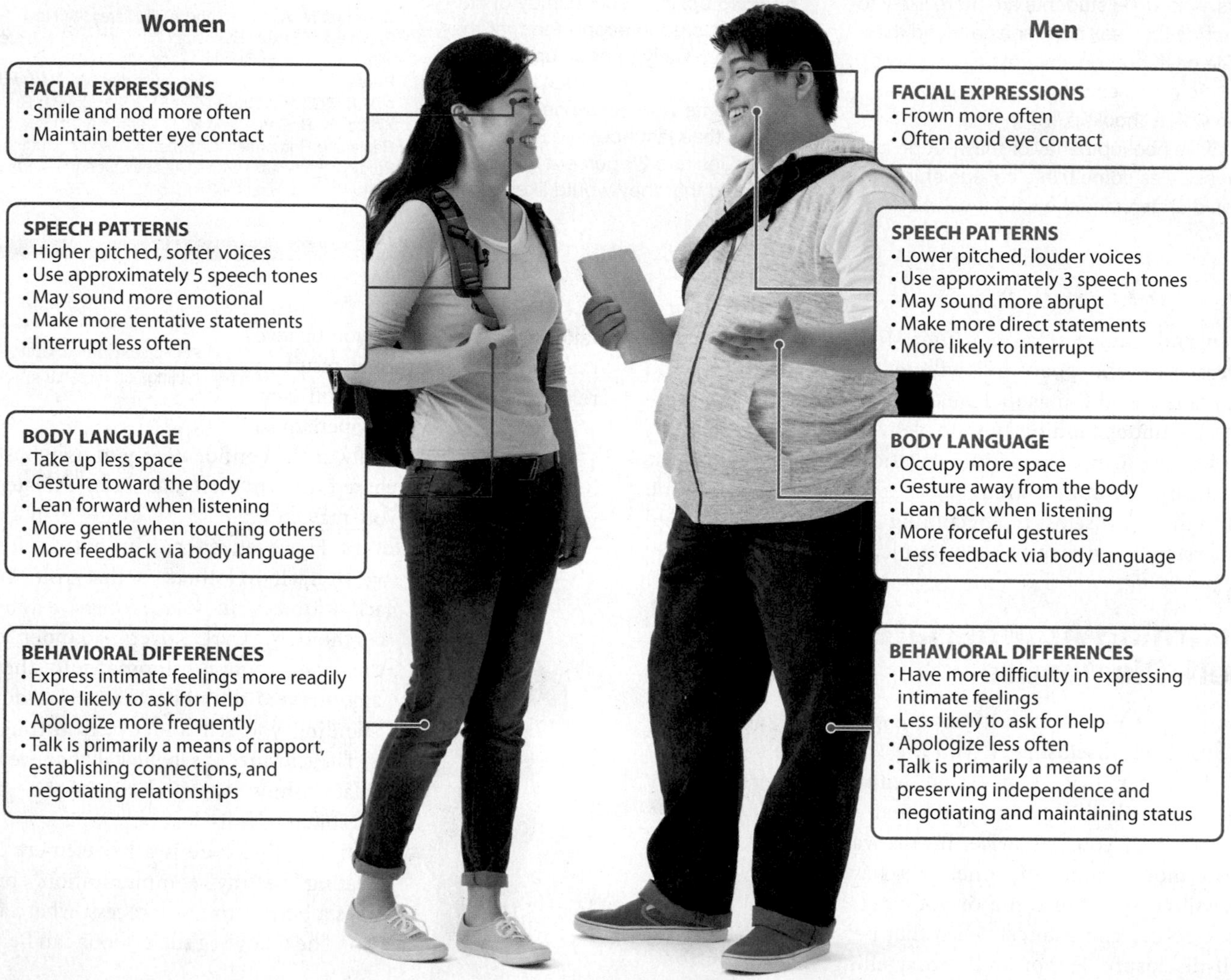

discussions of sex, so it's no wonder we find it hard to disclose our sexual past to those with whom we are intimate. However, with the triple threat of unintended pregnancy, sexually transmitted infections, and HIV/AIDS, it is important to discuss sexual history with a partner.

Women
FACIAL EXPRESSIONS
• Smile and nod more often
• Maintain better eye contact
SPEECH PATTERNS
• Higher pitched, softer voices
• Use approximately 5 speech tones
• May sound more emotional
• Make more tentative statements
• Interrupt less often
BODY LANGUAGE
• Take up less space
• Gesture toward the body
• Lean forward when listening
• More gentle when touching others
• More feedback via body language
BEHAVIORAL DIFFERENCES
• Express intimate feelings more readily
• More likely to ask for help
• Apologize more frequently
• Talk is primarily a means of rapport, establishing connections, and negotiating relationships
Men
FACIAL EXPRESSIONS
• Frown more often
• Often avoid eye contact
SPEECH PATTERNS
• Lower pitched, louder voices
• Use approximately 3 speech tones
• May sound more abrupt
• Make more direct statements
• More likely to interrupt
BODY LANGUAGE
• Occupy more space
• Gesture away from the body
• Lean back when listening
• More forceful gestures
• Less feedback via body language
BEHAVIORAL DIFFERENCES
• Have more difficulty in expressing intimate feelings
• Less likely to ask for help
• Apologize less often
• Talk is primarily a means of preserving independence and negotiating and maintaining status

- **Choose a safe context for self-disclosure.** When and where you make such disclosures and to whom may greatly influence the response you receive. Choose a setting in which you feel safe to let yourself be heard.
- **Be thoughtful about self-disclosure via social media.** Self-disclosure can be an effective method of building

STUDENT HEALTH TODAY

LIFE IS AN OPEN (FACE)BOOK

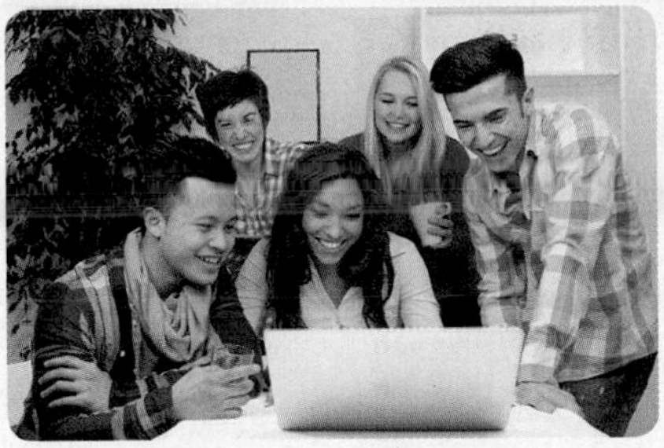

Headlines such as "Prince Harry Parties Naked in Las Vegas" and "Gay Students Accidentally Outed to Parents via Facebook" remind us that we cannot expect privacy in a world where nearly everyone has a camera and an Internet connection. We are a photo tag away from a family member or potential employer seeing us in less than flattering circumstances or knowing information we'd prefer kept secret.

"Social media screening," the practice of searching out all possible information on a prospective employee (sometimes to the point of asking for a Facebook password at an interview) is practiced by a third of employers. Their biggest concerns are inappropriate photos, evidence of drug or alcohol use or abuse, and poor writing skills.

If you are concerned about your privacy, make sure your publicly available information is what you want prospective employers, family, and other people to see. Tighten your privacy settings and untag yourself in photos you don't want people to see. Due to cached sites and reposts, you can't erase everything, so you may need to prepare an explanation for past posts, photos, and other information. Don't "overshare." As our "private" lives get more public all the time, we may have to accept Facebook founder Mark Zuckerberg's philosophy, that "privacy is no longer a social norm."

Sources: N. Messieh, "Survey: 37% of Your Prospective Employers Are Looking You up on Facebook," News: Social Media, *The Next Web*, Blog, April 18, 2012, http://thenextweb.com; B. Johnson, "Privacy No Longer a Social Norm, Says Facebook Founder," *The Guardian,* January 10, 2010, www.guardian.co.uk; N. Evans, "Back to Face the Music? Prince Harry Flies Home After Las Vegas Naked Photos Scandal," *Mirror News* Online, August 22, 2012, www.mirror.co.uk; G. Fowler, "When the Most Personal Secrets Get Outed on Facebook," *The Wall Street Journal*, October 13, 2012, http://online.wsj.com.

intimacy with another person, but not with large groups. Sharing information that is too personal on Facebook or Twitter may cause you to feel vulnerable or embarrassed later. (See the **Student Health Today** box for more on online privacy.)

Becoming a Better Listener

Listening is a vital part of interpersonal communication. Improving listening skills will enhance our relationships, improve our grasp of information, and allow us to interpret more effectively what others say. We listen best when (1) we believe that the message is somehow important and relevant to us; (2) the speaker holds our attention through humor, dramatic effect, or other techniques; and (3) we are in the mood to listen (free of distractions and worries). See the **Skills for Behavior Change** box for suggestions on improving your listening skills.

The Three Basic Listening Modes There are three main ways in which we listen:

- **Competitive listening** happens when we are more interested in explaining our own point of view than in understanding someone else's.[11]
- **Passive listening** occurs when we are listening, but not providing either verbal or nonverbal feedback to the speaker. The speaker may feel unsure if the message is being received.[12]
- **Active listening** is when we not only hear the words, but we try to understand what is really being said. The listener confirms understanding by restating or paraphrasing the speaker's message before responding. By actively listening, we show genuine interest in what the other person is thinking and feeling.[13]

SKILLS FOR BEHAVIOR CHANGE

LEARNING TO REALLY LISTEN

To become a better listener, practice the following skills on a daily basis:

- To avoid distractions, turn off the TV, shut your laptop lid, and put your phone away.
- Be present in the moment. Good listeners participate and acknowledge what the other person is saying through nonverbal cues such as nodding or smiling and asking questions at appropriate times.
- Ask for clarification. If you aren't sure what the speaker means, say that you don't completely understand or paraphrase what you think you heard.
- Control that deadly desire to interrupt. Try taking a deep breath for 2 seconds, then hold your breath for another second, and really listen to what is being said as you slowly exhale.
- Resist the temptation to "set the other person straight."
- Focus on the speaker. Hold back the temptation to launch into a story of your own experience in a similar situation.

nonverbal communication Unwritten and unspoken messages, both intentional and unintentional.

conflict Emotional state that arises when opinions differ or the behavior of one person interferes with the behavior of another.

conflict resolution Concerted effort by all parties to constructively resolve differences or points of contention.

Using Nonverbal Communication

Understanding what someone is saying often involves much more than listening and speaking. Often, what is not actually said may speak louder than any words could. Rolling the eyes, looking at the floor or ceiling rather than maintaining eye contact, body movements and hand gestures—all these nonverbal clues influence the way we interpret messages. **Nonverbal communication** includes all unwritten and unspoken messages, both intentional and unintentional. Ideally, our nonverbal communication matches and supports our verbal communication, but this is not always the case. Research shows that when verbal and nonverbal communication doesn't match, we are more likely to believe the nonverbal cues.[14] This is one reason it is important to be aware of the nonverbal cues we use regularly and to understand how others might interpret them.

Nonverbal communication can include the following:[15]

- **Touch.** This can be a handshake, a warm hug, a hand on the shoulder, or a kiss on the cheek.
- **Gestures.** These can include gestures that replace words, such as a thumbs-up or a wave hello or good-bye, or movements that augment verbal communication, such as indicating with your hands how big the fish was that got away. Gestures can also be rude, such as glancing at one's watch to indicate a wish to escape or rolling one's eyes to indicate disdain for what has been said.
- **Interpersonal space.** This is the amount of physical space that separates two people.
- **Body language.** This includes movements such as folding your arms across your chest, indicating defensiveness, or leaning forward in your chair to show interest.
- **Tone of voice.** This refers not to what you say, but how you say it—including the pitch and volume of your voice and speed of your speech.
- **Facial expressions.** These signal moods and emotions, such as smiling when you are happy.

Facial expressions are believed to have near universal meaning; however, most other body language is culturally specific. A gesture of agreement in one culture can be offensive in another. To communicate as effectively as possible, it is important to recognize and use appropriate nonverbal cues that support and help clarify your verbal messages. Awareness and practice of your verbal and nonverbal communication will also enhance your skills in interpreting messages.

WHY SHOULD I CARE?

Why is developing communication skills so important? Unless you decide to be a hermit, there is hardly a career or life path you might choose that won't require communicating and cooperating with others. Develop good communication skills now, and you'll be poised for success.

Managing Conflict through Communication

A **conflict** is an emotional state that arises when the behavior of one person interferes with that of another. Conflict is inevitable whenever people live or work together. Not all conflict is bad; in fact, airing feelings and coming to some form of resolution over differences can sometimes strengthen relationships. **Conflict resolution** and successful conflict management form a systematic approach to resolving differences fairly and constructively, rather than allowing them to fester. The goal of conflict resolution is to solve differences peacefully and creatively.

Prolonged conflict can destroy relationships unless the parties agree to resolve points of contention constructively. As two people learn to negotiate and compromise on their differences, the number and intensity of conflicts should diminish. Conflict resolution can therefore be a growth process as people learn to recognize problems and find solutions based on past experience.

Here are some strategies for conflict resolution:[16]

1. **Identify the problem or issue.** Talk with each other to clarify exactly what the conflict or problem is. Try to understand both sides of the problem. In this first stage, you must say what you want and listen to what the other person

SKILLS FOR BEHAVIOR CHANGE

COMMUNICATING WHEN EMOTIONS RUN HIGH

How many times have you struggled to find just the right words in an emotionally charged situation? The following guidelines can help you express your feelings more effectively:

- Try to be specific rather than general about how you feel.
- If you have mixed feelings, say so; express each feeling and explain what it is about.
- Use "I" messages rather than "you" statements that can cast blame. By using "I" messages, you take responsibility for communicating your own feelings, thoughts, and beliefs.
- During a heated conflict, pause before responding and consider the possible impact of your comment. Wait to discuss a problem if you can't remain calm.
- When you ask for feedback, be prepared for an honest answer.
- Be careful when trying to communicate or interpret emotionally charged messages via e-mail or text. It can be hard to interpret their intended meaning without the nonverbal support of tone of voice and body language.

wants. Focus on using "I" messages and avoid "you" messages. Be an active listener: Repeat what the other person has said and ask questions for clarification. See the **Skills for Behavior Change** box on the previous page for some guidelines on how to express difficult feelings.

2. **Generate several possible solutions.** Base your search for solutions on the goals and interests identified in the first step. Come up with several different alternatives, and avoid evaluating any of them until you have finished brainstorming.
3. **Evaluate the alternative solutions.** Narrow solutions to one or two that seem to work for both parties. Be honest with each other about a solution that feels unsatisfactory, but also be open to compromise.
4. **Decide on the best solution.** Choose an alternative that is acceptable to both parties. You both need to be committed to the decision for this solution to be effective.
5. **Implement the solution.** Discuss how the decision will be carried out. Establish who is responsible to do what and when. The solution stands a better chance of working if you agree on how it will be implemented.
6. **Follow up.** Evaluate whether the solution is working. Check in with the other person to see how he or she feels about it. Are you satisfied with the way the solution is working out? If something is not working as planned, or if circumstances have changed, discuss revising the plan. Remember that both parties must agree to any changes to the plan, as they did with the original idea.

WHAT DO YOU THINK?

How well do you manage conflict in your personal relationships?

- What could you improve about the way you resolve conflicts?

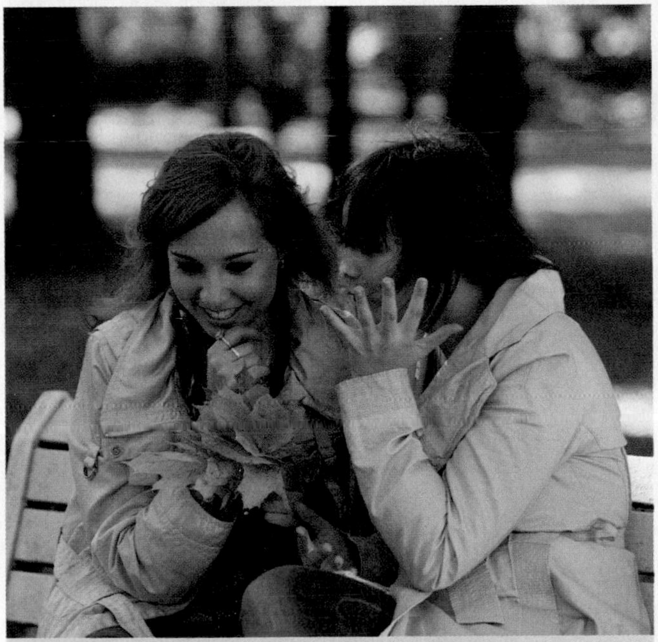

One way to communicate better is to pay attention to your body language. Much of our message is conveyed by nonverbal cues. Laughing, smiling, and gesturing all help convey meaning and assure your partner that you are actively engaged in the conversation.

LO 4 | COMMITTED RELATIONSHIPS

Compare and contrast the different types of committed relationships.

Commitment in a relationship means that one intends to act over time in a way that perpetuates the well-being of the other person, oneself, and the relationship. Polls show that the vast majority of Americans strive to develop a committed relationship, whether in the form of marriage, cohabitation, or partnerships.[17]

Marriage

In many societies, traditional committed relationships take the form of marriage. In the United States, marriage means entering into a legal agreement that includes shared finances, property, and responsibility for raising children. Many Americans also view marriage as a religious sacrament that emphasizes certain rights and obligations for each spouse. Marriage is socially sanctioned and highly celebrated in American culture, so there are numerous incentives for couples to formalize their relationship in this way.

Historically, close to 90 percent of Americans married at least once during their lifetime, and at any given time, about 50 percent of U.S. adults are married (**FIGURE 4.3**). However,

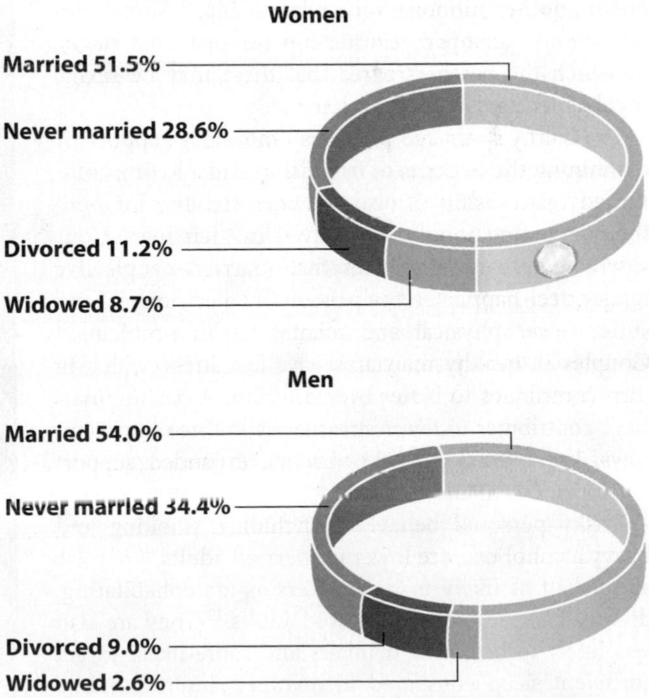

FIGURE 4.3 Marital Status of the U.S. Population by Sex

Note: The figure does not list the percentages for married men and women with a spouse absent and separated.

Source: U.S. Census Bureau, "Table A1. Marital Status of People 15 Years and Over, by Age, Sex, Personal Earnings, Race, and Hispanic Origin: 2013," America's Families and Living Arrangements, 2013, www.census.gov.

monogamy Exclusive sexual involvement with one partner.

serial monogamy Series of monogamous sexual relationships.

open relationship A relationship in which partners agree that sexual involvement can occur outside the relationship.

cohabitation Intimate partners living together without being married.

common-law marriage Cohabitation lasting a designated period of time (usually 7 years) that is considered legally binding in some states.

in recent years Americans have become less likely to marry. Since 1960, the annual number of marriages has steadily declined.[18] This decrease may be due to several factors, including delay of first marriages, an increase in cohabitation, and a small decrease in the number of divorced persons who remarry. In 1960, the median age for first marriage was 23 years for men and 20 years for women; today, the median age for first marriage has risen to 29 years for men and 26 years for women.[19]

88% OF AMERICANS LIST **LOVE** AS THE MOST IMPORTANT REASON TO MARRY.

Many Americans believe that marriage involves **monogamy,** or exclusive sexual involvement with one partner. However, the lifetime pattern for many Americans appears to be **serial monogamy,** which means a person has a monogamous sexual relationship with one partner before moving on to another monogamous relationship.[20] Some couples choose an **open relationship** (or open marriage), in which the partners agree that there may be sexual involvement outside their relationship.

A healthy marriage provides emotional support by combining the benefits of friendship and a loving committed relationship. It also provides stability for both the couple and for those involved in their lives. Considerable research indicates that married people live longer, feel happier, remain mentally alert longer, and suffer fewer physical and mental health problems.[21] Couples in healthy marriages have less stress, which in turn contributes to better overall health. A healthy marriage contributes to lower stress levels in three important ways: improved personal behaviors, expanded support networks, and financial stability.

Risky personal behaviors, including smoking and heavy alcohol use, are lower in married adults. They are about half as likely to be smokers as are cohabitating, divorced, separated, or widowed adults.[22] They are also less likely to be heavy drinkers and more likely to get sufficient sleep compared to divorced adults.[23] While it may be that marriage causes the improved behaviors, it may also be that people who engage in healthier behaviors are just more likely to get married. One negative health indicator for married people is body weight in men. Married men are far more likely than never-married men to be overweight, but no more likely than divorced or separated men. Married women, however, are less likely than divorced women to be overweight or obese.[24] Marriage additionally provides the opportunity for strong integration into a network of family and friends to provide assistance and help couples cope when stressors inevitably arise. Finally, marriage is strongly related to economic well-being, which can impact both health status and stress levels. See the **Money & Health** box for more on how marriage contributes to financial health.

Cohabitation

Cohabitation is a relationship in which two unmarried people with an intimate connection live together in the same household. For a variety of reasons, more Americans are choosing cohabitation. In some states, cohabitation that lasts a designated number of years (usually 7) legally constitutes a **common-law marriage** for purposes of purchasing real estate and sharing other financial obligations.

Cohabitation can offer many of the same benefits as marriage: love, sex, companionship, and the opportunity to know a partner better over time. In addition to emotional and physical benefits, some people may live together for practical reasons, such as the opportunity to share bills and housing costs. Over the past 20 years, there has been a large increase in the number of persons who have cohabited. In fact, cohabitation is increasingly the first coresidential partnership for

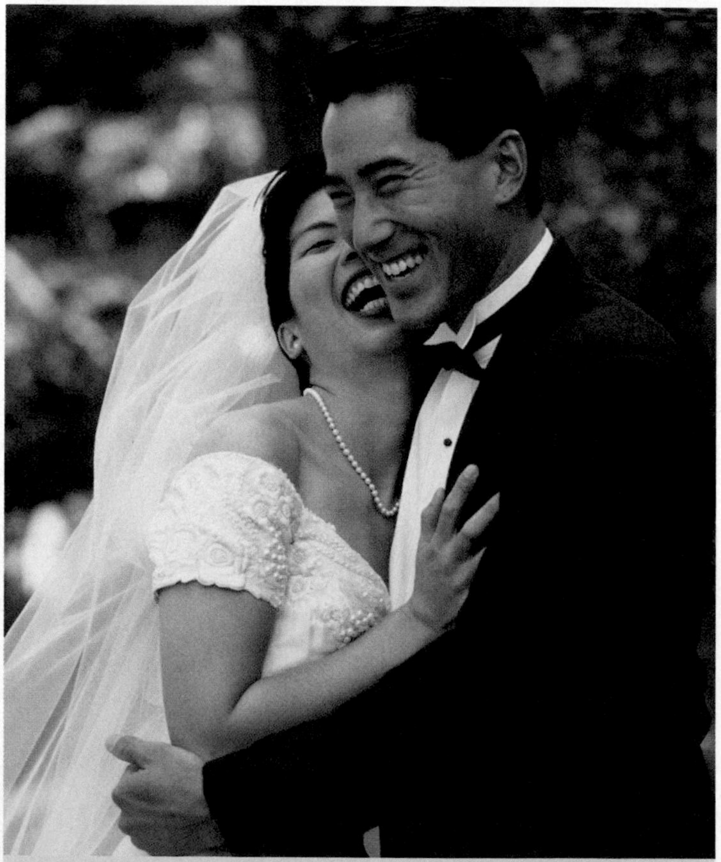

For many, weddings or commitment ceremonies serve as the ultimate symbol of a long-term, exclusive relationship between two people.

MONEY & HEALTH | FOR RICHER OR FOR POORER?

If you want to retire rich, stay married! Jay Zagorsky, an Ohio State University researcher, found that a person who gets married and stays married accumulates almost twice as much personal wealth as a person who gets divorced or never marries. Using the National Longitudinal Survey of Youth, Zagorsky followed 9,055 people for 15 years, finding that married people accumulated 77 percent more wealth than did divorced people.

This accumulation of wealth is attributed to a number of factors. It is cheaper to run one household of two than two households of one. Married people share items and buy them in larger quantities, which usually cost less. Additionally, because of task sharing, they are able to produce more in the same time as a couple than they could individually. For example, if one does laundry and the other vacuums, in the same time they have accomplished two tasks. There are also Social Security and tax advantages for married couples.

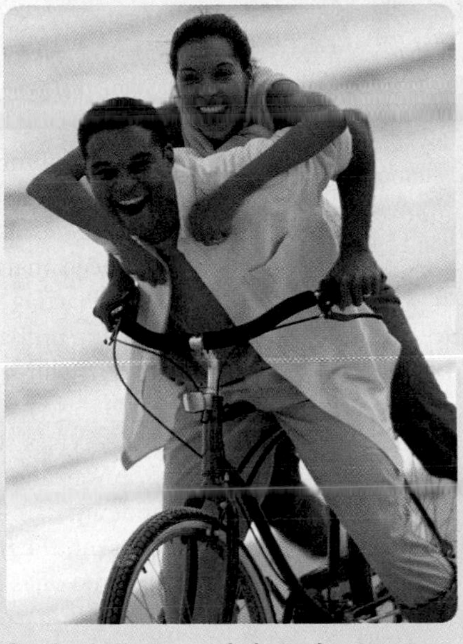
Studies indicate married people may experience higher levels of health and wealth than their unmarried counterparts.

Married people also behave differently: They work longer hours, advance further in their jobs, and they save more money. They are more likely to own homes and stocks. Financial stability is one more reason to invest in our relationships, as according to Zagorsky, "Divorce is as crushing to finances, as it is to emotions."

Sources: J. Zagorsky, "Marriage and Divorce's Impact on Wealth," *Journal of Sociology* 41 (2005): 406–24; *Forbes Magazine,* "Five Ways Love and Marriage Can Make You Wealthier," February 7, 2013, www.forbes.com/sites/financialfinesse/2013/02/07/5-ways-love-and-marriage-can-make-you-wealthier.

young adults, and the majority of young couples now live together before marriage.[25] On average, the first cohabitation before marriage for people over age 20 lasts about 18 months, with about 40 percent of couples transitioning into marriage within 3 years.[26]

Cohabitation before marriage has been a controversial issue for decades. While some voiced moral objections, other concerns were related to higher divorce rates among couples who cohabited before marriage. However, according to recent research based on more than 7,000 respondents to the National Survey of Family Growth, cohabitation before marriage is no longer a predictor for divorce.[27]

23 | IS THE AGE AFTER WHICH COUPLES MARRIED OR MOVED IN TOGETHER ARE LESS LIKELY TO **DIVORCE**.

While cohabitation can serve as a prelude to marriage, for some people, it is an alternative to marriage. Cohabitation is more common among those of lower socioeconomic status, those who are less religious, people who have been divorced, and those who have experienced parental divorce or high levels of parental conflict during childhood. Although cohabitation has advantages, it also has drawbacks. Perhaps the greatest disadvantage is the lack of societal validation for the relationship, especially if the couple subsequently has children. Many cohabitants must deal with pressures from parents and friends, difficulties in obtaining insurance and tax benefits, and legal issues over property.

Gay and Lesbian Marriage/Partnerships

The 2011 American Community Survey identified an estimated 605,472 same-sex couples in the United States, 25 percent of whom are legally married.[28] Whether they are gay or straight, male or female, most adults want intimate, committed relationships. Lesbians and gay men seek the same things in primary relationships that heterosexual partners do: love, friendship, communication, validation, companionship, and a sense of stability.

In addition to facing the same challenges to successful relationships as heterosexual couples, lesbian and gay couples often face discrimination and difficulties dealing with social, religious, and legal issues. For lesbian and gay couples, obtaining the same level of marriage benefits, such as tax deductions, power-of-attorney rights, partner health insurance, and child custody rights, has been challenging. However, over the last few years, changes in policies of the federal government have been improving the status of married homosexual

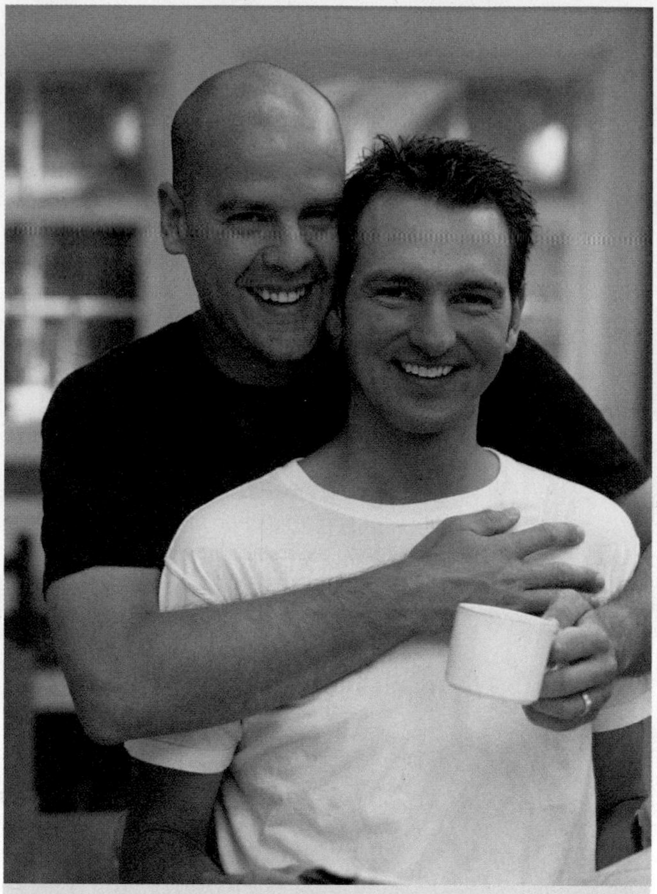

Most adults want to form committed, lasting relationships regardless of their sexual orientation.

couples. In early 2014, the U.S. Justice Department extended the same rights in legal matters to married same-sex couples as married heterosexual couples receive under federal law. This announcement follows policy changes made in 2013, when the U.S. Supreme Court overturned a portion of the Defense of Marriage Act (DOMA) that prevented married homosexual couples from being legally recognized by the federal government. This allowed married homosexual couples to be eligible for federal benefit programs. DOMA was originally established in 1996 to normalize heterosexual marriage on a federal level and to permit each state to decide whether or not to recognize same-sex unions.

At the time of this writing in 2014, Alaska, Arizona, California, Colorado, Connecticut, Delaware, Hawaii, Idaho, Illinois, Indiana, Iowa, Maine, Maryland, Massachusetts, Minnesota, Nevada, New Hampshire, New Jersey, New Mexico, New York, North Carolina, Oklahoma, Oregon, Pennsylvania, Rhode Island, Utah, Vermont, Virginia, Washington, West Virginia, Wisconsin, Wyoming, and the District of Columbia grant same-sex couples full marriage equality. Three other states have broad relationship-recognition laws that extend to same-sex couples all, or nearly all, the state rights and responsibilities of married heterosexual couples, whether labeled "civil unions" or "domestic partnerships."[29] Worldwide, the number of countries that have legalized same-sex marriages or that approve civil unions or registered domestic partnerships for same-sex couples continues to grow. As of the spring of 2014, 17 countries allow same-sex marriage.[30]

LO 5 | STAYING SINGLE

Describe the demographic trends related to remaining single.

Increasing numbers of adults of all ages are electing to marry later or to remain single. According to data from the most recent U.S. Census, 57 percent of women aged 20 to 34 had never been married. Likewise, men in this age group postponed marriage in increasing numbers, with 67 percent remaining unmarried.[31]

Singles clubs, social outings arranged by communities and religious groups, extended family environments, and many social services support the single lifestyle. Many singles live rich, rewarding lives and maintain a large network of close friends and family. Although sexual intimacy may or may not be present, the intimacy achieved through other interactions with loved ones is a key aspect of the single lifestyle.

LO 6 | CHOOSING WHETHER TO HAVE CHILDREN

Examine the factors that affect decisions related to whether or when to have children.

If you decide to raise children, your relationship with your partner will change. Resources of time, energy, and money are split many ways, and you will no longer be able to give each other undivided attention. Babies and young children do not time their requests for food, sleep, and care for the convenience of adults. Therefore, if your own basic needs for security, love, and purpose are met before becoming parents, you will be better prepared for meeting the needs of a child.

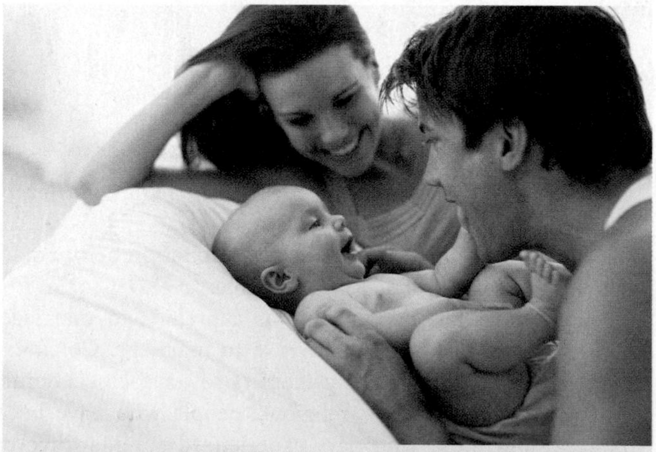

For many people, becoming parents is one of the greatest joys of their lives.

Any stresses existing in your relationship will be further accentuated when parenting is added to your responsibilities. Having a child does not save a bad relationship—in fact, it seems only to compound the problems that already exist. A child cannot and should not be expected to provide the parents with self-esteem and security.

Changing patterns in family life affect the environment in which children are raised. For instance, in modern society, it is not always clear which partner will adjust his or her work schedule to provide the primary care of children. And today, the blended family is increasingly common, creating instant families for stepparents and stepchildren.[32]

You could also be among the increasing numbers of individuals choosing to have children in a family structure other than a heterosexual marriage. Single women or lesbian couples can choose adoption or alternative insemination as a way to create a family. Single men or gay couples can choose to adopt or obtain the services of a surrogate mother. According to the U.S. Census Bureau, in 2012 over 28 percent of all children under age 18 were living in families headed by a man or woman raising a child alone, reflecting a growing trend in America.[33] Regardless of the structure of the family, certain factors remain important to the well-being of the unit: consistency, communication, affection, and mutual respect. Good parenting does not necessarily come naturally.

DID YOU KNOW?

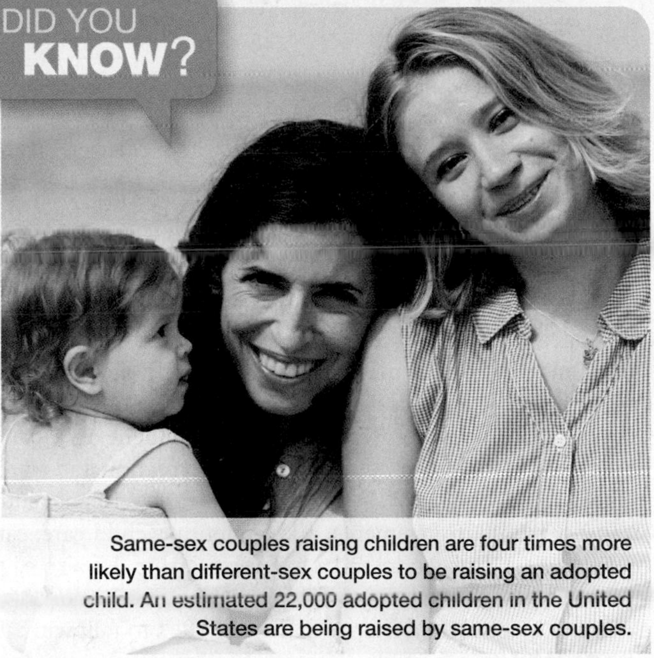

Same-sex couples raising children are four times more likely than different-sex couples to be raising an adopted child. An estimated 22,000 adopted children in the United States are being raised by same-sex couples.

Source: G. J. Gates, "LGBT Parenting in the United States," The Williams Institute, February 2013, http://williamsinstitute.law.ucla.edu/wp-content/uploads/LGBT-Parenting.pdf.

TABLE 4.1 | Common Parenting Styles

Authoritarian "Giving orders"	Parents use a set of rules that are clear and unbending. Obedience is highly valued and rewarded. Misbehavior is punished. Children may behave for a reward or out of fear of punishment. Children are not encouraged to think for themselves or to question those in authority.
Permissive "Giving in"	Parents take a hands-off approach. Children are allowed great freedom with few boundaries, minimal guidance, and little discipline. Without limits and expectations, children often struggle with impulse control, poor choices, and insecurity, and have trouble taking responsibility for their actions.
Assertive-Democratic "Giving choices"	Parents have clear expectations for children, clarify issues, and give reasons for limits. Children are given lots of practice in making choices and are guided to see the consequences of their decisions. Encouragement and acknowledgment of good behavior form the focal point of this style. Misbehavior is handled with an appropriate consequence or by problem solving with the child.

Source: S. Dinwiddie, *Effective Parenting Styles: Why Yesterday's Models Won't Work Today*, Accessed February 2014, www.kidsource.com/better.world.press/parenting.html. Copyright © 2009 Sue Dinwiddie. Reprinted by permission of the author.

Many people parent as they were parented (see **TABLE 4.1**). This strategy may or may not align with sound child-rearing principles. Establishing a positive, respectful parenting style sets the stage for healthy family growth and development.

Finally, as a potential parent you must consider the financial implications of deciding to have a child. It is estimated that a family with a child born in 2012 can expect to spend an average of about $240,000 for food, clothing, shelter, education, and other necessities for the child over the next 17 years. Keep in mind that these numbers do not include the cost of childbearing or the costs of a college education.[34]

Compared to 1975, when only 39 percent of women with children under the age of 5 worked outside the home, today about 65 percent of mothers with young children balance a job along with parenting.[35] Most families rely on a network of day care workers, family members, friends, neighbors, and nannies to provide child care. The price of day care can be shocking: In 2012, the average annual cost of full-time infant care ranged from about $4,863 in Mississippi to $16,430 in Massachusetts. Put another way, it can cost as much to send a baby to full-time day care as it does to send a child to college.[36]

Given that 51 percent of pregnancies in the United States are unintended, it's safe to say that many people become parents without a lot of forethought.[37] Some children are born into a relationship full of conflict or a relationship that doesn't last. No matter the circumstances, parents must take responsibility for their own emotions and make it clear to children that they are not the reason for conflict.

LO 7 | WHEN RELATIONSHIPS FALTER

Explain why relationships end and how to cope when they do.

Breakdowns in relationships often begin with a change in communication, however subtle. Either partner may stop listening and cease to be emotionally present for the other. In turn, the other feels ignored, unappreciated, or unwanted. Unresolved conflicts increase, and unresolved anger can cause problems in sexual relations, which can further increase communication difficulties.

College students, particularly those who are socially isolated and far from family and hometown friends, may be particularly vulnerable to staying in unhealthy relationships. They may become emotionally dependent on a partner for everything from eating meals to recreation and study time. Mutual obligations, such as shared rental, financial, or transportation arrangements, and sometimes child care, can complicate a decision to end a bad relationship. It's also easy to mistake sexual advances for physical attraction or love. Without a network of friends and supporters to talk with, to obtain validation for feelings, or to share concerns, a student can feel stuck in an unhealthy relationship.

Honesty and verbal affection are usually positive aspects of a relationship. In a troubled relationship, however, they can be used to cover up irresponsible or hurtful behavior. Saying "at least I was honest" is not an acceptable substitute for acting in a trustworthy way, and claiming "but I really do love you" is not a license for being inconsiderate or rude. Relationships that are lacking in mutual respect and consideration can become physically or emotionally abusive. (See **Chapter 19** for more information on intimate partner violence.)

jealousy Aversive reaction evoked by a real or imagined relationship involving a person's partner and a third person.

Confronting Couples Issues

Couples seeking a long-term relationship must confront a number of issues that can either enhance or diminish their chances of success. These issues can involve jealousy, gender roles, power sharing, and communication about unmet expectations.

Jealousy

Jealousy is a negative reaction evoked by a real or imagined relationship involving one's partner and a third person. Contrary to what many people believe, jealousy is not a sign of intense devotion. Instead, jealousy often indicates underlying problems, such as insecurity or possessiveness, which are significant barriers to a healthy relationship. Often, jealousy is rooted in a past relationship in which an individual experienced deception and loss. Other causes of jealousy typically include the following:

- **Overdependence on the relationship.** People who have few social ties and who rely exclusively on their partners tend to be overly fearful of losing them.
- **Severity of the threat.** People may feel uneasy if someone with stunning good looks and a great personality appears to be interested in their partner.
- **High value on sexual exclusivity.** People who believe that sexual exclusivity is a crucial indicator of love are more likely to become jealous.
- **Low self-esteem.** People who think poorly of themselves are more likely to fear that someone else will gain their partner's affection.
- **Fear of losing control.** Some people need to feel in control of every situation. Feeling that they may be losing control over a partner can cause jealousy.

In both men and women, jealousy is related to believing it would be difficult to find another relationship if the current one ends. Although a certain amount of jealousy can be expected in any loving relationship, it doesn't have to threaten the relationship as long as partners communicate openly about it.[38]

Changing Gender Roles

Throughout history, women and men have taken on various roles in relationships. In colonial America, gender roles and tasks were rigid and determined by tradition, while our modern society has very few gender-specific roles. Both women and men work, care for children, drive, run businesses, manage family finances, and perform equally well in the tasks of daily living. Rather than taking on traditional female and male roles, many couples find it makes more sense to divide tasks on the basis of schedule, convenience, and preference. However, the division is rarely equal. Even when women work full time, they tend to bear heavy family and household responsibilities. Today, many working women balance the responsibilities of being a partner, mother, and a full-time professional and find their never-ending duties to be overwhelming. The Bureau of Labor Statistics estimates that 20 percent of men did housework on an average day in 2012, compared to 48 percent of women, and 65 percent of women prepared meals compared to 39 percent of men.[39] Over time, if couples are unable to communicate how they feel about any unequal division of household responsibilities and arrive at an equitable solution, the relationship is likely to suffer.

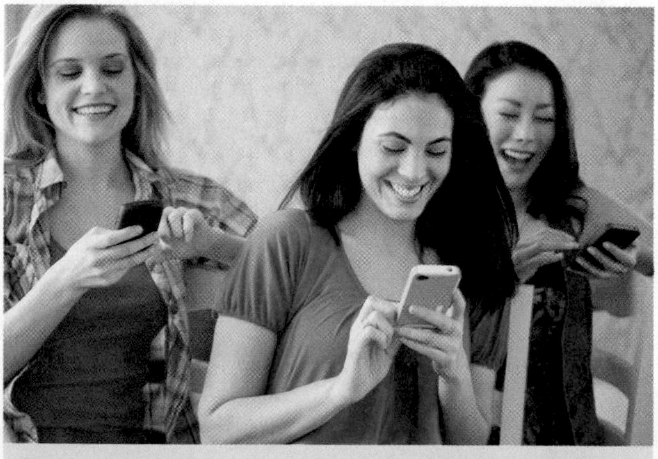

Though entertaining, spending too much time texting can cause you to miss valuable in-person interactions where ears, eyes, and body language can improve communication.

Sharing Power **Power** can be defined as the ability to make and implement decisions. In traditional relationships, men were the wage earners and consequently, had decision-making power. Women exerted much influence, but ultimately, they needed a man's income for survival. As increasing numbers of women have entered the workforce and generated their own financial resources, the power dynamics between women and men have shifted considerably. The increase in the divorce rate in the past century was partly due to working women gaining the ability to support themselves by choice rather than remaining in difficult or abusive relationships solely for financial reasons.

In successful relationships, partners share responsibilities, power, and control. Even when both partners are financially equal, power in other areas may be an issue. If one partner always has the final say in deciding social plans, for example, the unequal distribution of power in that area may affect the quality of the relationship.

Unmet Expectations We all have expectations—how we will spend our time and our money, how we will express love and intimacy, and how we will grow together as a couple. Expectations are an extension of our values, beliefs, hopes, and dreams for the future. When communicated and agreed upon, these expectations help relationships thrive. If we are unable to communicate our expectations, we set ourselves up for disappointment and hurt. Partners in healthy relationships can communicate wants and needs and have honest discussions when things aren't going as expected or as planned.

WHAT DO YOU THINK?

What factors do you think contribute most to divorce?

- What factors contribute most to couples staying together?
- Is divorce sometimes the best resort when a marriage experiences difficulties?

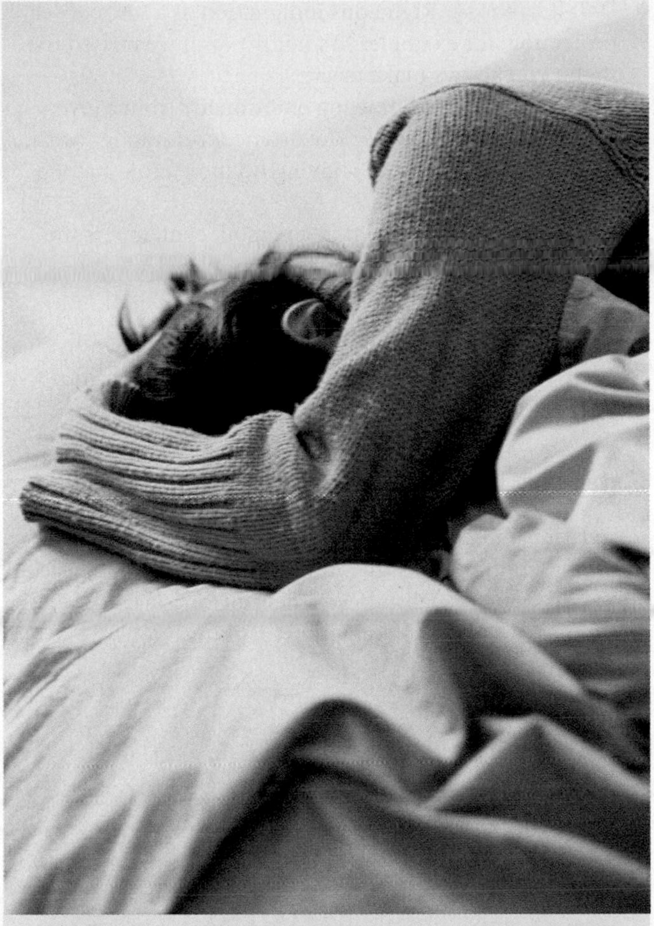

It may feel as if there is no end to the sorrow, anger, and guilt that often accompany a difficult breakup, but time is a miraculous healer. Acknowledging your feelings and finding healthful ways to express them will help you deal with the end of a romantic relationship.

When and Why Relationships End

Often we hear in the news that 50 percent of American marriages end in divorce. This number is based on comparing the annual marriage rate with the annual divorce rate. This is misleading, because in any given year, the people who are divorcing are not the same people who just got married.

It is more accurate to look at the total number of married people and calculate how many of them eventually divorce. Using this calculation, the divorce rate in the United States has never exceeded 40 percent.[40] Although this number is still high, it should be noted that the divorce rate in the United States shot up in the 1970s, peaked in the early 1980s, and has since declined to about 30 percent.[41] This decrease may be related to an increase in the age at which persons first marry as well as a higher level of education among those who are marrying—as both contribute to marital stability.[42] The risk of divorce is lower for college-educated people marrying for the first time and lower still for people who wait to marry until their mid-twenties and who haven't lived with multiple partners prior to marriage.[43]

SEE IT! VIDEOS

Is being gay in the spotlight no big deal? Watch **Celebrities Coming Out, Casually** available on MasteringHealth.™

Why do relationships end? There are many reasons, including physical or mental illness, financial concerns, career problems, and personality conflicts. Many people enter a relationship with certain expectations about how they and their partner will behave. Failure to communicate these beliefs can lead to resentment and disappointment. Differences in sexual needs may also contribute to the demise of a relationship. Under stress, communication and cooperation between partners can break down. Conflict, negative interactions, and a general lack of respect between partners can erode even the most loving relationship.

power Ability to make and implement decisions.

What behaviors signal that trouble is coming? Based on 35 years of research and couples therapy, John Gottman has identified four behavior patterns in couples that predict future divorce with 85 percent or better accuracy.

- **Criticism:** Phrasing complaints in terms of a partner's defect; for example: "You never talk about anyone but yourself. You are self-centered."

- **Defensiveness:** Righteous indignation as a form of self-protection; for example: "It's not my fault we missed the flight; you always make us late."
- **Stonewalling:** Withdrawing emotionally from a given interaction; for example: The listener seems to ignore the speaker as she speaks, giving no indication that the speaker was heard.
- **Contempt:** Talking down to a person, contempt is the biggest predictor of divorce; for example: "How could you be so stupid?"[44]

While these behaviors do not guarantee that an individual couple will divorce, they are "red flags" for relationships that are at great risk for failure.

Coping with Failed Relationships

No relationship comes with a guarantee. Losing a love is as much a part of life as falling in love. That being said, uncoupling can be very painful. Whenever we risk getting close to another, we also risk being hurt if things don't work out. Remember that knowing, understanding, and feeling good about oneself before entering a relationship are very important. Consider the following tips for coping with a failed relationship:[45]

- **Acknowledge that you've gone through a rough spot.** You may feel grief, loneliness, rejection, anger, guilt, relief, sadness, or all of these. Remember, it's good to reach out to others to deal with these feelings. Seek out trusted friends and, if needed, professional help.
- **Let go of negative thought patterns and habits.** Engage in activities that make you happy. Take a walk, read, listen to music, go to the movies or a concert, spend time with fun friends, volunteer with a community organization, or write in a journal. Find your joy!
- **Make a promise to yourself: no new relationships until you have moved past the last one.** You need time to resolve your experience rather than escape from it. It can be difficult to be trusting and intimate in a new relationship if you are still working on getting over a past relationship. Heal first, before looking for love again.

STUDY PLAN

Customize your study plan—and master your health!—in the Study Area of **MasteringHealth**.

ASSESS **YOURSELF**

Do your communication skills need improvement? Want to find out? Take the **How Well Do You Communicate?** assessment available on MasteringHealth.™

Need help creating a plan? Follow the strategies in the **Your Plan for Change** box for short- and long-term improvements to your health.

YOUR PLAN FOR **CHANGE**

The **ASSESS YOURSELF** activity "How Well Do You Communicate?" is available in MasteringHealth. This activity gives you the chance to look at how you communicate. After completing the activity and considering your responses, you can take steps toward becoming a better communicator and improving your relationships.

TODAY, YOU CAN:

- ☐ Call a friend you haven't talked to in a while or arrange a coffee date with a new acquaintance you'd like to get to know better.
- ☐ Start a journal and keep track of communication and relationship issues that arise. Look for trends and think about ways you can change your behavior to address them.

WITHIN THE NEXT 2 WEEKS, YOU CAN:

- ☐ Spend some time letting the people you care about know how important they are to you.
- ☐ If there is someone with whom you have a conflict, arrange a time to talk about the issues. Be sure to meet in a neutral setting away from distractions.

BY THE END OF THE SEMESTER, YOU CAN:

- ☐ Think about the ways you communicate with a sexual partner. Consider removing yourself from an unhappy relationship or improving communication with a partner to reach a satisfying relationship.
- ☐ Consider your behavior patterns with a partner. Do either of you display any of the patterns that Gottman reports predict divorce?

CHAPTER REVIEW

To hear an MP3 Tutor Session, scan here or visit the Study Area in **MasteringHealth.**

LO 1 | Intimate Relationships

- Characteristics of intimate relationships include behavioral interdependence, need fulfillment, emotional attachment, and emotional availability. Intimate relationships help us fulfill our needs for intimacy, social integration, nurturance, assistance, and affirmation. Family, friends, and partners provide the most common opportunities for intimacy. Each relationship may include healthy and unhealthy characteristics that can affect daily functioning.

LO 2 | Strategies for Successful Relationships

- There are many strategies for building better relationships. Examining one's own behaviors to determine what to change and how to change is an important ingredient of success. Characteristics of successful relationships include good communication, intimacy, friendship, and trust.

LO 3 | Communicating: A Key to Good Relationships

- To improve our communication skills, we need to develop our skills in using self-disclosure, listening effectively, conveying and interpreting nonverbal communication, and managing and resolving conflicts.

LO 4 | Committed Relationships

- For most people, commitment is an important part of a successful relationship. Types of committed relationships include marriage, cohabitation, and gay and lesbian partnerships (which can involve either marriage or cohabitation). Success in committed relationships requires understanding the elements of a good relationship.

LO 5 | Staying Single

- Remaining single is more common than ever before. Most single people lead healthy, happy, and well-adjusted lives.

LO 6 | Choosing Whether to Have Children

- Life decisions such as whether to marry or have children require serious consideration. Having children can be part of a rewarding, productive life as long as parents make the decision with full awareness and acceptance of the demands and responsibilities of parenting.

LO 7 | When Relationships Falter

- Factors that can cause relationship problems include breakdowns in communication, erosion of mutual respect, jealousy, differences over gender roles, power struggles, and unmet expectations. Before relationships fail, warning signs often appear. By recognizing these signs and taking action to change behaviors, partners may save and enhance their relationship.

POP QUIZ

Visit **MasteringHealth** to personalize your study plan with Chapter Review Quizzes and Dynamic Study Modules.

LO 1 | Intimate Relationships

1. Intimate relationships fulfill our psychological need for someone to listen to our worries and concerns. This is known as our need for
   a. dependence.
   b. social integration.
   c. enjoyment.
   d. spontaneity.
2. According to anthropologist Helen Fisher, attraction and falling in love follow a pattern based on
   a. lust, attraction, and attachment.
   b. intimacy, passion, and commitment.
   c. imprinting, attraction, attachment, and the production of a cuddle chemical.
   d. fascination, exclusiveness, sexual desire, giving the utmost, and being a champion.

LO 2 | Strategies for Successful Relationships

3. Predictability, dependability, and faith are three fundamental elements of
   a. trust.
   b. friendship.
   c. attraction.
   d. attachment.
4. One important factor in choosing a partner is *proximity*, which refers to
   a. mutual regard.
   b. attitudes and values.
   c. physical attraction.
   d. being in the same place at the same time.

LO 3 | Communicating: A Key to Good Relationships

5. The goal of conflict resolution is to
   a. constructively resolve points of contention.
   b. declare a winner and a loser.
   c. ensure that couples argue as little as possible.
   d. set a time limit on discussion of difficult issues.
6. One of the most important ways to express difficult feelings is to
   a. be specific rather than general about how you feel.
   b. express anger and resentment so the other person feels your heartache.
   c. point your finger at the other person.
   d. blame the other person for the difficulty you are experiencing.

LO 4 | Committed Relationships

7. A relationship in which two unmarried people with an

intimate connection share the same household is known as
a. monogamy.
b. cohabitation.
c. common-law household.
d. co-housemates.

LO 5 | Staying Single

8. Sofia is 30 years old and she decides to stay single rather than get married. Which of the following is *true* regarding Sofia's decision?
   a. Sofia needs to seek out sexual intimacy to stay content throughout life.
   b. Sofia is giving up any opportunity to become a parent if she's single.
   c. Sofia is in the minority of women ages 20 to 34, as most are married.
   d. Sofia can obtain intimacy through relationships with family and friends.

LO 6 | Choosing Whether to Have Children

9. The parenting style where parents take a hands-off approach to parenting and allow their children great freedom with few boundaries is known as
   a. permissive.
   b. assertive-democratic.
   c. authoritarian.
   d. democratic.

LO 7 | When Relationships Falter

10. All of the following are typical causes of jealousy *except*
    a. overdependence on the relationship.
    b. low self-esteem.
    c. a past relationship that involved deception.
    d. belief that relationships can easily be replaced.

Answers to the Pop Quiz can be found on page A-1. If you answered a question incorrectly, review the section identified by the Learning Outcome. For even more study tools, visit MasteringHealth.

THINK ABOUT IT!

LO 1 | Intimate Relationships

1. What are the characteristics of intimate relationships? What are behavioral interdependence, need fulfillment, emotional attachment, and emotional availability, and why is each important in relationship development?
2. What problems can form barriers to intimacy? What actions can you take to reduce or remove these barriers?

LO 2 | Strategies for Successful Relationships

3. What are common elements of good relationships? What are some warning signs of trouble? What actions can you take to improve your own interpersonal relationships?
4. How can you tell the difference between a love relationship and one that is based primarily on attraction? What characteristics do love relationships share?

LO 3 | Communicating: A Key to Good Relationships

5. What is nonverbal communication, and why is it important to develop skills in this area? Give examples of some things you do to communicate without words.

LO 4 | Committed Relationships

6. What are the different types of committed relationships? How are they different? What does it take for any kind of committed relationship to succeed?

LO 5 LO 6 | Staying Single and Choosing Whether to Have Children

7. Name some common misconceptions about people who choose to remain single and about couples who choose not to have children. Do you want to have children? Why or why not? What characteristics show that a couple is ready to have children?

LO 7 | When Relationships Falter

8. What are some of the common warning signs that a relationship is going to fail? What are some actions people can take to change behaviors to save or even enhance a troubled relationship?

ACCESS YOUR HEALTH ON THE INTERNET

Visit **MasteringHealth** for links to the websites and RSS feeds.

The following websites explore further topics and issues related to personal health.

National Center for Health Statistics. This division of the Centers for Disease Control and Prevention has up-to-date statistics on trends in marriage, divorce, and cohabitation. **www.cdc.gov/nchs**

The Gottman Institute. This organization helps couples directly and provides training to therapists. The website includes research information, self-help tips for relationship building, and a relationship quiz. **www.gottman.com**

The National Gay and Lesbian Task Force. This organization works toward lesbian, gay, bisexual, and transgender (LGBT) equality and provides research and policy analysis to create social change. **www.thetaskforce.org**

National Healthy Marriage Resource Center. A clearinghouse for news and research related to healthy marriages. **www.healthymarriageinfo.org**

The Hotline. This site provides information about domestic violence, including how to recognize abuse and how to get help in your local area. Phone support is available 24/7 at 1-800-799-SAFE (7233). **www.thehotline.org**

5 Understanding Your Sexuality

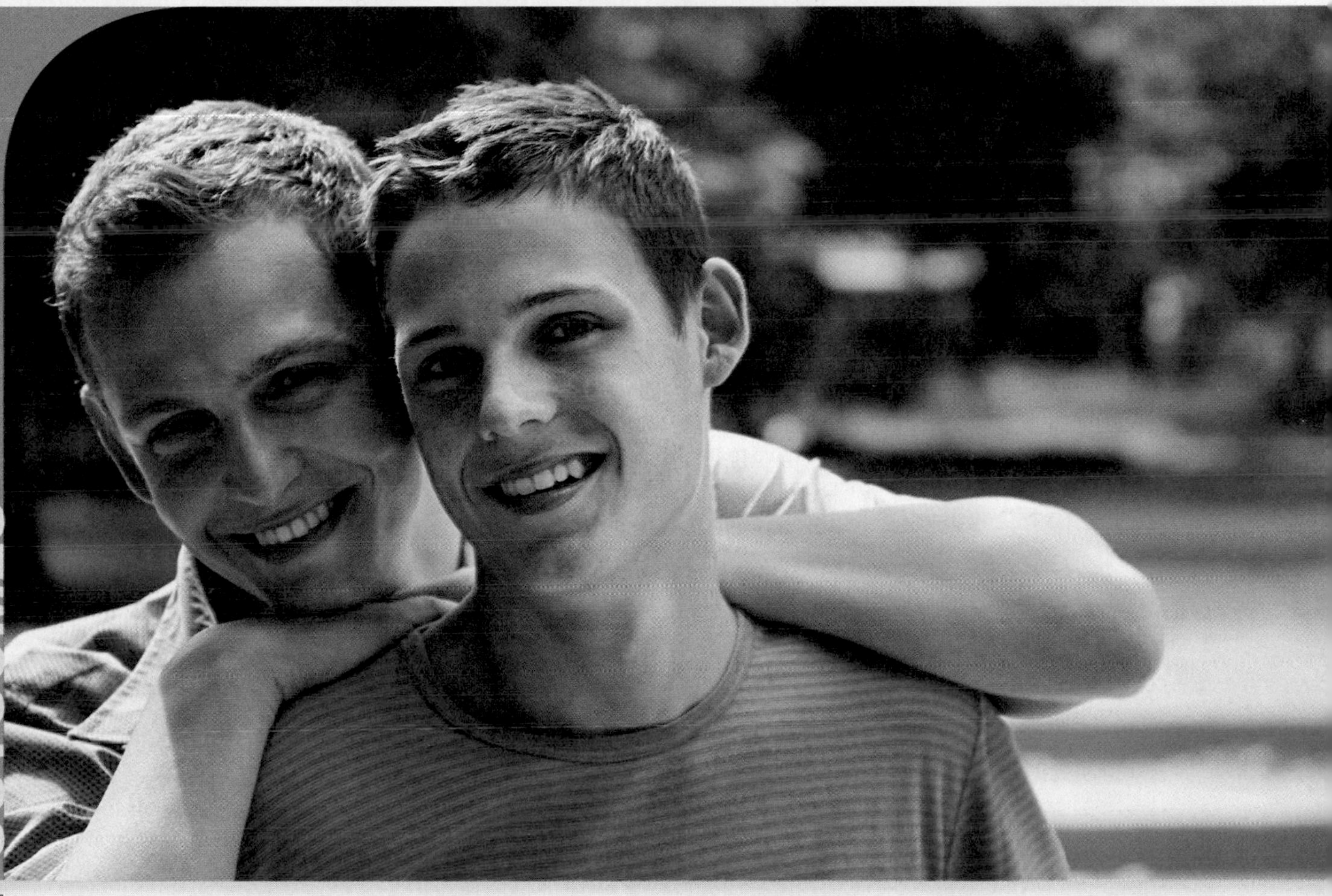

LEARNING OUTCOMES

1 Define *sexual identity* and discuss its major components, including biology, gender identity, gender roles, and sexual orientation.
2 Identify the primary structures of male and female sexual anatomy and explain the functions of each.
3 List and describe the stages of the human sexual response and what factors may influence these.
4 Explain the options available for the expression of one's sexuality.
5 Classify sexual dysfunctions, describe major disorders, and discuss treatment options.
6 Explain the effects of various drugs on sexual behavior.
7 Describe the state of the sex industry in the United States and related health concerns.

Do you see yourself as a sexual person? Do you identify as gay or straight? Are you comfortable in your own skin? Do you know enough about sexual anatomy and physiology to maximize your sexual pleasure and control your fertility? Human sexuality is complex and involves physical health, personal values, and interpersonal relationships, as well as cultural traditions, social norms, new technologies, current research findings, and changing political agendas. **Sexuality** is much more than sexual feelings or intercourse. Rather, it includes all the thoughts, feelings, and behaviors associated with being male or female, experiencing attraction, being in love, and being in relationships that include sexual intimacy. Elements of sexuality include the following:

- **Sensuality.** Awareness and feelings about your body and others' bodies, especially that of your sexual partner. Sensuality enables us to feel good about how our bodies look and feel and to enjoy the pleasure they can give to us and others.
- **Intimacy.** The ability to have a positive, close relationship with another human being.
- **Sexual identity.** The recognition and acknowledgment of oneself as a sexual being, including gender identity.
- **Sexual health and reproduction.** Attitudes and behaviors related to the health of the sexual organs, the ability to have children, and the health consequences of sexual behavior.
- **Sexualization.** The use of sexuality to influence or manipulate others in ways that may be harmful or exploitative.

Our sexuality is central to who we are as humans. In this chapter, we will focus on sexual identity and aspects of sexual health, reproduction, and sexual behaviors. Having a comprehensive understanding of your sexuality will help you make responsible and satisfying decisions about your life and your interpersonal relationships.

sexuality Thoughts, feelings, and behaviors associated with being male or female, experiencing attraction, being in love, and being in relationships that include sexual intimacy.

sexual identity Recognition of oneself as a sexual being; a composite of biological sex characteristics, gender identity, gender roles, and sexual orientation.

intersexuality Not exhibiting exclusively male or female sex characteristics; also known as disorders of sexual development (DSD).

gonads Reproductive organs that produce germ cells and sex hormones; in males, the testes, and in females, the ovaries.

puberty Period of sexual maturation.

pituitary gland Endocrine gland that controls the release of hormones from the gonads.

secondary sex characteristics Characteristics associated with sex but not directly related to reproduction, such as vocal pitch, amount of body hair, breasts, and location of fat deposits.

gender Characteristics and actions associated with being feminine or masculine as defined by the society or culture in which one lives.

gender roles Expression of maleness or femaleness in everyday life that conforms to society's expectations.

SEE IT! VIDEOS

Is being gay in the spotlight no big deal? Watch **Celebrities Coming Out, Casually** available on MasteringHealth.™

LO 1 | YOUR SEXUAL IDENTITY: MORE THAN BIOLOGY

Define *sexual identity* and discuss its major components, including biology, gender identity, gender roles, and sexual orientation.

Sexual identity, the recognition and acknowledgment of oneself as a sexual being, is determined by a complex interaction of genetic, physiological, environmental, and social factors. The beginning of sexual identity occurs at conception with the combining of chromosomes that determine sex. All eggs carry an X chromosome; sperm may carry either an X or a Y chromosome. If a sperm carrying an X chromosome fertilizes an egg, the resulting combination of sex chromosomes (XX) produces a female. If a sperm carrying a Y chromosome fertilizes an egg, the XY combination produces a male.

On rare occasions, chromosomes are added, lost, or rearranged in this process and the sex of the offspring is not clear. For example, a girl may have a large clitoris, but not have a vaginal opening. This condition is known as **intersexuality**. *Disorders of sexual development* (*DSDs*) is a less confusing term that has been recommended to refer to intersex conditions, which occur in an estimated 1 in 4,500 live births (see the **Health in a Diverse World** box).[1]

The genetic instructions included in the sex chromosomes lead to the development of male and female **gonads** (reproductive organs) at about the eighth week of fetal life. Once the male gonads (testes) and the female gonads (ovaries) develop, they play a key role in all future sexual development because the gonads are responsible for the production of sex hormones. The primary female sex hormones are estrogen and progesterone. The primary male sex hormone is testosterone. The release of testosterone in a maturing fetus stimulates the development of a penis and other male genitals. If no testosterone is produced, female genitals form.

At the time of **puberty**, sex hormones again play major roles in development. Hormones released by the **pituitary gland**, called *gonadotropins*, stimulate the testes and ovaries to make appropriate sex hormones. Increased estrogen production in females and testosterone production in males lead to the development of **secondary sex characteristics**. Male secondary sex characteristics include deepening of the voice, development of facial and body hair, and growth of the skeleton and musculature. Female characteristics include growth of the breasts, widening of the hips, and the development of pubic and underarm hair.[2]

In addition to a person's biological status as a male or female, another important component of sexual identity is gender. **Gender** refers to characteristics and actions typically associated with men or women (masculine or feminine) as defined by the culture in which one lives, while **gender roles** are the behaviors and activities we use to express masculinity

HEALTH IN A DIVERSE WORLD

DISORDERS OF SEXUAL DEVELOPMENT

At the 2012 Summer Olympics in London, the South African flag was carried into the Opening Ceremonies by middle-distance runner Caster Semenya, one of the fastest women on earth. Her silver-medal finish was impressive, but most news reports focused on her sex, not her achievements.

Previously, after Semenya won the gold medal in the 800-meter race at the 2009 World Championships, she was required to undergo gender testing and was subsequently barred from competition. Officials at the International Association of Athletics Federations (IAAF) wanted to determine whether Semenya has a disorder of sexual development (DSD) resulting in testosterone levels that give her an unfair athletic advantage over other female competitors. In July 2010, the IAAF announced that Semenya was again eligible to compete. The decision of the IAAF council was the culmination of an 18-month-long review by an expert working group that has studied issues relating to the participation of female athletes with hyperandrogenism, a condition involving overproduction of male sex hormones. The ruling by the IAAF states a female with hyperandrogenism who is recognized as a female in law will be eligible to compete in women's competition in athletics, provided that she has androgen levels below the male range (measured by reference to testosterone levels in serum) or, if she has androgen levels within the male range, she also has an androgen resistance such that she derives no competitive advantage from such levels.

Many people considered it an invasion of privacy when runner Caster Semenya was required to submit to gender testing before being allowed to return to competition.

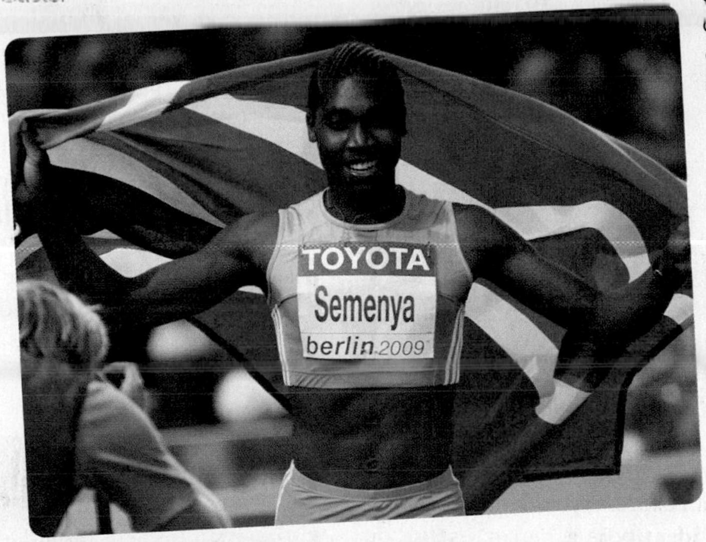

The details of Semenya's test results and whether she received medical treatment to regain her eligibility remain confidential; however, Semenya's case highlights the challenges facing people with DSDs. People with DSDs are born with various levels of male and female biological characteristics, ranging from different chromosomal arrangements to altered hormone production to variation in primary and secondary sex characteristics. While most people are born with either XX or XY chromosomes, some are born with XXY or XO chromosomes (where O signifies a missing or damaged chromosome). In some people, gonads do not develop fully into ovaries or testicles, although there may be no external signs to indicate this, and in others, external genitalia may be ambiguous.

Many, but not all, DSDs require some degree of medical intervention, whether hormonal or surgical, to ensure a person's physical health. It is also necessary to "assign" a gender to all children as early as possible to ensure their psychological health. If this assignment is later found to be inconsistent with the child's own sense of gender, he or she may choose to adopt a different gender identity. Most people born with DSDs today are allowed to grow up, establish their own gender identity, and choose as adults whether to have additional surgeries to alter any sexual tissues they feel are incongruent with their gender. To find out more about DSDs, visit the website of Accord Alliance at www.accordalliance.org.

Sources: Peter Lee et al., "Consensus Statement on Management of Intersex Disorders," *Pediatrics* 118 (2006): e488–e500; "IAFF Approves New Rules on Hyperandrogenism," *The Guardian,* April 12, 2011, www.guardian.co.uk/sport/2011/apr/12/iaaf-athletics-rules-hyperandrogenism-caster-semenya; J. Ellison, "Caster Semenya and the IOC's Olympics Gender Bender," *The Daily Beast*, July 26, 2012, www.thedailybeast.com/articles/2012/07/26/caster-semenya-and-the-ioc-s-olympics-gender-bender.html.

or femininity in ways that conform to society's expectations. Our sense of masculine and feminine traits is largely a result of **socialization** during our childhood. For example, your parents may have influenced your perception of gender roles by the toys they gave you (trucks vs. dolls) or chores they assigned you (cooking vs. yard work).

For some, gender roles can be confining when they lead to stereotypes. Bounds established by **gender-role stereotypes** can make it difficult to express one's true sexual identity. In the United States, men are traditionally expected to be independent, aggressive, logical, and always in control of their emotions, while women are traditionally expected to be passive, nurturing, intuitive, sensitive, and emotional. **Androgyny** refers to the combination of traditional masculine and feminine traits in a single person. Androgynous people do not always follow traditional gender roles, but instead choose behaviors based on a given situation.

socialization Process by which a society communicates behavioral expectations to its members.

gender-role stereotypes Generalizations concerning how men and women should express themselves and the characteristics each possess.

androgyny Combination of traditional masculine and feminine traits in a single person.

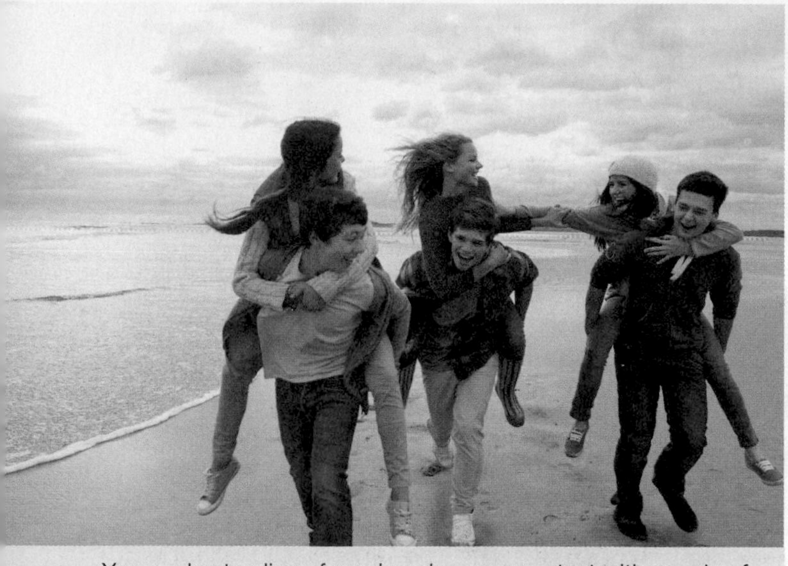

Your understanding of gender roles, your contact with people of various gender identities or sexual orientations, and your own degree of emotional maturity can all affect your sense of sexual identity.

Whereas gender roles are an expression of cultural expectations for behavior, **gender identity** is a person's sense or awareness of being masculine or feminine. A person's gender identity does not always match his or her biological sex: This is called being **transgender**. There is a broad spectrum of expression among transgender persons that reflects the degree of dissatisfaction they have with their sexual anatomy. Some transgender persons are very comfortable with their bodies and are content simply to dress and live as the other gender. *Transvestism,* more commonly referred to as cross-dressing, is the term used to describe the practice of wearing the clothing traditional of the opposite sex.

While cross-dressers are usually happy with their biologically assigned sex, **transsexuals** feel trapped in the wrong body.[3] Many opt for therapeutic interventions, such as sex reassignment surgery. In short, a transsexual wears clothes of the opposite sex because those clothes are associated with the gender they feel they were meant to be, whereas a cross-dresser wears clothes of the opposite sex because those clothes are associated with the opposite gender. For more, see the **Health in a Diverse World** box.

gender identity Personal sense or awareness of being masculine or feminine, a male or a female.

transgender Having a gender identity that does not match one's biological sex.

transsexual Person who is psychologically of one sex but physically of the other.

sexual orientation A person's enduring emotional, romantic, or sexual attraction to other persons.

heterosexual Experiencing primary attraction to and preference for sexual activity with people of the opposite sex.

homosexual Experiencing primary attraction to and preference for sexual activity with people of the same sex.

bisexual Experiencing attraction to and preference for sexual activity with people of both sexes.

gay Sexual orientation involving primary attraction to people of the same sex.

lesbian Sexual orientation involving attraction of women to other women.

sexual prejudice Negative attitudes and hostile actions directed at those with a different sexual orientation.

Sexual Orientation

Sexual orientation refers to a person's enduring emotional, romantic, or sexual attraction to others. You may be primarily attracted to members of the opposite sex (**heterosexual**), the same sex (**homosexual**), or both sexes (**bisexual**). Many homosexuals prefer the terms **gay**, queer, or **lesbian** to describe their sexual orientation. *Gay* and *queer* can apply to both men and women, but *lesbian* refers specifically to women.

Gay and bisexual people are often targets of **sexual prejudice**. Sexual prejudice refers to negative attitudes and hostile actions directed at members of a particular social group. Hate crimes, discrimination, and hostility

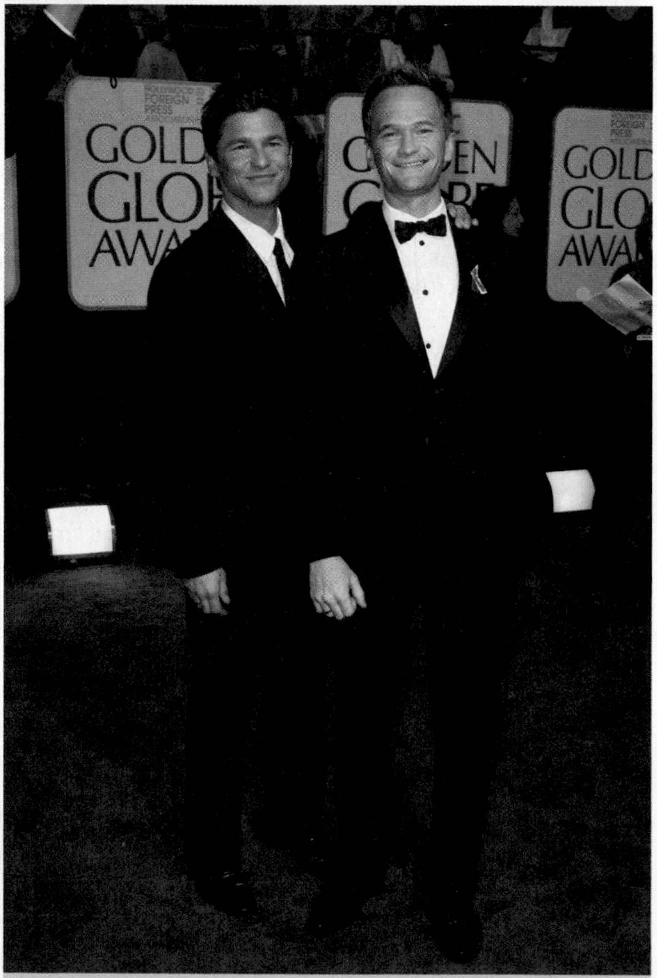

The presence of gay and lesbian celebrities in the media—such as Actor Neil Patrick Harris and his partner David Burtka—contributes to the increasing acceptance of gay relationships in everyday life.

HEALTH IN A DIVERSE WORLD

LIVING BETWEEN GENDERS

For most people, the checkbox on forms asking "male or female" is easy to complete. For people who are transgender, this is just one of many challenges: which box to check on forms, which bathroom or locker room to use, or which college dormitory to sign up for.

Recent policy progress, some forced on institutions by law and some adopted by choice, are efforts to make these choices easier, such as the following:

- A California law requiring public schools to allow transgender K through 12th-grade students access to the restroom and locker room of their choice and the choice to play boys' or girls' sports based on their self-perception of gender regardless of birth gender.
- Facebook now provides more than 50 gender identity options rather than just male or female, including transgender male, transgender female, gender questioning, and two spirit.
- More than 100 colleges and universities have gender-inclusive housing in which students can have a roommate of any gender.
- More than 150 colleges have created gender-neutral bathrooms.

Where do you stand?

- How do you feel about these accommodations for transgender persons? Are they a move in the right direction? What do you think motivates your feelings?
- How do you think it feels to be a person who doesn't neatly fit in the male/female categories?
- How can society protect the dignity of transgender persons while also protecting the privacy of people who may feel uncomfortable with these policy changes?

Sources: CBSNews, "California Law Allows Transgender Students to Pick Bathrooms, Sports Teams They Identify With," August 12, 2013, www.cbsnews.com/news/california-law-allows-transgender-students-to-pick-bathrooms-sports-teams-they-identify-with; ReadWrite Editors, "Facebook Provides 56 New Gender Identity Options," February 13, 2014, http://readwrite.com/2014/02/13/facebook-provides-56-new-gender-identity-options#awesm=~oCGUpaYfdpSNmP; Campus Pride, "Campus Pride Trans Policy Clearinghouse," 2014, www.campuspride.org/tpc.

toward sexual minorities are evidence of ongoing sexual prejudice.[4] Recent data from the Department of Justice indicated that bias regarding sexual orientation is the motivation for 20 percent of all hate crimes in the United States.[5]

Most researchers today agree that sexual orientation is best understood using a model that incorporates biological, psychological, and socioenvironmental factors. Biological explanations focus on research into genetics, hormones, and differences in brain anatomy. Psychological and socioenvironmental explanations examine parent–child interactions, sex roles, and early sexual and interpersonal interactions. Collectively, this growing body of research suggests that the origins of homosexuality, like heterosexuality, are complex.[6] To diminish the complexity of sexual orientation to "a choice" is a clear misrepresentation of current research. Homosexuals do not "choose" their sexual orientation any more than heterosexuals do.

To better understand sexual orientation as a continuum rather than discreet categories, psychiatrist Fritz Klein developed the Sexual Orientation Grid. This scale takes into account not only who you are attracted to and actually have sex with, but also factors such as which individuals you feel close to emotionally, who you enjoy socializing with, and in which "community" you feel most comfortable. It then places you on a continuum from exclusively opposite-sex attraction to exclusively same-sex attraction. This questionnaire is available as the **Assess Yourself** activity "What Are Your Sexual Attitudes?" in MasteringHealth. Completing the questionnaire may help you understand that there are not just three static sexual orientations (homosexual, heterosexual, or bisexual), but a whole range of complex, interacting, and fluid factors that influence your sexuality over time.

2% | OF COLLEGE STUDENTS REPORT BEING **UNSURE** OF THEIR SEXUAL ORIENTATION.

LO 2 | SEXUAL ANATOMY AND PHYSIOLOGY

Identify the primary structures of male and female sexual anatomy and explain the functions of each.

Understanding the functions of the male and female reproductive systems will help you derive pleasure and satisfaction from your sexual relationships, be sensitive to your partner's wants and needs, and make responsible choices regarding your own sexual health.

Female Sexual Anatomy and Physiology

The female reproductive system includes two major groups of structures, the external genitals and the internal organs

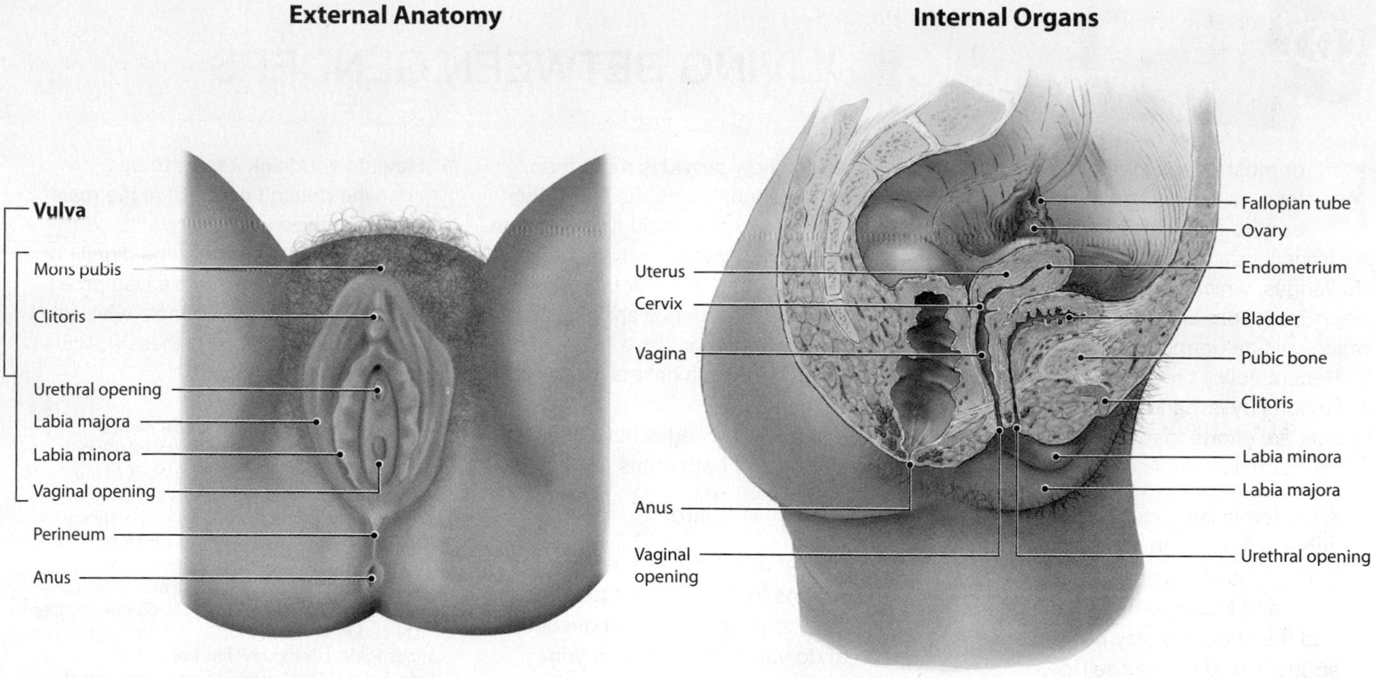

FIGURE 5.1 Female Sexual Anatomy

vulva External female genitalia.

mons pubis Fatty tissue covering the pubic bone in females; in physically mature women, the mons is covered with coarse hair.

labia majora "Outer lips," or folds of tissue covering the female sexual organs.

labia minora "Inner lips," or folds of tissue just inside the labia majora.

clitoris Pea-sized nodule of tissue located at the top of the labia minora; central to sexual arousal and pleasure in women.

urethral opening Opening through which urine is expelled.

hymen In some women, a thin tissue covering the vaginal opening.

perineum Tissue that forms the "floor" of the pelvic region, found between the vulva and the anus.

vagina Muscular, tube-shaped organ in females that serves as a passageway connecting the vulva to the uterus.

uterus (womb) Hollow, pear-shaped muscular organ whose function is to house a developing fetus.

endometrium Soft, spongy matter that makes up the uterine lining.

cervix Lower end of the uterus that opens into the vagina.

ovaries Almond-sized organs that house developing eggs and produce hormones.

(**FIGURE 5.1**). The external female genitals are collectively known as the **vulva** and include all structures that are outwardly visible: the mons pubis, the labia minora and majora, the clitoris, the urethral and vaginal openings, and the vestibule of the vagina and its glands. The **mons pubis** is a pad of fatty tissue covering and protecting the pubic bone; after the onset of puberty, it becomes covered with coarse hair. The **labia majora** are folds of skin and erectile tissue that enclose the urethral and vaginal openings; the **labia minora**, or inner lips, are folds of mucous membrane found just inside the labia majora.

The **clitoris** is located at the upper end of the labia minora and beneath the mons pubis, and its only known function is to provide sexual pleasure. Directly below the clitoris is the **urethral opening** through which urine is expelled from the body. Below the urethral opening is the vaginal opening. In some women, the vaginal opening is covered by a thin membrane called the **hymen**. It is a myth that an intact hymen is proof of virginity, as the hymen is not present in all women and is sometimes stretched or torn by physical activity.

The **perineum** is the area of smooth tissue found between the vulva and the anus. Although not technically part of the external genitalia, the tissue in this area has many nerve endings and is sensitive to touch; it can play a part in sexual excitement.

The internal female genitals include the vagina, uterus, fallopian tubes, and ovaries. The **vagina** is a muscular, tube-shaped organ that serves as a passageway from the uterus to the outside of the body. This passage allows menstrual flow to exit from the uterus during a woman's monthly cycle, receives the penis during intercourse, and serves as the birth canal during childbirth. The **uterus (womb)** is a hollow, muscular, pear-shaped organ. Hormones acting on the inner lining of the uterus (the **endometrium**) either prepare the uterus for implantation and development of a fertilized egg or signal that no fertilization has taken place, in which case the endometrium deteriorates and becomes menstrual flow.

The lower end of the uterus, the **cervix**, extends downward into the vagina. The **ovaries**, almond-sized organs suspended on either side

WHY SHOULD I CARE?

It is more difficult to please a partner sexually or to describe to a partner how to please you if you don't understand basic sexual anatomy. For example, the clitoris in females is very responsive to touch and when stimulated often leads to orgasm. The urethral opening located nearby is not. You should know the difference.

of the uterus, have two main functions: producing hormones (estrogen, progesterone, and small amounts of testosterone) and serving as the reservoir for immature eggs. All the eggs a woman will ever have are present in her ovaries at birth. Eggs mature and are released from the ovaries in response to hormone levels. Extending from the upper end of the uterus are two thin, flexible tubes called the **fallopian tubes** (also known as oviducts). The fallopian tubes, which do not actually touch the ovaries, capture eggs as they are released from the ovaries during ovulation, and they are the site where sperm and egg meet and fertilization takes place. The fallopian tubes then serve as the passageway to the uterus, where the fertilized egg becomes implanted and development continues.

The Onset of Puberty and the Menstrual Cycle With the onset of puberty, the female reproductive system matures, and the development of secondary sex characteristics transforms young girls into young women. The first sign of puberty is the beginning of breast development, which generally occurs around age 10.[7] The pituitary gland, the **hypothalamus**, and the ovaries all secrete hormones that act as chemical messengers. Working in a feedback system, hormonal levels in the bloodstream act as the trigger mechanism for releasing a certain type or amount of hormone.

Around age 9½ to 11½, the hypothalamus receives the message to begin secreting *gonadotropin-releasing hormone* (*GnRH*). The release of GnRH in turn signals the pituitary gland to release hormones called *gonadotropins.* Two gonadotropins, *follicle-stimulating hormone* (*FSH*) and *luteinizing hormone* (*LH*), signal the ovaries to start producing **estrogens** and **progesterone**. Estrogens regulate the menstrual cycle, and increased estrogen levels assist in the development of female secondary sex characteristics. Progesterone helps the endometrium develop in preparation for nourishing a fertilized egg and helps maintain pregnancy.

The normal age range for the onset of the first menstrual period, or **menarche**, is 10 to 18 years, with the average age falling between 12 and 13 years.[8] Body fat heavily influences the onset of puberty, and increasing rates of obesity in children may account for the fact that girls seem to be reaching puberty much earlier than in the past.[9] Other theories attempting to explain early menarche include family disruption, high stress levels, and endocrine disruptors in the food supply.[10]

The average menstrual cycle lasts 28 days and consists of three phases: the proliferative phase, the secretory phase, and the menstrual phase (**FIGURE 5.2**). The *proliferative phase* begins with the end of menstruation. During this time, the endometrium develops or "proliferates." How does this process work? By the end of menstruation, the hypothalamus senses very low levels of estrogen and progesterone in the blood. In response, it increases its secretions of GnRH, which in turn triggers the pituitary gland to release FSH. When FSH reaches the ovaries, it signals several **ovarian follicles** to begin maturing. Normally, only one of the follicles, the **graafian follicle**, reaches full maturity in the days preceding ovulation. While the follicles mature, they begin producing estrogen, which in turn signals the endometrial lining of the uterus to proliferate. If fertilization occurs, the endometrium will become a nesting place for the developing embryo. High estrogen levels signal the pituitary gland to slow down FSH production and increase release of LH. Under the influence of LH, the ovarian follicle ruptures and releases a mature **ovum** (plural: *ova*), a single mature egg cell, near a fallopian tube (around day 14). This is the process of **ovulation**. The other ripening follicles degenerate and are reabsorbed by the body. Occasionally, two ova mature and are released during ovulation. If both are fertilized, fraternal (nonidentical) twins develop. Identical twins develop when one fertilized ovum (called a *zygote*) divides into two separate zygotes.

The phase following ovulation is called the *secretory phase.* The ruptured graafian follicle, which has remained in the ovary, is transformed into the **corpus luteum** and begins secreting large amounts of estrogen and progesterone.

fallopian tubes Tubes that extend from near the ovaries to the uterus; site of fertilization and passageway for fertilized eggs.

hypothalamus Area of the brain located near the pituitary gland; works in conjunction with the pituitary gland to control reproductive functions.

estrogens Hormones secreted by the ovaries that control the menstrual cycle and assist in the development of female secondary sex characteristics.

progesterone Hormone secreted by the ovaries; helps the endometrium develop and helps maintain pregnancy.

menarche The first menstrual period.

ovarian follicles Areas within the ovary in which individual eggs develop.

graafian follicle Mature ovarian follicle that contains a fully developed egg (ovum).

ovum Single mature egg cell.

ovulation The point of the menstrual cycle at which a mature egg ruptures through the ovarian wall.

corpus luteum Cells that form from the remains of the graafian follicle following ovulation; it secretes estrogen and progesterone during the second half of the menstrual cycle.

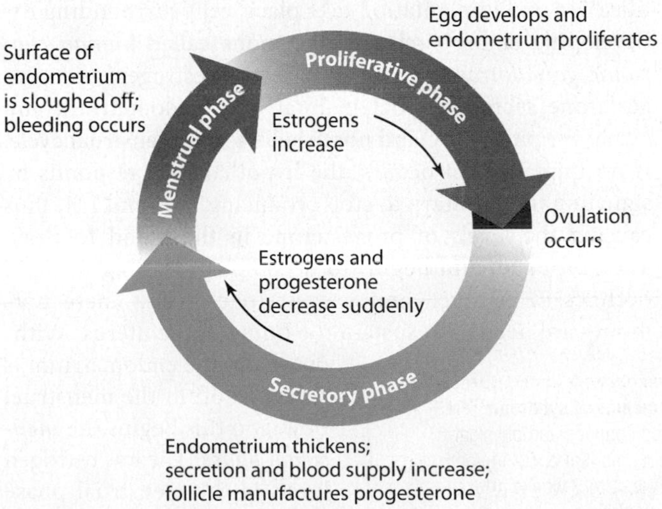

FIGURE 5.2 The Three Phases of the Menstrual Cycle

Source: Rathus et al., *Human Sexuality in a World of Diversity,* 6th ed., © 2009. Figure "The Three Phases of the Menstrual Cycle," © 2005 Allyn & Bacon. Reproduced with permission of Pearson Education, Inc.

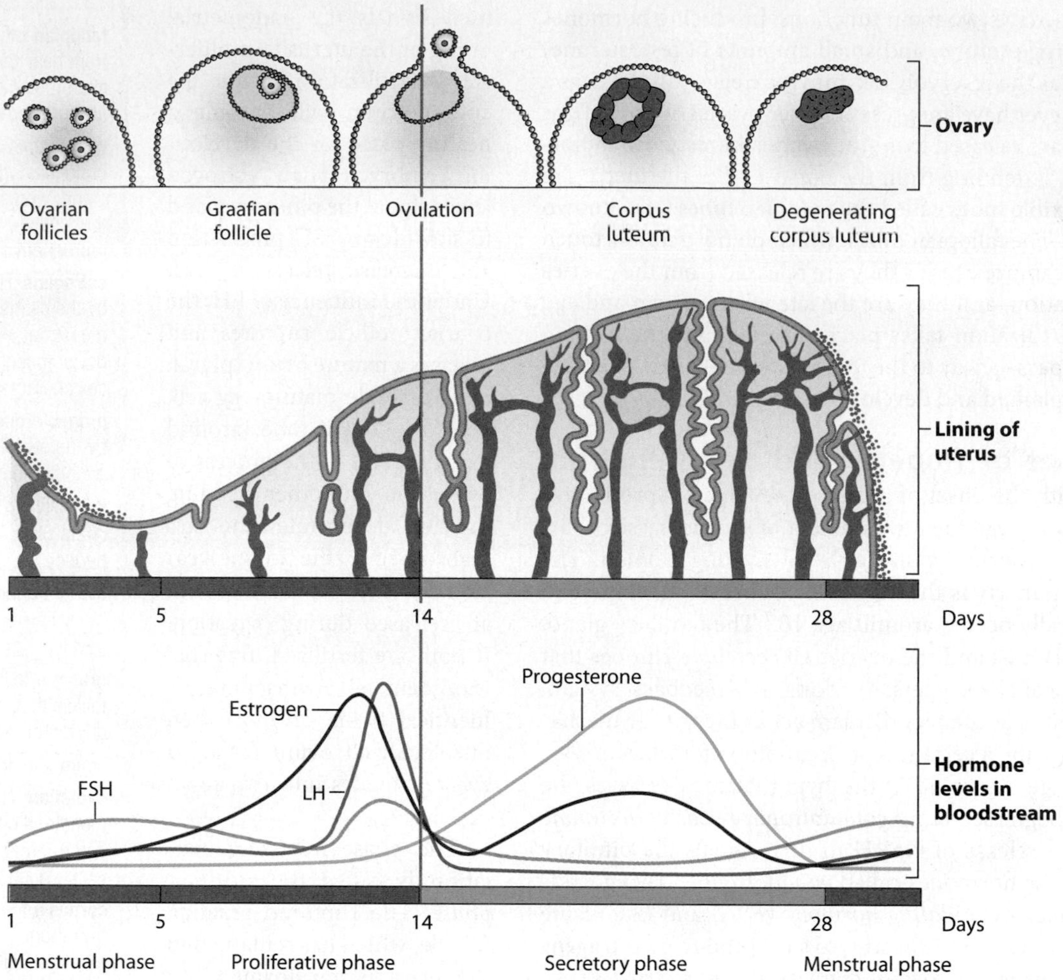

FIGURE 5.3 Hormonal Control and Phases of the Menstrual Cycle

These hormone secretions peak around day 20 or 21 of the average cycle and cause the endometrium to thicken. If fertilization and implantation take place, cells surrounding the developing embryo release a hormone called *human chorionic gonadotropin* (*HCG*), increasing estrogen and progesterone secretions that maintain the endometrium and signal the pituitary gland not to start a new menstrual cycle. If no implantation occurs, the hypothalamus responds by signaling the pituitary to stop producing FSH and LH, thus causing the levels of progesterone in the blood to peak. The corpus luteum begins to decompose, leading to rapid declines in estrogen and progesterone levels. These hormones are needed to sustain the lining of the uterus. Without them, the endometrium is sloughed off in the menstrual flow, and this begins the *menstrual phase.* The low estrogen levels of the menstrual phase signal the hypothalamus to release GnRH, which acts on the pituitary gland to secrete FSH, and the cycle (shown in **FIGURE 5.3**) begins again.

premenstrual syndrome (PMS) Mood changes and physical symptoms that occur in some women 1 to 2 weeks prior to menstruation.

premenstrual dysphoric disorder (PMDD) Group of symptoms similar to but more severe than PMS, including severe mood disturbances.

Menstrual Problems

Premenstrual syndrome (PMS) is a term used for a collection of physical, emotional, and behavioral symptoms that many women experience 7 to 14 days prior to their menstrual period. The most common symptoms are tender breasts, bloating, food cravings, fatigue, irritability, and depression. It is estimated that 85 percent of menstruating women experience at least one symptom of PMS each month.[11] For the majority of women, these disappear as their period begins, but for a small subset of women (5 to 8 percent), their symptoms are severe enough to affect their daily routines and activities to the point of being disabling. This severe form of PMS has its own diagnostic category in the *DSM-5*, **premenstrual dysphoric disorder (PMDD)**, with symptoms that include severe depression, hopelessness, anger, anxiety, low self-esteem, difficulty concentrating, irritability, and tension.[12]

There are several natural approaches to managing PMS that can also help PMDD. These strategies include eating more carbohydrates (whole grains, fruits, and vegetables), reducing caffeine and salt intake, exercising regularly, and taking measures to reduce stress. Recent investigation into methods of controlling severe emotional swings has led to the use of antidepressants for treating PMDD, primarily selective serotonin reuptake inhibitors (SSRIs; e.g., Prozac, Paxil, and Zoloft).[13]

Dysmenorrhea is a medical term for menstrual cramps, the pain or discomfort in the lower abdomen that many women experience just before or during menstruation. Along with cramps, some women experience nausea and vomiting, loose stools, sweating, and dizziness. Menstrual cramps can be classified as primary or secondary dysmenorrhea. Primary dysmenorrhea doesn't involve any physical abnormality and usually begins 6 months to a year after a woman's first period, while secondary dysmenorrhea has an underlying physical cause such as endometriosis or uterine fibroids.[14] You can reduce the discomfort of primary dysmenorrhea by using over-the-counter nonsteroidal anti-inflammatory drugs (NSAIDs) such as aspirin, ibuprofen (Advil or Motrin), or naproxen (Aleve). Other self-care strategies, such as soaking in a hot bath or using a heating pad on your abdomen, may also ease your cramps. For severe cramping, your health care provider may recommend a low-dose oral contraceptive to prevent ovulation. Without ovulation, there are fewer **prostaglandins** to trigger muscle contractions, thus reducing the severity of the cramps caused by the muscle contractions. Managing secondary dysmenorrhea involves treating the underlying cause.

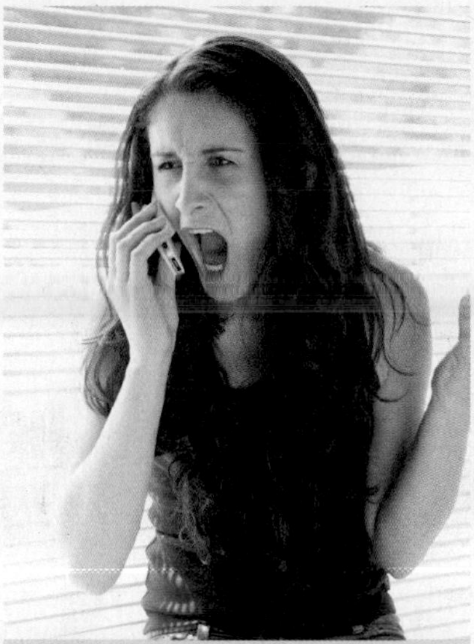

For most women, PMS symptoms—which can include irritability and moodiness, fatigue, bloating, breast tenderness, and food cravings—are mild and short-lived. Stress reduction, regular exercise, and a healthy diet are all good strategies for coping.

Toxic shock syndrome (TSS), although rare, is still something women should be aware of. It is caused by a bacterial infection facilitated by the use of a tampon, diaphragm, or contraceptive sponge (see **Chapter 6**). Symptoms occur during a woman's period or a few days afterward and are sometimes hard to recognize because they mimic the flu. They include sudden high fever, vomiting, diarrhea, dizziness, fainting, or a rash that looks like sunburn. Proper treatment usually assures recovery in 2 to 3 weeks.

Menopause Just as menarche signals the beginning of a woman's potential reproductive years, **menopause**—the permanent cessation of menstruation—signals the end. *Perimenopause* refers to the 4 to 6 years preceding menopause when hormonal changes take place and menstrual cycles and flow can become irregular. Menopause generally occurs between the ages of 45 and 55, with the average age of 51 among U.S. women. Menopausal changes result in decreased estrogen levels, which may produce troublesome symptoms in some women. Decreased vaginal lubrication, hot flashes, night sweats, headaches, dizziness, and joint pain are often associated with the onset of menopause.

Synthetic forms of estrogen and progesterone have long been prescribed as **hormone replacement therapy** (HRT) to relieve menopausal symptoms and reduce the risk of heart disease and osteoporosis. (The National Institutes of Health prefers use of the term **menopausal hormone therapy,** because hormone therapy is not a replacement and does not restore the physiology of youth.) However, recent findings, including results from the Women's Health Initiative (WHI), a large-scale study by the National Institutes of Health, suggest that hormone therapy using synthetic hormones may actually do more harm than good. In fact, the WHI terminated research studies on synthetic hormone use ahead of schedule due to concerns about participants' increased risk of breast cancer, heart attack, stroke, blood clots, and other health problems.[15] New data, however, indicate that these risks may have been related to the age at which women began treatment and the form (pill or patch) utilized.[16] Conflicting research such as this highlights the need for all women to discuss the risks and benefits of menopausal hormone therapy with their health care provider to make an informed decision. Adopting a lifestyle including regular exercise, a healthy diet, and adequate calcium intake can also help protect postmenopausal women from heart disease and osteoporosis.

Male Sexual Anatomy and Physiology

The structures of the male reproductive system are divided into external and internal genitals (**FIGURE 5.4**, page 140). The external genitals are the penis and the scrotum. The internal male genitals include the testes, epididymides, vasa deferentia, ejaculatory ducts, urethra, and other structures—the seminal vesicles, the prostate gland, and the Cowper's glands—that secrete components that, with sperm, make up semen. These three structures are sometimes referred to as the *accessory glands.*

The **penis** is the organ that deposits sperm in the vagina during intercourse. (See the **Health in a Diverse World** box on page 141 for a discussion of circumcision). The urethra, a tube that passes through the center of the penis, acts as the passageway for both semen and urine to exit the body. During sexual arousal, the spongy tissue in the penis becomes filled with blood, making

dysmenorrhea Condition of pain or discomfort in the lower abdomen just before or during menstruation.

prostaglandin Hormone-like substance associated with muscle contraction and inflammation.

menopause Permanent cessation of menstruation; generally occurs between the ages of 45 and 55.

hormone replacement therapy (menopausal hormone therapy) Use of synthetic estrogens and progesterone to compensate for hormonal changes in a woman's body during menopause.

penis Male sexual organ that releases sperm into the vagina.

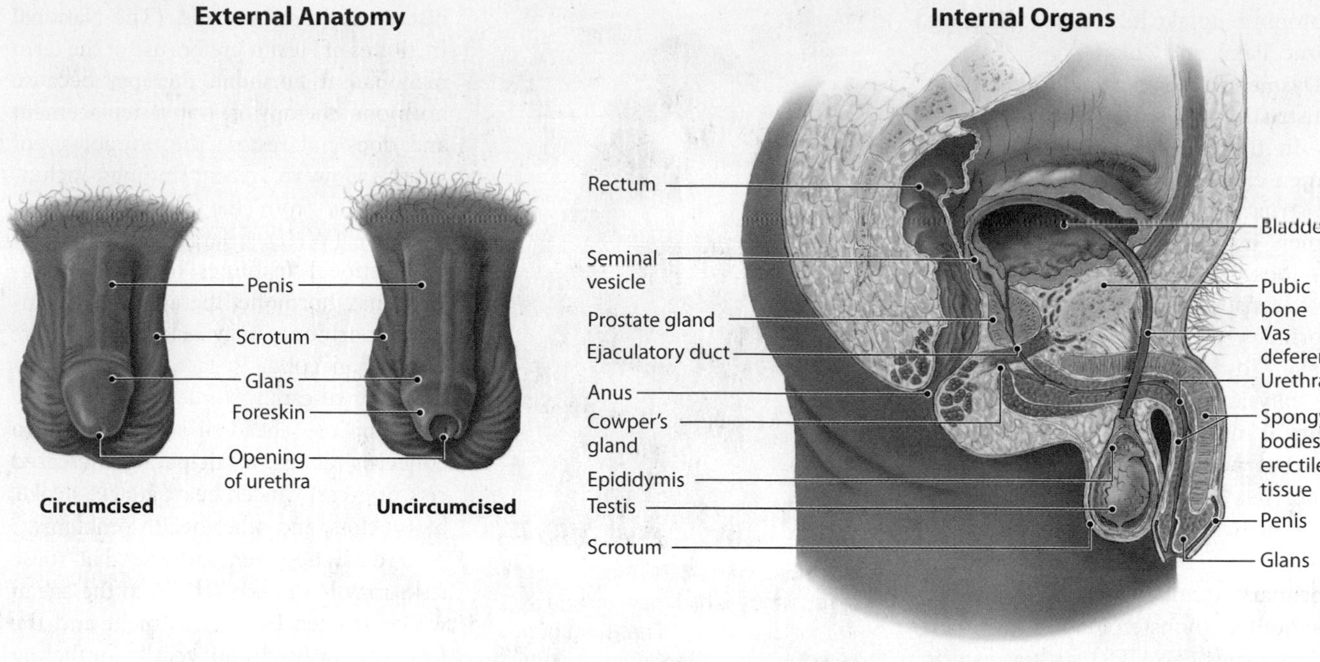

FIGURE 5.4 Male Sexual Anatomy

ejaculation Propulsion of semen from the penis.

scrotum External sac of tissue that encloses the testes.

testes Male sex organs that manufacture sperm and produce hormones.

testosterone Male sex hormone manufactured in the testes.

spermatogenesis The development of sperm.

epididymis Duct system where sperm mature and are stored.

vas deferens Tube that transports sperm from the epididymis to the ejaculatory duct.

seminal vesicles Glandular ducts that secrete nutrients for the semen.

semen Fluid containing sperm and nutrients that increase sperm viability and neutralize vaginal acid.

ejaculatory duct Tube formed by the junction of the seminal vesicle and the vas deferens that carries semen to the urethra.

prostate gland Gland that secretes chemicals that help sperm fertilize an ovum and secretes neutralizing fluids into the semen.

Cowper's glands Glands that secrete a pre-ejaculate fluid that lubricates the urethra and neutralizes any acid remaining in the urethra after urination.

the organ stiff (erect). Further sexual excitement leads to **ejaculation,** a series of rapid, spasmodic contractions that propel semen out of the penis.

Situated behind the penis is a sac called the **scrotum**. The scrotum protects the testes and helps control their internal temperature, which is vital to proper sperm production. The **testes** (singular: *testis*) manufacture sperm and **testosterone,** the hormone responsible for the development of male secondary sex characteristics.

The development of sperm is referred to as **spermatogenesis**. Like the maturation of eggs in the female, this process is governed by the pituitary gland. Follicle-stimulating hormone (FSH) is secreted into the bloodstream to stimulate the testes to manufacture sperm. Immature sperm are released into a comma-shaped structure on the back of each testis called the **epididymis** (plural: *epididymides*), where they ripen and reach full maturity.

Each epididymis contains coiled tubules that gradually straighten out to become the **vas deferens** (plural: *vasa deferentia*). These make up the tubular transportation system whose sole function is to store and move sperm. Along the way, the **seminal vesicles** provide sperm with nutrients and other fluids that comprise **semen**.

The vasa deferentia eventually connect each epididymis to the **ejaculatory ducts**, which pass through the prostate gland and empty into the urethra. The **prostate gland** contributes more fluids to the semen, including chemicals that help the sperm fertilize an ovum and neutralize the acidic environment of the vagina to make it more conducive to sperm motility (ability to move) and potency (potential for fertilization). Just below the prostate gland are two pea-shaped nodules called the **Cowper's glands.** The Cowper's glands secrete a pre-ejaculate fluid that lubricates the urethra and neutralizes any acid that may remain in the urethra after urination. In this process, urine and semen never come into contact with each other, as during ejaculation of semen, a small valve closes off the tube to the urinary bladder.

Andropause Whether or not men actually go through a form of male menopause, known as *andropause*, is the subject of much debate. While testosterone levels in men vary greatly, men do experience a gradual decline in testosterone levels as they age, similar to the declining hormone levels in women, particularly if they are obese or smoke cigarettes.[17] Men, however, do not experience a rapid hormone decline in middle age that affects their reproductive capacity as women do during menopause. Instead, men typically experience a gradual decline in testosterone levels throughout adulthood, about 1 percent a year on average after age 30.[18] Many doctors use the term *andropause* to describe age-related hormone changes in

HEALTH IN A DIVERSE WORLD

CIRCUMCISION *Risk Versus Benefit*

Debate continues over the practice of *circumcision,* the surgical removal of a fold of skin, known as the *foreskin,* covering the end of the penis. While nearly universal in the United States decades ago, only about 55 percent of baby boys are now circumcised, mostly for religious or cultural reasons or because of hygiene concerns.

While prescribed in Jewish and Muslim faiths worldwide, circumcision is not required in the Christian faith. Only in the United States do Christians regularly circumcise, although they do so with less frequency today.

Recent research supports claims that circumcision yields medical benefits, including decreased risk of urinary tract infections in the first year, decreased risk of penile cancer (although cancer of the penis is very rare), and decreased risk of sexual transmission of human papillomavirus (HPV) and human immunodeficiency virus (HIV).

However, strong arguments against circumcision include a lack of medical necessity, a possible reduction in sexual sensitivity, and the possibility of bleeding, infection, and surgical complications. The American Academy of Pediatrics recently took a stand on the issue stating that scientific evidence shows potential medical benefits of newborn male circumcision, but that the evidence is not currently strong enough to recommend routine circumcision.

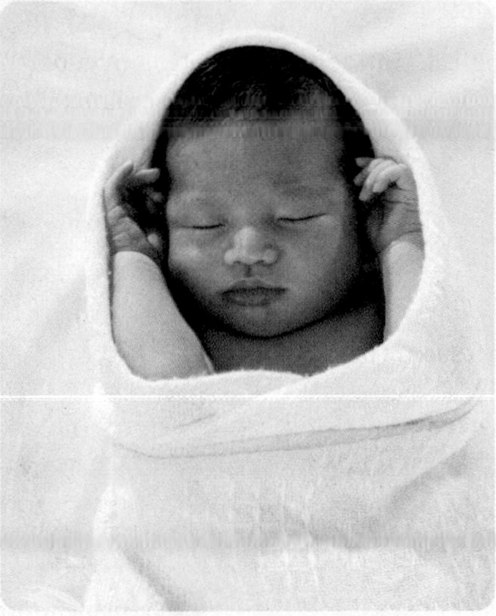

Arguments against Circumcision

- It is a surgical procedure that may cause pain to the infant, and there are potential complications such as bleeding, infection, improper healing, or cutting the foreskin too long or too short.
- Much of the research on the relationship between circumcision and sexually transmitted infections was done in developing countries and may not be indicative of outcomes in developed nations.
- Men lose a degree of sexual pleasure and stimulation when the foreskin is removed. Many unique nerve endings—found only in the foreskin—are lost forever.

Arguments for Circumcision

- Circumcised males have a lower risk of penile cancer.
- Circumcised males have a lower risk of urinary tract infections during their first year, easier genital hygiene, and a lower risk of foreskin infections.
- In developing countries, circumcision has been shown to have a protective effect against human immunodeficiency virus (HIV), herpes simplex virus 2 (HSV-2), and human papillomavirus (HPV) transmission in males.
- Families may have religious or cultural reasons for wishing to circumcise their sons (in the Jewish faith, for example, circumcision is performed in a ceremony called a *bris*, and it represents the covenant God made with the patriarch Abraham).

Where Do You Stand?

- If you had a son, what decision would you make regarding circumcising him?
- What factors—religious, cultural, aesthetic, or health-related—would have the most influence on your decision?
- If your faith requires circumcision, how do you weigh the medical factors against the religious and cultural factors?

Sources: M. Owings and S. Uddin, "Trends in Circumcision for Male Newborns in U.S. Hospitals: 1979–2010," National Center for Health Statistics, 2013) www.cdc.gov/nchs/data/hestat/circumcision_2013/circumcision_2013.htm; Mayo Clinic Staff, "Circumcision (Male): Why It's Done," September 2012, www.mayoclinic.com; American Academy of Pediatrics, "2012 Technical Report, Male Circumcision," *Pediatrics* 130, no. 3 (2012): e756–e785, DOI: 10.1542/peds.2012-1990.

men. Some men with lower testosterone levels do not experience signs and symptoms. Those who do may experience the following:[19]

- **Changes in sexual function.** These may include reduced sexual desire, fewer spontaneous erections—such as during sleep—and infertility. Testes may become smaller, as well.
- **Changes in sleep patterns.** Low testosterone may cause insomnia or other sleep disturbances.
- **Physical changes.** Various physical changes may occur, including increased body fat, reduced muscle bulk and strength, and decreased bone density. Abnormal enlargement of the male breasts (gynecomastia) and hair loss are possible.
- **Emotional changes.** Low testosterone levels may contribute to a decrease in motivation or self-confidence, cause sadness or depression, or interfere with concentration or memory.[20]

Treatment is available for age-related low testosterone levels, but it is not without controversy. For some men, testosterone therapy relieves the symptoms. For others, especially older men, the benefits aren't clear. And there are risks; testosterone therapy may increase the risk of prostate cancer or other health problems.

LO 3 | HUMAN SEXUAL RESPONSE

List and describe the stages of the human sexual response and what factors may influence these.

Many factors, both physical and psychological, influence sexual response and sexual desire. Thus, a person's sexual response may be vastly different from one sexual experience to another or from one partner to another.

Sexual response is a physiological process that generally follows a pattern that can be roughly divided into four stages: excitement/arousal, plateau, orgasm, and resolution (**FIGURE 5.5**). Regardless of the type of sexual activity (stimulation by a partner or self-stimulation), the response stages are the same; however, researchers agree that each individual

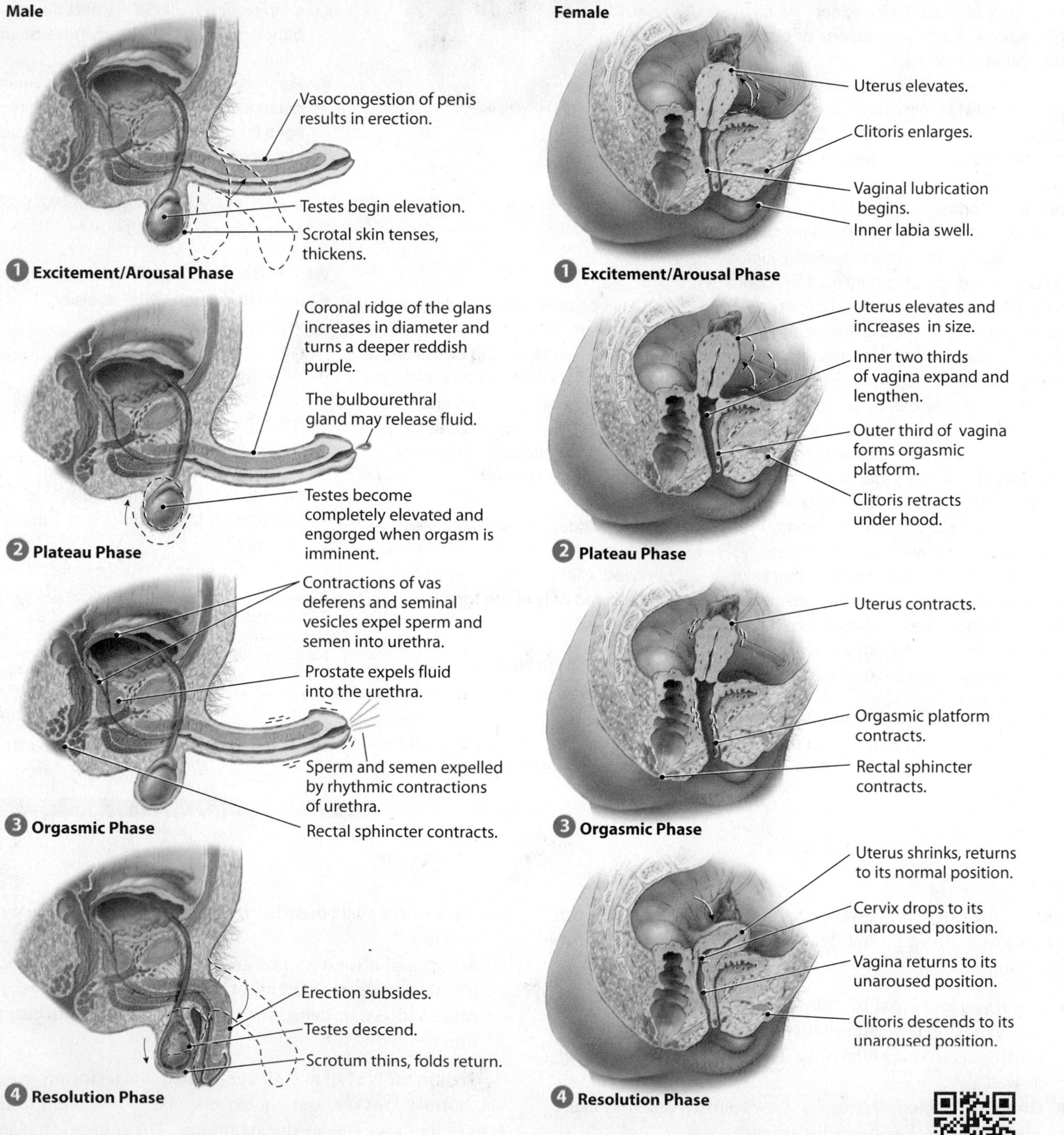

Male
Vasocongestion of penis results in erection.
Testes begin elevation.
Scrotal skin tenses, thickens.
1 Excitement/Arousal Phase
Coronal ridge of the glans increases in diameter and turns a deeper reddish purple.
The bulbourethral gland may release fluid.
Testes become completely elevated and engorged when orgasm is imminent.
2 Plateau Phase
Contractions of vas deferens and seminal vesicles expel sperm and semen into urethra.
Prostate expels fluid into the urethra.
Sperm and semen expelled by rhythmic contractions of urethra.
Rectal sphincter contracts.
3 Orgasmic Phase
Erection subsides.
Testes descend.
Scrotum thins, folds return.
4 Resolution Phase
Female
Uterus elevates.
Clitoris enlarges.
Vaginal lubrication begins.
Inner labia swell.
1 Excitement/Arousal Phase
Uterus elevates and increases in size.
Inner two thirds of vagina expand and lengthen.
Outer third of vagina forms orgasmic platform.
Clitoris retracts under hood.
2 Plateau Phase
Uterus contracts.
Orgasmic platform contracts.
Rectal sphincter contracts.
3 Orgasmic Phase
Uterus shrinks, returns to its normal position.
Cervix drops to its unaroused position.
Vagina returns to its unaroused position.
Clitoris descends to its unaroused position.
4 Resolution Phase

FIGURE 5.5 Comparison of Male and Female Sexual Response

VIDEO TUTOR Male and Female Sexual Response

has a personal response pattern that may or may not exactly conform to these phases.

During the first stage, *excitement/arousal*, **vasocongestion** (increased blood flow that causes swelling in the genitals) stimulates male and female genital responses. The vagina begins to lubricate, and the penis becomes partially erect. Both sexes may exhibit a "sex flush" or light blush all over their bodies. Excitement/arousal can be generated through fantasy or by touching parts of the body, kissing, viewing erotic images, or reading erotic literature.

26%

OF COLLEGE STUDENTS REPORT HAVING HAD MORE THAN ONE **SEX PARTNER** IN THE PAST 12 MONTHS.

During the *plateau phase*, the initial responses intensify. Voluntary and involuntary muscle tensions increase. A woman's nipples become erect, as does a man's penis. The penis secretes a few drops of preejaculatory fluid, which may contain sperm.

During the *orgasmic phase*, vasocongestion and muscle tensions reach their peak, and rhythmic contractions occur through the genital regions. In women, these contractions are centered in the uterus, outer vagina, and anal sphincter. In men, the contractions occur in two stages. First, contractions within the prostate gland begin propelling semen through the urethra. In the second stage, the muscles of the pelvic floor, urethra, and anal sphincter contract. Semen usually, but not always, is ejaculated from the penis. In both sexes, spasms in other major muscle groups also occur, particularly in the buttocks and abdomen. Feet and hands may also contract, and facial features often contort.

Muscle tension and congested blood subside in the *resolution phase* as the genital organs return to their prearousal states. Both sexes usually experience deep feelings of well-being and profound relaxation. Many women can experience multiple orgasms during the orgasmic phase. Some men experience a refractory period, during which their systems are incapable of subsequent arousal. This refractory period may last from a few minutes to several hours and tends to lengthen with age.

WHAT DO YOU THINK?

Why do we place so much importance on orgasm?

- Can sexual pleasure and satisfaction be achieved without orgasm?
- What is the role of desire in sexual response?

Men and women experience the same stages in the sexual response cycle; however, the length of time spent in any one stage varies. Thus, one partner may be in the plateau phase while the other is in the excitement or orgasmic phase. Such variations in response rates are entirely normal. Some couples believe that simultaneous orgasm is desirable for sexual satisfaction. Although simultaneous orgasm is pleasant, so are orgasms achieved at different times.

Sexual pleasure and satisfaction are also possible without orgasm or even intercourse. Expressing sexual feelings for another person involves many pleasurable activities, of which intercourse and orgasm may be only a part.

Sexual Responses among Older Adults

Older adults are commonly stereotyped as being uninterested or incapable of sexual relations. The truth is, though we do experience some physical changes as we age, they generally do not cause us to stop enjoying sex.

In women, the most significant physical changes follow menopause. Skin becomes less elastic; most internal sexual organs, including the uterus and cervix, shrink somewhat; the vaginal walls become thinner; and vaginal lubrication during sexual arousal may decrease. The resulting increased friction during penetration can be painful, although the use of artificial lubricants usually resolves this problem. Women who remain sexually active as they age report fewer problems with age-related changes in sexual functioning.

vasocongestion Engorgement of the genital organs with blood.

Although men do not experience menopause, their bodies do change as a result of the aging process. They require more direct and prolonged stimulation to achieve an erection, and erections become less firm. They are slower to reach orgasm, and their refractory periods are longer. Older men also experience a decrease in the intensity of ejaculation, as semen is less forcefully expelled over time.

The majority of healthy older men and women enjoy a regular and satisfying sex life. Among the advantages experienced by adults at this stage of life are a level of comfort with and appreciation of their body as well as no longer needing contraception (although protection from sexually transmitted infections (STIs) is still necessary if there are new or multiple partners).

LO 4 | EXPRESSING YOUR SEXUALITY

Explain the options available for the expression of one's sexuality.

Finding healthy ways to express your sexuality is an important part of sexual maturity. Many avenues of sexual expression are available.

Sexual Behavior: What Is "Normal"?

How do we know which sexual behaviors are considered normal? What or whose criteria should we use? These are not easy questions.

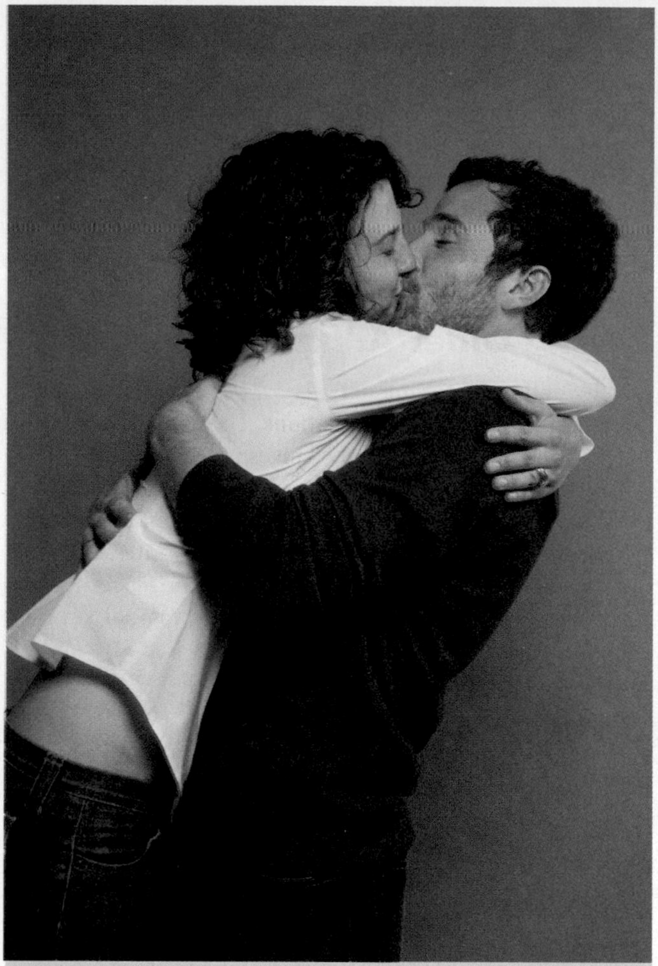

As with any other human behavior, the idea of "normal" sexual behavior varies from person to person and from society to society, usually along a spectrum of perceived acceptability or appropriateness.

Every society sets standards and attempts to normalize sexual behavior. Boundaries arise that distinguish good from bad or acceptable from unacceptable and result in criteria used to establish what is viewed as normal or abnormal. Some of the common standards for sexual behavior in Western culture today include the following:[21]

- **The coital standard.** Penile–vaginal intercourse (coitus) is viewed as the ultimate sex act.
- **The orgasmic standard.** Sexual interaction should lead to orgasm.
- **The two-person standard.** Sex is an activity to be experienced by two people.
- **The romantic standard.** Sex should be related to love.
- **The safer-sex standard.** If we choose to be sexually active, we should act to prevent unintended pregnancy or disease transmission.

celibacy State of not engaging in sexual activity.
autoerotic behaviors Sexual self-stimulation.
sexual fantasies Sexually arousing thoughts and dreams.
masturbation Self-stimulation of genitals.

These are not laws or rules, but rather social scripts that have been adopted over time. Sexual standards often shift through the years, and some people choose to ignore them altogether. Rather than making blanket judgments about normal versus abnormal, we might ask the following questions:[22]

- Is a sexual behavior healthy and fulfilling for a particular person?
- Is it safe?
- Does it involve the exploitation of others?
- Does it take place between responsible, consenting adults?

In this way, we can view behavior along a continuum that takes into account many individual factors. As you read about the options for sexual expression in the sections ahead, use these questions to explore your feelings about what is normal for you.

Options for Sexual Expression

The range of human sexual expression is virtually infinite. What you find enjoyable may not be an option for someone else (see the **Health in a Diverse World** box for a discussion of sexuality and disability). The ways you choose to meet your sexual needs today may be very different from what they were 2 weeks ago or will be 2 years from now. Accepting yourself as a sexual person with individual desires and preferences is the first step in achieving sexual satisfaction.

Celibacy

Celibacy is abstention from sexual activities with others. Some people choose celibacy for religious or moral reasons. Others may be celibate for a period of time due to illness, the breakup of a long-term relationship, or lack of an acceptable partner. For some, celibacy is a lonely, agonizing state, but others find it an opportunity for introspection, values assessment, and personal growth. While celibacy and abstinence are related terms, abstinence usually refers to the avoidance of intercourse, while celibacy usually refers to abstention from all sexual activities whatsoever. No good estimates of celibacy exist, but about 30 percent of college students report being abstinent (no sexual partners) in the past year.[23]

Autoerotic Behaviors

Autoerotic behaviors involve self-stimulation. The two most common are sexual fantasy and masturbation.

Sexual fantasies are sexually arousing thoughts and dreams. Fantasies may reflect real-life experiences, forbidden desires, or the opportunity to practice new or anticipated sexual experiences. The fact that you fantasize about a particular sexual experience does not necessarily mean that you want to, or have to, act out that experience. Sexual fantasies are just that—fantasy.

Masturbation is self-stimulation of the genitals. Although many people are uncomfortable discussing masturbation, it is a common sexual practice across the life span. Mas-

HEALTH IN A DIVERSE WORLD

SEXUALITY AND DISABILITY

Many of us tend to think of disabled people as asexual. It may be difficult to understand what sex would be like as or with a disabled person, but disabled people are not asexual, and it is possible for a disabled person to have a fulfilling sex life. However, beyond any physical limitations, there are many hurdles to overcome, including cultural standards of beauty and perfection and misconceptions about what disabled people can and can't do sexually.

The challenges a disabled person faces with respect to having a satisfying sexual relationship include both physical and psychological difficulties. Being disabled means that a person has certain limitations in physical function. That can mean many things, and the disability may or may not directly affect sexual function. For example, someone who is deaf is legally disabled, but sexually functional. A person who is paralyzed from the neck down may still be able to have an orgasm, in spite of being unable to move.

Some disabilities can be very socially isolating, though. For example, a single person who is paralyzed has obstacles to overcome in finding a romantic or sexual partner. Help may be needed for travel, and the number of people the person meets will be limited by how often he or she can get out socially. Help may be needed with various tasks of daily life. He or she may not be able to move to touch and arouse a partner. The psychological challenges for disabled people in finding a romantic or sexual partner can also be significant and may include overcoming anger or feelings that they don't measure up in the estimation of other people.

Whether able-bodied or disabled, we are all sexual beings deserving of intimacy and fulfilling sexual relationships.

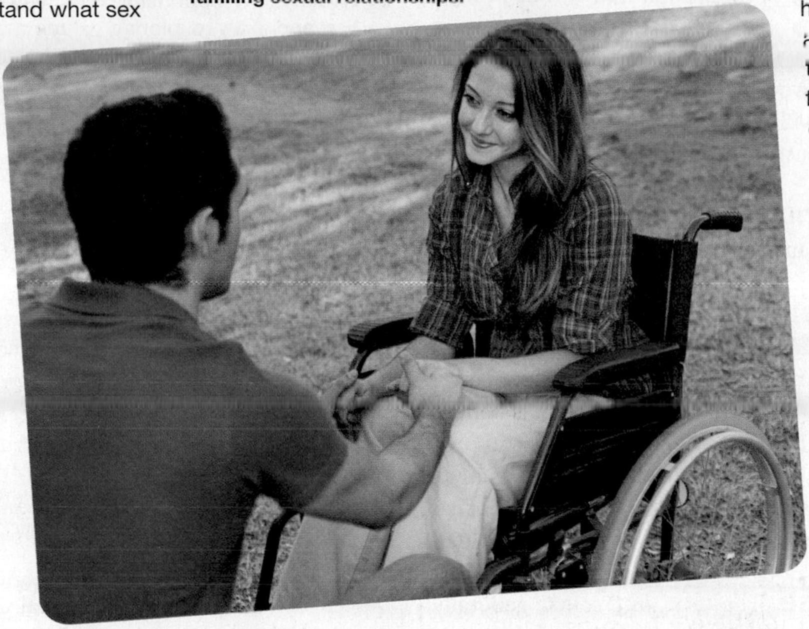

For anyone with a disability, counseling or therapy to deal with sexuality issues can help. Cognitive therapy and sex therapy—the treatment of sexual dysfunction, lack of sexual confidence, and other sexual problems—may help, or the person may want to see a certified sex surrogate. Surrogates offer therapeutic exercises to help the patient. These may include relaxation techniques, intimate communication, social skills, and sexual touching. One or a combination of these methods may help disabled people who want to explore the sexual side of their life. Resources such as www.surrogatetherapy.org/ can help those who want more information about sexuality and disability.

Each disabled person is unique, and it's important to consider his or her specific challenges, desires, and feelings involved in addressing his or her sexuality.

Sources: Christopher and Dana Reeve Foundation, "Sexual Health for Men," www.christopherreeve.org/site/c.mtKZKgMWKwG/b.4453431/k.A0C5/Sexuality_for_Men.htm; International Professional Surrogates Association, "What Is Surrogate Partner Therapy?," www.surrogatetherapy.org/what-is-surrogate-partner-therapy.

turbation is a natural pleasure-seeking behavior in infants and children. It is a valuable and important means for adolescents, as well as adults, to explore sexual feelings and responsiveness. In one survey of college students, 48 percent of women and 92 percent of men reported that they have masturbated.[24]

Kissing and Erotic Touching Kissing and erotic touching are two very common forms of nonverbal sexual communication. Both men and women have **erogenous zones**, areas of the body that when touched lead to sexual arousal. Erogenous zones may include genital and nongenital areas, such as the earlobes, mouth, nipples, and inner thighs. Almost any area of the body can be conditioned to respond erotically to touch. Spending time with your partner to explore and learn about his or her erogenous areas is another pleasurable, safe, and satisfying means of sexual expression.

Manual Stimulation Both men and women can be sexually aroused and achieve orgasm through manual stimulation of the genitals by a partner. For many women, orgasm is more likely to be achieved through manual stimulation than through intercourse. *Sex toys* include a wide variety of objects that can be used for sexual stimulation alone or with a

erogenous zones Areas of the body that, when touched, lead to sexual arousal.

cunnilingus Oral stimulation of a woman's genitals.

fellatio Oral stimulation of a man's genitals.

vaginal intercourse Insertion of the penis into the vagina.

anal intercourse Insertion of the penis into the anus.

partner. Vibrators and dildos are two common types of toys and can be found in a variety of shapes, styles, and sizes. Sex toys can be used both to enhance the sexual experience and also as therapeutic devices to help with issues such as orgasmic difficulty and erectile dysfunction. For women who may not reach orgasm through intercourse, they can provide another option for sexual satisfaction. (Note that toys must be cleaned after each use.)

Oral–Genital Stimulation **Cunnilingus** refers to oral stimulation of a woman's genitals and **fellatio** to oral stimulation of a man's genitals. Many partners find oral stimulation intensely pleasurable. In the most recent National College Health Assessment (NCHA), 43.6 percent of college students reported having oral sex in the past month.[25] For some people, oral sex is not an option because of moral or religious beliefs. Remember, HIV and other STIs can be transmitted via unprotected oral–genital sex just as they can through intercourse. Use of an appropriate barrier device is strongly recommended if either partner's disease status is unknown.

Vaginal Intercourse The term *intercourse* generally refers to **vaginal intercourse** (*coitus,* or insertion of the penis into the vagina), which is the most frequently practiced form of sexual expression. In the latest NCHA survey, 47.4 percent of college students reported having vaginal intercourse in the past month.[26] Coitus can involve a variety of positions, including the missionary position (man on top facing the woman), woman on top, side by side, or man behind (rear entry). Many partners enjoy experimenting with different positions. Knowledge of yourself and your body, along with your ability to communicate effectively, will play a large part in determining the enjoyment and meaning of intercourse for you and your partner. Also, it is easier to relax and enjoy sex when you know that you are protected from disease and unintended pregnancy. (See **Chapter 14** for more about safer sex.)

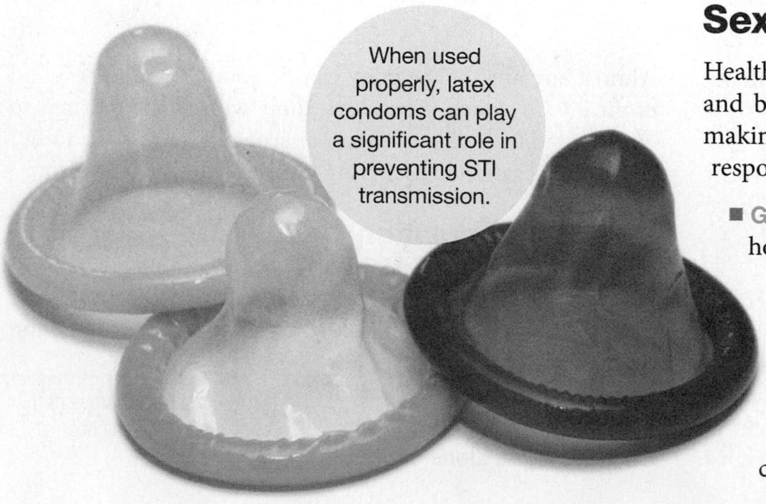

When used properly, latex condoms can play a significant role in preventing STI transmission.

SKILLS FOR BEHAVIOR CHANGE

TAKING STEPS TOWARD HEALTHY SEXUALITY

Healthy and responsible sexuality means having information and skills, exploring values and beliefs, and making responsible and informed choices. The following tips can help:

- Give some thought to your own sexuality. Do you choose to be sexually active now, or are you more comfortable waiting?
- Get to know your body and how you respond sexually to make communicating easier and sex better.
- If you have a partner now, sit down and talk about your sexual relationship. Are you both comfortable and satisfied with all aspects of the relationship? Discuss what you like and don't like.
- Explore and address any questions and feelings you may have about your gender identity or your sexual orientation.

Anal Intercourse The anal area is highly sensitive to touch, and some couples find pleasure in stimulation. **Anal intercourse** is the insertion of the penis into the anus. Research indicates that 5.4 percent of college-aged men and women have had anal sex in the past month.[27] Stimulation of the anus by mouth, fingers, or sex toys is also practiced. As with all forms of sexual expression, anal stimulation or intercourse is not for everyone. If you enjoy this form of sexual expression, note that condom use is especially important, as the delicate tissues of the anus are more likely to tear than vaginal tissues, significantly increasing the risk of transmission of HIV and other STIs. Also, anything inserted into the anus should not then be directly inserted into the vagina without cleaning, as bacteria commonly found in the anus can cause vaginal infections.

Responsible and Satisfying Sexual Behavior

Healthy sexuality is a product of assimilating information and building skills, of exploring values and beliefs, and of making responsible and informed choices. Healthy and responsible sexuality includes the following:

- **Good communication as the foundation.** Open and honest communication with your partner is the basis for establishing respect, trust, and intimacy. Do you communicate with your partner in caring and respectful ways? Can you share your thoughts and emotions freely with your partner? Can you share your sexual history with your partner? Do you discuss contraception and disease prevention? Are you able to communicate what you like and don't like? These are all

TECH & HEALTH | BETTER THAN SEXTING

Most people realize that "sexting," or sending sexual texts, photos, or videos on your cell phone, has the potential for loss of privacy and embarrassment. However, many still do it. Why? According to some students, sexting is a way for couples to express their feelings even if they are apart; for others, sexting is considered a "safe" way to be sexual, where you don't run the risk of unintended pregnancy or infection with a STI. In a recent survey, 78 percent of college students said they've received a sexually suggestive text message and 56 percent said they have received an intimate picture. Two-thirds of the students said they had sent messages, most of which (73%) were sent to a romantic partner.

While it's easy to send a "sext" without thinking too much about it, it's also easy for the recipient to pass it on. In fact, about 20 percent of the pictures get passed to a person beyond the intended recipient. When that happens, the person who sent the text is open to a variety of consequences, including embarrassment and harassment.

Former Congressman Anthony Weiner was forced to resign after he posted lewd photos of himself on Twitter and admitted to sexting with several women.

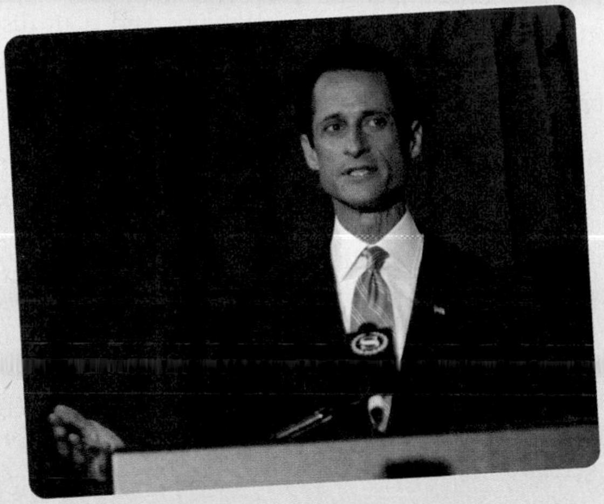

Instead of using your phone for sexting, consider using it for learning something about sex. There are hundreds of apps and websites that can help improve your knowledge, your confidence, and your sex life. Here are a few to check out:

- *SexPositive* is shame-free sex education app that teaches about relationships, sex, and sexuality.
- Looking to spice up your love life? *Adult Wheel of Foreplay* is a simple app that can suggest some new ways to express your affection.
- Worried about STI symptoms? Send a picture to *STD Triage* and a group of dermatologists will let you know if you should seek treatment.
- If you are diagnosed with an STI, *So They Can Know* allows you to anonymously contact former partners via e-mail so you can be responsible and let them know to seek treatment without being embarrassed.
- Speaking of being responsible, *Online Buddies* allows users the option to identify their HIV status upfront, making it easier to have a conversation about HIV risk with a potential partner.

If you are interested in learning more about sexual health, some of the best podcasts include Kinsey Confidential, Personal Life Media, and RH Reality Check.

Sources: B. Luscombe, "4 out of 5 College Students Sext," *Time Magazine*, July 25, 2011, http://healthland.time.com/2011/07/25/how-many-college-kids-sext-four-out-of-five.

components of the open communication that is necessary for healthy, responsible sexuality.

- **Acknowledging that you are a sexual person.** People who can see and accept themselves as sexual beings are more likely to make informed decisions and take responsible actions. If you see yourself as a potentially sexual person, you will plan ahead for contraception and disease prevention. If you are comfortable being a sexually active person, you will not need or want your sexual experiences to be clouded by alcohol or other drug use. If you choose not to be sexually active, you do so consciously, as a personal decision. Even if you are not sexually active, it is important to acknowledge that sex is a natural aspect of our lives and to recognize that you are in charge of your own decisions about your sexuality.
- **Understanding sexual structures and their functions.** If you understand how the human body works, sexual pleasure and response will not be mysterious events. You will be better able to pleasure yourself and communicate to your partner how best to pleasure you. You will understand how pregnancy and STIs can be prevented. You will be able to recognize sexual dysfunction and take responsible actions to address the problem.
- **Accepting and embracing your gender identity and your sexual orientation.** "Being comfortable in your own skin" is an old saying that is particularly relevant when it comes to sexuality. It is difficult to feel sexually satisfied if you are conflicted about your gender identity or sexual orientation. You should explore and address questions and feelings you may have. Good communication skills, acknowledging that you are a sexual person, and understanding your sexual anatomy and its functions will allow you to complete this task.

See the **Skills for Behavior Change** box on the previous page for tips on taking steps toward healthy sexuality, and check out the **Tech & Health** box for ways you can use technology for better sexual health.

variant sexual behavior A sexual behavior that is not commonly practiced.

sexual dysfunction Problems associated with achieving sexual satisfaction.

sexual performance anxiety Sexual difficulties caused by anticipating some sort of problem during a sex act.

libido Sexual drive or desire.

inhibited sexual desire Lack of sexual appetite or lack of interest and pleasure in sexual activity.

Variant Sexual Behavior

Although attitudes toward sexuality have changed substantially, some behaviors are still considered to be outside the norm. People who study sexuality prefer to use the neutral term **variant sexual behavior** to describe less common sexual behaviors, for example:

- **Group sex.** Sexual activity involving more than two people. Participants in group sex run a higher risk of exposure to HIV and other STIs than that associated with a sexual encounter with only one partner.
- **Swinging.** Also known as partner-swapping, increases the risk of exposure to HIV and other STIs.
- **Fetishism.** Using inanimate objects to heighten sexual arousal. Objects of fetishes often enhance one of the senses, such as silky clothing or lingerie, food with pleasant smells, or fancy shoes.

Some variant sexual behaviors can be harmful to the individual, to others, or to both. Some of the following activities are illegal in certain states:

- **Exhibitionism.** Exposing one's genitals to strangers in public places. Most exhibitionists are seeking a reaction of shock or fear. Exhibitionism is a minor felony in most states.
- **Voyeurism.** Observing other people for sexual gratification. Most voyeurs are men who attempt to watch women undressing or bathing. Voyeurism is an invasion of privacy and is illegal in most states.
- **Sadomasochism.** Sexual activities in which gratification is achieved by inflicting pain (verbal or physical abuse) on a partner or by being the object of such infliction. A sadist is a person who enjoys inflicting pain, and a masochist enjoys experiencing pain. These activities are legal when they involve consenting partners.
- **Pedophilia.** Sexual activity or attraction between an adult and a child. Any sexual activity involving a minor, including possession of child pornography, is illegal in all states.
- **Autoerotic asphyxiation.** The practice of reducing or eliminating oxygen to the brain, usually by tying a cord around one's neck while masturbating to orgasm. Tragically, deaths have occurred when individuals unintentionally strangle themselves.

LO 5 | SEXUAL DYSFUNCTION

Classify sexual dysfunctions, describe major disorders, and discuss treatment options.

Research indicates that **sexual dysfunction,** the term used to describe problems that can hinder sexual functioning, is quite common. Sexual dysfunction can be divided into four categories: desire disorders, arousal disorders, orgasmic disorders, and pain disorders. (See **TABLE 5.1**.) All can be treated successfully.

Both men and women can experience **sexual performance anxiety** when they anticipate some sort of problem during a sexual experience. A man may become anxious and unable to maintain an erection (an arousal disorder), or he may experience premature ejaculation (an orgasmic disorder). A woman may be unable to achieve orgasm (an arousal disorder) or to allow penetration because of the involuntary contraction of vaginal muscles (a pain disorder). Both men and women can overcome sexual performance anxiety by learning to focus on immediate sensations and pleasures rather than on orgasm.

Sexual Desire Disorders

Libido is a person's sexual drive or desire. A common reason people seek out a sex therapist is **inhibited sexual desire,** or the lack of interest and pleasure in sexual activity. A low sex drive (decreased libido) may be caused by hormonal imbalances in women or by low testosterone in both men and women. Fatigue, stress, and common conditions such as depression and anxiety can cause decreased libido. Antidepressant medications (e.g., Prozac, Zoloft, Paxil) are well

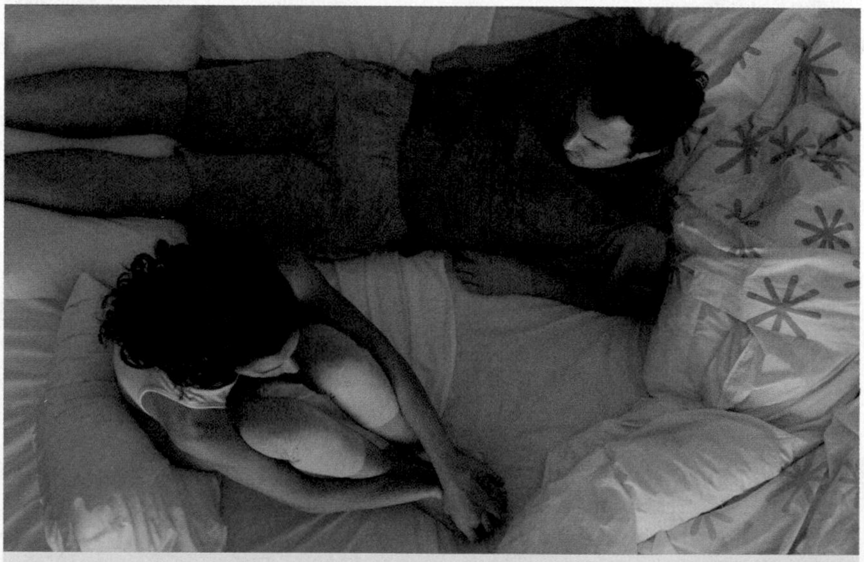

Sexual disorders can have both physical and psychological roots and can occur as a result of stress, fatigue, depression, or anxiety. They frequently have a physiological origin, such as overall poor health, chronic disease, or the use of alcohol or drugs.

TABLE 5.1 | Types of Sexual Dysfunction

	Description
Desire Disorders	
Inhibited sexual desire	Lack of interest in sexual activity
Sexual aversion disorder	Phobias (fears) or anxiety about sexual contact
Arousal Disorders	
Erectile dysfunction	Inability to maintain an erection
Female sexual arousal disorder	Inability to remain sexually aroused
Orgasmic Disorders	
Premature ejaculation	Reaching orgasm rapidly or prematurely
Delayed ejaculation	Difficulty reaching orgasm despite normal desire and stimulation
Female orgasmic disorder	Inability to have an orgasm or difficulty or delay in reaching orgasm
Pain Disorders	
Dyspareunia	Pain during or after sex
Vaginismus	Forceful contraction of the vaginal muscles that prevents penetration from occurring

known for reducing sexual desire in both men and women.[28] **Sexual aversion disorder** is another type of desire dysfunction, characterized by sexual phobias (unreasonable fears) and anxiety about sexual contact. The psychological stress related to a punitive upbringing, a rigid religious background, or a history of physical or sexual abuse may be sources of desire disorders.

Sexual Arousal Disorders

The most common sexual arousal disorder is **erectile dysfunction (ED)**—difficulty in achieving or maintaining an erection sufficient for intercourse. At some time in his life, every man experiences erectile dysfunction. The majority of arousal disorders are caused by the same lifestyle issues that increase the risk of high cholesterol, hypertension, and chronic diseases such as cardiovascular disease and diabetes—in turn affecting blood flow. Other risks for ED include certain medical conditions, treatments, and medications; using tobacco; being overweight; injuries; psychological conditions; drug and alcohol use; and prolonged bicycling.[29] Some 30 million men in the United States, half of them under age 65, suffer from ED. The condition generally becomes more of a problem as men age, affecting 1 in 5 men in their sixties.[30] Seeing a doctor to determine possible causes is essential. Lifestyle changes are usually key to risk reduction. The FDA has also approved several drugs, such as Viagra (sildenafil citrate), Levitra (vardenafil hydrochloride), and Cialis (tadalafil), to treat ED. These drugs work by relaxing the smooth muscle cells in the penis, allowing for increased blood flow to the erectile tissues. However, the best prevention for ED is to maintain overall physical and mental health.

WHAT DO YOU THINK?

Why do we find it so difficult to discuss sexual dysfunction?

- Do you think it is more difficult for men than for women? Or vice versa?

Orgasmic Disorders

Premature ejaculation (also known as *early ejaculation*)—ejaculation that occurs prior to or very soon after the insertion of the penis into the vagina—affects up to 70 percent of men at some time in their lives.[31] Treatment first involves a physical examination to rule out physiological causes. If the cause is not physiological, therapy is available to help a man learn how to control the timing of his ejaculation. **Delayed ejaculation** is persistent difficulty in reaching orgasm despite normal desire and stimulation. Fatigue, stress, performance pressure, and alcohol use can all contribute to orgasmic disorders in men.

In a woman, the inability to achieve orgasm is called **female orgasmic disorder.** A woman with this disorder often learns to fake orgasm to avoid embarrassment or to preserve her partner's ego. Contributing factors include a conservative upbringing, performance anxiety, lack of trust, relationship issues, and difficulty seeing oneself as a sexual being. Again, the first step in treatment is a physical exam to rule out physiological causes. Often the problem is solved by simple self-exploration to learn more about what forms of stimulation are arousing enough to produce orgasm. Through masturbation, a woman can learn how her body responds to various types of touch. Once she has become orgasmic through masturbation, she can then learn to communicate her needs to her partner.

Sexual Pain Disorders

Two common disorders in this category are dyspareunia and vaginismus. **Dyspareunia** is pain experienced by a woman during intercourse that may be caused by conditions such as endometriosis, uterine tumors, chlamydia, gonorrhea, or urinary tract infections. Childbirth trauma and insufficient lubrication during intercourse may also cause discomfort. Dyspareunia can also be psychological in origin. **Vaginismus** is the involuntary

sexual aversion disorder Desire dysfunction characterized by sexual phobias and anxiety about sexual contact.

erectile dysfunction (ED) Difficulty in achieving or maintaining an erection sufficient for intercourse.

premature ejaculation Ejaculation that occurs prior to or almost immediately following penile penetration of the vagina; also known as *early ejaculation*.

delayed ejaculation Persistent difficulty in reaching orgasm despite normal desire and stimulation.

female orgasmic disorder A woman's inability to achieve orgasm.

dyspareunia Pain experienced by women during intercourse.

vaginismus State in which the vaginal muscles contract so forcefully that penetration cannot occur.

contraction of vaginal muscles, making penile insertion painful or impossible. Most cases of vaginismus are related to fear of intercourse or unresolved sexual conflicts. As with other sexual problems, these disorders can be treated.

Seeking Help for Sexual Dysfunction

While sexual dysfunction can happen at any age, the incidence of dysfunction increases during the menopause years in women and after age 50 in men.[32] Many treatment models can help people with sexual dysfunction. It is important not to be afraid to talk to a sex educator, counselor, or health care provider. If you are looking for a qualified professional, the American Association of Sex Educators, Counselors, and Therapists (AASECT) can help. AASECT has been in the forefront of establishing criteria for certifying sex therapists. Their website provides information on how to locate a certified professional in your community.

LO 6 | DRUGS AND SEX

Explain the effects of various drugs on sexual behavior.

Because psychoactive drugs affect the body's overall physiological functioning, it is only logical that they also affect sexual behavior. Promises of increased pleasure make drugs tempting to people seeking greater sexual satisfaction. But if drugs are necessary to increase sexual feelings, it is likely that partners are being dishonest about their feelings for each other. Good sex should not depend on chemical substances. Alcohol is notorious for reducing inhibitions and promoting feelings of well-being and desirability. At the same time, alcohol inhibits sexual response; thus, the mind may be willing, but not the body. When drugs become central to sexual activities, they inevitably damage the relationship. A common danger associated with the use of drugs during sex is the tendency to blame alcohol or drugs for negative behavior or unsafe or undesired sexual activity.

An increasing number of young men have begun experimenting with the recreational use of drugs intended to treat erectile dysfunction (e.g., Viagra). Young men who take this type of medication are hoping to increase their sexual stamina or counteract performance anxiety or the effects of alcohol or other drugs. However, these drugs probably have only a placebo effect in men with normal erections, and combining them with other drugs, such as ketamine, amyl nitrate (poppers), or methamphetamine, can lead to potentially fatal drug interactions. In particular, when combined with amyl nitrate, these drugs can lead to a sudden drop in blood pressure and possible cardiac arrest.[33]

pornography Visual or literary depictions of sexual activity intended to be sexually arousing.

DID YOU **KNOW?**

According to a survey of American college students, nearly 23 percent of college men and 18 percent of college women who drank alcohol in the past year reported having unprotected sex as a consequence of their drinking.

Source: Data from American College Health Association, *American College Health Association—National College Health Assessment II (ACHA-NCHA II) Reference Group Data Report, Spring 2013* (Baltimore, MD: American College Health Association, 2013).

"Date rape" drugs such as Rohypnol or gamma-hydroxybutyrate (GHB) have been a growing concern in recent decades. (See more detail on these drugs in chapters covering drugs and violence—**Chapters 12** and **19,** respectively.) On college campuses, they are most often introduced to an unsuspecting woman through alcoholic drinks, often rendering her unconscious and vulnerable to rape. This problem is so serious that the U.S. Congress passed the Drug-Induced Rape Prevention and Punishment Act of 1996 to increase federal penalties for using drugs to facilitate sexual assault. However, it is important to note that while Rohypnol and GHB are dangerous, alcohol is far more commonly associated with sexual assault than are "date rape" drugs.[34]

LO 7 | THE SEX INDUSTRY

Describe the state of the sex industry in the United States and related health concerns.

Throughout history, sex has been a prominent theme in art, literature, and the media. But when do depictions of the human body and human sexual behaviors cross the line from art to pornography, from story to exploitation, or from sales tool to public perversion? These are difficult distinctions to make. Two particularly controversial aspects of the sex industry are pornography and prostitution.

Pornography refers to any visual or literary depictions of sexual activity intended to be sexually arousing. Availability of pornography has increased with the growth of the Inter-

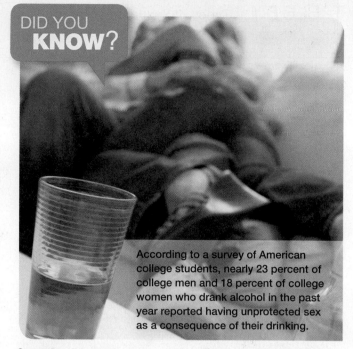

net; pornographic websites make up about 14 percent of all searches and 4 percent of all websites.[35] The pornography industry—which includes websites, video sales and rentals, cable, pay-per-view, phone sex, exotic dance clubs, computer games, and magazines—generates estimated revenues of approximately $14 billion annually in the United States, the biggest fraction of which comes from online revenue.[36] Clearly, pornography is a booming industry supported by millions of consumers. Why, then, is it so controversial?

The fear many people have is that viewing pornographic materials leads to negative attitudes toward women, sexual aggression, and sexual violence. However, current evidence suggests that pornography does not lead to sexual violence, predatory behavior, or major changes in individuals' sexual behaviors in normal, healthy adults. However, in those individuals who have preexisting negative attitudes toward women, this may be a legitimate concern.[37] Other concerns include preliminary research showing that pornography may have a negative impact on relationships, sexual satisfaction, and body image in both males and females.[38]

Prostitution, the practice of engaging in sexual acts for money, is a widespread industry around the world. Estimating the revenue generated by the U.S. prostitution industry is difficult, as most activity is illegal. However, a recent Department of Justice study investigating the sex trade in eight major U.S. cities found Dallas, Texas, to have an annual sex trade worth almost $100 million, and Atlanta, Georgia's, annual trade to be nearly $300 million, indicating that nationally, prostitution is a multibillion-dollar industry.[39] To curb the underground sex trade, several countries, including France and Germany, have legalized prostitution. In the United States, prostitution is legal only in selected counties in the state of Nevada. Illegal sex workers often struggle with substance abuse, physical and sexual violence, and STIs. Some countries that have legalized prostitution have made progress in regulating the industry and reducing these risks.

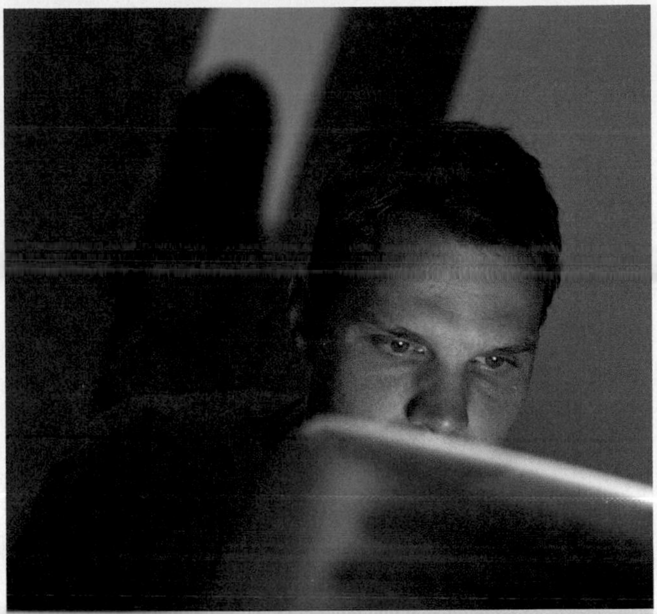
Internet pornography is a large part of the multibillion-dollar porn industry.

Findings from the Department of Justice indicate that the Internet has fueled the growth of illegal prostitution in the United States, allowing pimps new opportunities to connect with both recruits and clientele, and providing new marketing options in online classifieds and social media.[40]

prostitution Practice of engaging in sexual acts for money.

STUDY PLAN

Customize your study plan—and master your health!—in the Study Area of **MasteringHealth**.

ASSESS YOURSELF

How well do you understand your sexuality? Take the **What Are Your Sexual Attitudes?** assessment available on MasteringHealth.™

Need help creating a plan? Follow the strategies in the **Your Plan for Change** box for short- and long-term improvements to your health.

YOUR PLAN FOR CHANGE

If you were surprised or unhappy with any of your responses to the **ASSESS YOURSELF** activity, consider ways to change the attitudes you want to work on.

TODAY, YOU CAN:

- ☐ Develop a plan. Review your responses to the questionnaire and think about attitudes you would like to change. Evaluate your behavior and identify patterns and specific things you are doing. What can you change now? What can you change in the near future?
- ☐ Think about the level of sexual prejudice on campus. Consider joining or starting a group such as the Gay-Straight Alliance that works against sexual prejudice.

WITHIN THE NEXT 2 WEEKS, YOU CAN:

- ☐ Establish a time to sit down with the person with whom you are having a sexual relationship and have an honest and open discussion about sex. Before the discussion, think about what you would like to talk about and how you will bring it up. Are there sexual issues between you that need to be addressed? Are both you and your partner satisfied with the nature of your sexual relationship?
- ☐ Take steps to be more responsible about your sexuality. If you have had unprotected sex, make an appointment to be tested for STIs. If you have found yourself without contraception, stop by a drugstore and purchase several packages of condoms. If you feel your sexual decision making is sometimes impaired by drugs or alcohol, set goals to limit and control your use of these substances.

BY THE END OF THE SEMESTER, YOU CAN:

- ☐ Develop a greater understanding of and tolerance for people with different sexual values and lifestyles. Learn about different viewpoints by doing research, attending meetings on campus, or getting to know sexually diverse people.
- ☐ Expand your sense of gender identity. Consider taking a class or workshop in an activity or subject area that you traditionally associate with the opposite gender. Volunteer with a group that focuses on issues relating to the opposite gender.

CHAPTER REVIEW

LO 1 Your Sexual Identity: More than Biology

- *Sexual identity* is determined by the interaction of genetic, physiological, and environmental factors. Biological sex, gender identity, gender roles, and sexual orientation are all blended into our sexual identity.
- *Sexual orientation* refers to a person's enduring emotional, romantic, or sexual attraction to others. Gay, lesbian, and bisexual persons are repeatedly the targets of sexual prejudice. *Sexual prejudice* refers to negative attitudes and hostile actions directed at members of a particular social group.

LO 2 Sexual Anatomy and Physiology

- The major structures of female sexual anatomy include the mons pubis, labia minora and majora, clitoris, vagina, uterus, cervix, fallopian tubes, and ovaries. The major structures of male sexual anatomy are the penis, scrotum, testes, epididymides, vasa deferentia, ejaculatory ducts, urethra, and the accessory glands (seminal vesicles, prostate gland, and Cowper's glands).

LO 3 Human Sexual Response

- Physiologically, both males and females experience four stages of sexual response: excitement/arousal, plateau, orgasm, and resolution.

LO 4 Expressing Your Sexuality

- People can express themselves sexually in a variety of ways, including celibacy, autoerotic behaviors, kissing and erotic touch, manual stimulation, oral-genital stimulation, vaginal intercourse, and anal intercourse. Variant sexual behaviors are those that are less common. Some variant sexual behaviors are potentially harmful to others and are therefore illegal in some states.
- Responsible and satisfying sexuality involves good communication, acknowledging yourself as a sexual being, understanding sexual structures and functions, and accepting your gender identity and sexual orientation.

LO 5 Sexual Dysfunction

- Sexual dysfunctions can be categorized into four classes: desire disorders, arousal disorders, orgasmic disorders, and pain disorders. Stress, relationship issues, lack of exercise, smoking, alcohol and drug use, and other lifestyle choices can lead to sexual dysfunction.

LO 6 Drugs and Sex

- Alcohol and other psychoactive drugs can affect sexual behavior. Drug use can decrease inhibitions and lead people to engage in unsafe sexual activity.

LO 7 The Sex Industry

- Sex is a multibillion-dollar industry in the United States and throughout the world. Pornography and prostitution are two aspects of the sex industry that have varying degrees of legality in different countries. In the United States, prostitution is only legal in selected counties in Nevada.

POP QUIZ

Visit **MasteringHealth** to personalize your study plan with Chapter Review Quizzes and Dynamic Study Modules.

LO 1 Your Sexual Identity: More than Biology

1. Your personal inner sense of maleness or femaleness is known as your
   a. sexual identity.
   b. sexual orientation.
   c. gender identity.
   d. gender.
2. Individuals who are sexually attracted to both men and women are identified as
   a. heterosexual.
   b. bisexual.
   c. homosexual.
   d. intersex.

LO 2 Sexual Anatomy and Physiology

3. The most sensitive part of the female genital region is the
   a. mons pubis.
   b. vagina.
   c. clitoris.
   d. labia.
4. When a woman is ovulating,
   a. she has released an egg.
   b. she is experiencing menstrual bleeding.
   c. an egg has been fertilized and she is pregnant.
   d. she is experiencing PMS.
5. What is the role of testosterone in the male reproductive system?
   a. It is used to produce sperm for reproduction.
   b. It is the hormone that stimulates development of secondary male sex characteristics.
   c. It allows the penis to harden during sexual arousal.
   d. It secretes the seminal fluid preceding ejaculation.

LO 3 Human Sexual Response

6. Which of the following is *true* regarding the first stage of the human sexual response?
   a. In men, testes become completely engorged.
   b. In men and women, the rectal sphincter contracts.
   c. In men, the Cowper's gland may release fluid.
   d. In men and women, vasocongestion occurs.

LO 4 | **Expressing Your Sexuality**

7. Fellatio is the oral stimulation of the
   a. male genitals.
   b. female genitals.
   c. anal region.
   d. mouth and tongue.

LO 5 | **Sexual Dysfunction**

8. The pain that a woman may experience during sexual intercourse due to involuntary contraction of vaginal muscles is called
   a. dysmenorrhea.
   b. amenorrhea.
   c. dyspareunia.
   d. vaginismus.

LO 6 | **Drugs and Sex**

9. What is the effect of alcohol on sex?
   a. It promotes feelings of aversion.
   b. It promotes greater sexual satisfaction.
   c. It inhibits sexual response.
   d. It inhibits pregnancy.

LO 7 | **The Sex Industry**

10. Why is pornography a legitimate concern in our society?
    a. It may lead to problems in relationships.
    b. It increases the rate of sexual disorders.
    c. It turns otherwise healthy adults into sexual predators.
    d. It makes people prone to sadomasochism.

Answers to the Pop Quiz can be found on page A-1. If you answered a question incorrectly, review the section identified by the Learning Outcome. For even more study tools, visit MasteringHealth.

THINK ABOUT IT!

LO 1 | **Your Sexual Identity: More than Biology**

1. How have gender roles changed over your lifetime? Do you view the changes as positive for both men and women?
2. If scientists are able to establish the combination of factors that interact to produce homosexual, heterosexual, or bisexual orientation, will that put an end to prejudice against gays? Why or why not?

LO 2 | **Sexual Anatomy and Physiology**

3. Have you ever discussed with your friends what it was like going through puberty? Did you understand what was happening to you physically and emotionally and why?

LO 3 | **Human Sexual Response**

4. What makes a person's sexual response to one human vastly different from that to another human or from one sexual experience to another with the same partner?

LO 4 | **Expressing Your Sexuality**

5. What criteria do you use to determine "normal" sexual behavior? What criteria should we use to determine healthy sexual practices?

LO 5 | **Sexual Dysfunction**

6. How can we remove the stigma that surrounds sexual dysfunction so that individuals feel more comfortable seeking help? Are men and women affected differently by sexual dysfunction?

LO 6 | **Drugs and Sex**

7. What is the role of alcohol in the sex lives of your peers? How does it both improve and lessen the sexual experience?

LO 7 | **The Sex Industry**

8. Have you ever viewed pornography? What prompted you to do this? How did you feel about the experience?

ACCESS YOUR HEALTH ON THE INTERNET

Visit **MasteringHealth** for links to the websites and RSS feeds.

The following websites explore further topics and issues related to personal health.

American Association of Sex Educators, Counselors, and Therapists (AASECT). AASECT is a professional organization that provides standards of practice for treatment of sexual issues and disorders and provides referrals to local counselors and clinics. www.aasect.org

SmarterSex.org. This site, created by the peer education group BACCHUS network, presents user-friendly information on sexual health targeted at 18- to 24-year-olds. www.smartersex.org

Go Ask Alice. Columbia University Health Services provides this interactive question-and-answer resource. "Alice" is available to answer questions about any health-related issues, including relationships, nutrition and diet, exercise, drugs, sex, alcohol, and stress. www.goaskalice.columbia.edu

Sexuality Information and Education Council of the United States (SIECUS). SIECUS provides information, guidelines, and materials for advancement of healthy and proper sex education. www.siecus.org

Advocates for Youth. Here you can find current news, policy updates, research, and other resources about the sexual health of and choices particular to high school and college-aged students. www.advocatesforyouth.org

6 Considering Your Reproductive Choices

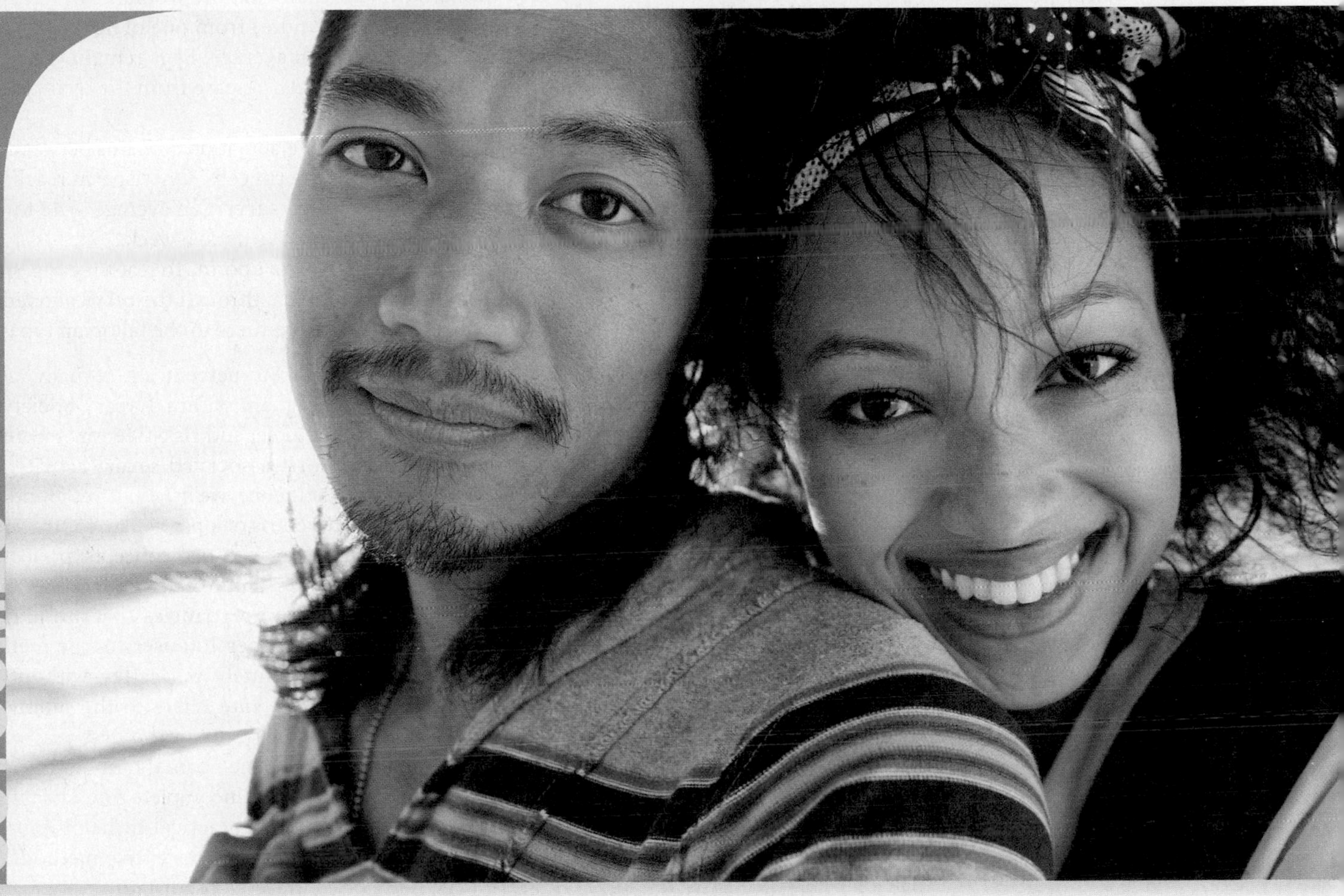

LEARNING OUTCOMES

1. Explain the process of conception and describe how the effectiveness of contraception is measured.
2. Compare and contrast the advantages, disadvantages, and effectiveness of different barrier methods in preventing pregnancy and sexually transmitted infections.
3. Compare the advantages, risks, and effectiveness of different hormonal methods in preventing pregnancy.
4. Describe the effectiveness, advantages, and disadvantages of intrauterine contraceptives.
5. Describe emergency contraception and how it is used.
6. Explain how behavioral methods of contraception work and compare their effectiveness to other methods of birth control.
7. Describe surgical methods of birth control and discuss their advantages and disadvantages.
8. Identify questions you should consider when choosing a method of contraception.
9. Summarize the political issues surrounding abortion and the various types of abortion procedures.
10. Explain key issues to consider when planning a pregnancy.
11. Describe fetal development and explain the importance of prenatal care.
12. Explain the basic stages of childbirth and complications that can arise during pregnancy, labor, and delivery.
13. Review primary causes of and possible solutions for infertility.

Today, we not only understand the inti mate details of reproduction, but we also possess technologies that can control or enhance our **fertility**. Along with information and technological advances comes choice, which goes hand in hand with responsibility. Choosing whether and when to have children is one of our greatest responsibilities. Children transform people's lives. They require a lifelong personal commitment of love and nurturing. Before having children, a person should ask: Am I mature enough physically, emotionally, and financially to care for another human being?

One measure of maturity is the ability to discuss reproduction and birth control with your sexual partner before engaging in sexual activity. Men often assume that their partners are taking care of birth control. Women sometimes feel that broaching the topic implies that they are promiscuous. Both may feel that bringing up the subject might interfere with romance and spontaneity.

Too often, neither partner brings up the topic, resulting in unprotected sex. In a recent survey, only 56 percent of college women and 50 percent of college men reported having used a method of contraception the last time they had vaginal intercourse.[1] This ambivalence toward contraceptives has serious consequences. Fifty-one percent of all pregnancies in the United States—more than 3 million a year—are unintended. In young women, the rates are even higher; in women aged 18 to 19, 77 percent of pregnancies are unintended, and in women aged 20–24, 64 percent are.[2] Additionally, each year there are 20 million new cases of sexually transmitted infections—half of which occur in 15- to 24-year-olds (see **Chapter 14** for more information).[3]

Discussing this topic with your health care provider or your sexual partner will be easier and less embarrassing if you understand human reproduction and contraception and honestly consider your attitudes toward these matters. Here we discuss important information for you to think about as you contemplate your own sexual and reproductive choices.

fertility A person's ability to reproduce.

birth control (contraception) Methods of preventing conception.

conception Fertilization of an ovum by a sperm.

perfect-use failure rate The number of pregnancies (per 100 users) likely to occur in the first year of use of a particular birth control method if the method is used consistently and correctly.

typical-use failure rate The number of pregnancies (per 100 users) likely to occur in the first year of use of a particular birth control method if the method's use is not consistent or always correct.

barrier method Contraceptive methods that block the meeting of egg and sperm by means of a physical barrier (such as condom, diaphragm, or cervical cap), a chemical barrier (such as spermicide), or both.

hormonal methods Contraceptive methods that introduce synthetic hormones into a woman's system to prevent ovulation, thicken cervical mucus, or prevent a fertilized egg from implanting.

surgical methods Surgically altering a man's or woman's reproductive system to permanently prevent pregnancy.

behavioral methods Temporary or permanent abstinence or planning intercourse in accordance with fertility patterns.

LO 1 | BASIC PRINCIPLES OF BIRTH CONTROL

Explain the process of conception and describe how the effectiveness of contraception is measured.

The term **birth control (also called contraception)** refers to methods of preventing conception. **Conception** occurs when a sperm fertilizes an egg. This usually takes place in a woman's fallopian tube. The following conditions are necessary for conception:

1. **A viable egg.** A sexually mature woman will release one egg (sometimes more) from one of her two ovaries once every 28 days, on average. Eggs remain viable for 24 to 36 hours after their release from the ovary into the fallopian tube.
2. **A viable sperm.** Each ejaculation contains between 200 and 500 million sperm cells. Once sperm reach the fallopian tubes, they survive an average of 48 to 72 hours—and can survive up to a week.
3. **Access to the egg by the sperm.** To reach the egg, sperm must travel up the vagina, through the cervical opening into the uterus, and from there to the fallopian tubes.

Without birth control, 85 percent of sexually active women would become pregnant within 1 year.[4] Society has searched for a simple, infallible, and risk-free way to prevent pregnancy since people first associated sexual activity with pregnancy. Outside of abstinence, we have not yet found one.

To evaluate the effectiveness of a particular contraceptive method, you must be familiar with two concepts: perfect-use failure rate and typical-use failure rate. **Perfect-use failure rate** refers to the number of pregnancies that are likely to occur in the first year of use (per 100 users of the method) if the method is used absolutely perfectly—without any error. The **typical-use failure rate** refers to the number of pregnancies that are likely to occur in the first year of use with typical use—that is, with the normal number of errors, memory lapses, and incorrect or incomplete use. The typical-use information is much more practical in helping people make informed decisions about contraceptive methods.

Present methods of contraception fall into several categories. **Barrier methods** block the egg and sperm from joining. **Hormonal methods** introduce synthetic hormones into the woman's system that prevent ovulation, thicken cervical mucus, or prevent a fertilized egg from implanting. **Surgical methods** can prevent pregnancy permanently. **Behavioral methods** may involve temporary or permanent abstinence or planning intercourse in accordance with fertility patterns. **TABLE 6.1** lists the most popular forms of contraception among sexually active college students.

Some contraceptive methods can also protect, to some degree,

HEAR IT! PODCASTS

Want a study podcast for this chapter? Download **Birth Control, Pregnancy, and Childbirth: Managing Your Fertility** available on MasteringHealth.™

TABLE 6.1 | Top Reported Means of Contraception Sexually Active College Students or Their Partners Used the Last Time They Had Intercourse

Method	Male	Female	Total
Male condom	70%	62%	64%
Birth control pills (monthly or extended cycle)	66%	62%	63%
Withdrawal	28%	31%	30%
Fertility awareness (calendar, mucus, basal body temperature)	5%	7%	6%
Intrauterine device	5%	6%	5%
Cervical ring	5%	4%	4%
Birth control shots	5%	4%	4%
Spermicide (foam, jelly, cream)	6%	3%	4%

Note: Survey respondents could select more than one method.
Source: Data from American College Health Association, *American College Health Association—National College Health Assessment II: Reference Group Data, Spring 2013* (Baltimore, MD: American College Health Association, 2013).

against **sexually transmitted infections (STIs)**. This is an important factor to consider when choosing a contraceptive. TABLE 6.2 on the next page summarizes the effectiveness, STI protection, frequency of use, and cost of various methods.

99% OF U.S. WOMEN WHO HAVE EVER BEEN SEXUALLY ACTIVE REPORT HAVING USED AT LEAST ONE FORM OF **BIRTH CONTROL.**

LO 2 | BARRIER METHODS

Compare and contrast the advantages, disadvantages, and effectiveness of different barrier methods in preventing pregnancy and sexually transmitted infections.

Barrier methods work on the simple principle of preventing sperm from ever reaching the egg by use of a physical or chemical barrier during intercourse. Some barrier methods prevent semen from having any contact with the woman's body, and others prevent sperm from going past the cervix. In addition, many barrier methods contain or are used in combination with a substance that kills sperm.

Male Condom

The **male condom** is a thin sheath designed to cover the erect penis and catch semen, preventing it from entering the vagina. Most male condoms are made of latex, although condoms made of polyurethane or lambskin also are available. Condoms come in a wide variety of styles and may be purchased in pharmacies, supermarkets, some public bathrooms, and many health clinics. A new condom must be used for each act of vaginal, oral, or anal intercourse.

A condom must be rolled onto the penis before the penis touches the vagina, and it must be held in place when removing the penis from the vagina after ejaculation to prevent slippage (see FIGURE 6.1). Condoms come with or without **spermicide** and with or without lubrication. If desired, users can lubricate their own condoms with contraceptive foams, creams, and jellies or other water-based lubricants.

sexually transmitted infections (STIs) Infectious diseases caused by pathogens transmitted through some form of sexual contact.

male condom Single-use sheath of thin latex or other material designed to fit over an erect penis and to catch semen upon ejaculation.

spermicide Substance designed to kill sperm.

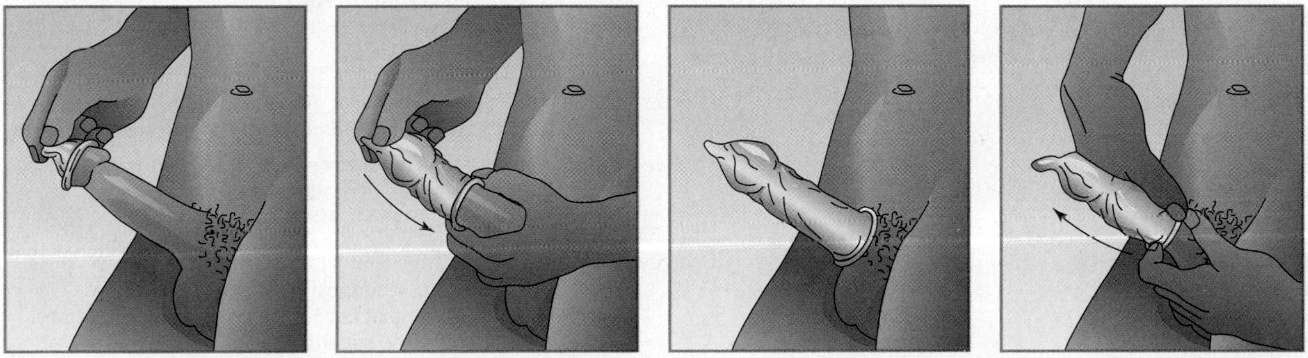

1 Pinch the air out of the top half-inch of the condom to allow room for semen.

2 Holding the tip of the condom with one hand, use the other hand to unroll it onto the penis.

3 Unroll the condom all the way to the base of the penis, smoothing out any air bubbles.

4 After ejaculation, hold the condom around the base until the penis is totally withdrawn to avoid spilling any semen.

FIGURE 6.1 How to Use a Male Condom

VIDEO TUTOR Choosing Contraception

TABLE 6.2 | Contraceptive Effectiveness, STI Protection, Frequency of Use, and Costs

Method	Failure Rate: Typical Use	Failure Rate: Perfect Use	STI Protection	Frequency of Use	Cost
Continuous abstinence	0	0	Yes	N/A	None
Implanon	0.05	0.05	No	Inserted every 3 years	$400–$800/exam, device, and insertion; $100–$300 for removal
Male sterilization	0.15	0.1	No	Done once	$350–$1,000/interview, counseling, examination, operation, and follow-up sperm count
Female sterilization	0.5	0.5	No	Done once	$1,500–$6,000/interview, counseling, examination, operation, and follow-up
IUD (intrauterine device)					
ParaGard (copper T)	0.8	0.6	No	Inserted every 10 years	$500–$1,000/exam, insertion, and follow-up visit
Mirena/Skyla	0.2	0.2	No	Inserted every 3–5 years	$500–$1,000/exam, insertion, and follow-up visit
Depo-Provera	6	0.2	No	Injected every 12 weeks	$30–$100/3-month injection; $35–$175 for initial exam; $20–$40 for further visits to clinic for shots
Oral contraceptives (combined pill and progestin-only pill)	9	0.3	No	Take daily	$15–$50 monthly pill pack at drugstores, often less at clinics; check for family planning programs in your student health center, $35–$250 for initial exam
Ortho Evra patch	9	0.3	No	Applied weekly	$15–$80/month at drugstores; often less at clinics, $35–$250 for initial exam
NuvaRing	9	0.3	No	Inserted every 4 weeks	$15–$80/month at drugstores, often less at clinics; $35–$250 for initial exam
Cervical cap (FemCap) (with spermicidal cream or jelly)					
Women who have never given birth	14	4	Some	Used every time	$60–$75 for cap; $50–$200 for initial exam; $8–$17/supplies of spermicide jelly or cream
Women who have given birth	32	No data	Some	Used every time	
Male condom (without spermicides)	18	2	Some	Used every time	$1.00 and up/condom—some family planning or student health centers give them away or charge very little. Available in drugstores, family planning clinics, some supermarkets, and from vending machines
Diaphragm (with spermicidal cream or jelly)	12	6	Some	Used every time	$15–$75 for diaphragm; $50–$200 for initial exam; $8–$17/supplies of spermicide jelly or cream
Today sponge					
Women who have never given birth	12	9	No	Used every time	$9.00–$15/package of three sponges. Available at family planning centers, drugstores, online, and in some supermarkets
Women who have given birth	24	20	No	Used every time	
Female condom (without spermicides)	21	5	Some	Used every time	$2–$4/condom. Available at family planning centers, drugstores, and in some supermarkets
Fertility awareness–based methods	24	0.04–5.0	No	Followed every month	$10–$12 for temperature kits. Charts and classes often free in health centers and churches
Withdrawal	22	4	No	Used every time	None
Spermicides (foams, creams, gels, vaginal suppositories, and vaginal film)	28	18	No	Used every time	$8/applicator kits of foam and gel ($4–$8 refills). Film and suppositories are priced similarly. Available at family planning clinics, drugstores, and some supermarkets
No method	85	85	No	N/A	None
Emergency contraceptive pill	Treatment initiated within 72–120 hours after unprotected intercourse reduces the risk of pregnancy by 75%–89% (with no protection against STIs). Costs depend on what services are needed: $39–$60/Plan B-One Step, available over the counter to women 17 and older; $20–$50/one pack of combination pills; $50–$70/two packs of progestin-only pills; $35–$150/visit with health care provider; $10–$20/pregnancy test; ella $77–$97/in addition to visit with health care provider				

Note: "Failure Rate" refers to the number of unintended pregnancies per 100 women during the first year of use. "Typical Use" refers to failure rates for men and women whose use is not consistent or always correct. "Perfect Use" refers to failure rates for those whose use is consistent and always correct.

Some family planning clinics charge for services and supplies on a sliding scale according to income.

Sources: Adapted from R. Hatcher et al., *Contraceptive Technology*, 20th rev. ed. (New York: Ardent Media, 2011); R. Hatcher et al., *Contraceptive Technology*, 19th rev. ed. Copyright © 2007 Contraceptive Technology Communications, Inc. Reprinted by permission of Ardent Media, LLC; Planned Parenthood, "Birth Control," 2013, www.plannedparenthood.org.

Never use products such as baby oil, cold cream, petroleum jelly, vaginal yeast infection medications, or body lotion with a condom. These products contain substances that will cause the latex to disintegrate.

Condoms are less effective and more likely to break during intercourse if they are old or improperly stored. To maintain effectiveness, store them in a cool place (not in a wallet or glove compartment), and inspect them for small tears before use. Lightly squeeze the package before opening to feel that air is trapped inside and the package has not been punctured. Discard all condoms that have passed their expiration date.

Advantages When used consistently and correctly, condoms can be up to 98 percent effective.[5] The condom is the only temporary means of birth control available for men, and latex and polyurethane condoms are the only barriers that effectively prevent the spread of some STIs and HIV. (Skin condoms, made from lamb intestines, are not effective against STIs.) Many people choose condoms because they are inexpensive and readily available without a prescription, and their use is limited to times of sexual activity, with no negative health effects. Some men find condoms help them stay erect longer or help prevent premature ejaculation.

Disadvantages There is considerable potential for user error; as a result, the typical use effectiveness of condoms in preventing pregnancy is around 82 percent.[6] Improper use of a condom can lead to breakage, leakage, or slippage, potentially exposing the users to STI transmission or an unintended pregnancy. For example, if the penis is not removed from the vagina before it becomes flaccid (soft), semen may leak out of the condom. Even when used perfectly, a condom doesn't protect against STIs that may have external areas of infection (e.g., herpes).

For some people, a condom ruins the spontaneity of sex because stopping to put it on may break the mood. Others report that the condom decreases sensation. These inconveniences and perceptions contribute to improper use or avoidance of condoms altogether. Partners who put on a condom as part of foreplay are generally more successful with this form of birth control. As a new condom is required for each act of intercourse, some users find it difficult to be sure to have a condom available when needed.

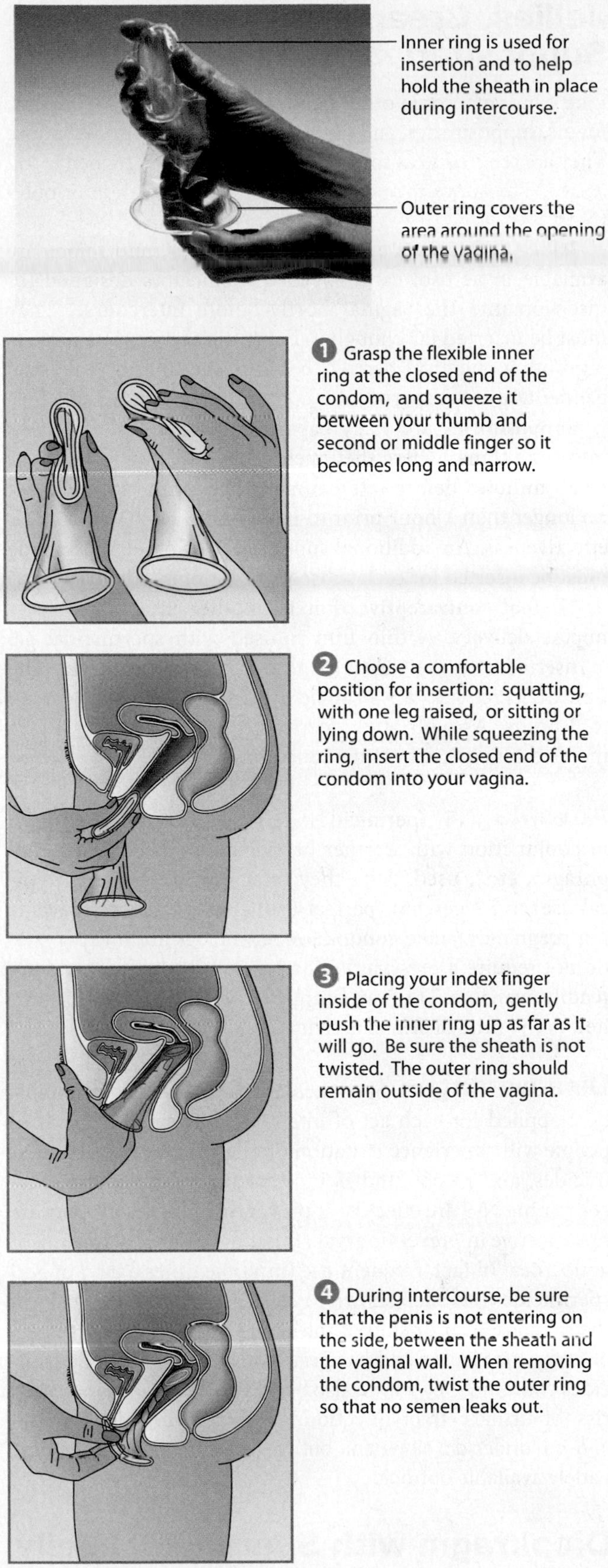

Inner ring is used for insertion and to help hold the sheath in place during intercourse.
Outer ring covers the area around the opening of the vagina.
1 Grasp the flexible inner ring at the closed end of the condom, and squeeze it between your thumb and second or middle finger so it becomes long and narrow.
2 Choose a comfortable position for insertion: squatting, with one leg raised, or sitting or lying down. While squeezing the ring, insert the closed end of the condom into your vagina.
3 Placing your index finger inside of the condom, gently push the inner ring up as far as it will go. Be sure the sheath is not twisted. The outer ring should remain outside of the vagina.
4 During intercourse, be sure that the penis is not entering on the side, between the sheath and the vaginal wall. When removing the condom, twist the outer ring so that no semen leaks out.

FIGURE 6.2 How to Use a Female Condom

Female Condom

female condom (FC2) Single-use nitrile sheath for internal use during vaginal intercourse to catch semen upon ejaculation.

The **female condom (FC2)** is a single-use, soft, lubricated, loose-fitting sheath meant for internal vaginal use. The newest, improved versions are made from nitrile rather than polyurethane. The sheath has a flexible ring at each end. One ring lies inside the sheath to serve as an insertion mechanism and hold the condom in place over the cervix. The other ring remains outside the vagina once the condom is inserted and protects the labia and the base of the penis from exposure to STIs. **FIGURE 6.2** shows the proper use of the female condom.

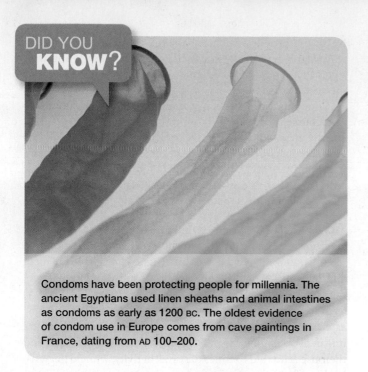

DID YOU **KNOW?**

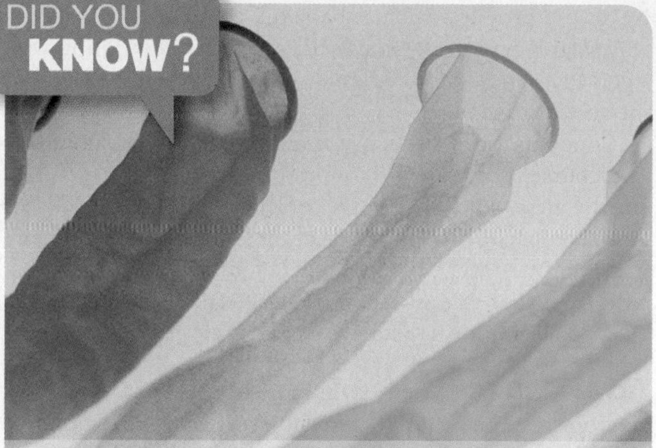

Condoms have been protecting people for millennia. The ancient Egyptians used linen sheaths and animal intestines as condoms as early as 1200 BC. The oldest evidence of condom use in Europe comes from cave paintings in France, dating from AD 100–200.

Advantages Used consistently and correctly, female condoms are 95 percent effective at preventing pregnancy.[7] They also can prevent the spread of HIV and other STIs, including those that can be transmitted by external genital contact. The female condom can be inserted in advance, so its use doesn't have to interrupt lovemaking. Some women choose to use the female condom because it gives them more personal control over pregnancy prevention and STI protection or because they cannot rely on their partner to use a male condom. Because the nitrile material is thin and pliable, there is less loss of sensation with the female condom than there is with the latex male condom. The female condom is relatively inexpensive, readily available without a prescription, and causes no negative health effects.

Disadvantages As with the male condom, there is potential for user error with the female condom, including possible slipping or leaking, both of which could lead to STI transmission or an unintended pregnancy. Because of the potential problems, the typical use effectiveness of the female condom is 79 percent.[8] Some people dislike using the female condom because they feel it is disruptive, noisy, odd looking, or difficult to use. Some women have reported external or vaginal irritation from using the female condom. As with the male condom, a new condom is required for each act of intercourse, so users may not always have one available when needed. Remember that male and female condoms should never be used simultaneously.

jellies and creams Spermicide packaged in tubes and inserted into the vagina with an applicator.

foams Spermicide packaged in aerosol cans and inserted into the vagina with an applicator.

suppositories Waxy capsules that are inserted deep into the vagina, where they melt and release a spermicide.

vaginal contraceptive film A thin film infused with spermicidal gel that is inserted into the vagina so that it covers the cervix.

diaphragm Latex, cup-shaped device designed to cover the cervix and block access to the uterus; should always be used with spermicide.

Jellies, Creams, Foams, Suppositories, and Film

Like condoms, some other barrier methods—jellies, creams, foams, suppositories, and film—do not require a prescription. They are referred to as spermicides—substances designed to kill sperm. The active ingredient in most of them is nonoxynol-9 (N-9).

Jellies and creams are packaged in tubes, and **foams** are available in aerosol cans. All have applicators designed for insertion into the vagina shortly before intercourse. They must be inserted far enough to cover the cervix, thus providing both a chemical barrier that kills sperm and a physical barrier that stops sperm from continuing toward an egg.

Suppositories are waxy capsules that are inserted deep into the vagina, where they melt. They must be inserted 10 to 20 minutes before intercourse to have time to melt, but no longer than 1 hour prior to intercourse, or they lose their effectiveness. An additional suppository or other spermicide must be inserted for each subsequent act of intercourse.

Vaginal contraceptive film is another method of spermicide delivery. A thin film infused with spermicidal gel is inserted into the vagina so that it covers the cervix. The film dissolves into a spermicidal gel that is effective for up to 3 hours. As with other spermicides, a new film must be inserted for each act of intercourse.

Advantages Spermicides are most effective when used in conjunction with another barrier method (condom, diaphragm, etc.); used alone they offer only 72 percent (typical use) to 82 percent (perfect use) effectiveness at preventing pregnancy.[9] Like condoms, spermicides are inexpensive, do not require a prescription or pelvic examination, and are readily available. They are simple to use, and their use is limited to the time of sexual activity.

Disadvantages Spermicides can be messy and must be reapplied for each act of intercourse. A small number of people will experience irritation or allergic reactions to spermicides, and recent studies indicate that while spermicides containing N-9 are effective at preventing pregnancy, they are not effective in preventing transmission of HIV, chlamydia, or gonorrhea. In fact, frequent use (multiple times a day) of N-9 spermicides has been shown to cause irritation and breaks in the mucous layer or skin of the genital tract, creating a point of entry for viruses and bacteria that cause disease. Spermicides containing N-9 have also been associated with increased risk of urinary tract infection.[10] New spermicides without N-9 are under development, but N-9 spermicides are the only widely available options.

Diaphragm with Spermicidal Jelly or Cream

Invented in the mid-nineteenth century, the **diaphragm** was the first widely used birth control method for women. The device is a soft, shallow cup made of thin latex rubber. Its

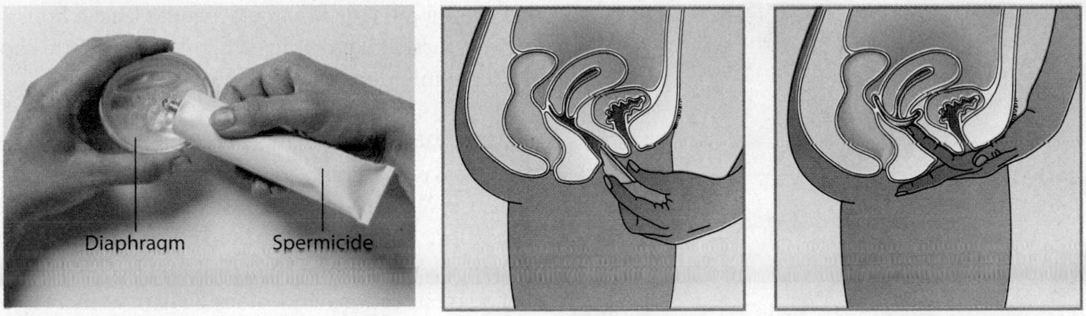

1 Place spermicidal jelly or cream inside the diaphragm and all around the rim.

2 Fold the diaphragm in half and insert dome-side down (spermicide-side up) into the vagina, pushing it along the back wall as far as it will go.

3 Position the diaphragm with the cervix completely covered and the front rim tucked up against your pubic bone; you should be able to feel your cervix through the rubber dome.

FIGURE 6.3 Proper Use and Placement of a Diaphragm

flexible, rubber-coated ring is designed to fit snugly behind the pubic bone in front of the cervix and over the back of the cervix on the other side so it blocks access to the uterus. Diaphragms must be used with spermicidal cream or jelly, which is applied to the inside of the diaphragm before it is inserted, up to 6 hours before intercourse. The diaphragm holds the spermicide in place, creating a physical and chemical barrier against sperm (**FIGURE 6.3**). Diaphragms are manufactured in different sizes and must be fitted to the woman by a trained health care provider, who should make sure the user knows how to insert her diaphragm correctly before leaving the provider's office.

Advantages If used consistently and correctly, diaphragms can be 94 percent effective in preventing pregnancy.[11] Due to its shape, when used with spermicidal jelly or cream, the diaphragm also offers some protection against gonorrhea and possibly chlamydia and human papillomavirus (HPV). After the initial prescription and fitting, the only ongoing expense involved with diaphragm use is spermicide. Because the diaphragm can be inserted up to 6 hours in advance and be used for multiple acts of intercourse, some users find it less disruptive than other barrier methods.

Disadvantages Although the diaphragm can be left in place for multiple acts of intercourse, additional spermicide must be applied each time, and the diaphragm must then stay in place for 6 to 8 hours after intercourse to allow the chemical to kill any sperm remaining in the vagina. Some women find inserting the device awkward at first. When inserted incorrectly, diaphragms are much less effective. It is also possible for a diaphragm to slip out of place, be difficult to remove, or require refitting by a health care provider (e.g., following a pregnancy or a significant weight gain or loss).

Cervical Cap with Spermicidal Jelly or Cream

One of the oldest methods used to prevent pregnancy, early **cervical caps** were made from beeswax, silver, or copper. The currently available *FemCap* is a clear silicone cup that fits snugly over the entire cervix. It comes in three sizes and must be fitted by a health care provider. The FemCap is designed for use with spermicidal jelly or cream. It is held in place by suction created during application and works by blocking sperm from the uterus.

cervical cap Small cup made of silicone that is designed to fit snugly over the entire cervix; should always be used with spermicide.

Advantages Cervical caps can be reasonably effective (up to 86%) with typical use.[12] They also may offer some protection against transmission of gonorrhea and possibly chlamydia and HPV. They are relatively inexpensive, as the only ongoing cost is the spermicide.

The FemCap can be inserted up to 6 hours prior to intercourse. The device must be left in place for 6 to 8 hours afterward, but after that time period, can be removed, cleaned,

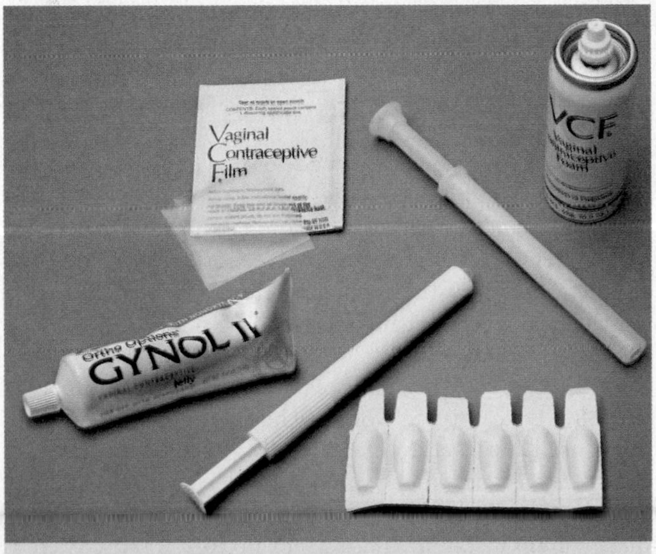

Spermicides come in many forms, including jellies, creams, films, foam, and suppositories.

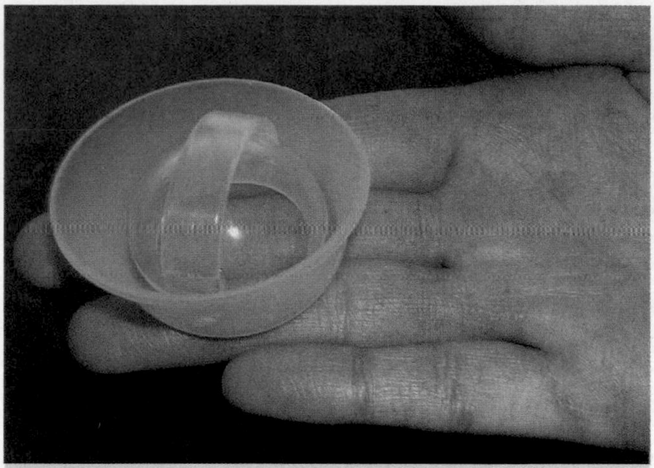

FemCap is used in conjunction with spermicide and is positioned to cover the cervix. It is shaped like a sailor's cap and has a loop to aid in removal.

and reinserted immediately. Because the FemCap is made of surgical-grade silicone, it is a suitable alternative for people who are allergic to latex.

Disadvantages The FemCap is somewhat more difficult to insert than a diaphragm because of its smaller size. Like a diaphragm, it requires an initial fitting and may require subsequent refitting if a woman's cervix size changes (e.g., after giving birth). Because the FemCap can become dislodged during intercourse by heavy thrusting or certain sexual positions, placement must be periodically checked. The device cannot be used during the menstrual period or for longer than 48 hours because of the risk of **toxic shock syndrome (TSS)**. Some women report unpleasant vaginal odors after use.

toxic shock syndrome (TSS) Potentially life-threatening disease that occurs when specific bacterial toxins multiply and spread to the bloodstream, most commonly through improper use of tampons, diaphragms, or cervical caps.

contraceptive sponge Contraceptive device made of polyurethane foam and containing nonoxynol-9 that fits over the cervix to create a barrier against sperm.

Contraceptive Sponge

The **contraceptive sponge** is made of polyurethane foam and contains nonoxynol-9 (sold in the United States as the *Today Sponge*). Prior to insertion, the sponge must be moistened with water to activate the spermicide. It is then folded and inserted deep into the vagina, where it fits over the cervix and creates a barrier against sperm.

Advantages The sponge is fairly effective (91% perfect use; 88% typical use in women who have never given birth) when used consistently and correctly.[13] A main advantage of the sponge is convenience, because it does not require a trip to a health care provider for fitting. Protection begins immediately upon insertion and lasts for up to 24 hours. There is no need to reapply spermicide or insert a new sponge for any subsequent acts of intercourse within the same 24-hour period; it must be left in place for at least 6 hours after the last intercourse. Like the diaphragm and cervical cap, the sponge offers limited protection from some STIs.

Disadvantages The sponge is less effective for women who have previously given birth (80% perfect use; 76% typical use).[14] Allergic reactions, such as irritation of the vagina, are more common with the sponge than with other barrier methods. Should the vaginal lining become irritated, the risk of yeast infections and other STIs may increase. The sponge should not be used during menstruation. Some cases of TSS have been reported in women using the sponge; the same precautions should be taken as with the diaphragm and cervical cap. Some women find the sponge difficult or messy to remove.

LO 3 | HORMONAL METHODS

Compare the advantages, risks, and effectiveness of different hormonal methods in preventing pregnancy.

The term *hormonal contraception* refers to birth control that contains synthetic estrogen, progestin, or both. These ingredients are similar to the hormones estrogen and progesterone that a woman's ovaries produce naturally for the process of ovulation and the menstrual cycle. In recent years, hormonal contraception has become available in a variety of forms (transdermal, injection, and oral). All forms require a prescription from a health care provider.

Hormonal contraception uses synthetic estrogen or progestin (synthetic progesterone) to alter a woman's biochemistry, prevent ovulation (release of the egg), and produce changes that make it more difficult for the sperm to reach the egg if ovulation does occur. Synthetic estrogen works to prevent the ovaries from releasing an egg. If no egg is released, there is nothing to be fertilized by the sperm and pregnancy cannot occur. Progestin thickens the cervical mucus, which hinders the movement of the sperm, inhibits the egg's ability to travel through the fallopian tubes, and suppresses the

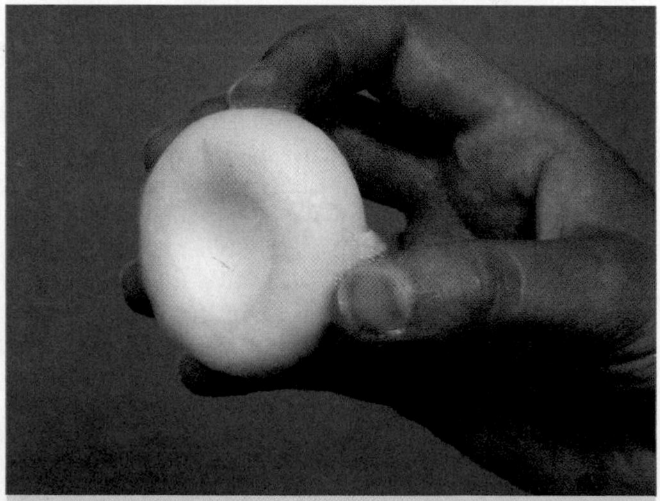

The Today sponge is a barrier method with spermicide that is most effective when used in conjunction with male condoms.

sperm's ability to unite with the egg. Progestin also thins the uterine lining, making it unlikely that a fertilized egg would be able to implant in the uterine wall.

Oral Contraceptives

Oral contraceptive pills were first marketed in the United States in 1960. Their convenience quickly made them the most widely used reversible method of fertility control. Most modern pills are more than 99 percent effective at preventing pregnancy with perfect use.[15] Today, oral contraceptives are the most commonly used birth control method among college women.[16]

Most oral contraceptives work through the combined effects of synthetic estrogen and progestin (*combination pills*). Combination pills are taken in a cycle. At the end of each 3-week cycle, the user stops taking pills or takes placebo pills for 1 week. The resultant drop in hormone level causes the uterine lining to shed, and the user will have a menstrual period, usually within 1 to 3 days. Menstrual flow is generally lighter than it is for women who don't use the pill, because the hormones in the pill prevent thick endometrial buildup.

Several newer brands of pills have extended cycles, such as the 91-day *Seasonale* and *Seasonique*. A woman using this regimen takes active pills for 12 weeks, followed by 1 week of placebos. On this cycle, women can expect to have a menstrual period every 3 months. Data indicate that women have an increased occurrence of spotting or bleeding in the first few months of an extended cycle pill.[17] *Lybrel*, another extended-cycle pill, supplies an active dose of hormones every day for 365 days. This eliminates menstruation completely during the time a woman takes it. While the idea of never having a period may be unsettling to some women, there is no physiological need for a woman to have a monthly period, and there are no known risks associated with its avoidance.

Advantages

Combination pills are highly effective at preventing pregnancy: more than 99 percent with perfect use and 91 percent with typical use.[18] It is easier to achieve perfect use with pills than it is with barrier contraceptives, as user error is less likely. Aside from its effectiveness, much of the pill's popularity is due to its convenience and ability to be used discreetly. Users like the fact that it does not interrupt or interfere with lovemaking, which can lead to enhanced sexual enjoyment.

In addition to preventing pregnancy, the pill may lessen menstrual difficulties, such as cramps and premenstrual syndrome (PMS). Oral contraceptives also lower the risk of several health conditions, including endometrial and ovarian cancers, noncancerous breast disease, osteoporosis, ovarian cysts, pelvic inflammatory disease (PID), and iron-deficiency anemia.[19] Many different brands of combination pills are on the market; some contain progestin, which offers additional benefits, such as reducing acne or minimizing fluid retention. With extended-cycle pills, the major additional benefit is the reduction in or absence of menstruation and any associated cramps or PMS symptoms. Users of these pills also like that they don't need to remember when to stop or start a cycle of pills or when to use placebos. Less-expensive generic versions are available for many brands.

Disadvantages

Although estrogen in combination pills is associated with increased risk of several serious health problems among older women, the risk is low for most healthy women under 35 who do not smoke. Problems include increased risk for blood clots (which can lead to strokes or heart attacks) and higher risk for increased blood pressure, thrombotic stroke, and myocardial infarction. These risks increase with age and cigarette smoking. Early warning signs of complications associated with oral contraceptives include severe abdominal, chest, or leg pain; severe headache; and/or eye problems.[20]

oral contraceptives Pills containing synthetic hormones that prevent ovulation by regulating hormones.

Different brands of pills have varying minor side effects. Some of the most common are spotting between periods (particularly with extended cycle regimens), breast tenderness, nausea, and vomiting. With most pills, these side effects clear up within a few months. Other, less common potential side effects include acne, weight gain, hair loss or growth, and a change in sexual desire. Because there are so many brands available, most women who wish to use the pill are able to find one that works for them without causing unpleasant side effects.

Apart from its risk factors and potential side effects, the pill's greatest disadvantage is that it must be taken every day (see the **Tech & Health** box on the next page). If a woman misses a pill, she should use a backup method of contraception for the remainder of that cycle. A backup method of

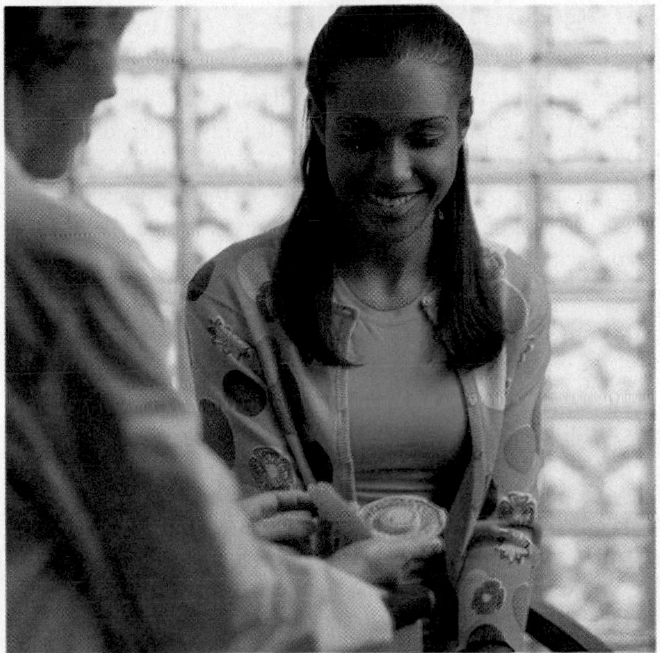

Studies show that college-age women are most familiar with the birth control pill and the male condom; talk to your health care provider about other options available to you and your partner.

TECH & HEALTH | BIRTH CONTROL, PREGNANCY, AND NEWBORNS *Apps for All Occasions*

The difference between the "perfect use" failure rates and "typical use" failure rates is most often human error. It is easy to leave your pills at home when you go out of town, to run out of condoms, or to forget to schedule an appointment to get your shot. Apps can help reduce this error and provide other resources for pregnancy and parenting.

Reminder apps, such as *myPill* and *iPill*, send text messages or sound discreet alarms to remind you to take your pill, schedule your shot, or visit the pharmacy to buy more pills.

For women trying to get pregnant, *Maybe Baby* and *FemiCycle* help predict fertility cycles based on fertility awareness methods. While not perfect, because ovulation is not always predictable, they do simplify charting basal temperatures and predicting fertile periods.

Once pregnant, there are many apps to choose from, such as *I'm Expecting* and *Baby Bump.* These apps provide many great tools, such as pregnancy countdowns, week-by-week information about fetal growth and development, and details on what a woman (and man) should expect from each week of pregnancy.

When the baby arrives, you can download all kinds of apps to chart growth, play white noise, and track nursing times and diaper changes. Just don't forget to put down your phone and cuddle the baby!

Ortho Evra Patch that releases hormones similar to those in oral contraceptives; each patch is worn for 1 week.

contraception is also necessary during the first week of use. After a woman discontinues the pill, return of fertility may be delayed, but the pill is not known to cause infertility. Another drawback is that the pill does not protect against STIs.

The costs associated with the pill (and all other hormonal contraceptives) have long been reported as a barrier to use, but the Affordable Care Act is changing that (see the **Money & Health** box).

Progestin-Only Pills

Progestin-only pills (or minipills) contain small doses of progestin and no estrogen. These pills are available in 28-day packs of active pills (menstruation usually occurs during the fourth week even though the active dose continues through the entire month). Ovulation may occur, but the progestin prevents pregnancy by thickening cervical mucus and interfering with implantation of a fertilized egg.

Advantages Progestin-only pills are a good choice for women who are at high risk for estrogen-related side effects or who cannot take estrogen-containing pills because of diabetes, high blood pressure, or other cardiovascular conditions. They also can be used safely by women who are older than age 35 and by women who are currently breast-feeding. The effectiveness rate of these pills is more than 99 percent with perfect use and 91 percent with typical use.[21]

Progestin-only pills share some of the health benefits associated with combination pills, and they carry no estrogen-related cardiovascular risks. Also, some of the typical side effects of combination pills, including nausea and breast tenderness, usually do not occur with progestin-only pills, and menstrual periods generally become lighter or cease.

Disadvantages Because of the lower dose of hormones in progestin-only pills, it is especially important that women take them at the same time each day. If a woman takes a pill 3 or more hours later than usual, she will need to use a backup method of contraception for the next 48 hours.[22] The most common side effect of progestin-only pills is irregular menstrual bleeding or spotting. Less common side effects include headaches and changes in mood or sex drive. As with all oral contraceptives, progestin-only pills do not protect against STIs.

Contraceptive Skin Patch

Ortho Evra is a square transdermal (through the skin) adhesive patch, which is as thin as a plastic strip bandage. It is worn for 1 week and is replaced on the same day of the week for 3 consecutive weeks; during the fourth week, no patch is worn. Ortho Evra works by delivering continuous levels of estrogen and progestin through the skin and into the bloodstream. The patch can be worn on one of four areas of the body: buttocks, abdomen, upper torso (front or back, exclud-

Ortho Evra is an adhesive patch that delivers estrogen and progestin through the skin for 1 week. Patches are changed weekly and worn for 3 out of 4 weeks.

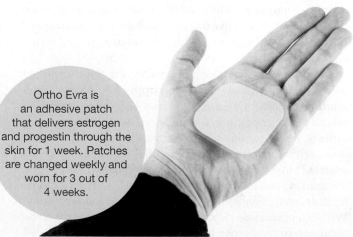

MONEY & HEALTH | HEALTH CARE REFORM AND CONTRACEPTIVES

In March 2010, President Obama signed the Patient Protection and Affordable Care Act (ACA) into law, which requires new private health insurance plans to cover "preventive services" with no co-payments or deductibles. Preventive services include birth control, yearly "wellness visits" (physical exams), breast-feeding counseling and supplies, and screening for domestic violence and sexually transmitted infections. Abortions are not included, but emergency contraception is.

Family planning experts anticipate that in coming years the law will significantly impact unintended pregnancy and abortion rates in two ways. One, women who have been unable to afford birth control will now have access. Half of all young adult women report having been unable to afford birth control consistently at some point, and when women have to choose between paying the heat bill and paying for birth control, birth control usually loses. Two, this coverage will enable women to "upgrade" their birth control to a more reliable method. Women who would prefer to use an IUD or implant to reduce the risk of "user error," but have been unable to because of the high upfront costs ($175–$1,000), will now be able to get one. The CHOICE study offered ACA-like benefits in St. Louis, Missouri, in advance of the implementation of the Affordable Care Act and researchers found significant reductions in unintended pregnancies, first abortions, and repeat abortions when women were given their choice of birth control method at no cost.

The implementation of the new law has not been without debate. The Obama administration created a firestorm of controversy by limiting the religious institutions exempt from offering these "preventive services" to include only churches themselves, not religious-affiliated charities, hospitals, or universities. The debate boiled down to this question: Should institutions with religious ties (like Catholic hospitals) be required to offer insurance plans covering birth control despite their objection to its use? Those wanting to reduce unintended pregnancies and provide broad preventive health services to all women argued that it shouldn't matter where a woman works, she should have equal access to birth control. Religious leaders argued that the requirement was an infringement on First Amendment rights and on religious liberty.

Nearly 200 Catholic institutions have filed multiple federal lawsuits, arguing that the mandate's exception for religious groups is too narrow and charging that requiring most religious employers to provide health insurance that includes birth-control services violates their right to religious freedom. The lawsuits remain unsettled, and likely will for some time.

While birth control remains a highly contentious political topic, it is one that almost all Americans have a stake in, as 99 percent of American women use birth control at some point in their lives, including 98 percent of Catholic women. In the meantime, the benefits of birth control, including a reduction in unintended pregnancies, a reduction in abortions, and more opportunities for women, are ones that most of us can agree upon.

Sources: U.S. Centers for Medicaid and Medicare Services, "What are my Birth Control Benefits?," Accessed May 2014, www.healthcare.gov/what-are-my-birth-control-benefits/; Planned Parenthood, "Key Facts on Birth Control Coverage," Accessed May 2014, www.plannedparenthood.org/files/PPFA/Myth_V_Fact_on_Birth_Control_coverage.pdf; A. Raphel, The Shorenstein Center, "The Affordable Care Act, Contraceptives, Abortion and Unintended-Pregnancy Rates," September 24, 2013, http://journalistsresource.org/studies/government/health-care/unintended-pregnancies-free-contraception#; Associated Press, "Catholic Group Challenging Affordable Care Act Because of Birth Control," March 12, 2014, www.cleveland.com/nation/index.ssf/2014/03/catholic_group_challenging_aff.html.

ing the breasts), or upper outer arm. It should not be used by women over age 35 who smoke cigarettes and is less effective in women who weigh more than 198 pounds.[23]

Advantages Ortho Evra is 99.7 percent effective with perfect use and 91 percent with typical use.[24] As with other hormonal methods, there is less room for user error than with barrier methods. Women who choose to use the patch often do so because they find it easier to remember to replace it weekly than to take a daily pill. Ortho Evra is not yet shown to, but likely offers, similar potential health benefits as combination pills (reduction in risk of certain cancers and diseases, lessening of PMS symptoms, etc.). Like other hormonal methods, the patch regulates a woman's menstrual cycle.

Disadvantages Using the patch requires an initial exam and prescription, weekly patch changes, and the ongoing expense of patch purchases. A backup method is required during the first week of use. Similar to other hormonal birth control methods, the patch offers no protection against HIV or other STIs. Some women experience minor side effects such as those associated with combination pills. The estrogen in the patch is associated with cardiovascular risks, particularly in women who smoke and women over the age of 35. Amid evidence that the patch may increase the risk of life-threatening blood clots, the U.S. Food and Drug Administration (FDA) mandated an additional warning label explaining that patch use exposes women to about 60 percent more estrogen than they would receive if they were taking a typical combination pill.[25]

Vaginal Contraceptive Ring

NuvaRing is a soft, flexible plastic hormonal contraceptive ring about 2 inches in diameter. The user inserts a ring into the vagina, leaves it in place for 3 weeks, then removes it for 1 week, during which she will have a menstrual period. Once the ring is inserted, it releases a steady flow of estrogen and progestin.

Advantages When used properly, the ring is 99.7 percent effective and 91 percent effective with typical use.[26] Advantages of NuvaRing include lower risk of user error, protection against pregnancy for 1 month, no pill to take daily or patch to change weekly, no need to be fitted by a health care provider, and rapid return of fertility when use is stopped. It also exposes the user to a lower dosage of estrogen than do the patch and some combination pills, so it may have fewer estrogen-related side effects. It likely offers some of the same potential health benefits as combination pills, and like other hormonal contraceptives, it regulates the menstrual cycle.

NuvaRing Soft, flexible ring inserted into the vagina that releases hormones, preventing pregnancy.

Depo-Provera, Depo-subQ Provera Injectable method of birth control that lasts for 3 months.

Nexplanon (Implanon) A plastic capsule inserted in a woman's upper arm that releases a low dose of progestin to prevent pregnancy.

Disadvantages NuvaRing requires an initial exam and prescription, monthly ring changes, and the ongoing expense of purchasing the ring (there is currently no generic version). A backup method must be used during the first week, and the ring provides no protection against STIs. Like combination pills, the ring poses possible minor side effects and potentially serious health risks for some women. Possible side effects unique to the ring include increased vaginal discharge and vaginal irritation or infection. Oil-based vaginal medicines to treat yeast infections cannot be used when the ring is in place, and a diaphragm or cervical cap cannot be used as a backup method for contraception.

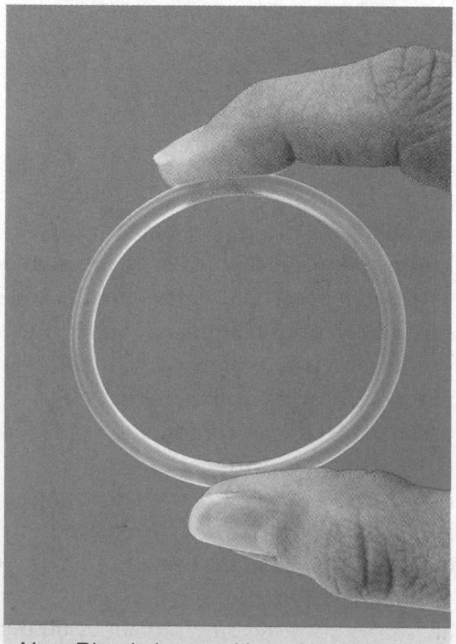

NuvaRing is inserted into the vagina, where it releases estrogen and progestin for 3 weeks.

Contraceptive Injections

Depo-Provera (injected intramuscularly) and the newer **Depo-subQ Provera** (injected just below the skin in a lower dose) are long-acting synthetic progesterones that are injected every 3 months by a health care provider. Both prevent ovulation, thicken cervical mucus, and thin the uterine lining, all of which prevent pregnancy.

Advantages Depo-Provera and Depo-subQ Provera take effect within 24 hours of the first shot, so there is usually no need to use a backup method. There is little room for user error as a health care provider administers the injection every 3 months. With perfect use, the shot is 99.8 percent effective, and with typical use it is 94 percent effective.[27] Some women feel that Depo-Provera encourages sexual spontaneity because they do not have to remember to take a pill or insert a device. With continued use of this method, a woman's menstrual periods become lighter and may eventually cease. There are no estrogen-related health risks associated with Depo-Provera, and it offers the same potential health benefits as progestin-only pills. Unlike estrogen-containing hormonal methods, Depo-Provera can be used by women who are breast-feeding.

Disadvantages Using Depo-Provera or Depo-subQ Provera requires an initial exam and prescription, then a follow-up visit every 3 months to have the shot administered. It offers no protection against STIs. The main disadvantage of Depo-Provera use is irregular bleeding, which can be troublesome at first, but within a year, most women are amenorrheic (have no menstrual periods). Weight gain is commonly reported. Prolonged use of Depo-Provera has been linked to loss of bone density.[28] Other possible side effects include dizziness, nervousness, and headache. Unlike other methods of contraception, this method cannot be stopped immediately if problems arise, and the drug and its side effects may linger for up to 6 months after the last shot. A disadvantage for women who want to get pregnant is that fertility may not return for up to 1 year after the final injection.

Contraceptive Implants

A single-rod implantable contraceptive, **Nexplanon** (formerly called **Implanon**) is a small, soft plastic capsule (about the size of a matchstick) that is inserted just beneath the skin on the inner side of a woman's upper underarm by a health care provider. Implanon continually releases a low, steady dose of progestin for up to 3 years, suppressing ovulation during that time.

Advantages After insertion, Nexplanon is generally not visible, making it a discreet method of birth control. Its main advantages are being highly effective (99.95%), not subject to user error, and only needing to be replaced every 3 years.[29] It has benefits similar to other progestin-only forms of contraception, in-cluding the lightening or cessation of menstrual periods, the lack of estrogen-related side effects, and safety for use by breast-feeding women. Fertility usually returns immediately after removal of the implant.

Disadvantages Insertion and removal of Nexplanon must be performed by a health care provider. There is a higher initial cost for this method, and it may not be covered by all health plans. Potential minor side effects include irritation, allergic reaction, and swelling or scarring around the area of insertion, and there is a possibility of infection or complications with removal. Nexplanon may be less effective in women who are overweight.[30] As with other progestin-only contraceptives, users can experience irregular bleeding. Implanon offers no protection against STIs, and it may require a backup method during the first week of use.

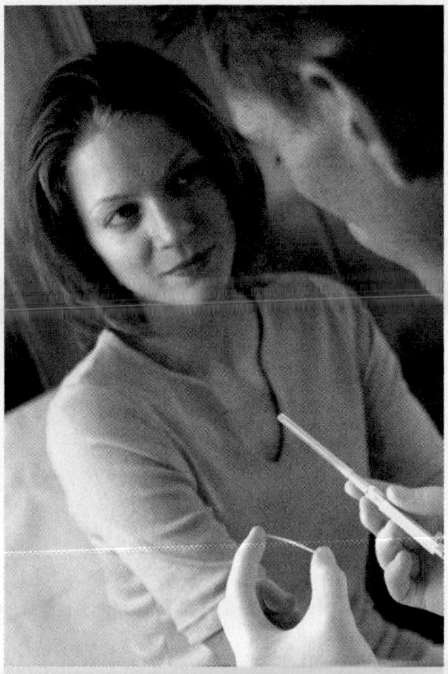
Implanon is inserted by a health care provider beneath the skin of a woman's arm, where it releases progestin for up to 3 years.

LO 4 | INTRAUTERINE CONTRACEPTIVES

Describe the effectiveness, advantages, and disadvantages of intrauterine contraceptives.

The **intrauterine device (IUD)** is a small plastic, flexible device with a nylon string attached. It is placed in the uterus through the cervix and provides protection from pregnancy for 3 to 10 years. The exact mechanism by which it works is not clearly understood, but researchers believe that IUDs affect the way sperm and eggs move, thereby preventing fertilization and/or affecting the lining of the uterus to prevent a fertilized ovum from implanting.

The IUD was once extremely popular in the United States; however, in the 1970s most brands were removed from the market because of serious complications, such as pelvic inflammatory disease and infertility. Redesigned for safe use, the IUD is again very popular with women around the world and is experiencing a resurgence of popularity among U.S. women.[31]

Three IUDs are currently available in the United States. *ParaGard* is a T-shaped plastic device with copper around the shaft. It does not contain any hormones and can be left in place for 10 years. *Mirena* is effective for 5 years and releases small amounts of progestin. The newest IUD, *Skyla*, is a lower dose and smaller-sized version of Mirena. It was tested with and is designed for women who have not yet had a baby, and it is effective for 3 years.

A health care provider must fit and insert an IUD. One or two strings extend from the IUD into the vagina so the user can periodically check to make sure that the device is in place. While IUDs were initially not recommended for women who had never had a baby, the American Congress of Obstetricians and Gynecologists supports their use for women of all ages.[32]

Advantages

The IUD is a safe, discreet, and highly effective method (more than 99%) of birth control.[33] It is effective immediately and needs to be replaced only every 3 to 10 years. ParaGard has the benefit of containing no hormones and so has none of the potential negative health impacts of hormonal contraceptives. Skyla and Mirena, on the other hand, likely offer some of the same potential health benefits as other progestin-only methods. All three IUDs can be used by breast-feeding women. With Mirena, periods become lighter or stop completely. The IUDs are fully reversible; after removal, there is usually no delay in return of fertility. IUDs offer sexual spontaneity, as there is no need to keep supplies on hand or to interrupt lovemaking. A health care provider can remove the IUD at any time.

intrauterine device (IUD) A device, often T-shaped, that is implanted in the uterus to prevent pregnancy.

SEE IT! VIDEOS

Why are IUDs gaining popularity? Watch **New Support for IUDs** available on MasteringHealth.™

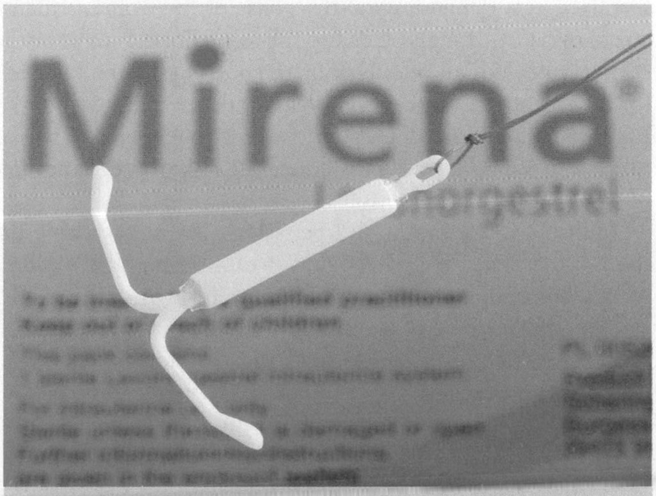

The Mirena IUD is a flexible plastic device inserted by a health care provider into a woman's uterus, where it releases progestin for up to 5 years.

Disadvantages

Disadvantages of IUDs include possible discomfort during insertion, the cost of insertion, and potential complications. Also, the IUD does not protect against STIs. In some women, the device can cause heavy menstrual flow and severe cramps for the first few months. Other negative side effects include acne, headaches, nausea, breast tenderness, mood changes, uterine cramps, and backache, which seem to occur most often in women who have never been pregnant. Women using IUDs also have a higher risk of benign ovarian cysts.

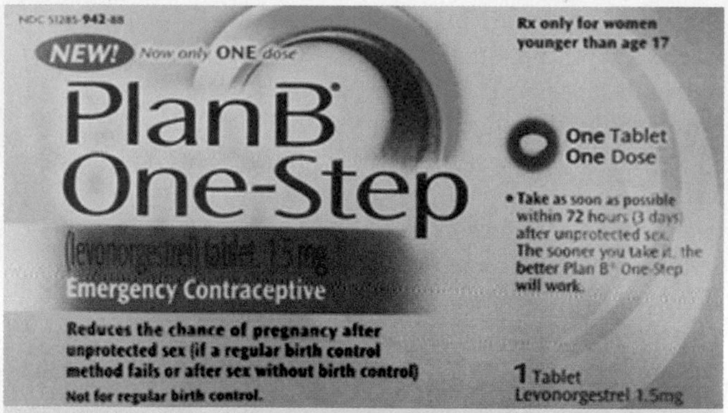

Emergency contraception pills contain hormones and are used after an act of unprotected intercourse. When taken within 72 hours of unprotected intercourse, ECPs reduce the risk of pregnancy by up to 95 percent.

LO 5 | EMERGENCY CONTRACEPTION

Describe emergency contraception and how it is used.

Emergency contraception is the use of a contraceptive to prevent pregnancy after unprotected intercourse, a sexual assault, or the failure of another birth control method. Combination estrogen-progestin pills and progestin-only pills are two common types of **emergency contraceptive pills (ECPs)**, sometimes referred to as "morning-after pills." Morning after pills are not the same as the "abortion pill," although the two are often confused. ECPs contain the same type of hormones as regular birth control pills and are used after unprotected intercourse but before a woman misses her period. A woman taking ECPs does so to prevent pregnancy; the method will not work if she is already pregnant, nor will it harm an existing pregnancy. In contrast, Mifeprex or mifepristone (formerly known as RU-486), the *early abortion pill,* is used to terminate a pregnancy that is already established—it is taken after a woman is sure she is pregnant (having taken a pregnancy test with a positive result). It and other abortion methods are discussed in detail later in the chapter.

ECPs prevent pregnancy the same way that other hormonal contraceptives do, by delaying or inhibiting ovulation, inhibiting fertilization, or blocking implantation of a fertilized egg, depending on the phase of the woman's menstrual cycle. Although ECPs use the same hormones as birth control pills, not all brands of birth control pills can be used for emergency contraception. When taken within 24 hours, ECPs reduce the risk of pregnancy by up to 95 percent; when taken 2 to 5 days later, ECPs reduce the risk of pregnancy by 88 percent.[34]

Multiple name-brand and generic ECPs are available in the United States including Plan B One-Step, Take Action, Next Choice One Dose, and My Way, all of which are available without a prescription and must be taken within 72 hours (3 days) of intercourse. The FDA has more recently approved ella. Unlike other ECPs, ella is only available by prescription. A progesterone receptor modulator, ella works by inhibiting or preventing ovulation. It can prevent pregnancy when taken up to 120 hours (5 days) after unprotected intercourse.)

emergency contraceptive pills (ECPs) Drugs taken within 3 to 5 days after unprotected intercourse to prevent pregnancy.

withdrawal Contraceptive method that involves withdrawing the penis from the vagina before ejaculation; also called *coitus interruptus.*

Although ECPs are no substitute for taking proper precautions before having sex (such as using a condom), widespread availability of emergency contraception has the potential to significantly reduce the rates of unintended pregnancies and abortions, particularly among young women. The 2013 federal court decision requiring the FDA to make emergency contraception available over the counter to all ages was a major win for reproductive health advocates because it removed two barriers for users: the potential embarrassment of asking the pharmacist for ECP and the need to have proper identification to prove age.[35]

LO 6 | BEHAVIORAL METHODS

Explain how behavioral methods of contraception work and compare their effectiveness to other methods of birth control.

Some methods of contraception rely on one or both partners altering their sexual behavior. In general, these methods require more self-control, diligence, and commitment, making them more prone to user error than hormonal and barrier methods.

Withdrawal

Withdrawal, also called *coitus interruptus,* involves removing the penis from the vagina just before ejaculation. In the 2013 *American College Health Association's National College Health Assessment (ACHA-NCHA),* 30 percent of respondents reported that withdrawal was the method of birth control they used the last time they had sexual intercourse.[36] This statistic is startlingly high, considering the very high risk of both pregnancy (78% with typical use) and STI transmission associated with this method of birth control.[37]

Advantages and Disadvantages Although withdrawal can be practiced when absolutely no other contraceptive available, and it is better than using no contraceptive at all, it is highly unreliable, even with "perfect" use, because there are a half million sperm in just the drop of pre-ejaculate fluid released *before* ejaculation. Timing withdrawal is also difficult, and males concentrating on accurate timing may not be able to relax and enjoy intercourse. Withdrawal offers no protection against STIs and requires a high degree of self-control, experience, and trust.

Abstinence and "Outercourse"

Strictly defined, *abstinence* means "deliberately avoiding intercourse." This definition would allow one to engage in forms of sexual intimacy such as massage, kissing, and masturbation. Couples who go beyond fondling and kissing to activities such as oral sex and mutual masturbation, but not vaginal or anal sex, are sometimes said to be engaging in "outercourse."

Advantages and Disadvantages Abstinence is the only method of avoiding pregnancy that is 100 percent effective. It is also the only method that is 100 percent effective against transmitting disease. Like abstinence, outercourse can be 100 percent effective for birth control as long as the male does not ejaculate near the vaginal opening. Unlike abstinence, however, outercourse is not 100 percent effective against STIs. Oral–genital contact can transmit disease, although the practice can be made safer by using a condom on the penis or a latex barrier, such as a dental dam, on the vaginal opening. Both abstinence and outercourse require discipline and commitment for couples to sustain over long periods of time.

Fertility Awareness Methods

Fertility awareness methods (FAMs) of birth control rely on altering sexual behavior during certain times of the month (FIGURE 6.4).

Fertility awareness methods are rooted in an understanding of basic physiology. A released ovum can survive about 36 hours after ovulation, and sperm can live for about 5 days in the reproductive tract. These techniques require observing female fertile periods and abstaining from sexual intercourse (or any penis–vagina contact) during the times when a sperm and egg could meet. Some of the more common forms include the following:

- **Cervical mucus method.** This method requires women to examine the consistency and color of their normal vaginal secretions. Prior to ovulation, vaginal mucus becomes slippery, thin, and stretchy, and normal vaginal secretions may increase. To prevent pregnancy, partners must avoid sexual activity involving penis–vagina contact while this mucus is present and for several days afterward.
- **Body temperature method.** This method relies on the fact that a woman's **basal body temperature** rises between 0.4 and 0.8 degrees after ovulation has occurred. For this method to be effective, a woman must chart her temperature for several months to learn to recognize her body's temperature fluctuations. To prevent pregnancy, partners must abstain from penis–vagina contact before the temperature rise until several days after the temperature rise is observed.
- **Calendar method.** This method requires the woman to record the exact number of days in her menstrual cycle. Because few women menstruate with complete regularity, this method involves keeping a record of the menstrual cycle for 12 months, during which time some other method of birth control must be used. This method assumes that ovulation occurs during the midpoint of the cycle. To prevent pregnancy, the couple must abstain from penis–vagina contact during the fertile time.

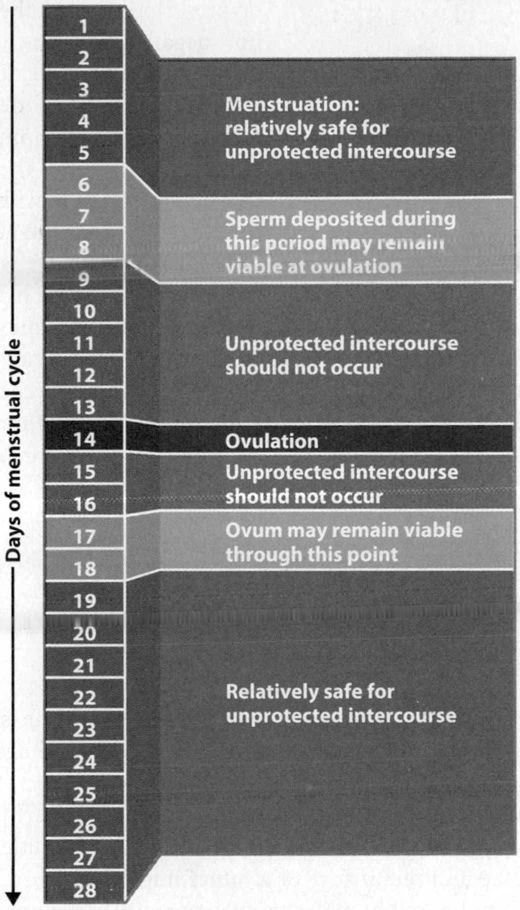

FIGURE 6.4 The Fertility Cycle

Fertility awareness methods (FAMs) can combine the use of a calendar, the cervical mucus method, and body temperature measurements to identify the fertile period. It is important to remember that most women do not have a consistent 28-day cycle.

fertility awareness methods (FAMs) Several types of birth control that require alteration of sexual behavior rather than chemical or physical intervention in the reproductive process.

basal body temperature The lowest temperature the body reaches, usually during sleep.

Advantages and Disadvantages Fertility awareness methods are the only forms of birth control that comply with certain religious teachings, including those of the Roman Catholic Church. They don't require a medical visit

sterilization Permanent fertility control achieved through surgical procedures.

tubal ligation Sterilization of a woman that involves cutting and tying off or cauterizing the fallopian tubes.

hysterectomy Surgical removal of the uterus.

vasectomy Male sterilization procedure that involves cutting and tying off the vasa deferentia.

or prescription, and there are no negative health effects. The effectiveness of fertility awareness methods depends on diligence, commitment, and self-discipline; they are 76 percent effective with typical use.[38] Women who attempt to use these methods without proper training run a high risk of unintended pregnancy; anyone interested in using FAMs is advised to take a class. Free classes are often offered by health centers and churches, and there is only minimal expense for supplies. These methods offer no STI protection, and they may not work for women with irregular menstrual cycles.

LO 7 | SURGICAL METHODS

Describe surgical methods of birth control and discuss their advantages and disadvantages.

In the United States, **sterilization** has become the second leading method of contraception for women of all ages and the leading method of contraception among married women and women over age 30.[39] Because sterilization is permanent, anyone considering it should think through possibilities such as divorce and remarriage or a future improvement in financial status that might make pregnancy realistic or desirable.

Female Sterilization

One method of sterilization for women is **tubal ligation**, a surgical procedure in which the fallopian tubes are sealed shut to block the sperm's access to released eggs (see **FIGURE 6.5**). The operation is usually done laparoscopically on an outpatient basis. The procedure usually takes less than an hour, and the patient is usually allowed to return home within a short time.

A tubal ligation does not affect ovarian and uterine function. The woman's menstrual cycle continues, and released eggs simply disintegrate and are absorbed by the lymphatic system. As soon as her incision heals, the woman may resume sexual intercourse with no fear of pregnancy.

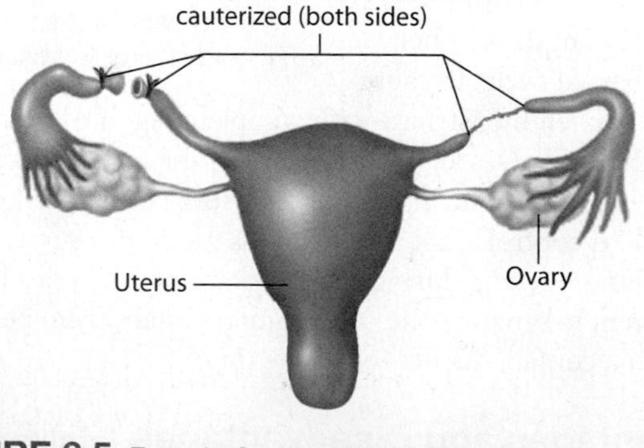

FIGURE 6.5 **Female Sterilization: Tubal Ligation**
In a tubal ligation, both fallopian tubes are cut and tied or sealed shut. This surgery is usually performed laparoscopically.

A newer sterilization procedure, *Essure*, involves the placement of small microcoils into the fallopian tubes via the vagina. The entire procedure takes about 35 minutes and can be performed in a physician's office. Once in place, the microcoils expand to the shape of the fallopian tubes. The coils promote the growth of scar tissue around the coils and lead to a blockage in the fallopian tubes. Like traditional forms of tubal ligation, Essure is permanent. It is recommended for women who cannot have a tubal ligation because of chronic health conditions such as obesity or heart disease.

Adiana is another minimally invasive method of blocking a woman's fallopian tubes. A soft insert about the size of a grain of rice is placed into each fallopian tube. Scar tissue begins to grow on and around the insert and eventually blocks the fallopian tubes. The insertion can be performed in a physician's office in about 15 minutes.

A **hysterectomy**, or removal of the uterus, is a method of sterilization requiring major surgery. It is usually done only when a woman's uterus is diseased or damaged, not as a primary means of female sterilization.

Advantages The main advantage to female sterilization is that it is highly effective (99.5%) and permanent.[40] After the one-time expense of the procedure, there is no other cost or ongoing action required. Sterilization has no negative effect on a woman's sex drive. A potential advantage of the Essure and Adiana methods is that they do not require an incision.

Disadvantages As with any surgery, there are risks involved with a tubal ligation. Although rare, possible complications include infection, pulmonary embolism, hemorrhage, anesthesia complications, and ectopic pregnancy. Essure and Adiana do not require an incision, so the immediate risks are lower; however, because these are relatively new techniques, the long-term risks are unknown. Sterilization offers no protection against STIs, and it is initially expensive if not covered by your insurance plan. The procedure is permanent and should be used only if both partners are certain they do not want more children.

Male Sterilization

Sterilization in men is less complicated than it is in women. A **vasectomy** is frequently done on an outpatient basis, using a local anesthetic (see **FIGURE 6.6**). This procedure involves making a small incision in the side of the scrotum to expose a vas deferens, cutting the vas deferens and either tying off or cauterizing the ends, then repeating the procedure on the other side.

WHAT DO YOU THINK?

Who do you think is responsible for deciding which method of contraception should be used in a sexual relationship?

- What are some examples of good opportunities for you and your partner to discuss contraceptives?
- What do you think are the biggest barriers in our society to the use of condoms?

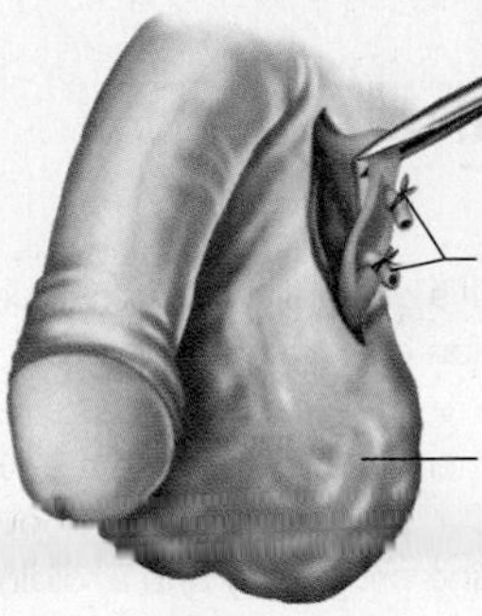

FIGURE 6.6 Male Sterilization: Vasectomy
In a vasectomy, the surgeon makes an incision in the scrotum, then locates and cuts the vasa deferentia, either sealing or tying both sides shut.

Many men are reluctant to consider sterilization because they fear the operation will affect their sexual performance or sex drive. However, a vasectomy in no way affects sexual response. Because sperm constitute only a small part of the semen (about 2%), the amount of ejaculate is not changed significantly. The testes continue to produce sperm, but the sperm can no longer enter the ejaculatory duct. Any sperm that are manufactured disintegrate and are absorbed into the lymphatic system.

Advantages A vasectomy is a highly effective and permanent means of preventing pregnancy. After 1 year, the pregnancy rate in women whose partners have had vasectomies is 0.15 percent (or about 1 in 1,500).[41] A vasectomy is a fairly simple outpatient procedure requiring minimal recovery time, and after the one-time expense, there is no other cost or ongoing action required.

Disadvantages Male sterilization offers no protection against STI transmission. Also, a vasectomy is not immediately effective in preventing pregnancy. Because sperm are stored in other areas of the reproductive system besides the vasa deferentia, couples must use alternative birth control methods for at least 1 month after the vasectomy. A physician will do a semen analysis to determine when unprotected intercourse can take place. As with any surgery, there are some risks involved with a vasectomy. In a small percentage of cases, serious complications occur, such as formation of a blood clot in the scrotum, infection, or inflammatory reactions. Very infrequently, the vasa deferentia may create a new path, negating the procedure. Sterilization is initially expensive if not covered by your insurance plan.

LO 8 | CHOOSING A METHOD OF CONTRACEPTION

Identify questions you should consider when choosing a method of contraception.

With all the options available, how does a person or a couple decide what method of contraception is best? Take some time to research the various methods, ask questions of your health care provider, and be honest with yourself about your own preferences. Questions to ask yourself are included below. Also, see the **Student Health Today** boxes on the next two pages: one for tips on talking about contraception with your partner and the other on men's involvement in making choices about contraception.

- **How comfortable would I be using a particular method?** If you aren't at ease with a method, you may not use it consistently, and it probably will not be a reliable choice for you. Think about whether the method may cause discomfort for you or your partner and consider your own comfort level with touching your body. For women, some methods, such as the diaphragm, sponge, or NuvaRing, require inserting a device into the vagina and taking it out. For men, using a condom requires rolling it onto the penis.
- **Will this method be convenient for me and my partner?** Some methods require more effort than others. Be honest with yourself about how likely you are to use the method consistently. Are you willing to interrupt lovemaking, to abstain from sex during certain times of the month, or to take a pill at the same time every day? You may feel condoms are easy and convenient to use, or you may prefer something that requires little ongoing thought, such as Nexplanon or an IUD.
- **Am I at risk for the transmission of STIs?** If you have multiple sex partners or are uncertain about the sexual history or disease status of your current sex partner, then you are at risk of contracting HIV or other STIs. Condoms (male and female) are the *only* birth control method that protects against STIs and HIV (although some other barrier methods offer limited protection).
- **Do I want to have a biological child in the future?** If you are unsure about your plans for future childbearing, you should use a temporary birth control method rather than a permanent one such as sterilization. Keep in mind that you may regret choosing a permanent method if you are young, if you have few or no children, or if you are choosing this method because you feel pressured by your partner. If you know you want to have children in the future, consider how soon that will be, as some methods, such as Depo-Provera, will cause a delay in return to fertility.
- **How would an unplanned pregnancy affect my life?** If an unplanned pregnancy would be a potentially devastating event for you or would have a serious impact on your plans for the future, then you should choose a highly effective birth control method, such as abstinence, the pill, patch, ring, implant, or IUD. If, however, you are in a stable relationship, have a reliable source of income, are planning to have children in the future, and would embrace a pregnancy should it occur now, then you may be comfortable with a less reliable method, such as condoms, fertility awareness, the diaphragm, cervical cap, or spermicides.
- **What are my religious and moral values?** If your beliefs prevent you from considering other birth control methods,

STUDENT HEALTH TODAY

LET'S TALK ABOUT (SAFER) SEX!

Communication is key to a healthy relationship, especially for those who are sexually intimate. It can be challenging to talk to your partner about using protection, but don't let embarrassment put your health at risk. The person that you're thinking about having sex with may or may not initially agree about using a condom or dental dam, so it's helpful to be prepared to discuss your concerns ahead of time. Remember: Communicating about sex is all about getting the most from your sex life and doing so safely.

Don't let embarrassment put your health at risk! Talking about safer sex may be uncomfortable, but it is worth the effort.

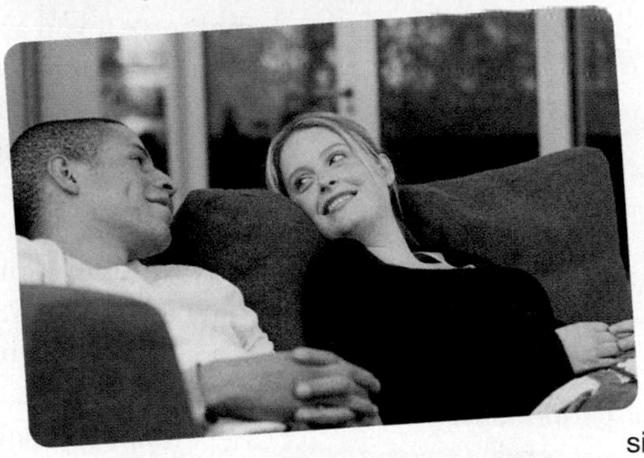

Why Communicating about Sex Is Essential

Open communication about sexual health is a sign of care and respect for your own body and your partner's. It empowers both of you to be assertive about your needs, likes, limits, and desires in the sexual relationship. Open communication also creates a safe environment to ask about your partner's sexual history, STI testing, and expectations.

If you are concerned that talking about sex beforehand is going to make your partner think you don't trust him or her, take some time to examine the strength of your relationship. Trust is about being open and honest. If you're afraid to talk with your partner, is it possible that you lack trust in him or her? If so, you might want to examine if this is a healthy relationship for you.

Finding the Time and Place for Sexual Communication

Find a convenient time and a place where you are both comfortable and free of distractions. It's generally better to have this conversation outside of the bedroom, so that you're not pressured by the heat of the moment to skip the conversation. And remember, you need to think about both preventing pregnancy and avoiding STIs.

Finding the Words for Condom/Dental Dam Negotiation

The table below lists some examples of how you can address potential excuses from your partner when you talk about using a condom or dental dam. While there is no perfect response for every situation, these may provide some helpful suggestions.

Excuse	Response
Don't you trust me?	It's not an issue of trust; people can have sexually transmitted infections and not know it.
It doesn't feel as good with a condom/dental dam.	I'll feel more relaxed; if I'm more relaxed, I can make it feel better for you. We can also use lubricant to increase sensation for both of us.
I don't have a condom with me.	I do.
It's up to you.	It's your health too, so it should be your decision, too.
I'm on the pill; you don't need a condom.	I'd like to use one anyway. It will help to protect us from infections that we may not know we have.
Putting it on interrupts everything.	Not if we put it on together.
I guess you don't really love me.	I do, but I'm not willing to risk our futures to prove it.
I will pull out in time.	Pre-ejaculate can still cause pregnancy and spread STIs.
I'm allergic to latex.	No problem, Student Health Services has a selection of nonlatex condoms and dental dams that we can get for free.
But I love you.	Then you'll help us protect ourselves.
Just this once.	Once is all it takes.

fertility awareness methods are a good option. When both partners are motivated to use these methods, they can be successful at preventing unintended pregnancy. If you are considering this option, sign up for a class to get specific training for using the method effectively.

- **How much will the birth control method cost?** Some contraceptive methods involve an initial outlay of money and few continuing costs (e.g., sterilization, IUD), whereas others are fairly inexpensive but must be purchased repeatedly (e.g., condoms, spermicides, monthly pills). You should consider whether a method will be cost-effective for you in the long run. Remember that any prescription methods require routine checkups, which may involve some cost to you. Be sure to check your health insurance to determine if the Affordable Care Act's requirement to cover "preventive services" makes hormonal contraceptives available to you at no cost.
- **Do I have any health factors that could limit my choice?** Hormonal birth control methods can pose potential health risks to women with certain preexisting conditions, such as high blood pressure, a history of stroke or blood clots, liver disease, migraines, or diabetes.

STUDENT HEALTH TODAY

HOW CAN MEN BE MORE INVOLVED IN BIRTH CONTROL?

The sexual health needs of young men have been largely overlooked in the field of reproductive health. Much of the focus on preventing teen pregnancy, sexually transmitted infections (STIs), and HIV/AIDS has been directed at young women.

On college campuses and in student health centers, the emphasis is also usually on women, leading to missed opportunities to emphasize the importance of shared responsibility for sexual health.

There are many reasons for the disparity: Men seek health care less often; it is sometimes incorrectly assumed that men are not interested in sexual health issues; and since women carry the baby, they are often seen as having a bigger stake in pregnancy prevention. However, healthy sexual relationships and ongoing reproductive health require that both partners be stakeholders. So, how can men be more involved in responsible sexual decision making?

Some men are more comfortable discussing reproductive health issues with male health care providers.

- Initiate discussions with your partner about contraception and your sexual health histories.
- Take an active role in discussing and deciding what type of contraception is best for you and your partner.
- Buy and use condoms every time you have sex.
- Help pay for contraceptive costs.
- If an unintended pregnancy occurs, share in the responsibility and decision making about the best way to handle the situation.

You should discuss this issue with your health care provider when considering birth control methods. In addition, women who smoke or are over age 35 are at risk of complications from combination hormonal contraceptives. Breast-feeding women can use progestin-only methods, but should avoid methods containing estrogen.

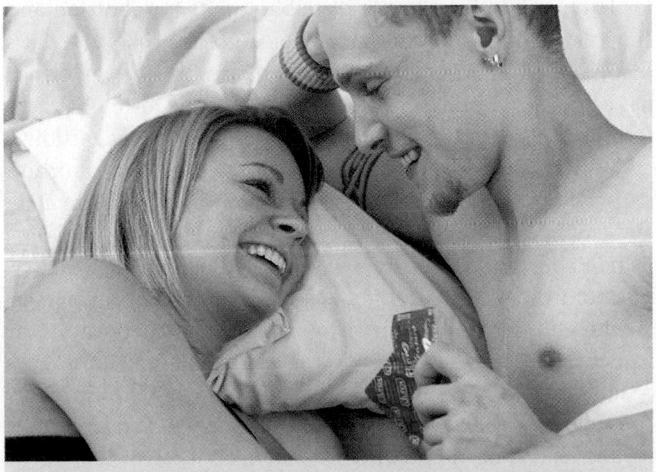

Different methods of birth control on the market include: barrier methods, hormonal methods, and other options (including surgery as a permanent option). When you choose a method, consider the cost, your comfort level, convenience, and health risks.

Men and women with latex allergies can use barrier methods made of polyurethane, silicone, or other materials, rather than latex condoms.

- **Are there any additional benefits I'd like from my contraceptive?** Hormonal birth control methods may have desirable secondary effects, such as the reduction of acne or the lessening of premenstrual symptoms. Some hormonal birth control methods have been associated with reduced risks of certain cancers. Extended-cycle pills and some progestin-only methods cause menstrual periods to be less frequent or to stop altogether, which some women find desirable. Condoms carry the added health benefit of protecting against STIs.

LO 9 | ABORTION

Summarize the political issues surrounding abortion and the various types of abortion procedures.

Women obtain abortions for a variety of reasons. The vast majority of abortions occur because of unintended pregnancies, as even the best birth control methods can fail.[42] In addition, some pregnancies are terminated because they are a consequence of rape or incest. Other reasons commonly cited are not being ready financially or emotionally to care for a child.[43] When an unintended pregnancy does occur, a woman must decide whether to terminate the pregnancy,

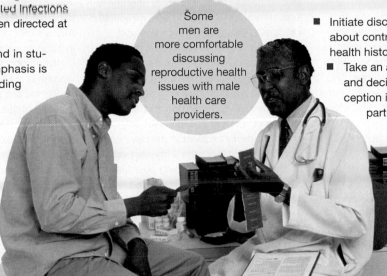

HEALTH IN A DIVERSE WORLD

CONTRACEPTIVE AVAILABILITY AND ABORTION IN THE DEVELOPING WORLD

While American women wrestle with the choice of which birth control to use, women in developing countries often struggle to access contraceptives at all. More than 220 million women in developing countries (26%) are unable to access modern birth control methods. Annually, in those 220 million women, there are an estimated 80 million unintended pregnancies, which translate into an estimated 30 million unplanned births, 40 million abortions, and 10 million miscarriages.

Unintended pregnancies in the developing world take a great toll. Of those 80 million women with unintended pregnancies, an estimated 104,000 will die from pregnancy-related causes, and of the babies born to those women, 600,000 will die in the first month and another 500,000 will die before their first birthday.

Unintended pregnancy is the primary driver of abortion in the United States and around the world, but whether abortion is legal or not has little to do with its overall incidence. The abortion rate in Africa, where abortion is illegal in most countries, is higher than the rate in Western Europe, where abortion is generally legal (29 per 1,000 women of childbearing age in Africa vs. 12 per 1,000 women of childbearing age in Western Europe). Not only are abortions more frequent in the developing world, they are less safe. Fifty-six percent of all abortions in developing countries are defined as "unsafe," compared with just 6 percent in the developed world. An estimated 47,000 women died from unsafe abortions last year, nearly all in developing nations where abortion is illegal. To put that risk in perspective, worldwide, women are 350 times more likely to die from unsafe abortions than from a legal abortion in the United States. When abortion is legalized, it becomes safer. After the legalization of abortion in 1997, South Africa experienced a 91 percent reduction in abortion-related deaths!

When contraceptives are unavailable, women often turn to abortion to end an unwanted pregnancy, even when death is a potential risk. Access to voluntary family planning services, including contraception, is essential in helping to reduce the number of unintended pregnancies and the incidence of abortion—and save the lives of mothers and babies in the developing world.

Sources: S. Singh and J. E. Darroch, *Adding It Up: Costs and Benefits of Contraceptive Services—Estimates for 2012* (New York, NY: Guttmacher Institute and United Nations Population Fund, 2012); Guttmacher Institute, "In Brief: Facts on Induced Abortion Worldwide," January 2012, www.guttmacher.org/pubs/fb_IAW.html.

abortion Termination of a pregnancy by expulsion or removal of an embryo or fetus from the uterus.

carry to term and keep the baby, or carry to term and give the baby up for adoption. This is a personal decision that each woman must make based on her personal beliefs, values, and resources and after carefully considering all alternatives.

In 1973, the landmark U.S. Supreme Court decision in *Roe v. Wade* stated that the "right to privacy ... founded on the Fourteenth Amendment's concept of personal liberty ... is broad enough to encompass a woman's decision whether or not to terminate her pregnancy."[44] The decision maintained that during the first trimester of pregnancy a woman and her health care provider have the right to terminate the pregnancy through **abortion** without legal restrictions. It allowed individual states to set conditions for second-trimester abortions. Third-trimester abortions were ruled illegal unless the mother's life or health was in danger. Prior to the legalization of abortions, women wishing to terminate a pregnancy had to travel to a country where the procedure was legal, consult an illegal abortionist, or perform their own abortions. These procedures sometimes led to infertility from internal scarring or death from hemorrhage or infection.

The Abortion Debate

Abortion is a highly charged and politically thorny issue in American society. In a recent national poll, 53 percent of people reported that *Roe v. Wade* should be kept in place, 29 percent felt it should be overturned, and 18 percent had no opinion.[45] Pro-choice individuals feel that it is a woman's right to make decisions about her own body and health, including the decision to continue or terminate a pregnancy. On the other side of the issue, pro-life individuals believe that the embryo or fetus is a human being with rights that must be protected. The political debate continues as pro-life groups lobby for laws prohibiting the use of public funds for abortion and abortion counseling while pro-choice groups lobby for laws that make abortions more widely available. At times, violence has arisen as a result of this controversy in the form of attacks on clinics or on individual physicians who perform abortions.

In the 40 years since *Roe v. Wade* legalized abortion nationwide, hundreds of laws have been passed at the state and federal level to narrow or expand its limits. In 2013 alone, 70 new abortion-related laws were passed in the United States, most of which focused on regulation of abortion providers or facilities, limitations on provision of medication abortions, or bans on private insurance coverage of abortion. These types of laws make abortions more difficult and costly to provide, consequently reducing the number of clinics and providers willing and able to provide abortion services. Thus, while abortion remains legal in all 50 states, for many women, due to difficulty accessing abortion services, abortion availability is severely limited.[46]

For a discussion of contraception and abortion access in developing countries, see the **Health in a Diverse World** box.

Emotional Aspects of Abortion

The best scientific evidence available indicates that among adult women who have an unplanned pregnancy, the risk of mental health problems is no greater if they have an abortion than if they deliver a baby. Although a variety of feelings such as regret, guilt, sadness, relief, and happiness are normal, no evidence has shown that an abortion causes long-term negative mental health outcomes.[47] Researchers found that the best predictor of a woman's emotional well-being following an abortion was her emotional well-being prior to the procedure.[48] The factors that place a woman at higher risk for negative psychological responses following an abortion include the following: perception of stigma, need for secrecy, low levels of social support for the abortion decision, prior history of mental health issues, low self-esteem, and avoidance and denial coping strategies.[49] The majority of women who have an abortion are able to view an abortion in context as one of life's events. Certainly, the presence of a support network and the assistance of mental health professionals are helpful to any woman who is struggling with the emotional aspects of her abortion decision.

Methods of Abortion

The choice of abortion procedure is determined by how many weeks the woman has been pregnant. Length of pregnancy is calculated from the first day of her last menstrual period.

Surgical Abortions

The majority of abortions performed in the United States today are surgical. If performed during the first trimester, abortion presents a relatively low health risk to the mother. About 88 percent of abortions occur during the first 12 weeks of pregnancy (see **FIGURE 6.7**).[50] The most commonly used method of first-trimester abortion is **suction curettage**, also called vacuum aspiration or dilation and curettage (D&C) (**FIGURE 6.8**). The vast majority of abortions in the United States are done using this procedure, which is usually performed under local anesthesia. The cervix is dilated with instruments or by placing laminaria, a sterile seaweed product, in the cervical canal. The laminaria is left in place for a few hours or overnight and slowly dilates the cervix. After the laminaria is removed, a long tube is inserted through the cervix and into the uterus, and gentle suction removes fetal tissue from the uterine walls.

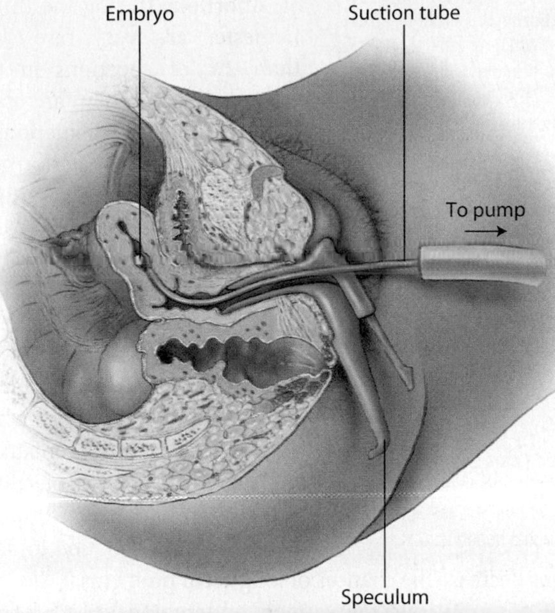

FIGURE 6.8 Suction Curettage Abortion

This procedure, in which a long tube with gentle suction is used to remove fetal tissue from the uterine walls, can be performed until the twelfth week of pregnancy.

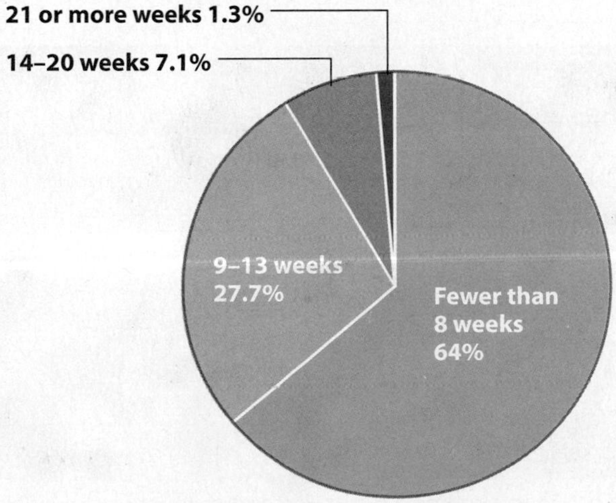

FIGURE 6.7 When Women Have Abortions (in weeks from the last menstrual period)

Source: K. Pazol et al., "Abortion Surveillance—United States 2009," *Surveillance Summaries* 61, no. SS08 (2012): 1–44, www.cdc.gov.

47% OF AMERICANS DESCRIBE THEMSELVES AS **"PRO-CHOICE,"** 46% AS **"PRO-LIFE."**

Pregnancies that progress into the second trimester (after week 12) are usually terminated through **dilation and evacuation (D&E)**. For this procedure, the cervix is dilated for 1 to 2 days, and a combination of instruments and vacuum aspiration is used to scrape and suck fetal tissue from the uterus. Second-trimester abortions may be done under general anesthesia. The D&E can be performed on an outpatient basis (usually in a physician's office), with or without pain medication. Generally, however, the woman is given a mild tranquilizer to help her relax. This procedure may cause moderate to severe uterine cramping and blood loss. After a D&E, a return visit to the clinic is an important follow-up.

suction curettage Abortion technique that uses gentle suction to remove fetal tissue from the uterus.

dilation and evacuation (D&E) Abortion technique that uses a combination of instruments and vacuum aspiration.

induction abortions Abortion technique in which chemicals are injected into the uterus through the uterine wall; labor begins, and the woman delivers a dead fetus.

intact dilation and extraction (D&X) Late-term abortion procedure in which the body of the fetus is extracted up to the head and then the contents of the cranium are aspirated.

medical abortion Termination of a pregnancy during the first 9 weeks using hormonal medications that cause the embryo to be expelled from the uterus.

preconception care Medical care received prior to becoming pregnant that helps a woman assess and address potential health issues.

Abortions during the third-trimester are very rare (less than 2% of abortions in the U.S.).[51] When they are performed, a D&E or saline **induction abortion** can be performed. The much debated, **intact dilation and extraction (D&X)**, often referred to as "partial birth abortion," is no longer legal in the United States.

The risks associated with surgical abortion include infection, incomplete abortion (when parts of the placenta remain in the uterus), excessive bleeding, and cervical and uterine trauma. Follow-up and attention to danger signs decrease the chances of long-term problems.

The mortality rate for women undergoing first-trimester abortions in the United States averages 1 death per every 1 million procedures at 8 or fewer weeks. The risk of death increases with the length of pregnancy. At 16 to 20 weeks, the mortality rate is 1 per 29,000; at 21 weeks or more, it increases to 1 per 11,000.[52] This higher rate later in the pregnancy is due to the increased risk of uterine perforation, bleeding, infection, and incomplete abortion; these complications occur because the uterine wall becomes thinner as the pregnancy progresses.

Medical Abortions

Unlike surgical abortions, a **medical abortion** (also called medication abortion) is performed without entering the uterus. Mifepristone, formerly known as RU-486 and currently sold in the United States under the brand name Mifeprex, is a steroid hormone that induces abortion by blocking the action of progesterone, the hormone produced by the ovaries and placenta that maintains the uterine lining. As a result, the lining and embryo are expelled from the uterus, terminating the pregnancy.

Mifepristone's nickname, "the abortion pill," may imply an easy process; however, this treatment actually involves more steps than a suction curettage abortion, which takes approximately 15 minutes followed by a physical recovery of about 1 day. With mifepristone, an initial visit to the clinic involves a physical exam and a dose of mifepristone and antibiotics, which may cause minor side effects such as nausea, headaches, weakness, and fatigue. The patient returns 2 to 3 days later for a dose of prostaglandins (misoprostol), which causes uterine contractions that expel the fertilized egg. The patient is required to stay under observation at the clinic for 4 hours and to make a follow-up visit within 2 weeks.[53]

More than 99 percent of women who use mifepristone early in pregnancy will experience a complete abortion.[54] The side effects are similar to those reported during heavy menstruation and include cramping, minor pain, and nausea. Less than 1 percent have more serious outcomes requiring a blood transfusion because of severe bleeding or the administration of intravenous antibiotics.[55]

LO 10 | LOOKING AHEAD TO PREGNANCY AND PARENTHOOD

Explain key issues to consider when planning a pregnancy.

The many methods available to control fertility give you choices that did not exist when your parents—and even you—were born. Today, sexually active people are able to choose if and when they want to have children. Some will remain childless by choice. Others will utilize birth control as a way to delay and space their desired number of children. As you approach the decision of whether or not to have children, or when to do so, take the time to evaluate your emotions, physical health, and finances.

Considering Parenthood

First and foremost, consider why you may want to have a child. To fulfill an inner need to carry on the family? To share love? To give your parents grandchildren? Because it's expected? Then, consider the responsibilities involved with becoming a parent. Are you ready to make all the sacrifices necessary to bear and raise a child? Can you care for this new human being in a loving and nurturing manner? Do you have a strong social support system? This emotional preparation for parenthood can be as important as the physical preparation.

Physical Health: Maternal Health

The birth of a healthy baby depends in part on the mother's **preconception care**. Maternal factors that can affect a fetus or infant include drug use (illicit or otherwise), alcohol consumption, and whether the mother smokes or is obese. To promote preconception health, get the best medical care you can, practice healthy behaviors, build a strong support network, and encourage safe environments at home and at work.[56]

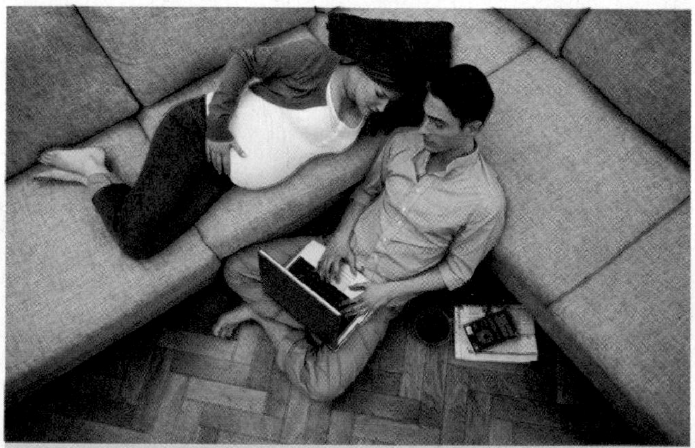

Preparing to become a parent requires thoughtful evaluation of one's emotional, physical, social, and financial well-being. Prospective mothers and fathers should be willing to implement healthy change where needed to prepare themselves for bringing a child into the world.

During a preconception care visit, a health care provider performs a thorough medical evaluation and talks with the woman about any conditions she might have, such as diabetes or high blood pressure. The health care provider will also determine if the woman has had any problems with prior pregnancies, if any genetic disorders run in the family, and if the woman's immunizations are up-to-date. If, for example, she has never had rubella (German measles), a woman needs to be immunized prior to becoming pregnant. A rubella infection can kill the fetus or cause blindness or hearing disorders in the infant. The health care provider will encourage the woman to eliminate alcohol consumption and tobacco use and may adjust some medications, such as antidepressants, to safer levels.

Nutrition counseling is another important part of preconception care. Among the many important nutrition issues is folic acid (folate) intake. When consumed the month before conception and during early pregnancy, folate reduces the risk of spina bifida, a congenital birth defect resulting from failure of the spinal column to close.

Why is preconception care so important? Beginning prenatal care at week 11 or 12 of a pregnancy is often late to prevent a variety of health problems for both child and mother. The fetus is most susceptible to developing certain problems in the first 4 to 10 weeks after conception, before prenatal care is normally initiated. Since many women don't realize they are pregnant until later, they often can't reduce health risks unless intervention had begun before conception.[57]

For suggestions on preparing for a healthy pregnancy, see the **Skills for Behavior Change** box.

SKILLS FOR BEHAVIOR CHANGE

PREPARING FOR PREGNANCY

Before becoming pregnant, parents-to-be should assess and improve their own health to help ensure the health of their child. Among the most important factors to consider are the following:

FOR WOMEN:

- If you smoke, drink alcohol, or use drugs, stop.
- Reduce your caffeine intake or avoid it altogether.
- Maintain a healthy weight; lose or gain weight if necessary.
- Avoid X-rays and environmental chemicals such as herbicides and pesticides.
- Get checked for sexually transmitted infections and seek treatment if you have one.
- Take prenatal vitamins, which are especially important for providing adequate folic acid.

FOR MEN:

- If you smoke, quit.
- Drink alcohol only in moderation, and avoid drug use.
- Get checked for sexually transmitted infections and seek treatment if you have one.
- Avoid exposure to toxic chemicals in your home, work, and school environment.
- Maintain a healthy weight; lose or gain weight if necessary.

16% OF COLLEGE STUDENTS REPORT HAVING **UNPROTECTED** SEX AFTER DRINKING ALCOHOL IN THE LAST 12 MONTHS.

Physical Health: Paternal Health

It is common knowledge that mothers-to-be, even before they become pregnant, should steer clear of toxic chemicals that can cause birth defects, should eat a healthy diet, and should stop smoking and drinking alcohol. Today, similar precautions are recommended for fathers-to-be as, by one route or another, dozens of chemicals studied so far (from occupational exposures to by-products of cigarette smoke) appear to harm sperm.[58] Chemical exposure can reduce the number of sperm, reduce the sperms' ability to fertilize an egg, cause miscarriage, or cause birth defects.[59] A fathers' age may also play a role; recent research shows a relationship between older fathers and autism, ADHD, bipolar disorder, and schizophrenia.[60]

WHAT DO YOU THINK?

Have you thought about whether and when to have children?

- Is there a certain age at which you feel you will be ready to be a parent?
- What goals do you hope to achieve before undertaking parenthood?
- What are your biggest concerns about parenthood?

Financial Evaluation

Finances are another important consideration. Are you willing to go out to dinner less often, forgo a new pair of shoes, or drive an older car? These are important questions to ask when considering the financial aspects of being a parent. Can you afford to give your child the life you would like him or her to enjoy?

It is important to check whether your medical insurance provides maternity benefits. If not, you can expect to pay, on average, $18,000 for a normal delivery and up to $28,000 for a cesarean section, including prenatal care. Complications during delivery can increase the cost substantially.[61] Both partners should investigate their employers' policies concerning parental leave, including length of leave available and conditions for returning to work.

The U.S. Department of Agriculture estimates that it will cost an average of $241,080 to raise a child born in 2010 to

human chorionic gonadotropin (HCG) Hormone detectable in blood or urine samples of a mother within the first few weeks of pregnancy.

age 18, not including college tuition.[62] While housing costs and food are the two largest expenditures, quality child care is also expensive. According to the National Association of Child Care Resource and Referral Agencies (NACCRRA), full-time child care costs for an infant range from $4,863 a year in Mississippi to $16,430 a year in Massachusetts.[63]

Contingency Planning

A final consideration is how to provide for your child should something happen to you and your partner. If both of you were to die, do you have relatives or close friends who could raise your child? If you have more than one child, would they have to be split up or could they be kept together? Although unpleasant to think about, this sort of contingency planning is crucial. Children who lose their parents are heartbroken and confused. A prearranged plan of action can smooth their transition into new families; without one, a judge will usually decide who will raise them.

LO 11 | PREGNANCY

Describe fetal development and explain the importance of prenatal care.

Pregnancy is an important event in a woman's life. The actions taken before as well as behaviors engaged in during pregnancy can significantly affect the health of both infant and mother.

The Process of Pregnancy

The process of pregnancy begins the moment a sperm fertilizes an ovum in the fallopian tubes (**FIGURE 6.9**). From there, the single fertilized cell, now called a *zygote*, multiplies and becomes a sphere-shaped cluster of cells called a *blastocyst* that travels toward the uterus, a journey that may take 3 to 4 days. Upon arrival, the embryo burrows into the thick, spongy endometrium (implantation) and is nourished from this carefully prepared lining.

Pregnancy Testing

A pregnancy test scheduled with your health care provider or at a local family planning clinic will confirm a pregnancy. Women who wish to know imme-

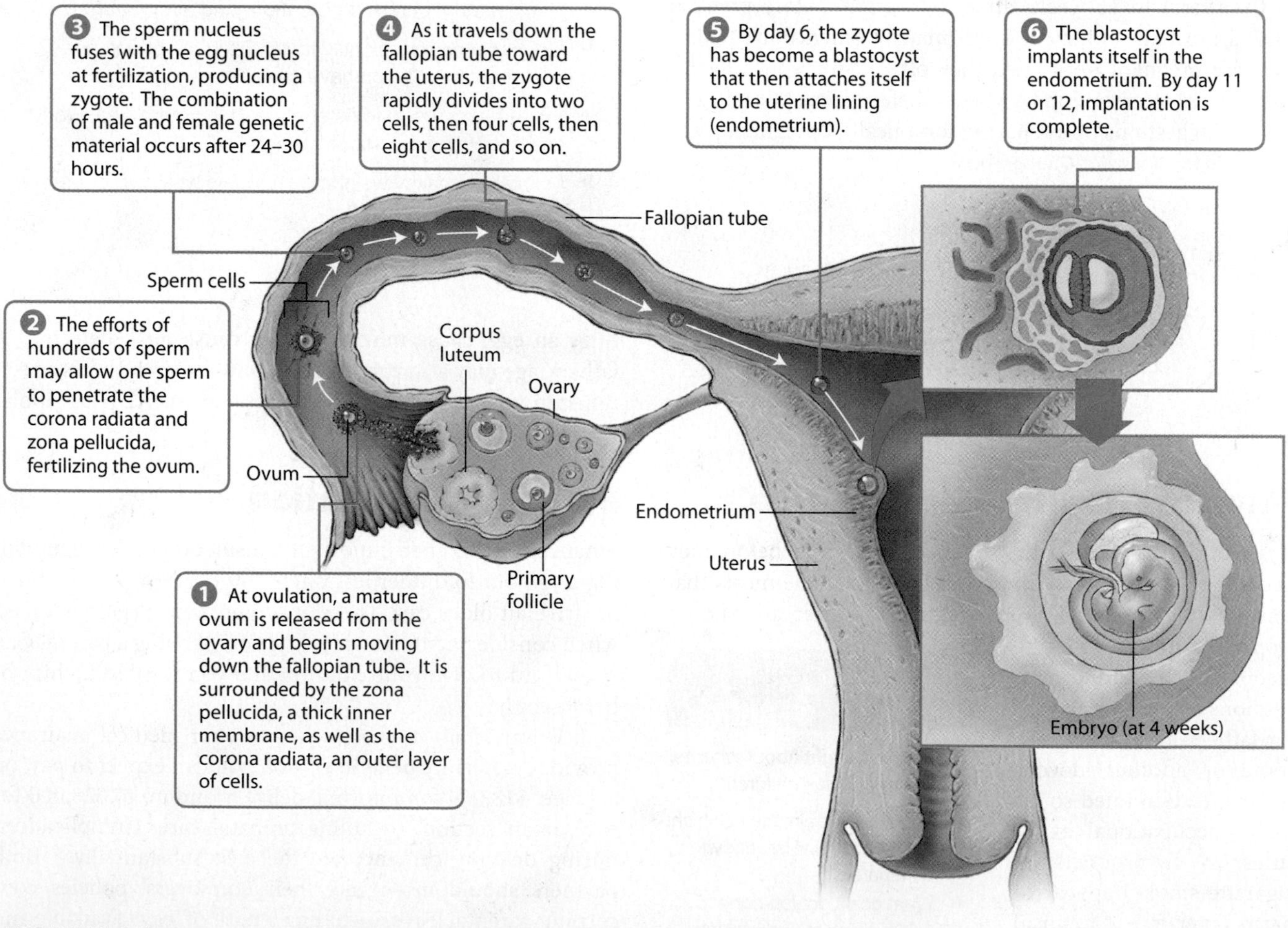

3 The sperm nucleus fuses with the egg nucleus at fertilization, producing a zygote. The combination of male and female genetic material occurs after 24–30 hours.
4 As it travels down the fallopian tube toward the uterus, the zygote rapidly divides into two cells, then four cells, then eight cells, and so on.
5 By day 6, the zygote has become a blastocyst that then attaches itself to the uterine lining (endometrium).
6 The blastocyst implants itself in the endometrium. By day 11 or 12, implantation is complete.
Fallopian tube
Sperm cells
2 The efforts of hundreds of sperm may allow one sperm to penetrate the corona radiata and zona pellucida, fertilizing the ovum.
Corpus luteum
Ovary
Ovum
Endometrium
Uterus
Primary follicle
1 At ovulation, a mature ovum is released from the ovary and begins moving down the fallopian tube. It is surrounded by the zona pellucida, a thick inner membrane, as well as the corona radiata, an outer layer of cells.
Embryo (at 4 weeks)

FIGURE 6.9 Fertilization Fertilization usually occurs in the upper third of the fallopian tube, and implantation in the uterus takes place about 6 days later.

diately can purchase home pregnancy test kits sold over the counter in drugstores. A positive test is based on the secretion of **human chorionic gonadotropin (HCG)**, which is found in the woman's urine.

Home pregnancy tests vary, but some can be used as early as a week after conception and many are 99 percent reliable.[64] Instructions must be followed carefully. If the test is done too early in the pregnancy, it may show a false negative. Other causes of false negatives are unclean testing devices, ingestion of certain drugs, and vaginal or urinary tract infections. Accuracy also depends on the quality of the test itself and the user's ability to follow directions. Blood tests administered and analyzed in a doctor's office are more accurate than home tests.

Early Signs of Pregnancy A woman's body undergoes substantial changes during a pregnancy (**FIGURE 6.10**). The first sign of pregnancy is usually a missed menstrual period (although some women "spot" in early pregnancy, which may be mistaken for a period). Other signs include breast tenderness, emotional upset, extreme fatigue, sleeplessness, nausea, and vomiting (especially in the morning).

Pregnancy typically lasts 40 weeks and is divided into three phases, or **trimesters**, of approximately 3 months each. The due date is calculated from the expectant mother's last menstrual period.

trimester A 3-month segment of pregnancy.

embryo Fertilized egg from conception through the eighth week of development.

The First Trimester During the first trimester, few noticeable changes occur in the mother's body. She may urinate more frequently and experience morning sickness, swollen breasts, or undue fatigue. These symptoms may not be frequent or severe, so women often do not realize they are pregnant right away.

During the first 2 months after conception, the **embryo** differentiates and develops its various organ systems, beginning with the nervous and circulatory systems. At the start of the third month, the embryo is called a **fetus**, indicating

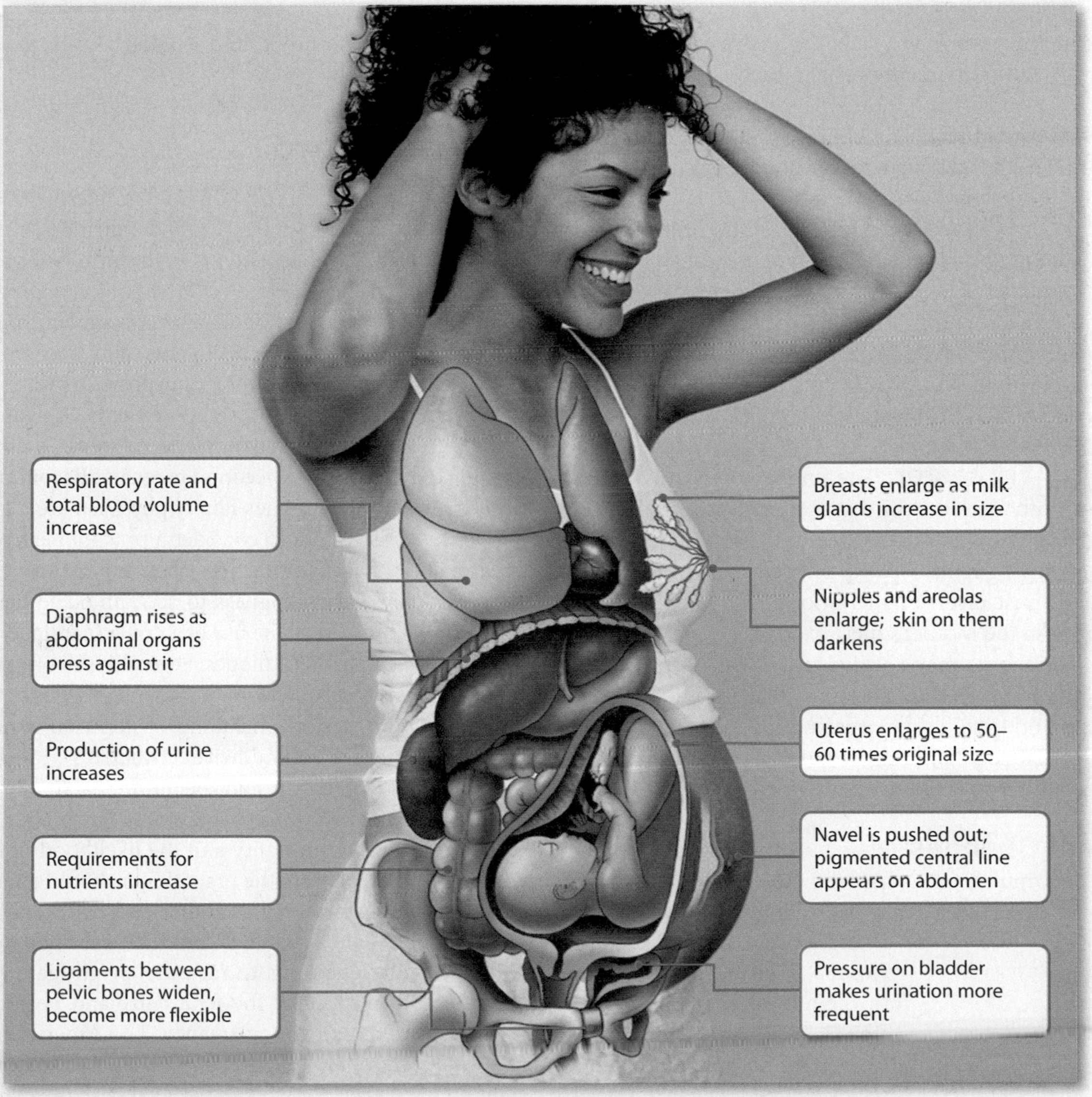

Respiratory rate and total blood volume increase
Diaphragm rises as abdominal organs press against it
Production of urine increases
Requirements for nutrients increase
Ligaments between pelvic bones widen, become more flexible
Breasts enlarge as milk glands increase in size
Nipples and areolas enlarge; skin on them darkens
Uterus enlarges to 50–60 times original size
Navel is pushed out; pigmented central line appears on abdomen
Pressure on bladder makes urination more frequent

FIGURE 6.10 Changes in a Woman's Body during Pregnancy

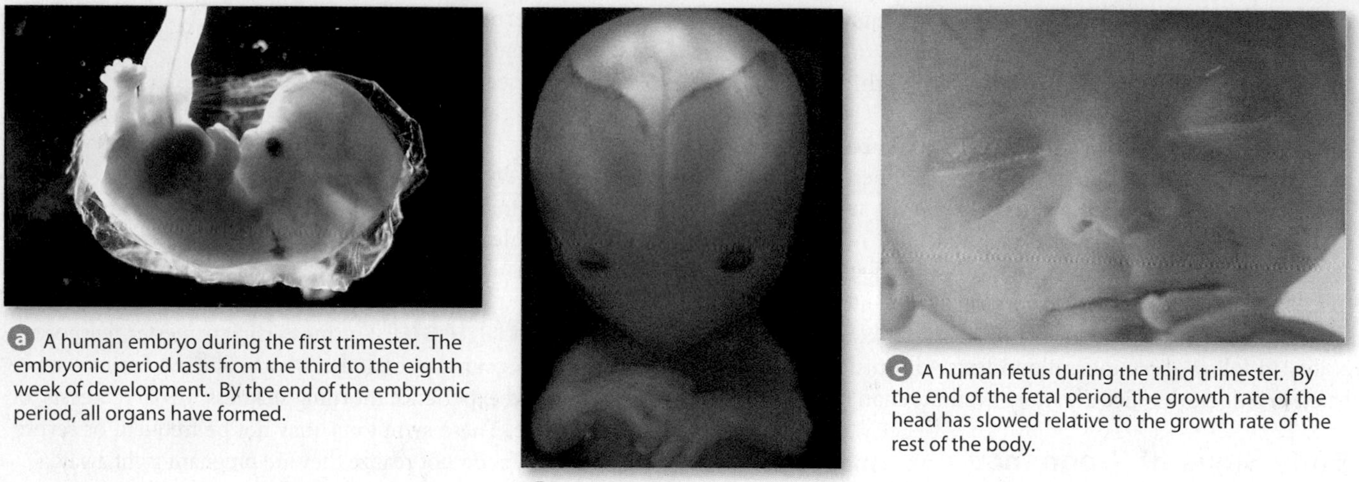

a A human embryo during the first trimester. The embryonic period lasts from the third to the eighth week of development. By the end of the embryonic period, all organs have formed.

b A human fetus during the second trimester. Growth during the fetal period is very rapid.

c A human fetus during the third trimester. By the end of the fetal period, the growth rate of the head has slowed relative to the growth rate of the rest of the body.

FIGURE 6.11 Fetoscopic Photographs Showing Development in the First, Second, and Third Trimesters of Pregnancy

that all organ systems are in place. For the rest of the pregnancy, growth and refinement occur in each body system so that at birth they can function independently, yet in coordination with all the others. The photos in **FIGURE 6.11** illustrate physical changes during fetal development.

The Second Trimester

At the beginning of the second trimester, the fourth through sixth months of pregnancy, physical changes in the mother become more visible. Her breasts swell and her waistline thickens. During this time, the fetus makes greater demands on the mother's body. In particular, the **placenta**, the network of blood vessels that carries nutrients and oxygen to the fetus and fetal waste products to the mother, becomes well established.

The Third Trimester

The end of the sixth month through the ninth mark the third trimester. This is the period of greatest fetal growth, when the fetus gains most of its weight. The growing fetus depends entirely on its mother for nutrition and must receive large amounts of calcium, iron, and protein from the mother's diet.

Although the fetus may survive if it is born during the seventh month, it needs the layer of fat it acquires during the eighth month and time for the organs (especially the respiratory and digestive organs) to develop fully. Infants born prematurely usually require intensive medical care.

Emotional Changes

Of course, the process of pregnancy involves much more than the changes in a woman's body and the developing fetus. Many important emotional changes occur from the time a woman learns she is pregnant through the *postpartum period* (the first 6 weeks after her baby is born). Throughout pregnancy, women may experience fear of complications, anxiety about becoming a parent, and wonder and excitement over the developing baby.

fetus Developing human from the ninth week until birth.

placenta Network of blood vessels connected to the umbilical cord that transports oxygen and nutrients to a developing fetus and carries away fetal wastes.

Prenatal Care

A successful pregnancy depends on a mother who takes good care of herself and her fetus. Good nutrition and exercise; avoiding drugs, alcohol, and other harmful substances; and regular medical checkups from the beginning of pregnancy are all essential. Early detection of fetal abnormalities, identification of high-risk mothers and infants, and screening for possible complications are the major purposes of prenatal care.

A woman should carefully choose the health care provider who will attend her pregnancy and delivery. If possible, she should do this before she becomes pregnant. Recommendations from friends and from one's family physician are a good starting point. She should also consider a practitioner's philosophy about pain management during labor, experience in handling complications, and willingness to accommodate her personal beliefs on issues such as the use of a doula (a trained childbirth assistant) or Lamaze techniques. Several types of practitioners are qualified to care for a woman through pregnancy, birth, and the postpartum period, including obstetrician-gynecologists, family practitioners, and midwives (**TABLE 6.3**).

Ideally, a woman should begin prenatal appointments within the first 3 months of becoming pregnant. This early care reduces infant mortality and the likelihood of low birthweight. On the first visit, the practitioner should obtain a complete medical history of the mother and her family and note any hereditary conditions that could put a woman or her fetus at risk. Regular checkups to measure weight gain and blood pressure and to monitor the fetus's size and position should continue throughout the pregnancy. The American Congress of Obstetricians and Gynecologists recommends seven or eight prenatal visits for women with low-risk pregnancies.

TABLE 6.3 | Choosing a Prenatal Care Provider

Provider/Description	Advantages	Disadvantages
Obstetrician/Gynecologist: Medical doctor (MD) who specializes in obstetrics (care of a woman and child during pregnancy, birth, and the postpartum period) and gynecology (care of the reproductive system of women)	Trained to handle all types of pregnancy- and delivery-related emergencies.	Generally can perform deliveries only in a hospital setting. Cannot serve as the baby's physician after birth.
Family Practitioner: MD or nurse practitioner who provides comprehensive care for people of all ages	No need to change physicians; can refer to a specialist if necessary, can serve as the baby's physician after birth.	Some provide pregnancy care only to low-risk pregnancies; rarely perform home births.
Midwife: Experienced practitioner who can assist with pregnancies and deliveries. Midwives can oversee delivery of babies in nonhospital birthing sites, such as home deliveries or birthing centers. Most strive to help women have a natural childbirth experience.		
Certified Nurse Midwife: Registered Nurse (RN) or Nurse Practitioner (NP) with specialized training in pregnancy and delivery; most work in private practice or in conjunction with physicians.	Certified nurse midwives have formal training and accreditation. They may work with physicians and have access to traditional medical facilities, but are often able to offer more personal attention than an MD could.	RNs cannot provide medication without physician approval, but NPs can in many states; need to refer to physician when the pregnancy is deemed high risk
Lay Midwives: Uncertified or unlicensed midwife who was educated through informal routes such as self-study or apprenticeship rather than through a formal program.	Midwives tend to view pregnancy and childbirth as a family event. They usually offer low intervention, highly personalized birth plans. Home birth can lower costs.	Cannot administer any medication; would need to refer to a physician. May not have extensive training in handling an emergency. Women should carefully evaluate the credentials of a prospective lay midwife and seriously consider the risks related to delivery outside a hospital.

Nutrition and Exercise Despite "eating for two," pregnant woman only need about 300 additional calories a day. Special attention should be paid to getting enough folic acid (found in dark leafy greens, citrus fruits, and beans), iron (dried fruits, meats, legumes, liver, egg yolks), calcium (nonfat or low-fat dairy products and some canned fish), and fluids. While vitamin supplements can correct some deficiencies, there is no substitute for a well-balanced diet. Babies born to poorly nourished mothers run high risks of substandard mental and physical development.

Weight gain during pregnancy helps nourish a growing baby. For a woman of normal weight before pregnancy, the recommended gain during pregnancy is 25 to 35 pounds.[65] For overweight women, weight gain of 15 to 25 pounds is recommended, and for obese women, 11 to 20 pounds is recommended. Underweight women should gain 28 to 40 pounds, and women carrying twins should gain about 35 to 45 pounds. Gaining too much or too little weight can lead to complications. With higher weight gains, women may develop gestational diabetes, hypertension, or increased risk of delivery complications. Gaining too little increases the chance of a low birthweight baby.

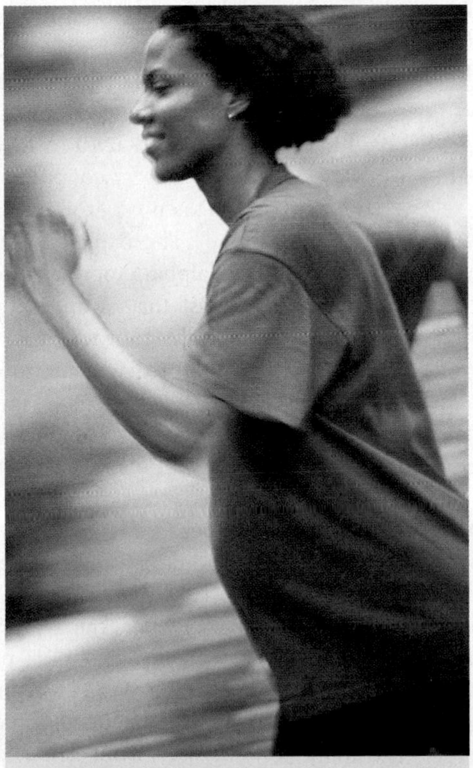

A doctor-approved exercise program during pregnancy can help control weight, make delivery easier, and have a healthy effect on the fetus.

As in all other stages of life, exercise is an important factor in overall health during pregnancy. Regular exercise is recommended for pregnant women; however, they should consult with their health care provider before starting any exercise program. Exercise can help control weight, make labor easier, and help with a faster recovery due to increased strength and endurance. Women can usually maintain their customary level of activity during most of the pregnancy, although there are some cautions: Pregnant women should avoid exercise that puts them at risk of falling or having an abdominal injury, such as horseback riding, soccer, or skiing, and in the third trimester, exercises that involve lying on the back should be avoided as they can restrict blood flow to the uterus.

Drugs and Alcohol A woman should consult with a health care provider regarding the safety of any drugs she might use during pregnancy. Even too much of common over-the-counter medications such as aspirin can damage a developing fetus. During the first 3 months of pregnancy, the fetus is especially subject to the **teratogenic** (birth defect–causing) effects of drugs, environmental chemicals, X-rays, or diseases. The fetus can also develop an addiction to or tolerance for drugs that the mother is using.

Maternal consumption of alcohol is detrimental to a growing fetus. Birth defects associated with **fetal alcohol syndrome (FAS)** include developmental disabilities, neural and cardiac impairments, and cranial and facial deformities. The exact amount of alcohol that causes FAS is not known; therefore, the American Congress of Obstetricians and Gynecologists recommends completely avoiding alcohol during pregnancy.[66]

Smoking Tobacco use, and smoking in particular, harms every phase of reproduction. Women who smoke have more difficulty becoming pregnant and have a higher risk of being infertile. Women who smoke during pregnancy have a greater chance of miscarriage, complications, premature births, low birthweight infants, stillbirth, and infant mortality specifically due to sudden infant death syndrome (SIDS).[67] Smoking restricts the blood supply to the developing fetus and thus limits oxygen and nutrition delivery and waste removal. Tobacco use also appears to be a significant factor in the development of cleft lip and palate.

teratogenic Causing birth defects; may refer to drugs, environmental chemicals, radiation, or diseases.

fetal alcohol syndrome (FAS) Pattern of birth defects, learning, and behavioral problems in a child caused by the mother's alcohol consumption during pregnancy.

toxoplasmosis Disease caused by an organism found in cat feces that, when contracted by a pregnant woman, may result in stillbirth or birth defects.

Down syndrome A genetic disorder caused by the presence of an extra chromosome that results in mental disabilities and distinctive physical characteristics.

ultrasonography (ultrasound) Common prenatal test that uses sound waves to create a visual image of a developing fetus.

chorionic villus sampling (CVS) Prenatal test that involves snipping tissue from the fetal sac to be analyzed for genetic defects.

triple marker screen (TMS) Common maternal blood test that can be used to identify fetuses with certain birth defects and genetic abnormalities.

amniocentesis Medical test in which a small amount of fluid is drawn from the amniotic sac to test for Down syndrome and other genetic abnormalities.

Other Teratogens A pregnant woman should avoid exposure to X-rays, toxic chemicals, heavy metals, pesticides, gases, and other hazardous compounds. She should also avoid cleaning litter boxes, if possible, because cat feces can contain organisms that cause **toxoplasmosis.** If a pregnant woman contracts this disease, the baby may be stillborn or suffer mental disabilities or other birth defects.

Maternal Age The average age at which a woman has her first child has been creeping up (from 21 in 1970 to almost 26 today), so a woman who becomes pregnant after age 35 has plenty of company. Although births to women in their twenties are declining, the rate of first births to women between the ages of 30 and 39 is the highest reported in four decades, and births to women over 39 have continued to increase slightly over the years.[68]

Statistically, the chances of having a baby with birth defects rise after the age of 35. Researchers believe this is due to a decline in the quality of eggs after this age. Two specific age-related risks are miscarriage and **Down syndrome.** The risk of miscarriage nearly doubles for women 35 to 45 compared to women under 35.[69] Another concern is that a woman's fertility begins to decline as she ages. Less than 10 percent of women in their early twenties have issues with infertility, compared to nearly 30 percent of women in their early forties.

While some risks increase with age, many doctors note that older mothers bring some advantages to their pregnancies: They tend to follow medical advice during pregnancy more thoroughly, are more mature psychologically, better prepared financially, and generally more ready to care for an infant than are some younger women.

Prenatal Testing and Screening Modern technology enables medical practitioners to detect health defects in a fetus as early as the fourteenth to eighteenth weeks of pregnancy. One common test is **ultrasonography** or **ultrasound,** which uses high-frequency sound waves to create a *sonogram,* or visual image, of the fetus in the uterus. The sonogram is used to determine the fetus' size and position. Knowing the baby's position helps health care providers perform other tests and safely deliver the infant. Sonograms can also detect birth defects in the nervous and digestive systems.

Chorionic villus sampling (CVS) involves snipping tissue from the developing fetal sac. Chorionic villus sampling can be used at 10 to 12 weeks of pregnancy. This is an attractive option for couples who are at high risk for having a baby with Down syndrome or a debilitating hereditary disease.

The **triple marker screen** (often called the TMS or AFT [alpha-fetoprotein] test) is a commonly used maternal blood test that is optimally conducted between the sixteenth and eighteenth weeks of pregnancy. The TMS is a screening test, not a diagnostic tool; it can detect susceptibility for a birth defect or genetic abnormality, but it is not meant to confirm a diagnosis of any condition. A *quad screen test* (or AFP-plus test) is also available. Because it screens for an additional protein in maternal blood, it is more accurate than the triple marker screen. Even more precise is the *integrated screen,* which used the quad screen, plus results from an earlier blood test, plus ultrasound, to screen for abnormalities.

Amniocentesis is a common testing procedure that is

WHAT DO YOU THINK?

Would you want to know if you or your partner were carrying a child with a genetic birth defect or other abnormality?

- Would you consider having your genes tested before starting a family?
- What would you do if both you and your partner were carriers of a genetic disorder that could be passed to your children?

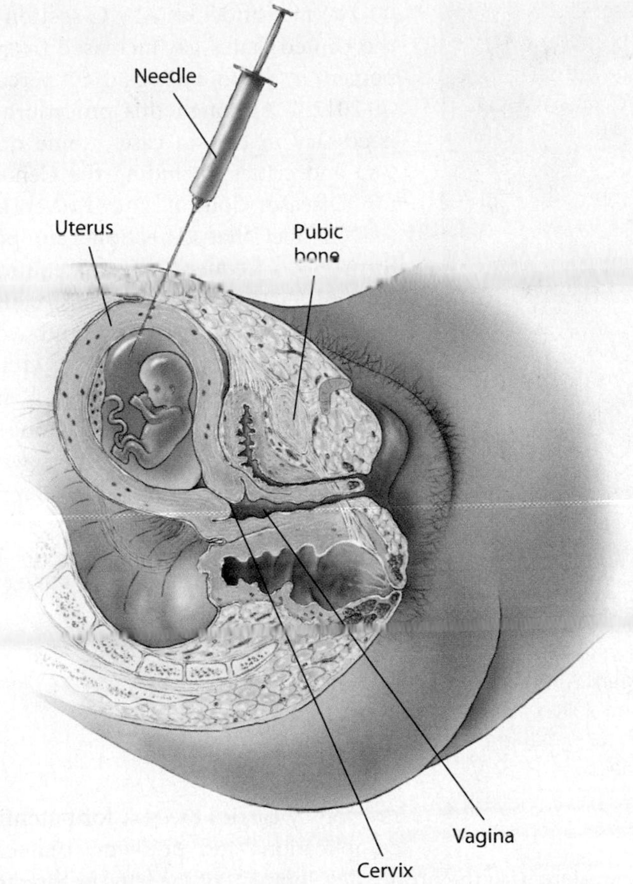

FIGURE 6.12 **Amniocentesis** The process of amniocentesis, in which a long needle is used to withdraw a small amount of amniotic fluid for genetic analysis, can detect certain congenital problems as well as the fetus's sex.

strongly recommended for women over age 35. This test involves inserting a long needle through the mother's abdominal and uterine walls into the **amniotic sac**, the protective pouch surrounding the fetus. The needle draws out 3 to 4 teaspoons of fluid, which is analyzed for genetic information about the baby (**FIGURE 6.12**). Amniocentesis can be performed between weeks 14 and 18.

If any of these tests reveals a serious birth defect, parents are advised to undergo genetic counseling. In the case of a chromosomal abnormality such as Down syndrome, the parents are usually offered the option of a therapeutic abortion. Some parents choose this option; others research the condition and decide to continue the pregnancy.

LO 12 | CHILDBIRTH

Explain the basic stages of childbirth and complications that can arise during pregnancy, labor, and delivery.

Prospective parents need to make several key decisions before the baby is born. These include where to have the baby, whether to use pain medication during labor and delivery, which childbirth method to choose, and whether to breast-feed or use formula. Answering these questions in advance will help to smooth the passage into parenthood.

Labor and Delivery

During the few weeks preceding delivery, the baby normally shifts to a head-down position, and the cervix begins to dilate (widen). The junction of the pubic bones loosens to permit expansion of the pelvic girdle during birth. The exact mechanisms that initiate labor are unknown. A change in the hormones in the fetus and mother cause strong uterine contractions to occur, signaling the beginning of labor. Another common early signal is the breaking of the amniotic sac, which causes a rush of fluid from the vagina (commonly referred to as "water breaking").

amniotic sac Protective pouch surrounding the fetus.

The birth process has three stages, shown in **FIGURE 6.13**, which can last from several hours to more than a day.

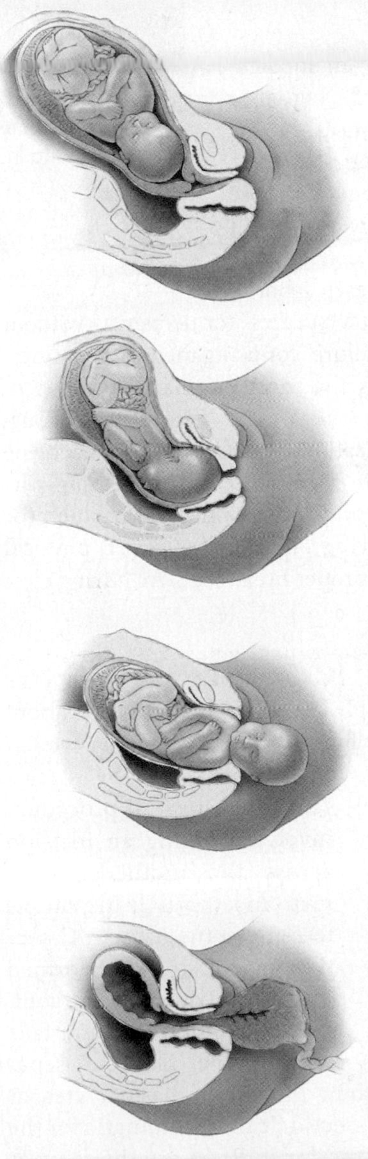

❶ **Stage I: Dilation of the cervix** Contractions in the abdomen and lower back push the baby downward, putting pressure on the cervix and dilating it. The first stage of labor may last from a couple of hours to more than a day for a first birth, but it is usually much shorter during subsequent births.

❷ **End of Stage I: Transition** The cervix becomes fully dilated, and the baby's head begins to move into the vagina (birth canal). Contractions usually come quickly during transition, which generally lasts 30 minutes or less.

❸ **Stage II: Expulsion** Once the cervix has become fully dilated, contractions become rhythmic, strong, and more intense as the uterus pushes the baby headfirst through the birth canal. The expulsion stage lasts 1 to 4 hours and concludes when the infant is finally pushed out of the mother's body.

❹ **Stage III: Delivery of the placenta** In the third stage, the placenta detaches from the uterus and is expelled through the birth canal. This stage is usually completed within 30 minutes after delivery.

FIGURE 6.13 **The Birth Process**
The entire process of labor and delivery usually takes from 2 to 36 hours. Labor is generally longer for a woman's first delivery and shorter for subsequent births.

In some cases, toward the end of the second stage, the attending health care provider may perform an *episiotomy*, a straight incision in the mother's perineum (the area between the vulva and the anus), to prevent the baby's head from tearing vaginal tissues and to speed the baby's exit from the vagina. Upon exit, the baby takes its first breath, which is generally accompanied by a loud wail. After delivery, the attending provider assesses the baby's overall condition, clears the baby's mucus-filled breathing passages, and ties and severs the umbilical cord. The mother's uterus continues to contract in the third stage of labor until the placenta is expelled.

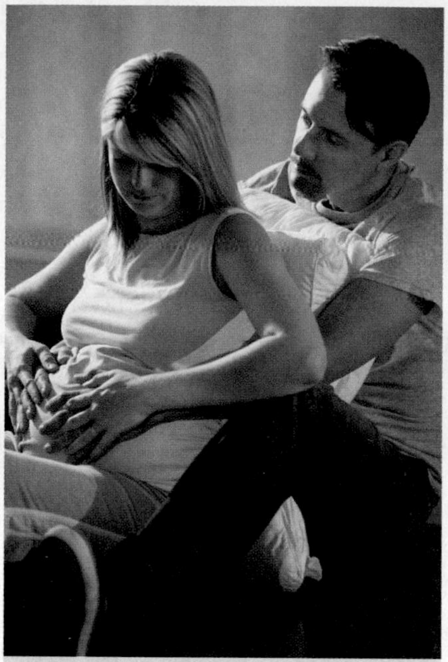
Expectant parents often take part in childbirth classes to learn what to expect during labor and delivery and to practice techniques for breathing and relaxation during labor.

Managing Labor Pain medication given to the mother during labor can cause sluggish responses in the newborn and other complications. For this reason, some women choose a drug-free labor and delivery—but it is important to keep a flexible attitude about pain relief, because each labor is different. One person is not a "success" for delivering without medication or another a "failure" for using medical measures.

The Lamaze method is the most popular technique of childbirth preparation in the United States. It discourages the use of pain medication. Prelabor classes teach the mother to control her pain through special breathing patterns, focusing exercises, and relaxation. The partner (or labor coach) assists by giving emotional support, physical comfort, and coaching for proper breath control during contractions.

Cesarean Section (C-Section) If labor lasts too long or if a baby is in physiological distress or is about to exit the uterus any way but headfirst, a **cesarean section (C-section)** may be necessary. This surgical procedure involves making an incision across the mother's abdomen and through the uterus to remove the baby. A C-section may also be performed if labor is extremely difficult, maternal blood pressure falls rapidly, the placenta separates from the uterus too soon, the mother has diabetes, or other problems occur. A C-section can be traumatic for the mother if she is not prepared for it. Risks are the same as for any major abdominal surgery, and recovery from birth takes considerably longer after a C-section.

cesarean section (C-section) Surgical birthing procedure in which a baby is removed through an incision made in the mother's abdominal wall and uterus.

preeclampsia Pregnancy complication characterized by high blood pressure, protein in the urine, and edema.

The rate of delivery by C-section in the United States has increased from 5 percent in the mid-1960s to 33 percent in 2012.[70] Although this procedure is necessary in certain cases, some doctors and critics, including the Centers for Disease Control and Prevention (CDC), feel that C-sections are performed too frequently in this country. Natural birth advocates suggest that hospitals, driven by profits and worried about malpractice, are too quick to intervene in the birth process. Some doctors say that the increase is due to maternal demand: busy mothers want to schedule their deliveries.[71] Parents need to be aware that inducing labor early can have negative impacts on the baby's health and should be avoided unless essential.

Complications of Pregnancy and Childbirth

Pregnancy carries the risk for potential complications and problems that can interfere with the proper development of the fetus or threaten the health of the mother and child. Some complications may result from a preexisting health condition of the mother, such as diabetes or an STI, and others can develop during pregnancy and may result from physiological problems, genetic abnormalities, or exposure to teratogens.

Preeclampsia and Eclampsia **Preeclampsia** is a condition characterized by high blood pressure, protein in the urine, and edema (fluid retention), which usually causes swelling of the hands and face. Symptoms may include sudden weight gain, headache, nausea or vomiting, changes in vision, racing pulse, mental confusion, and stomach or right shoulder pain. If preeclampsia is not treated, it can cause strokes and seizures, a condition called *eclampsia*. Potential problems can include liver and kidney damage, internal bleeding, stroke, poor fetal growth, and fetal and maternal death.

Preeclampsia tends to occur in the late second or third trimester. The cause is unknown; however, the incidence is higher in first-time mothers; women over 40 or under 18 years of age; women carrying multiple fetuses; and women with a history of chronic hypertension, diabetes, kidney disorder, or previous history of preeclampsia. Family history of preeclampsia is also a risk factor, whether the history is on the father's or mother's side. Treatment for preeclampsia ranges from bed rest and monitoring for mild cases to hospitalization and close monitoring for more severe cases.

Miscarriage

Even when a woman does everything "right," not every pregnancy ends in delivery. In fact, in the United States, between 15 to 20 percent of known pregnancies end in **miscarriage** (also referred to as *spontaneous abortion*).[72] Most miscarriages occur during the first trimester.

Reasons for miscarriage vary. In some cases, the fertilized egg has failed to divide correctly. In others, genetic abnormalities, maternal illness, or infections are responsible. Maternal hormonal imbalance may also cause a miscarriage, as may a weak cervix, toxic chemicals in the environment, or physical trauma to the mother. In most cases, the cause is not known.

Rh Factor

A rare blood incompatibility between mother and fetus can cause **Rh factor** problems, sometimes resulting in miscarriage. Rh is a blood protein, and problems occur when the mother is Rh-negative and the fetus is Rh-positive. During a first birth, some of the baby's blood passes into the mother's bloodstream. An Rh-negative mother may manufacture antibodies to destroy the Rh-positive blood introduced into her bloodstream at the time of birth. Her first baby will be unaffected, but subsequent babies with positive Rh factor will be at risk for a severe anemia called *hemolytic disease,* because the mother's Rh antibodies will attack the fetus's red blood cells. Prevention is preferable to treatment. Women with Rh-negative blood should be injected with a medication called RhoGAM within 72 hours after any birth, miscarriage, or abortion. The injection prevents the mother from developing Rh antibodies.

Ectopic Pregnancy

The implantation of a fertilized egg outside the uterus, usually in the fallopian tube or occasionally in the pelvic cavity, is called an **ectopic pregnancy.** Because these structures are not capable of expanding and nourishing a developing fetus, the pregnancy must be terminated surgically or a miscarriage will occur. Ectopic pregnancy is generally accompanied by pain in the lower abdomen or aching in the shoulders as blood flows upward toward the diaphragm. If bleeding is significant, blood pressure drops, and the woman can go into shock. If an ectopic pregnancy progresses undiagnosed and untreated, the fallopian tube will rupture, which puts the woman at great risk of hemorrhage, peritonitis (infection in the abdomen), and even death. Ectopic pregnancy occurs in about 2 percent of pregnancies in North America and is a leading cause of maternal mortality in the first trimester.[73] Ectopic pregnancy is a potential side effect of pelvic inflammatory disease, which has become increasingly common. The scarring or blockage of the fallopian tubes that occurs with this disease prevents a fertilized egg from passing to the uterus.

Stillbirth

One of the most traumatic events a couple can face is a **stillbirth.** Stillbirth is the death of a fetus *after* the twentieth week of pregnancy but before delivery. A stillborn baby is born dead, often for no apparent reason. Each year in the United States, there is about 1 stillbirth in every 160 births.[74] Birth defects, placental problems, poor fetal growth, infections, and umbilical cord accidents are known contributing factors.

miscarriage Loss of the fetus before it is viable; also called *spontaneous abortion.*

Rh factor Antigen present in the red blood cells of 85 percent of people; those with the Rh factor are known as Rh positive (Rh^+); those without it are Rh negative (Rh^-).

ectopic pregnancy Dangerous condition that results from the implantation of a fertilized egg outside the uterus, usually in a fallopian tube.

stillbirth Fetus that is dead at birth.

postpartum depression Mood disorder experienced by women who have given birth; involves depression, fatigue, and other symptoms and may last for weeks or months.

The Postpartum Period

The postpartum period lasts 6 weeks after delivery. During this period, many women experience fluctuating emotions. For many new mothers, the physical stress of labor, dehydration and blood loss, and other stresses challenge their stamina. Many new mothers experience what is called the "baby blues," characterized by periods of sadness, anxiety, headache, sleep disturbances, and irritability. For most women, these symptoms disappear after a short while. About 1 in 7 new mothers experience **postpartum depression,** a more disabling syndrome characterized by mood swings, lack of energy, crying, guilt, and depression. It can happen anytime within the first year after childbirth. Mothers who experience postpartum depression should seek professional treatment. Counseling is the most common type of treatment, but sometimes medication is recommended.[75]

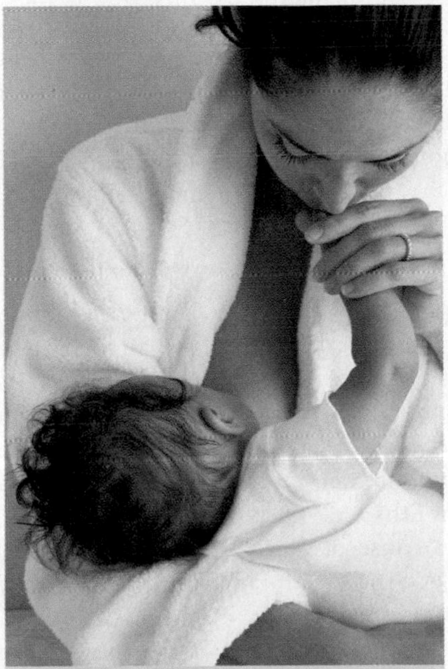

In addition to its numerous health benefits, breast-feeding enhances the development of intimate bonds between mother and child.

Breast-Feeding

Although the new mother's milk will not begin to flow for 2 or more days after delivery, her breasts secrete a yellow fluid called *colostrum* beginning immediately after birth. Because colostrum contains vital antibodies to help fight infection and boost the baby's immune system, all newborns should be allowed to suckle.

The American Academy of Pediatrics strongly recommends that infants be exclusively breast-fed for 6 months and breast-fed as a supplement until 12 months of age. Scientific findings indicate there are many advantages to breast-feeding. Breast milk is perfectly matched to babies' nutritional needs as they grow. Breast-fed babies have fewer illnesses and a much lower hospitalization rate because breast milk contains maternal antibodies and immunological cells that stimulate the infant's immune system. When breast-fed babies do get sick, they recover more quickly. They are also less likely to be obese later in life than are babies fed formula, and they have fewer allergies. They may even be more intelligent: A recent study found that the longer a baby was breast-fed, the higher the IQ in adulthood. Researchers theorize that breast milk contains substances that enhance brain development.[76] Breast-feeding also has the added benefit of helping mothers lose weight after birth because the production of milk burns hundreds of calories a day. Breast-feeding also causes the hormone oxytocin to be released, which makes the uterus return to its normal size faster.

sudden infant death syndrome (SIDS) Sudden death of an infant under 1 year of age for no apparent reason.

infertility Inability to conceive after a year or more of trying.

Breast milk is not the only way to nourish a baby. Some women are unable or unwilling to breast-feed; women with certain medical conditions or taking certain medications are advised not to breast-feed. Prepared formulas can provide nourishment that allows a baby to grow and thrive. When deciding whether to breast-feed or formula-feed, mothers must consider their own desires and preferences, too. Both feeding methods can supply the physical and emotional closeness essential to the parent–child relationship.

WHY SHOULD I CARE?

Even if you use another method for contraception, it's a good idea to also use a condom for protection against STIs. You don't want to get an STI—not only can they be unpleasant right now, but some STIs can stay with you for life, causing lasting harm to your health and your fertility, not to mention wreaking havoc on your love life!

Infant Mortality After birth, infant death can be caused by birth defects, low birthweight, injuries, or unknown causes. In the United States, the unexpected death of a child under 1 year of age, for no apparent reason, is called **sudden infant death syndrome (SIDS)**. SIDS is responsible for about 2,500 deaths a year. It is the leading cause of death for children age 1 month to 1 year and most commonly occurs in babies less than 6 months old.[77] It is not a specific disease; rather, it is ruled a cause of death after all other possibilities are ruled out. A SIDS death is sudden and silent; death occurs quickly, often during sleep, with no signs of suffering.

The exact cause of SIDS is unknown, but a few risk factors are known. For example, babies placed to sleep on their stomachs are more likely to die from SIDS than those placed on their backs, as are babies who are placed on or covered by soft bedding; however, breast-feeding and avoiding exposure to tobacco smoke are known protective factors.[78]

Birthweight When a baby is born weighing less than 5½ pounds, it is considered low birthweight. About 1 in 12 babies in the United States is low birthweight. While some low birthweight babies are born healthy despite their size, others develop serious health problems. Low birthweight babies are more likely than babies with normal weight to have respiratory distress syndrome, bleeding in the brain, vision loss, and heart problems.[79]

LO 13 | INFERTILITY

Review primary causes of and possible solutions for infertility.

For the couple desperately wishing to conceive, the road to parenthood may be frustrating. An estimated 1 in 10 American couples experiences **infertility**, usually defined as the inability to conceive after trying for a year or more. Although the focus is often on women, in about 20 percent of cases, infertility is due to a cause involving only the male partner, and in about 30 to 40 percent of cases, infertility is due to causes involving both partners.[80] Because of this, it is important for both partners to be medically evaluated.

Reasons for the high level of infertility in the United States include the trend toward delaying childbirth (as a woman gets older, she is less likely to conceive), endometriosis, the rising incidence of pelvic inflammatory disease, and low sperm count. Environmental contaminants known as *endocrine disrupters*, including some pesticides and emissions from burning plastics, appear to affect fertility in both men and women. Stress and anxiety (in general and about fertility) can also interfere with getting pregnant. Obesity and diabetes, increasingly common in the United States today, also have reproductive implications.

Causes in Women

Most cases of infertility in women result from problems with ovulation. The most common cause for female infertility is polycystic ovary syndrome (PCOS). A woman's ovaries have follicles, which are tiny, fluid-filled sacs that hold the eggs. When an egg is mature, the follicle breaks open to release the egg so it can travel to the fallopian tubes for fertilization. In women with PCOS, immature follicles bunch together to form large cysts or lumps. The eggs mature within the bunched follicles, but the follicles don't break open to release them. As a result, women with PCOS often don't have menstrual periods, or they have periods infrequently. Because eggs are not released, most women with PCOS have trouble getting pregnant. Researchers estimate that 5 to 10 percent of women of childbearing age—as many as 5 million women in the United States—have PCOS.[81]

While obesity doesn't cause infertility, it is a risk factor for PCOS. It also increases the level of estrogen in the

SEE IT! VIDEOS

Infertility can be troubling issue. Watch **What Are the Reasons for Infertility?** available on MasteringHealth.™

body and can cause ovulatory disorders, both of which interfere with getting pregnant.[82]

In some women, the ovaries stop functioning before natural menopause, a condition called *premature ovarian failure*. Other causes of infertility include **endometriosis**. With this very painful disorder, parts of the lining of the uterus implant outside the uterus, blocking the fallopian tubes. The disorder can be treated surgically or with hormonal therapy.

Pelvic inflammatory disease (PID) is a serious infection that scars the fallopian tubes and blocks sperm migration. (See **Chapter 14** for more on PID.) Infection-causing bacteria (chlamydia or gonorrhea) can invade the fallopian tubes, causing normal tissue to turn into scar tissue. This scar tissue blocks or interrupts the normal movement of eggs into the uterus. If the fallopian tubes are totally blocked by scar tissue, a woman becomes infertile. Infertility also can occur if the fallopian tubes are partially blocked or even slightly damaged. About 1 in 10 women with PID becomes infertile, and if a woman has multiple episodes of PID, her chance of becoming infertile increases.[83]

Causes in Men

Among men, the single largest fertility problem is **low sperm count**.[84] Although only one viable sperm is needed for fertilization, research has shown that all the other sperm in the ejaculate aid in the fertilization process. There are normally 60 to 80 million sperm per milliliter of semen. When the count drops below 20 million, fertility declines.

Low sperm count may be attributable to environmental factors (such as exposure of the scrotum to intense heat or cold, radiation, certain chemicals, or altitude), being overweight, or wearing excessively tight underwear or clothing. Other factors, such as the mumps virus, can damage the cells that make sperm, or varicocele (enlarged veins on a man's testicle) can heat the testicles and damage the sperm.[85]

Infertility Treatments

Medical procedures can identify the cause of infertility in about 90 percent of cases.[86] Once the cause has been determined, the chances of becoming pregnant range from 30 to 70 percent, depending on the reason for infertility.[87] The numerous tests and the invasion of privacy that are often involved in efforts to conceive can put stress on an otherwise strong, healthy relationship. A good physician or fertility team will take the time to ascertain a couple's level of motivation and coping skills.

Workups to determine the cause of infertility can be expensive, and the costs are not usually covered by health insurance. Fertility workups for men include a sperm count, a test for sperm motility, and an analysis of any disease processes present. Women are thoroughly examined by an obstetrician-gynecologist to determine the composition of cervical mucus and evidence of tubal scarring or endometriosis.

Fertility Drugs Fertility drugs stimulate ovulation in women who are not ovulating. Of women who use these drugs, 60 to 80 percent will begin to ovulate; of those who ovulate, about half will conceive.[88] Fertility drugs can have many side effects, including headaches, depression, fatigue, fluid retention, and abnormal uterine bleeding. Women using fertility drugs are also at increased risk of developing multiple ovarian cysts (fluid-filled growths) and liver damage. The drugs sometimes trigger the release of more than one egg. As many as 1 in 3 women treated with fertility drugs will become pregnant with more than one child.[89]

Alternative Insemination Another treatment option is **alternative insemination** (also known as *artificial insemination*) of a woman with her partner's sperm. The couple may also choose insemination by an anonymous donor through a sperm bank. Donated sperm are medically screened, classified according to the donor's physical characteristics (such as hair and eye color), and then frozen for future use.

Assisted Reproductive Technology Assisted reproductive technology (ART) includes several different medical procedures that help a woman become pregnant. The most common is **in vitro fertilization (IVF)**. During IVF, eggs and sperm are mixed in a laboratory dish to fertilize, and some of the fertilized eggs (zygotes) are then transferred to the woman's uterus.

Other types of assisted reproductive technologies include the following:

- Intracytoplasmic sperm injection (ICSI), which involves the injection of a single sperm into an egg. The fertilized egg is then placed in the woman's uterus or fallopian tube. Used with IVF, ICSI is often a successful treatment for men with impaired sperm.
- Gamete intrafallopian transfer (GIFT), which involves collecting eggs from the ovaries, then placing them into a thin flexible tube with the sperm. This mixture is then injected into the woman's fallopian tubes, where fertilization takes place.
- Zygote intrafallopian transfer (ZIFT), which combines IVF and GIFT. Eggs and sperm are mixed outside the body. The fertilized eggs (zygotes) are then returned to the fallopian tubes, through which they travel to the uterus.

endometriosis Disorder in which endometrial tissue establishes itself outside the uterus.

pelvic inflammatory disease (PID) Inflammation of the female genital tract that may cause scarring or blockage of the fallopian tubes, resulting in infertility.

low sperm count Sperm count below 20 million sperm per milliliter of semen.

alternative insemination Fertilization procedure accomplished by depositing semen from a partner or donor into a woman's vagina via a thin tube.

in vitro fertilization (IVF) Fertilization of an egg in a nutrient medium and subsequent transfer back to the mother's body.

Other Infertility Treatments In *nonsurgical embryo transfer,* a donor egg is fertilized by the man's sperm and implanted in the woman's uterus. In *embryo transfer,* an ovum from a donor is artificially inseminated by the man's sperm, allowed to stay in the donor's body for a time, and then transplanted into the woman's body. Infertile couples have another alternative—embryo adoption programs. Fertility treatments such as IVF often produce excess fertilized eggs that couples may choose to donate for other infertile couples to adopt.

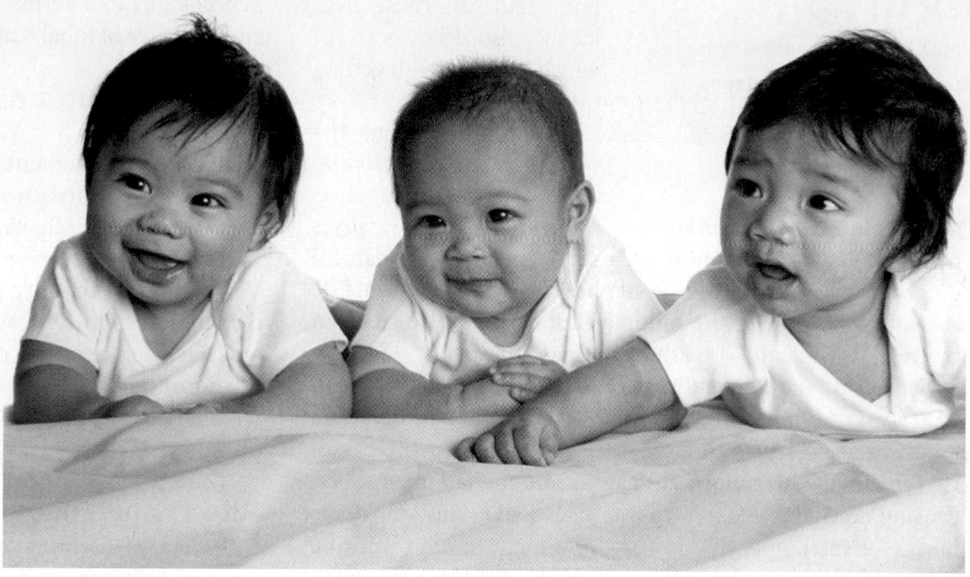

In addition to helping infertile couples, these technologies can also help young women who are not yet ready to have a baby, but who are concerned about future infertility. A woman can have her eggs frozen to be fertilized in the future when she is ready for a child.

There are many ethical and moral questions surrounding infertility treatments. Before deciding on a treatment, you must ask yourself important questions: Has infertility been confirmed? Have all alternatives and potential risks been considered? Have you examined your attitudes, values, and beliefs about conceiving a child in this manner? Finally, will you tell your child about the method of conception, and if so, how?

Surrogate Motherhood

Many infertile couples are able to conceive after treatment. Those who cannot conceive may choose to live without children, or they may decide to adopt or to pursue surrogate motherhood. With surrogacy, a woman is hired to carry another person's pregnancy to term, at which point the intended parents gain custody. In traditional surrogacy, the gestational carrier is also the biological mother of the child. In gestational surrogacy, the surrogate is not the biological mother; instead an embryo is created via IVF using the couple's own (or donor) egg and sperm. In the United States, an estimated 750 children a year are born via surrogate.[90] The practice has become increasingly popular in the past decade; not only does it help infertile couples, but gay male couples can also use a surrogate to carry one partner's biological child. Couples considering surrogate motherhood are advised to consult a lawyer before entering into this type of contract.

Adoption

Adoption serves several important purposes. It provides a way for individuals and couples who may not be able to have a biological child to form a legal parental relationship with a child who needs a home. As such, it benefits children whose birth parents are unable or unwilling to raise them and provides adults who are unable to conceive or carry a pregnancy to term a means to create a family. It is estimated that approximately 2 percent of the U.S. adult population has adopted children.[91]

There are two types of adoption: *confidential* and *open.* In confidential adoption, the birth parents and the adoptive parents never know each other. Adoptive parents are given only basic information about the birth parents, such as medical background that they need to care for the child. In open adoption, birth parents and adoptive parents know some information about each other. There are different levels of openness. Both parties must agree to this plan, and it is not available in every state.

Increasingly, couples are choosing to adopt children from other countries. In 2013, U.S. families adopted more than 9,000 foreign-born children.[92] The cost of overseas adoption varies widely, but can cost more than $30,000, including agency fees, dossier and immigration processing fees, travel, and court costs.[93] However, it may be a good alternative for many couples, especially those who want to adopt an infant rather than an older child. Some families find it beneficial to serve as foster parents prior to deciding to adopt, and others choose to adopt older children from the foster system in the United States rather than wait for an infant placed through international adoption.

STUDY PLAN

Customize your study plan—and master your health!—in the Study Area of **MasteringHealth.**

ASSESS **YOURSELF**

Is your current method of contraception right for you? Want to find out? Take the **Are You Comfortable with Your Contraception?** assessment available on MasteringHealth.™

Need help creating a plan? Follow the strategies in the **Your Plan for Change** box for short- and long-term improvements to your health.

YOUR PLAN FOR **CHANGE**

The **ASSESS YOURSELF** activity gave you the chance to look at your contraception preferences and habits. After completing the activity, you may want to to explore new contraception options.

TODAY, YOU CAN:

- ☐ Visit your local drugstore and study the forms of contraception that are available without a prescription. Think about those you would consider using and why.
- ☐ If you are not currently using any contraception or are not in a sexual relationship now, but might be in the future, purchase a package of condoms (or pick up free samples from your campus health center) to keep on hand just in case.

WITHIN THE NEXT 2 WEEKS, YOU CAN:

- ☐ Make an appointment for a checkup with your health care provider. Be sure to ask him or her any questions you have about contraception.
- ☐ Sit down with your partner and discuss contraception. Talk about how your current method is working for both of you, if the effectiveness level of the method you are using is high enough, and if you aren't using birth control consistently, what you can do together to improve.

BY THE END OF THE SEMESTER, YOU CAN:

- ☐ Periodically reevaluate whether your new or continued contraception is still effective for you. Review your experiences, and take note of any consistent problems you may have encountered.
- ☐ Always keep a backup form of contraception on hand. Check this supply periodically and throw out and replace any supplies that have expired.

CHAPTER REVIEW

To hear an MP3 Tutor Session, scan here or visit the Study Area in **MasteringHealth.**

LO 1 Basic Principles of Birth Control

- Birth control, or contraception, prevents conception, the fertilization of an egg by sperm. Types of contraception include barrier, hormonal, surgical, and behavioral methods.

LO 2 Barrier Methods

- Latex or polyurethane male and female condoms, when used correctly for oral sex or intercourse, provide the most effective protection in preventing sexually transmitted infections (STIs). Other barrier contraceptive methods include spermicides, the diaphragm, the cervical cap, and the contraceptive sponge.

LO 3 Hormonal Methods

- Oral contraceptives, Ortho Evra, NuvaRing, Depo-Provera, and Nexplanon are examples of hormonal contraceptives containing synthetic estrogen and/or progestin.

LO 4 Intrauterine Contraceptives

- Intrauterine devices are small devices that can be placed in the uterus through the cervix and left for 3 to 10 years.

LO 5 Emergency Contraception

- Emergency contraception may be used after unprotected intercourse or the failure of another contraceptive method.

LO 6 Behavioral Methods

- Fertility awareness methods rely on altering sexual practices to avoid pregnancy, as do abstinence, outercourse, and withdrawal.

LO 7 Surgical Methods

- While most methods of contraception are reversible, sterilization is permanent.

LO 8 Choosing a Method of Contraception

- Choosing a method of contraception involves taking time to research the various options, asking questions of your health care provider, being honest with yourself, and having open conversations with potential partners.

LO 9 Abortion

- Abortion is legal in the United States, but strongly opposed by many Americans. Abortion methods include suction curettage, dilation and evacuation (D&E), and medical abortions. Intact dilation and extraction (D&X) is no longer legal in the United States.

LO 10 Looking Ahead to Pregnancy and Parenthood

- Parenting is a demanding job that requires careful planning. Prospective parents must consider emotional health, maternal and paternal health, and financial resources.

LO 11 Pregnancy

- Full-term pregnancy has three trimesters. Prenatal care includes a complete physical exam within the first trimester, follow-up checkups throughout the pregnancy, healthy nutrition and exercise, and avoidance of all substances that could have teratogenic effects on the fetus, such as alcohol and drugs, tobacco smoke, X-rays, and harmful chemicals. Prenatal tests, including ultrasonography, chorionic villus sampling, triple marker screen, and amniocentesis, can be used to detect birth defects.

LO 12 Childbirth

- Childbirth occurs in three stages. Partners should jointly choose a labor method early in the pregnancy to be better prepared when labor occurs. Possible complications of pregnancy and childbirth include preeclampsia and eclampsia, miscarriage, Rh factor problems, ectopic pregnancy, and stillbirth.

LO 13 Infertility

- Infertility in women may be caused by pelvic inflammatory disease (PID) or endometriosis. In men, it may be caused by low sperm count. Treatments may include fertility drugs, alternative insemination, in vitro fertilization (IVF), assisted reproductive technology (ART), embryo transfer, and embryo adoption programs. Surrogate motherhood and adoption are also options.

POP QUIZ

Visit **MasteringHealth** to personalize your study plan with Chapter Review Quizzes and Dynamic Study Modules.

LO 1 Basic Principles of Birth Control

1. What is meant by the *failure rate* of contraceptive use?
   a. The number of times a woman fails to get pregnant when she wanted to
   b. The number of times a woman gets pregnant when she did not want to
   c. The number of pregnancies that occur in women using a particular method of birth control
   d. The number of times a couple fails to use birth control

LO 2 Barrier Methods

2. Which type of lubricant could you safely use with a latex condom?
   a. Mineral oil
   b. Water-based lubricant
   c. Body lotion
   d. Petroleum jelly

3. Which of the following is a barrier contraceptive?
   a. Seasonale
   b. FemCap
   c. Ortho Evra
   d. Contraceptive patch

LO **3** | **Hormonal Methods**

4. Hormonal birth control methods contain estrogen and/or
   a. oxytocin.
   b. testosterone.
   c. cortisol.
   d. progestin.

LO **4** | **Intrauterine Contraceptives**

5. An IUD is placed in a woman's
   a. fallopian tube.
   b. ovary.
   c. uterus.
   d. vagina.

LO **5** | **Emergency Contraception**

6. Emergency contraception is up to 88 percent effective when used within how many days of unprotected intercourse?
   a. 1
   b. 2–5
   c. 5–7
   d. 7–14

LO **6** | **Behavioral Methods**

7. Mariana and David want to practice a method of avoiding pregnancy that is 100 percent effective. What method would you recommend?
   a. abstinence
   b. calendar method
   c. cervical mucus method
   d. condoms

LO **7** | **Surgical Methods**

8. Benjamin wants to be sterilized. The male sterilization process his health care provider will perform is called
   a. suction curettage.
   b. tubal ligation.
   c. hysterectomy.
   d. vasectomy.

LO **8** | **Choosing a Method of Contraception**

9. Emily wants to use a contraception method that also protects against STIs. She should use
   a. Ortho Evra.
   b. condoms.
   c. a contraceptive sponge.
   d. an IUD.

LO **9** | **Abortion**

10. What is the most commonly used method of first-trimester abortion?
    a. Suction curettage
    b. Dilation and evacuation (D&E)
    c. Medical abortion
    d. Induction abortion

LO **10** | **Looking Ahead to Pregnancy and Parenthood**

11. At which stage of life should women have preconception care?
    a. When becoming sexually active
    b. Before becoming pregnant
    c. In the second trimester of pregnancy
    d. During childbirth

LO **11** | **Pregnancy**

12. Toxic chemicals, pesticides, X-rays, and other hazardous compounds that cause birth defects are referred to as
    a. carcinogens.
    b. teratogens.
    c. mutants.
    d. environmental assaults.
13. What is the recommended pregnancy weight gain for a woman who is at a healthy weight before pregnancy?
    a. 15 to 20 pounds
    b. 20 to 30 pounds
    c. 25 to 35 pounds
    d. 30 to 45 pounds
14. Which prenatal test involves snipping tissue from the developing fetal sac?
    a. Triple marker screen
    b. Ultrasound
    c. Amniocentesis
    d. Chorionic villus sampling

LO **12** | **Childbirth**

15. In an ectopic pregnancy, the fertilized egg implants in the woman's
    a. fallopian tube.
    b. uterus.
    c. vagina.
    d. ovaries.

LO **13** | **Infertility**

16. The number of American couples who experience infertility is
    a. 1 in 10.
    b. 1 in 24.
    c. 1 in 60.
    d. 1 in 100.

Answers to the Pop Quiz can be found on page A-1. If you answered a question incorrectly, review the section identified by the Learning Outcome. For even more study tools, visit MasteringHealth.

THINK ABOUT IT!

LO **1** | **Basic Principles of Birth Control**

1. How, in general, do contraceptives work? What is the difference between "perfect use" and "typical use" failure rates? Which do you think is a better predictor of effectiveness?

LO **2** | **Barrier Methods**

2. What are the options for barrier birth control methods? What are their major advantages and disadvantages?

LO **3** | **Hormonal Methods**

3. What benefits can hormonal methods of birth control provide beyond preventing pregnancy?

How could a person go about deciding which of the many hormonal methods to try?

LO 4 Intrauterine Contraceptives

4. How quickly does fertility return after the removal of an IUD? Can women who have not yet had a child use an IUD?

LO 5 Emergency Contraception

5. What recent court decision has changed the availability of ECPs? Can you imagine using ECPs if you had a contraceptive failure?

LO 6 Behavioral Methods

6. Do your religious views impact your sexual behavior or choice of birth control methods? If so, how do they impact your family planning decisions?

LO 7 Surgical Methods

7. Do you think there should be an age limit on surgical methods so people don't give up their fertility too early? How do you think you will decide when you are done having children?

LO 8 Choosing a Method of Contraception

8. List the most effective contraceptive methods. What are their drawbacks? What medical conditions would keep a person from using each one? Which methods do you think would be most effective for you? Why?

LO 9 Abortion

9. What are the various methods of abortion? What are the two opposing viewpoints concerning abortion? What is *Roe v. Wade*, and what impact has it had on the abortion debate in the United States?

LO 10 Looking Ahead to Pregnancy and Parenthood

10. What are the most important considerations in deciding whether the time is right to become a parent? If you choose to have children, what factors will you consider in regard to the right time to have them and the number to have?

LO 11 Pregnancy

11. Discuss the growth of the fetus through the three trimesters. What medical checkups or tests should be done during each trimester?
12. Discuss the emotional aspects of pregnancy. What types of emotional reactions are common during each trimester and the postpartum period?

LO 12 Childbirth

13. Discuss some of the many decisions related to childbirth, including choice of provider, whether to use pain medication, whether to breastfeed, etc.
14. What are some of the complications that can occur during pregnancy and childbirth? What actions can we take to prevent these complications?

LO 13 Infertility

15. If you and your partner are unable to have children, what alternative methods of conception would you consider? Would you consider adoption?

ACCESS YOUR HEALTH ON THE INTERNET

Visit **MasteringHealth** for links to the websites and RSS feeds.

Use the following websites to further explore topics and issues related to reproductive health.

Guttmacher Institute. This is a nonprofit organization focusing on sexual and reproductive health research, policy analysis, and public education. **www.guttmacher.org**

Association of Reproductive Health Professionals. This organization was originally founded by Alan Guttmacher as the educational arm of Planned Parenthood. Now an independent organization, it provides education for health care professionals and the general public. The *Patient Resources* portion of the website includes information on various methods of birth control and an interactive tool to help you choose a method that will work for you. **www.arhp.org**

Planned Parenthood. This site offers a range of up-to-date information on sexual health issues, such as birth control, the decision of when and whether to have a child, sexually transmitted infections, abortion, and safer sex. **www.plannedparenthood.org**

The American Pregnancy Association. This is a national organization offering a wealth of resources to promote reproductive and pregnancy wellness. The website includes educational materials and information on the latest research. **www.americanpregnancy.org**

Centers for Disease Control and Prevention. The CDC provides up-to-date information on preconception care, pregnancy, breast-feeding, infant care, infertility, and contraception, all in one well-organized website. **www.cdc.gov/ncbddd/pregnancy_gateway/index.html**

American College of Nurse-Midwives. If the concept of midwifery is new to you, learn more about it at their website. **www.mymidwife.org**

International Council on Infertility Information Dissemination. This site includes current research and information on infertility. **www.inciid.org**

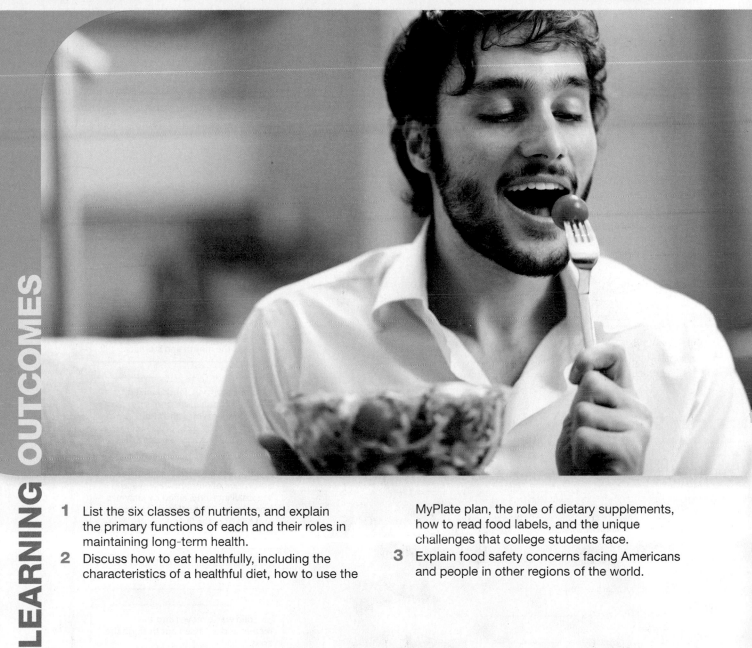

7 Nutrition: Eating for a Healthier You

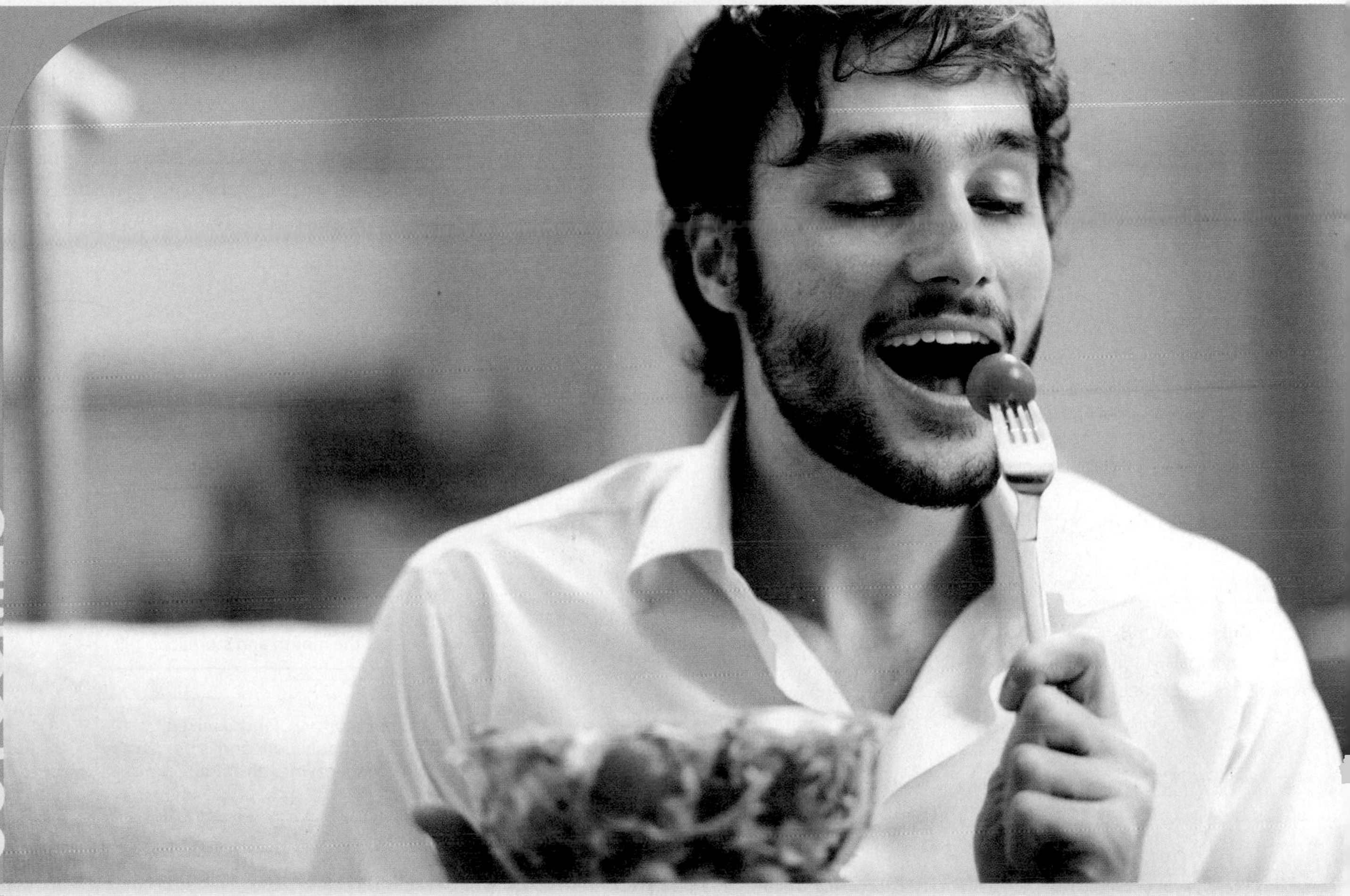

LEARNING OUTCOMES

1. List the six classes of nutrients, and explain the primary functions of each and their roles in maintaining long-term health.
2. Discuss how to eat healthfully, including the characteristics of a healthful diet, how to use the MyPlate plan, the role of dietary supplements, how to read food labels, and the unique challenges that college students face.
3. Explain food safety concerns facing Americans and people in other regions of the world.

Advice about food comes at us from all directions: from the Internet, popular magazines, television, friends, and neighbors. Even when this advice is backed by research, it can be contradictory. For example, some studies indicate that a balanced high-fat diet can be healthful, whereas other studies support consuming a low-fat diet. Choosing what to eat and how much to eat from this media-driven array of food advice can be mind-boggling. For some, this can cause unnecessary anxiety about eating and lead to a lifetime of cycling on and off diets.[1] Why does something that can be a source of pleasure end up being a problem for so many of us? What influences our eating habits, and how can we learn to eat more healthfully?

The answers to these questions aren't as simple as they may seem. When was the last time you ate because you felt truly hungry? True **hunger** occurs when our brains initiate a physiological response that prompts us to seek food for the energy and **nutrients** that our bodies require to maintain proper functioning. Often, people in the United States don't eat in response to hunger—instead, we eat because of **appetite,** a learned psychological desire to consume food. Hunger and appetite are not the only forces influencing our desire to eat. Cultural factors, food advertising, perceived nutritional value, social interaction, emotions, and financial means are other factors.

Nutrition is the science that investigates the relationship between physiological function and the essential elements of the foods we eat. With an understanding of nutrition, you

hunger The physiological impulse to seek food.

nutrients The constituents of food that sustain humans physiologically: water, proteins, carbohydrates, fats, vitamins, and minerals.

appetite The learned desire to eat; normally accompanies hunger but is more psychological than physiological.

nutrition The science that investigates the relationship between physiological function and the essential elements of foods eaten.

HEAR IT! PODCAST

Want a study podcast for this chapter? Download **Nutrition: Eating for Optimum Health** available on MasteringHealth.™

Mouth

Salivary glands

Esophagus

Liver

Stomach

Pancreas

Small intestine

Large intestine

Rectum

Anus

❶ Your mouth prepares for the food by increasing production of saliva, which aids in chewing and swallowing and contains an enzyme that begins breaking down some carbohydrates.

❷ From the mouth, the food passes down the esophagus, a tube that connects the mouth and stomach.

❸ In the stomach, food is mixed by muscular contractions and is broken down with enzymes and stomach acids.

❹ Further digestive activity and absorption of nutrients take place in the small intestine, aided by enzymes from the small intestine and pancreas, and bile from the liver.

❺ Water and salts are reabsorbed into the system by the large intestine.

❻ Solid waste moves into the rectum and is passed out through the anus.

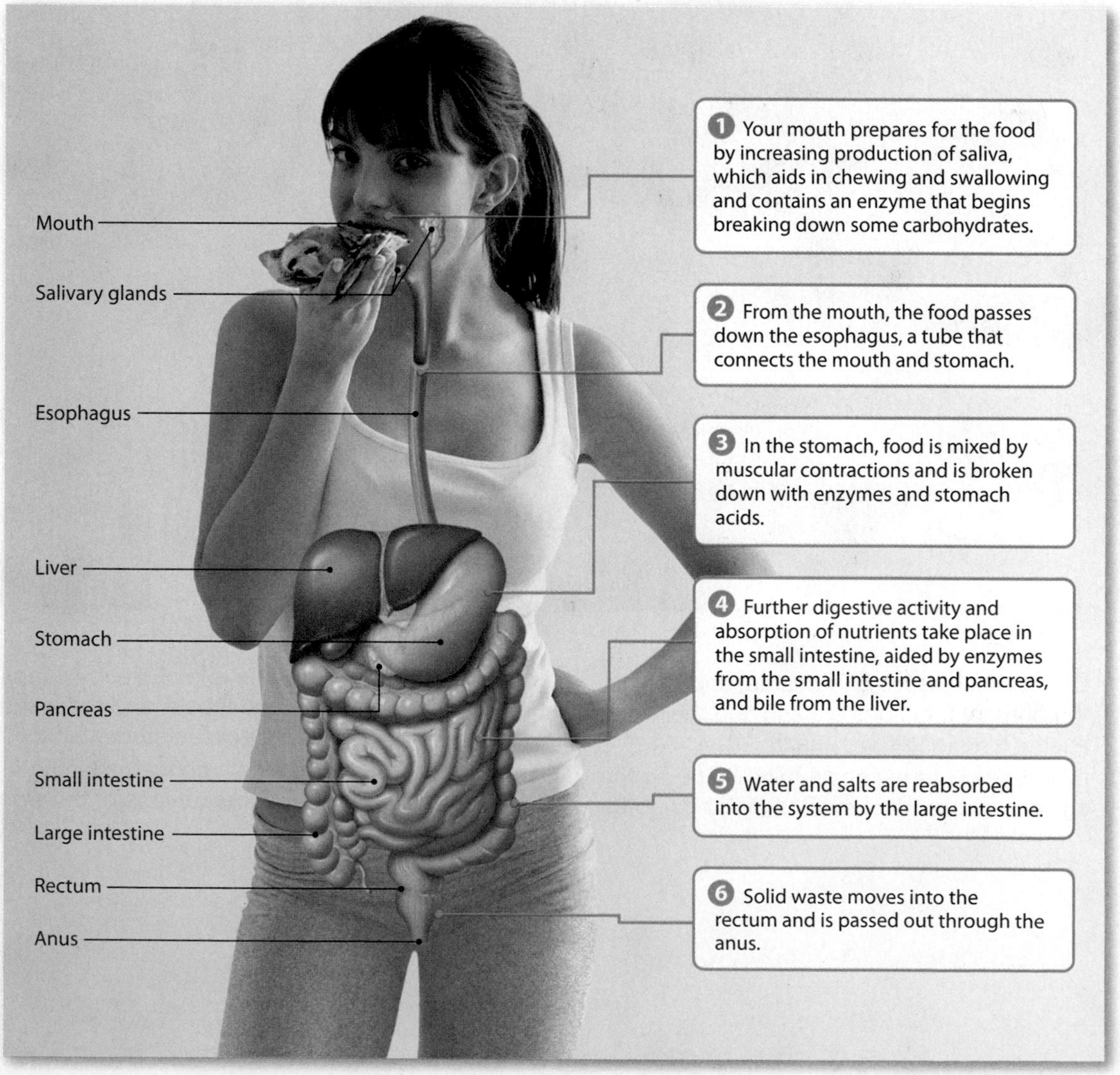

FIGURE 7.1 The **Digestive Process** The entire digestive process takes approximately 24 hours.

will be able to make more informed choices about your diet. Your health depends largely on what you eat, how much you eat, and the amount of exercise that you get throughout your life. The next few chapters focus on fundamental principles of nutrition, weight management, and exercise.

LO 1 | ESSENTIAL NUTRIENTS FOR HEALTH

List the six classes of nutrients, and explain the primary functions of each and their roles in maintaining long-term health.

Food provides the chemicals we need for activity and body maintenance. Our bodies cannot synthesize certain *essential nutrients* (or cannot synthesize them in adequate amounts); we must obtain them from the foods we eat. Of the six groups of essential nutrients, the four we need in the largest amounts—water, proteins, carbohydrates, and fats—are called *macronutrients*. The other two groups—vitamins and minerals—are needed in smaller amounts, so they are called *micronutrients*.

Before the body can use foods, the digestive system must break down larger food particles into smaller, more usable forms. The **digestive process** is the sequence of functions by which the body breaks down foods into molecules small enough to be absorbed and excretes the wastes. (See **FIGURE 7.1**.)

Recommended Intakes for Nutrients

In the next sections, we discuss each nutrient group and identify how much of each you need. These recommended amounts are known as the **Dietary Reference Intakes (DRIs)** and are published by the Food and Nutrition Board of the Institute of Medicine. The DRIs establish the amount of each nutrient needed to prevent deficiencies or reduce the risk of chronic disease, as well as identify maximum safe intake levels for healthy people. The DRIs are umbrella guidelines and include the following categories:

- **Recommended Dietary Allowances (RDAs)** are daily nutrient intake levels meeting the nutritional needs of 97 to 98 percent of healthy individuals.
- **Adequate Intakes (AIs)** are daily intake levels assumed to be adequate for most healthy people. AIs are used when there isn't enough research to support establishing an RDA.
- **Tolerable Upper Intake Levels (ULs)** are the highest amounts of a nutrient that an individual can consume daily without risking adverse health effects.
- **Acceptable Macronutrient Distribution Ranges (AMDRs)** are ranges of protein, carbohydrate, and fat intake that provide adequate nutrition, and they are associated with a reduced risk for chronic disease.

Whereas the RDAs, AIs, and ULs are expressed as amounts—usually milligrams (mg) or micrograms (μg)—AMDRs are expressed as percentages. The AMDR for protein, for example, is 10 to 35 percent, meaning that no less than 10 percent and no more than 35 percent of the calories you consume should come from proteins. But that raises a new question: What are calories?

DO IT! NUTRITOOLS
Complete the **Know Your Protein Sources** activity available on MasteringHealth.™

Calories

A *kilocalorie* is a unit of measure used to quantify the amount of energy in food. On nutrition labels and in consumer publications, the term is shortened to **calorie**. *Energy* is defined as the capacity to do work. We derive energy from the energy-containing nutrients in the foods we eat. These energy-containing nutrients—proteins, carbohydrates, and fats—provide calories. Vitamins, minerals, and water do not. **TABLE 7.1** shows the caloric needs for various individuals.

digestive process The process by which the body breaks down foods and either absorbs or excretes them.

Dietary Reference Intakes (DRIs) Set of recommended intakes for each nutrient published by the Institute of Medicine.

calorie A unit of measure that indicates the amount of energy obtained from a particular food.

TABLE 7.1 | Estimated Daily Calorie Needs

	Calorie Range		
	Sedentary[a]		Active[b]
Children			
2–3 years old	1,000	→	1,400
Females			
4–8 years old	1,200	→	1,800
9–13	1,400	→	2,200
14–18	1,800	→	2,400
19–30	1,800	→	2,400
31–50	1,800	→	2,200
51+	1,600	→	2,200
Males			
4–8 years old	1,200	→	2,000
9–13	1,600	→	2,600
14–18	2,000	→	3,200
19–30	2,400	→	3,000
31–50	2,200	→	3,000
51+	2,000	→	2,800

[a]A lifestyle that includes only the light physical activity associated with typical day-to-day life.

[b]A lifestyle that includes physical activity equivalent to walking more than 3 miles per day at 3 to 4 miles per hour, in addition to the light physical activity associated with typical day-to-day life.

Source: U.S. Department of Agriculture and U.S. Department of Health and Human Services, *Dietary Guidelines for Americans, 2010*, 7th ed. (Washington, DC: U.S. Government Printing Office).

Water: A Crucial Nutrient

Humans can survive for several weeks without food but only for about 1 week without water. **Dehydration**, a state of abnormal depletion of body fluids, can develop within a single day, especially in a hot climate. Too much water can also pose a serious risk to your health. This condition, *hyponatremia,* is characterized by low sodium levels.

The human body consists of 50 to 70 percent water by weight. The water in our system bathes cells; aids in fluid, electrolyte, and acid-base balance; and helps regulate body temperature. Water is the major component of our blood, which carries oxygen, nutrients, and hormones and other substances to body cells and removes metabolic wastes.

dehydration Abnormal depletion of body fluids; a result of lack of water.

proteins Large molecules made up of chains of amino acids; essential constituents of all body cells.

amino acids The nitrogen-containing building blocks of protein.

essential amino acids The nine basic nitrogen-containing building blocks of human proteins that must be obtained from foods.

complete proteins Proteins that contain all nine of the essential amino acids.

incomplete proteins Proteins that lack one or more of the essential amino acids.

Individual needs for water vary drastically according to dietary factors, age, size, overall health, environmental temperature and humidity levels, and exercise. We usually get the fluids we need each day through the water and other beverages we consume, as well as through the food we eat. In fact, fruits and vegetables are 80 to 95 percent water, meats are more than 50 percent water, and even dry bread and cheese are about 35 percent water! Contrary to popular opinion, caffeinated drinks, including coffee, tea, and soda, also count toward total fluid intake. Consumed in moderation, caffeinated beverages have not been found to dehydrate people whose bodies are used to caffeine.[2]

There are situations in which a person needs additional fluids in order to stay properly hydrated. It is important to drink extra fluids when you have a fever or an illness involving vomiting or diarrhea. Anyone with kidney function problems or who tends to develop kidney stones may need more water, as may people with diabetes or cystic fibrosis. The elderly and very young also may have increased water needs. When the weather heats up, or when you exercise, work, or engage in other activities in which you sweat profusely, extra water is needed to keep your body's core temperature within a normal range. If you are an athlete and wonder about water consumption, visit the American College of Sports Medicine's website (www.acsm.org) to download its brochure, "Selecting and Effectively Using Hydration for Fitness."[3]

Proteins

Next to water, **proteins** are the most abundant substances in the human body. Proteins are major components of living cells and are called the "body builders" because of their role in developing and repairing bone, muscle, skin, and blood cells. They are the key elements of antibodies that protect us from disease, enzymes that control chemical activities in the body, and many hormones that regulate body functions. Proteins also supply an alternative source of energy to cells when fats and carbohydrates are not available. Specifically, every gram of protein you eat provides 4 calories. (There are about 28 grams in an ounce.) Adequate protein in the diet is vital to many body functions and ultimately to survival.

Your body breaks down proteins into smaller nitrogen-containing molecules known as **amino acids,** the building blocks of protein. Nine of the 20 different amino acids needed by the body are termed **essential amino acids,** which means the body must obtain them from the diet; the other 11 amino acids are considered nonessential because the body can make them. Dietary protein that supplies all the essential amino acids is called **complete protein.** Typically, protein from animal products is complete.

Nearly all proteins from plant sources are **incomplete proteins** that lack one or more of the essential amino acids. However, it is easy to combine plant foods to produce a complete protein meal (**FIGURE 7.2**). Plant foods rich in incomplete

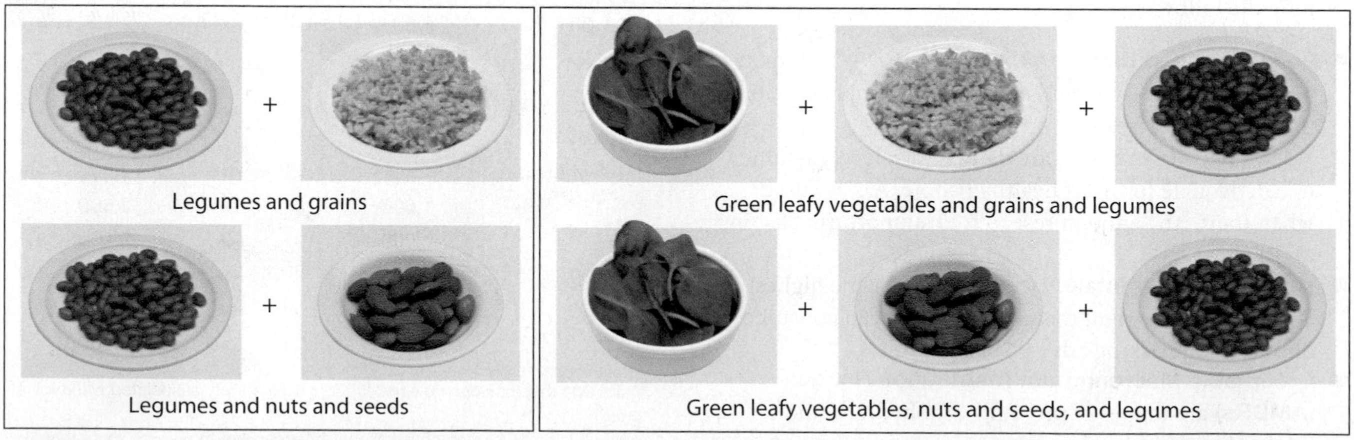

Legumes and grains
Green leafy vegetables and grains and legumes
Legumes and nuts and seeds
Green leafy vegetables, nuts and seeds, and legumes

FIGURE 7.2 Foods Providing Complementary Amino Acids Complementary combinations of plant-based foods can provide all essential amino acids. In some cases, you might need to combine three sources of protein to supply all nine; however, the foods do not necessarily have to be eaten in the same meal. Here, two of the limited amino acids in leafy green vegetables are supplied by either grains or nuts and seeds, and the third is found in legumes.

HEALTH IN A DIVERSE WORLD

GLOBAL MALNUTRITION

Are Insects the Answer?

Worldwide, 842 million people—about 1 in 8—do not have enough to eat. Inadequate protein intake is especially dangerous, and it is common in impoverished children. To reduce malnutrition, some experts in public health are recommending the breeding and harvesting of more than 1,400 species of edible, high-protein insects for food. Sound disgusting? Here are the facts:

- Insects are high in protein, ranging from 45 to 80 percent of their body weight.
- Many insects are also good sources of fats, certain B vitamins, zinc, and iron.
- Insects are more environmentally friendly to raise than cattle and pigs because they reproduce quickly, take little space to grow, require less feed and less water, and produce significantly less waste.

In many countries, insects are already a common food source. This vendor is selling insects in Rizhao, China.

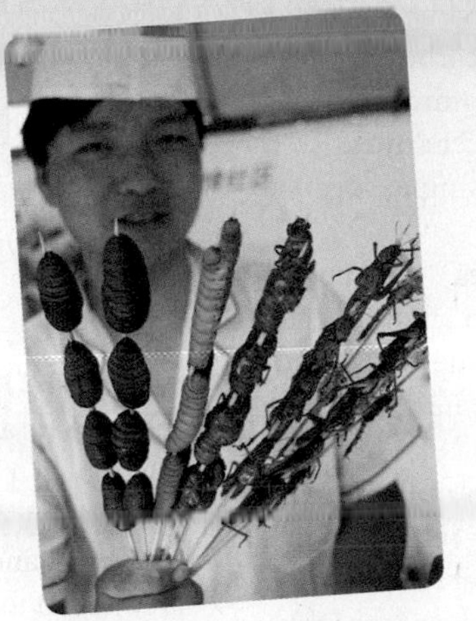

The practice of consuming bugs, called *entomophagy,* is already common in areas of Africa, Asia, and Mexico. Mopani worms and termites are popular snacks in Nigeria. Japanese restaurants serve boiled wasp larvae called *hachi-no-ko* or fried cicada called *semi*. Grasshoppers, known as *chapulinos,* are popular in Mexico.

Entomophagy is still considered socially unacceptable in the United States and Europe, although most Westerners unknowingly consume about a pound of insects a year that are accidently mixed into processed foods. Will Americans ever accept insects as part of a healthy diet? Perhaps if they could be processed into more conventional food forms. Bug Butter, anyone?

Sources: Food and Agriculture Organization of the United Nations, "The State of Food Insecurity in the World, 2012," FAO, 2013, www.fao.org/publications/sofi/en/; Department of Entomology, University of Kentucky College of Agriculture, 2010, www.ca.uky.edu/entomology/dept/bugfood2.asp; M. Dickie and A. Van Huis, "The Six Legged Meat of the Future," *Wall Street Journal*, 2011, http://online.wsj.com/article/SB10001424052748703293204576106072340020728.html.

proteins include *legumes* (beans, lentils, peas, peanuts, and soy products); *grains* (e.g., wheat, corn, rice, and oats); and *nuts and seeds.* Certain vegetables, such as leafy green vegetables and broccoli, also contribute valuable plant proteins. Consuming a variety of foods from these categories will provide all the essential amino acids.

Although protein deficiency poses a threat to the global population (see the **Health in a Diverse World** box), few Americans suffer from protein deficiencies. In fact, the average American consumes more than 79 grams of protein daily, much of it from high-fat animal flesh and dairy products.[4] The AMDR for protein is 10 to 35 percent of calories. Adults should consume about 0.8 gram (g) per kilogram (kg) of body weight.[5] To calculate your protein needs, divide your body weight in pounds by 2.2 to get your weight in kilograms, then multiply by 0.8. The result is your recommended protein intake per day. For example, a woman who weighs 130 pounds should consume about 47 grams of protein each day. A 6-ounce steak provides 53 grams of protein—more than she needs!

People who need to eat extra protein include pregnant women and patients fighting a serious infection, recovering from surgery or blood loss, or recovering from burns. In these instances, proteins that are lost to cellular repair and development need to be replaced. Athletes also require more protein to build and repair muscle fibers.[6] In addition, a sedentary person may find it easier to stay in energy balance when consuming a diet with a higher percentage of protein and a lower percentage of carbohydrate. Why? Because proteins make a person feel full for a longer period of time.

WHY SHOULD I CARE?

The nutritional choices you make during college can have both immediate and lasting effects on your health. Thousands of studies associate what we eat with chronic diseases such as diabetes, heart disease, hypertension, stroke, and many types of cancer.

carbohydrates Basic nutrients that supply the body with glucose, the energy form most commonly used to sustain normal activity.

Carbohydrates

Carbohydrates supply us with the energy we need to sustain normal daily activity. In comparison to proteins or fats, carbohydrates are broken down more quickly and efficiently, yielding a fuel called glucose. All body cells can burn glucose for fuel; moreover, glucose is the only fuel that red blood cells can use and is the primary fuel for the brain. Carbohydrates are the best fuel for moderate to intense

DO IT! NUTRITOOLS

Complete the **Know Your Carbohydrate Sources** activity available on MasteringHealth.™

exercise because they can be readily broken down to glucose even when we're breathing hard and our muscle cells are getting less oxygen.

Like proteins, carbohydrates provide 4 calories per gram. The RDA for adults is 130 grams of carbohydrate per day.[7] There are two major types: simple and complex.

Simple Carbohydrates

Simple carbohydrates or *simple sugars* are found naturally in fruits, many vegetables, and dairy. The most common form of simple carbohydrates is *glucose*. Fruits and berries contain *fructose* (commonly called *fruit sugar*). Glucose and fructose are **monosaccharides.** Eventually, the human body converts all types of simple sugars to glucose to provide energy to cells.

> **simple carbohydrates** A carbohydrate made up of only one sugar molecule, or of two sugar molecules bonded together; also called simple sugars.
>
> **monosaccharides** Simple sugars that contain only one molecule of sugar.
>
> **disaccharides** Combinations of two monosaccharides.
>
> **complex carbohydrates** A carbohydrate consisting of long chains of sugar molecules; also called a polysaccharide.
>
> **starches** Polysaccharides that are the storage forms of glucose in plants.
>
> **glycogen** The polysaccharide form in which glucose is stored in the liver and, to a lesser extent, in muscles.
>
> **fiber** The indigestible portion of plant foods that helps move food through the digestive system and softens stools by absorbing water.
>
> **whole grains** Grains that are milled in their complete form and thus include the bran, germ, and endosperm, with only the husk removed.

Disaccharides are combinations of two monosaccharides. Perhaps the best-known example is *sucrose* (granulated table sugar). *Lactose* (milk sugar), found in milk and milk products, and *maltose* (malt sugar) are other examples of common disaccharides. Disaccharides must be broken down into monosaccharides before the body can use them.

Sugar is found in high amounts in a wide range of processed food products. A classic example is the amount of sugar in one can of soda: more than 10 teaspoons per can! Moreover, such diverse items as ketchup, barbecue sauce, and flavored coffee creamers derive 30 to 65 percent of their calories from sugar. Read food labels carefully before purchasing. If *sugar* or one of its aliases (including *high fructose corn syrup* and *cornstarch*) appears near the top of the ingredients list, then that product contains a lot of sugar and is probably not your best nutritional bet. Also, most labels list the amount of sugar as a percentage of total calories.

Complex Carbohydrates: Starches and Glycogen

Complex carbohydrates are found in grains, cereals, legumes, and other vegetables. Also called *polysaccharides*, they are formed by long chains of monosaccharides. Like disaccharides, they must be broken down into simple sugars before the body can use them. *Starches, glycogen,* and *fiber* are the main types of complex carbohydrates.

Starches make up the majority of complex carbohydrates and come mostly from flours, breads, pasta, rice, corn, oats, and barley, as well as from legumes, potatoes, and other vegetables. The body breaks down these complex carbohydrates into glucose, which can be easily absorbed by cells and used as energy.

THE AVERAGE AMERICAN CONSUMES

15.9 grams

OF **FIBER** DAILY—MUCH LESS THAN THE RECOMMENDED 25 TO 38 GRAMS PER DAY.

When not needed for energy, glucose can be stored in body muscles and the liver as a polysaccharide called **glycogen.** When the body requires a sudden burst of energy, it breaks glycogen back down into glucose.

Complex Carbohydrates: Fiber

Sometimes referred to as "bulk" or "roughage," **fiber** is the indigestible portion of plant foods that helps move foods through the digestive system, delays absorption of cholesterol and other nutrients, and softens stools by absorbing water. Dietary fiber is found only in plant foods, such as fruits, vegetables, nuts, and grains.[8]

Fiber is either *soluble* or *insoluble*. Soluble fibers, such as pectins, gums, and mucilages, dissolve in water, form gel-like substances, and can be digested easily by bacteria in the colon. Major food sources of soluble fiber include citrus fruits, berries, oat bran, dried beans, and some vegetables. Insoluble fibers, such as lignins and cellulose, typically do not dissolve in water and cannot be fermented by bacteria in the colon. They are found in most fruits and vegetables and in **whole grains**, such as brown rice, wheat, bran, and whole-grain breads and cereals (see **FIGURE 7.3**). The AMDR for

A kernel of wheat

Bran	Germ	Endosperm
• High fiber • B vitamins • Phytochemicals • Minerals	• Vitamin E • Healthy unsaturated fats • Antioxidants • Phytochemicals • Minerals • B vitamins	• Starch • Protein • B vitamins

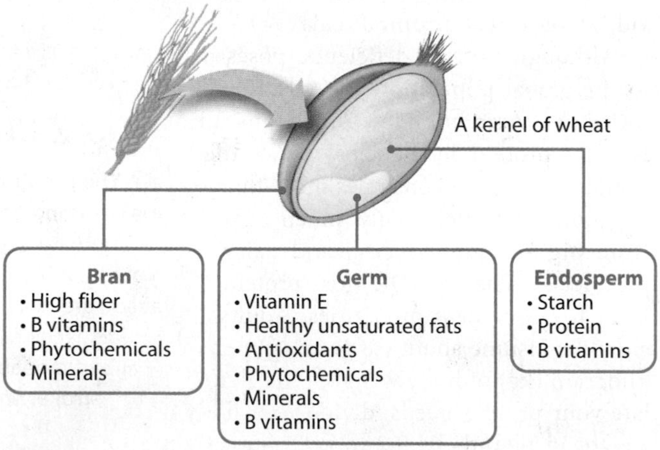

FIGURE 7.3 Anatomy of a Whole Grain Whole grains are more nutritious than refined grains because they contain the bran, germ, and endosperm of the seed—sources of fiber, vitamins, minerals, and beneficial phytochemicals (chemical compounds that occur naturally in plants).

Source: Adapted from Joan Salge Blake, Kathy D. Munoz, and Stella Volpe, *Nutrition: From Science to You,* 1st ed. © 2010, page 138. Printed and electronically reproduced by permission of Pearson Education, Inc., Upper Saddle River, New Jersey.

STUDENT HEALTH TODAY

WHY FIBER IS YOUR FRIEND

Fiber may seem like something only your grandparents need to be concerned about. However, getting the recommended amount of fiber in your diet can help you feel your best right now and avoid problems in the future. Research supports many benefits of fiber:

- **Protection against constipation.** When consumed with adequate fluids, fiber absorbs moisture and produces softer, bulkier stools that are more easily passed.
- **Protection against diverticulosis.** *Diverticulosis* is a condition in which pressure generated to pass compacted stools causes tiny bulges or pouches to form in the wall of the large intestine. These bulges can become irritated and infected and cause intense pain. Adequate fiber intake helps to prevent constipation and diverticulosis.
- **Protection against heart disease.** Many studies indicate that fiber helps delay or reduce the absorption of dietary cholesterol, a factor in heart disease.
- **Protection against type 2 diabetes.** Studies suggest that soluble fiber slows the movement of food through the digestive tract and thereby slows the release of glucose into the bloodstream. This helps the body control blood glucose levels and may reduce the risk for type 2 diabetes. A recent analysis of over four decades of studies involving more than 400,000 participants found that the risk of type 2 diabetes decreased by 6 percent for every 2 gram/day increase in fiber intake.
- **Protection against obesity.** Because most high-fiber foods are low in fat, they help control caloric intake. Many take longer to chew, which slows you down at the table. Because fiber stays in the digestive tract longer than other nutrients, making you feel full longer, fiber can help you succeed in your weight-loss efforts.
- **May reduce the risk of colorectal cancer.** One of the leading causes of cancer deaths in the United States, colorectal cancer is much less common in countries whose populations eat diets high in fiber and low in animal fat. Although some studies have not found an association between fiber-rich diets and reduced risk for colorectal cancer, other studies have. Recently, an analysis of 20 studies involving more than 10,000 people found support for the hypothesis that high dietary fiber intake is associated with a reduced colorectal cancer risk.

Below are some ways for you to incorporate more fiber into your daily diet:

- Whenever possible, select whole-grain breads, especially those that are low in fat and sugars. Choose breads with 3 or more grams of fiber per serving. Read labels—just because bread is brown doesn't mean it is better for you.
- Eat whole, unpeeled fruits and vegetables rather than drinking their juices.
- Substitute whole-grain pastas, bagels, and pizza crust for the refined, white flour versions.

Cereal can be a good source of whole grains and fiber.

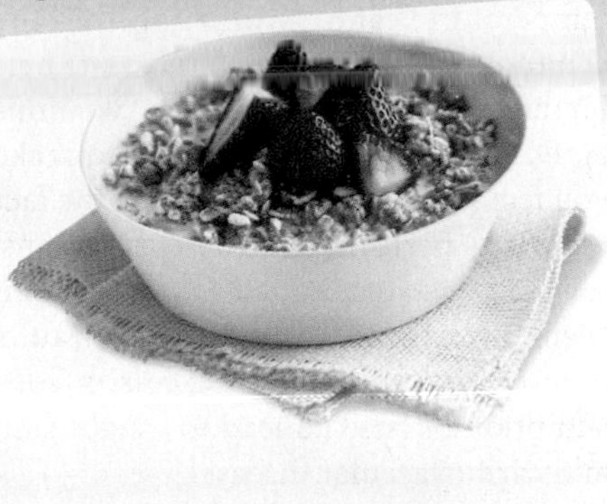

- Add wheat crumbs or grains to meat loaf and burgers to increase fiber intake.
- Enhance your fiber intake with quinoa, an edible seed that is also high in protein.
- Toast grains to bring out their nutty flavor and make foods more appealing.
- Sprinkle ground flaxseed on cereals, yogurt, and salads, or add to casseroles, burgers, and baked goods. Flaxseed has a mild flavor and is also high in essential fatty acids.

Sources: K. Maki et al., "Whole-Grain Ready-to Eat Oat Cereal, as Part of a Dietary Program for Weight Loss, Reduces Low-Density Lipoprotein Cholesterol in Adults with Overweight and Obesity More than a Dietary Program Including Low-Fiber Control Foods," *Journal of the American Dietetic Association* 110, no. 2 (2010): 205–14; B. Yao et al., "Dietary Fiber Intake and Risk of Type 2 Diabetes: A Dose-Response Analysis of Prospective Studies," *European Journal of Epidemiology* 29, no. 2 (2014): 79–88, DOI:10.1007/s10654-013-9876-x; Q. Ben et al., "Dietary Fiber Intake Reduces Risk for Colorectal Adenoma: A Meta-Analysis," *Gastroenterology* 146, no. 3 (2014): 689–99.

carbohydrates is 45 to 60 percent of total calories, and health experts recommend that the majority of this intake be fiber-rich carbohydrates. Find out more about the benefits of fiber in the **Student Health Today** box.

Despite growing evidence supporting the benefits of whole grains and high-fiber diets, intake among the general public remains low. Most experts believe that Americans should double their current consumption of dietary fiber. The AI for fiber is 25 grams per day for women and 38 grams per day for men.[9]

What's the best way to increase your intake of dietary fiber? Eat fewer refined carbohydrates in favor of more fiber-rich carbohydrates, including whole-grain breads and cereals, fresh fruits, legumes and other vegetables, nuts, and seeds. As with most nutritional advice, however, too much of a good thing can pose problems. A sudden increase in dietary fiber may cause flatulence (intestinal gas), cramping, or bloating. Consume plenty of water or other (sugar-free!) liquids to reduce such side effects.

Fats

Fats, perhaps the most misunderstood nutrient, are the most energy dense, providing 9 calories per gram. Fats are a

fats Essential nutrients needed for energy, cell function, insulation of body organs, maintenance of body temperature, and healthy skin and hair.

significant source of our body's fuel. The body can store only a limited amount of carbohydrate, so the longer you exercise, the more fat your body burns. Fats also play a vital role in maintaining healthy skin and hair, insulating body organs against shock, maintaining body temperature, and promoting healthy cell function. Fats make foods taste better and carry the fat-soluble vitamins A, D, E, and K to cells. They also make you feel full after eating. Despite the fact that fats perform all these functions, we are constantly urged to cut back on them, because some fats are less healthy than others and because excessive consumption of fats can lead to weight gain and cardiovascular disease.

Triglycerides make up about 95 percent of total body fat and are the most common form of fat in foods. When we consume too many calories from any source, the liver converts the excess into triglycerides, which are stored in fat cells throughout our bodies. Another oily substance in foods derived from animals is **cholesterol.** We don't need to consume any dietary cholesterol because our liver can make all that we need. Moreover, cholesterol contributes to a buildup of fatty plaque inside our blood vessels, the first stage of heart disease. Thus, the recommended intake for cholesterol is less than 300 milligrams a day (one egg contains about 215 milligrams).[10]

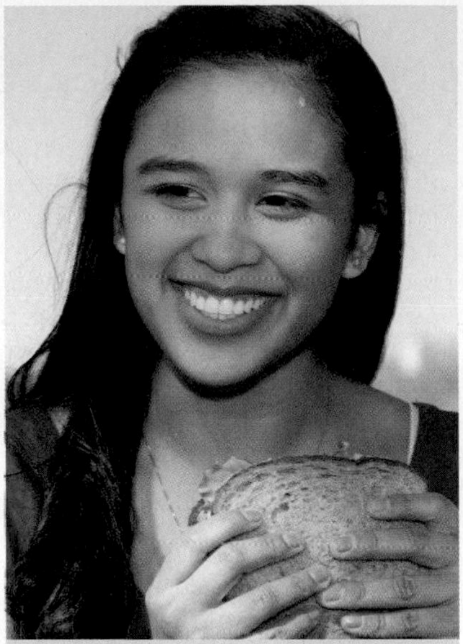

Studies have shown that eating 2.5 servings of whole grains per day can reduce cardiovascular disease risk by as much as 21%. But are people getting the message? One nutrition survey showed that only 8% of U.S. adults consume 3 or more servings of whole grains each day, and 42% ate no whole grains at all on a given day.

Sources: Dietary Guidelines Advisory Committee 2010, "What is the Relationship Between Whole Grain Intake and Cardiovascular Disease?," U.S. Department of Agriculture Nutrition Evidence Library, 2010, www.nutritionevidencelibrary.com/evidence.cfm?evidence_summary_id=250214.

triglycerides The most common form of fat in our food supply and in the body; made up of a molecule called glycerol and three fatty acid chains.

cholesterol A lipid found in foods and synthesized by the body. Although essential to functioning, cholesterol circulating in the blood can accumulate on the inner walls of blood vessels.

high-density lipoproteins (HDLs) Compounds that facilitate the transport of cholesterol in the blood to the liver for metabolism and elimination from the body.

low-density lipoproteins (LDLs) Compounds that transport cholesterol in the blood to the body's cells.

saturated fats Fats that are unable to hold any more hydrogen in their chemical structure; derived mostly from animal sources; solid at room temperature.

unsaturated fats Fats with one or more chemical bonds that exclude hydrogen; derived mostly from plants; liquid at room temperature.

Because oil and water don't mix, neither triglycerides nor cholesterol can travel independently in the bloodstream. Instead, they are "packaged" inside protein coats to form compounds called lipoproteins (*lipo-* refers to lipids, a diverse group of oily substances). The levels of two types of lipoproteins in a blood sample help clinicians determine the patient's risk for heart disease.

High-density lipoproteins (HDLs) are relatively high in protein and low in cholesterol and triglycerides. A high level of HDLs in the blood is healthful because HDLs remove cholesterol from dying cells and from plaques within blood vessels. Their cholesterol load is eventually transported to the liver and eliminated from the body.

Low-density lipoproteins (LDLs) are much higher in both cholesterol and triglycerides than HDLs. They travel in the bloodstream delivering cholesterol to body cells; however, LDLs not taken up by cells degrade and release their cholesterol into the bloodstream. This cholesterol can then stick to the lining of blood vessels, contributing to the plaque that causes heart disease. (See **Chapter 15** for more on the role cholesterol plays in cardiovascular health.)

Types of Dietary Fats Triglycerides contain *fatty acid* chains of oxygen, carbon, and hydrogen atoms. Fatty acid chains that cannot hold any more hydrogen in their chemical structure are called **saturated fats.** They generally come from animal sources, such as meat, dairy, and poultry products, and are solid at room temperature. **Unsaturated fats** have room for additional hydrogen atoms in their chemical structure, and are liquid at room temperature. They generally come from plants and include most vegetable oils.

The terms *monounsaturated fatty acids* (*MUFAs*) and *polyunsaturated fatty acids* (*PUFAs*) refer to the relative number of hydrogen atoms that are missing in a fatty acid chain. Peanut, canola, and olive oils are high in monounsaturated fats, which appear to lower LDL levels and increase HDL levels. Corn, sunflower, and safflower oils are high in polyunsaturated fats. For a breakdown of the types of fats in common vegetable oils, see **FIGURE 7.4**.

Two specific types of polyunsaturated fatty acids essential to a healthful diet are *omega-3 fatty acids* (found in many types of fatty fish; dark green, leafy vegetables; walnuts; and flaxseeds) and *omega-6 fatty acids* (found in corn, soybean, peanut, sunflower, and cottonseed oils). Both are classified as *essential fatty acids*—that is, those we must receive from our diets—because the body cannot synthesize them yet requires them for functioning. The most important fats within these groups are *linoleic acid*, an omega-6 fatty acid, and *alpha-linolenic acid,* an omega-3 fatty acid. The body needs these to make hormone-like compounds that control immune function, pain perception, and inflammation, to name a few key benefits. You may also have heard of EPA (eicosapentaenoic acid)

DO IT! NUTRITOOLS

Complete the **Know Your Fat Sources** activity available on MasteringHealth.™

and DHA (docosahexaenoic acid). These are derivatives of alpha-linolenic acid that are found abundantly in oily fish such as salmon and tuna and are associated with a reduced risk for heart disease.[11]

The AMDR for fats is 20 to 35 percent of calories, with 5 to 10 percent coming from essential fatty acids. Within this range, we should minimize our intake of saturated fats.

WHY SHOULD I CARE?

Cholesterol can accumulate on the inner walls of arteries and narrow the channels through which blood flows. This buildup, called plaque, is a major cause of atherosclerosis, a component of cardiovascular disease.

Avoiding *Trans* Fatty Acids For decades, Americans shunned butter, cream, and other foods high in saturated fats. What they didn't know is that some processed foods low in animal fats, such as margarine, could be just as harmful. These processed foods contain ***trans* fatty acids**. Research shows that just a 2 percent caloric intake of these fats is associated with a 23 percent increased risk for heart disease and a 47 percent increased chance of sudden cardiac death.[12]

Although a small amount of *trans* fatty acids do occur in some animal products, the great majority are in processed foods made with partially hydrogenated oils (PHOs).[13] PHOs are produced when food manufacturers add hydrogen to a plant oil, solidifying it, helping it resist rancidity, and giving the food in which it is used a longer shelf life. The hydrogenation process straightens out the fatty acid chain so that it is more like a saturated fatty acid, and it has similar harmful effects, lowering HDLs and raising LDLs. *Trans* fats have been used in margarines, many commercial baked goods, and restaurant deep-fried foods.

In 2013, the U.S. Food and Drug Administration (FDA) issued a preliminary determination that PHOs are no longer recognized as safe for consumption. If it is finalized, foods containing PHOs will no longer be sold legally in the United States.[14] In the meantime, *trans* fats are being removed from most foods, and if they are present, they must be clearly indicated on food packaging. If you see the words *partially*

***trans* fats (*trans* fatty acids)** Fatty acids that are produced when polyunsaturated oils are hydrogenated to make them more solid.

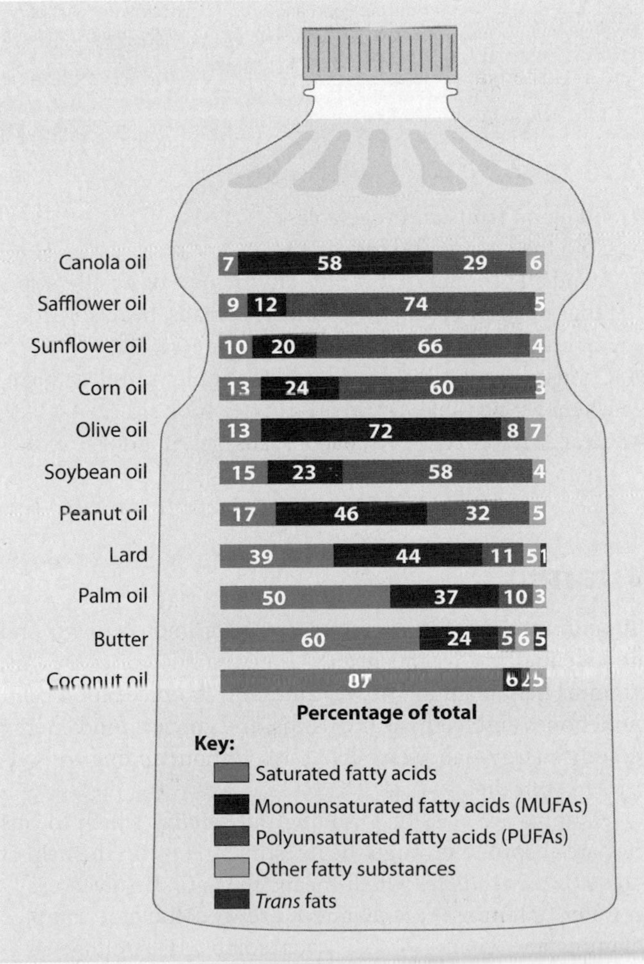

FIGURE 7.4 **Percentages of Saturated, Polyunsaturated, Monounsaturated, and *Trans* Fats in Common Vegetable Oils**

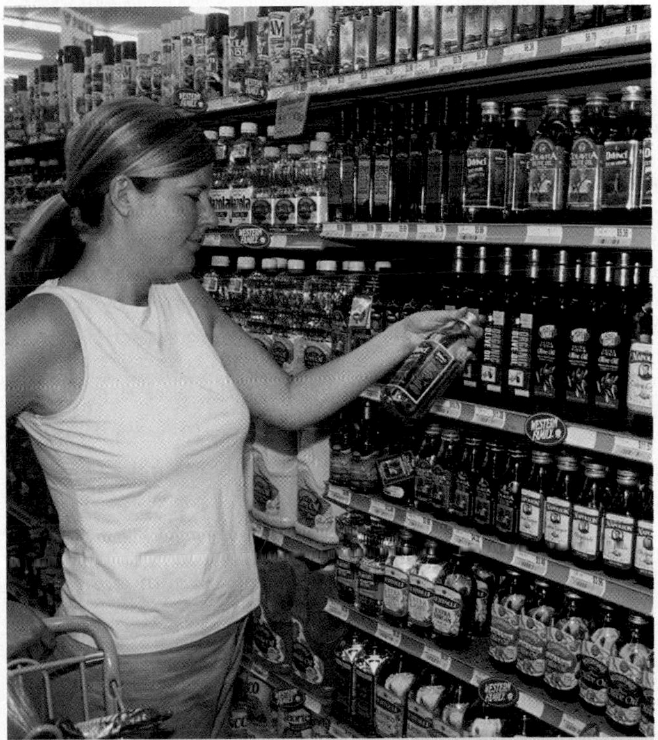

All fats are not the same, and your body needs some fat to function. Try to reduce saturated fats, which are in meat, full-fat dairy, and poultry products, and avoid *trans* fats, which typically come in stick margarines, commercially baked goods, and deep-fried foods. Replace these with unsaturated fats, such as those in plant oils, fatty fish, and nuts and seeds.

STUDENT HEALTH TODAY

TOWARD SUSTAINABLE SEAFOOD

The 2010 MyPlate food guidance system recommends consuming fish twice a week to reduce saturated fat and cholesterol levels and to increase omega-3 fatty acid levels. However, there are many environmental concerns surrounding the seafood industry today that call into question the sustainability and safety of such consumption. More than 70 percent of the world's natural fishing grounds have been overfished, and whole stretches of the oceans are, in fact, dead zones where fish and shellfish can no longer live. The FDA is also keeping a close eye on the safety of fish and shellfish affected by oil spills. Fish and shellfish from areas not affected by oil disasters are considered safe for consumers to eat.

To counteract the loss of wild fish populations, increasing numbers of fish are being farmed, which poses additional health risks and environmental concerns. Some farmed fish are laden with antibiotics. Other fish farms allow highly concentrated levels of parasites and bacteria from runoff to enter the ocean and rivers. Some farmed fish are fed wild fish, resulting in a net loss of fish from the sea.

At the same time that fish populations are threatened, high levels of toxins are being found in many of the fish available on the market. Mercury, a waste product of many industries, binds to proteins and stays in an animal's body, accumulating as it moves up the food chain; in humans, mercury can damage the nervous system and kidneys and cause birth defects and developmental problems in fetuses and children. Polychlorinated biphenyls (PCBs), chemicals that can build up in the fatty tissue of fish, are another cause of major concern.

So what is a savvy fish consumer to do? Know where your fish are caught and the methods by which they are caught. Several environmental groups have developed guides to inform consumers of safe and sustainable seafood choices. The Monterey Bay Aquarium in California provides a national guide for seafood available for purchase in the United States. You can find the guide online at www.montereybayaquarium.org/cr/cr_seafoodwatch/download.aspx. This guide is also available as a free iPhone or Android application, or it can be accessed on other mobile devices at http://mobile.seafoodwatch.org. Another great resource is the FishPhone service offered by the Blue Ocean Institute. Simply send a text message to 30644 with the word FISH and the type of fish you want to know about, and it will send you information about whether it is safe to eat.

Remember: Your consumer choices make a difference. Purchasing seafood from environmentally responsible sources will support fisheries and fish farms that are healthier for you and the environment.

Source: Food and Drug Administration, "Gulf of Mexico Oil Spill: Questions and Answers," Updated April 22, 2013, www.fda.gov/Food/RecallsOutbreaksEmergencies/Emergencies/ucm221563.htm.

vitamins Essential organic compounds that promote metabolism, growth, and reproduction and help maintain life and health.

hydrogenated oils, fractionated oils, shortening, lard, or *hydrogenation* on a food label, then *trans* fats are present.

New Fat Advice: Is More Fat Ever Better?

Some researchers worry that we have gone too far in our antifat frenzy. In fact, some studies have shown that balanced high-fat diets produce significant improvements in weight loss, blood fat, and blood glucose measures.[15]

Balance is the key. No more than 7 to 10 percent of your total calories should come from saturated fat, and no more than 35 percent should come from all forms of fat.[16] Follow these guidelines to add more healthy fats to your diet:

- Eat fatty fish (bluefish, herring, mackerel, salmon, sardines, or tuna) at least twice weekly. The **Student Health Today** box provides tips for making sustainable seafood choices.
- Use olive, peanut, soy, and canola oils instead of butter or lard.
- Add healthy amounts of green leafy vegetables, walnuts, walnut oil, and ground flaxseed to your diet.

Follow these guidelines to reduce your overall intake of less-healthy fats:

- Read the Nutrition Facts on food labels to find out how much fat is in your food.
- Chill meat-based soups and stews, scrape off any fat that hardens on top, and then reheat to serve.
- Fill up on fruits and vegetables.
- Hold the creams and sauces.
- Avoid all products with *trans* fatty acids. For healthy toppings on your bread, try vegetable spreads, bean spreads, nut butters, sugar-free jams, fat-free cheese, etc.
- Choose lean meats, fish, or skinless poultry. Broil or bake whenever possible. Drain off fat after cooking.
- Choose fewer cold cuts, bacon, sausages, hot dogs, and organ meats.
- Select nonfat and low-fat dairy products.

Vitamins

Vitamins are organic compounds that promote growth and are essential to life and health. Every minute of every day, vitamins help maintain nerves and skin, produce blood cells, build bones and teeth, heal wounds, and convert food energy to body energy—and they do all this without adding any calories to your diet.

Vitamins are classified as either *fat soluble,* which means they are absorbed through the intestinal tract with the help of fats, or *water soluble,* which means they are dissolved easily in water. Vitamins A, D, E, and K are fat soluble; B-complex vitamins and vitamin C are water soluble. Fat-soluble vitamins tend to be stored in the body, and toxic levels can accumulate if people regularly consume more than the UL. Excesses of water-soluble vitamins generally are excreted in the urine and rarely cause toxicity problems. See **TABLE 7.2**

TABLE 7.2 | A Guide to Water-Soluble Vitamins

Vitamin Name	Primary Functions	Recommended Intake	Reliable Food Sources	Toxicity/Deficiency Symptoms
Thiamin (vitamin B_1)	Required as enzyme cofactor for carbohydrate and amino acid metabolism	RDA: Men: 1.2 mg/day Women: 1.1 mg/day	Pork, fortified cereals, enriched rice and pasta, peas, tuna, legumes	*Toxicity*: none known *Deficiency*: beriberi; fatigue, apathy, decreased memory, confusion, irritability, muscle weakness
Riboflavin (vitamin B_2)	Required as enzyme cofactor for carbohydrate and fat metabolism	RDA: Men: 1.3 mg/day Women: 1.1 mg/day	Beef liver, shrimp, milk and other dairy foods, fortified cereals, enriched breads and grains	*Toxicity*: none known *Deficiency*: ariboflavinosis; swollen mouth and throat; seborrheic dermatitis; anemia
Niacin, nicotinamide, nicotinic acid	Required for carbohydrate and fat metabolism Plays role in DNA replication and repair and cell differentiation	RDA: Men: 16 mg/day Women: 14 mg/day UL: 35 mg/day	Beef liver, most cuts of meat/fish/poultry, fortified cereals, enriched breads and grains, canned tomato products	*Toxicity*: flushing, liver damage, glucose intolerance, blurred vision differentiation *Deficiency*: pellagra; vomiting, constipation, or diarrhea; apathy
Pyridoxine, pyridoxal, pyridoxamine (vitamin B_6)	Required as enzyme cofactor for carbohydrate and amino acid metabolism Assists synthesis of blood cells	RDA: Men and women aged 19–50: 1.3 mg/day Men aged >50: 1.7 mg/day Women aged >50: 1.5 mg/day UL: 100 mg/day	Chickpeas (garbanzo beans), most cuts of meat/fish/poultry, fortified cereals, white potatoes	*Toxicity*: nerve damage, skin lesions *Deficiency*: anemia; seborrheic dermatitis; depression, confusion, and convulsions
Folate (folic acid)	Required as enzyme cofactor for amino acid metabolism Required for DNA synthesis Involved in metabolism of homocysteine	RDA: Men: 400 µg/day Women: 400 µg/day UL: 1,000 µg/day	Fortified cereals, enriched breads and grains, spinach, legumes (lentils, chickpeas, pinto beans), greens (spinach, romaine lettuce), liver	*Toxicity*: masks symptoms of vitamin B_{12} deficiency, specifically signs of nerve damage *Deficiency*: macrocytic anemia; neural tube defects in a developing fetus; elevated homocysteine levels
Cobalamin (vitamin B_{12})	Assists with formation of blood Required for healthy nervous system function Involved as enzyme cofactor in metabolism of homocysteine	RDA: Men: 2.4 µg/day Women: 2.4 µg/day	Shellfish, all cuts of meat/fish/poultry, milk and other dairy foods, fortified cereals and other fortified foods	*Toxicity*: none known *Deficiency*: pernicious anemia; tingling and numbness of extremities; nerve damage; memory loss, disorientation, and dementia
Pantothenic acid	Assists with fat metabolism	AI: Men: 5 mg/day Women: 5 mg/day	Meat/fish/poultry, shiitake mushrooms, fortified cereals, egg yolk	*Toxicity*: none known *Deficiency*: rare
Biotin	Involved as enzyme cofactor in carbohydrate, fat, and protein metabolism	RDA: Men: 30 µg/day Women: 30 µg/day	Nuts, egg yolk	*Toxicity*: none known *Deficiency*: rare
Ascorbic acid (vitamin C)	Antioxidant in extracellular fluid and lungs Regenerates oxidized vitamin E Assists with collagen synthesis Enhances immune function Assists in synthesis of hormones, neurotransmitters, and DNA Enhances iron absorption	RDA: Men: 90 mg/day Women: 75 mg/day Smokers: 35 mg more per day than RDA UL: 2,000 mg	Sweet peppers, citrus fruits and juices, broccoli, strawberries, kiwi	*Toxicity*: nausea and diarrhea, nosebleeds, increased oxidative damage, increased formation of kidney stones in people with kidney disease *Deficiency*: scurvy; bone pain and fractures, depression, and anemia

Note: RDA, Recommended Dietary Allowance; UL, upper limit; AI, Adequate Intake.

TABLE 7.3 | A Guide to Fat-Soluble Vitamins

Vitamin Name	Primary Functions	Recommended Intake	Reliable Food Sources	Toxicity/Deficiency Symptoms
A (retinol, retinal, retinoic acid)	Required for ability of eyes to adjust to changes in light Protects color vision Assists cell differentiation Required for sperm production in men and fertilization in women Contributes to healthy bone Contributes to healthy immune system	RDA: Men: 900 μg Women: 700 μg UL: 3,000 μg/day	Preformed retinol: beef and chicken liver, egg yolks, milk Carotenoid precursors: spinach, carrots, mango, apricots, cantaloupe, pumpkin, yams	*Toxicity*: fatigue; bone and joint pain; spontaneous abortion and birth defects of fetuses in pregnant women; nausea and diarrhea; liver damage; nervous system damage; blurred vision; hair loss; skin disorders *Deficiency*: night blindness and xerophthalmia; impaired growth, immunity, and reproductive function
D (cholecalciferol)	Regulates blood calcium levels Maintains bone health Assists cell differentiation	RDA: Adult aged 19–70: 600 IU/day Adult aged >70: 800 IU/day UL: 4,000 IU/day	Canned salmon and mackerel, fortified milk and milk alternatives, fortified cereals	*Toxicity*: hypercalcemia *Deficiency*: rickets in children; osteomalacia and/or osteoporosis in adults
E (tocopherol)	As a powerful antioxidant, protects cell membranes, polyunsaturated fatty acids, and vitamin A from oxidation Protects white blood cells Enhances immune function Improves absorption of vitamin A	RDA: Men: 15 mg/day Women: 15 mg/day UL: 1,000 mg/day	Sunflower seeds, almonds, vegetable oils, fortified cereals	*Toxicity*: rare *Deficiency*: hemolytic anemia; impairment of nerve, muscle, and immune function
K (phylloquinone, menaquinone, menadione)	Serves as a coenzyme during production of specific proteins that assist in blood coagulation and bone metabolism	AI: Men: 120 μg/day Women: 90 μg/day	Kale, spinach, turnip greens, brussels sprouts	*Toxicity*: none known *Deficiency*: impaired blood clotting; possible effect on bone health

Note: RDA, Recommended Dietary Allowance; UL, upper limit; AI, Adequate Intake.

and TABLE 7.3 for recommended intake amounts, food sources, functions, and potential dangers of specific vitamins.

Vitamin D Vitamin D, the sunshine vitamin, is formed from a compound in the skin when exposed to the sun's ultraviolet rays. In most people, an adequate amount of vitamin D can be synthesized with 5 to 30 minutes of sun on the face, neck, hands, arms, and legs twice a week, without sunscreen.[17] However, the sun is not high enough in the sky during late fall to early spring in northern climates to allow for vitamin D synthesis. For people who cannot rely on the sun to meet their daily vitamin D needs, consuming vitamin D–fortified milk, yogurt, soy milk, cereals, and fatty fish, such as salmon, can also supply this vitamin.

Vitamin D is essential for the body's regulation of calcium, the primary mineral component of bone. It also assists in the process of calcification by which bone minerals are crystallized. For these reasons, a deficiency of vitamin D can promote loss of bone density and strength, a condition called *osteoporosis*. Two other bone disorders, *rickets* in children, and its adult version, *osteomalacia,* both of which cause softening and distortion of the bones, can also be prevented with adequate intake of vitamin D.[18] Vitamin D also helps fight infections, lowers blood pressure, reduces the risk of developing diabetes mellitus, and may reduce the growth of cancer cells. Breast and prostate cancer, heart disease, and stroke have also been connected to inadequate vitamin D.

More is not always better, however. Too much vitamin D, generally from excessive intake of vitamin D supplements, can reduce appetite and cause nausea, vomiting, and constipation. Excess vitamin D can also affect the nervous system, cause depression, and deposit calcium in the soft tissues of the kidneys, lungs, blood vessels, and heart.[19]

Folate One of the B vitamins, folate is needed for the production of compounds necessary for DNA synthesis in body cells. It is also particularly important for proper cell division during embryonic development; folate deficiencies during the first few weeks of pregnancy, typically before a woman even realizes she is pregnant, can prompt a *neural tube defect (NTD)*, in which the primitive tube that eventually forms the brain and spinal cord fails to close properly. A common NTD is *spina bifida*, a birth defect in which a portion of the bones of the vertebral column do not completely enclose the spinal cord. In 1998, the FDA began requiring that all bread, cereal, rice, and pasta products sold in the United States be fortified with folic acid, the synthetic form of folate, to reduce the incidence of spina bifida and other neural tube defects.

Minerals

Minerals are inorganic, indestructible elements that aid physiological processes within the body. Without minerals, vitamins could not be absorbed. Minerals are readily excreted and, with a few exceptions, are usually not toxic. *Major minerals* are the minerals that the body needs in fairly large amounts: sodium, calcium, phosphorus, magnesium, potassium, sulfur, and chloride. *Trace minerals* include iron, zinc, manganese, copper, fluoride, selenium, chromium, and iodine. Only very small amounts of trace minerals are needed, and serious problems may result if excesses or deficiencies occur (see **TABLE 7.4** and **TABLE 7.5**).

minerals Inorganic, indestructible elements that aid physiological processes.

TABLE 7.4 | A Guide to Major Minerals

Mineral Name	Primary Functions	Recommended Intake	Reliable Food Sources	Toxicity/Deficiency Symptoms
Sodium	Fluid balance Acid–base balance Transmission of nerve impulses Muscle contraction	AI: Adults: 1.5 g/day (1,500 mg/day)	Table salt, pickles, most canned soups, snack foods, cured luncheon meats, canned tomato products	*Toxicity*: water retention, high blood pressure, loss of calcium *Deficiency*: muscle cramps, dizziness, fatigue, nausea, vomiting, mental confusion
Potassium	Fluid balance Transmission of nerve impulses Muscle contraction	AI: Adults: 4.7 g/day (4,700 mg/day)	Most fresh fruits and vegetables: potatoes, bananas, tomato juice, orange juice, melons	*Toxicity*: muscle weakness, vomiting, irregular heartbeat *Deficiency*: muscle weakness, paralysis, mental confusion, irregular heartbeat
Phosphorus	Fluid balance Bone formation Component of ATP, which provides energy for our bodies	RDA: Adults: 700 mg/day	Milk/cheese/yogurt, soy milk and tofu, legumes (lentils, black beans), nuts (almonds, peanuts and peanut butter), poultry	*Toxicity*: muscle spasms, convulsions, low blood calcium *Deficiency*: muscle weakness, muscle damage, bone pain, dizziness
Chloride	Fluid balance Transmission of nerve impulses Component of stomach acid (HCl) Antibacterial	AI: Adults: 2.3 g/day (2,300 mg/day)	Table salt	*Toxicity*: none known *Deficiency*: dangerous blood acid–base imbalances, irregular heartbeat
Calcium	Primary component of bone Acid–base balance Transmission of nerve impulses Muscle contraction	RDA: Adults aged 19 to 50 and men aged 51–70: 1,000 mg/day Women aged 51–70 and adults aged >70: 1,200 mg/day UL for adults 19–50: 2,500 mg/day UL for adults aged 51 and above: 2,000 mg/day	Milk/yogurt/cheese (best-absorbed form of calcium), sardines, collard greens and spinach, calcium-fortified juices and milk alternatives	*Toxicity*: mineral imbalances, shock, kidney failure, fatigue, mental confusion *Deficiency*: osteoporosis, convulsions, heart failure
Magnesium	Component of bone Muscle contraction Assists more than 300 enzyme systems	RDA: Men aged 19–30: 400 mg/day Men aged >30: 420 mg/day Women aged 19–30: 310 mg/day Women aged >30: 320 mg/day UL: 350 mg/day	Greens (spinach, kale, collard greens), whole grains, seeds, nuts, legumes (navy and black beans)	*Toxicity*: none known *Deficiency*: low blood calcium, muscle spasms or seizures, nausea, weakness, increased risk for chronic diseases, such as heart disease, hypertension, osteoporosis, and type 2 diabetes
Sulfur	Component of certain B-vitamins and amino acids Acid–base balance Detoxification in liver	No DRI	Protein-rich foods	*Toxicity*: none known *Deficiency*: none known

Note: RDA, Recommended Dietary Allowance; UL, upper limit; AI, Adequate Intake; DRI, Dietary Reference Intake.

TABLE 7.5 | A Guide to Trace Minerals

Mineral Name	Primary Functions	Recommended Intake	Reliable Food Sources	Toxicity/Deficiency Symptoms
Selenium	Required for carbohydrate and fat metabolism	RDA: Adults: 55 μg/day UL: 400 μg/day	Nuts, shellfish, meat/fish/poultry, whole grains	*Toxicity*: brittle hair and nails, skin rashes, nausea and vomiting, weakness, liver disease *Deficiency*: specific forms of heart disease and arthritis, impaired immune function, muscle pain and wasting, depression, hostility
Fluoride	Development and maintenance of healthy teeth and bones	RDA: Men: 4 mg/day Women: 3 mg/day UL: 2.2 mg/day for children aged 4–8; 10 mg/day for children aged >8	Fish, seafood, legumes, whole grains, drinking water (variable)	*Toxicity*: fluorosis of teeth and bones *Deficiency*: dental caries, low bone density
Iodine	Synthesis of thyroid hormones Temperature regulation Reproduction and growth	RDA: Adults: 150 μg/day UL: 1,100 μg/day	Iodized salt, saltwater seafood	*Toxicity*: goiter *Deficiency*: goiter, hypothyroidism, cretinism in infant of mother who is iodine deficient
Chromium	Glucose transport Metabolism of DNA and RNA Immune function and growth	AI: Men aged 19–50: 35 μg/day Men aged >50: 30 μg/day Women aged 19–50: 25 μg/day Women aged >50: 20 μg/day	Whole grains, brewer's yeast	*Toxicity*: none known *Deficiency*: elevated blood glucose and blood lipids, damage to brain and nervous system
Manganese	Assists many enzyme systems Synthesis of protein found in bone and cartilage	AI: Men: 2.3 mg/day Women: 1.8 mg/day UL: 11 mg/day for adults	Whole grains, nuts, leafy vegetables, tea	*Toxicity*: impairment of neuromuscular system *Deficiency*: impaired growth and reproductive function, reduced bone density, impaired glucose and lipid metabolism, skin rash
Iron	Component of hemoglobin in blood cells Component of myoglobin in muscle cells Assists many enzyme systems	RDA: Adult men: 8 mg/day Women aged 19–50: 18 mg/day Women aged >50: 8 mg/day	Meat/fish/poultry (best-absorbed form of iron), fortified cereals, legumes, spinach	*Toxicity*: nausea, vomiting, and diarrhea; dizziness, confusion; rapid heartbeat, organ damage, death *Deficiency*: iron-deficiency microcytic (small red blood cells), hypochromic anemia
Zinc	Assists more than 100 enzyme systems Immune system function Growth and sexual maturation Gene regulation	RDA: Men: 11 mg/day Women: 8 mg/day UL: 40 mg/day	Meat/fish/poultry (best-absorbed form of zinc), fortified cereals, legumes	*Toxicity*: nausea, vomiting, and diarrhea; headaches, depressed immune function, reduced absorption of copper *Deficiency*: growth retardation, delayed sexual maturation, eye and skin lesions, hair loss, increased incidence of illness and infection
Copper	Assists many enzyme systems Iron transport	RDA: Adults: 900 μg/day UL: 10 mg/day	Shellfish, organ meats, nuts, legumes	*Toxicity*: nausea, vomiting, and diarrhea; liver damage *Deficiency*: anemia, reduced levels of white blood cells, osteoporosis in infants and growing children

Note: RDA, Recommended Dietary Allowance; UL, upper limit; AI, Adequate Intake.

SKILLS FOR BEHAVIOR CHANGE

SHAKE YOUR SALT HABIT

Take simple steps today to reduce your sodium intake:

- When buying packaged foods, choose low-sodium or sodium-free products.
- At the movies, order popcorn without salt.
- Use kosher salt—it has 25 percent less sodium than regular table salt.
- Avoid adding salt to foods during cooking or at the table; instead, try using fresh or dried herbs and spices to season foods.

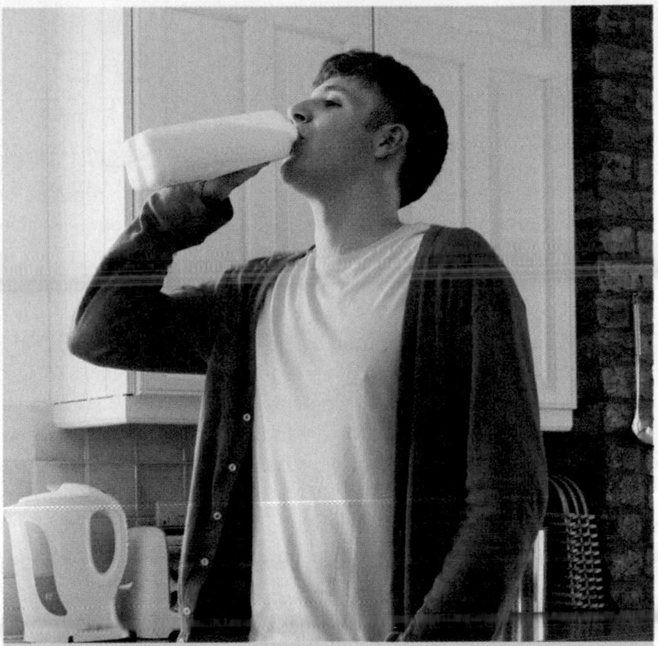

Milk is a great source of calcium and other nutrients. If you don't like milk or can't drink it, make sure to get enough calcium—at least 1,000 milligrams a day—through other sources.

Sodium Sodium is necessary for the regulation of blood volume and blood pressure, fluid balance, transmission of nerve impulses, heart activity, and certain metabolic functions. It enhances flavors, acts as a preservative, and tenderizes meats, so it's often present in high quantities in the foods we eat. A common misconception is that table salt and sodium are the same thing: Table salt is a compound containing both sodium and chloride. It accounts for only 15 percent of our sodium intake. The majority of sodium in our diet comes from processed foods that are infused with sodium to enhance flavor and preservation. Pickles, fast foods, salty snacks, processed cheeses, canned and dehydrated soups, frozen dinners, many breads and bakery products, and smoked meats and sausages often contain several hundred milligrams of sodium per serving.

The AI for sodium is just 1,500 milligrams, which is about 0.65 of a teaspoon.[20] The latest National Health and Nutrition Examination Survey (NHANES) estimated that the average American over 2 years of age consumes 3,463 milligrams of sodium per day, or about 1.5 teaspoons.[21]

Both the Institute of Medicine and the American Heart Association recommend consuming no more than the AI for sodium.[22] Why is high sodium intake a concern? Salt-sensitive individuals respond to a high-sodium diet with an increase in blood pressure (hypertension), which contributes to heart disease and strokes. Although the cause of the majority of cases of hypertension is unknown, lowering sodium intake reduces the risk. See the **Skills for Behavior Change** box for tips on how to reduce your sodium intake.

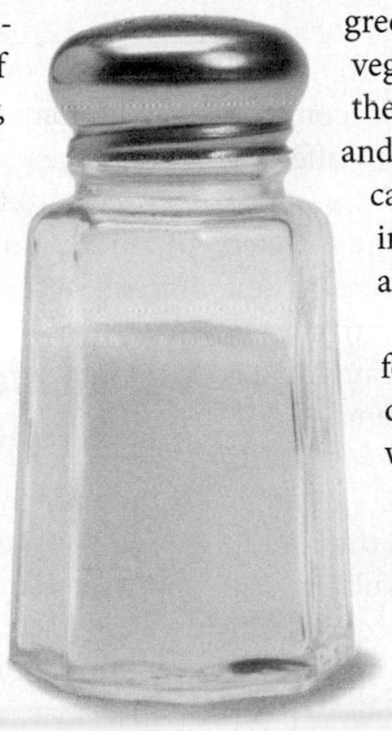

Even if you never use table salt, you still may be getting excess sodium in your diet.

Calcium Calcium is the primary mineral component of bones and teeth. It is also essential for muscle contraction, nerve impulse transmission, and regulation of the heartbeat. An alkaline mineral, calcium is an important buffer, reducing blood acidity and helping to maintain pH balance. It's also important for blood clotting and other functions. The issue of calcium consumption has gained national attention with the rising incidence of osteoporosis among older adults. Most Americans do not consume the recommended 1,000 to 1,200 milligrams of calcium per day.[23]

Dairy products, as well as calcium-fortified juices and milk alternatives, are excellent sources of calcium. So are many leafy green vegetables, including broccoli, collard greens, and kale. Although the amount of calcium vegetables provide is lower, it is better absorbed than the calcium from dairy products. Spinach, chard, and beet greens are not particularly good sources of calcium because they contain oxalic acid, which interferes with calcium absorption. Many peas and beans also offer good supplies.

For optimal absorption, consume calcium-rich foods and beverages throughout the day. Many dairy products and milk alternatives are fortified with vitamin D, which is necessary for calcium regulation. Avoid taking calcium as supplements unless you cannot meet your calcium requirements from foods and beverages.[24] Constipation and bloating are common side effects, and supplements are associated with an increased risk for the formation of kidney stones. Some research has also raised concerns about an increased risk for cardiovascular disease with their use.[25]

HEALTH HEADLINES

HEALTH CLAIMS OF SUPERFOODS

Functional foods contain both nutrients and other active compounds that may improve overall health, reduce the risk for certain diseases, or delay aging. If the term "functional foods" strikes you as a bit stodgy, you're not alone. In food advertisements, fitness and food magazines, and even among health care organizations, these foods are increasingly being referred to as "superfoods." For instance, Harvard Medical School recently published a list of 12 superfoods, including broccoli, beans, salmon, oatmeal, Greek yogurt, and dark chocolate. Do superfoods live up to their new name? Let's look at a few.

Salmon is a rich source of the omega-3 fatty acids EPA and DHA, which combat inflammation, improve HDL/LDL blood profiles, and reduce the risk for cardiovascular disease. DHA may also promote a healthy nervous system, reducing the risk for age-related dementia.

Yogurt makes it onto most superfood lists because, like other fermented milk products, it contains living, beneficial bacteria called probiotics. You will see their genus name, for example, *Lactobacillus* or *Bifidobacterium,* in the list of ingredients on the product's label. Probiotics colonize the large intestine, where they help complete digestion, produce certain vitamins, and are thought to reduce the risk of diarrhea and other bowel disorders, boost immunity, and help regulate body weight.

Cocoa is particularly rich in a class of chemicals called flavonols that have been shown in many studies to reduce the risk for cardiovascular disease, diabetes, and even arthritis. Dark chocolate has a higher level of flavonols than milk chocolate.

Given such claims, it's easy to get carried away by the idea that superfoods, like superheros, have superpowers. But eating a square of dark chocolate won't rescue you from the ill effects of a fast-food burger and fries. What matters is your whole diet. Focus on including superfoods as components of a varied diet rich in fresh fruits, legumes and other vegetables, whole grains, lean sources of protein, and nuts and seeds. These are the "everyday heroes" of a super-healthful diet.

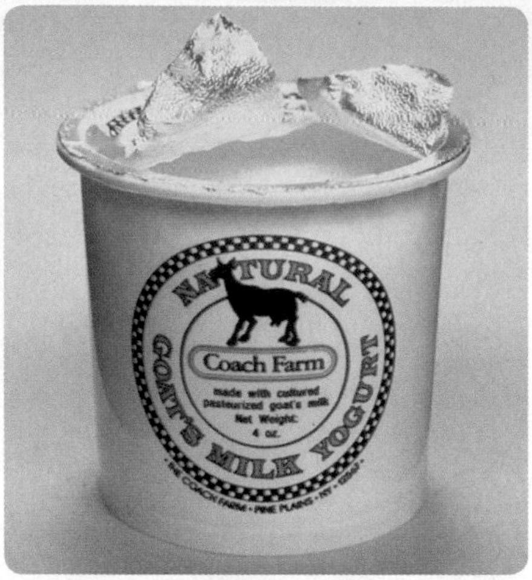

Yogurt and kefir (a fermented milk drink) are dairy products containing beneficial bacteria called *probiotics*.

Sources: Academy of Nutrition and Dietetics, "Position of the Academy of Nutrition and Dietetics: Functional Foods" *Journal of the Academy of Nutrition and Dietetics* 113 (2013):1096–1103; G. M. Cole and S. A. Frautschy, "DHA May Reduce Age-Related Dementia," *Journal of Nutrition* 140, no. 4 (2010): 869–74; D. Swanson, R. Block, and S .A. Mousa, "Omega-3 Fatty Acids EPA and DHA: Health Benefits Throughout Life," *Advances in Nutrition* 3, no. 1 (2012): 1–7; P. Hemarajata and J. Versalovic, "Effects of Probiotics on Gut Microbiota: Mechanisms of Intestinal Immunomodulation and Neuromodulation," *Therapeutic Advances in Gastroenterology* 6, no. 1 (2013): 39–51, Available at www.ncbi.nlm.nih.gov/pmc/articles/PMC3539293/; R. Krajmalnik-Brown et al., "Effects of Gut Microbes on Nutrient Absorption and Energy Regulation," *Nutrition in Clinical Practice* 27, no. 2 (2012): 201–14; L. Hooper et al., "Effects of Chocolate, Cocoa, and Flavanols on Cardiovascular Health: A Systematic Review and Meta-Analysis of Randomized Trials," *American Journal of Clinical Nutrition* 95, no. 3, (2012): 740–53, DOI: 10.3945/ajcn.111.023457; D. Grassi et al., "Protective Effects of Flavanol-Rich Dark Chocolate on Endothelial Function and Wave Reflection During Acute Hyperglycemia," *Hypertension* 60, no. 3 (2012): 827–32, DOI: 10.1161/HYPERTENSIONAHA.112.193995; S. Ramos-Romero et al., "Effect of a Cocoa Flavonoid-Enriched Diet on Experimental Autoimmune Arthritis," *British Journal of Nutrition* 107, no. 4 (2012): 523–32, DOI: 10.1017/S000711451100328X.

anemia Condition that results from the body's inability to produce adequate hemoglobin.

functional foods Foods believed to have specific health benefits beyond their basic nutrients.

Iron Worldwide, iron deficiency is the most common nutrient deficiency, affecting nearly 30 percent of the world's population.[26] In the United States, iron deficiency is less prevalent, but it is still the most common micronutrient deficiency.[27] Women aged 19 to 50 need about 18 milligrams of iron per day, and men aged 19 to 50 need about 8 milligrams.

Iron deficiency can lead to *iron-deficiency anemia.* **Anemia** results from the body's inability to produce adequate amounts of hemoglobin (the oxygen-carrying component of the blood). Anemia can also result from blood loss, cancer, ulcers, and other conditions. When iron-deficiency anemia occurs, body cells receive less oxygen. As a result, the iron-deficient person feels tired. Iron is also important for energy metabolism, DNA synthesis, and other body functions.

Iron overload or iron toxicity due to ingesting too many iron-containing supplements is the leading cause of accidental poisoning in small children in the United States. Symptoms of toxicity include nausea, vomiting, diarrhea, rapid heartbeat, weak pulse, dizziness, shock, and confusion. Excess iron intake from high meat consumption, iron fortification, and supplementation is also associated with problems such as cardiovascular disease and cancer.[28]

Beneficial Non-Nutrient Components of Foods

Increasingly, nutrition research is focusing on components of foods that interact with nutrients to promote human health, rather than solely as sources of macro- and micronutrients.[29] Foods that may confer health benefits beyond the nutrients they contribute to the diet—

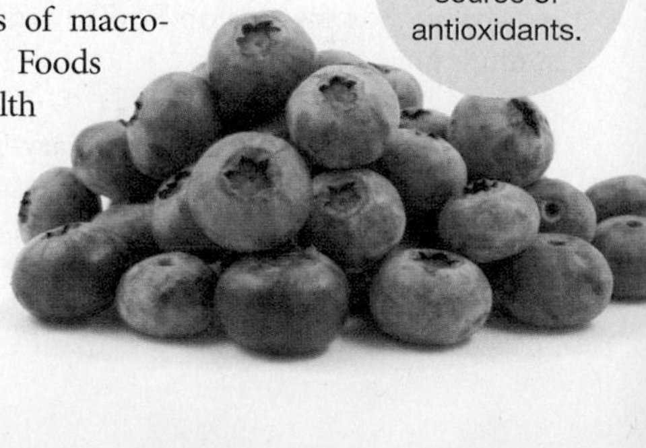

Blueberries are a great source of antioxidants.

whole foods, fortified foods, enriched foods, or enhanced foods—are called **functional foods**. When functional foods are included as part of a varied diet, they have the potential to positively impact health.[30]

Some of the most popular functional foods today are those containing **antioxidants.** These substances appear to protect against oxidative stress, a complex process in which *free radicals* (atoms with unpaired electrons) destabilize other atoms and molecules, prompting a chain reaction that can damage cells, cell proteins, or genetic material in the cells. Free radical formation is a natural process that cannot be avoided, but antioxidants combat it by donating their electrons to stabilize free radicals, activating enzymes that convert free radicals to less damaging substances, or reducing or repairing the damage they cause.

Among the more commonly cited antioxidants are vitamins C and E, as well as the minerals copper, iron, manganese, selenium, and zinc. Other potent antioxidants are **phytochemicals,** compounds that occur naturally in plants and are thought to protect them against ultraviolet radiation, pests, and other threats. Common examples include the *carotenoids,* pigments found in red, orange, and dark green fruits and vegetables. Beta-carotene, the most researched carotenoid, is a precursor of vitamin A, meaning that vitamin A can be produced in the body from beta-carotene. Both vitamin A and beta-carotene have antioxidant properties. Phenolic phytochemicals, which include a group known as flavonoids, are found in an array of fruits and vegetables as well as soy products, tea, and chocolate. Like carotenoids, they are thought to have antioxidant properties that may prevent cardiovascular disease.[31]

To date, many such claims about the health benefits of antioxidant nutrients and phytochemicals have not been fully investigated. However, studies do show that individuals deficient in antioxidant vitamins and minerals have an increased risk for age-related diseases, and that antioxidants consumed in whole foods, mostly fruits and vegetables, may reduce these individuals' risks. In contrast, antioxidants consumed as supplements do not confer such a benefit, and may be harmful.[32] For example, researchers have long theorized that because many cancers result from DNA damage, and because vitamin E appears to protect against such damage, vitamin E would also reduce cancer risk. Surprisingly, the great majority of studies have demonstrated no effect or, in some cases, a negative effect.[33]

Foods rich in nutrients and phytochemicals are increasingly being referred to as "superfoods." Do they live up to their name? See the **Health Headlines** box.

LO 2 | HOW CAN I EAT MORE HEALTHFULLY?

Discuss how to eat healthfully, including the characteristics of a healthful diet, how to use the MyPlate plan, the role of dietary supplements, how to read food labels, and the unique challenges that college students face.

Today, Americans continue to consume high numbers of calories (see **FIGURE 7.5**). In 2010, the average person consumed 2,044 calories per day.[34] In general, it isn't the actual amount of food, but the number of calories in the foods we choose to eat that has increased. When these trends are combined with our increasingly sedentary lifestyle,

antioxidants Substances believed to protect against oxidative stress and resultant tissue damage.

phytochemicals Naturally occurring non-nutrient plant chemicals believed to have beneficial health effects.

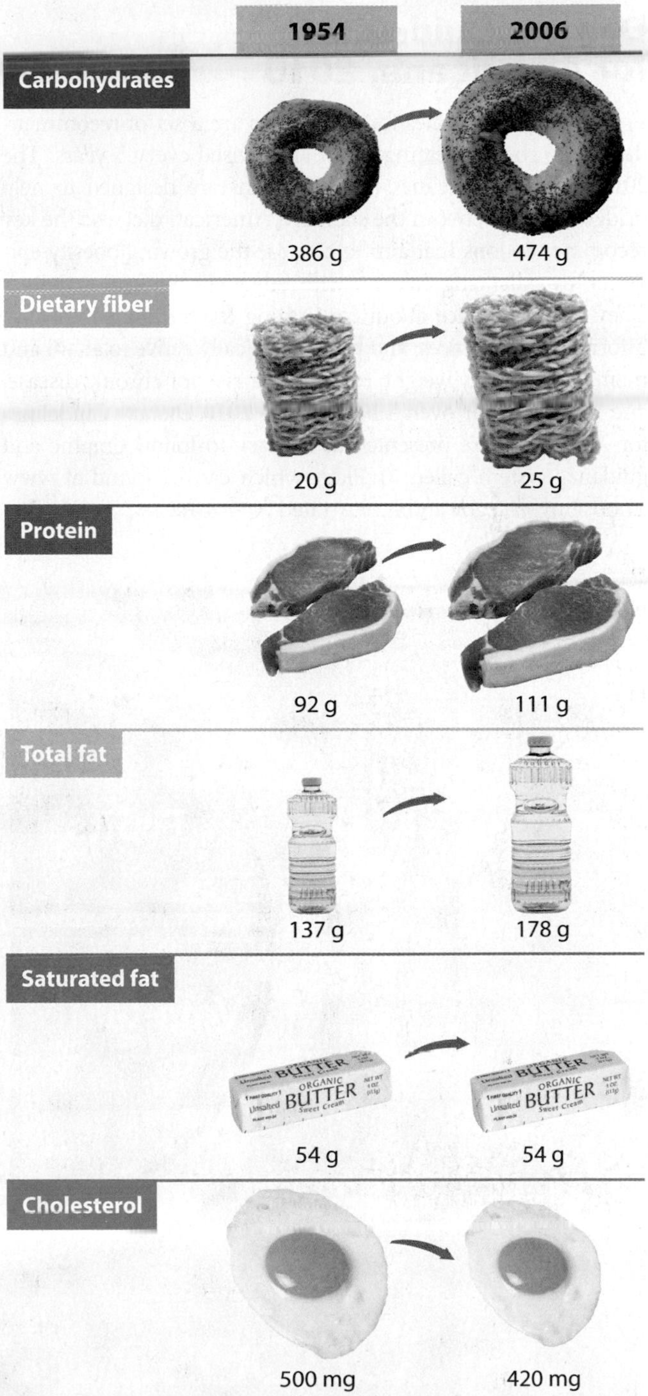

FIGURE 7.5 **Trends in Per Capita Nutrient Consumption**
Since 1954, Americans' daily caloric intake has increased by about 25%, as has daily consumption of carbohydrates, fiber, and protein. Daily total fat intake has increased by 30%.

Source: Data are from USDA Economic Research Service, Food Availability (Per Capita) Data System (FADS), updated June 2014, www.ers.usda.gov/data-products/food-availability-(per-capita)-data-system/.aspx#26715.

it is not surprising that we have seen a dramatic rise in obesity.[35]

The Center for Nutrition Policy and Promotion at the U.S. Department of Agriculture publishes two dietary tools created for consumers to make healthy eating easy: the Dietary Guidelines for Americans and the MyPlate food guidance system.

Dietary Guidelines for Americans, 2010

The Dietary Guidelines for Americans are a set of recommendations for healthy eating. They are revised every 5 years. The 2010 Dietary Guidelines for Americans are designed to help bridge the gap between the standard American diet and the key recommendations that aim to combat the growing obesity epidemic by balancing calories with adequate physical activity.[36] They provide advice about consuming fewer calories, making informed food choices, and being physically active to attain and maintain a healthy weight, reduce your risk for chronic disease, and improve your overall health. The 2010 Dietary Guidelines for Americans are presented as an easy-to-follow graphic and guidance system called MyPlate, which can be found at www.choosemyplate.gov and is illustrated in **FIGURE 7.6**.

MyPlate Food Guidance System

The MyPlate food guidance system takes into consideration the dietary and caloric needs for a wide variety of individuals, such as pregnant or breast-feeding women, those trying to lose weight, and adults with different activity levels. When you visit the interactive website, you can create personalized dietary and exercise recommendations based on the information you enter.

MyPlate also encourages consumers to eat for health through three general areas of recommendation:

1. Balance calories:
   - Enjoy your food, but eat less.
   - Avoid oversized portions.
2. Increase foods:
   - Fill half your plate with fruits and vegetables.
   - Make at least half your grains whole.
   - Switch to fat-free or 1 percent milk.
3. Reduce foods:
   - Compare sodium in foods such as soup, bread, and frozen meals, and choose the foods with lower numbers.
   - Drink water instead of sugary drinks.

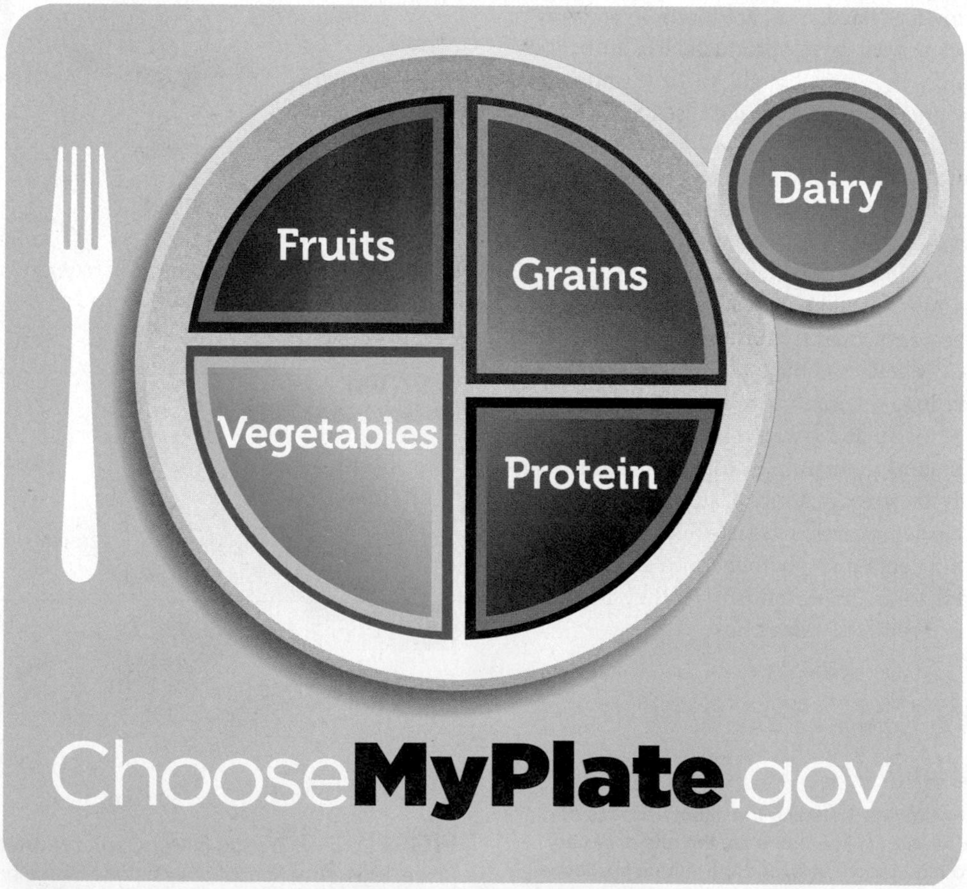

FIGURE 7.6 MyPlate Plan The USDA MyPlate food guidance system takes a new approach to dietary and exercise recommendations. Each colored section of the plate represents a food group, and an interactive tool at www.choosemyplate.gov helps you analyze and track your foods and physical activity, and provides helpful tips to personalize your plan.

Source: U.S. Department of Agriculture, 2013, www.choosemyplate.gov.

Understand Serving Sizes MyPlate presents personalized dietary recommendations based on servings of particular nutrients. But how much is one serving? Is it different from a portion? Although these two terms are often used interchangeably, they actually mean very different things. A *serving* is the recommended amount you should consume, whereas a *portion* is the amount you choose to eat at any one time. Many people select portions that are much bigger than recommended servings. See **FIGURE 7.7** for a handy pocket guide with tips on recognizing serving sizes.

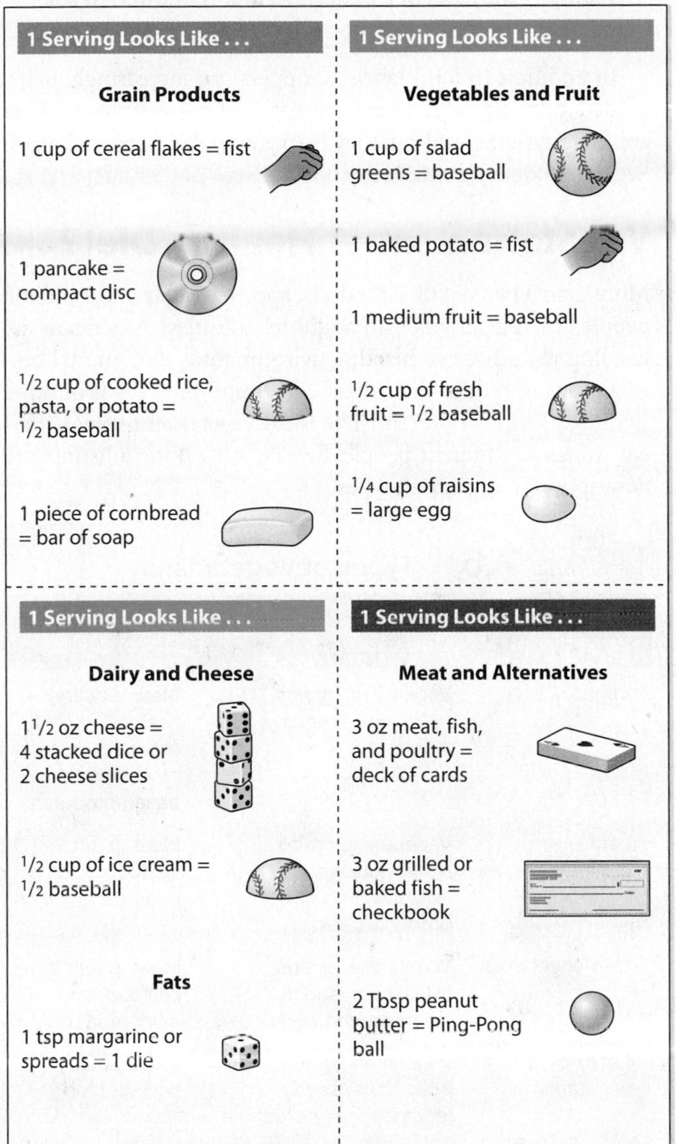

1 Serving Looks Like . . .
Grain Products
1 cup of cereal flakes = fist
1 pancake = compact disc
1/2 cup of cooked rice, pasta, or potato = 1/2 baseball
1 piece of cornbread = bar of soap
1 Serving Looks Like . . .
Vegetables and Fruit
1 cup of salad greens = baseball
1 baked potato = fist
1 medium fruit = baseball
1/2 cup of fresh fruit = 1/2 baseball
1/4 cup of raisins = large egg
1 Serving Looks Like . . .
Dairy and Cheese
1 1/2 oz cheese = 4 stacked dice or 2 cheese slices
1/2 cup of ice cream = 1/2 baseball
Fats
1 tsp margarine or spreads = 1 die
1 Serving Looks Like . . .
Meat and Alternatives
3 oz meat, fish, and poultry = deck of cards
3 oz grilled or baked fish = checkbook
2 Tbsp peanut butter = Ping-Pong ball

FIGURE 7.7 Serving Size Card One of the challenges of following a healthy diet is judging how big a portion size should be and how many servings you are really eating. The comparisons on this card can help you recall what a standard food serving looks like. For easy reference, photocopy or cut out this card, fold on the dotted lines, and keep it in your wallet. You can even laminate it for long-term use.

Source: National Heart, Lung and Blood Institute, "Serving Size Card," accessed April 2010, http://hp2010.nhlbihin.net/portion/servingcard7.pdf.

Unfortunately, we don't always get a clear picture from food producers and advertisers about what a serving really is. Consider a bottle of chocolate milk: The food label may list one serving size as 8 fluid ounces and 150 calories. However, note the size of the entire bottle. If it holds 16 ounces, drinking the whole thing serves up 300 calories.

SEE IT! VIDEOS

Cut back on sugar while satisfying your sweet tooth! Watch **Ditching Sugar** available on MasteringHealth.™

Eat Nutrient-Dense Foods Although eating the proper number of servings from MyPlate is important, it is also important to recognize that there are large caloric, fat, and energy differences among foods within a given food group. For example, salmon and hot dogs provide vastly different nutrient levels per calorie. Salmon is rich in essential fatty acids and is considered nutrient dense. Hot dogs are loaded with saturated fats, cholesterol, and sodium—all substances we should limit. It is important to eat foods that have a high nutritional value for their caloric content.

Reduce Empty Calorie Foods Avoid *empty calories*, that is, calories that have little or no nutritional value. Sugar is sugar, but when you eat it in a piece of fruit, you're getting dietary fiber, lots of vitamins and minerals, and phytochemicals. In contrast, when you drink a 12-ounce soft drink, you're getting nearly 200 empty calories. Don't be fooled by fruit drinks, either. Unless the label states that they're 100 percent juice, they may also be loaded with added sugar. Even 100 percent fresh-squeezed orange juice has 20 grams (5 teaspoons!) of naturally occurring sugar in an 8-ounce serving. Bottled coffees, teas, and energy drinks usually are even higher in sugar and empty calories.

47.5%

OF ADULTS DRINK AT LEAST ONE **SUGARY** DRINK A DAY.

MyPlate recommends we limit our intake of sugary drinks as well as the following sugar- and fat-laden items:[37]

- **Cakes, cookies, pastries, and donuts:** One slice of chocolate cake contains 77 percent empty calories.
- **Cheese:** Switching from whole milk mozzarella cheese to nonfat mozzarella cheese saves you 76 empty calories per ounce.
- **Pizza:** One slice of pepperoni pizza adds 139 empty calories to your meal.
- **Ice cream:** More than 75 percent of the 275 calories in ice cream are empty calories.
- **Sausages, hot dogs, bacon, and ribs:** Adding a sausage link to your breakfast adds 96 empty calories.

- **Wine, beer, and all alcoholic beverages:** A whopping 155 empty calories are consumed with each 12 fluid ounces of beer.
- **Refined grains, including crackers, cookies, and white rice:** Switching to whole wheat versions can save you 25 fat-laden empty calories per serving.

Physical Activity Strive to be physically active for at least 30 minutes daily, preferably with moderate to vigorous activity levels on most days. Physical activity does not mean you have to go to the gym, jog 3 miles a day, or hire a personal trainer. Any activity that gets your heart pumping counts, including gardening and other yard work, playing basketball, and dancing. MyPlate personalized plans offer recommendations for weekly physical activity. (For more on physical fitness, see **Chapter 9**.)

% Daily Values (%DVs) Percentages listed as "% DV" on food and supplement labels; identify how much of each listed nutrient or other substance a serving of food contributes to a 2,000 calorie/day diet.

vegetarian A person who follows a diet that excludes some or all animal products.

Read Food Labels

How do you know what nutrients the packaged foods you eat are contributing to your diet? To help consumers evaluate the nutritional values of packaged foods, the FDA and the USDA developed the Nutrition Facts label that is typically displayed on the side or back of packaged foods. One of the most helpful items on the label is the **% daily values (%DVs)** list, which tells you how much of an average adult's allowance for a particular substance (fat, fiber, calcium, etc.) is provided by a serving of the food. The %DV is calculated based on a 2,000 calorie per day diet, so your values may be different from those listed on a label. The label also includes information on the serving size and calories. In 2014, the FDA announced plans to make the data on the label more helpful for consumers by identifying the calories per serving in much larger type, and adjusting the serving size so that it better reflects the amount of the food that people typically eat.[38] **FIGURE 7.8** walks you through a typical Nutrition Facts label. For the latest information on the new label, go to www.FDA.gov and search "Nutrition Facts label."

35%

OF COLLEGE STUDENTS FREQUENTLY READ **NUTRITION LABELS**.

Food labels contain other information as well, such as the name and manufacturer of the product, an ingredients list, and sometimes claims about the product's contents or effects. The FDA allows three types of claims on the packages of foods and dietary supplements:[39]

- Health claims describe a relationship between a food product and health promotion or disease prevention. These must be approved by the FDA and supported by evidence. For example, an approved health claim on a package of whole-grain bread may state, "In a low-fat diet, whole-grain foods like this bread may reduce the risk of heart disease."
- Nutrient content claims indicate a specific nutrient is present at a certain level. For example, a product label might say "High in fiber" or "Low in fat" or "This product contains 100 calories per serving." Nutrient content claims can use the following words: *more, less, fewer, good source of, free, light, lean, extra lean, high, low, reduced.*
- Structure and function claims describe the effect that a component in the food product has on the body. For example, the label of a carton of milk is allowed to state, "Calcium builds strong bones."

In addition to food labels, shoppers are increasingly being guided in their food choices by nutritional rating systems. What are these systems, and can they help you make smarter choices? See the **Student Health Today** box on page 214 for answers.

Vegetarianism: A Healthy Diet?

More than 3 percent of U.S. adults, approximately 4 to 9 million people, are vegetarians.[40] In addition, countless Americans are heeding the advice of health, environmental, and animal ethics groups to reduce their meat consumption in favor of other "faceless" forms of protein. The word **vegetarian** means different things to different people. See **TABLE 7.6** for a listing and description of vegetarian types.

TABLE **7.6** | Types of Vegetarians

Type of Vegetarian	Does Eat	Doesn't Eat
Vegan	Vegetables, grains, fruits, nuts, seeds, and legumes	Meat, poultry, seafood, dairy products, eggs, any other animal-based products
Lacto-vegetarian	Vegetables, grains, fruits, nuts, seeds, legumes, and dairy products	Meat, poultry, seafood, and eggs
Ovo-vegetarian	Vegetables, grains, fruits, nuts, seeds, legumes, and eggs	Meat, poultry, seafood, and dairy products
Lacto-ovo-vegetarian	Vegetables, grains, fruits, nuts, seeds, legumes, dairy products, and eggs	Meat, poultry, and seafood
Pesco-vegetarian	Vegetables, grains, fruits, nuts, seeds, legumes, dairy products, eggs, and seafood	Meat and poultry
Semi-vegetarian (or "non–red meat eater")	Vegetables, grains, fruits, nuts, seeds, legumes, dairy products, eggs, seafood, and poultry (occasional)	Red meat

Sample Label for Macaroni and Cheese

Nutrition Facts

Serving size 1 cup (228g)
Servings Per Container 2

Amount Per Serving

Calories 250	Calories from Fat 110
	% Daily Value*
Total Fat 12g	**18%**
Saturated Fat 3g	**15%**
Trans Fat 1.5g	
Cholesterol 30mg	**10%**
Sodium 470mg	**20%**
Total Carbohydrate 31g	**10%**
Dietary Fiber 0g	**0%**
Sugars 5g	
Protein 5g	
Vitamin A	4%
Vitamin C	2%
Calcium	20%
Iron	4%

* Percent Daily Values are based on a 2,000 calorie diet. Your Daily Values may be higher or lower depending on your calorie needs:

	Calories:	2,000	2,500
Total Fat	Less than	65g	80g
Sat Fat	Less than	20g	25g
Cholesterol	Less than	300mg	300mg
Sodium	Less than	2,400mg	2,400mg
Total Carbohydrate		300g	375g
Dietary Fiber		25g	30g

Start here. The size of the serving on the food package influences the number of calories and all the nutrient amounts listed on the top part of the label. Pay attention to the serving size, especially how many servings there are in the food package. Then ask yourself, "How many servings am I consuming?"

Limit these nutrients. The nutrients listed first are the ones Americans generally eat in adequate amounts, or even too much of. Eating too much fat, saturated fat, *trans* fat, cholesterol, or sodium may increase your risk of certain chronic diseases, such as heart disease, some cancers, or high blood pressure.

Get enough of these nutrients. Most Americans don't get enough dietary fiber, vitamin A, vitamin C, calcium, and iron in their diets. Eating enough of these nutrients can improve your health and help reduce the risk of some diseases and conditions.

The footnote is not specific to the product. It shows recommended dietary advice for all Americans. The Percent Daily Values are based on a 2,000-calorie diet, but the footnote lists daily values for both a 2,000- and 2,500-calorie diet.

Pay attention to calories (and calories from fat). Many Americans consume more calories than they need. Remember: The number of servings you consume determines the number of calories you actually eat (your portion amount). Dietary guidelines recommend that no more than 30% of your daily calories consumed come from fat.

5% DV or less is low and 20% DV or more is high. The % DV helps you determine if a serving of food is high or low in a nutrient, whether or not you consume the 2,000-calorie diet it is based on. It also helps you make easy comparisons between products (just make sure the serving sizes are similar).

Note that a few nutrients—*trans* fats, sugars, and protein—do not have a % DV. Experts could not provide a reference value for *trans* fat, but it is recommended that you keep your intake as low as possible. There are no recommendations for the total amount of sugar to eat in one day, but check the ingredient list to see information on added sugars, such as high fructose corn syrup. A % DV for protein is required to be listed if a claim is made (such as "high in protein") or if the food is meant for infants and children under 4 years old. Otherwise, none is needed.

FIGURE 7.8 Reading a Food Label

Source: Center for Food Safety and Applied Nutrition, "A Key to Choosing Healthful Foods: Using the Nutrition Facts on the Food Label," Updated March 2013, www.fda.gov/Food/ResourcesForYou/Consumers/ucm079449.htm

VIDEO TUTOR
Understanding Food Labels

Common reasons for pursuing a vegetarian lifestyle include concern for animal welfare, the environmental costs of meat production, food safety, personal health, weight loss, and weight maintenance. Generally, people who follow a balanced vegetarian diet weigh less and have better cholesterol levels, fewer problems with irregular bowel movements (constipation and diarrhea), and a lower risk of heart disease than do nonvegetarians. A recent analysis of 29 studies involving a total of more than 20,000 participants found that people who follow a vegetarian diet have an average blood pressure several points lower than that of nonvegetarians.[41] Some studies suggest that vegetarianism may also reduce the risk of some cancers, particularly colon cancer.[42]

With proper meal planning, vegetarianism provides a healthful alternative to a meat-based diet. Eating a variety of healthful foods throughout the day helps to ensure proper nutrient intake. Vegan diets are of greater concern than diets that include dairy products and eggs. Vegans may be deficient in vitamins B_2 (riboflavin), B_{12}, and D, as well as calcium, iron, zinc, and other minerals; however, many foods are fortified with these nutrients, or vegans can obtain them from supplements. Vegans also have to pay more attention to the amino acid content of their foods, but eating a variety of types of plant foods throughout the day will provide adequate amounts of protein. Pregnant women, older adults, sick people, and families with young children who are vegans need to take special care to ensure that their diets are adequate. In all cases, seek advice from a health care professional if you have questions.

WHAT DO YOU THINK?

Why are so many people becoming vegetarians?

- How easy is it to be a vegetarian on your campus?
- What concerns about vegetarianism do you have, if any?

STUDENT HEALTH TODAY

NUTRITION RATING SYSTEMS

Next time you're at the grocery store, take a close look at the tags on the store shelves. Do you see anything different—stars, perhaps, or numbers inside blue hexagons? If so, you're looking at one of several new nutrition rating systems. These systems were designed by nutrition scientists and physicians to help consumers quickly locate healthful foods. Three of the most popular systems in American markets are as follows:

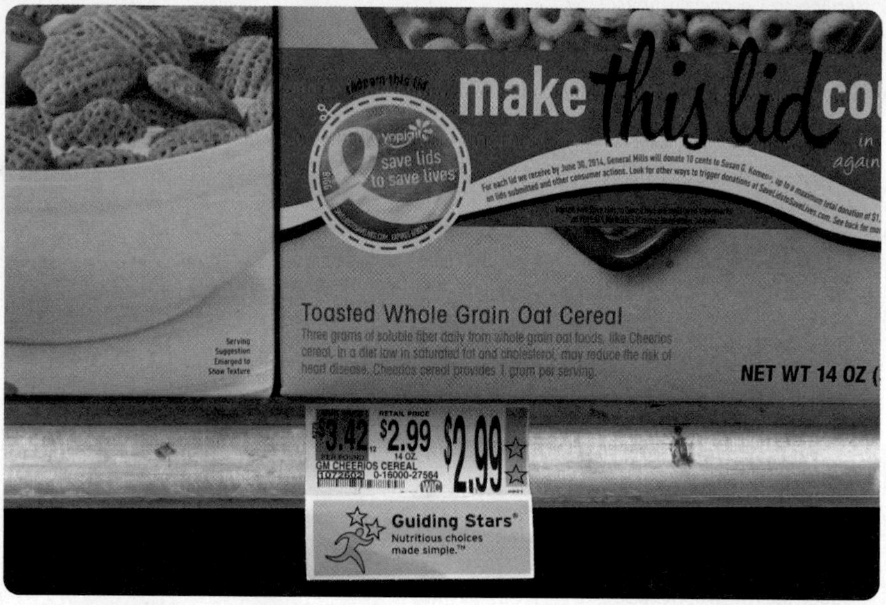

- **Guiding Stars.** This system rates the nutritional quality of foods using information from the Nutrition Facts label and the food's ingredients list. Foods are rated with from zero to three stars, with three indicating the highest nutritional quality. A fresh tomato, for example, gets three stars. When the program was implemented, all foods sold by the participating retailers were evaluated, and less than one-fourth earned even a single star. What the system lacks in subtlety it makes up for in simplicity—even consumers who haven't been introduced to it can almost instantly understand the basic message behind it: The product with the most stars "wins."
- **NuVal.** The NuVal System uses a scale of 1 to 100. The higher the number, the higher the nutritional quality. In rating each food, the system considers more than 30 dietary components—not just nutrients, but fiber, antioxidants, and other food components known to affect health. In this system, a tomato gets a top score of 100 points. The 100-point rating scale allows consumers to make more subtle distinctions between very similar foods; for example, two brands of whole-grain bread get scores of 48 versus 29. Although the consumer doesn't need to stop and research the food, the ranking suggests real differences, and in fact, the bread with the higher score is lower in calories and sodium, higher in calcium, and has twice the dietary fiber per slice.
- **Aggregate Nutrient Density Index (ANDI).** This index ranks foods based on the number of micronutrients per calorie and takes into account as many known beneficial phytochemicals as possible. It does not, however, consider macronutrient density, such as the amount of high-quality protein or essential fatty acids in the food. A top score is 1,000. How does this system rate our tomato? It gets just 164 points! In contrast, kale gets a top score of 1,000. Again, the difference is in the calorie/micronutrient ratio: A medium-sized tomato and two thirds of a cup of kale have about the same number of calories, yet the kale has about 7 times as much vitamin A and 3.5 times as much vitamin C.

Do these ranking systems prompt shoppers to choose more healthful foods? Research suggests they just might. An evaluation in the *American Journal of Clinical Nutrition* found that the systems reduce the time and effort consumers spend in making food choices, as compared with more detailed labels, and have the potential to help them choose more healthful foods. That's important because, as an evaluation of the NuVal system from the Harvard School of Public Health found, people who eat food with higher scores have a lower risk of cardiovascular disease and diabetes, and may even enjoy a longer life.

Sources: S. A. Gerrior, "Nutrient Profiling Systems: Are Science and the Consumer Connected?," *American Journal of Clinical Nutrition* 91, no. 4 (2010): 1116S–7S; L. M. Fischer et al., "Development and Implementation of the Guiding Stars Nutrition Guidance Program," *American Journal of Health Promotion* 26, no. 2 (2011): e55–63, DOI: 10.4278/ajhp.100709-QUAL-238; S. E. Chiuve, L. Sampson, and W. C. Willett, "The Association between a Nutritional Quality Index and Risk of Chronic Disease," *American Journal of Preventive Medicine* 40, no. 5 (2011):505–13, DOI: 10.1016/j.amepre.2010.11.022.

Supplements: Research on the Daily Dose

Dietary supplements are products containing one or more dietary ingredients taken by mouth and intended to supplement existing diets. Ingredients range from vitamins, minerals, and herbs, to enzymes, amino acids, fatty acids, and organ tissues. They can come in tablet, capsule, liquid, powder, and other forms. Because of dietary supplements' potential for influencing health, their sales have skyrocketed.

It is important to note that dietary supplements are not regulated like foods or drugs. The FDA does not evaluate the safety and efficacy of supplements prior to their marketing, and it can take action to remove a supplement from the

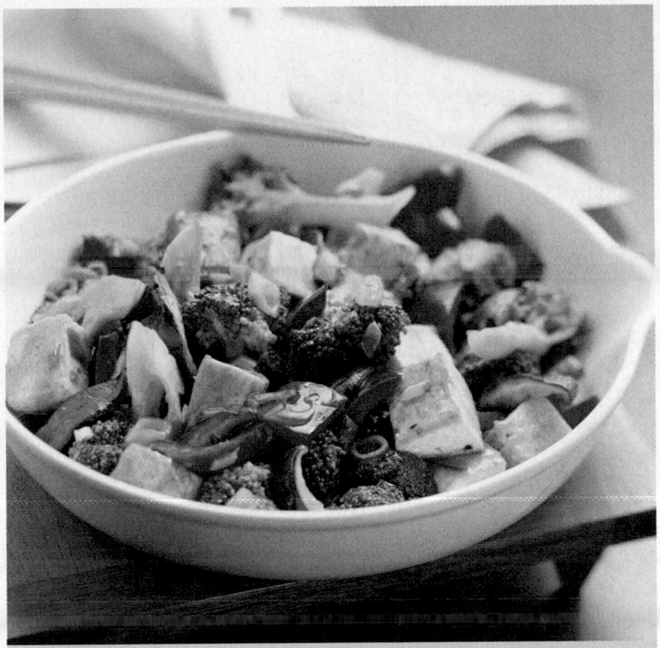

Adopting a vegetarian diet can be a very healthy way to eat. Take care to prepare your food healthfully by avoiding added sugars and excessive sodium. Make sure you get complementary essential amino acids throughout the day. Meals like this tofu and vegetable stir-fry can be further enhanced by adding a whole grain, such as brown rice.

market only after the product has been proved harmful. Currently, the United States has no formal guidelines for supplement marketing and safety, and supplement manufacturers are responsible for self-monitoring their activities.

Do you really need to take dietary supplements? The Office of Dietary Supplements, part of the National Institutes of Health, states that some supplements may help ensure that you get adequate amounts of essential nutrients if you don't consume a variety of foods, as recommended in the Dietary Guidelines for Americans. However, dietary supplements are not intended to prevent or treat disease, and recently the U.S. Preventive Services Task Force concluded that there is insufficient evidence to recommend that healthy people take multivitamin/mineral supplements to prevent cardiovascular disease or cancer.[43] Populations who may benefit from using multivitamin/mineral supplements include pregnant and breast-feeding women, older adults, vegans, people on a very low-calorie weight-loss diets, alcohol-dependent individuals, and patients with malabsorption problems or other significant health problems.

The wisdom of taking other types of supplements, as opposed to consuming nutrients in whole foods, is also unproven. For example, the benefit of fish consumption in reducing the risk for cardiovascular disease is well-established, but studies have shown conflicting results about fish-oil supplements.[44]

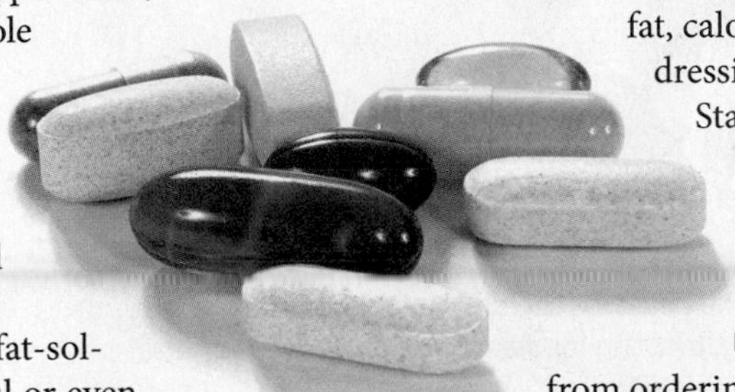

Taking high-dose supplements of the fat-soluble vitamins A, D, and E can be harmful or even fatal. Too much vitamin A, for example, can damage the liver, and excessive vitamin E increases the risk for a stroke.[45] The Academy of Nutrition and Dietetics recommends that, though some people benefit from taking supplements, a healthy diet is the best way to give your body what it needs.[46]

COLLEGE **MALES** SPEND AN AVERAGE OF

$99.17

AND COLLEGE **FEMALES** SPEND AN AVERAGE OF

$52.11

ON FAST FOOD IN A MONTH.

Eating Well in College

Many college students find it hard to fit a well-balanced meal into the day, but breakfast and lunch are important if you are to keep energy levels up and get the most out of your classes. Eating a complete breakfast that includes fiber-rich carbohydrates, protein, and healthy unsaturated fat (such as a banana, peanut butter, and whole-grain bread sandwich or a bowl of oatmeal topped with dried fruit and nuts) is key. If you are short on time, bring a container of yogurt and some trail mix to your morning class.

dietary supplements Products taken by mouth and containing dietary ingredients such as vitamins and minerals that are intended to supplement existing diets.

If your campus is like many others, your lunchtime options include a variety of fast-food restaurants. Generally speaking, you can eat more healthfully and for less money if you bring food from home or eat at your campus dining hall. If you must eat fast food, follow the tips below to get more nutritional bang for your buck:

- Ask for nutritional analyses of menu items. Most fast-food chains now have them. Calories of individual items are often noted on the menu.
- Order salads, but be careful about what you add to them. Taco salads and Cobb salads are often high in fat, calories, and sodium. Ask for low-fat dressing on the side, and use it sparingly. Stay away from high-fat add-ons, such as bacon bits, croutons, and crispy noodles.
- If you crave french fries, try baked "fries," which may be lower in fat.
- Avoid giant sizes, and refrain from ordering extra sauce, bacon, cheese, and other toppings that add calories, sodium, and fat.

DO IT! NUTRITOOLS

Ever wondered how your favorite meal stacks up, nutrition-wise? Complete the **Build a Meal, Build a Salad, Build a Pizza,** and **Build a Sandwich** activities available on MasteringHealth.™

- Limit sodas and other beverages that are high in added sugars.
- At least once per week, swap a vegetable-based meat substitute into your fast-food choices. Most fast-food restaurants now offer veggie burgers and similar products, which provide excellent sources of protein and often have less fat and fewer calories than typical meaty meals.

In the dining hall, try these ideas:

- Choose lean meats, grilled chicken, fish, or vegetable dishes. Avoid fried chicken, fatty cuts of red meat, or meat dishes smothered in creamy or oily sauce.
- Hit the salad bar and load up on leafy greens, beans, tuna, or tofu. Choose items such as avocado or nuts for "good" fat. Go easy on the dressing, or substitute vinaigrette or low-fat dressings.
- When choosing items from a made-to-order food station, ask the preparer to hold the butter or oil, mayonnaise, sour cream, or cheese- or cream-based sauces.
- Avoid going back for seconds and consuming large portions.
- If there is something you'd like but don't see in your dining hall, speak to your food service manager and provide suggestions.
- Pass on high-calorie, low-nutrient foods such as sugary cereals, ice cream, and other sweet treats. Choose fruit or low-fat yogurt to satisfy your sweet tooth.

Between classes, avoid vending machines. Reach into your backpack for an apple, banana, some dried fruit and nuts, a single serving of unsweetened applesauce, or whole-grain crackers spread with peanut butter. Energy bars can be a nutritious option if you choose right. Check the Nutrition Facts label for bars that are below 200 calories and provide at least 3 grams of dietary fiber. Cereal bars usually provide less protein than energy bars; however, they also tend to be much lower in calories and sugar, and high in fiber.

Maintaining a nutritious diet within the confines of student life can be challenging. However, if you take the time to plan healthy meals, you will find that you are eating better, enjoying it more, and actually saving money. The **Skills for Behavior Change** box boils down healthy eating into some simple tips to follow. The **Money & Health** box examines ways to include fruits and vegetables in your diet without breaking the bank.

SKILLS FOR BEHAVIOR CHANGE

HEALTHY EATING SIMPLIFIED

Does all this information leave you scratching your head about how to eat healthfully? When it all starts to feel too complicated, here are some simple tips to follow:

- You don't need foods from fancy packages to improve your health. Fruits, vegetables, and whole grains should make up the bulk of your diet. Shop the perimeter of the store and the bulk foods aisle.
- Let the MyPlate method guide you. Your meal should be mostly vegetables and grains. Less than a quarter of your meal should be lean protein. Include a calcium-rich beverage. A serving of fruit should be dessert.
- Avoid or limit processed and packaged foods. This will help you limit added sodium, sugar, and fat. If you can't make sense of the ingredients, don't eat it.
- Eat natural snacks such as fresh or dried fruit, nuts, string cheese, yogurt without added sugar, hard-boiled eggs, and vegetables.
- Be mindful of your eating. Eat until you are satisfied but not overfull.
- Bring healthful foods with you when you head out the door. Whether to class, on a road trip, or going to work, you can control the foods that are available. Don't put yourself in a position to buy from a vending machine or convenience store.

Source: M. Pollan, *Food Rules: An Eater's Manual* (New York: Penguin Books, 2010).

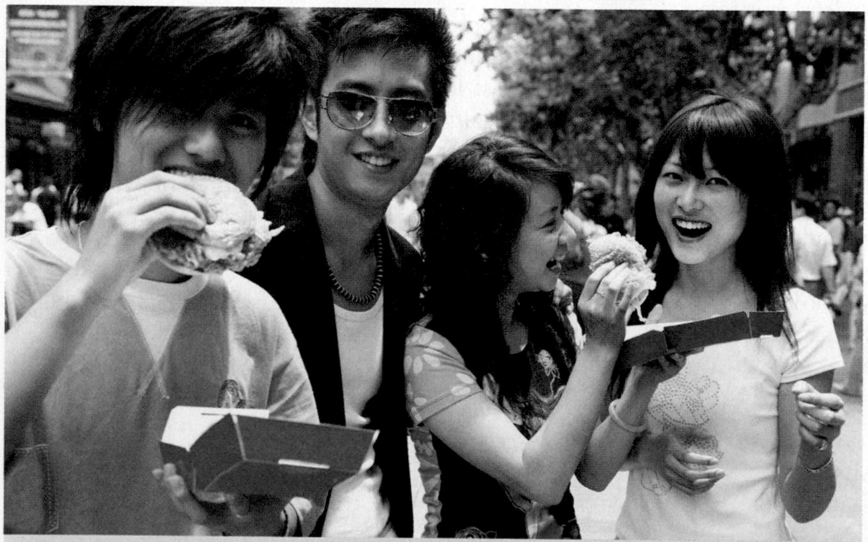

Meals like this one may be convenient, but they are high in saturated fat, sodium, refined carbohydrates, and calories. Even when you are short on time and money, it is possible—and worthwhile—to make healthier choices. If you are ordering fast food, opt for foods prepared by baking, roasting, or steaming; ask for the leanest meat option; and request that sauces, dressings, and gravies be served on the side.

MONEY & HEALTH | ARE FRUITS AND VEGGIES BEYOND YOUR BUDGET?

Many people on a tight budget, including college students, think that fruits and vegetables are beyond their budget. Maybe a carton of orange juice and a package of carrots are affordable, but five to nine servings a day? No way.

If that sounds like you, it's time for some facts. In 2011, the U.S. Department of Agriculture published data showing that the average American family spends more money on food than is necessary to consume a nutritious diet—one that includes the recommended servings of fruits and vegetables. The report concluded that, contrary to popular opinion, people on a tight budget can eat healthfully, including plenty of fruits and vegetables, and spend less on food.

So how do you do it? Here are some tips:

- Focus on five fresh favorites. Throughout the United States, five of the least expensive, perennially available fresh vegetables are carrots, eggplant, lettuce, potatoes, and summer squash. Five fresh fruit options are apples, bananas, pears, pineapple, and watermelon.
- Buy small amounts frequently. Most items of fresh produce keep only a few days, so buy amounts that you know you'll be able to eat or freeze.
- Celebrate the season. From apples to zucchini, when fruits and veggies are in season, they cost less. If you can freeze them, stock up. If not, enjoy them fresh while you can.
- Do it yourself. Avoid prewashed, precut fruits and vegetables, including salad greens. They cost more and often spoil faster. Also choose frozen 100 percent juice concentrate and add the water yourself.
- Buy canned or frozen on sale, in bulk. Canned and frozen produce, especially when it's on sale, may be much less expensive than fresh. Most frozen items are just as nutritious as fresh, and can be even more so, depending on how long ago the fresh food was harvested. For canned items, choose fruits without added sugars and vegetables without added salt or sauces. Bear in mind that beans are legumes and count as a vegetable choice. Low-sodium canned beans are one of the most affordable, convenient, and nutritious foods you can buy. If you can't find low-sodium beans, just rinse them before heating.
- Fix and freeze. Make large batches of homemade soup, vegetable stews, and pasta sauce and store them in single-serving containers in your freezer.
- Grow your own. All it takes is one sunny window, a pot, soil, and a packet of seeds. Lettuce, spinach, and fresh herbs are particularly easy to grow indoors in small spaces.

Sources: U.S. Department of Agriculture, *Eating Healthy on a Budget: The Consumer Economics Perspective*, September 2011, www.choosemyplate.gov/food-groups/downloads/ConsumerEconomicsPerspective.pdf; U.S. Department of Agriculture, Center for Nutrition Policy and Promotion, *Smart Shopping for Veggies and Fruits,* September 2011, www.choosemyplate.gov/food-groups/downloads/TenTips/DGTipsheet9SmartShopping.pdf; U.S. Centers for Disease Control and Prevention, Fruits & Veggies: More Matters, *30 Ways in 30 Days to Stretch Your Fruit & Vegetable Budget,* September 2011, www.fruitsandveggiesmatter.gov/downloads/Stretch_FV_Budget.pdf.

Choosing Organic or Locally Grown Foods

organic Grown without use of toxic and persistent pesticides, chemicals, or hormones.

Concerns about the health effects of chemicals used to grow and produce food have led many people to turn to foods that are **organic**—foods and beverages developed, grown, or raised without the use of toxic and persistent pesticides or fertilizers, antibiotics, or hormones. Any food sold in the United States as organic has to meet criteria set by the USDA under the National Organic Rule and can carry a USDA seal verifying products as "certified organic." Under this rule, a product that is certified may carry one of the following terms: "100 percent Organic" (100% compliance with organic criteria), "Organic" (must contain at least 95% organic materials), "Made with Organic Ingredients" (must contain at least 70% organic ingredients), or "Some Organic Ingredients" (contains less than 70% organic ingredients—usually listed individually). To be labeled with any of the above terms, the foods also must be produced without genetic modification or germ-killing radiation. However, reliable monitoring systems to ensure credibility are still under development.

U.S. FDA label for organic foods.

The market for organic foods has been increasing faster than food sales in general for many years. Whereas only a small subset of the population once bought organic, 81 percent of all U.S. families are now buying organic foods at least occasionally.[47] In 2010, annual organic food sales were estimated to be $31 billion.[48]

Is buying organic food really better for you, though? That depends on what aspect of the food is being studied, and how the research is conducted. Two recent review studies, both of which examined decades of research into the nutrient quality of organic versus traditionally grown foods, reached opposite conclusions: one found organic foods more nutritious, and the other did not.[49] However, we do know that pesticide residues remain on conventionally grown produce. The U.S. Environmental Protection Agency warns that food pesticides can lead to health problems like cancer, nerve damage, and birth defects.[50] In 2013, the USDA reported that 3.7 percent of food samples harvested in 2011 had pesticide residues that exceeded the established tolerance level or had residues of pesticides for which no tolerance level has been established.[51] Both agencies advise consumers to wash fruits and vegetables before cooking or consuming them.

The word **locavore** has been coined to describe people who eat mostly food grown or produced locally, usually within close proximity to their homes. Farmers' markets or homegrown foods or those grown by independent farmers are thought to be fresher and to require far fewer resources to get them to market and keep them fresh for longer periods of time. Locavores believe that locally grown organic food is preferable to foods produced by large corporations or supermarket-based organic foods, as they make a smaller impact on the environment.

locavore A person who primarily eats food grown or produced locally.

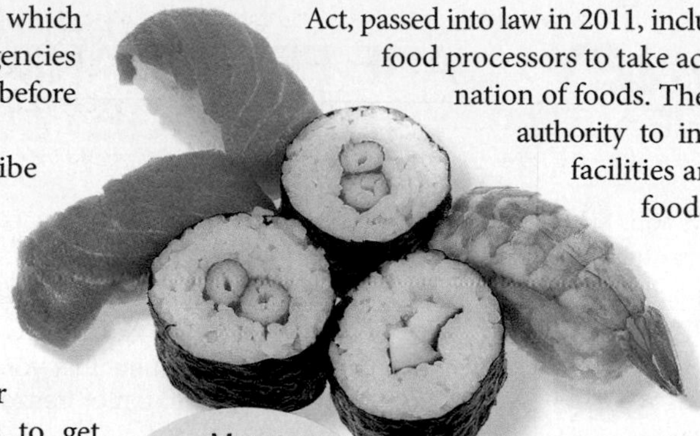

Many people worldwide enjoy sashimi and sushi. Use caution when eating, however, as raw fish can be a breeding ground for dangerous microbes.

LO 3 | FOOD SAFETY: A GROWING CONCERN

Explain food safety concerns facing Americans and people in other regions of the world.

Eating unhealthy food is one thing. Eating food that has been contaminated with a microorganism, toxin, or other harmful substance is quite another. As outbreaks of foodborne illness (commonly called food poisoning) make the news, the food industry has come under fire. The Food Safety Modernization Act, passed into law in 2011, included new requirements for food processors to take actions to prevent contamination of foods. The act gave the FDA greater authority to inspect food-manufacturing facilities and to recall contaminated foods.[52]

Foodborne Illnesses

Are you concerned that the chicken you are buying doesn't look pleasingly pink or your "fresh" fish smells a little *too* fishy? You may have good reason to be worried. Scientists estimate that foodborne illnesses sicken 1 in 6 Americans (over 48 million people) and cause some 128,000 hospitalizations and 3,000 deaths in the United States annually.[53] Although the incidence of infection with certain microbes has declined, current data from the U.S. Centers for Disease Control and Prevention (CDC) show a lack of recent progress in reducing foodborne infections and highlight the need for improved prevention.[54]

TABLE 7.7 lists some of the most common microbial culprits behind foodborne illness. Foodborne illness can be caused by multiplication of the microbe itself or by the presence in the food of a toxin that was originally produced by a microbe. These toxins can produce illness even if the microbes that produced them are no longer there. For example, botulism is caused by a deadly toxin produced by the bacterium *Clostridium botulinum*. This bacterium is widespread in soil, water,

TABLE 7.7 | Five Most Common Foodborne Illnesses

Microbe	Illnesses per Year	Description
Norovirus	5.4 million	Transmitted through contact with the vomit or stool of infected people, norovirus is the most common cause of foodborne illness in the United States annually. Symptoms include nausea, vomiting, and diarrhea. Most cases are self-limiting, but about 800 Americans die of infection each year. There is no treatment, but washing hands and all kitchen surfaces can help prevent transmission.
Salmonella	1 million	Commonly found in the intestines of birds, reptiles, and mammals, it can spread to humans through foods of animal origin. Infection by *Salmonella* usually consists of fever, diarrhea, and abdominal cramps. Salmonellosis can be life threatening if the bacteria invade the bloodstream, as is more likely in people with poor underlying health or weakened immune systems.
Clostridium perfringens	966,000	Bacterial species found in the intestinal tracts of humans and animals, as well as in the environment. Infection causes abdominal cramping and diarrhea.
Campylobacter	845,000	Most raw poultry has *Campylobacter* in it, and this bacterial infection most frequently results from eating undercooked chicken, raw eggs, or foods contaminated with juices from raw chicken. Shellfish and unpasteurized milk are also sources. Infection causes fever, diarrhea, and abdominal cramps.
Staphylococcus aureus	241,000	*Staph* lives on human skin, in infected cuts, and in the nose and throat. Infection causes severe nausea, vomiting, and diarrhea that lasts 1–3 days.

Source: Data are from Centers for Disease Control and Prevention, CDC Estimates of Foodborne Illness in the United States, "CDC 2011 Estimates: Findings," Updated January 8, 2014, from www.cdc.gov/foodborneburden/2011-foodborne-estimates.html.

SEE IT! VIDEOS

Are whole grain product labels telling the truth? Watch **Grain Labels Do Not Reflect "Whole" Truth** available on MasteringHealth.™

plants, and intestinal tracts, but it can grow only in environments with limited or no oxygen. Potential food sources include improperly canned food and vacuum-packed or tightly wrapped foods. Though rare, botulism is fatal if untreated.

Signs of foodborne illnesses vary tremendously but usually include diarrhea, nausea, abdominal cramping, and vomiting. Depending on the amount and virulence of the microbe, symptoms may appear as early as 30 minutes after eating contaminated food or as long as several days or weeks later. Most of the time, symptoms occur 5 to 8 hours after eating and last only a day or two. For certain populations, such as the very young; older adults; or people with severe illnesses such as cancer, diabetes, kidney disease, or AIDS, foodborne diseases can be fatal.

Several factors contribute to foodborne illnesses. Since fresh foods are not in season much of the year, the United States imports $18 billion in fresh fruits and vegetables from other countries, often from great distances. These countries include Mexico (36% of imports), several Central and South American countries (about 25%), and China (8%).[55] Although we are told when we travel to developing and transitioning countries to "boil it, peel it, or don't eat it," we bring these imported foods into our kitchens at home and eat them, often without washing them.

Food can become contaminated in the field by being watered with tainted water, fertilized with animal manure, or harvested by people who have not washed their hands properly after using the toilet. Food-processing equipment, facilities, or workers may contaminate food, or it can become contaminated if not kept clean and cool during transport or on store shelves. To give you an idea of the implications, studies have shown that the bacterium *Escherichia coli* can survive in cow manure for up to 70 days and can multiply in crops grown with manure unless heat or additives such as salt or preservatives are used to kill the microbes.[56] There are no regulations that prohibit farmers from using animal manure to fertilize crops. In addition, *E. coli* quickly reproduces in summer months as cattle await slaughter in crowded, overheated pens. This increases the chances of meat coming to market already contaminated.

Avoiding Risks in the Home

Part of the responsibility for preventing foodborne illness lies with consumers—more than 30 percent of all foodborne illnesses result from unsafe handling of food at home. Four basic steps reduce the likelihood of contaminating your food (see **FIGURE 7.9**). Among the most basic precautions are to wash your hands and to wash all produce before eating it. Also, avoid cross-contamination in the kitchen by using separate cutting boards and utensils for meats and produce. Temperature control is also important—refrigerators must be set at 40°F or lower. Cook meats to the recommended temperature to kill contaminants before eating. Keep hot foods hot and cold foods cold to avoid unchecked bacterial growth. Eat leftovers within 3 days, and if you're unsure how long something has been sitting in the fridge, don't take chances. When in doubt, throw it out. See the **Skills for Behavior Change** box for more tips about reducing the risk of foodborne illness.

SKILLS FOR BEHAVIOR CHANGE

REDUCE YOUR RISK FOR FOODBORNE ILLNESS

- When shopping, put perishable foods in your cart last. Check for cleanliness throughout the store, especially at the salad bar and at the meat and fish counters. Never buy dented cans of food. Check the "sell by" or "use by" date on foods.
- Once you get home, put dairy products, eggs, meat, fish, and poultry in the refrigerator immediately. If you don't plan to eat meats within 2 days, freeze them. You can keep an unopened package of hot dogs or luncheon meats for about 2 weeks.
- When refrigerating or freezing raw meats, make sure their juices can't spill onto other foods.
- Never thaw frozen foods at room temperature. Put them in the refrigerator to thaw or thaw in the microwave, following manufacturer's instructions.
- Wash your hands with soap and warm water before preparing food. Wash fruits and vegetables before peeling, slicing, cooking, or eating them—but not meat, poultry, or eggs! Wash cutting boards, countertops, and other utensils and surfaces with detergent and hot water after food preparation.
- Use a meat thermometer to ensure that meats are completely cooked. To find out proper cooking temperatures for different types of meat, visit http://foodsafety.gov/keep/charts/mintemp.html.
- Refrigeration slows the secretion of bacterial toxins into foods. Never leave leftovers out for more than 2 hours. On hot days, don't leave foods out for longer than 1 hour.

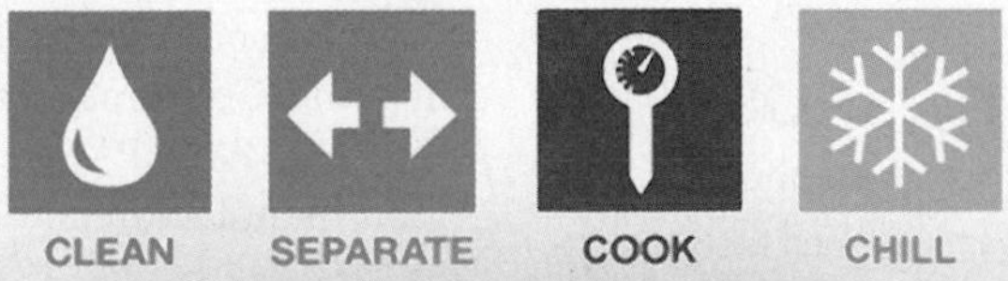

FIGURE 7.9 The Core Four Practices This logo reminds consumers how to prevent foodborne illness.

Source: Partnership for Food Safety Education, http://www.fightbac.org/safe-food-handling.

Food Irradiation

Food irradiation is a process that exposes foods to low doses of radiation, or ionizing energy, to break down the DNA of harmful bacteria, destroying them or keeping them from reproducing. Essentially, the rays pass through the food without leaving any radioactive residue.[57]

USDA label for irradiated foods.

Irradiation lengthens food products' shelf life and prevents the spread of deadly microorganisms, particularly in high-risk foods such as ground beef and pork. Thus, the minimal costs of irradiation result in lower overall costs to consumers and reduce the need for toxic chemicals to preserve foods. Use of food irradiation is limited because of consumer concerns about safety and because irradiation facilities are expensive to build. Still, food irradiation is now common in over 40 countries. Foods that have been irradiated are marked with the "radura" logo.

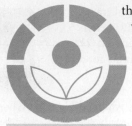

food irradiation Exposing foods to low doses of radiation to kill microorganisms or keep them from reproducing.

food allergy Overreaction by the immune system to normally harmless proteins, which are perceived as allergens. In response, the body produces antibodies, triggering allergic symptoms.

celiac disease An inherited immune disorder causing malabsorption of nutrients from the small intestine and triggered by the consumption of gluten, a protein found in certain grains.

food intolerance Adverse effects that result when people who lack the digestive chemicals needed to break down certain substances eat those substances.

Food Sensitivities

About 33 percent of people today *think* they have a food allergy; however, it is estimated that only 5 percent of children and 4 percent of adults actually do.[58] Still, the prevalence of reported food allergies is on the rise. Data suggest the prevalence of peanut allergies among children tripled between 1997 and 2008.[59]

A **food allergy**, or hypersensitivity, is an abnormal response to a component—usually a protein—in food that is triggered by the immune system. Symptoms of an allergic reaction vary in severity and may include a tingling sensation in the mouth; swelling of the lips, tongue, and throat; difficulty breathing; skin hives; vomiting; abdominal cramps; and diarrhea. Approximately 100 to 200 deaths per year occur as a result of more severe reactions called *anaphylaxis* that cause widespread inflammation and cardiovascular problems such as a sudden drop in blood pressure. Anaphylaxis may occur within seconds to hours after eating the foods to which one is allergic.[60]

SEE IT! VIDEOS

How accurate are restaurant calorie counts? Watch **Menu Calorie Counts** available on MasteringHealth.™

The Food Allergen Labeling and Consumer Protection Act (FALCPA) requires food manufacturers to label foods clearly to indicate the presence of (or possible contamination by) any of the eight major food allergens: milk, eggs, peanuts, wheat, soy, tree nuts (walnuts, pecans, cashews, pistachios, etc.), fish, and shellfish. Although over 160 foods have been identified as allergy triggers, these eight foods account for 90 percent of all food allergies in the United States.[61]

Celiac disease is an immune disorder that causes malabsorption of nutrients from the small intestine in genetically susceptible people. It is thought to affect over 2 million Americans, most of whom are undiagnosed.[62] When a person with celiac disease consumes gluten—a protein found in wheat, rye, and barley—the person's immune system responds with inflammation. This degrades the lining of the small intestine and reduces nutrient absorption. Pain, abdominal cramping, often diarrhea, and other symptoms follow in the short term. Untreated, celiac disease can lead to long-term health problems, such as nutritional deficiencies, tissue wasting, osteoporosis, seizures, liver disease, and cancer of the small intestine. Individuals diagnosed with celiac disease are encouraged to consult a dietitian for help designing a gluten-free diet.

Food intolerance can cause you to have symptoms of digestive upset, but the upset is not the result of an immune system response. Probably the best example of a food intolerance is *lactose intolerance,* a problem that affects about 1 in every 10 American adults. Lactase is an enzyme produced by the small intestine that degrades lactose, the sugar in dairy products. If you don't have enough lactase, you cannot digest lactose, and it remains in the gut to be used by bacteria. Gas is formed, and you experience bloating, abdominal pain, and sometimes diarrhea. Americans of European descent typically have rates of lactose intolerance as low as 2 to 3 percent, whereas 24 percent or more of minority populations are lactose intolerant.[63] Food intolerance also occurs in response to some food additives, such as the flavor enhancer monosodium glutamate (MSG), certain dyes, sulfites, gluten, and other substances. In some cases, the food intolerance may have psychological triggers.

If you suspect that you have a food allergy, celiac disease, or a food intolerance, see your doctor. Because these diseases

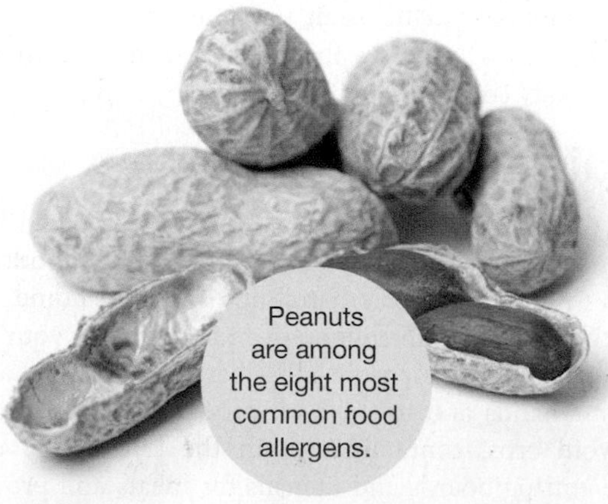

Peanuts are among the eight most common food allergens.

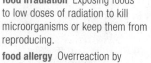

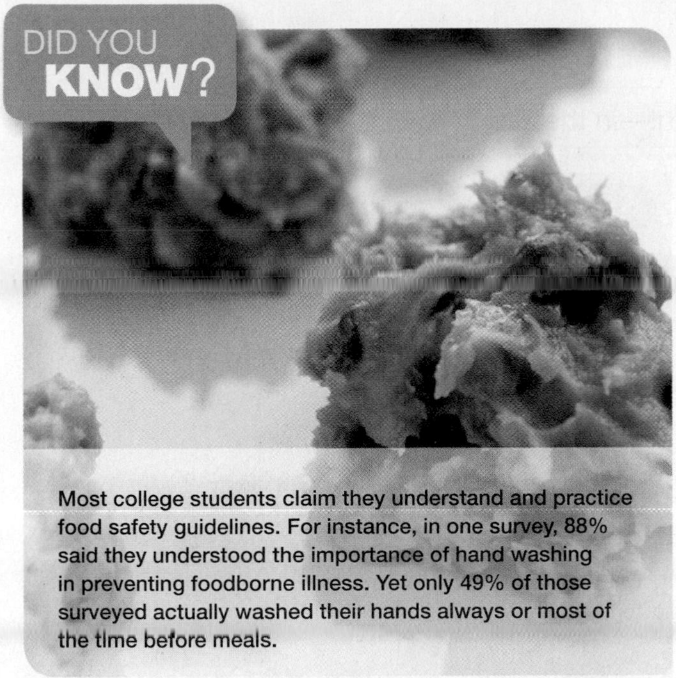

Most college students claim they understand and practice food safety guidelines. For instance, in one survey, 88% said they understood the importance of hand washing in preventing foodborne illness. Yet only 49% of those surveyed actually washed their hands always or most of the time before meals.

Source: Data are from B.A. Miko et al., "Personal and Household Hygiene, Environmental Contamination, and Health in Undergraduate Residence Halls in New York City, 2011," *PLoS One* 8, no. 11 (2013): e81460.

can have some common symptoms, as well as share symptoms with other gastrointestinal disorders, clinical diagnosis is essential.

Genetically Modified Food Crops

Genetic modification involves the insertion or deletion of genes into the DNA of an organism. In the case of **genetically modified (GM) foods**, usually this genetic cutting and pasting is done to enhance production, for example, by making disease- or insect-resistant plants, improving yield, or controlling weeds. In addition, GM foods are sometimes created to improve the color and appearance of foods or to enhance specific nutrients. For example, in regions where rice is a staple and vitamin A deficiency and iron-deficiency anemia are leading causes of morbidity and mortality, GM technology has been used to create varieties of rice high in vitamin A and iron. Another use under development is the production and delivery of vaccines through GM foods.

SEE IT! VIDEOS
Is organic produce better for you? Watch **Organic Produce** available on MasteringHealth.™

Farmers in the United States have widely accepted GM crops.[64] Soybeans and cotton are the most common GM crops, followed by corn. On supermarket shelves, an estimated 75 percent of processed foods are genetically modified.[65]

The long-term safety of GM foods—for humans and other species—is still in question. Although the genetic engineering of insect-resistant crops has reduced the use of insecticides, it has simultaneously increased the use of herbicides (which kill weeds). This has not only led to the evolution of so-called "superweeds," but has also killed off beneficial weeds such as milkweed.[66] As a result, butterfly populations that depend on these weeds, particularly the monarch butterfly, have been decimated.[67] In addition, unintentional transfer of potentially allergy-provoking proteins has occurred, and although rigorous, validated tests of crops are performed to screen for known allergens, there is a potential for the transfer of new, unknown allergens.[68] However, the American Association for the Advancement of Science reports that foods containing genetically modified (GM) ingredients are no more a risk than are the same foods com posed of crops modified over time with conventional plant breeding techniques, and the World Health Organization states that no adverse effects on human health have been shown from consumption of GM foods in countries that have approved their use.[69] Thus, the debate surrounding the risks and benefits of GM foods is not likely to end soon.

genetically modified (GM) foods Foods derived from organisms whose DNA has been altered using genetic engineering techniques.

STUDY PLAN

Customize your study plan—and master your health!—in the Study Area of **MasteringHealth**.

ASSESS YOURSELF

Do you eat healthfully? Want to find out? Take the **How Healthy Are Your Eating Habits?** assessment available on MasteringHealth.™

Need help creating a plan? Follow the strategies in the **Your Plan for Change** box for short- and long-term improvements to your health.

YOUR PLAN FOR **CHANGE**

The **ASSESS YOURSELF** activity "How Healthy Are Your Eating Habits?" is available at MasteringHealth.™ This activity gives you the chance to evaluate your current nutritional habits. Once you have considered these results, you can decide whether you need to make changes in your daily eating for long-term health.

TODAY, YOU CAN:

- ☐ Start keeping a more detailed food log. The easy-to-use SuperTracker at www.supertracker.usda.gov can help you keep track of your food intake and analyze what you eat. Take note of the nutritional content of the various foods you eat and write down particulars about the number of calories, grams of saturated fat, grams of sugar, milligrams of sodium, and so on of each food. Try to find specific weak spots: Are you consuming too many calories or too much salt or sugar? Do you eat too little calcium or iron? Use the SuperTracker to plan a healthier food intake to overcome these weak spots.
- ☐ Take a field trip to the grocery store. Forgo your fast-food dinner and instead spend time in the produce section of the supermarket. Purchase your favorite fruits and vegetables, and try something new to expand your tastes.

WITHIN THE NEXT 2 WEEKS, YOU CAN:

- ☐ Plan at least three meals that you can make at home or in your dorm room, and purchase the ingredients you'll need ahead of time. Something as simple as a chicken sandwich on whole-grain bread will be more nutritious, and probably cheaper, than heading out for a fast-food meal.
- ☐ Start reading labels. Be aware of the amount of calories, sodium, sugars, and saturated fats in prepared foods; aim to buy and consume those that are lower in all of these and are higher in micronutrients and fiber.

BY THE END OF THE SEMESTER, YOU CAN:

- ☐ Get in the habit of eating a healthy breakfast every morning. Combine whole grains, proteins, and fruit in your breakfast—for example, eat a bowl of cereal with soy milk and bananas or a cup of low-fat yogurt with granola and berries. Eating a healthy breakfast will jump-start your metabolism, prevent drops in blood glucose levels, and keep your brain and body performing at their best through your morning classes.
- ☐ Commit to one or two healthful changes to your eating patterns for the rest of the semester. You might resolve to eat five servings of fruits and vegetables every day, to switch to low-fat or nonfat dairy products, to stop drinking soft drinks, or to use only olive oil in your cooking. Use your food diary to help you spot places where you can make healthier choices on a daily basis.

CHAPTER REVIEW

To hear an MP3 Tutor Session, scan here or visit the Study Area in **MasteringHealth.**

LO 1 Essential Nutrients for Health

- The Recognizing that we eat for more reasons than just survival is a step toward improving our eating habits.
- The Dietary Reference Intakes (DRIs) are recommended nutrient intakes for healthy people.
- The essential nutrients include water, proteins, carbohydrates, fats, vitamins, and minerals. Water makes up 50 to 60 percent of our body weight and is necessary for nearly all life processes. Proteins are major components of our cells and tissues and are key elements of antibodies, enzymes, and hormones. Carbohydrates are our primary sources of energy. Fats provide energy while we are at rest and for long-term activity. They also play important roles in maintaining body temperature, cushioning and protecting organs, and promoting healthy cell function. Vitamins are organic compounds, and minerals are inorganic elements. We need these micronutrients in small amounts to maintain healthy body structure and function.
- The Dietary Guidelines for Americans and the MyPlate food guidance system provide guidelines for healthy eating.

LO 2 How Can I Eat More Healthfully?

- The Nutrition Facts label on food labels identifies the serving size, number of calories per serving, and amounts of various nutrients, as well as the %DV, which is the percentage of recommended daily values those amounts represent.
- With a little menu planning, vegetarianism can be a healthful lifestyle choice, providing plenty of nutrients, plus fiber and phytochemicals, typically with less saturated fat and fewer calories.
- College students face unique challenges in eating healthfully. Learning to make better choices, to eat healthfully on a budget, and to eat nutritionally in the dorm are all possible when you use the information in this chapter.
- Organic foods are grown and produced without the use of toxic and persistent synthetic pesticides, fertilizers, antibiotics, hormones, or genetic modification. The USDA offers certification of organic farms and regulates claims regarding organic ingredients used on food labels.

LO 3 Food Safety: A Growing Concern

- Foodborne illnesses can be traced to contamination of food at any point from fields to the consumer's kitchen. To keep food safe at home, follow four steps: clean, separate, cook, and chill.
- Food irradiation, food allergies, celiac disease, food intolerances, GM foods, and other food safety and health concerns are becoming increasingly important to health-wise consumers. Recognizing potential risks and taking steps to prevent problems are part of a sound nutritional plan.

POP QUIZ

Visit **MasteringHealth** to personalize your study plan with Chapter Review Quizzes and Dynamic Study Modules.

LO 1 Essential Nutrients for Health

1. Triglycerides
   a. provide 4 calories per gram.
   b. are the primary component of the plaque that clogs blood vessels and leads to cardiovascular disease.
   c. are only found in meat, dairy, and poultry products.
   d. include saturated fats, unsaturated fats, and *trans* fats.
2. Which of the following foods would be considered a healthy, *nutrient-dense* food?
   a. Nonfat milk
   b. Cheddar cheese
   c. Soft drink
   d. Potato chips
3. What is the most crucial nutrient for life?
   a. Water
   b. Protein
   c. Minerals
   d. Starch
4. Which of the following substances helps move food through the digestive tract?
   a. Folate
   b. Fiber
   c. Minerals
   d. Starch
5. Which of the following nutrients is critical for the repair and growth of body tissue?
   a. Carbohydrates
   b. Proteins
   c. Vitamins
   d. Fats
6. What substance provides energy, promotes healthy skin and hair, insulates body organs, helps maintain body temperature, and contributes to healthy cell function?
   a. Fats
   b. Fibers
   c. Proteins
   d. Carbohydrates
7. What is the most common nutrient deficiency worldwide?
   a. Fat deficiency
   b. Iron deficiency
   c. Fiber deficiency
   d. Calcium deficiency
8. Which of the following fats is a healthier fat to include in the diet?
   a. *Trans* fat
   b. Saturated fat
   c. Unsaturated fat
   d. Hydrogenated fat

LO 2 How Can I Eat More Healthfully?

9. Carrie eats dairy products and eggs, but she does not eat fish, poultry, or meat. Carrie is considered a(n)
   a. vegan.
   b. lacto-ovo-vegetarian.
   c. ovo-vegetarian.
   d. pesco-vegetarian.

LO 3 Food Safety: A Growing Concern

10. Lucas's doctor diagnoses him with celiac disease. Which of the following foods should Lucas cut out of his diet to eat gluten free?
    a. shellfish
    b. eggs
    c. peanuts
    d. wheat

Answers to the Pop Quiz can be found on page A-1. If you answered a question incorrectly, review the section identified by the Learning Outcome. For even more study tools, visit MasteringHealth.

THINK ABOUT IT!

LO 1 Essential Nutrients for Health

1. Which factors influence a person's dietary patterns and behaviors? What factors have been the greatest influences on your eating behaviors?
2. What are the major types of nutrients that you need to obtain from the foods you eat? What happens if you fail to get enough of some of them? Are there significant differences between men and women in particular areas of nutrition?

LO 2 How Can I Eat More Healthfully?

3. What are the major food groups in the MyPlate plan? From which groups do you eat too few servings? What can you do to increase or decrease your intake of selected food groups?
4. Distinguish between the different types of vegetarianism. Which types are most likely to lead to nutrient deficiencies? What can be done to ensure that even the most strict vegetarian receives enough of the major nutrients?
5. What are the major problems that many college students face when trying to eat the right foods? List five actions that you and your classmates could take immediately to improve your eating.

LO 3 Food Safety: A Growing Concern

6. What are the major risks for foodborne illnesses, and what can you do to protect yourself?
7. How does a food intolerance differ from a food allergy?

ACCESS YOUR HEALTH ON THE INTERNET

Visit **MasteringHealth** for links to the websites and RSS feeds.

The following websites explore further topics and issues.

Academy of Nutrition and Dietetics. The Academy provides information on a full range of dietary topics, including sports nutrition, healthful cooking, and nutritional eating; the site also links to scientific publications and information on scholarships and public meetings. **www.eatright.org**

U.S. Food and Drug Administration (FDA). The FDA provides information for consumers and professionals in the areas of food safety, supplements, and medical devices. There are links to other sources of information about nutrition and food. **www.fda.gov**

Food and Nutrition Information Center. This site offers a wide variety of information related to food and nutrition. **http://fnic.nal.usda.gov**

National Institutes of Health: Office of Dietary Supplements. This is the site of the International Bibliographic Database of Information on Dietary Supplements (IBDIDS), updated quarterly. **http://dietary-supplements.info.nih.gov**

U.S. Department of Agriculture, USDA: Choose MyPlate. The USDA offers a personalized nutrition and physical activity plan based on the MyPlate program, sample menus and recipes, and a full discussion of the *Dietary Guidelines for Americans.* **www.choosemyplate.gov**

U.S. Department of Health and Human Services: Food Safety. This is the official gateway site to food safety information provided by the federal government, including recalls and alerts, news, and tips for reporting problems. **www.foodsafety.gov**

Linus Pauling Institute. This is a key U.S. research center for studies on macro- and micronutrients, and it is a leader in antioxidant research. **http://lpi.oregonstate.edu**

8 Reaching and Maintaining a Healthy Weight

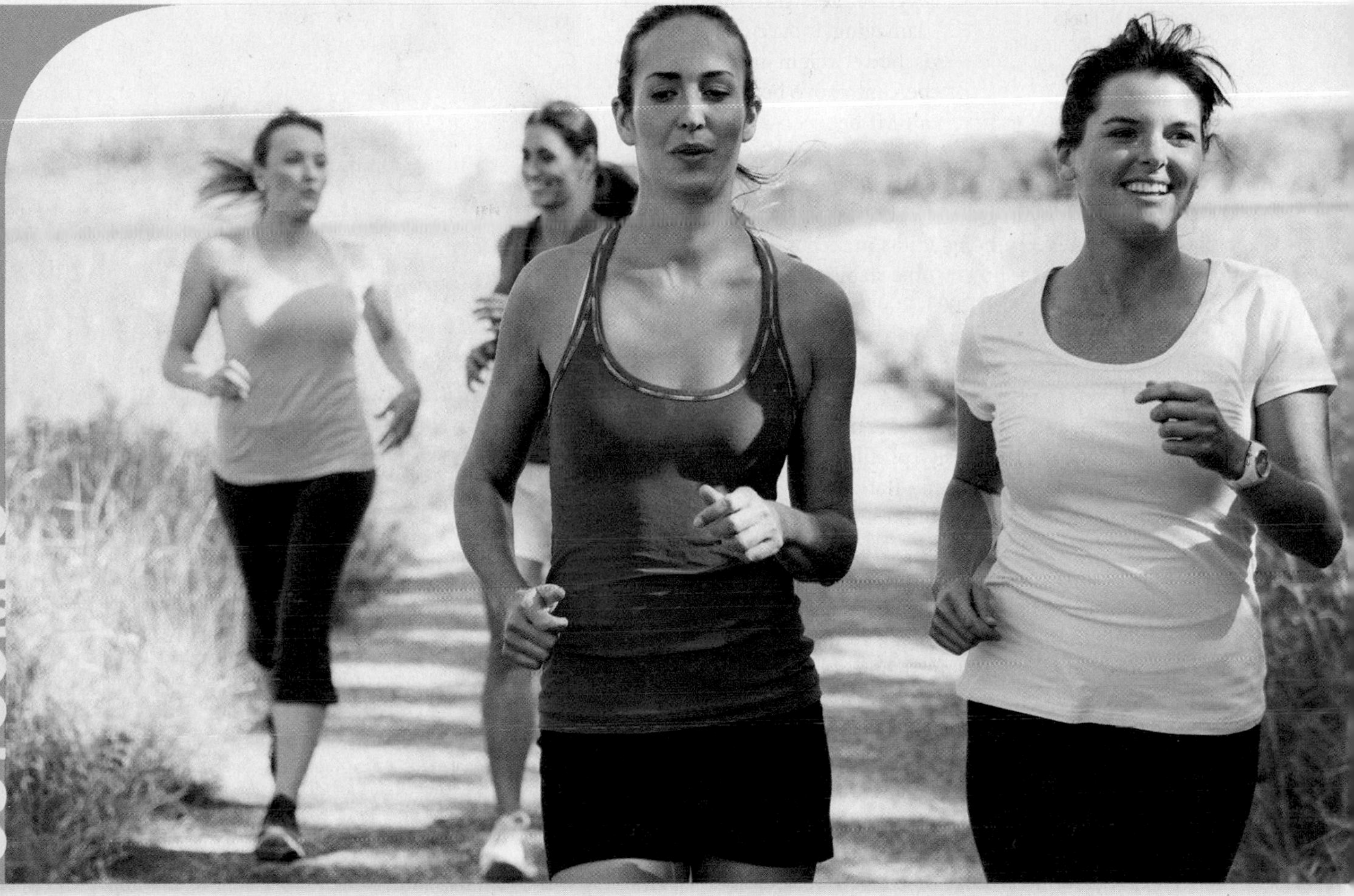

LEARNING OUTCOMES

1. Explain *overweight* and *obesity,* describe the current epidemic of overweight/obesity in the United States and globally, and demonstrate understanding of risk factors associated with weight problems. Describe factors that put people at risk for problems with obesity, distinguishing between controllable and uncontrollable factors.
2. Learn reliable options for determining your percentage of body fat and a healthy weight.
3. Explain the effectiveness and potential pros/cons of various weight control strategies, including exercise, diet, lifestyle modification, supplements/diet drugs, surgery, and other options.

The United States currently has the dubious distinction of being among the fattest nations on Earth. Young and old, rich and poor, rural and urban, educated and uneducated, Americans share one thing in common—they are fatter than virtually all previous generations.[1] The word **obesogenic**, meaning "characterized by environments that promote increased food intake, nonhealthful foods, and physical inactivity," has become an apt descriptor of our society. Obesogenic comes from the word *obesity*, meaning body weight that is more than 20 percent above recommended levels for health or a body mass index (BMI) over 30. Less extreme, but still damaging, is *overweight*, which is body weight more than 10 percent above healthy levels or a BMI between 25 and 29. The U.S. maps in **FIGURE 8.1** illustrate just how high levels of obesity have risen in the past two decades. Indeed, the prevalence of obesity has tripled among children and doubled among adults in recent decades.[2] While previous research has shown some stabilization in overweight and obesity rates between 2003–2004 and 2011–2012, current rates are still extremely high, with more than 68 percent of U.S. adults overall (over 170 million people) being overweight or obese.[3] Rates of obesity are 34.4 percent among men and 36.1 for women, and rates of extreme obesity are on the rise.[4]

obesogenic Characterized by environments that promote increased food intake, nonhealthful foods, and physical inactivity; refers to conditions that lead people to become excessively fat.

A bright spot in the obesity profile appears to be among the very youngest populations. Rates for 2- to 5-year-olds have dropped significantly, from a high of nearly 14 percent in 2003–2004 to just over 8 percent in 2011–2012![5] While the exact reasons for the declining rates in youth have not been determined, greater public awareness; more options for healthy foods in child care centers, restaurants, and grocery stores; improved labeling; improvements in physical activity programs; and decreases in sugar consumption are among suspected contributors.

Although smoking is still the leading cause of preventable death in the United States, obesity is rapidly gaining ground on this killer as associated health problems soar. Cardiovascular disease (CVD), stroke, cancer, hypertension, diabetes, depression, digestive problems, gallstones, sleep apnea, osteoarthritis, certain cancers, and other ailments lead the list of life-threatening, weight-related problems.

Consider the following facts about specific risks for obese individuals compared to their nonobese counterparts:[6]

- They have a 104 percent increase in risk of heart failure.
- BMI greater than 30 reduces their life expectancy by 2 to 4 years.
- BMI greater than 40 costs 8 to 10 years of life expectancy—similar to a long-term smoker.
- Obese adolescents have a 16-times increased risk of becoming severely obese adults, and at current prevalence rates, will result in 1.5 million life years lost.[7]

Research points to higher obesity rates and risks among some ethnic groups. Mexican American men (81 percent) and non-Hispanic whites (73 percent) are more likely to be overweight/obese than are non-Hispanic blacks (69 percent). Non-Hispanic black women (80 percent) and Mexican American women (78 percent) are more likely to be overweight or obese than are non-Hispanic white women (60 percent). In sharp contrast, nearly 58 percent of Asian populations are at a healthy weight.[8] Of youth aged 2 to 19, over 39 percent of Hispanics, Mexican Americans, and non-Hispanic blacks, as well as nearly 28 percent of non-Hispanic whites, are overweight/obese, with low parental education, low-income, and higher unemployment related to increased risk.[9]

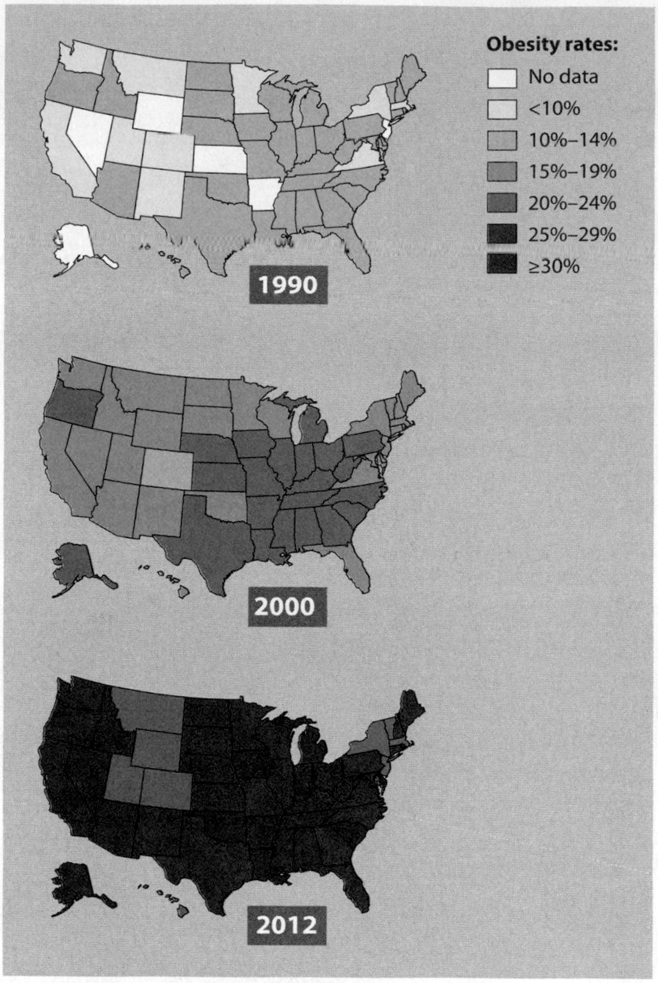

FIGURE 8.1 Obesity Trends among U.S. Adults, 1990, 2000, and 2012

Source: Centers for Disease Control and Prevention, "U.S. Obesity Trends: 1999–2010," 2012, www.cdc.gov/obesity/data/trends.html; CDC, "Prevalence of Self-Reported Obesity among U.S. Adults, 2013, www.cdc.gov/obesity/data/adult.html.

*Note: Historical maps are provided for reference only, as differences in the analysis of prevalence rates for 2011 make direct comparisons to previous years incompatible.

HEAR IT! PODCASTS

Want a study podcast for this chapter? Download **Managing Your Weight: Finding a Health Balance** available on MasteringHealth.™

14% TO 8%

THE DROP IN PREVALENCE RATES FOR **OBESITY** BETWEEN 2003–2004 AND 2011–2012 FOR YOUTH AGED 2 TO 5 YEARS.

Diabetes, strongly associated with overweight and obesity, is another major concern. Nearly 26 million Americans have diabetes, and another 79 million adults have prediabetes.[10] **Focus On: Minimizing Your Risk for Diabetes** discusses the devastating effects of obesity on diabetes-related risks and the benefits of prevention. (See the **Money & Health** box on the next page for information on the economics of obesity.)

CVD and chronic, killer diseases are not the only risks associated with overweight and obesity. The costs of social isolation, bullying in school, stigmatization, discrimination, and diminished quality of life can also be devastating. Obese individuals suffer more major disability and difficulty with activities of daily living (ADLs) than do their nonobese counterparts. They are also more likely to experience falls and injury, with the exception of morbidly obese individuals—who may fall less—perhaps because they are less active, and seem to be less prone to injury when they fall.[11] (**FIGURE 8.2** summarizes these and other potential health consequences of obesity.)

globesity Global rates of obesity.

The United States is not alone in the obesity epidemic. In fact, overweight and obesity has become the fifth-leading risk for global death, and nearly 1.5 billion adults aged 20 and over and 40 million children under the age of 5 are overweight/obese.[12] While obesity was once predominantly a problem in high-income countries, today increasing numbers of low- and middle-income countries have overweight/obesity problems.[13] The global epidemic of high rates of overweight and obesity in multiple regions of the world has come to be known as **globesity**. (The **Health in a Diverse World** box on page 229 looks at the problem of globesity.)

Of concern is that over 40 million of the world's children under the age of 5 were overweight in 2011. Children in low-income countries tend to have inadequate prenatal care and early nutrition and are increasingly exposed to high-fat,

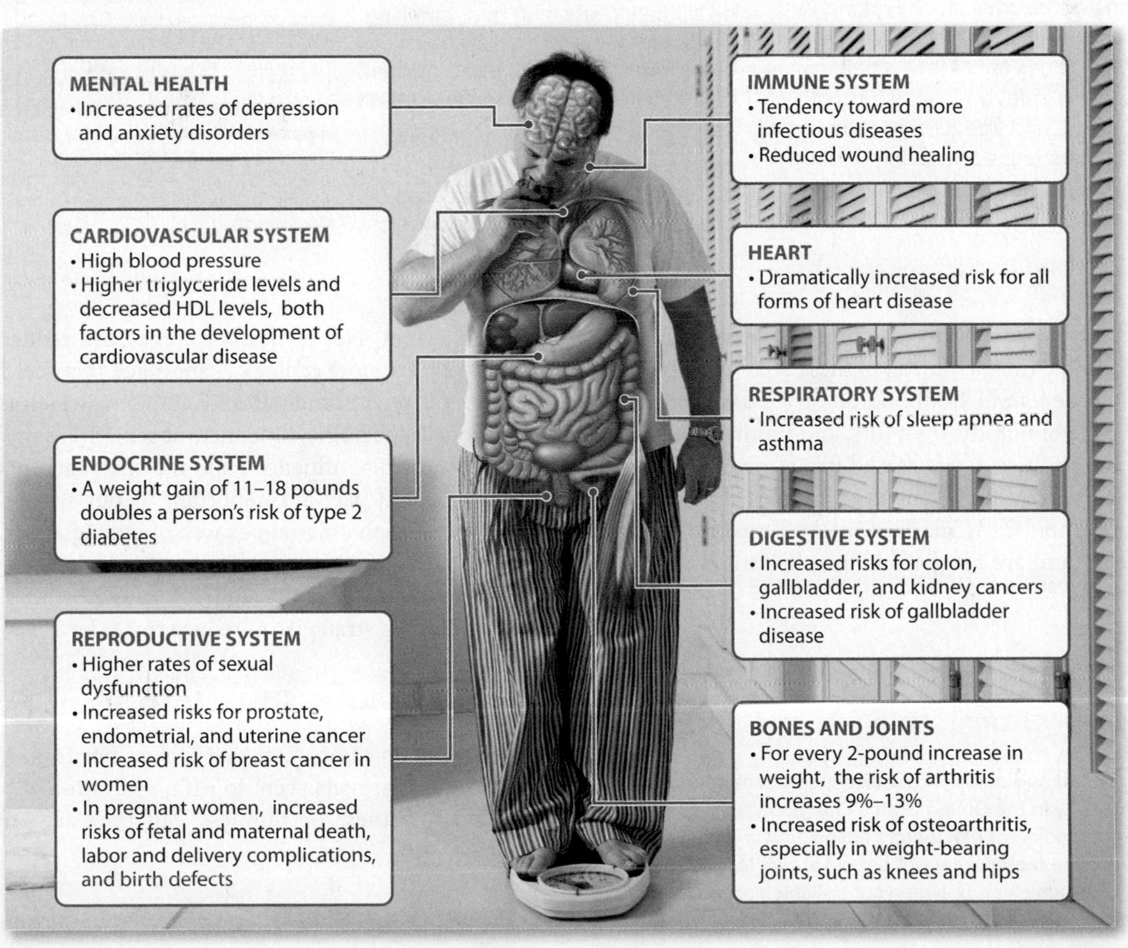

MENTAL HEALTH
• Increased rates of depression and anxiety disorders
CARDIOVASCULAR SYSTEM
• High blood pressure
• Higher triglyceride levels and decreased HDL levels, both factors in the development of cardiovascular disease
ENDOCRINE SYSTEM
• A weight gain of 11–18 pounds doubles a person's risk of type 2 diabetes
REPRODUCTIVE SYSTEM
• Higher rates of sexual dysfunction
• Increased risks for prostate, endometrial, and uterine cancer
• Increased risk of breast cancer in women
• In pregnant women, increased risks of fetal and maternal death, labor and delivery complications, and birth defects
IMMUNE SYSTEM
• Tendency toward more infectious diseases
• Reduced wound healing
HEART
• Dramatically increased risk for all forms of heart disease
RESPIRATORY SYSTEM
• Increased risk of sleep apnea and asthma
DIGESTIVE SYSTEM
• Increased risks for colon, gallbladder, and kidney cancers
• Increased risk of gallbladder disease
BONES AND JOINTS
• For every 2-pound increase in weight, the risk of arthritis increases 9%–13%
• Increased risk of osteoarthritis, especially in weight-bearing joints, such as knees and hips

FIGURE 8.2 Potential Negative Health Effects of Overweight and Obesity

VIDEO TUTOR Obesity Health Effects

MONEY & HEALTH | "LIVING LARGE" CAN BE INCREASINGLY COSTLY

"The startling economic costs of obesity, often borne by the non obese, could become the epidemic's second-hand smoke."

—Sharon Begley, "As America's Waistline Expands, Costs Soar," Reuters, April 30, 2012.

On top of the physical costs of overweight and obesity, many insurance companies are charging more for people who are overweight and refuse to participate in available "wellness" programs. In fact, the U.S. Patient Protection and Affordable Care Act in 2010 has a provision that allows employers to charge obese workers significantly higher premiums (between 30 and 50 percent more in some cases!) for their health insurance if they don't make a good faith effort to reduce their health risks. Is this fair? Many argue that such penalties unfairly reflect a form of obesity stigma and size discrimination, whereas others argue that those within a normal weight range shouldn't have to subsidize excess costs. Still others argue that this is a slippery slope on the way to paying more for factors like eating high-fat foods and having high cholesterol, having too many beers in a week, or even unintended pregnancy. Consider these recent statistics:

- According to new estimates, obesity now accounts for nearly 21 percent of U.S. health care costs, more than double previous estimates! By some estimates, morbidly obese individuals may cost between $6,500 and $15,000 more per year in additional health care costs when factors such as longer hospital stays, recovery, and increased medications are included.
- According to a new Mayo Clinic study, being obese adds more to health care costs than does smoking. For those who are morbidly obese, costs may be as much as 50 percent higher than for nonobese individuals.
- Another study indicates that obese individuals miss more work and are less productive in many instances because they don't have the physical stamina to handle demanding jobs. By some estimates, the annual cost attributable to obesity among full-time employees is believed to be in excess of $73 billion for those with a BMI over 35 percent.

Currently, there is much debate about these extra costs, even as many insurers and businesses implement policies and programs to motivate employees and members of insurance groups to take action, "or else." Stay tuned—the debate has just begun!

Sources: J. Cawley and C. Meyerhoefer, "The Medical Care Costs of Obesity: An Instrumental Variables Approach," *Journal of Health Economics* 31, no. 1 (2012): 219, DOI: 10.1016/j.jhealeco.2011.10.003; James P. Moriarty et al., "The Effects of Incremental Costs of Smoking and Obesity on Health Care Costs among Adults," *Journal of Occupational and Environmental Medicine* 54, no. 3 (2012): 286, DOI: 10.1097/JOM.0b013e318246f1f4; Mayo Clinic, "Mayo Clinic Study Obesity Outweighs Smoking in Employee Health Costs," May 2012, http://mayoclinichealthsystem.org; E. A. Finkelstein et al., "The Costs of Obesity in the Workplace," *Journal of Occupational and Environmental Medicine* 52, no. 10 (2012): 971–76.

high-sugar, high-calorie foods—often of poor nutritional value. At the same time, children in these areas are becoming increasingly sedentary. Childhood obesity is associated with a higher chance of obesity, disability, and premature death in adulthood. In addition to increased future risks, obese children have more breathing difficulties, increased risk of fractures, hypertension, early markers of cardiovascular disease, more diabetes, and are more likely to suffer stigma and bullying in schools.[14]

LO 1 | FACTORS CONTRIBUTING TO OVERWEIGHT AND OBESITY

Explain *overweight* and *obesity,* describe the current epidemic of overweight/obesity in the United States and globally, and demonstrate understanding of risk factors associated with weight problems. Describe factors that put people at risk for problems with obesity, distinguishing between controllable and uncontrollable factors.

The reasons for our soaring rates of overweight and obesity are complex, and not all of them are within easy individual control. Although diet and exercise are clearly two major contributors, other factors, including genetics and physiology, are also important. Newer thinking regarding reducing obesity risk involves a more ecological approach that seeks to change obesogenic environmental and contextual factors. Learned behaviors in the home; influences at school and in social environments; media influences; and the environments where we live, work, and play are important to our weight profiles.[15] Experts realize that a complex web of interactive factors influences what we eat, how much we eat, and when we eat, as well as how we expend energy. Figuring out what these factors are and developing strategies to reduce risk is key.[16]

Genetic and Physiological Factors

Are some people born to be fat? Genes, hormones, and other physiological aspects seem to influence some of our predisposition to fatness or thinness, but they are not the only culprits.

Genes: A Variety of Theories In spite of decades of research, the exact role of genes in one's predisposition toward obesity remains in question. Children whose parents are obese tend to be overweight. In fact, countless observational studies back up the theory that fat parents tend to have fat children. But is that due to their learned eating and exercise behaviors,

HEALTH IN A DIVERSE WORLD

COMBATING GLOBESITY

The United States has 87 million obese individuals—over 13 percent of the 671 million obese people in the world—yet our population only makes up 5 percent of the world's population. In short, we are the world's obesity leader. Nonetheless, virtually every nation on earth is experiencing expanding waistlines. In fact, the number of overweight and obese people globally rose from 857 million in 1980 to 2.1 billion in 2013, an increase of nearly 30 percent in nearly 35 years. Consider these global statistics:

- While rates of obesity in the U.S. are in the 30 to 34 percent range, some nations of the world have obesity rates over 50 percent. Tonga men and women and women in Kuwait, Libya, Samoa, and Micronesia top the 50 percent obese scale.
- Nearly 22 percent of girls and 24 percent of boys in developed countries are overweight or obese.

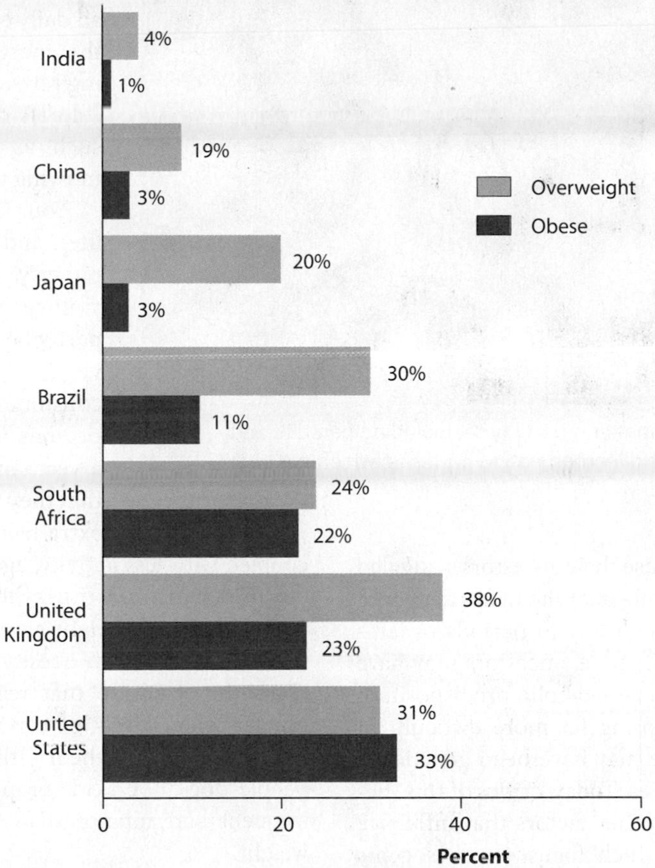

Source: Adapted from World Health Organization, "Global Database on Body Mass Index (BMI)," 2012, http://apps.who.int/bmi/index.jsp.

- While obesity is more prevalent in developed nations, less developed nations are gaining ground rapidly and consuming more high-sugar, high-calorie, high-fat foods. It's a surprising paradox that many of the hungriest nations also have high rates of obesity.

The World Health Organization (WHO) projects that by 2015 approximately 2.3 billion adults will be overweight and more than 700 million will be obese. The figure shows some of the world's most and least overweight countries. What factors do you think influence average weights in these nations? If we continue at our current rate, what do you think this graph will look like in another decade?

Sources: M. Ng, et al. "Global, Regional, and National Prevalence of Overweight and Obesity in Children and Adults during 1980–2013: A Systematic Analysis for the Global Burden of Disease Study, 2013. *The Lancet,* Early Online Publication, May 29, 2014: doi:10.1016/S0140-6736(14)60460-8; World Health Organization, "Obesity and Overweight," Fact Sheet no. 311, Updated March 2011, www.who.int/mediacentre/factsheets/fs311/en/index.html.

environmental cues, genes, or a combination of these factors? Early support for a genetic basis for obesity came as a result of research on twins. Researchers found that adopted individuals tend to be similar in weight to their biological parents and that identical twins are twice as likely to weigh the same as are fraternal twins, even if they are raised separately.[17] Subsequent research supported this theory and began to explore the fact that obesity involves complex gene-gene and gene-environmental interactions: One gene in particular, the *FTO* gene, may be among the most important.[18] Much of this work has centered on the role of genes in eating behavior. Specifically, people with certain genetic variations may tend to graze for food more often, eat more meals, and consume more calories every day, as well as display patterns of seeking out high-fat food groups. Also, different genes may influence weight gain at certain periods of life, particularly during adolescence and young adulthood.[19] Rather than acting individually, the effects of the genes may be in clusters, influencing the regulation of food intake through action in the central nervous system, as well as influencing fat cell synthesis and functioning.

So, if your genes play a key role in obesity tendencies, are you doomed to a lifelong battle with your weight? Probably not, based on exciting new research that points to the fact that even if obesity does run in your family, a healthy lifestyle can override "obesity" genes. Results of a major European study found that the effects of the *FTO* gene on obesity is over 30 percent less among physically active adults. Those who seemed to be beating their obesity tendencies exercised at least 90 minutes a day compared to those who exercised 30 minutes.[20]

One potential genetic basis for obesity was identified as a result of observational studies of certain Indian and African tribes. Labeled the *thrifty gene theory,* researchers noted higher body fat and obesity levels in some of these tribes than

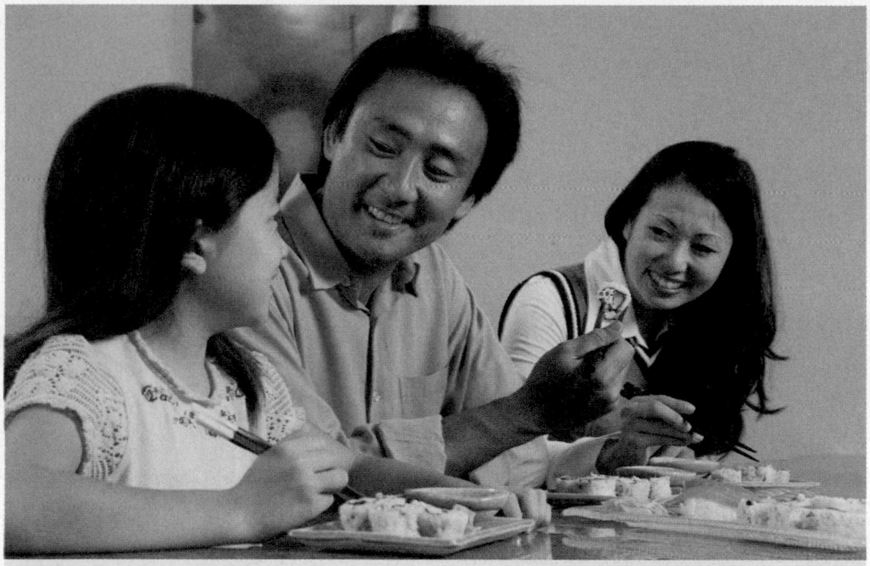

Many factors help determine weight and body type, including heredity and genetic makeup, environment, and learned eating patterns, which are often connected to family habits.

in the general population.[21] Because their ancestors struggled through centuries of famine, members of the tribes appear to have survived by adapting metabolically to periods of famine with slowed metabolism. Over time, ancestors may have passed on a genetic, hormonal, or metabolic predisposition toward fat storage that makes losing fat more difficult. In short, it was thought that people may have been genetically programmed to burn fewer calories. Today, critics of this theory believe that there are many other factors that influence obesity development, most of which focus on obesogenic behaviors and environments.

Metabolic Rates Several aspects of your metabolism also help determine whether you gain, maintain, or lose weight. Each of us has an innate energy-burning capacity called **basal metabolic rate (BMR)**—the minimum rate at which the body uses energy to maintain basic vital functions. A BMR for the average, healthy adult is usually between 1,200 and 1,800 calories per day. Technically, to measure BMR, a person would be awake, but all major stimuli (including stressors to the sympathetic nervous system and digestion) would be at rest. Usually, the best time to measure BMR is after 8 hours of sleep and after a 12-hour fast.

basal metabolic rate (BMR) The rate of energy expenditure by a body at complete rest in a neutral environment.

resting metabolic rate (RMR) The energy expenditure of the body under BMR conditions plus other daily sedentary activities.

exercise metabolic rate (EMR) The energy expenditure that occurs during exercise.

adaptive thermogenesis Theoretical mechanism by which the brain regulates metabolic activity according to caloric intake.

set point theory Theory that a form of internal thermostat controls our weight and fights to maintain this weight around a narrowly set range.

yo-yo diets Cycles in which people diet and regain weight.

A more practical way of assessing your energy expenditure levels is the **resting metabolic rate (RMR).** Slightly higher than the BMR, the RMR includes the BMR plus any additional energy expended through daily sedentary activities such as food digestion, sitting, studying, or standing. The **exercise metabolic rate (EMR)** accounts for the remaining percentage of all daily calorie expenditures and refers to the energy expenditure that occurs during physical activity. For most of us, these calories come from light daily activities, such as walking, climbing stairs, and mowing the lawn.

Your BMR and RMR fluctuate through life, and are highest during infancy, puberty, and pregnancy. Generally, the younger you are, the higher your BMR, partly because cells undergo rapid subdivision during periods of growth, and that consumes lots of energy. After age 30, a person's BMR slows down 1 to 2 percent a year, and older people commonly find that they must work harder to burn off an extra helping of ice cream. Slower BMR, coupled with less activity, age-related muscle loss, and shifting priorities from fitness to family and career obligations contribute to the weight-gain of many middle-aged people.

Other theories on obesity focus on the brain's hypothalamus—the structure that regulates appetite—which signals hunger when levels of certain nutrients in the blood fall. According to one theory, the monitoring system in obese people does not work properly, making cues to eat more frequent and intense than they are in people of normal weight.

Anyone who has ever lost weight to find a point at which, try as they might, they can't lose another ounce may be a victim of **adaptive thermogenesis,** whereby the brain slows metabolic activity and energy expenditure as a form of defensive protection against possible starvation. With increased weight loss may come increased hunger sensations, slowed energy expenditure, and a tendency to regain weight or make further weight loss more difficult.[22]

On the other side of the BMR equation is **set point theory,** which suggests that our bodies fight to maintain weight around a narrow range or set fat point. If we go on a drastic starvation diet or fast, BMR slows to conserve energy. Set point theory suggests that our own bodies may sabotage our weight loss efforts by holding on to calories, explaining why people tend to stay near a certain weight threshold and why moving to a different level of weight loss is difficult. The good news is that set points can be changed; however, these changes may take time to be permanent. A healthy diet, steady weight loss, and exercise appear to be the best methods of sustaining weight loss.

Yo-yo diets refer to when people cycle between periods of weight loss and gain. When dieters resume eating after their weight loss, BMR is reset lower due to earlier calorie restrictions, making it almost certain that they will regain the pounds they just lost. Repeated cycles of dieting and regaining weight may actually increase the likelihood of getting heavier over time.

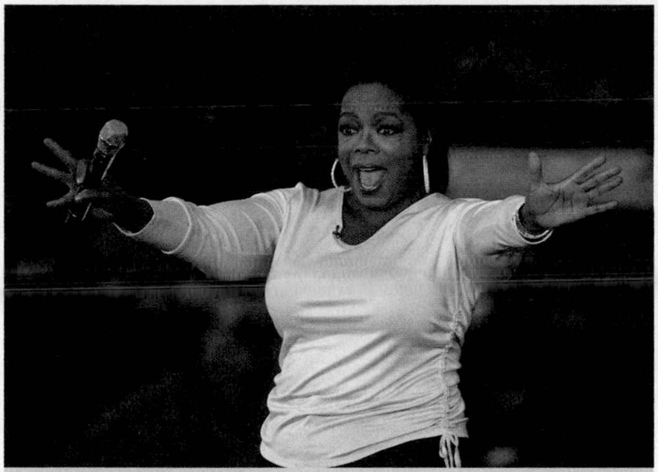

Just about any calorie-cutting diet can produce weight loss in the short term. However, without improved nutrition and sustained exercise, lost weight will return. Oprah Winfrey has been candid about her struggles with this pattern of weight cycling, or yo-yo dieting, which disrupts the body's metabolism and makes future weight loss more difficult to achieve and sustain.

Hormonal Influences: Ghrelin and Leptin

Obese people may be more likely than thin people to satisfy their appetite and eat for reasons other than nutrition.[23] Over the years, people have attributed obesity to thyroid gland problems and resultant hormone imbalances that cause fatigue, impede the way calories burn and energy is used, and a number of other functions. Many experts now believe that less than 2 percent of the obese population actually has thyroid issues.[24] Several other hormones, dietary proteins, and other chemicals can affect caloric expenditure and a person's ability to lose weight, control appetite, and sense fullness.

While hormones may have an impact on a person's ability to lose weight, control appetite, and sense fullness, the problem with overconsumption may be related more to **satiety** and to environmental cues than appetite or hunger. People generally feel satiated, or full, when they have satisfied their nutritional needs and their stomach signals "no more."

One hormone, produced in the stomach, that researchers suspect may influence satiety and play a role in keeping weight off is *ghrelin,* sometimes referred to as "the hunger hormone." Initial interest in ghrelin was the result of an early study that focused on a small group of obese people who had lost weight over a 6-month period.[25] They noted that ghrelin levels rose before every meal and fell drastically shortly afterward, suggesting that the hormone plays a role in appetite stimulation. Since then, ghrelin has been shown to be an important growth hormone that plays a key role in the regulation of appetite and food intake control, gastrointestinal motility, gastric acid secretion, endocrine and exocrine pancreatic secretions, glucose and lipid metabolism, and cardiovascular and immunological processes.[26]

Another hormone that has gained increased attention and research is *leptin,* an appetite regulator produced by fat cells in mammals. As fat tissue increases, levels of leptin in the blood increase, and when levels of leptin in the blood rise, appetite drops. Scientists believe leptin serves as a form of "adipostat" that signals you are getting full, slows food intake, and promotes energy expenditure.[27] Although obese individuals have enough leptin and leptin receptors, they do not always work to suppress appetite. While the exact reasons for this are unknown, it may be that environmental cues are stronger than biological signals in some individuals.

Fat Cells and Predisposition to Fatness

Some obese people may have excessive numbers of fat cells. An average-weight adult has approximately 25 to 35 billion fat cells, a moderately obese adult 60 to 100 billion, and an extremely obese adult as many as 200 billion.[28] This type of obesity, **hyperplasia,** usually appears in early childhood and perhaps, due to the mother's dietary habits, even prior to birth. The most critical periods for the development of hyperplasia are the last 2 to 3 months of fetal development, the first year of life, and the period between ages 9 and 13. Central to this theory is the belief that the number of fat cells in a body does not increase appreciably during adulthood. Based on this, nutrition and exercise during childhood appear key to future weight problems. However, the ability of each of these cells to swell **(hypertrophy)** and shrink does carry over into adulthood. People with large numbers of fat cells may be able to lose weight by decreasing the size of each cell in adulthood, but with the next calorie binge, the cells swell and sabotage weight-loss efforts. Weight gain may be tied to both the number of fat cells in the body and the capacity of individual cells to enlarge (**FIGURE 8.3**).

satiety The feeling of fullness or satisfaction at the end of a meal.

hyperplasia A condition characterized by an excessive number of fat cells.

hypertrophy The act of swelling or increasing in size, as with cells.

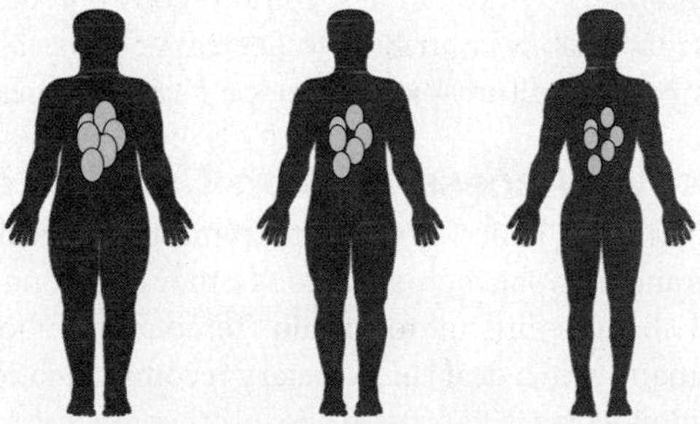

	Before body weight reduction	Initial weight reduction	Second weight reduction
Body weight	328 lb	227 lb	165 lb
Fat cell size	0.9 μg/cell	0.6 μg/cell	0.2 μg/cell
Fat cell number	75 billion	75 billion	75 billion

FIGURE 8.3 One Person at Various Stages of Weight Loss Note that, according to the hyperplasia theory, the number of fat cells remains constant, but their size decreases when weight is lost.

STUDENT HEALTH TODAY

BEWARE OF PORTION INFLATION AT RESTAURANTS

Would you be surprised to learn that today's serving portions are significantly larger than those of past decades? From burgers and fries to meat-and-potato or pasta meals, today's popular restaurant foods dwarf their earlier counterparts. For example, a 25-ounce prime rib dinner served at one local steak chain contains nearly 3,000 calories and 150 grams of fat! That's half the calories and more than three times the fat that most adults need in a whole day, and it's just part of the meal.

Many researchers believe that the main reason Americans are gaining weight is that people no longer recognize a normal serving size. "Biggie" size has become the new normal for many, with larger sizes equated with better value. The National Heart, Lung, and Blood Institute has developed a pair of "Portion Distortion" quizzes that show how today's portions compare with those of 20 years ago. Test yourself online at http://hp2010.nhlbihin.net/portion to see whether you can guess the differences between today's meals and those previously considered normal.

Today's bloated portions.

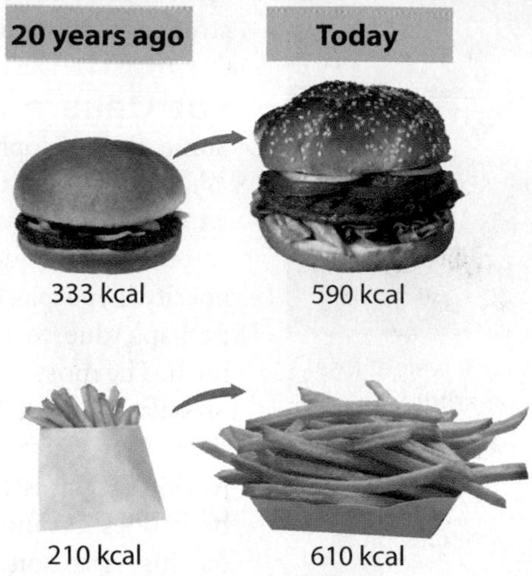

20 years ago
Today
333 kcal
590 kcal
210 kcal
610 kcal

To make sure you're not overeating when you dine out, follow these strategies:

- Order the smallest size available. Focus on taste, not quantity. Get used to eating less, eating slowly, and enjoying what you eat.
- Take your time, and let your fullness indicator have a chance to kick in while there is still time to quit.
- Dip your food in dressings, gravies, and sauces on the side rather than pouring extra calories over the top.
- Order a healthy appetizer as your main meal, and a small size salad or veggie.
- Split an entrée with a friend, and order a side salad for each of you. Alternately, put half of your meal in a take out box immediately, and finish the rest at the restaurant.
- Avoid buffets and all-you-can-eat establishments. If you go to them, use small plates and fill them with salads, veggies and other high-protein, low-calorie, low-fat options.

Source: Data are from National Heart, Lung, and Blood Institute, "Portion Distortion," May 8, 2012, http://hp2010.nhlbihin.net/portion.

Environmental Factors

Environmental factors have come to play a large role in weight maintenance. Automobiles, remote controls, desk jobs, and sedentary habits contribute to decreased physical activity and energy expenditure—a clear recipe for weight gain.

Greater Access to High-Calorie Foods Even though most Americans report trying to cut back on portion sizes and high-fat, high-sugar foods, they often find these behavioral changes difficult to sustain. Temptations abound, and far too many turn a deaf ear to dietary recommendations. Why? In addition to the factors listed above, other environmental factors prompt us to eat what we shouldn't and to eat too much:

- Because of constant advertising, we are bombarded with messages to eat, eat, eat, and taste often trumps nutrition.
- Super-sized portions of fast food and packaged products are touted as "more for your money," leading to increased calorie and fat intake. (See the **Student Health Today** box.)
- Widespread availability of high-calorie coffee and sugary drinks lure people in for a form of break/reward between meals, which really add up in calories over time.
- Families have increased reliance on restaurant and store-bought convenience foods, which tend to be higher in calories than food made from scratch.
- Bottle-feeding infants may increase energy intake relative to breast-feeding.
- Misleading food labels confuse consumers about serving sizes.

The good news is that although we still consume about 500 calories per day more today than we did in 1970, daily consumption of some foods appears to be declining in the last decade. For example, annual consumption of sugars, including *high fructose corn syrup*, was 119 pounds per person in 1970, increasing to 151 pounds per person in 1999. Today's consumption has decreased to 139 pounds per person.[29] Some believe that a greater awareness of the perils of consuming too many sugary drinks has caused people to cut consumption. Schools have made changes in available foods, and communities have taken aim at our sugar-laden products in the marketplace. If we are consuming less, why aren't we seeing major changes in obesity rates? One possibility is that we are exercising less than ever, thereby offsetting potential weight loss.[30]

U.S. ADULTS GET

11.3%

OF TOTAL DAILY CALORIES FROM **FAST FOODS.**

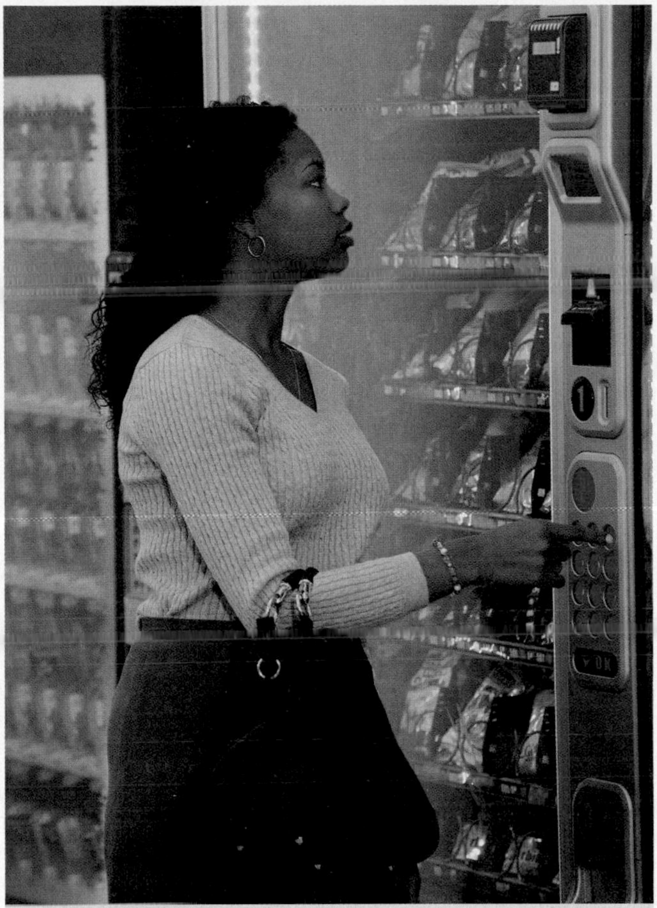
The easy availability of high-calorie foods, such as those found in most vending machines, is one of the environmental factors contributing to the obesity problem in the United States today.

Early Sabotage: A Youthful Start on Obesity

Children have always loved junk food. However, today's youth have easy access to a vast array of high-fat, high-calorie foods, have fewer physical education requirements in schools, and are more obese than ever before. While rates seem to be decreasing in the very young, nearly 32 percent of children and adolescents aged 2 to 19 are overweight/obese—three times higher than their parent's generation.[31] Sedentary activities, like using the Internet, playing video games, and watching television, have all but replaced physical play for many children. School policies have also been a factor in the growth of childhood obesity; for decades the trend was to eliminate physical education, while cafeterias were more likely to serve pizza and fries than healthy food.

In addition, youth are at risk because of factors that are only beginning to be understood. Epidemiological studies suggest that maternal nutrition, diabetes, and obesity may play a role in predisposing children to overweight or obesity prior to puberty and early onset puberty.[32] Research also shows that race and ethnicity seem to be intricately interwoven with environmental factors in increasing risks to young people.[33]

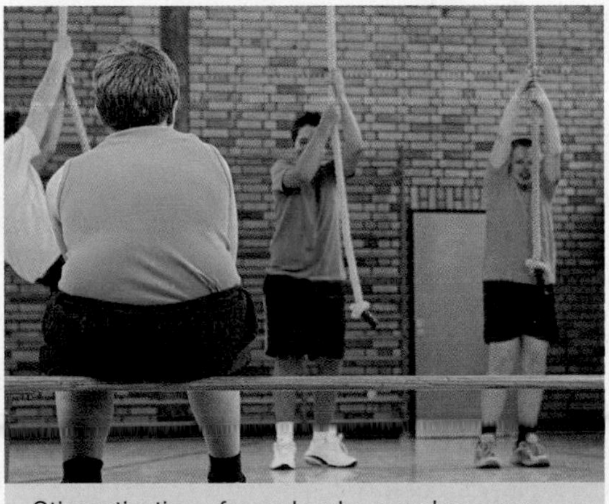
Stigmatization of people who are obese can contribute to depression and low self-esteem.

On top of potential physical problems of obesity, *obesity stigma* is a major threat to overweight and obese children's self-esteem; it increases risk of suicidal thoughts, anxiety, and depression; it contributes to low grades in school; and it decreases likelihood of physical activity. Obese youth may feel a lack of social acceptance, be bullied by classmates, and develop feelings of mistrust and fear of others.[34]

Psychosocial and Socioeconomic Factors

The relationship of weight problems to emotional insecurities, needs, and wants remains difficult to assess. What we do know is that eating tends to be a focal point of people's lives and is in part a social ritual associated with companionship, celebration, and enjoyment. *Comfort food* is also used to help you feel good when other things in life are not going well. Our friends and loved ones are often key influences in our eating behaviors. In fact, according to recent research, young adults who are overweight and obese tend to befriend and date overweight and obese people who like to socialize around food in much the same way that smokers or exercisers tend to hang out with other smokers or exercisers.[35] Your social circle may pose a major obstacle in the psychological battle to control food intake.

Socioeconomic status can have a significant effect on risk for obesity. When economic times are tough, people tend to eat more inexpensive, high-calorie processed foods. People living in poverty may have less access to fresh, nutrient-dense foods and have less time to cook nutritious meals due to shiftwork, longer commutes, or multiple jobs.[36] Additionally, unsafe neighborhoods and poor infrastructure, such as lack of sidewalks or parks, can make it difficult for less-affluent people to exercise.[37]

Lifestyle Factors

Although heredity, metabolism, and environment all have an impact on weight management, the way we live our lives is also responsible. In general, Americans are eating more and moving less than ever before—becoming overfat as a result. Weight management can be much harder when it feels like a chore.

For many, moderate or high-levels of physical activity are rare events. One big problem in determining real activity levels of Americans is that data are largely based on self-reporting, and people overestimate their daily exercise level and intensity. Complicating the problem further is a hodgepodge of terminology for determining activity levels and more than one fitness measure, so defining yourself as "active" can mean very different things for different people.

SKILLS FOR BEHAVIOR CHANGE

FINDING THE FUN IN HEALTHY EATING AND EXERCISE

With a little creativity, you can make healthy weight control a fun, positive part of your life. Here are some tips:

- Cook and eat with friends. Share the responsibility for making the meal while you spend time with people you like.
- Experiment with new foods—variety is the spice of life!
- Invite an international student over for dinner and cook together.
- Vary your exercise routine—the exercise itself or the location. Even small changes can breathe life into an old routine.
- Try something new: Join a team for the social aspects in addition to exercise, or run a 10K for the challenge, or learn how to skateboard for fun.

According to data from the 2012 Health Interview Survey, 30 percent of adults reported being inactive, 20 percent of adults reported being insufficiently active, and 50 percent reported sufficient levels of activity—mostly through physical activity during leisure time. Great variation in activity patterns exists by race and socioeconomic status. For more information on physical activity, see **Chapter 9**.[38]

The **Skills for Behavior Change** box offers some ideas for making exercising and healthy eating more fun.

LO 2 | ASSESSING BODY WEIGHT AND BODY COMPOSITION

Learn reliable options for determining your percentage of body fat and a healthy weight.

Everyone has his or her own ideal weight, based on individual variables such as body structure, height, and fat distribution. Traditionally, experts used measurement techniques such as height-weight charts to determine whether an individual was an ideal weight, overweight, or obese. These charts can be misleading because they don't take body composition—a person's ratio of fat to lean muscle—or fat distribution into account. In fact, weight can be a deceptive indicator. Many a muscular athlete or middle-aged woman who brags about weighing the same as in high school is shocked to find out that he or she has relatively high fat levels based on BMI. More accurate measures of evaluating healthy weight and disease risk focus on a person's percentage of body fat and how that fat is distributed in his or her body.

overweight Having a body weight more than 10 percent above healthy recommended levels; in an adult, having a BMI of 25 to 29.

obesity A body weight more than 20 percent above healthy recommended levels; in an adult, a BMI of 30 or more.

It's important to remember that fat isn't all bad. In fact, some fat is essential for healthy body functioning. Fat regulates body temperature, cushions and insulates organs and tissues, and is the body's main source of stored energy. Body fat is composed of two types: essential fat and storage fat. *Essential fat* is the fat necessary for maintenance of life and reproductive functions. *Storage fat,* the nonessential fat that many of us try to shed, makes up the remainder of our fat reserves.

WHAT DO YOU THINK?

Can you think of factors in your particular environment that might contribute to your own risks for obesity? Risks of your family and friends?

- What actions could you take to combat them?

Overweight and Obesity

In general, **overweight** is increased body weight due to excess fat that exceeds healthy recommendations, whereas **obesity** refers to body weight that greatly exceeds health recommendations. Traditionally, *overweight* was defined as being 1 to 19 percent above one's ideal weight, based on a standard height-weight chart, and *obesity* was defined as being 20 percent or more above one's ideal weight. Experts now usually define *overweight* and *obesity* in terms of BMI (discussed below) or percentage of body fat. Although opinion varies somewhat, most experts agree that men's bodies should contain between 8 and 20 percent total body fat, and women should be within the range of 20 to 30 percent. These ranges vary with ages and stages of life, with limits on the upper and lower end that reflect less than desirable weight levels (see **TABLE 8.1**).

DID YOU KNOW?

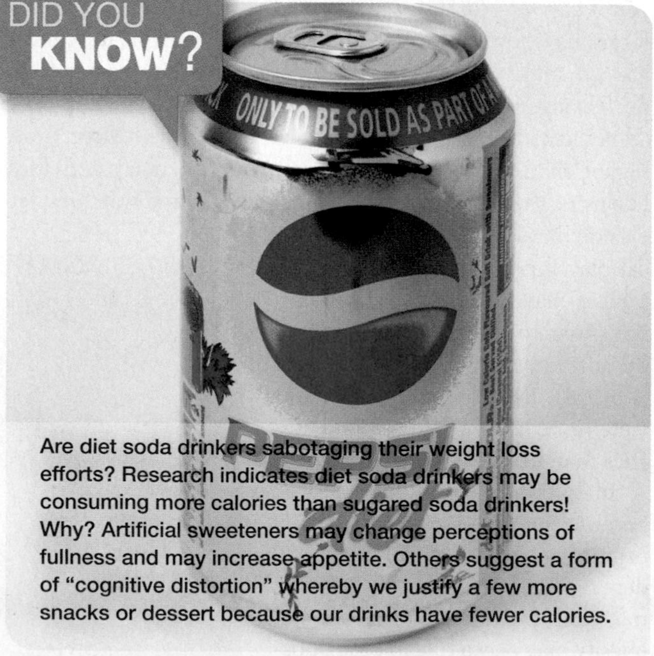

Are diet soda drinkers sabotaging their weight loss efforts? Research indicates diet soda drinkers may be consuming more calories than sugared soda drinkers! Why? Artificial sweeteners may change perceptions of fullness and may increase appetite. Others suggest a form of "cognitive distortion" whereby we justify a few more snacks or dessert because our drinks have fewer calories.

Source: S. N. Bleich, J. A. Wolfson, and S. Vine, "Diet-Beverage Consumption and Caloric Intake among US Adults, Overall and by Body Weight," *American Journal of Public Health* 104, no. 3 (2014): e72–e78.

TABLE 8.1 | Body Fat Percentage Norms for Men and Women[a]

Men Age	Very Lean	Excellent	Good	Fair	Poor	Very Poor
20–29	<7%	7%–10%	11%–15%	16%–19%	20%–23%	>23%
30–39	<11%	11%–14%	15%–18%	19%–21%	22%–25%	>25%
40–49	<14%	14%–17%	18%–20%	21%–23%	24%–27%	>27%
50–59	<15%	15%–19%	20%–22%	23%–24%	25%–28%	>28%
60–69	<16%	16%–20%	21%–22%	23%–25%	26%–28%	>28%
70–79	<16%	16%–20%	21%–23%	24%–25%	26%–28%	>28%
Women Age	**Very Lean**	**Excellent**	**Good**	**Fair**	**Poor**	**Very Poor**
20–29	<14%	14%–16%	17%–19%	20%–23%	24%–27%	>27%
30–39	<15%	15%–17%	18%–21%	22%–25%	26%–29%	>29%
40–49	<17%	17%–20%	21%–24%	25%–28%	29%–32%	>32%
50–59	<18%	18%–22%	23%–27%	28%–30%	31%–34%	>34%
60–69	<18%	18%–23%	24%–28%	29%–31%	32%–35%	>35%
70–79	<18%	18%–24%	25%–29%	30%–32%	33%–36%	>36%

[a]Assumes nonathletes. For athletes, recommended body fat is 5% to 15% for men and 12% to 22% for women. Please note that there are no agreed-upon national standards for recommended body fat percentage.

Source: Based on data from The Cooper Institute, Dallas, Texas, www.cooperinstitute.org.

Underweight

Men with only 3 to 7 percent body fat and women with approximately 8 to 15 percent are considered **underweight,** which can seriously compromise health. Extremely low body fat can cause hair loss, visual disturbances, skin problems, a tendency to fracture bones easily, digestive system disturbances, heart irregularities, gastrointestinal problems, difficulties in maintaining body temperature, and amenorrhea (in women). Today, fewer than 4 percent of children aged 2 to 5 years, youth aged 6 to 11, and adolescents aged 12 to 19 and 2 percent of adults aged 20 to 74 are underweight. These rates indicate a decline in the number of underweight individuals in recent decades as overweight and obesity percentages have increased.[39] (See **Focus On: Enhancing Your Body Image** beginning on page 249 for an in-depth discussion of eating disorders and body image issues.)

Body Mass Index (BMI)

Body mass index (BMI) is a description of body weight relative to height—numbers that are highly correlated with your total body fat. Find your BMI in inches and pounds in **FIGURE 8.4**, or calculate your BMI now by dividing your weight in kilograms by height in meters squared. The mathematical formula is

$$\text{BMI} = \text{weight (kg)}/\text{height squared (m}^2)$$

A BMI calculator is also available from the National Heart, Lung, and Blood Institute at www.nhlbi.nih.gov/guidelines/obesity/BMI/bmicalc.htm.

Desirable BMI levels may vary with age and by sex; however, most BMI tables for adults do not account for such variables. **Healthy weight** is defined as having a BMI of 18.5 to 24.9, the range of lowest statistical health risk.[40] A BMI of 25 to 29.9 indicates overweight and potentially significant health risks. A BMI of 30 to 39.9 is classified as obese. A BMI of 40 to 49.9 is **morbidly obese,** and a new category of BMI of 50 or higher has been labeled as **super obese.**[41] Nearly 3 percent of obese men and almost 7 percent of obese women are morbidly obese.[42]

Limitations of BMI Like other assessments of fatness, the BMI has its limitations. Water, muscle, and bone mass are not included in BMI calculations, and base metabolism index levels don't account for the fact that muscle weighs more than fat. BMI levels can be inaccurate for people who are under 5 feet tall, are highly muscled, or who are older and have little muscle mass. Although a combination of measures might be most reliable in assessing fat levels, BMI continues to be a quick, inexpensive, and useful tool for developing basic health recommendations.[43]

underweight Having a body weight more than 10 percent below healthy recommended levels; in an adult, having a BMI below 18.5.

body mass index (BMI) A number calculated from a person's weight and height that is used to assess risk for possible present or future health problems.

healthy weight Those with BMIs of 18.5 to 24.9, the range of lowest statistical health risk

morbidly obese Having a body weight 100 percent or more above healthy recommended levels; in an adult, having a BMI of 40 or more.

super obese Having a body weight higher than morbid obesity; in an adult, having a BMI of 50 or more.

Height (feet and inches)																	
4′6″	24	27	29	31	34	36	39	41	43	46	48	51	53	55	58	60	63
4′8″	22	25	27	29	31	34	36	38	40	43	45	47	49	52	54	56	58
4′10″	21	23	25	27	29	31	33	36	38	40	42	44	46	48	50	52	54
5′0″	20	22	23	25	27	29	31	33	35	37	39	41	43	45	47	49	51
5′2″	18	20	22	24	26	27	29	31	33	35	37	38	40	42	44	46	48
5′4″	17	19	21	22	24	26	28	29	31	33	34	36	38	40	41	43	45
5′6″	16	18	19	21	23	24	26	27	29	31	32	34	36	37	39	40	42
5′8″	15	17	18	20	21	23	24	26	27	29	30	32	33	35	37	38	40
5′10″	14	16	17	19	20	22	23	24	26	27	29	30	32	33	34	36	37
6′0″	14	15	16	18	19	20	22	23	24	26	27	29	30	31	33	34	35
6′2″	13	14	15	17	18	19	21	22	23	24	26	27	28	30	31	32	33
6′4″	12	13	15	16	17	18	20	21	22	23	24	26	27	28	29	30	32
6′6″	12	13	14	15	16	17	19	20	21	22	23	24	25	27	28	29	30
6′8″	11	12	13	14	15	17	18	19	20	21	22	23	24	25	26	28	29
6′10″	11	12	13	14	15	16	17	18	19	20	21	22	23	24	25	26	27
7′0″	10	11	12	13	14	15	16	17	18	19	20	21	22	23	24	25	26
	100		120		140		160		180		200		220		240		260

Weight (pounds)

Key:

- Underweight
- Normal weight
- Overweight
- Obese

FIGURE 8.4 Body Mass Index (BMI) Locate your height, read across to find your weight, and then read up to determine your BMI. Note that BMI values have been rounded off to the nearest whole number.

Youth and BMI Today, over 30 percent of youth in America are obese, three times higher than rates in the 1980s.[44] Although the labels *obese* and *morbidly obese* have been used for years for adults, there is growing concern that such labels increase bias and stigma against youth.[45] BMI ranges above a normal weight for children and teens are often labeled differently, as "at risk of overweight" and "overweight," to avoid the sense of shame such words may cause. In addition, BMI ranges for children and teens take into account normal differences in body fat between boys and girls and the differences in body fat that occur at various ages. Specific guidelines for calculating youth BMI are available at the Centers for Disease Control and Prevention website, www.cdc.gov.

Waist Circumference and Ratio Measurements

Knowing where your fat is carried may be more important than knowing how much you carry. Men and postmenopausal women tend to store fat in the upper regions of the body, particularly in the abdominal area. Premenopausal women

Underwater (hydrostatic) weighing:
Measures the amount of water a person displaces when completely submerged. Fat tissue is less dense than muscle or bone, so body fat can be computed within a 2%–3% margin of error by comparing weight underwater and out of water.

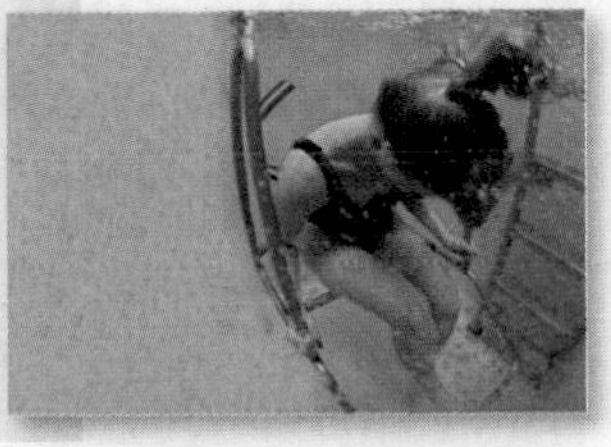

Skinfolds:
Involves "pinching" a person's fold of skin (with its underlying layer of fat) at various locations of the body. The fold is measured using a specially designed caliper. When performed by a skilled technician, it can estimate body fat with an error of 3%–4%.

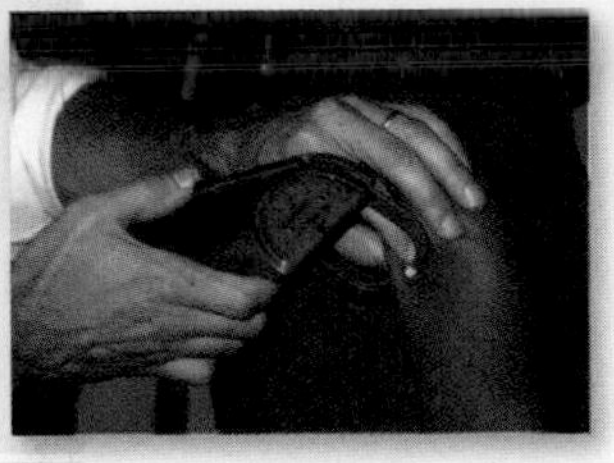

Bioelectrical impedance analysis (BIA):
Involves sending a very low level of electrical current through a person's body. As lean body mass is made up of mostly water, the rate at which the electricity is conducted gives an indication of a person's lean body mass and body fat. Under the best circumstances, BIA can estimate body fat with an error of 3%–4%.

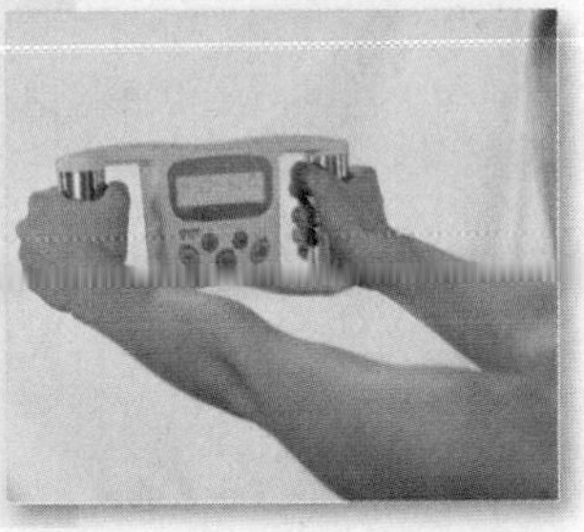

Dual-energy X-ray absorptiometry (DXA):
The technology is based on using very-low-level X ray to differentiate between bone tissue, soft (or lean) tissue, and fat (or adipose) tissue. The margin of error for predicting body fat is 2%–4%.

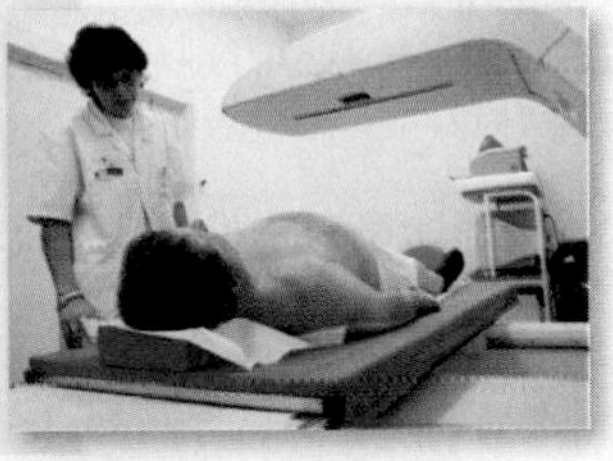

Bod Pod:
Uses air displacement to measure body composition. This machine is a large, egg-shaped chamber made from fiberglass. The person being measured sits in the machine wearing a swimsuit. The door is closed and the machine measures how much air is displaced. That value is used to calculate body fat, with a 2%–3% margin of error.

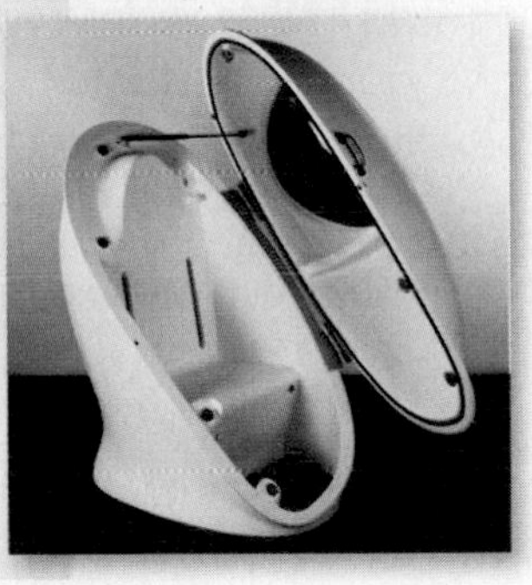

FIGURE 8.5 Overview of Various Body Composition Assessment Methods

Source: Adapted from J. Thompson and M. Manore, *Nutrition: An Applied Approach My Plate Edition*, 3rd edition, © 2012. Printed and electronically reproduced by permission of Pearson Education, Inc., Upper Saddle River, New Jersey.

usually store fat in the lower regions of their bodies, particularly the hips, buttocks, and thighs. Waist circumference measurements, including **waist circumference** (WC) only, the **waist circumference-to-hip ratio** (WHR), and the **waist circumference-to-height ratio** (WHtR), have all been used to measure abdominal fat as an indicator of obesity and health risk. Where you carry the weight may be of particular importance in determining whether you develop diabetes, cardiovascular disease, hypertension, or stroke.[46]

A waistline greater than 40 inches (102 centimeters) in men and 35 inches (88 centimeters) in women may be particularly indicative of greater health risk.[47] If a person is less than 5 feet tall or has a BMI of 35 or above, waist circumference standards used for the general population might not apply.

The waist circumference-to-hip ratio measures regional fat distribution. A waist-to-hip ratio greater than 1 in men and 0.8 in women indicates increased health risks.[48] Newer research has pointed to waist-to-hip ratio being more effective than waist circumference alone or BMI use when measuring body fat in children and adolescents.[49] A waist circumference-to-height ratio is a simple screening tool that says that your waist should be approximately one-half of your height; if you were 70 inches tall, your waist shouldn't be more than 35 inches. There is considerable debate over whether waist-to-hip or waist-to-height measures are better than BMI and whether one of these is better than the other.[50]

waist circumference Simple measure of circumference around waist, measured one inch above naval in inches or centimeters.

waist circumference-to-hip ratio Waist circumference divided by hip circumference; a high ratio indicates increased health risks due to unhealthy fat distribution.

waist circumference-to-height ratio Measure of a person's waist circumference, divided by their height; measures under .50 are desirable.

Measures of Body Fat

There are numerous ways to assess whether your body fat levels are too high. One low-tech way is simply to look in the mirror or consider how your clothes fit now compared with how they fit last year. For those who wish to take a more precise measurement of their percentage of body fat, more accurate techniques are available, several of which are described and depicted in **FIGURE 8.5**. These methods usually involve the help of a skilled professional and typically must be done in a lab or clinical setting. Before undergoing any procedure, make sure you understand the expense, potential for accuracy, risks, and training of the tester. Also, consider why you are seeking this assessment and what you plan to do with the results.

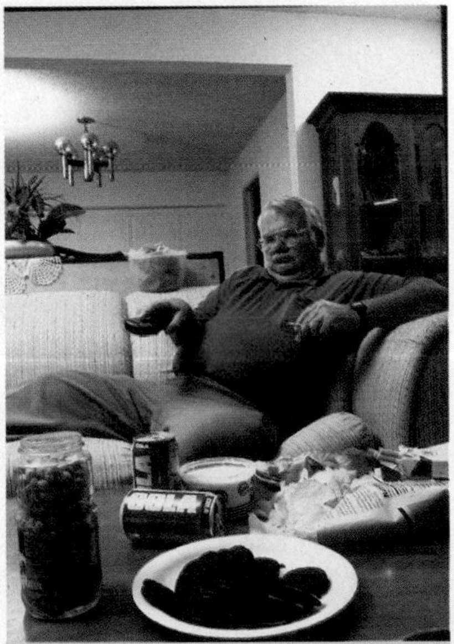

Abdominal obesity puts individuals at increased risk of CVD, stroke, and diabetes, particularly among men.

LO 3 | MANAGING YOUR WEIGHT

Explain the effectiveness and potential pros/cons of various weight control strategies, including exercise, diet, lifestyle modification, supplements/diet drugs, surgery, and other options.

At some point in our lives, almost all of us will decide to lose weight or modify our diet. Many will have mixed success. Failure is often related to thinking about losing weight in terms of short-term "dieting" rather than adjusting long-term behaviors. Drugs and intensive counseling can contribute to positive weight loss, but even then, many people regain weight after treatment. Maintaining a healthful body takes constant attention and nurturing over the course of your lifetime.

Improving Your Eating Habits

Before you can change an unhealthy eating habit, you must first determine what causes or triggers it. Keeping a detailed daily log of eating triggers—when, what, where, and how much you eat—for at least a week can give clues about what causes you to want food. Typically, these dietary triggers center on patterns and problems in everyday living rather than on real hunger pangs. Many people eat compulsively when stressed; however, for other people, the same circumstances diminish their appetite, causing them to lose weight. See the **Skills for Behavior Change** box for tips on healthy snacking, and see **FIGURE 8.6** for ways you can adjust your eating triggers and snack more healthfully in order to manage your weight.

If your trigger is . . . then	try this strategy . . .
A stressful situation	Acknowledge and address feelings of anxiety or stress, and develop stress management techniques to practice daily.
Feeling angry or upset	Analyze your emotions and look for a noneating activity to deal with them, such as taking a quick walk or calling a friend.
A certain time of day	Change your eating schedule to avoid skipping or delaying meals and overeating later; make a plan of what you'll eat ahead of time to avoid impulse or emotional eating.
Pressure from friends and family	Have a response ready to help you refuse food you do not want, or look for healthy alternatives you can eat instead when in social settings.
Being in an environment where food is available	Avoid the environment that causes you to want to eat: Sit far away from the food at meetings, take a different route to class to avoid passing the vending machines, shop from a list and only when you aren't hungry, arrange nonfood outings with your friends.
Feeling bored and tired	Identify the times when you feel low energy and fill them with activities other than eating, such as exercise breaks; cultivate a new interest or hobby that keeps your mind and hands busy.
The sight and smell of food	Stop buying high-calorie foods that tempt you to snack, or store them in an inconvenient place, out of sight; avoid walking past or sitting or standing near the table of tempting treats at a meeting, party, or other gathering.
Eating mindlessly or inattentively	Turn off all distractions, including phones, computers, television, and radio, and eat more slowly, savoring your food and putting your fork down between bites so you can become aware of when your hunger is satisfied.
Spending time alone in the car	Get a book on tape to listen to, or tape your class notes and use the time for studying. Keep your mind off food. Don't bring money into the gas station where snacks are tempting.
Alcohol use	Drink plenty of water and stay hydrated. Seek out healthy snack choices. After a night out, brush your teeth immediately upon getting home and stay out of the kitchen.
Feeling deprived	Allow yourself to eat "indulgences" in moderation, so you won't crave them; focus on balancing your calorie input to calorie output.
Eating out of habit	Establish a new routine to circumvent the old, such as taking a new route to class so you don't feel compelled to stop at your favorite fast-food restaurant on the way.
Watching television	Look for something else to occupy your hands and body while your mind is engaged with the screen: Ride an exercise bike, do stretching exercises, doodle on a pad of paper, or learn to knit.

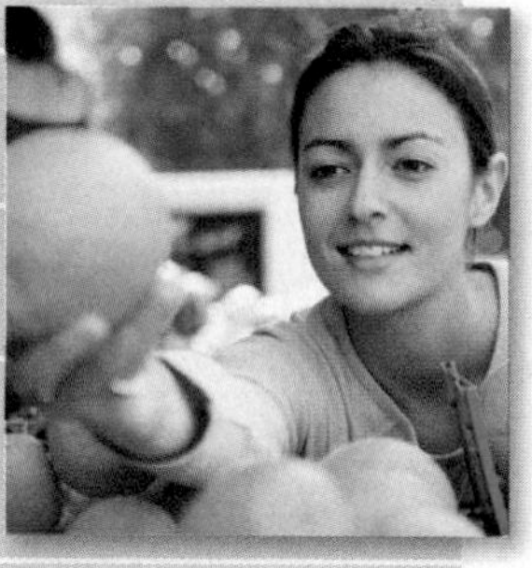

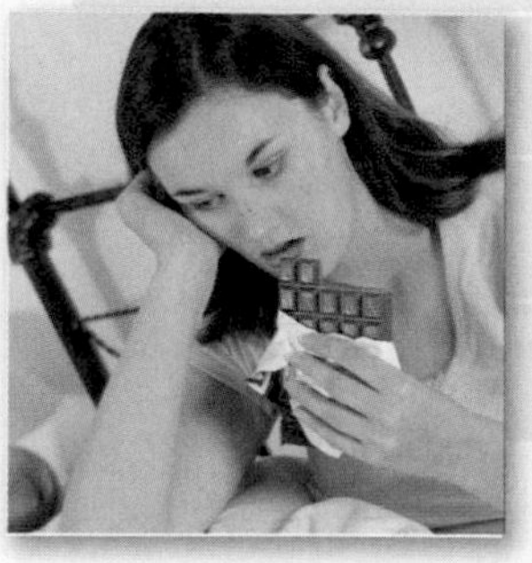

FIGURE 8.6 Avoid Trigger-Happy Eating Learn what triggers your "eat" response—and what stops it—by keeping a daily log.

SKILLS FOR BEHAVIOR CHANGE

TIPS FOR SENSIBLE SNACKING

- **Keep healthy munchies around.** Buy 100 percent whole wheat breads, and if you need something to spice that up, use low-fat or soy cheese, low-fat cream cheese, peanut butter, hummus, or other high-protein healthy favorites. Some baked or popped crackers are low in fat and calories and high in fiber.
- **Keep "crunchies" on hand.** Apples, pears, green or red pepper sticks, popcorn, snap peas, and celery all are good choices. Wash the fruits and vegetables and cut them up to carry with you; eat them when a snack attack comes on.
- **Choose natural beverages.** Drink plain water, 100 percent juice in small quantities, or other low-sugar choices to satisfy your thirst. Hot tea, coffee (black), or soup broths are also good choices.
- **Eat nuts instead of candy.** Although relatively high in calories, nuts are also loaded with healthy fats and are healthy when consumed in moderation.
- **If you must have a piece of chocolate, keep it small and dark.** Dark chocolate has more antioxidants.
- **Avoid high-calorie energy bars.** Eat these only if you are exercising hard and don't have an opportunity to eat a regular meal. Select ones with a good mixture of fiber and protein and that are low in fat, sugar, and calories.

Once you have evaluated your behaviors and determined your triggers, you can begin to devise a plan for improved eating by doing the following:

- Seeking assistance from reputable sources such as MyPlate (www.choosemyplate.gov), a registered dietitian (RD), some physicians, health educators, or exercise physiologists with nutritional training.
- Being wary of nutritionists or nutritional life coaches, since there is no formal credential for those titles.
- Avoiding weight-loss programs that promise quick, "miracle" results or that are run by "trainees," often people with short courses on nutrition and exercise that are designed to sell products or services.
- Assessing the nutrient value of any prescribed diet, verifying dietary guidelines are consistent with reliable nutrition research, and analyzing the suitability of the diet to your tastes, budget, and lifestyle.

Any diet that requires radical behavior changes or sets up artificial dietary programs through prepackaged products is likely to fail. The most successful plans allow you to make food choices in real-world settings and do not ask you to sacrifice everything you enjoy. See **TABLE 8.2** for an analysis of some popular diets marketed today. For information on other plans, check out the regularly updated list of reviews on the website of the Academy of Nutrition and Dietetics (formerly the American Dietetic Association) at www.eatright.org.

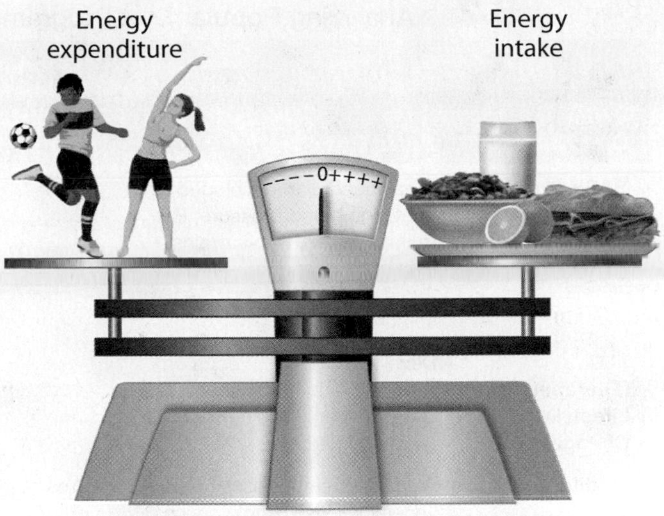

FIGURE 8.7 The Concept of Energy Balance If you consume more calories than you burn, you gain weight. If you burn more than you consume, you lose weight. If both are equal, your weight will not change.

WHY SHOULD I CARE?

It may be easy to grab a fast-food meal, but unless you are very physically active, your body will likely store that "super-sized" meal as fat, which is anything but easy to lose. Eating 500 extra calories a day—less than the average hamburger—can lead to a pound of weight gain in just a week's time.

Understanding Calories and Energy Balance

A *calorie* is a unit of measure that indicates the amount of energy gained from food or expended through activity. Each time you consume 3,500 calories more than your body needs to maintain weight, you gain a pound of storage fat. Conversely, each time your body expends an extra 3,500 calories, you lose a pound of fat. If you consume 140 calories (the amount in one can of regular soda) more than you need every single day and make no other changes in diet or activity, you would gain 1 pound in 25 days (3,500 calories ÷ 140 calories ÷ 1 day = 25 days). Conversely, if you walk for 30 minutes each day at a pace of 15 minutes per mile (172 calories burned) in addition to your regular activities, you would lose 1 pound in 20 days (3,500 calories ÷ 172 calories ÷ 1 day = 20.3 days). **FIGURE 8.7** illustrates the concept of energy balance.

Including Exercise

Any increase in the intensity, frequency, and duration of daily exercise can have a significant impact on total calorie expenditure because lean (muscle) tissue is more metabolically active than fat tissue. Exact estimates

TABLE 8.2 | Analyzing Popular Diet Programs

Diet Name	Basic Principles	Good for Diabetes and Heart Health?	Weight Loss Effectiveness	Pros, Cons, and Other Things to Consider
DASH (Dietary Approaches to Stop Hypertension)	A balanced plan developed to fight high blood pressure. Eat fruits, veggies, whole grains, lean protein, and low-fat dairy. Avoid sweets, fats, red meat, and sodium.	Yes	Not specifically designed for weight loss.	A safe and healthy diet, rated the #1 best diet overall by 2014 *U.S. News & World Report*. Although not designed for weight reduction, it is regarded as very effective in improving cholesterol levels and other biomarkers long term.
TLC (Therapeutic Lifestyle Change)	Developed by NIH. Focus on CVD risk reduction with fruits and veggies, lean protein, low fat, etc. Balanced and effective.	Yes	Weight loss likely; cholesterol key.	A safe and healthy diet rated #2 best diet overall by 2014 *U.S. News & World Report*.
Mediterranean	A plan that emphasizes fruits, vegetables, fish, whole grains, beans, nuts, legumes, olive oil, and herbs and spices. Poultry, eggs, cheese, yogurt, and red wine can be enjoyed in moderation, whereas sweets and red meat are saved for special occasions.	Yes	Effective	Widely considered to be one of the more healthy, safe, and balanced diets. Weight loss may not be as dramatic, but long-term health benefits have been demonstrated. Tied as one of the #3 best diets overall by 2014 *U.S. News & World Report*.
Weight Watchers	The program assigns every food a point value based on its nutritional values and how hard your body has to work to burn it off. Total points allowed depend on someone's activity level and their personal weight goals. In-person group meetings or online membership are options.	Yes (depending on individual choices).	Effective	Experts consider Weight Watchers effective and easy to follow for both short- and long-term weight loss. Other pluses include an emphasis on group support and room for occasional indulgences. But while not as expensive as some plans, there are membership fees. Tied as one of the #3 best diets overall by 2014 *U.S. News & World Report*.
Jenny Craig	Prepackaged meals do the work of restricting calorie intake. Members get personalized meal and exercise plans, plus weekly counseling sessions.	Yes	Effective short term, long-term results dependent on adopting healthful eating later.	Support and premade meals make weight loss easier; however, it may be difficult to maintain for long run. Cons include cost, which will run hundreds of dollars per month for food alone, plus membership fees. Lactose- and gluten-intolerant individuals cannot join due to available foods.
Biggest Loser	Four servings a day of fruits and vegetables, three of protein foods, two of whole grains, and no more than 200 calories of "extras" like desserts. Exercise, food journals, portion control, and calculating personal calorie allowances are all stressed.	Yes	Effective	This diet is effective at weight loss. Also helps reduce blood glucose levels and reduces other biomarkers such as cholesterol, triglycerides, etc.
Nutrisystem	Low-calorie, prepackaged meals are ordered online and delivered to your home.	No for heart health, but probably helps diabetics.	Effective short-term, long-term results dependent on adopting healthful eating later.	Nutrisystem is quite safe, easier to follow than many other diets, and has few nutritional deficiencies, according to experts. As a heart diet, it's off the mark. It is also expensive (similar to Jenny Craig) due to the cost of ordering food and may not help you learn to eat healthfully after diet is done.
Medifast	Dieters eat six meals a day, five of them 100-calorie Medifast products. After goal weight loss, people wean from Medifast food and gradually add back in starchy veggies, whole grains, fruit, and low-fat dairy products.	Likely yes	Effective in short term; long-term results unproven.	Medifast scored above average in short-term weight loss but gets lower marks for keeping weight off. Because of the extremely low calorie intakes on the program, it is hard to stay on the program for long; doesn't teach healthy eating as part of plan.

TABLE 8.2 | Analyzing Popular Diet Programs *(continued)*

Atkins	Carbs—sugars and "simple starches" like potatoes, white bread, and rice—are avoided in this plan and protein and fat from chicken, meat, and eggs are embraced.	Not likely with so much fat eaten	Effective in short term, mixed long-term results.	Atkins is extremely effective at short-term weight loss, but many experts worry that fat intake is up to three times higher than standard daily recommendations.
Paleo	Based on the theory that digestive systems have not evolved to deal with many modern foods such as dairy, legumes, grains and sugar, this plan emphasizes meats, fish, poultry, fruits, and vegetables.	Unknown (too few studies).	Unknown (too few studies).	Gets low marks by health and nutrition experts due to avoidance of grains, legumes, and dairy and higher fat than the government recommends. Missing essential nutrients, costly to maintain. It can be hard to follow long term and has had only a few very small studies done to document effectiveness.
Fast Diet (also known as the 5:2 diet or Intermittent Fasting Diet)	Based on the theory that by drastically reducing calories on two days (500 cal/day) each week and eating normally the other five, you will lose weight	Not likely as it doesn't follow guidelines for carbohydrates. Should talk with registered dietician or health care provider.	Effective, but weight loss is relatively slow unless calorie intake is monitored on non-fast days and exercise is part of regimen.	Exceeds dietary guidelines for fat and protein and falls short on carbohydrate recommendation. Does encourage fruits and veggies, but feast and famine regimen is hard to sustain.

Source: Opinions on diet pros and cons are based on *U.S. News & World Report*, "Best Diet Rankings," 2012, http://health.usnews.com. Dietary reviews are available online from registered dieticians at the Academy of Nutrition and Dietetics, 2014, http://www.eatright.org/dietreviews.

vary, but experts currently think that 2 to 50 more calories per day are burned per pound of muscle than each pound of fat tissue. Thus, the base level of calories needed to maintain a healthy weight varies greatly from person to person.

The number of calories spent through physical activity depends on three factors:

1. The number and proportion of muscles used
2. The amount of weight moved
3. The length of time the activity takes

An activity involving both the arms and legs burns more calories than one involving only the legs. An activity performed by a heavy person burns more calories than the same activity performed by a lighter person. And an activity performed for 40 minutes requires twice as much energy as the same activity performed for only 20 minutes.

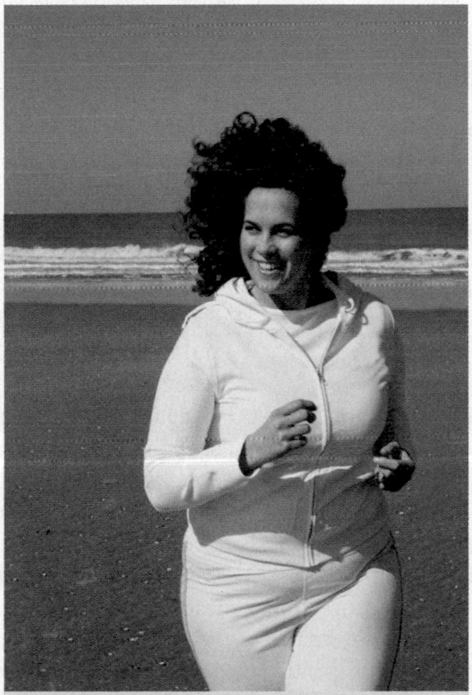

Participating in daily physical activity is key to managing your weight. Go for a jog on your own for some quiet time, or join a soccer game for social, fast-moving fun, but get out there and move!

Keeping Weight Control in Perspective

Weight loss is a struggle for many people, and many factors influence success or failure. Supportive friends, relatives, community resources, and policies that support healthy food choices and exercise options all increase the likelihood of success. People of the same age, sex, height, and weight can have resting metabolic rates that differ by as much as 1,000 calories a day. This may explain why one person's extra food intake and weight gain may lead to weight loss and hunger in another person. Depression, stress, cultural influences, and the availability of high-fat, high-calorie foods can also make weight loss harder.

To reach and maintain a healthy weight, develop a program of exercise and healthy eating behaviors that you can maintain. Remember, you didn't gain your weight in a week or two, and it is both unrealistic and potentially dangerous to take drastic weight loss measures. Instead, try to lose a healthy 1 to 2 pounds during the first week, and stay with this slow and easy regimen. Adding exercise and cutting back on calories to expend about 500 calories more than you consume each day will help you lose weight at a rate of 1 pound per week. You may find tracking your intake and activity easier with one of the apps described

TECH & HEALTH | TRACKING YOUR DIET OR WEIGHT LOSS? THERE'S AN APP FOR THAT

A recent study found people who kept detailed food journals lost more weight than people who did not. Today, there are many diet tracking applications for smart phones available for free or low cost. The best programs combine food and physical activity logs, so if you splurge on dessert, you can figure out how many miles you'll need to jog to burn it off. These apps often feature calculators for determining daily calorie intake goals as well as barcode scanners that allow you to quickly add packaged foods to your log. Here are just a few of the apps out there:

- **Lose It!** (Free: Android, iPhone, Nook tablet, PCs), www.loseit.com

  Simple to use, comprehensive database of foods and activities designed to help you log meals and track exercise.

- **Restaurant Weight Watcher.** (Modest cost; Android only), http://ellisapps.com

  Lists nutrition information for the menus of over 200 restaurants and continues to add new ones.

- **MyFitnessPal Calorie Counter & Diet Tracker** (Free: iPhone, Android, Blackberry, PCs) www.myfitnesspal.com

  A combination of diet and fitness goals as well as a nutritional analysis of what you are eating

- **MyNetDiary.** (Free trial of basic version, and modest cost for full features: Android, iPhone, Blackberry) www.mynetdiary.com

  A comprehensive food diary that allows you to scan bar codes on foods to add your daily favorites

- **Diet Point • Weight Loss** (Free: Android and iPhone) https://itunes.apple.com/us/app/diet-point-weight-loss/id582932885?mt=8

  Weight loss assistant that offers 55 unique diet plans, from low carb to vegan to paleo, including grocery lists, instructions, and reminders. Includes BMI and BMR calculator that tracks energy expenditure as well as exercise tracking.

in the **Tech & Health** box. See the **Skills for Behavior Change** box for strategies to help your weight management program succeed.

Considering Drastic Weight-Loss Measures?

When nothing seems to work, people often become frustrated and may take significant risks to lose weight. Dramatic weight loss may be recommended in cases of extreme health risk. Even in such situations, drastic dietary, pharmacological, or surgical measures should be considered carefully and discussed with several knowledgeable health professionals.

Very-Low-Calorie Diets

In severe cases of obesity that are not responsive to traditional dietary strategies, medically supervised, powdered formulas with daily values of 400 to 700 calories plus vitamin and mineral supplements may be given to patients. Such **very-low-calorie diets (VLCDs)** should never be undertaken without strict medical supervision. While significant, fast weight loss often occurs initially on these diets, many quickly re-gain weight, as individuals have not learned how to maintain losses. Today, a newer, less stringent version of fasting diets, known as "intermittent fasting" or the "5:2 diet" focuses on 2 days of fasting in the 500 calorie range per day followed by 5 days of normal eating. More research is necessary to analyze potential risks/benefits of this diet.

very-low-calorie diets (VLCDs) Diets with a daily caloric value of 400 to 700 calories.

More important, fasting, starvation diets, and other forms of VLCDs have been shown to cause significant health risks, including sugar imbalance, cold intolerance, constipation, decreased BMR, dehydration, diarrhea, emotional problems, fatigue, headaches, heart irregularities, kidney infections and failure, loss of lean body tissue, weakness, and the potential for coma and death.

One particularly dangerous potential complication of VLCDs or starvation diets is *ketoacidosis.* After a prolonged period of inadequate carbohydrate or food intake, the body will have depleted its immediate energy stores and will begin metabolizing fat stores through *ketogenesis* in order to supply the brain and nervous system with an alternative fuel known as *ketones.* Ketogenesis is one of the body's normal processes for metabolizing fat and may help provide energy to the brain during times of fasting, low carbohydrate intake, or vigorous exercise. However, ketones may also suppress appetite and cause dehydration at a time when a person should feel hungry and seek out food. The condition of having increased levels of ketones in the body is *ketosis*; if enough ketones accumulate in the blood, it may lead to *ketoacidosis,* in which the blood becomes more acidic. People with untreated type 1 diabetes and individuals with anorexia nervosa or bulimia nervosa are at risk of developing ketoacidotic symptoms as damage to body tissues begins.

SEE IT! VIDEOS

A new strategy to keep off the weight? Watch **Keeping It Off** available on MasteringHealth.™

SKILLS FOR BEHAVIOR CHANGE

KEYS TO SUCCESSFUL WEIGHT MANAGEMENT

MAKE A PLAN

- Establish short- and long-term plans. What are the diet and exercise changes you can make this week? Once you do 1 week, plot a course for 2 weeks, and so on.
- Look for balance. Remember it's calories taken in and burned over time that make the difference.

CHANGE YOUR HABITS

- Be adventurous. Expand your usual foods to enjoy a wider variety.
- Eat small portions, less often and savor the flavor.
- Notice whether you are hungry before starting a meal. Eat slowly, noting when you start to feel full, and *stop* before you are full.
- Eat breakfast, especially low-fat foods with whole grains and protein. This will prevent you from being too hungry and overeating at lunch.
- Keep healthful snacks on hand for when you get hungry.

INCORPORATE EXERCISE

- Be active and slowly increase your time, speed, distance, or resistance levels.
- Vary your physical activity. Find activities that you really love and try things you haven't tried before.
- Find an exercise partner to help you stay motivated.

If fasting continues, the body will turn to its last resort—protein—for energy, breaking down muscle and organ tissue to stay alive. As this occurs, the body loses weight rapidly. At the same time, it also loses significant water stores. Within approximately 10 days after the typical adult begins a complete fast, the body will have depleted its energy stores, and death may occur.

Weight Loss Supplements and Drug Treatment Thousands of over-the-counter supplements and drugs that claim to make weight loss fast and easy are available for purchase. It's important to note that U.S. Food and Drug Administration (FDA) approval is not required for over-the-counter "diet aids" or supplements, a situation that leaves consumers vulnerable to **dietary supplement fraud (DSF).** In contrast, **food fraud** is described as the "deliberate and intentional substitution, addition, tampering, or misrepresentation of food, food ingredients, or food packing, or false or misleading statements about a product."[51]

The lack of regular and continuous monitoring of supplements in the United States leaves consumers vulnerable to fraud and potentially toxic "remedies" as they desperately try to shed pounds. Recent FDA warnings have identified a growing trend of potentially harmful hidden ingredients in supposedly safe dietary supplements. According to the FDA, "*consumers may unknowingly take products laced with varying quantities of approved prescription drug ingredients, controlled substances, and untested and unstudied pharmaceutically active ingredients.*"[52] Most dietary supplements contain stimulants, such as caffeine, or diuretics, and their effectiveness in promoting weight loss has been largely untested and unproved by any scientific studies. In many cases, the only thing that users lose is money. Virtually all persons who used supplements and diet pills in review studies regained their weight once they stopped taking them.[53]

Historically, FDA-approved diet pills have been available only by prescription and are closely monitored. These lines were blurred in 2007 when the FDA approved the first over-the-counter weight loss pill—a half-strength version of the prescription drug *orlistat* (brand name *Xenical*), marketed as Alli. This drug inhibits the action of lipase, an enzyme that helps the body to digest fats, causing about 30 percent of fats consumed to pass through the digestive system undigested, leading to reduced overall caloric intake. Known side effects of orlistat include gas with watery fecal discharge; oily stools and spotting; frequent, often unexpected, bowel movements; and possible deficiencies of fat-soluble vitamins.

dietary supplement fraud A type of product fraud similar to food fraud but not controlled or monitored by the FDA as food or food additives would be.

food fraud The deliberate and intentional substitution, addition, tampering or misrepresentation of food, food ingredients or food packing, or false or misleading statements about a product.

In 2012, the FDA approved the first new weight loss drugs in nearly 13 years. These new drugs, *Belvig* and *Qsymia*, were met with much controversy and carry several warnings and restrictions. Qsymia is an appetite suppressant and antiseizure drug that reduces the desire for food. Belvig affects serotonin levels, helping patients feel full. Before taking any weight loss supplements and herbal remedies or prescription drugs, you should always discuss risks, benefits, and options with your doctor and carefully read FDA warnings.

In general, diet pills have been shown to be most effective when used as part of comprehensive lifestyle change, including diet and exercise. The challenge is to develop effective drugs that can be used over time without adverse effects or abuse. Several once-approved drugs have since been recalled due to a variety of problems like heart attacks, heart valve problems, stroke, and liver damage.

Other currently available diet drugs and supplements that you should view with caution include these:

- **Human chorionic gonadotropin (hCG).** This is a hormone produced by the placenta during pregnancy that, in prescription form, is also a federally approved treatment for some female fertility problems; it has recently become known as a crash-diet miracle drug. However, hCG has not been approved by the FDA for weight loss. In fact, after more than 50 years of extensive, double-blind research, results consistently show that hCG is no more effective for weight loss than cutting calories.[54]

- **Sibutramine (Meridia).** This prescription-only medication suppresses appetite by inhibiting the uptake of serotonin in the brain. It works best with a reduced-calorie diet and exercise, but side effects include dry mouth, headache, constipation, insomnia, and high blood pressure. Although research has shown positive effects on blood glucose control, the FDA has issued warnings about use of Meridia for people who have hypertension or heart disease.[55]
- ***Hoodia gordonii.*** This African cactus-like plant is a purported appetite suppressant. No convincing evidence has been shown for or against it; to date, it is not FDA approved and has not been tested in clinical trials.[56] Supplements containing *Hoodia gordonii* have become popular in recent years, and there are many off-market brands produced, including some that contain more unproven ingredients such as bitter orange and other stimulants.
- **Herbal weight-loss aids.** Products containing *ephedra* can cause rapid heart rate, tremors, seizures, insomnia, headaches, and raised blood pressure, all without significant effects on long-term weight control. *St. John's wort* and other alternative medicines reported to enhance serotonin, suppress appetite, and reduce the side effects of depression have not been shown to be effective in weight loss, either.

Surgery When all else fails, particularly for people who are severely overweight and have weight-related diseases such as diabetes or hypertension, a person may be a candidate for weight-loss surgery. Generally, these surgeries fall into one of two major categories: *restrictive surgeries,* such as gastric banding or lap banding, that limit food intake, and *malabsorption surgeries,* such as gastric bypass, which decrease the absorption of food into the body (**FIGURE 8.8**).

SEE IT! VIDEOS
What makes one diet plan work better than another? Watch **Best Diet Plan Apparently Works** available on MasteringHealth.™

To select the best option, a physician will consider that operation's benefits and risks, the patient's age, BMI, eating behaviors, obesity-related health conditions, mental history, dietary history, and previous operations. Like drugs prescribed for weight loss, surgery for obesity also carries risks for consumers.[57] Some health advocates have proposed that obesity be classified as a disability, which could potentially affect a physician's decision on recommending surgery.

In *adjustable gastric banding* and other restrictive surgeries, the surgeon uses an inflatable band to partition off part of the stomach. The band is wrapped around that part of the stomach and is pulled tight, like a belt, leaving only a small opening between the two parts of the stomach so the stomach is smaller and the person feels full more quickly. Food digestion slows so that the person also feels full longer. Although the bands are designed to stay in place, they can be removed surgically. They can also be inflated to different levels to adjust the amount of restriction. Although weight loss isn't as dramatic as with gastric bypass surgery, the risks are fewer. Vomiting may occur, and the band may slip out of place, leak, or result in infection. Sometimes more surgery is necessary to correct problems or reverse this surgery.

Sleeve gastrectomy is another form of restrictive weight loss that is often done laparoscopically. In this surgery, about 75 percent of the stomach is removed, leaving only a tube (about the size of a banana) or sleeve that is connected directly

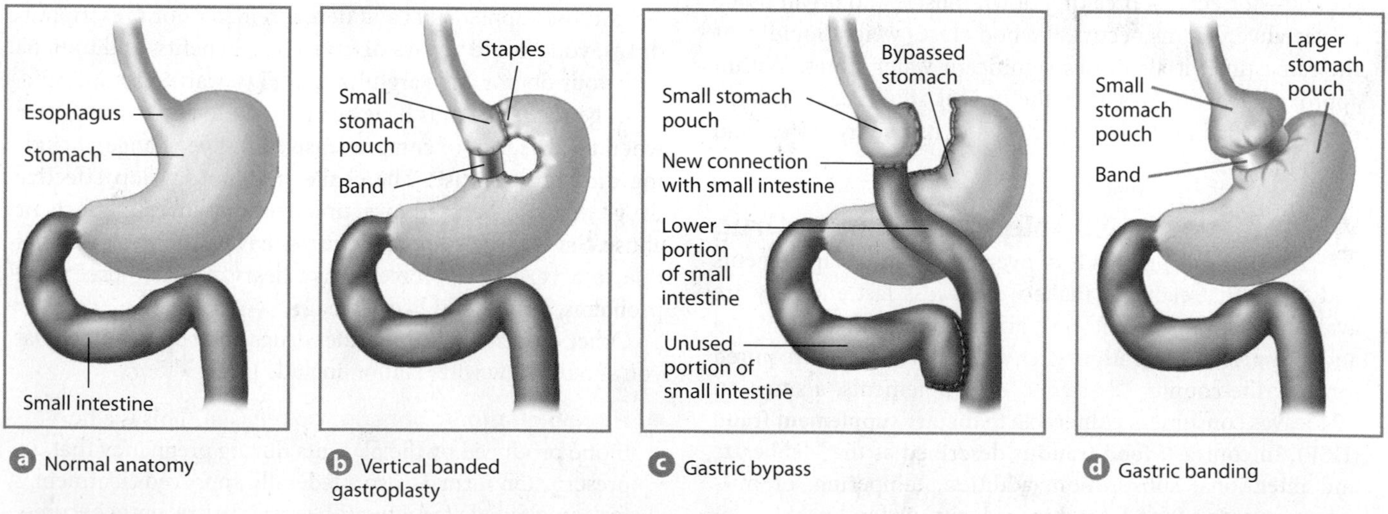

FIGURE 8.8 Weight-Loss Surgery Alters the Normal Anatomy of the Stomach

Source: Adapted from J. Thompson and M. Manore, *Nutrition: An Applied Approach,* 4th edition, © 2015. Printed and electronically reproduced by permission of Pearson Education, Inc., Upper Saddle River, New Jersey.

to the intestines. Usually, this procedure is done on extremely obese or ill patients who need an interim, less invasive procedure before more invasive gastric bypass. However, this procedure isn't reversible and potential risks may be higher.

Gastric bypass is one of the most common types of weight loss surgery and it combines restrictive and malabsorption elements. It can be done laparoscopically or via full open surgery. In this surgery, the stomach is drastically reduced by suturing off a major section (as much as 70%) of the stomach, restricting the amount of food you can eat and absorb. The remaining pouch is hooked up directly to the small intestine. Results are fast and dramatic, with health issues related to obesity, such as diabetes, high blood pressure, arthritis, sleep apnea, and other problems diminishing or being reduced drastically in a short time.

While weight loss tends to be maintained and health problems decline, there are many risks, including nutritional deficiencies, blood clots in the legs, a leak in a staple line in the stomach, pneumonia, infection, and although rare, even death. Another risk is rapid gastric emptying, commonly referred to as "dumping," in which undigested foods rush through the small intestine, causing cramping and problems with uncontrollable diarrhea.[58] Because the stomach pouch that remains after surgery is only the size of a lime, the person can drink only a few tablespoons of liquid and consume only a very small amount of food at a time. For this reason, other possible side effects include nausea, vitamin and mineral deficiencies, and dehydration. Additional risks include the potential for excess bleeding, ulcers, hernia, and the typical risks from anesthesia. These risks must be considered against the risks of obesity. Because the surgery and follow up is very expensive and insurance may or may not cover it, many people do not have the resources to have this procedure.

A technique gaining in popularity because it's even more effective than gastric bypass for rapid weight loss is the *biliopancreatic diversion* or *duodenal switch procedure,* which combines elements of restrictive and malabsorption surgeries. The patient receives a partial gastrectomy to reduce the size of the stomach (less than gastric bypass's reduction) while bypassing less of the small intestine. The pyloric valve remains intact, which helps prevent dumping syndrome, ulcers, blockages, and other problems that can occur with other techniques. This surgery is one of the most difficult and highest risk surgeries for patients, with the risk of death and other complications higher than those of other options.[59]

Aftercare for gastric surgery patients often includes counseling to help them cope with the urge to eat after the ability to eat normal portions has been removed, as well as other adjustment problems. Keep in mind that it is always best to lose weight by eating a healthy diet and getting regular physical activity. Ironically, even after undergoing surgery, people must learn to eat healthy foods and exercise, otherwise, they can continue to gain weight—even returning to their original weight.

Considerable research has demonstrated exciting, unexpected results from gastric surgeries: Even prior to weight loss, patients have shown complete remission of type 2 diabetes in the majority of cases, with drastic reductions in blood glucose levels in others.[60] While extremely promising, newer research indicates that about one-third of those who have gastric surgery with remission of diabetic symptoms will relapse and begin to show diabetic symptoms within 5 years after surgery. Those least likely to have remission of symptoms will be those who had diabetes for 15 years or more prior to surgery. Research to determine the mechanisms by which gastric surgery for weight reduction results in remission of diabetic symptoms is ongoing.[61] For those at high risk from these diseases, the choice of undergoing a high-risk surgery may ultimately be similar to the risk of maintaining their current weight.

Unlike restrictive and malabsorption surgeries, which facilitate overall weight loss, *liposuction* is a surgical procedure in which fat cells are removed from specific areas of the body. Generally, liposuction is considered cosmetic surgery rather than weight-loss surgery and is used for spot reducing and body contouring. Although this technique has garnered much attention, it is not without risk: Infections, severe scarring, and even death have resulted. In many cases, people who have liposuction regain fat in those areas or require multiple surgeries to repair lumpy, irregular surfaces from which the fat was removed.

Trying to Gain Weight

For some people, trying to gain weight is a challenge for a variety of metabolic, hereditary, psychological, and other reasons. If you are one of these individuals, the first priority is to determine why you cannot gain weight. Perhaps you're an athlete and you burn more calories than you manage to eat. Perhaps you're stressed out and skip meals to increase study time. Among older adults, senses of taste and smell may decline, making food less pleasurable to eat. Visual problems and other disabilities may make meals more difficult to prepare, and dental problems may make eating more difficult. People who engage in extreme energy-burning sports and exercise routines may be at risk for caloric and nutritional deficiencies, which can lead not only to weight loss, but also to immune system problems and organ dysfunction; weakness, which leads to falls and fractures; slower recovery from diseases; and a host of other problems as well. People who are too thin need to take the same steps as those who are overweight or obese to find out what their healthy weight is and attain that weight.

STUDY PLAN

Customize your study plan—and master your health!—in the Study Area of **MasteringHealth.**

ASSESS **YOURSELF**

Do you need to lose weight? Want to find out if you're ready? Take the **Are You Ready to Start a Weight-Loss Program?** assessment available on MasteringHealth.™

Need help creating a plan? Follow the strategies in the **Your Plan for Change** box for short- and long-term improvements to your health.

YOUR PLAN FOR **CHANGE**

The **ASSESS YOURSELF** identifies six areas of importance in determining your readiness for weight loss. If you wish to lose weight to improve your health, understanding your attitudes about food and exercise will help you succeed in your plan.

TODAY, YOU CAN:

- ☐ Set SMART goals for weight loss and give them a reality check: Are they **s**pecific, **m**easurable, **a**chievable, **r**elevant, and **t**ime oriented? For example, rather than aiming to lose 15 pounds this month (which probably wouldn't be healthy or achievable), set a comfortable goal to lose 5 pounds. Realistic goals will encourage weight-loss success by boosting your confidence in your ability to make lifelong healthy changes.
- ☐ Begin keeping a food log and identifying the triggers that influence your eating habits. Think about what you can do to eliminate or reduce the influence of your two most common food triggers.

WITHIN THE NEXT 2 WEEKS, YOU CAN:

- ☐ Get in the habit of incorporating more fruits, vegetables, and whole grains in your diet and eating less fat. The next time you make dinner, look at the proportions on your plate. If vegetables and whole grains do not take up most of the space, substitute 1 cup of the meat, non-whole grains, or cheese in your meal with 1 cup of legumes, salad greens, or a favorite vegetable. You'll reduce the number of calories while eating the same amount of food!
- ☐ Aim to incorporate more exercise into your daily routine. Visit your campus recreation center or a local gym and familiarize yourself with the equipment and facilities that are available. Try a new machine or sports activity, and experiment until you find a form of exercise you really enjoy.

BY THE END OF THE SEMESTER, YOU CAN:

- ☐ Get in the habit of grocery shopping every week and buying healthy, nutritious foods while avoiding high-fat, high-sugar, or overly processed foods. As you make healthy foods more available and unhealthy foods less available, you'll find it easier to eat better.
- ☐ Chart your progress and reward yourself as you meet your goals. If your goal is to lose weight and you successfully take off 10 pounds, reward yourself with a new pair of jeans or other article of clothing (which will likely fit better than before!).

CHAPTER REVIEW

To hear an MP3 Tutor Session, scan here or visit the Study Area in **MasteringHealth.**

LO 1 Factors Contributing to Overweight and Obesity

- Overweight, obesity, and weight-related health problems have reached epidemic levels. *Globesity,* or global rates of obesity, is also on the rise, particularly among developing regions of the world. Obesogenic behaviors in an obesogenic environment are key reasons for our weight-related problems.
- Societal costs from obesity include increased health care costs, lowered worker productivity, low self-esteem, increased depression, discrimination, and stigma. Individual health risks from overweight and obesity include increased chance of developing cardiovascular diseases, arthritis, stroke, diabetes, gastrointestinal problems, low back pain, and a number of other diseases. Overweight individuals are also at risk of struggling with depression, low self-esteem, and high levels of stress.
- It is important to consider environmental, cultural, and socioeconomic factors when working to prevent obesity. In addition to genetics, metabolism, hormonal influences, excess fat cells, and physical risks, key environmental influences, such as poverty, socioeconomic status, education level, and lack of access to nutritious food, and lifestyle factors, including sedentary lifestyle and high calorie consumption, all make weight loss challenging.

LO 2 Assessing Body Weight and Body Composition

- Percentage of body fat is a fairly reliable indicator for levels of overweight and obesity. There are many different methods of assessing body fat. Body mass index (BMI) is one of the most commonly accepted measures of weight based on height. *Overweight* is most commonly defined as a BMI of 25 to 29 and *obesity* as a BMI of 30 or greater. Waist circumference, or the amount of fat in the belly region, is believed to be related to the risk for several chronic diseases, particularly type 2 diabetes.

LO 3 Managing Your Weight

- Increased physical activity, a balanced, healthy diet that controls caloric intake, and other strategies are recommended for controlling your weight. When these options fail and risks increase, doctor-recommended prescription medications, weight loss surgery, and other strategies are used to maintain or lose weight. However, sensible eating behavior and aerobic exercise and exercise that builds muscle mass offer the best options for weight loss and maintenance.

POP QUIZ

Visit **MasteringHealth** to personalize your study plan with Chapter Review Quizzes and Dynamic Study Modules.

LO 1 Factors Contributing to Overweight and Obesity

1. The rate at which your body consumes food energy to sustain basic functions is your
   a. basal metabolic rate.
   b. resting metabolic rate.
   c. body mass index.
   d. set point.

LO 2 Assessing Body Weight and Body Composition

2. The proportion of your total weight that is made up of fat is called
   a. body composition.
   b. lean mass.
   c. percentage of body fat.
   d. BMI.
3. All of the following statements are true *except* which?
   a. A slowing basal metabolic rate may contribute to weight gain after age 30.
   b. Hormones are increasingly implicated in hunger impulses and eating behavior.
   c. The more muscles you have, the fewer calories you will burn.
   d. Overweight and obesity among young adults can have serious health consequences even before they reach middle age.
4. All of the following statements about BMI are true *except* which?
   a. BMI is based on height and weight measurements.
   b. BMI is accurate for everyone, including athletes with high amounts of muscle mass.
   c. Very low and very high BMI scores are associated with greater risk of mortality.
   d. BMI stands for "body mass index."
5. Which of the following BMI ratings is considered overweight?
   a. 20
   b. 25
   c. 30
   d. 35
6. Which of the following body circumferences is most strongly associated with risk of heart disease and diabetes?
   a. Hip circumference
   b. Chest circumference
   c. Waist circumference
   d. Thigh circumference

LO **3** | **Managing Your Weight**

7. One pound of additional body fat is created through consuming how many extra calories?
   a. 1,500 calories
   b. 3,500 calories
   c. 5,000 calories
   d. 7,000 calories
8. To lose weight, you must establish a(n)
   a. negative caloric balance.
   b. isocaloric balance.
   c. positive caloric balance.
   d. set point.
9. Successful weight maintainers are most likely to do which of the following?
   a. Eat two large meals a day before 1 P.M.
   b. Skip meals
   c. Drink diet sodas
   d. Eat high-volume but low-calorie density foods
10. Successful, healthy weight loss is characterized by
    a. a lifelong pattern of healthful eating and exercise.
    b. cutting out all fats and carbohydrates and eating a lean, mean, high-protein diet.
    c. never eating foods that are considered bad for you and rigidly adhering to a plan.
    d. a pattern of repeatedly losing and regaining weight.

Answers to the Pop Quiz can be found on page A-1. If you answered a question incorrectly, review the section identified by the Learning Outcome. For even more study tools, visit MasteringHealth.

THINK ABOUT IT!

LO 1 Factors Contributing to Overweight and Obesity

1. Discuss the pressures, if any, you feel to change your body's shape. Do these pressures come from media, family, friends, and other external sources, or from concern for your personal health?
2. List the risk factors for your being overweight or obese right now. Which seem most likely to determine whether you will be obese in middle age?
3. Why do you think that obesity rates are rising in both developed and less-developed regions of the world? What strategies can we take collectively and individually to reduce risks of obesity?

LO 2 Assessing Body Weight and Body Composition

4. Which measurement would you choose to assess your fat levels? Why?

LO 3 Managing Your Weight

5. Are you satisfied with your body weight? If so, what do you do to maintain a healthy weight? If not, what are some lifestyle changes you could make to improve your weight and overall health?

ACCESS YOUR HEALTH ON THE INTERNET

Visit **MasteringHealth** for links to the websites and RSS feeds.

The following websites explore further topics and issues related to personal health.

Academy of Nutrition and Dietetics. This site includes recommended dietary guidelines and other current information about weight control. **www.eatright.org**

Weight Control Information Network. This is an excellent resource for diet and weight-control information. **http://win.niddk.nih.gov/index.htm**

The Rudd Center for Foods Policy and Obesity. This website provides excellent information on the latest in obesity research, public policy, and ways we can stop the obesity epidemic at the community level. **www.yaleruddcenter.org**

FOCUS ON

Enhancing Your Body Image

Dissatisfaction with one's appearance and shape is an all-too-common feeling in today's society that can foster unhealthy attitudes and thought patterns, as well as disordered eating and exercising behaviors.

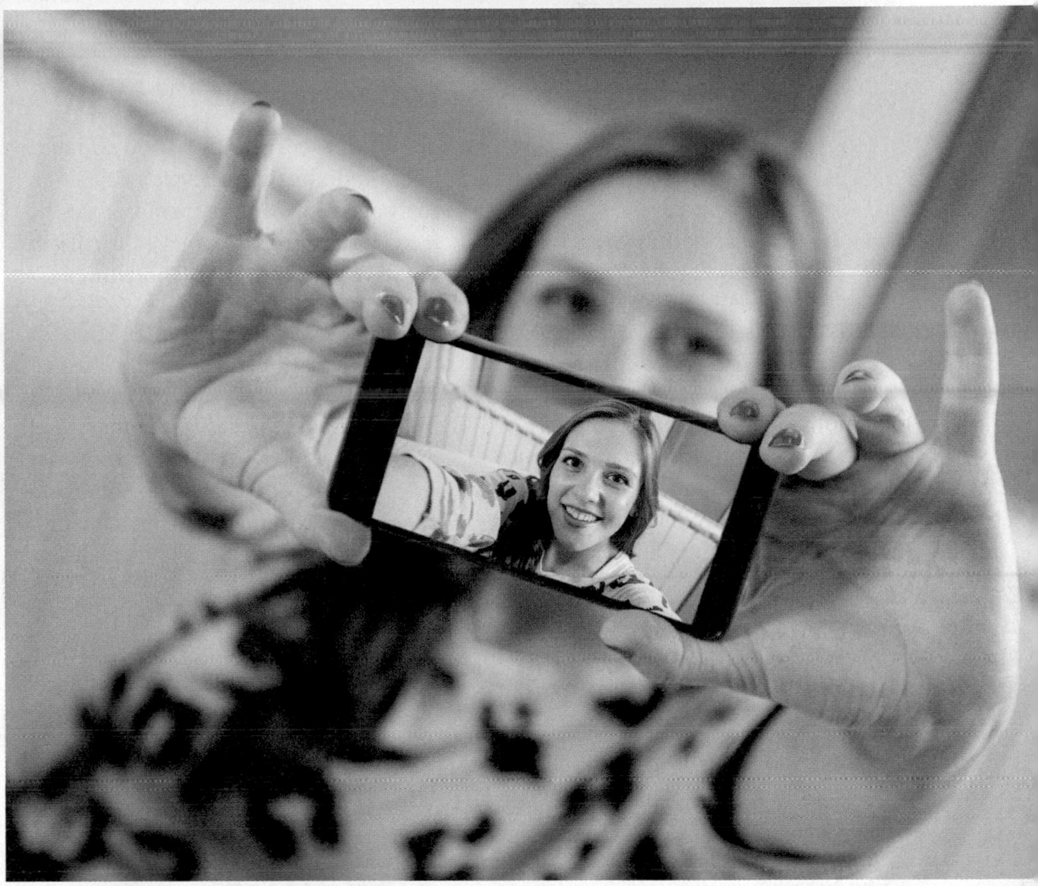

LEARNING OUTCOMES

1 Define body image, list the factors that influence it, and identify the difference between being dissatisfied with your appearance and body image disorders.

2 Describe the signs and symptoms of disordered eating, as well as the physical effects and treatment options for anorexia nervosa, bulimia nervosa, and binge-eating disorder.

3 List the criteria, symptoms, and treatment for exercise disorders such as muscle dysmorphia and female athlete triad.

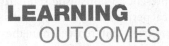

When you look in the mirror, do you like what you see? If you feel disappointed, frustrated, or even angry, you're not alone. Preoccupation with appearance and a distorted image of how we look is a major problem for a wide range of people. In a UK study, 93 percent of the women reported negative thoughts about their appearance during the past week and wanted to lose weight, even though the majority were in the underweight or normal weight ranges.[1] Concerns about weight seem to be central to many people's body dissatisfaction. As body mass increases, dissatisfaction increases, particularly during transitional periods in life, such as the transition from middle school to high school and from high school to adulthood. Females, in particular, seem to experience peak levels of body dissatisfaction during the transition from high school to young adulthood.[2] Tragically, being dissatisfied with your body can result in behaviors that disrupt your relationships, affect your mental health, and lead to life-threatening illness. Developing and maintaining a healthy body image can enhance your interactions with others, reduce stress, give you an increased sense of personal empowerment, and bring confidence and joy to your life.

80%

OF ADULT AMERICAN WOMEN REPORT **DISSATISFACTION** WITH THEIR APPEARANCE.

LO 1 | WHAT IS BODY IMAGE?

Define body image, list the factors that influence it, and identify the difference between being dissatisfied with your appearance and body image disorders.

Body image refers to what you believe or emotionally feel about your body's shape, weight, and general appearance. The term refers to more than what you see when you look in a mirror, including the following:

- How you see yourself in your mind
- What you believe about your own appearance (including your memories, assumptions, and generalizations)
- How you feel about your body, including your height, shape, and weight
- How you sense and control your body as you move

A *negative body image* is defined as either a distorted perception of your shape or feelings of discomfort, shame, or anxiety about your body. You may be convinced that only other people are attractive and that your own body is a sign of personal failure. In contrast, a *positive body image* is a true perception of your appearance: You see yourself as you really are. You understand that everyone is different, and you celebrate your uniqueness—including your perceived "flaws," which you know have nothing to do with your value as a person.[3]

Is your body image negative or positive—or somewhere in between? Researchers have developed a body image continuum that may help you decide (see **FIGURE 1**). Notice that the continuum identifies behaviors associated with particular states, from total dissociation with one's body to body not being an issue.

body image How you see yourself in your mind, what you believe about your appearance, and how you feel about your body.

Many Factors Influence Body Image

You're not born with a body image, but you do begin to develop one at an early age. Let's look more closely at the factors that probably played a role in the development of your body image.

The Media and Popular Culture

Images and celebrities in the media set the standard for what we find attractive, leading some people to go to dangerous extremes to have the biggest biceps or fit into size zero jeans. Most of us think of this obsession with appearance as a recent phenomenon. The truth is, it has long been part of American culture. During the early twentieth century, while men idolized the hearty outdoorsman President Teddy Roosevelt, women pulled their corsets ever tighter to achieve unrealistically tiny waists. In the 1920s and 1930s, men emulated the burly cops and robbers in gangster films, while women dieted and bound their breasts to achieve the boyish "flapper" look. By the 1960s, tough guys were the male ideal, whereas rail-thin supermodels embodied the nation's standard of female beauty. Today's societal obsession around appearance and idolizing thin celebrities such as Robert Pattinson and Keira Knightley isn't much different.

Most of the models you see in magazines and advertisements have been digitally altered to eliminate any perceived imperfection and very often to make them thinner. These pervasive images present an unrealistic standard of physical perfection that many adults, teens, and even children will nonetheless try to achieve.

SEE IT! VIDEOS
What does a "real" woman look like? Watch **A Real Look at Real Women** available on MasteringHealth.™

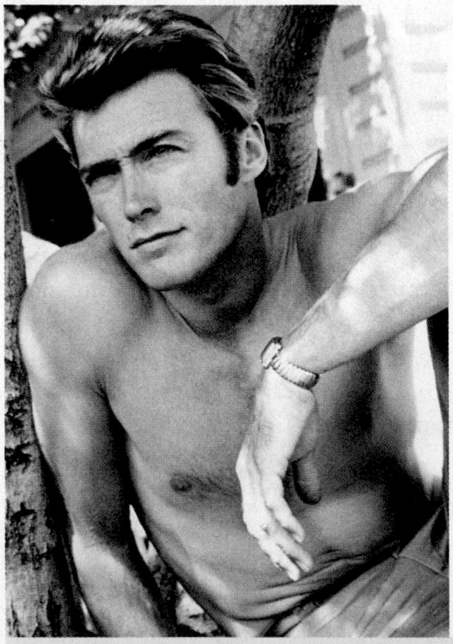

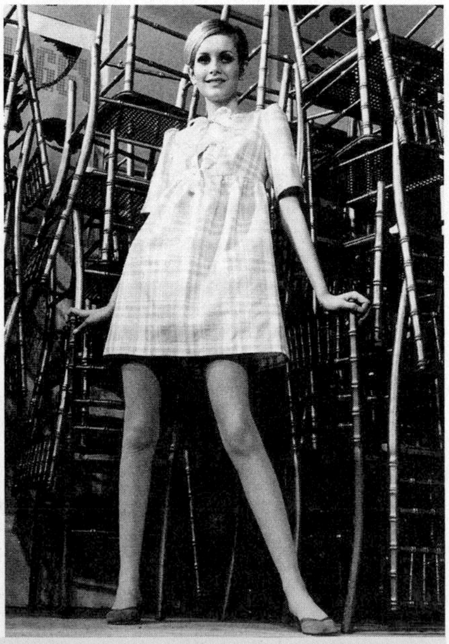

Although the exact nature of the "in" look may change from generation to generation, unrealistic images of both male and female celebrities are nothing new. For example, in the 1960s, images of brawny film stars such as Clint Eastwood and ultrathin models such as Twiggy dominated the media.

Body hate/ disassociation	Distorted body image	Body preoccupied/ obsessed	Body acceptance	Body is not an issue
I often feel separated and distant from my body—as if it belonged to someone else. I hate my body, and I often isolate myself from others. I don't see anything positive or even neutral about my body shape and size. I don't believe others when they tell me I look okay. I hate the way I look in the mirror.	I spend a significant amount of time exercising and dieting to change my body. My body shape and size keeps me from dating or finding someone who will treat me the way I want to be treated. I have considered changing (or have changed) my body shape and size through surgical means. I wish I could change the way I look in the mirror.	I weigh and measure myself a lot. I spend a significant amount of time viewing myself in the mirror. I compare my body to others. I have days when I feel fat. I accept society's ideal body shape and size as the best body shape and size. I'd be more attractive if I were thinner, more muscular, etc.	I pay attention to my body and my appearance because it is important to me, but it only occupies a small part of my day. I would like to change some things about my body, but I spend most of my time highlighting my positive features. My self-esteem is based on my personality traits, achievements, and relationships—not just my body image.	I feel fine about my body. I don't worry about changing my body shape or weight. I never weigh or measure myself. My feelings about my body are not influenced by society's concept of an ideal body shape. I know that the significant others in my life will always love me for who I am, not for how I look.

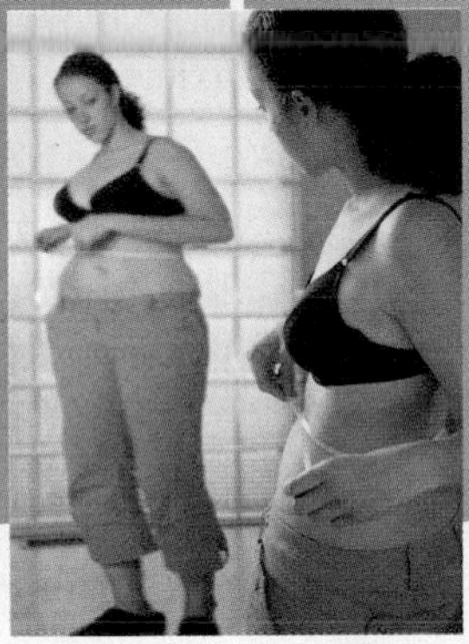

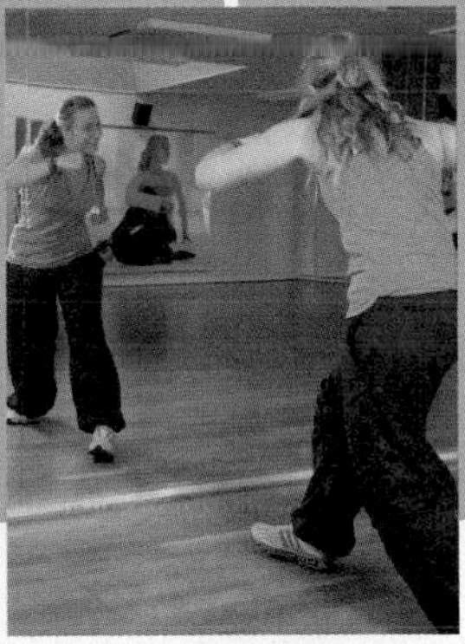

FIGURE 1 Body Image Continuum This continuum shows a range of attitudes and behaviors toward body image. Functioning at either extreme—not caring at all or being obsessed—leads to problems. When you are functioning in the "body acceptance" area, you are taking care of your body and emotions.

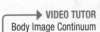

Source: Adapted from Smiley/King/Avery, "Eating Issues and Body Image Continuum," Campus Health Service 1996. Copyright © 1997 Arizona Board of Regents for University of Arizona.

VIDEO TUTOR
Body Image Continuum

The increase in popularity of social media has also increased concerns regarding negative body images.[4] Many social media sites actively warn against posts promoting or glorifying self-harm, but the message can still be hard to avoid and is often disguised as a type of encouragement—images of unrealistically thin bodies are coupled with catch phrases telling young people to get "thin," or avoid being "fat."[5]

Today, more than 69 percent of American adults 20 years and older are overweight or obese; thus, a significant disconnect exists between the media's idealized images of male and female bodies and the typical American body.[6] At the same time, the media are more pervasive than ever before, bombarding us with messages telling us that we just don't measure up. In fact, one study conducted with college women of multiple ethnicities found that female body dissatisfaction was attributed to perceptions of celebrity role models and Western culture's thin idealization.[7]

Family, Community, and Cultural Groups

The members of society with whom we most often interact—family, friends, and others—strongly influence the way we see ourselves. Parents are especially influential in body image development. For instance, it's common and natural for fathers of adolescent girls to experience feelings of discomfort related to their daughters' changing bodies. If they are able to navigate these feelings successfully and validate the acceptability of their daughters' appearance throughout puberty, it's likely that they'll help their daughters maintain a positive body image. In contrast, if they verbalize or indicate even subtle judgments about their daughters' changing bodies, girls may begin to question how members of the opposite sex view their bodies in general. In addition, mothers who model body acceptance or body ownership may be more likely to foster a similar positive body image in their daughters, whereas mothers who are frustrated with or ashamed of their own bodies may foster negative attitudes in their daughters.

Interactions with siblings and other relatives, peers, teachers, coworkers, and other community members can also influence body image development. For instance, peer harassment (teasing and bullying) is widely acknowledged to contribute to a negative body image. Associations within one's cultural group are also a factor. For example, studies have found that European American females experience the highest rates of body dissatisfaction, and as a minority group becomes more acculturated into the mainstream and exposed to media, the body dissatisfaction levels of women in that group increase.[8]

Body image also reflects the larger culture in which you live. In parts of Africa, for example, obesity has been associated with abundance, erotic desirability, and fertility. Girls in Mauritania traditionally were force-fed to increase their body size in order to signal a family's wealth, although the practice has recently become much less common.[9]

Physiological and Psychological Factors

Recent neurological research suggests that people who have been diagnosed with a body image disorder show differences in the brain's ability to regulate chemicals called *neurotransmitters,* which are linked to mood.[10] Poor regulation of neurotransmitters is also involved in depression and in anxiety disorders, including obsessive-compulsive disorder. One study linked distortions in body image, particularly the face, to a malfunction in the brain's visual processing region that was revealed by magnetic resonance imaging (MRI) scanning.[11]

How Can I Build a More Positive Body Image?

If you want to develop a more positive body image, your first step might be to challenge some commonly held myths and attitudes in contemporary society.[12]

Myth 1: How you look is more important than who you are. Do you think your weight is important in defining who you are? How much does it matter to you to have friends who are thin and attractive? How important do you think being thin is in trying to attract your ideal partner?

Myth 2: Anyone can be slender and attractive if they work at it. When you see someone who is extremely thin, what assumptions do you make about that person? When you see someone who is overweight or obese, what assumptions do you make? Have you ever berated yourself for not having the "willpower" to change some aspect of your body?

Myth 3: Extreme dieting is an effective weight-loss strategy. Do you believe in trying fad diets or "quick-weight-loss" products? How far would you be willing to go to attain the "perfect" body?

Myth 4: Appearance is more important than health. How do you evaluate whether a person is healthy? Do you believe it's possible for overweight people to be healthy? Is your desire to change some aspect of your body motivated by health reasons or by concerns about appearance?

To learn ways to bust these toxic myths and attitudes and to build a more positive body image, check out the **Skills for Behavior Change** box.

Some People Develop Body Image Disorders

Although most Americans are dissatisfied with some aspect of their appearance, very few have a true body image disorder. However, several diagnosable body image disorders affect a small percentage of the population. Two of the most common are body dysmorphic disorder and social physique anxiety.

Body Dysmorphic Disorder

Approximately 1 percent of people in the United States suffer from **body dysmorphic disorder (BDD).**[13] Persons with BDD are obsessively concerned with their appearance and have a distorted view of their own body shape,

body dysmorphic disorder (BDD) Psychological disorder characterized by an obsession with one's appearance and a distorted view of one's body or with a minor or imagined flaw in appearance.

DID YOU **KNOW?**

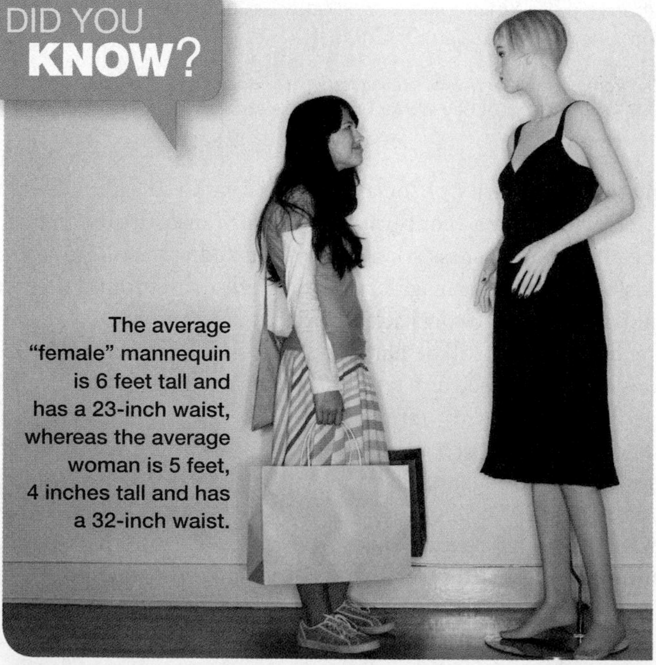

The average "female" mannequin is 6 feet tall and has a 23-inch waist, whereas the average woman is 5 feet, 4 inches tall and has a 32-inch waist.

Source: R. Duyff, American Dietetic Association Complete Food and Nutrition Guide, 4th ed. (Hoboken, NJ: John Wiley & Sons, Inc., 2012), 50; C. Fryar, Q. Gu, and C. Ogden, "Anthropometric Reference Data for Children and Adults: United States, 2007–2010," National Center for Health Statistics. *Vital and Health Statistics*, Series 11, no. 252 (2012), www.cdc.gov/nchs/data/series/sr_11/sr11_252.pdf.

SKILLS FOR BEHAVIOR CHANGE

TEN STEPS TO A POSITIVE BODY IMAGE

How do you turn negative thoughts positive? One way is to think about new ways to look more healthfully and happily at yourself and your body. The more you do that, the better you will feel about who you are and the body you naturally have.

- **Step 1.** Appreciate all that your body can do. Every day your body carries you closer to your dreams. Celebrate all of the amazing things your body does for you—running, dancing, breathing, laughing, dreaming.
- **Step 2.** Make a list of things you like about yourself—things that aren't related to how much you weigh or how you look. Read your list often. Add to it as you become aware of more things to like about yourself.
- **Step 3.** Remind yourself that true beauty is not skin deep. When you feel good about yourself and who you are, you carry yourself with a sense of confidence, self-acceptance, and openness that makes you beautiful. Beauty is a state of mind, not a state of body.
- **Step 4.** Look at yourself as a whole person. When you see yourself in a mirror or in your mind, choose not to focus on specific body parts. See yourself as others see you—as a whole person.
- **Step 5.** Surround yourself with positive people. It is easier to feel good about yourself when you are around others who are supportive and who recognize the importance of liking yourself as you naturally are.
- **Step 6.** Shut down those voices in your head that tell you your body is not "right" or that you are a "bad" person. You can overpower those negative thoughts with positive ones.
- **Step 7.** Wear comfortable clothes that make you feel good about your body. Work with your body, not against it.
- **Step 8.** Become a critical viewer of social and media messages. Pay attention to images, slogans, and attitudes that make you feel bad about your appearance. Protest these messages: Write a letter to the advertiser. Talk back to the image or message.
- **Step 9.** Do something nice for yourself—something that lets your body know you appreciate it. Take a bubble bath, make time for a nap, or find a peaceful place outside to relax.
- **Step 10.** Use the time and energy that you might have spent worrying about food, calories, and your weight to do something to help others. Reaching out to other people can help you feel better about yourself and make a positive change in our world.

Source: "10 Steps to Positive Body Image," from National Eating Disorders Association website, April 22, 2013. Copyright © 2013 National Eating Disorders Association. Reprinted with permission. For more information visit www.NationalEatingDisorders.org or call NEDA's helpline 1-800-931-2237.

size, weight, perceived lack of muscles, facial blemishes, size of body parts, etc. Although the cause of the disorder isn't known, an anxiety disorder such as obsessive-compulsive disorder is often present as well. (Anxiety disorders are discussed in **Chapter 2**.) Contributing factors may include genetic susceptibility, childhood teasing, physical or sexual abuse, low self-esteem, and rigid sociocultural expectations of beauty.[14]

People with BDD may try to fix their perceived flaws through abuse of steroids, excessive bodybuilding, repeated cosmetic surgeries, extreme tattooing, or other appearance-altering behaviors. It is estimated that 10 percent of people seeking dermatology or cosmetic treatments have BDD.[15] Not only do such actions fail to address the underlying problem, but they are also actually considered diagnostic signs of BDD. Psychiatric treatment, including psychotherapy and/or antidepressant medications, is often successful.

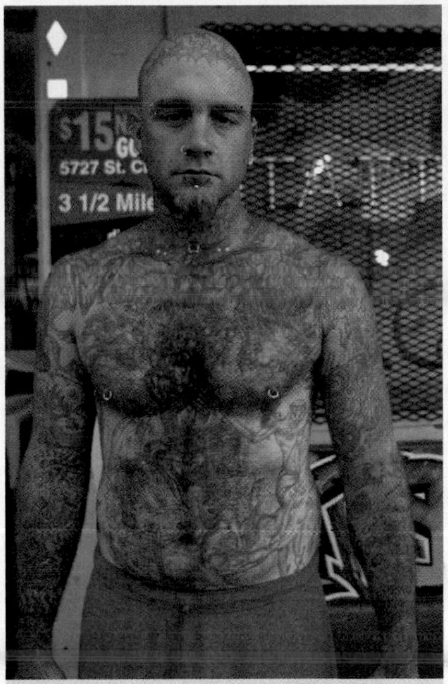

It's not always easy to spot people who are highly dissatisfied with their bodies, as they don't necessarily stick out in a crowd. For instance, people who cover their bodies with tattoos may have a strong sense of self-esteem. On the other hand, extreme tattooing can be an outward sign of a severe body image disturbance known as body dysmorphic disorder.

Social Physique Anxiety

An emerging problem, seen in both young men and women, is **social physique anxiety (SPA).** The desire to "look good" becomes so strong that it has a destructive and sometimes disabling effect on the person's ability to function effectively in relationships and interactions with others. People

social physique anxiety (SPA) A desire to look good that has a destructive effect on a person's ability to function well in social interactions and relationships.

suffering from SPA spend a disproportionate amount of time fixating on their bodies, working out, and performing tasks that are ego centered and self-directed, rather than focusing on interpersonal relationships and general tasks.[16] Experts speculate that this anxiety may contribute to disordered eating (discussed next).

disordered eating A pattern of atypical eating behaviors that is used to achieve or maintain a lower body weight.

LO 2 | WHAT IS DISORDERED EATING?

Describe the signs and symptoms of disordered eating, as well as the physical effects and treatment options for anorexia nervosa, bulimia nervosa, and binge-eating disorder.

People with a negative body image can fixate on a wide range of self-perceived "flaws." The "flaw" that distresses the majority of people with negative body image is feeling overweight.

Some people channel their anxiety about their weight into self-defeating thoughts and harmful behaviors. Check out the eating issues continuum in **FIGURE 2**: The far left identifies a pattern of thoughts and behaviors associated with **disordered eating.** These behaviors can include chronic dieting, rigid eating patterns, abusing diet pills and laxatives, self-induced vomiting, and many others.

Eating disordered	Disruptive eating patterns	Food preoccupied/ obsessed	Concerned in a healthy way	Food is not an issue
I worry about what I will eat or when I will exercise all the time. I follow a very rigid eating plan and know precisely how many calories, fat grams, or carbohydrates I eat every day. I feel incredible guilt, shame, and anxiety when I break my diet. I regularly stuff myself and then exercise, vomit, or use laxatives to get rid of the food. My friends and family tell me I am too thin, but I feel fat. I am out of control when I eat. I am afraid to eat in front of others. I prefer to eat alone.	My food and exercise concerns are starting to interfere with my school and social life. I use food to comfort myself. I have tried diet pills, laxatives, vomiting, or extra time exercising in order to lose or maintain my weight. I have fasted or avoided eating for long periods of time in order to lose or maintain my weight. If I cannot exercise to burn off calories, I panic. I feel strong when I can restrict how much I eat. I feel out of control when I eat more than I wanted to.	I think about food a lot. I'm obsessed with reading books and magazines about dieting, fitness, and weight control. I sometimes miss school, work, and social events because of my diet or exercise schedule. I divide food into "good" and "bad" categories. I feel guilty when I eat "bad" foods or when I eat more than what I feel I should be eating. I am afraid of getting fat. I wish I could change how much I want to eat and what I am hungry for.	I pay attention to what I eat in order to maintain a healthy body. Food and exercise are important parts of my life, but they only occupy a small part of my time. I enjoy eating, and I balance my pleasure with my concern for a healthy body. I usually eat three balanced meals daily, plus snacks, to fuel my body with adequate energy. I am moderate and flexible in my goals for eating well and being physically active. Sometimes I eat more (or less) than I really need, but most of the time I listen to my body.	I am not concerned about what or how much I eat. I feel no guilt or shame no matter what I eat or how much I eat. Exercise is not really important to me. I choose foods based on cost, taste, and convenience, with little regard to health. My eating is very sporadic and irregular. I don't worry about meals; I just eat whatever I can, whenever I can. I enjoy stuffing myself with lots of tasty food at restaurants, holiday meals, and social events.

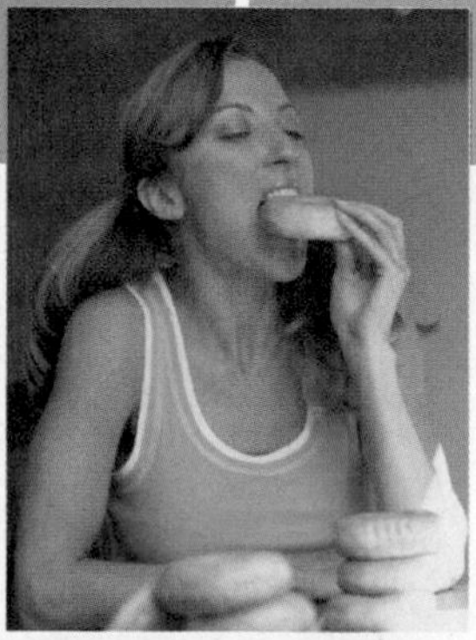

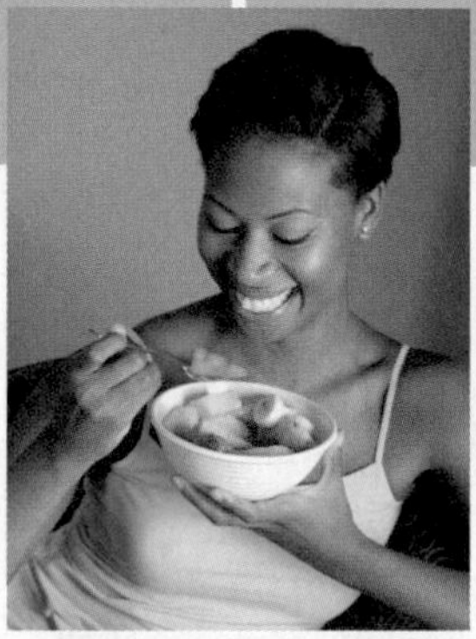

FIGURE 2 Eating Issues Continuum This continuum shows progression from eating disorders to normal eating. Being concerned in a healthy way is the goal, rather than functioning at either extreme.

Source: Adapted from Smiley/King/Avery, "Eating Issues and Body Image Continuum," Campus Health Service 1996. Copyright © 1997 Arizona Board of Regents for University of Arizona.

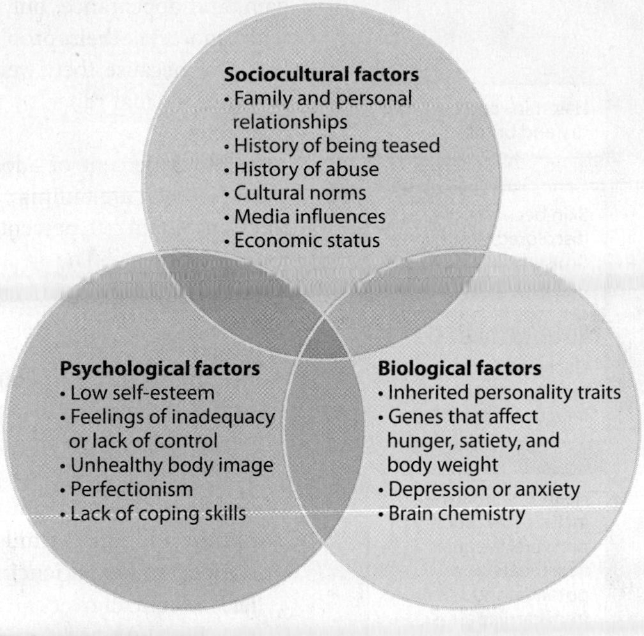

Sociocultural factors
• Family and personal relationships
• History of being teased
• History of abuse
• Cultural norms
• Media influences
• Economic status
Psychological factors
• Low self-esteem
• Feelings of inadequacy or lack of control
• Unhealthy body image
• Perfectionism
• Lack of coping skills
Biological factors
• Inherited personality traits
• Genes that affect hunger, satiety, and body weight
• Depression or anxiety
• Brain chemistry

FIGURE 3 Factors That Contribute to Eating Disorders

eating disorder A psychiatric disorder characterized by severe disturbances in body image and eating behaviors.

anorexia nervosa Eating disorder characterized by deliberate food restriction, self-starvation, or extreme exercising to achieve weight loss, and an extremely distorted body image.

Some People Develop Eating Disorders

Only some people who exhibit disordered eating patterns progress to a clinical **eating disorder.** The diagnosis of an eating disorder can be applied only by a physician to a patient who exhibits severe disturbances in thoughts, behavior, and body functioning—disturbances that can prove fatal. The eating disorders defined by the American Psychiatric Association (APA) in the *Diagnostic and Statistical Manual of Mental Disorders, Fifth Edition* (*DSM-5*) are *anorexia nervosa, bulimia nervosa, binge-eating disorder,* and a cluster of less distinct conditions collectively referred to as Other Specified Feeding or Eating Disorder (OSFED).[17]

At any given time, 10 percent or more of late adolescent and adult women in the United States report symptoms of eating disorders.[18] Although anorexia nervosa and bulimia nervosa used to affect people primarily in their teens and twenties, increasing numbers of children as young as 7 have been diagnosed, as have women as old as 80.[19] In 2013, 2.2 percent of college students reported that they were dealing with either anorexia or bulimia.[20] Disordered eating and eating disorders are also common among ballet dancers and athletes, particularly athletes in sports with an aesthetic component (e.g., figure skating or gymnastics) or are tied to a weight class (e.g., tae kwon do, judo, or wrestling).[21]

Eating disorders are on the rise among men, who currently represent up to 25 percent of anorexia and bulimia patients.[22] Many men suffering from eating disorders fail to seek treatment.

What factors put individuals at risk? Many people with eating disorders feel disenfranchised in other aspects of their lives and try to gain a sense of control through food. Many are clinically depressed, suffer from obsessive-compulsive disorder, or have other psychiatric problems. In addition, individuals with low self-esteem, negative body image, and a high tendency for perfectionism are at risk.[23] **FIGURE 3** shows how individual and social factors can interact to increase the risk of an eating disorder.

Anorexia Nervosa

Anorexia nervosa is a persistent, chronic eating disorder characterized by deliberate food restriction and severe, life-threatening weight loss. It involves self-starvation motivated by an intense fear of gaining weight and an extremely distorted body image. Initially, most people with anorexia nervosa lose weight by reducing total food intake, particularly of high-calorie foods. Eventually, they progress to restricting their intake of almost all foods. The little they do eat, they may purge through vomiting or using laxatives. Although they lose weight, people with anorexia nervosa never feel thin enough.

An estimated 0.3 percent of females suffer from anorexia nervosa in their lifetime.[24] The *DSM-5* criteria for anorexia nervosa are as follows:[25]

- Refusal to maintain body weight at or above a minimally normal weight for age and height
- Intense fear of gaining weight or becoming fat, even though considered underweight by all medical criteria

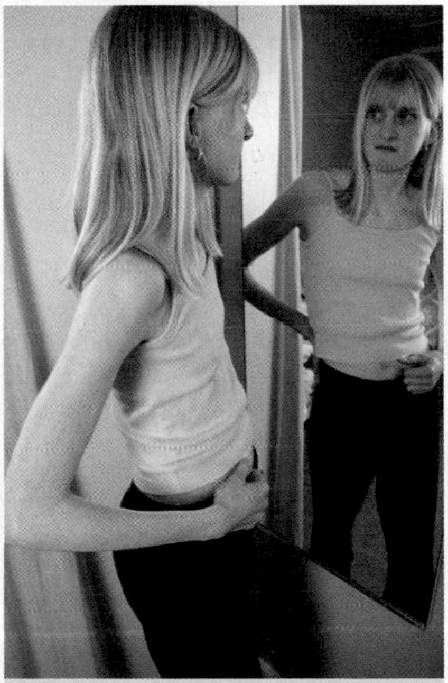

People with anorexia nervosa put themselves at risk of starving to death. In addition, people with anorexia nervosa or bulimia nervosa may die from sudden cardiac arrest caused by electrolyte imbalances. About 20 percent of people with a serious eating disorder die from it.

Source: National Eating Disorders Association, "Anorexia Nervosa," www.nationaleatingdisorders.org/anorexia-nervosa.

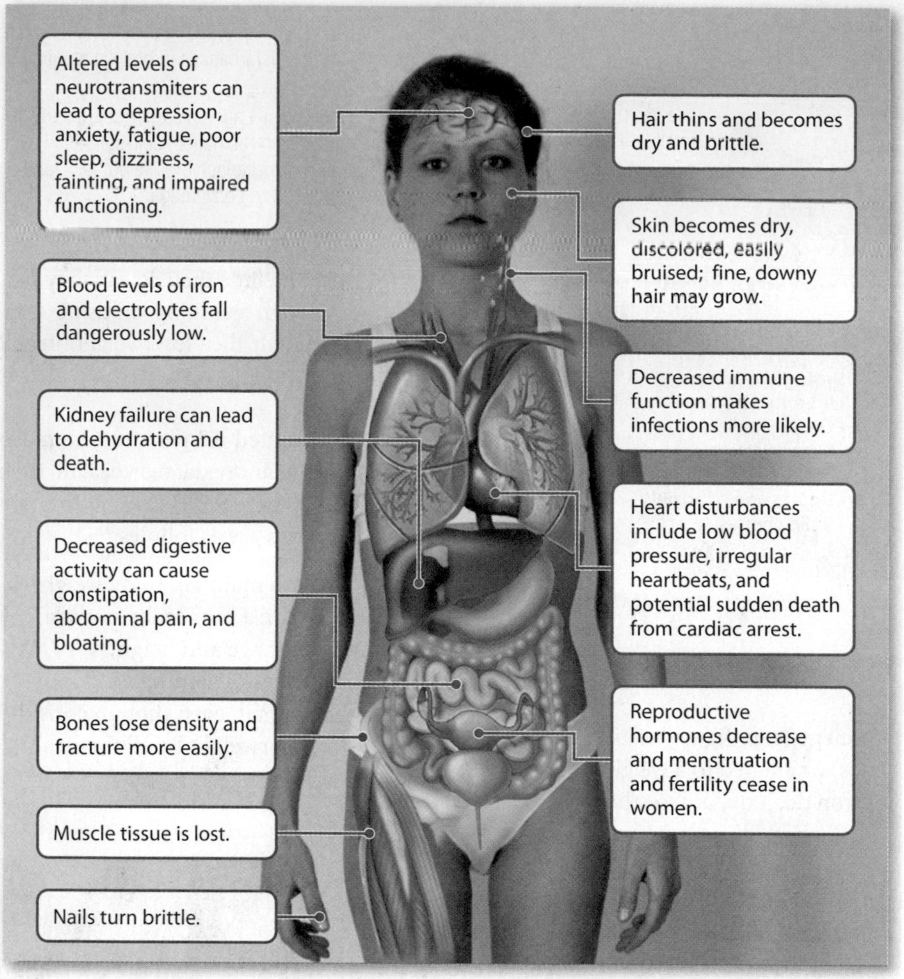

Altered levels of neurotransmiters can lead to depression, anxiety, fatigue, poor sleep, dizziness, fainting, and impaired functioning.
Blood levels of iron and electrolytes fall dangerously low.
Kidney failure can lead to dehydration and death.
Decreased digestive activity can cause constipation, abdominal pain, and bloating.
Bones lose density and fracture more easily.
Muscle tissue is lost.
Nails turn brittle.
Hair thins and becomes dry and brittle.
Skin becomes dry, discolored, easily bruised; fine, downy hair may grow.
Decreased immune function makes infections more likely.
Heart disturbances include low blood pressure, irregular heartbeats, and potential sudden death from cardiac arrest.
Reproductive hormones decrease and menstruation and fertility cease in women.

FIGURE 4 What Anorexia Nervosa Can Do to the Body

- Disturbance in the way in which one's body weight or shape is experienced, undue influence of body weight or shape on self-evaluation, or denial of the seriousness of the current low body weight

FIGURE 4 illustrates physical symptoms and negative health consequences associated with anorexia nervosa. Because it involves starvation and can lead to heart attacks and seizures, anorexia nervosa has the highest death rate (20%) of any psychological illness.[26] The causes of anorexia nervosa are complex and variable. Many people with anorexia have other coexisting psychiatric problems, including low self-esteem, depression, an anxiety disorder such as obsessive-compulsive disorder, and substance abuse. Some people have a history of being physically or sexually abused, and others have troubled interpersonal relationships with family members. Cultural norms that value appearance and glorify thinness as beauty are, of course, a factor, as are weight-based shame and peer comparisons and weight bias.[27] Physical factors are thought to include an imbalance of neurotransmitters and genetic susceptibility.[28]

bulimia nervosa Eating disorder characterized by binge eating followed by inappropriate purging measures or compensatory behavior, such as vomiting or excessive exercise, to prevent weight gain.

Bulimia Nervosa

Individuals with **bulimia nervosa** often binge on huge amounts of food and then engage in some kind of purging, or "compensatory behavior," such as vomiting, taking laxatives, or exercising excessively, to lose the calories they have just consumed. People with bulimia are obsessed with their bodies, weight gain, and appearance, but unlike those with anorexia, their problem is often "hidden" because their weight may fall within a normal range or they may be overweight.

Up to 3 percent of adolescents and young women are bulimic; rates among men are about 10 percent of the rate among women.[29] The *DSM-5* diagnostic criteria for bulimia nervosa are as follows:[30]

- Recurrent episodes of binge eating (defined as eating, in a discrete period of time, an amount of food that is larger than most people would eat during a similar period of time and under similar circumstances, and experiencing a sense of lack of control over eating during the episode)
- Recurrent inappropriate compensatory behavior to prevent weight gain, such as self-induced vomiting; misusing laxatives, diuretics, or other medications; fasting; or excessive exercise
- Binge eating and inappropriate compensatory behavior occurs on average at least once a week for 3 months
- Body shape and weight unduly influence self-evaluation

FIGURE 5 illustrates the physical symptoms and negative health consequences associated with bulimia nervosa. One of the more common symptoms is tooth erosion, which results from excessive vomiting. Bulimics who vomit are also at risk for electrolyte imbalances and dehydration, both of which can contribute to a heart attack and sudden death.

A combination of genetic and environmental factors is thought to cause bulimia nervosa.[31] A family history of obesity, an underlying anxiety disorder, and an imbalance in neurotransmitters are all possible contributing factors. In support of the role of neurotransmitters, a study showed that brain circuitry involved in regulating impulsive behavior seems to be less active in women with bulimia than in healthy women.[32] However, it is unknown whether such differences exist before bulimia develops or arise as a consequence of the disorder.

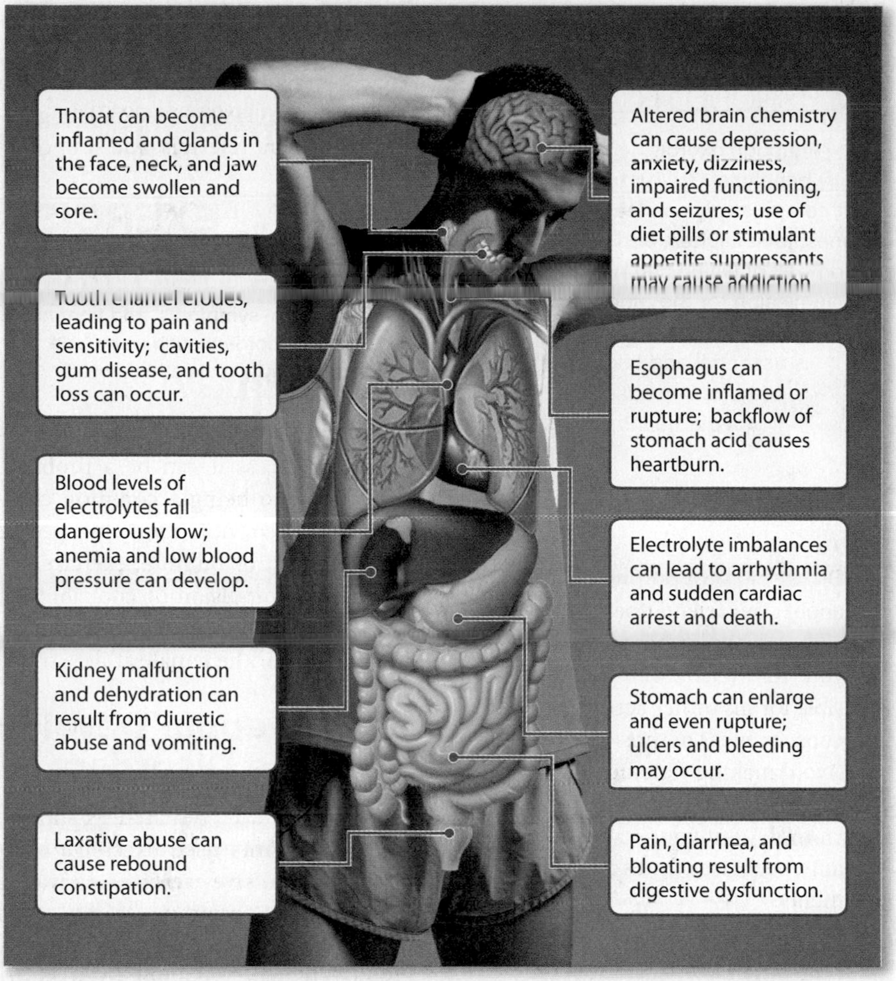

Throat can become inflamed and glands in the face, neck, and jaw become swollen and sore.
Tooth enamel erodes, leading to pain and sensitivity; cavities, gum disease, and tooth loss can occur.
Blood levels of electrolytes fall dangerously low; anemia and low blood pressure can develop.
Kidney malfunction and dehydration can result from diuretic abuse and vomiting.
Laxative abuse can cause rebound constipation.
Altered brain chemistry can cause depression, anxiety, dizziness, impaired functioning, and seizures; use of diet pills or stimulant appetite suppressants may cause addiction
Esophagus can become inflamed or rupture; backflow of stomach acid causes heartburn.
Electrolyte imbalances can lead to arrhythmia and sudden cardiac arrest and death.
Stomach can enlarge and even rupture; ulcers and bleeding may occur.
Pain, diarrhea, and bloating result from digestive dysfunction.

FIGURE 5 What Bulimia Nervosa Can Do to the Body

Binge-Eating Disorder

Individuals with **binge-eating disorder** gorge like their bulimic counterparts but do not take excessive measures to lose the weight that they gain. Thus, they are often clinically obese. Binge-eating episodes are typically characterized by eating large amounts of food rapidly, even when not feeling hungry, and feeling guilty or depressed after overeating.[33]

A national survey reported a lifetime prevalence of binge-eating disorder in the study participants of 1.4 percent.[34] The *DSM-5* criteria for binge-eating disorder are as follows:[35]

- Recurrent episodes of binge eating (defined as eating, in a discrete period of time, an amount of food that is larger than most people would eat during a similar period of time and under similar circumstances, and experiencing a sense of lack of control over eating during the episode)
- Binge-eating episodes are associated with three (or more) of the following: (1) eating much more rapidly than normal; (2) eating until feeling uncomfortably full; (3) eating large amounts of food when not feeling physically hungry; (4) eating alone because of embarrassment over how much one is eating; (5) feeling disgusted with oneself, depressed, or guilty after overeating.
- Experiencing marked distress regarding binge eating
- The binge eating occurs, on average, at least once a week for 3 months.
- The binge eating is not associated with the recurrent use of inappropriate compensatory behavior (e.g., purging) and does not occur exclusively during the course of bulimia nervosa or anorexia nervosa.

binge-eating disorder A type of eating disorder characterized by gorging on food once a week or more, but not typically followed by a purge.

other specified feeding or eating disorder (OSFED) Eating disorders that are a true psychiatric illness but that do not fit the strict diagnostic criteria for anorexia nervosa, bulimia nervosa, or binge-eating disorder.

Other Specified Feeding or Eating Disorder

The APA recognizes that some patterns of disordered eating qualify as a legitimate psychiatric illness but don't fit into the strict diagnostic criteria for anorexia, bulimia, or binge-eating disorder. Called **other specified feeding or eating disorders (OSFED),** this group of disorders includes five specific subtypes: night eating syndrome, purging disorder, binge-eating disorder of low frequency/limited duration, bulimia nervosa of low frequency/duration, and atypical anorexia nervosa. Atypical anorexia nervosa is defined in this category as displaying anorexic features without low weight.[36] All of these subtypes can cause remarkable distress or impairment but don't exhibit the full criteria of another feeding or eating disorder.

Treatment for Eating Disorders

Because eating disorders are caused by a combination of many factors, there are no simple solutions. Without treatment, approximately 20 percent of people with a serious eating disorder will die from it; with treatment, long-term full recovery rates range from 44 to 76 percent for anorexia nervosa and from 50 to 70 percent for bulimia nervosa.[37]

Treatment often focuses first on reducing the threat to life. Once the patient is stabilized, long-term therapy

WHAT DO YOU THINK?

Is attention to the national obesity epidemic likely to worsen problems with eating disorders? Why or why not?

- What do you think can be done to increase awareness of eating disorders in the United States?
- Can you think of ways to prevent eating disorders?

compulsive exercise Disorder characterized by a compulsion to engage in excessive amounts of exercise and feelings of guilt and anxiety if the level of exercise is perceived as inadequate.

focuses on the psychological, social, environmental, and physiological factors that have led to the problem. Through therapy, the patient works on adopting new eating behaviors, building self-confidence, and finding other ways to deal with life's problems. Support groups can help the family and the individual learn positive actions and interactions. Treatment of an underlying anxiety disorder or depression may also be a focus.

WHY SHOULD I CARE?

Although exercising is generally beneficial to your health, doing it compulsively can lead to broken bones, joint injuries, and even depression—all of which can put you out of commission for the other things you enjoy. Remember that moderation is essential and taking rest days is important to your health.

How Can You Help Someone with Disordered Eating?

Although every situation is different, there are several things you can do if you suspect someone you know is struggling with disordered eating:[38]

- **Learn** as much as you can about disordered eating through books, articles, brochures, and trustworthy websites.
- **Know the facts** about weight, nutrition, and exercise. Being armed with accurate information can help you reason against excuses used to maintain a disordered eating pattern.
- **Be honest.** Talk openly and honestly about your concerns.
- **Be caring, but be firm.** Caring about your friend does not mean allowing him or her to manipulate you. Your friend must be responsible for his or her actions and the consequences of those actions. Avoid making statements that you cannot or will not uphold.
- **Compliment** your friend's personality, successes, and accomplishments.
- **Be a good role model** for healthy eating, exercise, and self-acceptance.
- **Tell someone.** Don't wait until the situation is so severe that your friend's life is in danger. Addressing disordered eating patterns in their beginning stages offers your friend the best chance for working through these issues and becoming healthy again.

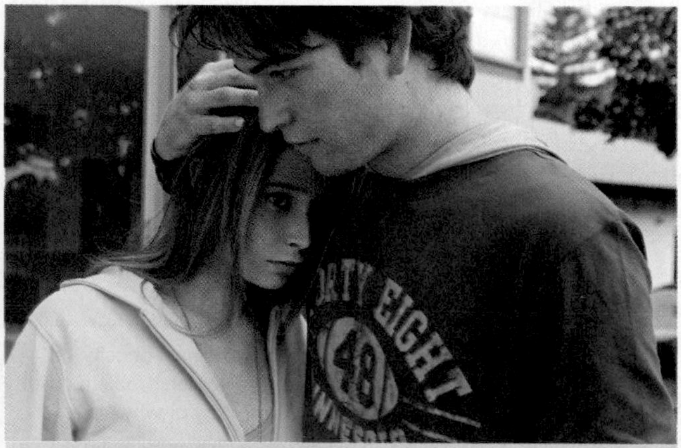

When talking to a friend about an eating disorder or disordered eating patterns, avoid casting blame, preaching, or offering unsolicited advice. Instead, be a good listener, let the person know that you care, and offer your support.

There are many resources for people who are considering seeking help or finding out if they are at risk for developing an eating disorder. The National Eating Disorders Association has a general online screening tool allowing individuals to assess their own patterns to determine if they should seek professional help, which is found at www.nationaleatingdisorders.org/online-eating-disorder-screening. They also have additional information and a Helpline (1-800-931-2237) for guidance, treatment referrals, and support.[39]

LO 3 | CAN EXERCISE BE UNHEALTHY?

List the criteria, symptoms, and treatment for exercise disorders such as muscle dysmorphia and female athlete triad.

Although exercise is generally beneficial, in excess it can be a problem. In addition to being a common compensatory behavior used by people with anorexia or bulimia, exercise can become a compulsion or contribute to more complex disorders such as muscle dysmorphia or the female athlete triad.

Some People Develop Exercise Disorders

In a recent study, researchers showed that participants used excessive exercise or **compulsive exercise** as a way to regulate their emotions.[40] Also called *anorexia athletica,* compulsive exercise is characterized not by a *desire* to exercise but a *compulsion* to do so; that is, the person struggles with guilt and anxiety if he or she doesn't work

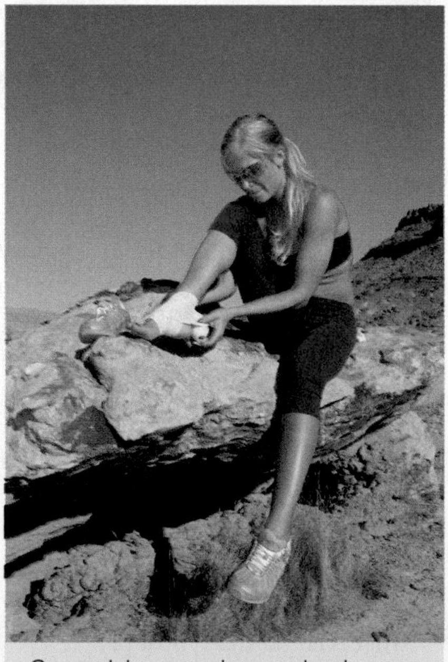

Compulsive exercise can lead to injuries and cause social and academic problems.

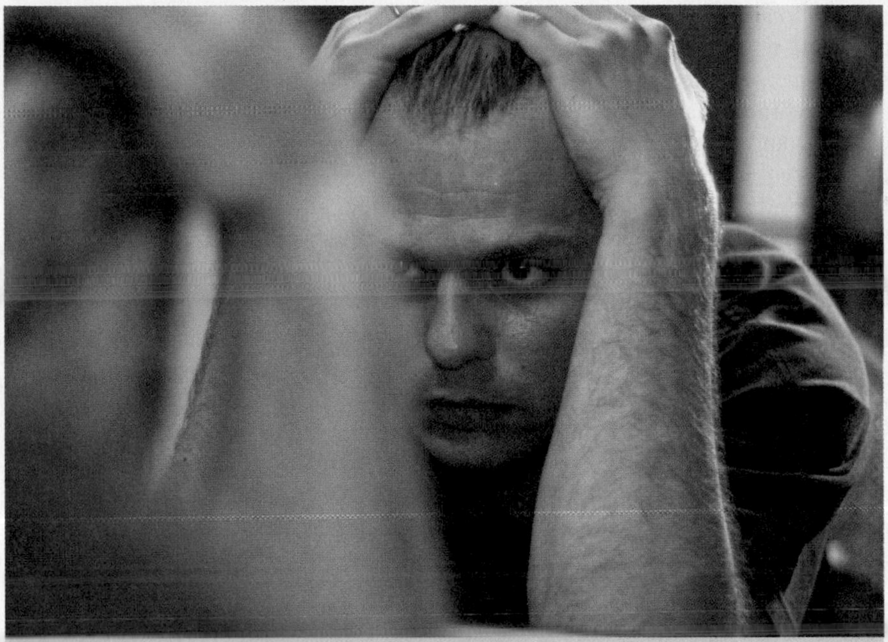

Men with muscle dysmorphia may have unusually muscular bodies but suffer from very low self-esteem.

out. Compulsive exercisers, like people with eating disorders, often define their self-worth externally. They over-exercise in order to feel more in control of their lives. Disordered eating or an eating disorder is often part of the picture.

Compulsive exercise can contribute to a variety of other injuries. It can also put significant stress on the heart, especially if combined with disordered eating. Psychologically, people who engage in compulsive exercise are often plagued by anxiety and/or depression. Their social life and academic success can suffer as they fixate more and more on exercise.

Muscle Dysmorphia

Muscle dysmorphia is a form of body image disturbance and exercise disorder in which a man believes that his body is insufficiently lean or muscular.[41] Men with muscle dysmorphia believe that they look "puny," when in reality they look normal or even unusually muscular. As a result of their adherence to a meticulous diet and time-consuming workout schedule, and their shame over their perceived appearance flaws, they may neglect important social or occupational activities.

Other behaviors characteristic of muscle dysmorphia include comparing oneself unfavorably to others, checking one's appearance in the mirror, and camouflaging one's appearance. Men with muscle dysmorphia also are likely to abuse anabolic steroids and dietary supplements.[42]

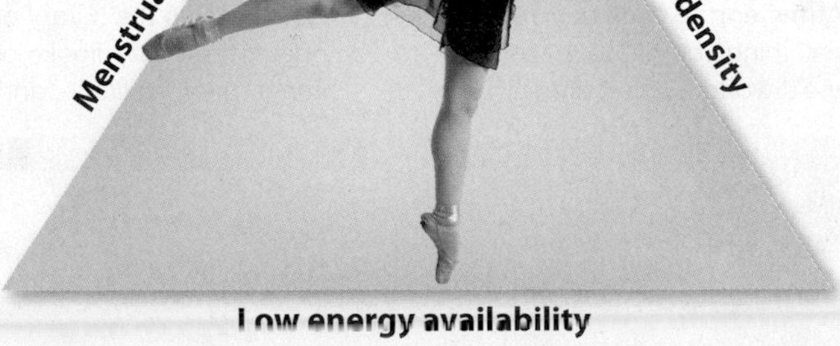

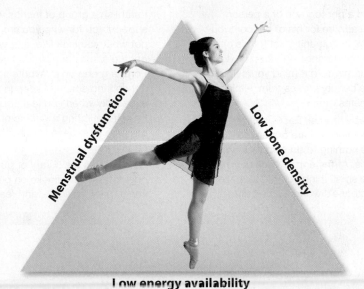

FIGURE 6 The Female Athlete Triad The female athlete triad is a cluster of three interrelated health problems.

SEE IT! VIDEOS

Can you go too far with extreme exercise? Watch **Young Boys Exercising to Extremes** available on MasteringHealth.™

The Female Athlete Triad

Female athletes in competitive sports often strive for perfection. In an effort to be the best, they may do more damage than good and put themselves at risk for a syndrome called the **female athlete triad** (see **FIGURE 6**). *Triad* means "three," and there are three interrelated problems:[43]

- Low energy intake, typically prompted by disordered eating behaviors
- Menstrual dysfunction, such as amenorrhea
- Poor bone density

How does the female athlete triad develop, and what makes it so dangerous? First, a chronic pattern of low energy (food) intake and intensive exercise alters normal body functions. For example, when an athlete restricts her eating, she can deplete her body stores of nutrients essential to health. At the same time, her body begins to burn its stores of

muscle dysmorphia Body image disorder in which men believe that their bodies are insufficiently lean or muscular.

female athlete triad A syndrome of three interrelated health problems seen in some female athletes: disordered eating, amenorrhea, and poor bone density.

1 MILLION

AMERICAN **MALES** ARE ESTIMATED TO STRUGGLE WITH SOME FORM OF EATING DISORDER.

fat tissue for energy. Adequate body fat is essential to maintaining healthy levels of the female reproductive hormone *estrogen*; when an athlete isn't getting enough food, estrogen levels decline. This can manifest as amenorrhea: The body is using all calories to keep the athlete alive, and nonessential body functions such as menstruation cease.

In addition, fat-soluble vitamins, calcium, and estrogen are all essential for dense, healthy bones, so their depletion weakens the athlete's bones, leaving her at high risk for fracture.

The female athlete triad is particularly prevalent in women who participate in highly competitive individual sports or activities that emphasize leanness and require body-contouring clothing. Gymnasts, figure skaters, cross-country runners, and ballet dancers are among those at highest risk for the female athlete triad.

Warning signs of the female athlete triad include dry skin; light-headedness/fainting; lanugo (fine, downy hair covering the body); multiple injuries; and muscle cramps, weakness, and fatigue.[44] Behaviors associated with the female athlete triad include preoccupation with food and weight, compulsive exercise, use and abuse of weight-loss products or laxatives, decreased ability to concentrate, self-criticism, anxiety, and depression. Treatment can be challenging, and it requires a multidisciplinary approach involving the athlete's coach and trainer, a sports medicine team, a psychologist, and other professionals, as well as family members and friends.

ASSESS **YOURSELF**

Could you be suffering from an eating or exercise disorder? Take the **Are Your Efforts to Be Thin Sensible?** assessment available on MasteringHealth.™

Need help creating a plan? Follow the strategies in the **Your Plan for Change** box for short- and long-term improvements to your health.

YOUR PLAN FOR **CHANGE**

The **ASSESS YOURSELF** activity gives you a chance to evaluate your feelings about your body and determine whether you might be engaging in eating or exercise behaviors that could undermine your health and happiness. Below are some steps you can take to improve your body image, starting today.

TODAY, YOU CAN:

- ☐ Talk back to the media. Write letters to advertisers and magazines that depict unhealthy and unrealistic body types. Boycott their products or start a blog commenting on harmful body image messages in the media.
- ☐ Just for today, eat the recommended number of servings from every food group at every meal (see Chapter 7). And don't count calories!

WITHIN THE NEXT 2 WEEKS, YOU CAN:

- ☐ Find a photograph of a person you admire for his or her contributions to humanity, not for his or her appearance. Put it up next to your mirror to remind yourself that true beauty comes from within and benefits others.
- ☐ Start a journal. Each day, record one thing you are grateful for that has nothing to do with your appearance. At the end of each day, record one small thing you did to make someone's world a little brighter.

BY THE END OF THE SEMESTER, YOU CAN:

- ☐ Establish a group of friends who support you for who you are, not what you look like, and who get the same support from you. Form a group on a favorite social-networking site, and keep in touch, especially when you feel troubled by self-defeating thoughts or have the urge to engage in unhealthy behaviors.
- ☐ Borrow from the library or purchase one of the many books on body image now available, and read it!

9 Improving Your Physical Fitness

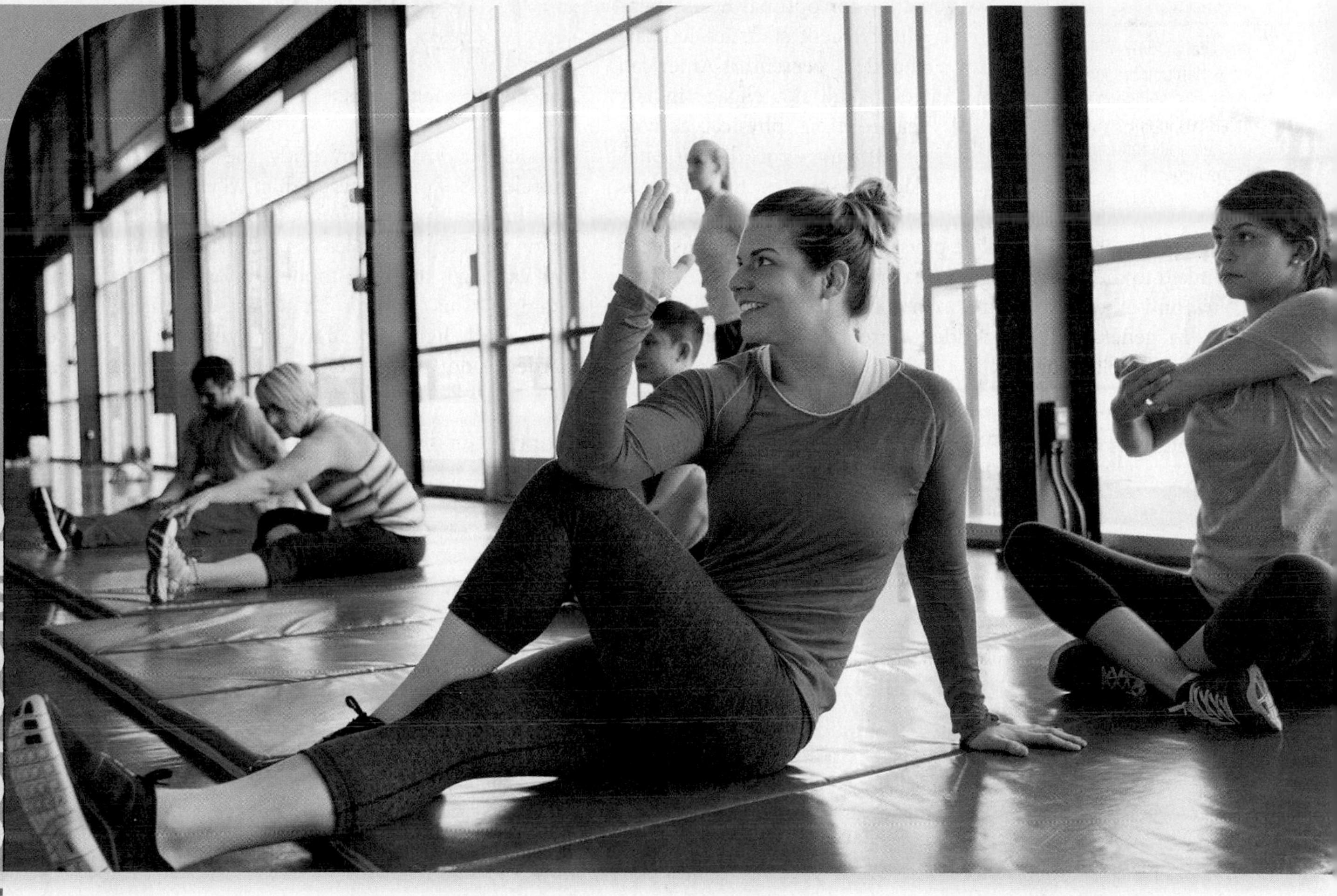

LEARNING OUTCOMES

1. Describe the health benefits of being physically active.
2. Distinguish between the physical activity required for health, fitness, and performance.
3. Identify lifestyle obstacles to physical activity, describe ways to surmount them, and make a commitment to getting physically fit.
4. Use the FITT guidelines (frequency, intensity, time, and type) to design a fitness program that meets your personal goals.
5. Devise a plan to implement your safe and effective fitness program.
6. Describe optimal foods and fluids consumption recommendations for exercise and recovery.
7. Explain how to prevent and treat common exercise injuries.

Most Americans are aware of the wide range of physical, social, and mental health benefits of physical activity—and that they should be more physically active. The physiological body changes that result from regular physical activity reduce the likelihood of coronary artery disease, high blood pressure, type 2 diabetes, obesity, and other chronic diseases. Furthermore, engaging in regular physical activity helps control stress, increase self-esteem, and contribute to that "feel-good" feeling.[1]

Despite knowing about the importance of physical activity for health and wellness, most people are not sufficiently active for optimal health benefits. Recent statistics indicate that 23.1 percent of American adults did not engage in any leisure time physical activity or activity done during one's "down" time in the previous month.[2] The growing percentage of Americans who live physically inactive lives has been linked to the current high incidences of obesity, type 2 diabetes, and other chronic and mental health diseases.[3]

physical activity Refers to all body movements produced by skeletal muscles resulting in substantial increases in energy expenditure, but generally refers to movement of the large muscle groups.

In general, college students are more physically active than are older adults, but a recent survey indicated that 52.2 percent of college women and 45.5 percent of college men do not meet recommended guidelines for engaging in moderate or vigorous physical activities.[4]

College is a great time to develop positive attitudes and behaviors that can increase the quality and quantity of your life. It may not be easy to change a sedentary lifestyle, but it is definitely worth every effort made. And if you are currently engaging in regular physical activity, stick with it! Getting up and moving is key to reaping the many health benefits from a physically active lifestyle.

LO 1 | PHYSICAL ACTIVITY FOR HEALTH

Describe the health benefits of being physically active.

Physical activity is any body movement that works your muscles, uses more energy than when resting, and enhances health.[5] Walking, swimming, strength training, dancing, and doing yoga are examples of physical activity. Physical activities can vary by light, moderate, or vigorous intensity. For example, walking on a flat surface at a casual pace requires little effort (light), while walking uphill is more intense and harder to do (moderate). Jogging and running are examples

TABLE 9.1 | Physical Activity Guidelines for Americans

	Key Guidelines for Health*	For Additional Fitness or Weight-Loss Benefits*	PLUS
Adults	150 min/week moderate-intensity physical activity	300 min/week moderate-intensity physical activity	Muscle strengthening activities for ALL the major muscle groups at least 2 days/week
	OR	OR	
	75 min/week of vigorous-intensity physical activity	150 min/week of vigorous-intensity physical activity	
	OR	OR	
	Equivalent combination of moderate- and vigorous-intensity (e.g., 100 min moderate-intensity + 25 min vigorous-intensity) physical activity	Equivalent combination of moderate- and vigorous-intensity (e.g., 200 min moderate-intensity + 50 min vigorous-intensity) physical activity	
		OR	
		More than the previously described amounts	
Older Adults	If unable to follow above guidelines, then as much physical activity as your condition allows	If unable to follow above guidelines, then as much physical activity as your condition allows	In addition to muscle strengthening activities, those with limited mobility should add exercises to improve balance and reduce risk of falling
Children and Youth	60 min or more of moderate- or vigorous-intensity physical activity daily	Add vigorous-intensity physical activities within the 60 daily minutes at least 3 days/week	Include muscle and bone strengthening activities within the 60 daily minutes at least 3 days/week Activities should be age-appropriate, enjoyable, and varied

*Avoid inactivity, some activity is better than none, accumulate physical activity in sessions of 10 minutes or more at one time, and spread activity throughout the week.

Source: Office of Disease Prevention and Health Promotion, U.S. Department of Health and Human Services, *2008 Physical Activity Guidelines for Americans: Be Active, Healthy, and Happy!*, ODPHP Publication no. U0036 (Washington, DC: U.S. Department of Health and Human Services, 2008), Available at www.health.gov/paguidelines.

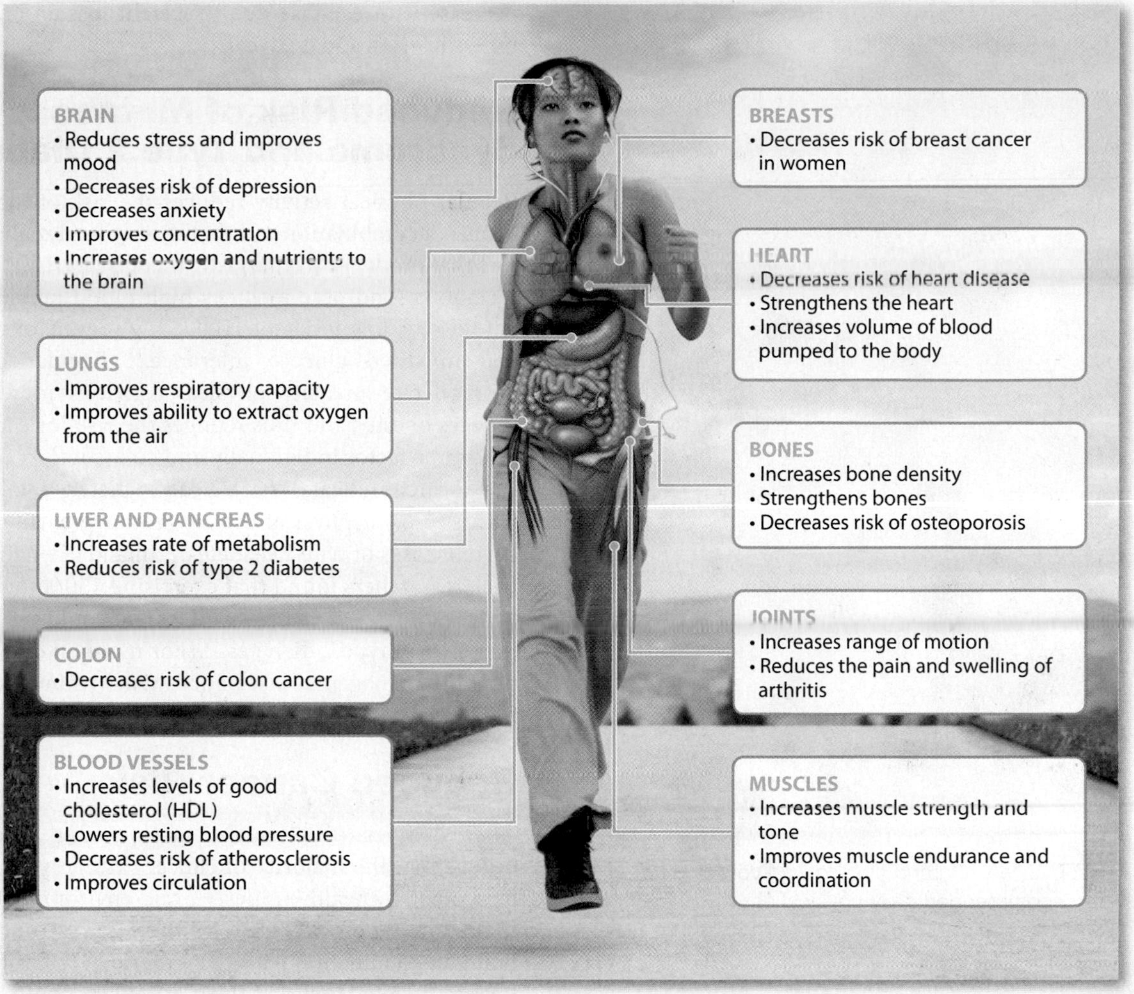

BRAIN
• Reduces stress and improves mood
• Decreases risk of depression
• Decreases anxiety
• Improves concentration
• Increases oxygen and nutrients to the brain
LUNGS
• Improves respiratory capacity
• Improves ability to extract oxygen from the air
LIVER AND PANCREAS
• Increases rate of metabolism
• Reduces risk of type 2 diabetes
COLON
• Decreases risk of colon cancer
BLOOD VESSELS
• Increases levels of good cholesterol (HDL)
• Lowers resting blood pressure
• Decreases risk of atherosclerosis
• Improves circulation
BREASTS
• Decreases risk of breast cancer in women
HEART
• Decreases risk of heart disease
• Strengthens the heart
• Increases volume of blood pumped to the body
BONES
• Increases bone density
• Strengthens bones
• Decreases risk of osteoporosis
JOINTS
• Increases range of motion
• Reduces the pain and swelling of arthritis
MUSCLES
• Increases muscle strength and tone
• Improves muscle endurance and coordination

FIGURE 9.1 Some Health Benefits of Regular Exercise

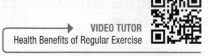

VIDEO TUTOR
Health Benefits of Regular Exercise

of vigorous-intensity physical activities. There are three general categories of physical activity defined by the purpose for which they are done: leisure time physical activity, occupational physical activity, and lifestyle physical activity.

Exercise is defined as planned, repetitive, and structured bodily movement undertaken to maintain or better any number of physical fitness components—for example, cardiorespiratory fitness, muscular strength or endurance, or flexibility. Although all exercise is physical activity, not all physical activity would be considered exercise. For example, walking from your car to class is physical activity, whereas going for a brisk 30-minute walk to maintain a healthy body weight is considered exercise.

From a major review of research on physical activity and health, researchers concluded that "there is irrefutable evidence of the effectiveness of regular physical activity in the primary and secondary prevention of several chronic diseases (e.g., cardiovascular disease, diabetes, cancer, hypertension, obesity, depression, and osteoporosis)."[6] Adding more physical activity to your day, like walking or cycling to school, can benefit your health.

In fact, it is estimated that if the number of adults meeting the 2008 Physical Activity Guidelines (see **TABLE 9.1**) increased by 25 percent, there would be 1.3 million fewer deaths per year and the life expectancy would increase. In the United Stated, it is estimated that physical inactivity is responsible for 6.7 percent of the cases of coronary heart disease, 8.3 percent of the cases of type 2 diabetes, 12.4 percent of the cases of breast cancer, and 12.0 percent of the cases of colon cancer. Furthermore, physical inactivity accounts for approximately 10.8 percent of deaths in the United States.[7]

Regular participation in physical activity improves more than 50 different physiological, metabolic, and psychological aspects of human life. **FIGURE 9.1** summarizes some of these major health-related benefits.

HEAR IT! PODCASTS

Want a study podcast for this chapter? Download **Personal Fitness: Improving Health through Exercise** available on MasteringHealth.™

exercise Planned, structured, and repetitive bodily movement done to improve or maintain one or more component of physical fitness.

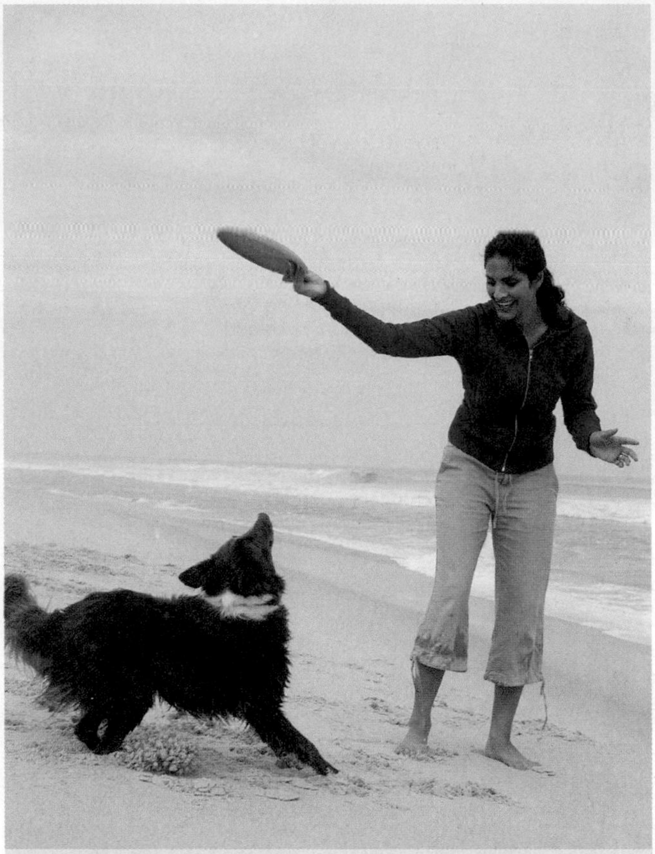
Activities such as walking and playing with your dog count toward your recommended daily physical activity.

Reduced Risk of Cardiovascular Diseases

Aerobic exercise is good for the heart and lungs and reduces the risk for heart-related diseases. It improves blood flow and eases the performance of everyday tasks. Regular exercise makes the cardiovascular and respiratory systems more efficient by strengthening the heart muscle, thus enabling more blood to be pumped with each stroke. The number of *capillaries* (small blood vessels that allow gas exchange between blood and surrounding tissues) in trained skeletal muscles is greater than in untrained ones, which allows enhanced blood flow to working muscles. Exercise also improves the respiratory system by increasing the amount of oxygen that is inhaled and distributed to body tissues.[8]

Regular physical activity can reduce hypertension, or chronic high blood pressure, a cardiovascular disease and a significant risk factor for coronary heart disease and stroke.[9] Regular aerobic exercise also improves the blood lipid profile. It typically increases high-density lipoproteins (HDLs, or "good" cholesterol), which are associated with lower risk for coronary artery disease because of their role in removing plaque built up in the arteries.[10] Triglycerides (a blood fat) typically decrease with aerobic exercise. Low-density lipoproteins (LDLs, or "bad" cholesterol) and total cholesterol often decrease with exercise due to weight loss and the improvements in HDL and triglycerides.

Reduced Risk of Metabolic Syndrome and Type 2 Diabetes

Regular physical activity reduces the risk of metabolic syndrome, a combination of heart disease and diabetes risk factors that produces a synergistic increase in risk.[11] Specifically, metabolic syndrome includes high blood pressure, abdominal obesity, low levels of HDLs, high levels of triglycerides, and impaired glucose tolerance.[12] Regular participation in moderate-intensity physical activities increases fitness, reduces obesity, and thus reduces the risk for each metabolic syndrome factor individually and collectively.[13]

Research indicates that a healthy dietary intake combined with sufficient physical activity could prevent many of the current cases of type 2 diabetes.[14] In a major national clinical trial, researchers found that exercising 150 minutes per week while eating fewer calories and less fat could prevent or delay the onset of type 2 diabetes.[15] (For more on diabetes prevention and management, see **Focus On: Minimizing Your Risk for Diabetes**).

Reduced Cancer Risk

After decades of research, most cancer epidemiologists believe that the majority of cancers are preventable and can be avoided by healthier lifestyle and environmental choices.[16] In fact, a report released by the World Cancer Research Fund, in conjunction with the American Institute for Cancer Research, stated that one-third of cancers could be prevented by being physically active and eating well.[17]

Regular physical activity appears to lower the risk for some specific cancers, particularly colon and rectal cancer.[18] Regular exercise is also associated with lower risk for breast cancer. Research on exercise and breast cancer risk has found that the earlier in life a woman starts to exercise, the lower her breast cancer risk.[19]

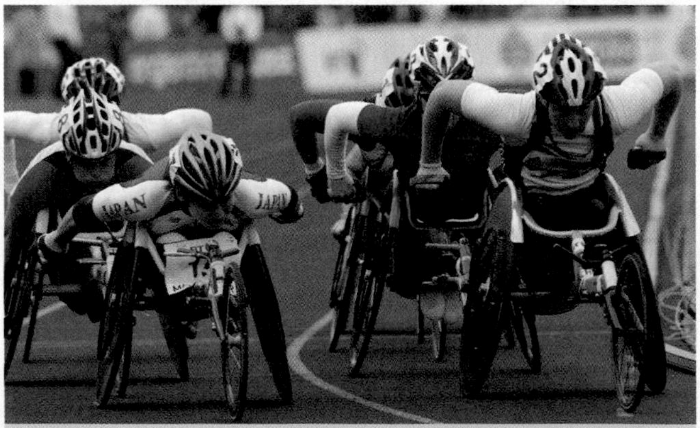

It is important for all people, including those with disabilities, to develop optimal levels of physical fitness to participate in physical activities they enjoy—including competitive sports.

Improved Bone Mass

Osteoporosis, a disease characterized by low bone mass, deterioration of bone tissue, and increased fracture risk, is becoming more prevalent among older populations. Regular weight-bearing and strength-building physical activities are recommended to maintain bone health and prevent osteoporotic fractures. Although men and women are both negatively affected by osteoporosis, it is more common in women. Both men and women have much to gain by being physically active and remaining physically active as they age—bone mass levels are significantly higher among active individuals than among sedentary persons.[20] However, it appears that the full bone-related benefits of physical activity can only be achieved with sufficient hormone levels (estrogen in women; testosterone in men) and adequate calcium, vitamin D, and total caloric intakes.[21]

Improved Weight Control

For many people, the desire to lose weight or maintain a healthy weight is the main reason for physical activity. On the most basic level, physical activity requires your body to generate energy through calorie expenditure; if calories expended exceed calories consumed over a span of time, the net result will be weight loss. Some activities are more intense or vigorous than others and result in more calories used. **FIGURE 9.2** shows the caloric cost of various activities when done for 30 minutes.

In addition to the calories expended during activity, physical activity has a direct positive effect on metabolic rate, keeping it elevated for several hours following vigorous physical activities. This increase in metabolic rate can lead to body composition changes that favor weight management. After weight loss, increased physical activity also improves your chances of maintaining the weight loss. If you are currently at a healthy body weight, regular physical activity can prevent significant weight gain.[22]

Improved Immunity

Research shows that regular moderate-intensity physical activity reduces individual susceptibility to disease.[23] Just how physical activity alters immunity is not well understood. We know that moderate-intensity physical activity temporarily increases the number of white blood cells (WBCs), which are responsible for fighting infection.[24] Often the relationship of physical activity to immunity, or more specifically to disease susceptibility, is described as a J-shaped curve. Susceptibility to disease decreases with moderate activity, but then increases as you move to extreme levels of physical activity or exercise or if you continue to exercise without adequate recovery time and/or dietary intake.[25] Athletes engaging in marathon-type events or very intense physical training programs have been shown to be at greater risk for upper respiratory tract infections (cold and flu), particularly in the 8 hours immediately after an intense exercise session.[26]

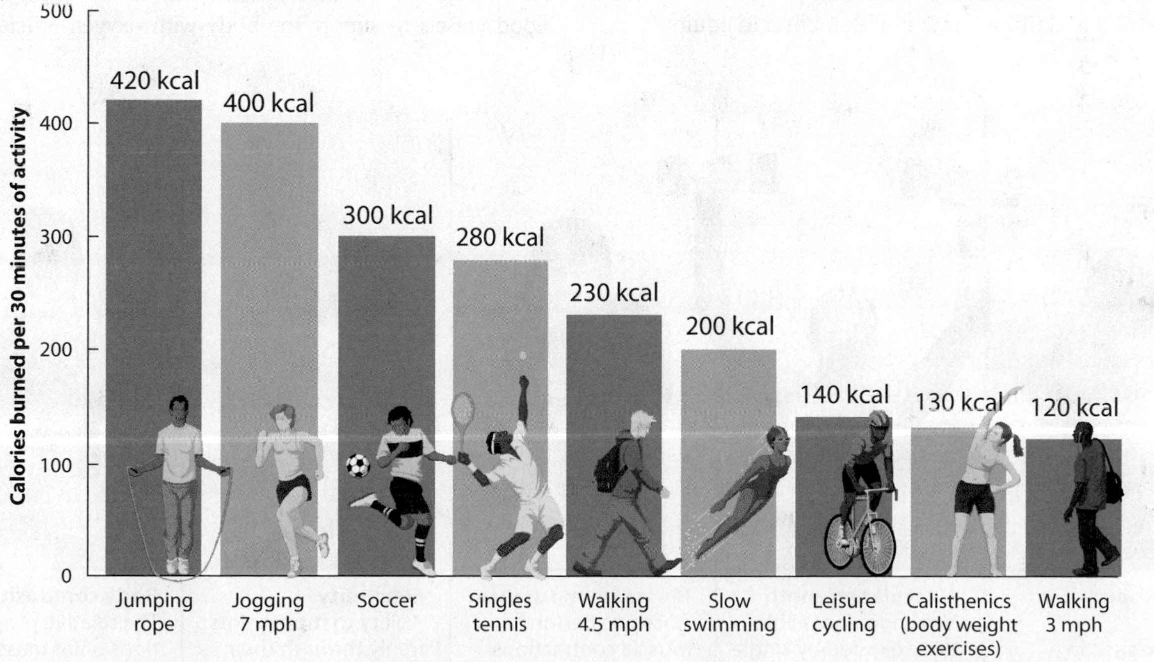

FIGURE 9.2 Calories Burned by Different Activities The harder you exercise, the more energy you expend. Estimated calories burned for various moderate and vigorous activities are listed for a 30-minute bout of activity. Note that the number of calories burned depends on body weight (generally, the higher your body weight, the greater the number of calories you'll burn).

Improved Mental Health and Stress Management

Most people who engage in regular physical activity are likely to notice psychological benefits, such as feeling better about themselves and an overall sense of well-being. Although these mental health benefits are difficult to quantify, they are frequently mentioned as reasons to be physically active.

Physical activity contributes to mental health in more than one way. Learning new skills, developing increased ability and capacity in recreational activities, and sticking with a physical activity plan all improve an individual's self-esteem. In addition, regular physical activity can improve a person's physical appearance, further increasing self-esteem.

physical fitness A balance of health-related attributes that allows you to perform moderate to vigorous physical activities on a regular basis and complete daily physical tasks without undue fatigue.

cardiorespiratory fitness The ability of the heart, lungs, and blood vessels to supply oxygen to skeletal muscles during sustained physical activity.

Regular aerobic activity can provide a break from stressors. It can improve the way the body handles stress through its effect on neurotransmitters associated with mood enhancement. Physical activity might also help the body recover from the stress response more quickly as fitness increases.[27]

There is increasing evidence that regular physical activity improves cognitive function across the lifespan. Research has associated regular activity with academic and standardized test performance in school.[28] Regular aerobic activity has also been associated with improved function in adults and with the prevention and improvement of dementia in adults.[29]

Longer Life Span

Experts have long debated the relationship between physical activity and longevity. Several studies indicate significant decreases in long-term health risk and increases in years lived, particularly among those who have several risk factors and who use physical activity as a means of risk reduction. Results from a study of nearly a million participants showed that the greatest benefits from physical activity occurred in sedentary individuals who added a little physical activity to their lives, with additional benefits added as physical activity levels were increased.[30]

LO 2 | PHYSICAL ACTIVITY FOR FITNESS AND PERFORMANCE

Distinguish between the physical activity required for health, fitness, and performance.

Physical fitness refers to a balance of physical attributes that are either health or skill related. The health-related attributes—cardiorespiratory fitness, muscular strength and endurance, flexibility, and body composition—allow you to perform moderate- to vigorous-intensity physical activities on a regular basis without getting too tired and with energy left over to handle physical or mental emergencies. **FIGURE 9.3** identifies the major health-related components of physical fitness.

Cardiorespiratory Fitness

Cardiorespiratory fitness is the ability of the heart, lungs, and blood vessels to supply the body with oxygen efficiently. The

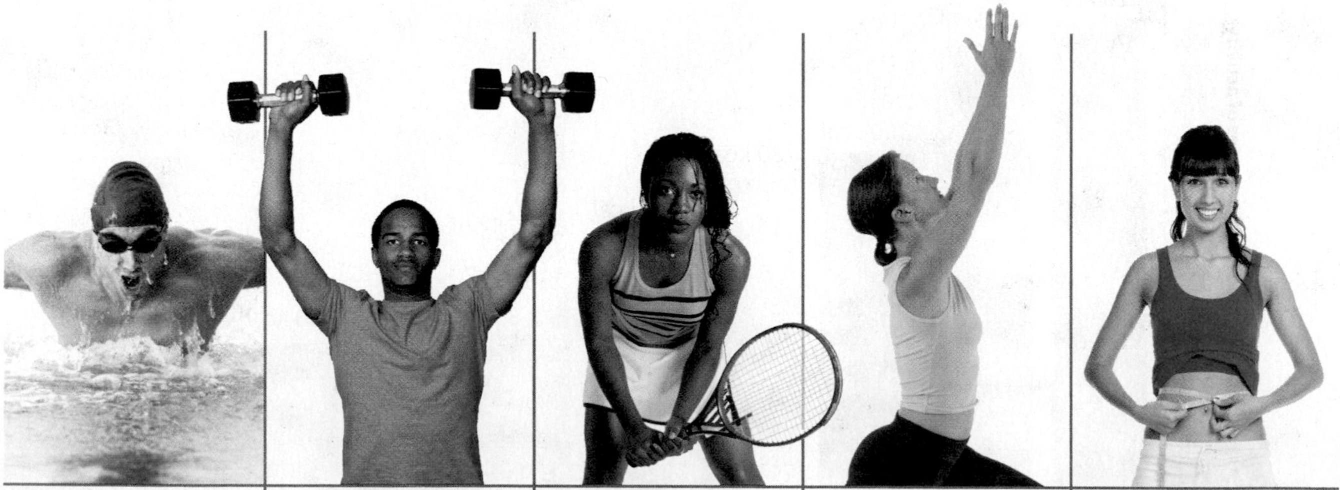

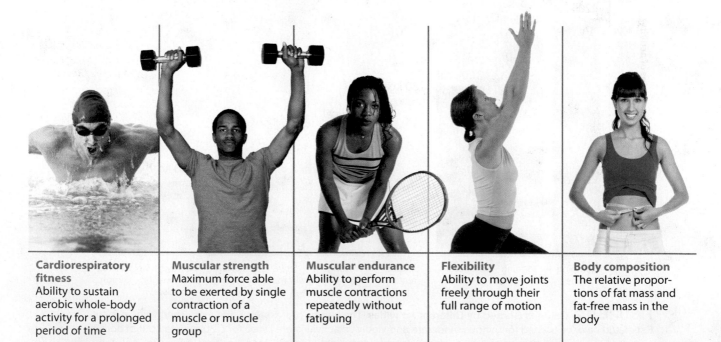

Cardiorespiratory fitness
Ability to sustain aerobic whole-body activity for a prolonged period of time

Muscular strength
Maximum force able to be exerted by single contraction of a muscle or muscle group

Muscular endurance
Ability to perform muscle contractions repeatedly without fatiguing

Flexibility
Ability to move joints freely through their full range of motion

Body composition
The relative proportions of fat mass and fat-free mass in the body

FIGURE 9.3 Health-Related Components of Physical Fitness

ONLY 20.8%

OF AMERICAN ADULTS MEET GUIDELINES FOR BOTH CARDIORESPIRATORY AND MUSCULAR **FITNESS**.

primary category of physical activity known to improve cardiorespiratory fitness is **aerobic exercise**. The word *aerobic* means "with oxygen" and describes any type of exercise that requires oxygen to make energy for prolonged activity. Aerobic activities, such as swimming, cycling, and jogging, are among the best exercises for improving or maintaining cardiorespiratory fitness.

Cardiorespiratory fitness is measured by determining **aerobic capacity** (or **power**), the volume of oxygen the muscles consume during exercise. Maximal aerobic power (commonly written as VO_{2max}) is defined as the volume of oxygen that the muscles consume per minute during maximal exercise. The most common measure of maximal aerobic capacity is a walk or run test on a treadmill. For greatest accuracy, this is done in a lab with specialized equipment and technicians to measure the precise amount of oxygen entering and exiting the body during the exercise session. To get a more general sense of cardiorespiratory fitness, submaximal tests performed in the classroom or field can predict maximal aerobic capacity. In a submaximal test of aerobic fitness, your performance during an exercise session is assessed to estimate your maximal aerobic capacity.

Muscular Strength and Endurance

Muscular strength refers to the amount of force a muscle or group of muscles is capable of exerting in one contraction. The most common way to assess the strength of a particular muscle group is to measure the maximum amount of weight you can move one time (and no more), or your one repetition maximum (1 RM).

Muscular endurance is the ability of a muscle or group of muscles to exert force repeatedly without fatigue or the ability to sustain a muscular contraction. The more repetitions you can perform successfully (e.g., push-ups) or the longer you can hold a certain position (e.g., wall sit), the greater your muscular endurance. General muscular endurance is most often measured from the number of curl-ups or push-ups an individual can do. The **Assess Yourself** questionnaire found online in MasteringHealth (see the box at the end of this chapter for details) describes these tests.

Flexibility and Body Composition

Flexibility refers to the range of motion, or the amount of movement possible, at a particular joint or series of joints. A larger range of motion in a joint means a greater level of flexibility in that particular body area. Various tests measure the flexibility of the body's joints. One of the most common measures of general flexibility is the sit-and-reach test, described in the online Assess Yourself questionnaire. **Body composition** is the fifth and final component of a comprehensive fitness program. Body composition describes the relative proportions and distribution of fat and fat-free (muscle, bone, water, organs) tissues in the body.

Skill-Related Components of Physical Fitness

In addition to the five health-related components of physical fitness, physical fitness for athletes also involves attributes that improve their ability to perform athletic tasks. These attributes, called the *skill-related components* of physical fitness, can also help recreational athletes and general exercisers increase

SEE IT! VIDEOS

Yoga is a great way to exercise your body and mind. Watch **Beginner's Guide to Yoga** available on MasteringHealth.™

WHY SHOULD I CARE?

Even the most consistent exercisers can have a setback due to injury, schedule, or a period of low motivation. Regardless of your current level of exercise, the information in this chapter can help you reduce your risk for injury and develop strategies to maintain your current level of exercise. Make sure you have a plan in place to stick with your exercise routine during finals or other stressful times.

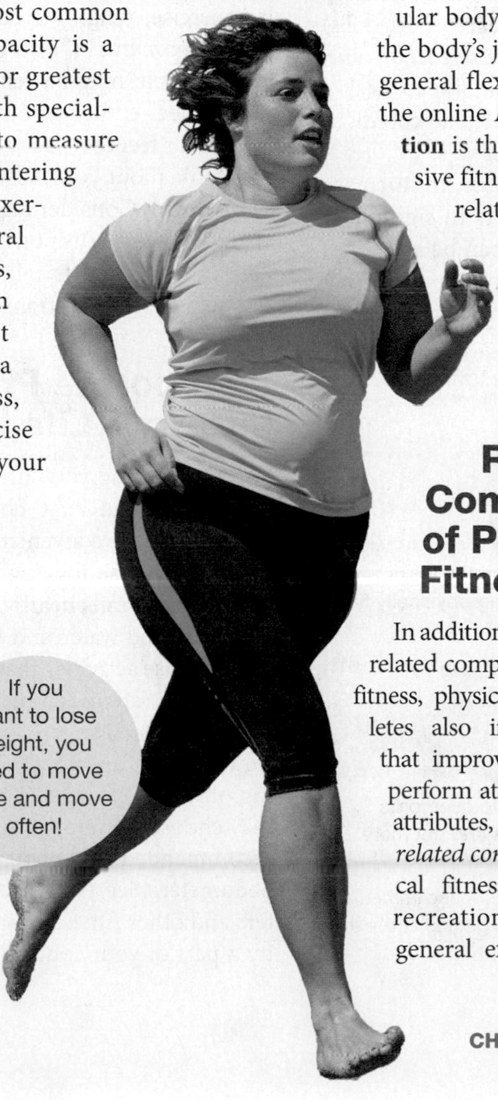

If you want to lose weight, you need to move more and move often!

aerobic exercise Prolonged exercise that requires oxygen to make energy for activity.

aerobic capacity (or power) The functional status of the cardiorespiratory system; refers specifically to the volume of oxygen the muscles consume during exercise.

muscular strength The amount of force that a muscle is capable of exerting in one contraction.

muscular endurance A muscle's ability to exert force repeatedly without fatiguing or the ability to sustain a muscular contraction for a length of time.

flexibility The range of motion, or the amount of movement possible, at a particular joint or series of joints.

body composition The relative proportions of fat and fat-free (muscle, bone, water, organs) tissues in the body.

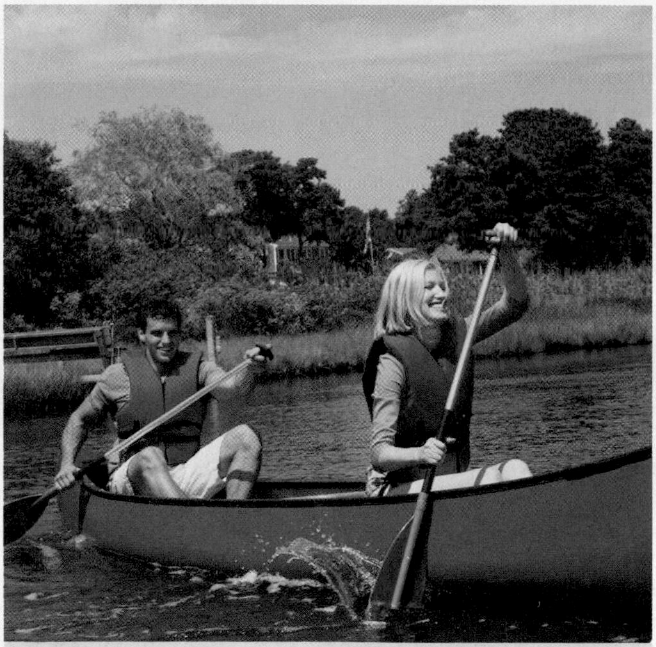

Although physical activity actually stimulates the stress response, a physically fit body adapts efficiently to the *eustress* of exercise—and as a result is better able to tolerate and effectively manage *stress* of all kinds.

fitness levels and their ability to perform daily tasks. The skill-related components of physical fitness (also called sport skills) are *agility*, *balance*, *coordination*, *power*, *speed*, and *reaction time*. Some of the skill-related fitness components can impact health. For example, consider the importance of balance and coordination for older adults who are at increased risk for falls.[31]

Athletes will undertake specific exercises to increase their sport skills, and regular training results in significant improvements. Improving your sport skills can be as easy as participating regularly in any sport or activity or performing drills that mimic a sport-specific skill or work specifically on any of the skill-related components of fitness. You can practice drills in group classes or work with a personal trainer.

LO 3 | COMMITTING TO PHYSICAL FITNESS

Identify lifestyle obstacles to physical activity, describe ways to surmount them, and make a commitment to getting physically fit.

To succeed at incorporating physical fitness into your life, you need to design a fitness program that takes obstacles into account and that is founded on the activities you enjoy most. Even regular exercisers can benefit from strategies to maintain motivation and overcome common obstacles.

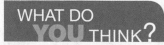

WHAT DO YOU THINK?

Why is it hard to overcome your obstacles and get more physically active?

- What would be the immediate "pay-off" to getting active this week?

What If I Have Been Inactive for a While?

If you have been physically inactive for the past few months or longer, you should start your program slowly. If you are inactive and also have risk factors for cardiovascular disease, such as obesity, high blood pressure, smoking, or a family history of heart disease, you should first make sure that your physician clears you for exercise before getting started. Once you are ready to begin, consider consulting a personal trainer or fitness instructor to help you get started. In this phase of your fitness program, the *initial conditioning stage,* you may begin at levels lower than those recommended for physical fitness. Starting slowly will ease you into a workout regime with a minimum of soreness. For example, you might start your cardiorespiratory program by simply moving more and reducing your sedentary time each day. Take the stairs instead of the elevator, walk farther from your car to the store, and plan for organized movement each day, such as a 10- to 15-minute walk. In addition, you can start your muscle fitness program with simple body weight exercises, emphasizing proper technique and body alignment before adding any resistance.

Overcome Common Obstacles to Physical Activity

People have real and perceived barriers that prevent regular exercise, ranging from personal ("I do not have time") to environmental ("I do not have a safe place to be active"). Some people may be reluctant to exercise if they are overweight, feel embarrassed to work out with their more "fit" friends, or feel they lack the knowledge and skills required.

Think about your obstacles to physical activity and write them down. Consider anything that gets in the way of exercising, however minor. Once you honestly evaluate why you are not as physically active as you want to be, review **TABLE 9.2** for suggestions on overcoming your hurdles.

Incorporate Physical Activity into Your Life

When designing your fitness program, there are several factors to consider. First, choose activities that are appropriate for you, that are convenient, and that you genuinely enjoy. For example, choose jogging because you like to run and there are beautiful trails nearby versus swimming when you do not really like the water and the pool is difficult to get to. Likewise, choose activities that are suitable for your current fitness level. If you are overweight or have not exercised in months, then do not sign up for advanced aerobics classes. Start slowly, plan fun activities, and progress to more challenging physical activities as your physical fitness improves. You may choose to simply walk more in an attempt to achieve the recommended goal of 10,000 steps per day; keep track with a pedometer. (See **TABLE 9.3** on page 270 for more on pedometers and other fitness equipment.) Try to make physical activity a part of your routine by incorporating it into something

TABLE 9.2 | Overcoming Obstacles to Physical Activity

Obstacle	Possible Solution
Lack of time	■ Look at your schedule. Where can you find 30-minute time slots? Perhaps you need to focus on shorter times (10 minutes or more) throughout the day. ■ Multitask. Read while riding an exercise bike or listen to lectures or podcasts while walking. ■ Be physically active during your lunch and study breaks as well as between classes. Skip rope or throw a Frisbee with a friend. ■ Select activities that require less time, such as brisk walking or jogging versus going to the gym for a class. ■ Ride your bike to class, or park (or get off the bus) farther from your destination.
Social influence	■ Invite family and friends to be active with you. ■ Join a class to meet new people. ■ Explain the importance of exercise and your commitment to physical activity to people who may not support your efforts. ■ Find a role model to support your efforts. ■ Plan for physically active dates—go dancing or bowling.
Lack of motivation, willpower, or energy	■ Schedule your workout time just as you would any other important commitment. ■ Enlist the help of an exercise partner to make you accountable for working out. ■ Give yourself an incentive. ■ Schedule your workouts when you feel most energetic. ■ Remind yourself that exercise gives you more energy. ■ Get things ready for your workout; for example, if you walk in the morning, set out your walking clothes the night before. Or pack your gym bag before going to bed.
Lack of resources	■ Select an activity that requires minimal equipment, such as walking, jogging, jumping rope, or calisthenics. ■ Identify inexpensive resources on campus or in the community. ■ Use active forms of transportation. ■ Take advantage of no-cost opportunities, such as playing catch in the park/green space on campus.

Source: Adapted from National Center for Chronic Disease Prevention and Health Promotion, "How Can I Overcome Barriers to Physical Activity?," Updated February 2011, www.cdc.gov/physicalactivity/everyone/getactive/barriers.html.

you already have to do—such as getting to class or work. See the **Health Headlines** box on page 271 for more on using your transportation for fitness.

LO 4 | CREATING YOUR OWN FITNESS PROGRAM

Use the FITT guidelines (frequency, intensity, time, and type) to design a fitness program that meets your personal goals.

The first step in creating a personal physical fitness program is identifying your goals. Take some time to reflect on your personal circumstances and desires regarding physical fitness. Do you want to be better at sports or feel better about your body? Is your goal to manage stress or reduce your risk of chronic diseases? Perhaps your most vital goal will be to establish a realistic schedule of diverse physical activities that you can maintain and enjoy throughout your life. Your physical fitness goals and objectives should be both achievable and in line with what you truly want. Achievable, truly desired goals increase motivation, and this, in turn, leads to a better chance of success.

Set SMART Goals

To set successful goals, try using the *SMART* system. SMART goals are **s**pecific, **m**easurable, **a**ction-oriented, **r**ealistic, and **t**ime-oriented.

A vague goal would be "Improve fitness by exercising more." A SMART goal would be as follows:

- **Specific**—"I'll participate in a resistance-training program that targets all of the major muscle groups 3–5 days per week."
- **Measurable**—"I'll improve my fitness classification from average to good."
- **Action-oriented**—"I'll meet with a personal trainer to learn how to safely do resistance exercises and to plan a workout for the gym and home."

TABLE 9.3 | Popular Fitness Equipment

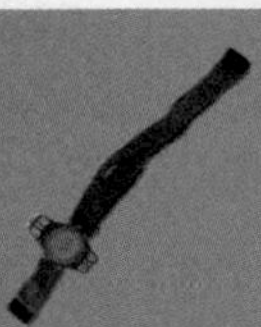

Heart Rate Monitor

A chest strap with a watch device that measures heart rate during training.

- Provides instant and continuous feedback about the intensity of your workout.
- Strap must fit well; can be uncomfortable (most women tuck the strap under the bottom strap of their sport bra).

Cost: $50–$200

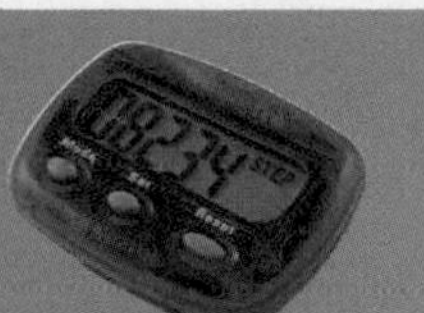

Pedometer

A battery-operated device, usually worn on your belt, that measures the number of steps taken. Some models also monitor calories, distance, and speed.

- Great motivation and feedback regarding the recommended 10,000 steps per day.
- Must be calibrated for your height, weight, and stride length.

Cost: $25–$50

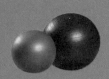

Stability Ball

Ball made of burst-resistant vinyl that can be used for strengthening core muscles or to improve flexibility.

- Balls must be inflated correctly to be most effective.

Cost: $25–$50

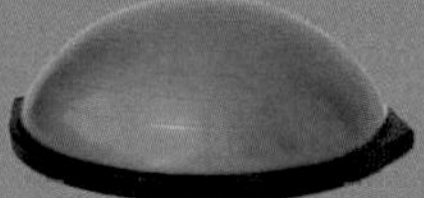

Balance Board

A board with a rounded bottom that can be used to improve balance, core muscle strength, and flexibility.

- Great for improving agility, coordination, reaction skills, and ankle strength.
- Can be difficult initially for new users. Caution new users with weak ankles, as there is risk of straining ligaments and tendons.

Cost: $40–$80

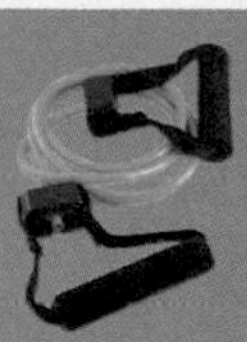

Resistance Band

Rubber or elastic material, sometimes with handles, that can be used to build muscular strength and endurance. Also can be used in yoga or Pilates to provide assistance in flexibility training.

- Improves muscular strength and endurance, balance, coordination, and flexibility.
- Lightweight, durable, and portable.
- Breaks down over time; need to inspect regularly to avoid injury if it breaks during use.

Cost: $5–$15

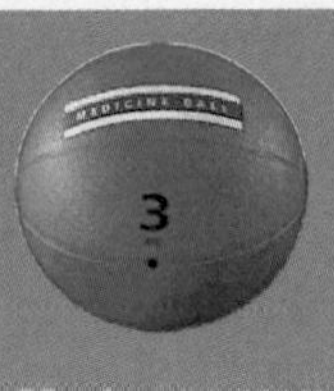

Medicine Ball

A heavy ball, about 14 inches in diameter, used in rehabilitation and strength training. Weight varies from 2 to 25 lb. Some made with handles.

- Can be used effectively to increase explosive power.
- Also used to develop core body strength.
- If used incorrectly, there is potential for lower back injuries.

Cost: $10–$150

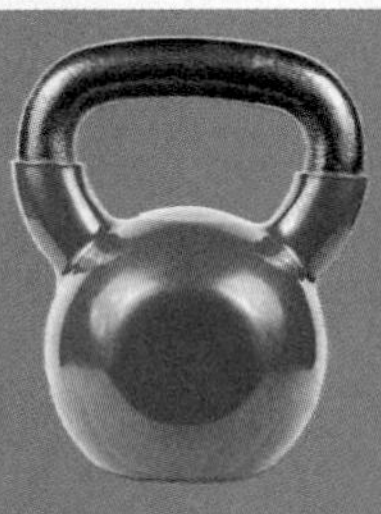

Kettlebell

A heavy ball with a handle used for full-body muscular strength and endurance exercises. Weight varies from 5 to 100 lb.

- Can be used effectively to increase muscular fitness, core strength, and explosive power.
- Movements can be complex, and if used incorrectly, there is potential for lower back and/or wrist injuries.

Cost: $10–$150

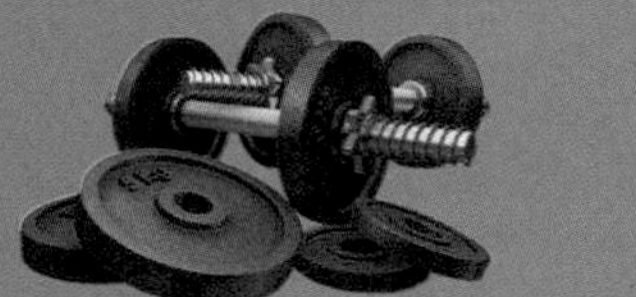

Free Weights

Rubber, plastic, or metal dumbbells or barbells, often with adjustable weight; can be used with a weight bench.

- Traditional method for building muscular strength and endurance.
- A full set allows you to increase resistance as you train, allowing for greater improvements in muscular strength.
- Potential for injury if form is incorrect; must concentrate on body alignment and ensuring sufficient core body strength.

Cost: $1–$300

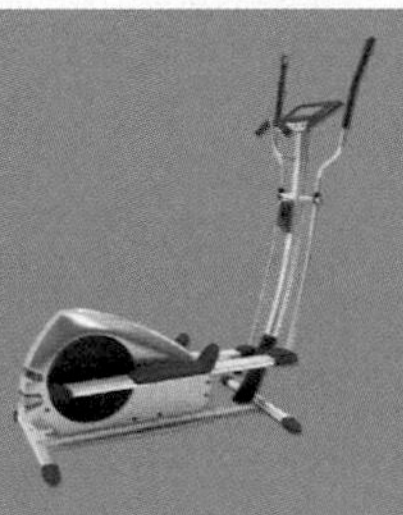

Elliptical Trainer

A stationary exercise machine that simulates walking or running without impact on the bones and joints. Some machines include arm movements.

- Nonimpact; less wear and tear on the joints and risk of shin splints.
- Readout and programs vary.

Cost: $300–$4,000

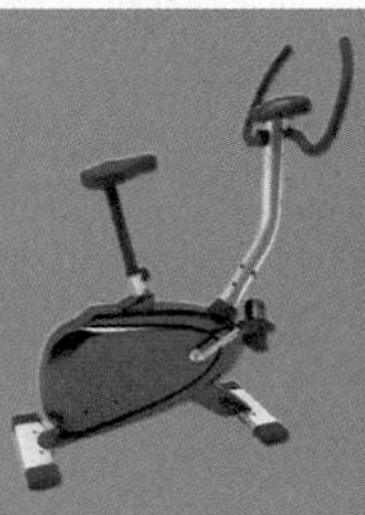

Stationary Bike

A lower-body exercise machine designed to simulate bike riding.

- Generally easy to use; does not require balance.
- Comes with varied resistance programs.
- Recumbent styles offer less strain on back and knees and are useful for individuals struggling with back pain.

Cost: $200–$2,000

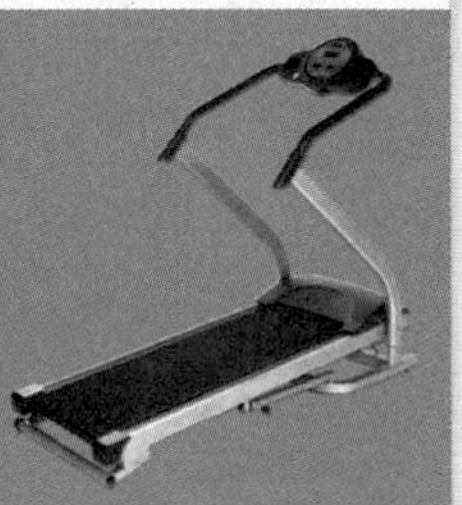

Treadmill

Exercise machine for walking or running on a moving platform while remaining in one place.

- Generally easy to use; comes with an emergency shutoff.
- Different models have varied readouts and programmability.
- Less impact on joints than running on most pavements.

Cost: $500–$4,000

@ HEALTH HEADLINES

TRANSPORT YOURSELF!

Before we became a car culture, much of our transportation was human powered. Historically, bicycling and walking were important means of transportation and recreation in the United States. These modes not only helped keep people in good physical condition, but they also had little impact on the environment. Since World War II, however, the development of automobile-oriented communities has led to a steady decline of bicycling and walking. Currently, only about 10 percent of trips are made by foot or bike.

The more we use our cars to get around, the more congested our roads, the more polluted our air, and the more sedentary we become. Many people are now embracing a movement toward more active transportation. *Active transportation* means using your own power to get from place to place—whether walking, riding a bike, skateboarding, or roller skating. Here are just a few of the many reasons to make active transportation a bigger part of your life:

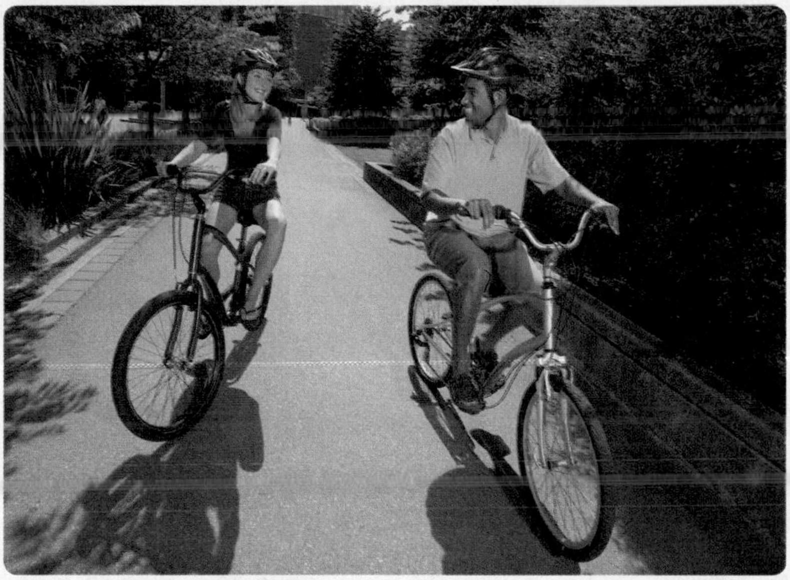

Hop on that bike and join the green revolution!

- **You will be adding more exercise into your daily routine.** People who use active forms of transportation to complete errands are more likely to meet physical activity guidelines.
- **Walking or biking can save you money.** With rising gas prices, parking rates, car maintenance costs, and insurance payments, fewer automobile trips could add up to considerable savings. During the course of a year, bicycle commuters who ride 5 miles to work can save about $500 on fuel and more than $1,000 on other expenses related to driving.
- **Walking or biking may save you time!** Cycling is usually the fastest mode of travel door to door for distances up to 6 miles in city centers. Walking is simpler and faster for distances of about a mile.
- **You will enjoy being outdoors.** Research is emerging on the physical and mental health benefits of nature and being outdoors. So much of what we do is inside, with recirculated air and artificial lighting, that our bodies are deficient in fresh air and sunlight.
- **You will make a significant contribution to reducing air pollution.** Leaving your car at home just 2 days a week will reduce greenhouse gas emissions by an average of 1,600 pounds per year.
- **You will help reduce traffic.** The average traveler now wastes the equivalent of a full work week stuck in traffic every year. More active commuters means fewer cars on the roads and less traffic congestion.
- **You will contribute to global environmental health.** Annually, personal transportation consumes approximately 136 billion gallons of gasoline and produces 1.2 billion tons of carbon dioxide. Reducing vehicle trips will help reduce overall greenhouse gas emissions and the need to source more fossil fuel.

Sources: T. Gotschi and K. Mills, *Active Transportation for America: The Case for Increased Federal Investment in Bicycling and Walking* (Washington, DC: Rails to Trails Conservancy, 2008), Available at www.railstotrails.org/ourwork/advocacy/active-transportation/makingthecase; D. Shinkle and A. Teigens, *Encouraging Bicycling and Walking: The State Legislative Role* (Washington, DC: National Conference of State Legislatures, 2008), Updated April 2009, Available at www.americantrails.org/resources/trans/Encourage-Bicycling-Walking-State-Legislative-Role.html; U.S. Environmental Protection Agency, "Climate Change: What You Can Do—On the Road," Updated September 2013, www.epa.gov/climatechange/wycd/road.html.

- **Realistic**—"I'll increase the weight I can lift by 20 percent."
- **Time-oriented**—"I'll try my new weight program for 8 weeks, then reassess."

Use the FITT Principle

Now that you've set realistic goals and are motivated to improve your physical fitness, the next step is to learn about the fitness recommendations and principles involved so that you can devise your own workout plan. What is the best approach to take? Where should you start? Assuming your intention is to improve your health-related physical fitness (although the principles can also be applied to performance-related physical fitness), the **FITT (frequency, intensity, time, and**

FITT Acronym for *frequency, intensity, time,* and *type,* the terms that describe the recommended levels of exercise to improve a health-related component of physical fitness.

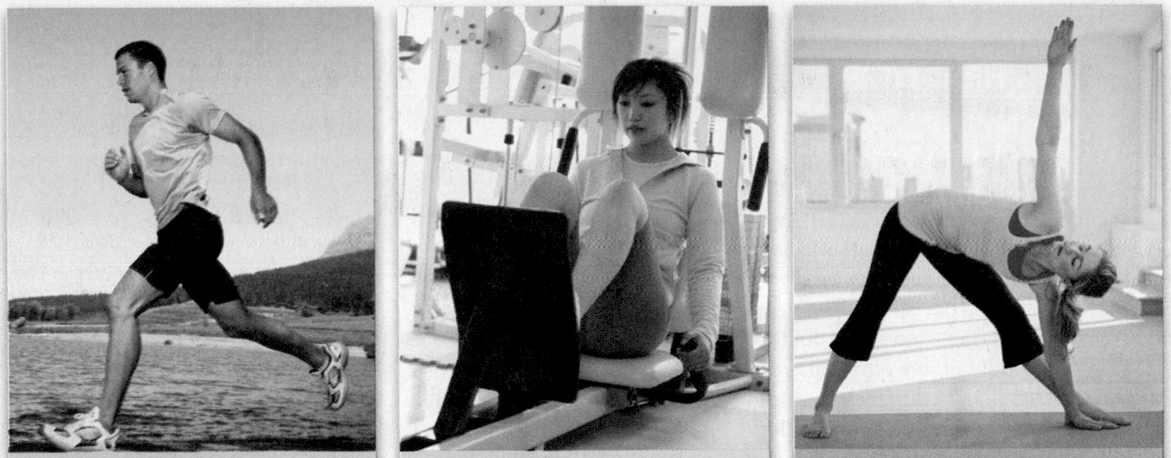

	Cardiorespiratory Endurance	Muscular Fitness	Flexibility
Frequency	3–5 days per week	2–3 days per week	Minimally 2–3 days per week
Intensity	64%–96% of maximum heart rate	60%–80% of 1 RM	To the point of mild tension
Time	20–60 minutes	8–10 exercises, 2–4 sets, 8–12 reps	10–30 seconds per stretch, 2–4 reps
Type	Any rhythmic, continuous, large muscle group activity	Resistance training (with body weight and/or external resistance) for all major muscle groups	Stretching, dance, or yoga exercises for all major muscle groups

FIGURE 9.4 The FITT Principle Applied to Cardiorespiratory Fitness, Muscular Strength and Endurance, and Flexibility

type) principle should be used to define your exercise program (**FIGURE 9.4**):

- Exercise **frequency** refers to the number of times per week you need to engage in particular exercises to achieve the desired level of physical fitness in a particular component.
- **Intensity** refers to how hard your workout must be to achieve the desired level of physical fitness.
- How much **time**, or the *duration*, refers to how many minutes or repetitions of an exercise are required at a specified intensity during any one session.
- **Type** refers to what kind of exercises should be performed to improve the various components of physical fitness.

frequency As part of the FITT prescription, refers to how many days per week a person should exercise.

intensity As part of the FITT prescription, refers to how hard or how much effort is needed when a person exercises.

time As part of the FITT prescription, refers to the duration of an exercise session.

type As part of the FITT prescription, refers to what kind of exercises a person should do.

The FITT Principle for Cardiorespiratory Fitness

The most effective aerobic exercises for building cardiorespiratory fitness are total body activities involving the large muscle groups of your body. The FITT prescription for cardiorespiratory fitness includes 3 to 5 days per week of vigorous, rhythmic, continuous activity at 64 to 95 percent of your estimated maximal heart rate for 20 to 60 minutes.[32]

Frequency The frequency of your program is related to your intensity. If you choose to do moderate-intensity exercises, you should aim for a frequency of at least 5 days (frequency drops to at least 3 days per week with vigorous-intensity activities). Newcomers to exercise can still improve by doing less intense exercise (light to moderate level), but doing it more days during a week. In this case, follow the recommendations from the Centers for Disease Control and Prevention (CDC) for moderate physical activity (refer to Table 9.1).

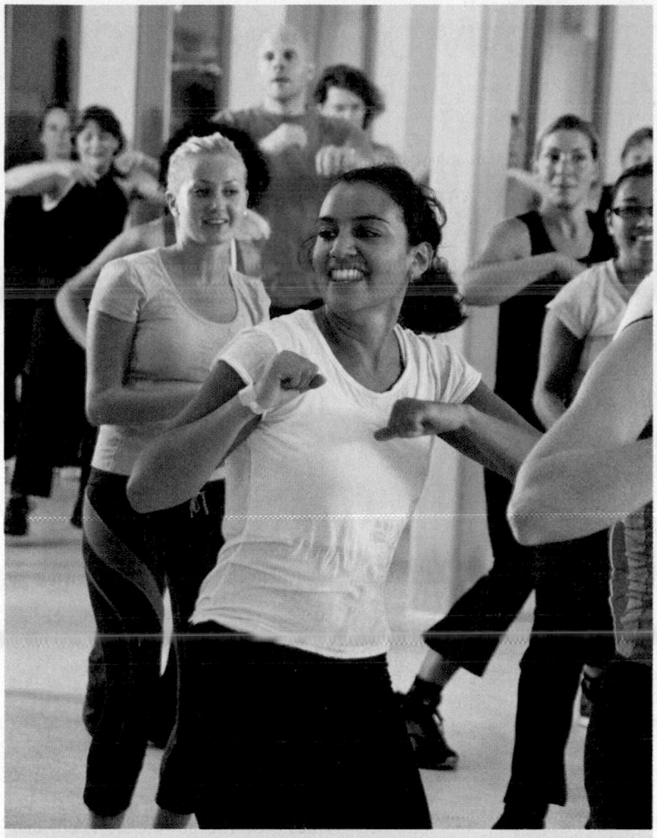

One great way to motivate yourself to get moving is to sign up for an exercise class. Find something that interests you—dance, yoga, aerobics, martial arts, acrobatics—and get involved. The structure, schedule, social interaction, and challenge of learning a new skill can be terrific motivators that make exercising and being physically active exciting and fun.

Intensity The most common methods used to determine the intensity of cardiorespiratory endurance exercises are target heart rate, rating of perceived exertion, and the talk test. The exercise intensity required to improve cardiorespiratory endurance is a heart rate between 64 and 94 percent of your maximum heart rate. Before calculating your **target heart rate**, you must first estimate your maximal heart rate with the formula [206.9 − 0.67(age)]. The example below is based on a 20-year-old. Substitute your age to determine your target heart rate training range, then multiply by 0.64 and 0.94 to determine the lower and upper limits of your target range. **FIGURE 9.5** shows a range of target heart rates for various ages.

1. 206.9 − 0.67 (20) = target heart rate for a 20-year-old
2. 206.9 − 13.4 = 193.5 (maximal heart rate)
3. 193.5 (0.64) = 123.8 (lower target limit)
4. 193.5 (0.94) = 181.89 (upper target limit)
5. Target range = 124–182 beats per minute

To determine how close you are to your target heart rate, take your pulse. Lightly place your index and middle fingers (not your thumb) over the carotid artery in your neck or on the radial artery on the inside of your wrist (**FIGURE 9.6**). Count your pulse while exercising, if possible, or start counting your pulse immediately after you stop exercising, as your

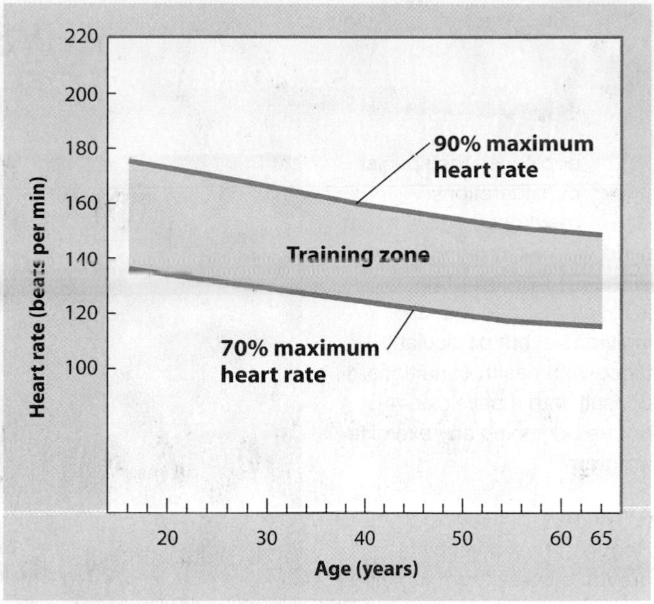

FIGURE 9.5 Target Heart Rate Ranges These ranges are based on calculating the maximum heart rate as [206.9 − 0.67 (age)] and the training zone as 64 percent to 96 percent of maximum heart rate. Individuals with low fitness levels should start below or at the low end of these ranges.

heart rate decreases rapidly when you stop. Using a watch or a clock, take your pulse for 10 seconds (the first pulse is "0" if you are starting a stopwatch, but 1 if you are using a watch that is already running) and multiply this number by 6 to get the number of beats per minute.

Another way to determine the intensity of cardiorespiratory exercise intensity is to use Borg's rating of perceived exertion (RPE) scale. **Perceived exertion** refers to how hard you feel you are working, which you might base on your heart rate, breathing rate, sweating, and level of fatigue. This scale uses a rating from 6 (no exertion at all) to 20 (maximal exertion).

target heart rate The heart rate range of aerobic exercise that leads to improved cardiorespiratory fitness (i.e., 64% to 96% of maximal heart rate).

perceived exertion The subjective perception of effort during exercise that can be used to monitor exercise intensity

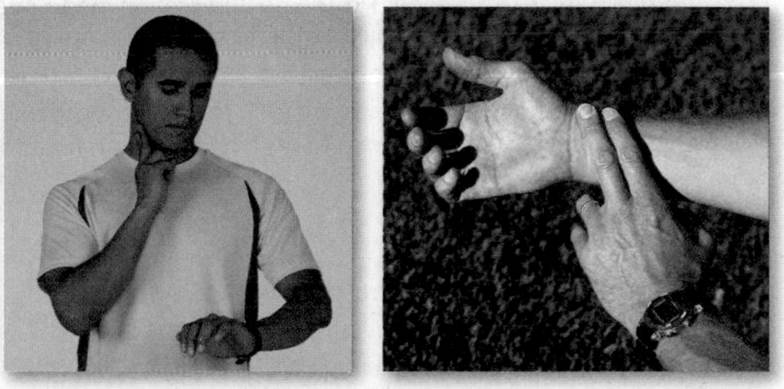

a Carotid pulse

b Radial pulse

FIGURE 9.6 Taking a Pulse Palpation of the carotid (neck) or radial (wrist) artery is a simple way to determine heart rate.

HEALTH IN A DIVERSE WORLD

PHYSICAL ACTIVITY AND EXERCISE FOR SPECIAL POPULATIONS

People with the special considerations mentioned below might need to make modifications to the FITT prescription. It is recommended that all individuals, but particularly those with health conditions, consult with a physician before beginning any exercise program.

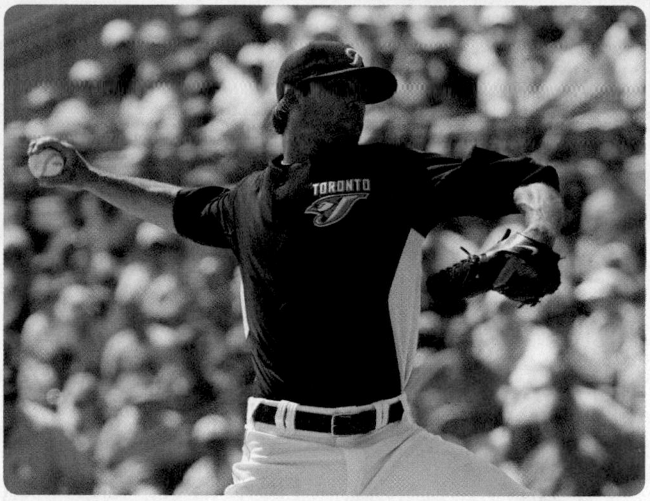

Athletes like Brandon Morrow, a Major League Baseball pitcher and a type 1 diabetic, are living proof that chronic conditions needn't prevent you from achieving your physical activity goals.

Asthma

Regular physical activity provides benefits for individuals with asthma. It strengthens the respiratory muscles, making it easier to breathe; improves immune system functioning; and helps maintain weight.

Before engaging in exercise, ensure that your asthma is under control. Ask about adjusting your medications (for example, your doctor may recommend you use your inhaler 15 minutes prior to exercise). Keep your inhaler nearby. Warm up and cool down properly; it is particularly important that you allow your lungs and breathing rate to adjust slowly. Protect yourself from your asthma triggers when exercising (e.g., pollution or cold environments). If you have symptoms while exercising, stop and use your inhaler; if an asthma attack persists, call 9-1-1.

Obesity

Obese individuals may have limitations such as heat intolerance, shortness of breath during physical activity, lack of flexibility, frequent musculoskeletal injuries, and difficulty with balance. Programs should emphasize physical activities that can be sustained for longer periods of time such as walking, swimming, or bicycling. Use caution when performing these activities in hot or humid environments. Although it is recommended to start slow (5 to 10 minutes of activity) and at a lower intensity (55% to 65% of maximal heart rate), the ultimate goal for weight loss and prevention of re-gain is to perform at least 30 to 60 minutes of exercise per day—150 to 300 minutes per week. Regardless of the amount of weight lost, evidence suggests that individuals who are obese improve their health with cardiorespiratory and resistance-training activities.

Coronary Heart Disease

Although regular physical activity reduces risk of coronary heart disease, vigorous-intensity activity acutely increases risk of sudden cardiac death and myocardial infarction (heart attack). Individuals with coronary heart disease must consult their physicians and might need to participate in a supervised exercise program for individuals with heart disease.

Hypertension

Using the FITT prescription, individuals who are hypertensive should engage in physical activity on most, if not all, days of the week, at a moderate intensity (12 to 13 on the Borg RPE scale), for 30 minutes or more.

Diabetes

Physical activity benefits individuals with diabetes in many ways. It controls blood glucose (for individuals with type 2) by improving transport into the cells, controls body weight, and reduces risk for heart disease.

Before people with type 1 diabetes engage in physical activity, they must learn how to manage their resting blood glucose levels. Individuals should have an exercise partner; eat 1 to 3 hours prior to the activity; eat complex carbohydrates after the activity; avoid late-evening exercise; and monitor their blood glucose before, during, and after activity.

One of the most important factors for individuals with type 2 diabetes is the time or length of their physical activity. Because a critical objective of the management of type 2 diabetes is to reduce body fat (obesity), the recommendations for time are longer—at least 30 minutes, working up to 60 minutes per session or 300 minutes per week. Multiple 10-minute sessions can be used to accumulate these totals. For sessions of this length, it is prudent to reduce the intensity of the activity to a target heart rate range of 40 to 60 percent of maximal heart rate.

Source: P. Williamson, *Exercise for Special Populations* (Philadelphia, Lippincott Williams & Wilkins, 2011).

An RPE of 12 to 16 is generally recommended for training the cardiorespiratory system.

The easiest method of measuring cardiorespiratory exercise intensity is the "talk test." A "moderate" level of exercise (heart rate at 64 to 76 percent of maximum) is a conversational level of exercise. At this level you are able to talk with a partner while exercising. If you can talk, but only in short fragments and not sentences, you may be at a "vigorous" level of exercise (heart rate at 76 to 96 percent of maximum). If you are breathing so hard that speaking at all is difficult, the intensity of your exercise may be too high. Conversely, if you are able to sing or laugh heartily while exercising, the intensity of your exercise is light and may be insufficient for maintaining or improving cardiorespiratory fitness.

Time For cardiorespiratory fitness benefits, the American College of Sports Medicine (ACSM) recommends that vigorous activities be performed for at least 20 minutes at a time, and moderate activities for at least 30 minutes.[33] See also the **Health in a Diverse World** box for recommendations for individuals with chronic diseases or conditions that require alterations to the FITT prescription. Free time for exercise can vary from day to day, so you can also set a time goal for the entire week as long as you keep your sessions to at least 10 minutes (150 minutes per week for moderate intensity, and 75 minutes per week for vigorous intensity).

30 MINUTES

OF PHYSICAL ACTIVITY A DAY—ALL AT ONE TIME OR IN THREE 10-MINUTE SESSIONS—PROVIDES SUBSTANTIAL HEALTH **BENEFITS**.

Type Any sort of rhythmic, continuous, and physical activity that can be done for 20 or more minutes will improve cardiorespiratory fitness. Examples include walking briskly, cycling, jogging, fitness classes, and swimming.

The FITT Principle for Muscular Strength and Endurance

The FITT prescription for muscular strength and endurance includes 2 to 3 days per week of exercises that train the major muscle groups, using enough sets, repetitions, and resistance to maintain or improve muscular strength and endurance.[34]

Frequency For frequency, performing eight to ten exercises that train the major muscle groups 2 to 3 days a week is recommended. It is believed that overloading the muscles, a normal part of resistance training described below, causes microscopic tears in muscle fibers, and the rebuilding process that increases the muscle's size and capacity takes about 24 to 48 hours. Thus, resistance training exercise programs should include at least 1 day of rest between workouts before the same muscles are overloaded again. But don't wait too long between workouts: One of the important principles of strength training is the idea of *reversibility*. Reversibility means that if you stop exercising, the body responds by deconditioning. Within 2 weeks, muscles begin to revert to their untrained state.[35] The saying "use it or lose it" applies!

Intensity To determine the intensity of exercise needed to improve muscular strength and endurance, you need to know the maximum amount of weight you can lift (or move) in one contraction. This value is called your **one repetition maximum (1 RM)**. Once your 1 RM is determined, it is used as the basis for intensity recommendations for improving muscular strength and endurance. Muscular strength is improved when resistance loads are greater than 60 percent of your 1 RM, whereas muscular endurance is improved using loads less than 50 percent of your 1 RM.

DID YOU **KNOW?**

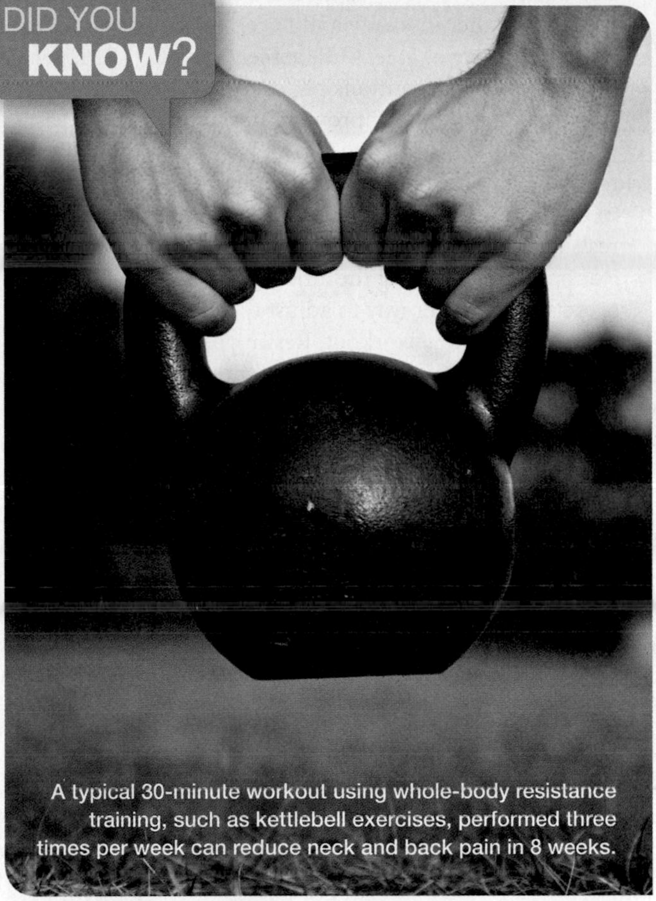

A typical 30-minute workout using whole-body resistance training, such as kettlebell exercises, performed three times per week can reduce neck and back pain in 8 weeks.

Source: K. Jay et al., "Kettlebell Training for Musculoskeletal and Cardiovascular Health: A Randomized Controlled Trial," *Scandinavian Journal of Work, Environment, and Health* 37, no. 3 (2011): 196–203.

Everyone begins a resistance training program at an initial level of strength. To become stronger, you must *overload* your muscles, that is, regularly create a degree of tension in your muscles that is greater than they are accustomed to. Overloading them forces your muscles to adapt by getting larger, stronger, and capable of producing more tension. If you "underload" your muscles, you will not increase strength. If you create too great an overload, you may experience muscle injury, muscle fatigue, and potentially a loss in strength. Once your strength goal is reached, no further overload is necessary; your challenge at that point is to maintain your level of strength by engaging in a regular (once or twice per week) total-body resistance exercise program.

one repetition maximum (1 RM) The amount of weight or resistance that can be lifted or moved only once.

Time The time recommended for muscular strength and endurance exercises is measured, not in minutes of exercise, but rather in repetitions and sets.

- **Repetitions and sets.** To increase muscular strength, you need higher intensity and fewer repetitions and sets: Use a resistance of at least 60 percent of your 1 RM, performing 8 to 12 repetitions per set, with two to four sets performed overall. If improving muscular endurance is your goal, use less resistance and more repetitions. The recommendations for improving muscular endurance are to perform one to two sets of 15 to 25 repetitions using a resistance that is less than 50 percent of your 1 RM.
- **Rest periods.** Varying the amount of rest between exercises is another way to adjust the intensity of your resistance-training workout. Resting between exercises is crucial to reduce fatigue and help with performance and safety in subsequent sets. A rest period of 2 to 3 minutes is recommended when using the guidelines for general health benefits. However, the rest period when working to develop strength or endurance will vary. Note that the rest period refers specifically to the muscle group being exercised, and it is possible to alternate muscle groups. For example, you can alternate a set of push-ups with curl-ups, as the muscle groups worked in one set can rest while you are working the other muscle groups.

Type To improve muscular strength or endurance, it is most often recommended that resistance training use either the body's weight or devices that provide a fixed or variable resistance (see **TABLE 9.4**). When selecting the type of strength-training exercises to do, there are three important principles to bear in mind: specificity, exercise selection, and exercise order. According to the *specificity principle,* the effects of resistance exercise training are specific to the muscles exercised; thus to improve total body strength, include exercises for all the major muscle groups.

The second important concept is *exercise selection.* It is important to select exercises that will meet your goals. Selecting eight to ten exercises targeting all major muscle groups is generally recommended and will ensure that exercises are balanced for opposing muscle groups.

Finally, for optimal training effects, pay attention to *exercise order.* When training all major muscle groups in a single workout, complete large muscle group exercises (e.g., the bench press or leg press) before small muscle group exercises, multiple-joint exercises before single-joint exercises (e.g., biceps curls, triceps extension), and high-intensity exercises before lower-intensity exercises.

The FITT Principle for Flexibility

Although often overshadowed by cardiorespiratory and muscular fitness training, flexibility is important. Improving your flexibility not only enhances the efficiency of your movements, it can enhance your sense of well-being, help manage stress effectively, and prevent or reduce joint pain. Furthermore, inflexible muscles are susceptible to injury, and flexibility training reduces the incidence and severity of lower back problems and muscle or tendon injuries.[36] Improved flexibility also means less tension and pressure on joints, resulting in less joint pain and joint deterioration.[37] This means that remaining flexible can help prevent the decreased physical function that often occurs with aging.[38] **FIGURE 9.7** illustrates some basic stretching exercises to increase flexibility.

TABLE **9.4** | Methods of Providing Muscular Resistance

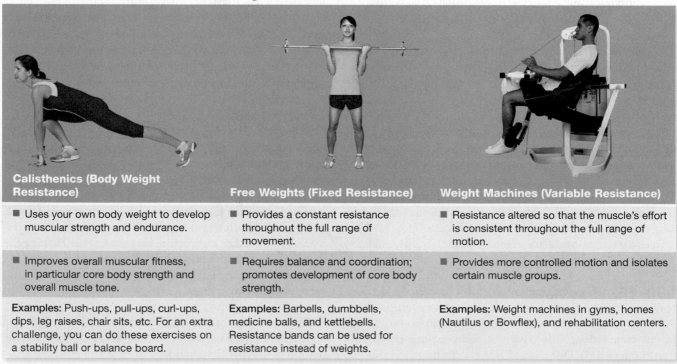

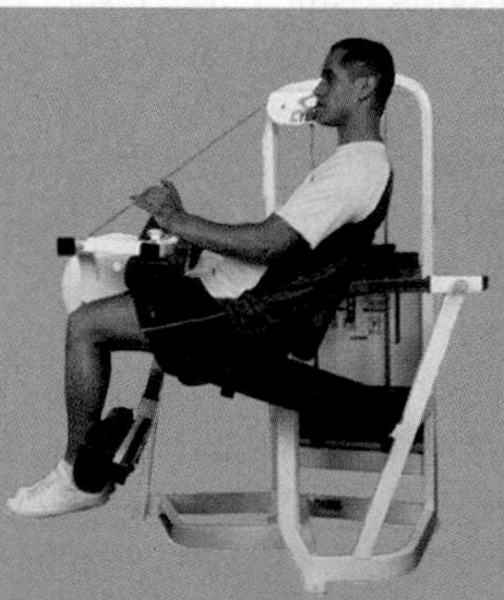

Calisthenics (Body Weight Resistance)	Free Weights (Fixed Resistance)	Weight Machines (Variable Resistance)
■ Uses your own body weight to develop muscular strength and endurance.	■ Provides a constant resistance throughout the full range of movement.	■ Resistance altered so that the muscle's effort is consistent throughout the full range of motion.
■ Improves overall muscular fitness, in particular core body strength and overall muscle tone.	■ Requires balance and coordination; promotes development of core body strength.	■ Provides more controlled motion and isolates certain muscle groups.
Examples: Push-ups, pull-ups, curl-ups, dips, leg raises, chair sits, etc. For an extra challenge, you can do these exercises on a stability ball or balance board.	**Examples:** Barbells, dumbbells, medicine balls, and kettlebells. Resistance bands can be used for resistance instead of weights.	**Examples:** Weight machines in gyms, homes (Nautilus or Bowflex), and rehabilitation centers.

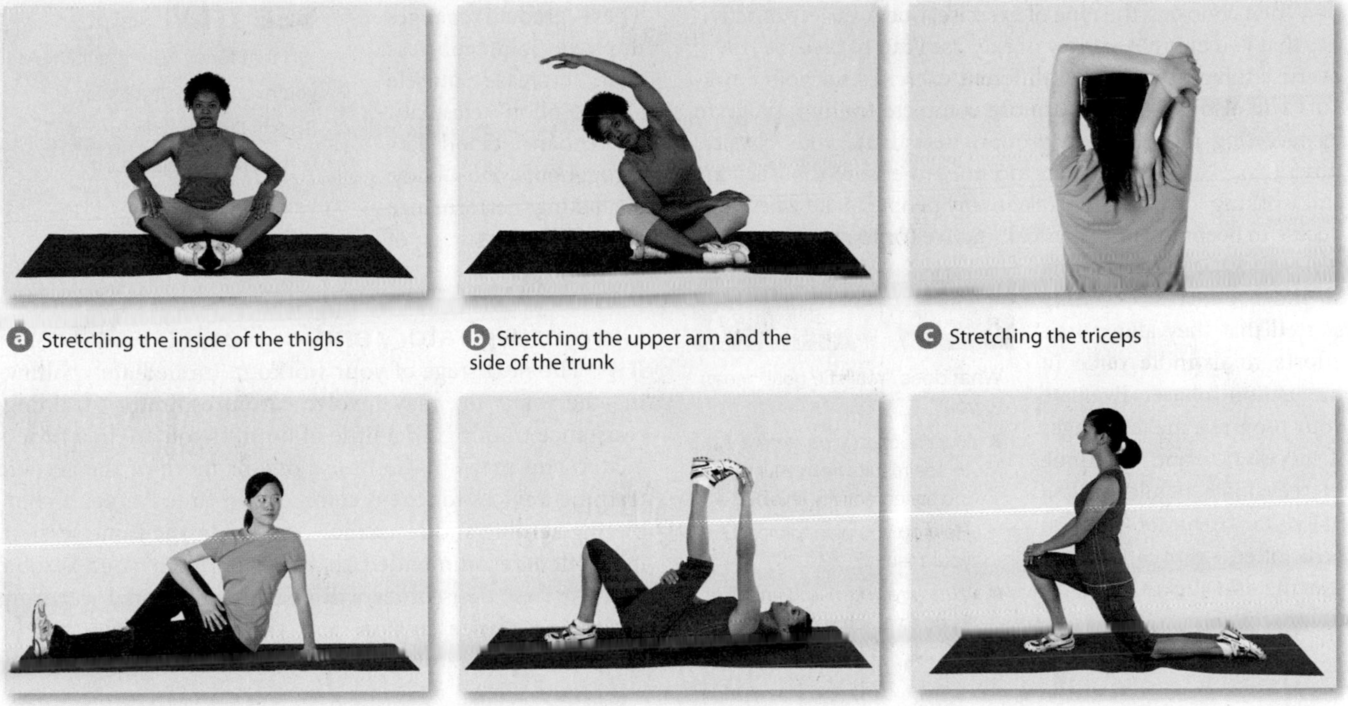

ⓐ Stretching the inside of the thighs

ⓑ Stretching the upper arm and the side of the trunk

ⓒ Stretching the triceps

ⓓ Stretching the trunk and the hip

ⓔ Stretching the hip, back of the thigh, and the calf

ⓕ Stretching the front of the thigh and the hip flexor

FIGURE 9.7 Stretching Exercises to Improve Flexibility Use these stretches as part of your cool-down. Hold each stretch for 10 to 30 seconds and repeat two to four times.

Frequency The FITT principle calls for a minimum of 2 to 3 days per week for flexibility training.

Intensity Flexibility has the least formal method for identifying the intensity required for improvement. Specifically, the recommendations are that you perform or hold stretching positions at an individually determined "point of mild tension." You should be able to feel tension or mild discomfort in the muscle(s) you are stretching, but the stretch should not hurt.[39]

Time The time recommended to improve flexibility is based upon time per stretch. Once you are in a stretching position, you should hold at the "point of tension" for 10 to 30 seconds for each stretch and repeat two to four times in close succession.[40]

Type The most effective exercises for increasing flexibility involve stretching the major muscle groups of your body when the body is already warm, such as after your cardiorespiratory workout. The safest exercises for improving flexibility involve **static stretching**. Static stretching techniques slowly and gradually lengthen a muscle or group of muscles and their tendons. The primary strategy is to decrease the resistance to stretch (tension) within a tight muscle targeted for increased range of motion.[41] To do this, you repeatedly stretch the muscle and its two tendons of attachment to elongate them. With each repetition of a static stretch, your range of motion improves temporarily due to the slightly lessened sensitivity of tension receptors in the stretched muscles; when done regularly, range of motion increases.[42]

LO 5 | IMPLEMENTING YOUR FITNESS PROGRAM

Devise a plan to implement your safe and effective fitness program.

As your physical fitness improves, you need to adjust the frequency, intensity, time, and type of your exercise to maintain or continue to improve your level of physical fitness.

Develop a Progressive Plan

Experts recommend that you begin an exercise regimen by picking an exercise and gradually increasing the frequency or time of your workouts. You should make gradual changes, and the intensity is the last component of your workout you will increase. For example, in week 1, you might exercise 3 days for 20 minutes per day, and then move to 4 days in week 3 or 4. Then, consider increasing your duration to 30 minutes per session over the next couple of weeks. In general, an increase of 5 to 10 minutes a session every 1 to 2 weeks is tolerated by most during the first month. Gradual increases in intensity are typically made once the duration and frequency goals are met.

static stretching Stretching techniques that slowly and gradually lengthen a muscle or group of muscles and their tendons.

When choosing the type of exercise, find a variety of activities that you enjoy. A variety of exercises can reduce the risk of overuse injuries. Choosing different exercises for your workouts will also provide for a more complete training program by targeting more muscle groups. Reevaluate your physical fitness goals and action plan monthly to ensure that they are still working for you. A mistake many people make when they decide to become more physically active (or to make any other behavior change) is putting so much effort into getting started that they allow their efforts to dwindle once in the action phase. Evaluate your progress, make changes if necessary, and continue to reevaluate regularly. The **Skills for Behavior Change** box offers more tips on starting and sticking with an exercise plan.

WHAT DO YOU THINK?

What does "realistic goal" mean to you?

- How soon do you expect to see results from your increased activity levels?
- How do you plan to measure your results?
- What are you willing and able to do to reach your goal?

SEE IT! VIDEOS

Will that fancy sports drink help you exercise better? Watch **Sports Drinks Science: Is It Hype?** available on MasteringHealth.™

Design Your Exercise Session

A well-designed exercise program should improve or maintain cardiorespiratory fitness, muscular strength and endurance, flexibility, and body composition. But what should you do when you begin your exercise routine? A comprehensive workout includes a warm-up, cardiorespiratory and/or resistance training, and then a cool-down to finish the session.

Warm-Up The warm-up prepares the body physically and mentally for cardiorespiratory and/or resistance training. A warm-up should involve large body movements, generally using light cardiorespiratory ac-tivities, followed by range-of-motion exercises of the muscle groups to be used during the exercise session. Usually 5 to 15 minutes long, a warm-up is shorter when you are geared up and ready to go and longer when you are struggling to get moving or your muscles are cold or tight. It's important to listen to your body and take the time you need to prepare for intense activity. The warm-up provides a transition from rest to physical activity by slowly increasing heart rate, blood pressure, breathing rate, and body temperature. These gradual changes improve joint lubrication, increase muscle and tendon elasticity, and enhance blood flow throughout the body, facilitating performance during the next stage of the workout.

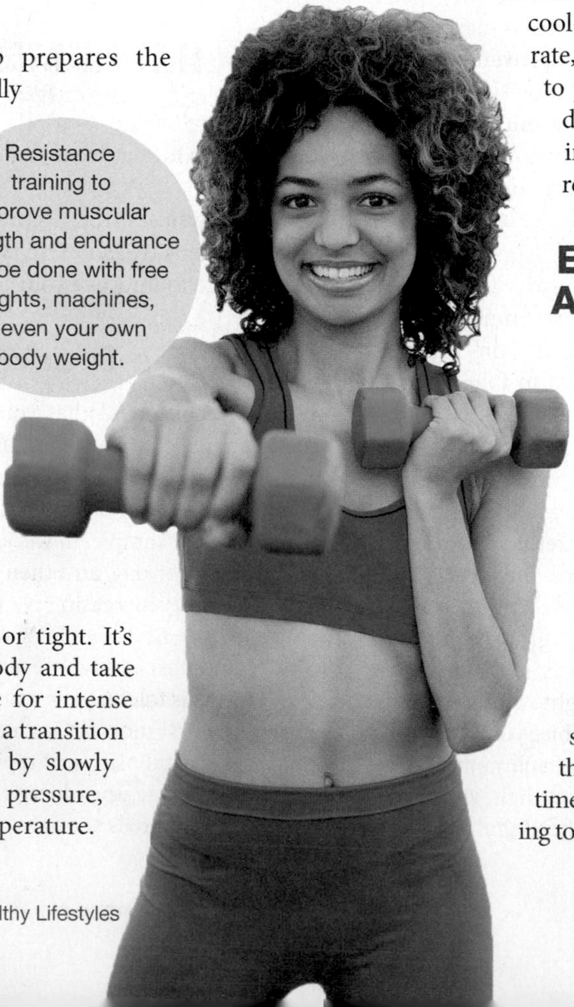

Resistance training to improve muscular strength and endurance can be done with free weights, machines, or even your own body weight.

Cardiorespiratory and/or Resistance Training The next stage of your workout, immediately following the warm-up, may involve cardiorespiratory training, resistance training, or a little of both. If you are in a fitness center, you may choose to use one or more of the aerobic training devices for the recommended time frame. If completing aerobic and resistance exercise in the same session, it is often recommended that you perform your aerobic exercise first. This order will provide additional warm-up for the resistance session, and your muscles will not be fatigued for the aerobic workout.

Cool-Down and Stretching Just as you ease into a workout with a warm-up, you should slowly transition from activity to rest. A cool-down is an essential component of a fitness program; it involves another 10 to 15 minutes of activity time. Start your cool-down with 5 to 10 minutes of moderate- to low-intensity activity, and follow it with approximately 5 to 10 minutes of stretching. Because of the body's increased temperature, the cool-down is an excellent time to stretch to improve flexibility. The purpose of the cool-down is to gradually reduce your heart rate, blood pressure, and body temperature to pre-exercise levels. In addition, the cool-down reduces the risk of blood pooling in the extremities and facilitates quicker recovery between exercise sessions.

Explore Fitness Activities

Some forms of activity have the potential to improve several components of physical fitness and thus improve your everyday functioning ("functional" exercises). For example, core strength training improves posture and can prevent back pain. In addition, yoga, tai chi, and Pilates improve flexibility, muscular strength and endurance, balance, coordination, and agility. They also develop the mind-body connection through concentration on breathing and body position. Some people see these activities as strongly connected to their spiritual health as well, particularly when time is spent relaxing, breathing deeply, and trying to quiet the mind.

SKILLS FOR BEHAVIOR CHANGE

PLAN IT, START IT, STICK WITH IT!

The most successful physical activity program is one that is realistic and appropriate for your skill level and needs.

- **Make it enjoyable.** Pick activities you like to do so you will make the effort and find the time to do it.
- **Start slowly.** If you have been physically inactive for a while or are a first-time exerciser, any type and amount of physical activity is a step in the right direction. Going to the fitness center or putting your sneakers on for a walk is already an achievement. Make sure you start slowly, letting your body adapt so that your new physical activity or exercise does not cause excess pain the next day (a real reaction to using muscles you have not used much or as intensely before). Do not be discouraged; you will increase your activity each week, and soon you will be on your way to meeting the physical activity recommendations and your personal goals!
- **Make only one lifestyle change at a time.** It is not realistic to change everything at once, as more than one major change at the same time is very difficult. For example, work on your time management skills and increase your lifestyle activity. Then, add a more structured exercise program. After making these changes you will likely be more motivated to change your diet or add resistance exercises. Success with one behavioral change will increase your confidence and encourage other positive changes.
- **Set reasonable expectations for yourself and your physical fitness program.** You will not become "fit" overnight. It takes several months to really feel the benefits of new physical activity. Be patient.
- **Choose a time to exercise and stick with it.** Set priorities and keep to a schedule. Try exercising at different times of the day to learn what works best for you. Yet be flexible, so if something comes up that you cannot work around, you will find time later that day or evening to do some physical activity. Be careful of an all-or-none attitude.
- **Keep a record of your progress.** Include the intensity, time, and type of physical activity, your emotions, and your personal achievements.
- **Take lapses in stride.** Sometimes life gets in the way. Start again and do not despair; your commitment to physical fitness has ebbs and flows like everything else in life.

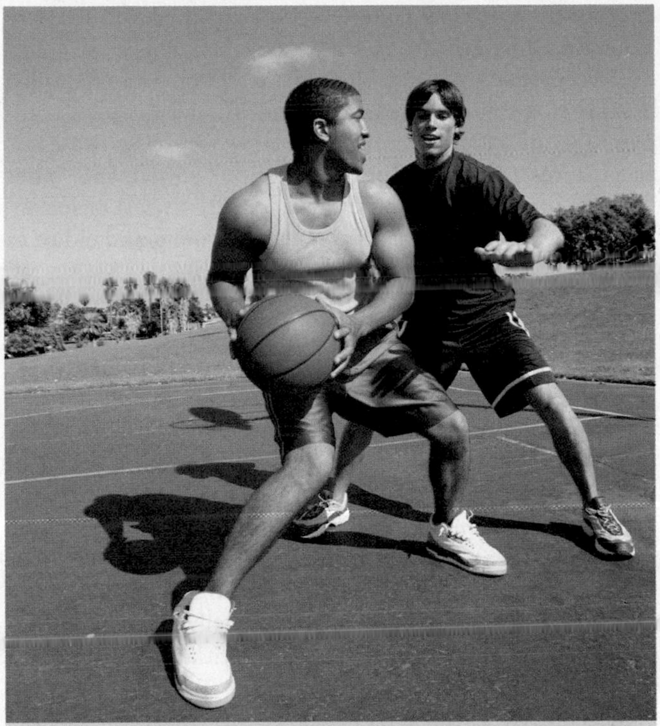

Your core muscles are essential for supporting your spine in everything you do—from standing to sitting, from dancing to playing basketball. Core muscles work together to effectively transmit forces between your upper and lower body, allowing you to twist, jump, lift, bend, and change directions. While weak core muscles can lead to back pain, strong core muscles can prevent back pain and improve physical performance in all of your activities.

Core Strength Training Before we explore yoga, tai chi, and Pilates, let's consider core strength for a moment. The body's core muscles are the foundation for all movement.[43] These muscles include the deep back, abdominal, and hip muscles that attach to the spine and pelvis. The contraction of these muscles provides the basis of support for movements of the upper and lower body and powerful movements of the extremities. A weak core generally results in poor posture, low back pain, and muscle injuries. A strong core provides a more stable center of gravity, and as a result, a more stable platform for movements, thus reducing the chance of injury.

You can develop core strength by doing various exercises, including calisthenics, yoga, or Pilates. Holding yourself in a front or reverse plank (an upward-facing version of a push-up position) or doing abdominal curl-ups are examples of exercises that increase core strength. Increased core strength does not happen from one single exercise, but rather from a structured regime of postures and exercises.[44] The use of instability devices (stability ball, wobble boards, etc.) and exercises to train the core have become popular.[45] Although research suggests instability training is effective for improving core strength and reducing back pain, it should not replace traditional programs completely; it should rather be used in conjunction with and become part of the FITT prescription.[46]

Yoga Yoga, based on ancient Indian practices, blends the mental and physical aspects of exercise—a union of mind and body that participants often find relaxing and satisfying. If done regularly, yoga improves flexibility, vitality, posture, agility, balance, coordination, and muscular strength and endurance. Many people also report an improved sense of general well-being.

The practice of yoga focuses attention on controlled breathing and physical exercise, and it incorporates a complex array of static stretching and balance exercises expressed as postures (*asanas*). During a session, participants move to different asanas and hold them for 30 seconds or longer. Asanas can be changed and adapted for young and old or to accommodate physical limitations or disabilities. Asanas can also be combined to provide well-conditioned athletes with a challenging workout.

Some forms of yoga are more meditative in their practice, whereas other forms, such as Ashtanga and Bikram, are more athletic. *Ashtanga yoga,* also called "power yoga," is an energetic form of yoga that focuses on a series of poses done in a continuous, repeated flow, with controlled breathing. *Bikram yoga,* also known as *hot yoga,* is unique in that classes are held in rooms heated to 105°F. The theory behind this practice is that performing yoga in a hot environment allows the muscles to easily stretch to their point of tension with a greater potential for increasing flexibility.

Tai Chi Tai chi is an ancient Chinese form of exercise that combines stretching, balance, muscular endurance, coordination, and meditation. It increases range of motion and flexibility while reducing muscular tension. Based on Qigong, a Taoist philosophy dedicated to spiritual growth and good health, tai chi was developed about AD 1000 by monks who wanted to defend themselves against bandits and warlords. It involves a series of positions called *forms* that are performed continuously. Tai chi is often described as "meditation in motion" because it promotes serenity through gentle movements that connect the mind and body.

Pilates Developed by Joseph Pilates in 1926, Pilates is an exercise style that combines stretching with movement against resistance, frequently aided by devices such as tension springs or heavy rubber bands. It teaches body awareness, good posture, and easy and graceful body movements while improving flexibility, coordination, core strength, muscle tone, and economy of motion.

Pilates differs from yoga and tai chi in that it includes a component specifically designed to increase strength. The method consists of a sequence of carefully performed movements. Some are carried out on specially designed equipment, whereas others can be performed on mats. Each exercise stretches and strengthens the muscles involved and has a specific breathing pattern associated with it.

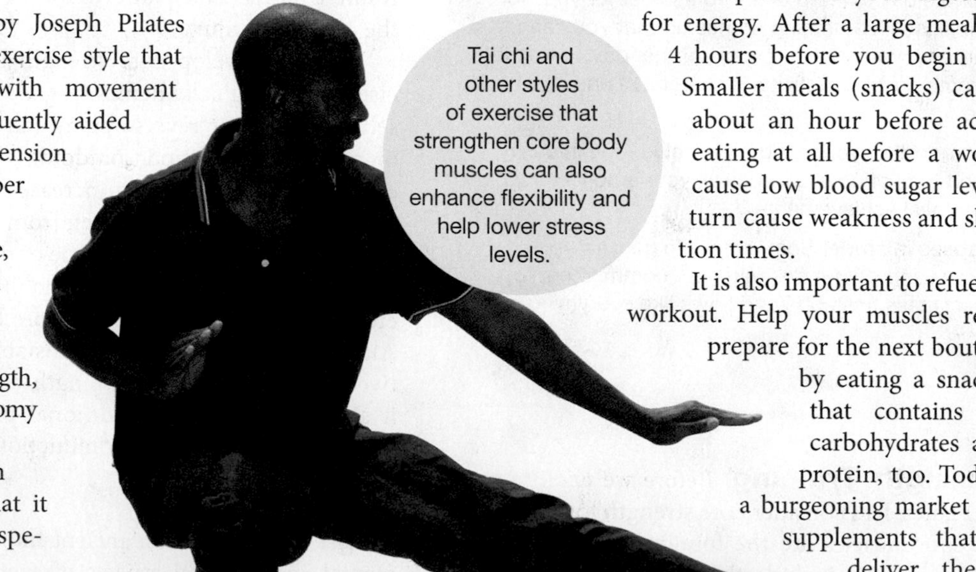

Tai chi and other styles of exercise that strengthen core body muscles can also enhance flexibility and help lower stress levels.

LO 6 | TAKING IN PROPER **NUTRITION** FOR EXERCISE

Describe optimal foods and fluids consumption recommendations for exercise and recovery.

It's important to evaluate your eating habits in light of your exercise habits. Whether you're a seasoned fitness buff or a beginner, the importance of proper nutrition for exercise can't be overstated.

Foods for Exercise and Recovery

To make the most of your workouts, follow the recommendations from the MyPlate plan, and make sure that you eat sufficient carbohydrates, the body's main source of fuel. Your body stores carbohydrates as glycogen primarily in the muscles and liver and then uses this stored glycogen for energy when you are physically active. Fats are also an important source of energy, packing more than double the energy per gram compared to carbohydrates. Protein plays a role in muscle repair and growth, but is not normally a source of energy.

When you eat is almost as important as what you eat. Eating a large meal before exercising can cause upset stomach, cramping, and diarrhea, because your muscles have to compete with your digestive system for energy. After a large meal, wait 3 to 4 hours before you begin exercising. Smaller meals (snacks) can be eaten about an hour before activity. Not eating at all before a workout can cause low blood sugar levels that in turn cause weakness and slower reaction times.

It is also important to refuel after your workout. Help your muscles recover and prepare for the next bout of activity by eating a snack or meal that contains plenty of carbohydrates and a little protein, too. Today, there is a burgeoning market for dietary supplements that claim to deliver the nutrients needed for muscle recovery, as well as additional "performance-enhancing" ingredients; see **TABLE 9.5** for some of the most popular performance-enhancing drugs and supplements, their purported benefits, and associated risks.

Fluids for Exercise and Recovery

In addition to eating well, staying hydrated is also crucial. How much fluid do you need? Keep in mind that the goal of fluid replacement is to prevent excessive dehydration (greater than 2% loss of body weight). The ACSM and the National Athletic Trainers Association recommend consuming 5 to 7 milliliters per kilogram of body weight (approximately 0.7 to 1.07 ounces per 10 pounds body weight) 4 hours prior to exercise.[47] Drinking fluids during exercise is also important, but it is difficult to provide guidelines for how much or when because intake should be based on time, intensity, and type of activity performed. A good way to monitor how much fluid you need to replace is to weigh yourself before and after your workout. The difference in weight is how much you should drink. So, for example, if you lost 2 pounds during a training session, you should drink 32 ounces of fluid.[48]

What are the best fluids to drink? For exercise sessions lasting less than 1 hour, plain water is sufficient for rehydration. If your exercise session exceeds 1 hour—and you sweat profusely—consider a sports drink containing electrolytes. The electrolytes in these products are minerals and ions such as sodium and potassium that are needed for proper functioning of your nervous and muscular systems. Replacing electrolytes is particularly important for endurance athletes.

TABLE **9.5** | Performance-Enhancing Dietary Supplements and Drugs—Their Uses and Effects

Supplement/Drug	Primary Uses	Side Effects
Creatine Naturally occurring compound that helps supply energy to muscle	■ Improve postworkout recovery ■ Increase muscle mass ■ Increase strength ■ Increase power	■ Weight gain, nausea, muscle cramps ■ Large doses can impair kidney function
Ephedra and ephedrine Stimulant that constricts blood vessels and increases blood pressure and heart rate *Illegal; banned by FDA in 2006; banned by sports organizations	■ Lose weight ■ Increase performance	■ Nausea, vomiting ■ Anxiety and mood changes ■ Hyperactivity ■ Rarely seizures, heart attack, stroke, psychotic episodes
Anabolic steroids Synthetic versions of the hormone testosterone *Nonmedical use is illegal; banned by major sports organizations	■ Improve strength, power, and speed ■ Increase muscle mass	■ In adolescents, stops bone growth; therefore reduced adult height ■ Masculinization of females; feminization of males ■ Mood swings ■ Severe acne, particularly on the back ■ Sexual dysfunction ■ Aggressive behavior ■ Potential heart and liver damage
Steroid precursors Substances that the body converts into anabolic steroids, for example, androstenedione (andro), dehydroepiandrosterone (DHEA) *Nonmedical use is illegal; banned by major sports organizations	■ Converted in the body to anabolic steroids to increase muscle mass	■ In addition to side effects noted with anabolic steroids: ■ Body hair growth, increased risk of pancreatic cancer
Human growth hormone Naturally occurring hormone secreted by the pituitary gland that is essential for body growth *Nonmedical use is illegal; banned by major sports organizations	■ Antiaging agent ■ Improve performance ■ Increase muscle mass	■ Structural changes to the face ■ Increased risk of high blood pressure ■ Potential for congestive heart failure

Sources: Mayo Clinic Staff, "Performance-Enhancing Drugs and Your Teen Athlete," MayoClinic.com, August 2013, www.mayoclinic.com/health/performance-enhancing-drugs/SM00045; Office of Diversion Control, Drug and Chemical Evaluation Section, "Drugs and Chemicals of Concern: Human Growth Hormone," August 2013, www.deadiversion.usdoj.gov/drug_chem_info/hgh.pdf; Office of Dietary Supplements, National Institutes of Health, "Ephedra and Ephedrine Alkaloids for Weight Loss and Athletic Performance," reviewed July 2004, http://ods.od.nih.gov/factsheets/EphedraandEphedrine.

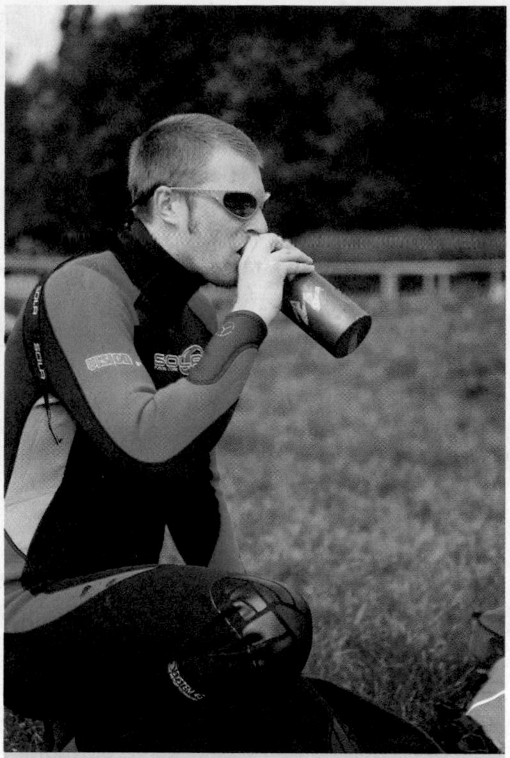

The American College of Sports Medicine and the National Athletic Trainers' Association recommend consuming 14 to 22 ounces of fluid several hours prior to exercise and about 6 to 12 ounces per 15 to 20 minutes during—assuming you are sweating.

In endurance events lasting more than 4 hours, an athlete's overconsumption of plain water can dilute the sodium concentration in the blood with potentially fatal results, an effect called **hyponatremia** or **water intoxication**.

What is the best choice to replenish fluids after a workout? Although water is the best choice in most cases, there are situations in which you might need to choose something different. Some people are likely to consume more when their drink is flavored, a point that may be significant in ensuring proper hydration. Recently, research has considered chocolate milk as a recovery drink.[49] Chocolate milk is a liquid that not only hydrates, but also is a source of sodium, potassium, carbohydrates, and protein. Consuming carbohydrates and protein immediately after exercise will help replenish muscle and liver glycogen stores and stimulate muscle protein synthesis for better recovery from exercise. The protein in milk, whey protein, is ideal because it contains all of the essential amino acids and is rapidly absorbed by the body. Low-fat chocolate milk is a good choice to hydrate and recover after exercise.

hyponatremia or water intoxication Overconsumption of water, which leads to a dilution of sodium concentration in the blood, with potentially fatal results.

traumatic injuries Injuries that are accidental and occur suddenly and violently.

overuse injuries Injuries that result from the cumulative effects of day-after-day stresses placed on tendons, muscles, and joints.

LO 7 | PREVENTING AND TREATING COMMON EXERCISE INJURIES

Explain how to prevent and treat common exercise injuries.

There are two basic types of exercise injuries: traumatic and overuse injuries. **Traumatic injuries** occur suddenly and violently, typically by accident. Typical traumatic injuries are broken bones, torn ligaments and muscles, contusions, and lacerations. Many traumatic injuries are unavoidable—for example, spraining your ankle by landing on another person's foot after jumping up for a rebound in basketball. Others are preventable through proper training, appropriate equipment and clothing, and common sense. If your traumatic injury causes a noticeable loss of function, immediate pain, or pain that does not go away after 30 minutes, consult a physician.

Doing too much intense exercise, too much exercise without variation, or not allowing for sufficient rest and recovery time increase the likelihood of **overuse injuries**. Overuse injuries occur because of cumulative, day-after-day stresses placed on tendons, muscles, and joints.

WHAT DO YOU THINK?

In what ways do your physical activities put you at risk of injury?

- What changes can you make in terms of your training program, equipment, or footwear to reduce these risks?

Common Overuse Injuries

Three of the most common overuse injuries are plantar fasciitis, shin splints, and runner's knee.

Plantar Fasciitis *Plantar fasciitis* is an inflammation of the plantar fascia, a broad band of dense, inelastic tissue (fascia) that runs from the heel to the toe on the bottom of your foot. The main function of the plantar fascia is to protect the nerves, blood vessels, and muscles of the foot from injury. In repetitive, weight-bearing physical activities such as walking and running, the plantar fascia may become inflamed. Common symptoms are pain and tenderness under the ball of the foot, at the heel, or at both locations.[50] The pain of plantar fasciitis is particularly noticeable during your first steps in the morning. If not treated properly, this injury may progress until weight-bearing activities are too painful to endure.

Shin Splints *Shin splints,* a general term for any pain that occurs on the front part of the lower legs, describes more than 20 different medical conditions. The most common type of shin splints occurs along the inner side of the tibia and is usually a combination of muscle irritation and irritation of the tissues that attach the muscles to the bone. Specific pain on the tibia or on the fibula (the adjacent smaller bone) should be examined for a possible stress fracture.

Sedentary people who start a new weight-bearing physical activity program are at the greatest risk for shin splints, although even well-conditioned aerobic exercisers who rapidly increase their distance or pace may be at risk.[51] Running and exercise classes are the most frequent cause of shin splints, but those who do a great deal of walking (such as postal carriers and restaurant workers) may also develop them.

Runner's Knee *Runner's knee* describes a series of problems involving the muscles, tendons, and ligaments of the knee. The most common cause is abnormal movements of the patella (or kneecap), and women are more commonly affected due to greater dynamic flexibility in their hips and knees. With runner's knee, abnormal patella movements irritate the cartilage on the back of the patella and nearby tendons and ligaments. The main symptom is pain experienced when downward pressure is applied to the kneecap after the knee is straightened fully. Additional symptoms include pain, swelling, redness, and tenderness around the patella, and a dull aching pain in the center of the knee.[52]

Prevent Exercise Injuries

To reduce your risk of overuse or traumatic injuries, use common sense and the proper gear and equipment. Vary your physical activities throughout the week, setting appropriate and realistic short- and long-term goals. Listen to your body when working out. Warning signs include muscle stiffness and soreness, bone and joint pains, and whole-body fatigue that simply does not go away.

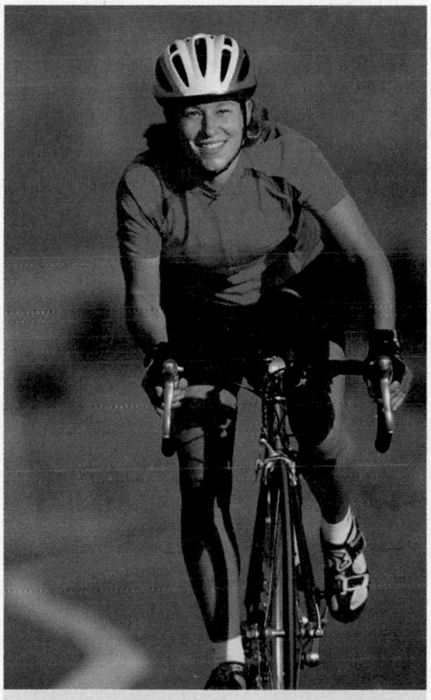

Reducing risk for exercise injuries requires common sense and some preventative measures. Wear protec-tive gear (helmets, knee pads, elbow pads, eyewear) and footwear that is appropriate for your activity. Vary your activities to avoid overuse injuries. Dress for the weather, try to avoid exercising in extreme condi-tions, and always stay properly hydrated. Finally, respect your personal physical limitations, listen to your body, and if needed, reevaluate and change your exercise program.

Appropriate Footwear Proper footwear can decrease the likelihood of foot, knee, or back injuries. Biomechanics research has revealed that running is a collision sport—with each stride, the runner's foot collides with the ground with a force three to five times the runner's body weight.[53] The force not absorbed by the running shoe is transmitted upward into the foot, leg, thigh, and back. Our bodies can absorb forces such as these, but may be injured by the cumulative effect of repetitive impacts (such as running 40 miles per week). Thus, the shoes' ability to absorb shock is critical—not just for runners, but for anyone engaged in weight-bearing activities.

In addition to absorbing shock, an athletic shoe should provide a good fit for maximal comfort and performance. To get the best fit, shop at a sports or fitness specialty store where there is a large selection and the salespeople are trained in properly fitting athletic shoes. Try on shoes later in the day when your feet are largest, and check to make sure there is a little extra room in the toe and that the width is appropriate. Because different activities place different stresses on your feet and joints, you should choose shoes specifically designed for your sport or activity. Shoes of any type should be replaced once they lose their cushioning. A common rule of thumb is to replace running shoes after 300 to 500 miles of usage, which is typically between 3 and 9 months depending on your activity level. Let your body be the judge. If you start to feel aches and pains that can't be attributed to other factors, it may be time to shop for a new pair of shoes.

Appropriate Protective Equipment It is essential to use well-fitted, appropriate protective equipment for your physical activities. For example, using the correct racquet with the proper tension helps prevent the general inflammatory condition known as tennis elbow. As another example, eye injuries can occur in virtually all physical activities, although some activities (such as baseball, basketball, and racquet sports) are more risky than others.[54] As many as 90 percent of eye injuries could be prevented by wearing appropriate eye protection, such as goggles with polycarbonate lenses.[55]

Wearing a helmet while bicycle riding is an important safety precaution. An estimated 66 to 88 percent of head injuries among cyclists can be prevented by wearing a helmet.[56] Of the college students who rode a bike in the past 12 months, 42.9 percent reported never wearing a helmet, and 22.7 percent said they wore one only sometimes or rarely.[57] The direct medical costs from cyclists' failure to wear helmets is an estimated $81 million a year.[58] Cyclists aren't the only ones who should be wearing helmets. People who skateboard, ski, in-line skate, snowboard, play contact sports, or use kick-scooters should also wear helmets. Look for helmets that meet the standards established by the American National Standards Institute or the Snell Memorial Foundation. (The **Money & Health** box on the next page offers suggestions for evaluating and choosing a fitness center, equipment, and fitness clothing.)

Exercising in the Heat Exercising in hot or humid weather increases your risk of a heat-related illness. In these conditions, your body's rate of heat production can exceed its ability to cool itself. The three different heat stress illnesses, progressive in their level of severity, are heat cramps, heat exhaustion, and heatstroke.

MONEY & HEALTH | INVESTING IN YOUR PHYSICAL HEALTH! *How to Shop for Fitness Facilities, Equipment, and Clothing*

To achieve your personal goals, all you need is a good pair of shoes, comfortable clothing to suit the environment you will be physically active in, your own body to use as resistance, and a safe place for activity. However, you may enjoy going to a fitness center or want to buy exercise equipment to enhance your workout, and you may need new exercise clothing. Use the following tips to help guide you through this process.

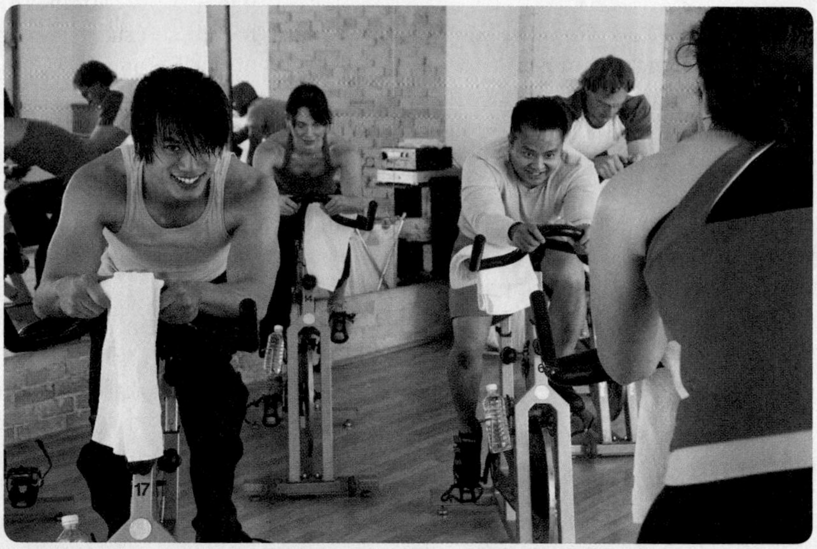

Before you sign on the dotted line, check out the classes, equipment, and personnel a fitness center offers.

Choosing a Facility

- Visit several facilities before making a decision, if possible during the time when you intend to use them (so you can see how busy or crowded they are at that time).
- Determine the location and hours of operation; are these convenient for you?
- Consider the exercise classes offered. What is the schedule? Can you try a class for free? Are classes included in the price of membership, or do they cost extra?
- Evaluate their equipment. Is it sufficient to cover your training needs (e.g., aerobic exercise machines, resistance-training equipment, mats, and other items to assist with stretching)? Is it kept clean and in good condition? Do they offer instruction in how to use the equipment?
- Consider the personnel (including training in first aid and CPR), options for working with a personal trainer, and how friendly and approachable they are.
- Consider the financial implications. What membership benefits, student rates, or other discounts are available? Steer clear of clubs that pressure you for a long-term commitment and do not offer trial memberships or grace periods that allow you to get a refund.

Buying Exercise Clothing

- Choose your exercise clothing based on comfort, not looks. It should be neither too loose nor too tight.
- Consider the environment (temperature, humidity, ventilation) when making your selection.
- Choose clothing that helps you to feel good about yourself and the activity you are undertaking.

heat cramps Involuntary and forcible muscle contractions that occur during or following exercise in hot and/or humid weather.

heat exhaustion A heat stress illness caused by significant dehydration resulting from exercise in hot and/or humid conditions.

heatstroke A deadly heat stress illness resulting from dehydration and overexertion in hot and/or humid conditions.

Heat cramps (heat-related involuntary and forcible muscle contractions that cannot be relaxed), the least serious problem, can usually be prevented by adequate fluid replacement and a dietary intake that includes the electrolytes lost through sweating.

Heat exhaustion is actually a mild form of shock, in which the blood pools in the arms and legs away from the brain and major organs of the body. Caused by excessive water loss from intense or prolonged exercise or work in a hot and/or humid environment, symptoms of heat exhaustion include nausea, headache, fatigue, dizziness and faintness, and, paradoxically, "goosebumps" and chills. When suffering from heat exhaustion, your skin will be cool and moist.

Heatstroke, often called *sunstroke,* is a life-threatening emergency condition with a high morbidity and mortality rate.[59] Heatstroke occurs during vigorous exercise when the body's heat production significantly exceeds its cooling capacities. Core body temperature can rise from normal (98.6°F) to 105°F to 110°F within minutes after the body's cooling mechanism shuts down. A rapid increase in core body temperature can cause brain damage, permanent disability, and death. Common signs of heatstroke are dry, hot, and usually red skin; very high body temperature; and rapid heart rate. If you experience any of the symptoms mentioned here, stop exercising immediately. Move to the shade or a cool spot to rest and drink plenty of cool fluids for heat cramps and exhaustion. If heatstroke is suspected, seek medical attention immediately.

Heat stress illnesses may also occur in situations in which the danger is not so obvious. Serious or fatal heat stroke may result from prolonged immersion in a sauna, hot tub, or steam bath or from exercising in a plastic or rubber head-to-toe "sauna suit." Similarly, exercising or training in the heat with lots of heavy clothing and equipment, such as a football uniform, including the helmet, puts an individual at risk.

To prevent heat stress, first, acclimatize yourself to hot or humid conditions. The process of heat acclimatization, which increases your body's cooling efficiency, requires about 10 to 14 days of gradually increased physical activity in the hot environment. Second, reduce your risk of dehydration by replacing fluids before, during, and after exercise. Third, wear clothing appropriate for the activity and the environment—for example, light-colored nylon shorts and a mesh tank top. Finally, use common sense—for example, on a day when the temperature is 85°F and the humidity is 80 percent, postpone your lunchtime run until the evening when it is cooler.

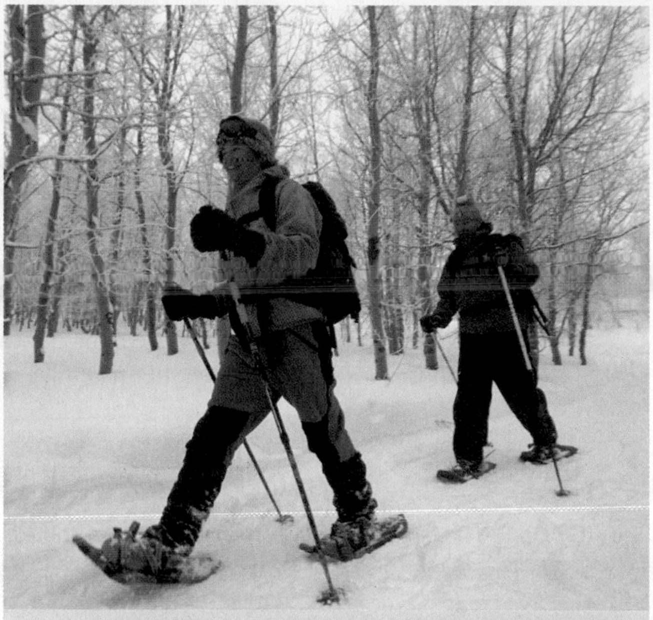

Staying with a friend and dressing in layers are two key tips for making cold weather exercise both safe and fun.

Exercising in the Cold When you exercise in cool weather, especially in windy conditions, your body's rate of heat loss is frequently greater than its rate of heat production. These conditions may lead to **hypothermia**—a condition where the body's core temperature drops below 95°F. Temperatures need not be frigid for hypothermia to occur; it can also result from prolonged, vigorous exercise in 40°F to 50°F temperatures, particularly if there is rain, snow, or a strong wind.

As body core temperature drops from its normal 98.6°F to about 93.2°F, shivering begins. Shivering—the involuntary contraction of nearly every muscle in the body—increases body temperature by using the heat given off by muscle activity. You may also experience cold hands and feet, poor judgment, apathy, and amnesia. Shivering ceases in most hypothermia victims as body core temperatures drop to between 87°F and 90°F, a sign that the body has lost its ability to generate heat. Death usually occurs at body core temperatures between 75°F and 80°F.

To prevent hypothermia, analyze weather conditions before engaging in outdoor physical activity. Remember that wind and humidity are as significant as temperature. Have a friend join you for safety when exercising outdoors in cold weather and wear layers of appropriate clothing to prevent excessive heat loss and frostbite. Keep your head, hands, and feet warm. Finally, do not allow yourself to become dehydrated.

Applying ice to an injury such as a sprain can help relieve pain and reduce swelling, but never apply the ice directly to the skin, as that could lead to frostbite.

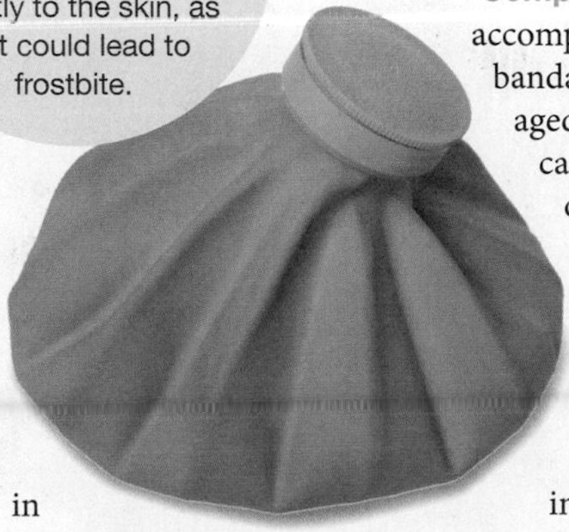

hypothermia Potentially fatal condition caused by abnormally low body core temperature.

RICE Acronym for the standard first-aid treatment for virtually all traumatic and overuse injuries: **r**est, **i**ce, **c**ompression, and **e**levation.

Treat Exercise Injuries

First-aid treatment for virtually all fitness-training related injuries involves **RICE**: rest, ice, compression, and elevation.

- Rest—is required to avoid further irritation of the injured body part.
- Ice—is applied to relieve pain and constrict the blood vessels to reduce internal or external bleeding. To prevent frostbite, wrap the ice or cold pack in a layer of wet toweling or elastic bandage before applying it to your skin. A new injury should be iced for approximately 20 minutes every hour for the first 24 to 72 hours.
- Compression—of the injured body part can be accomplished with a 4- or 6-inch-wide elastic bandage; this applies indirect pressure to damaged blood vessels to help stop bleeding. Be careful, though, that the compression wrap does not interfere with normal blood flow. Throbbing or pain indicates that the compression wrap should be loosened.
- Elevation—of an injured extremity above the level of your heart also helps control internal or external bleeding by making the blood flow upward to reach the injured area.

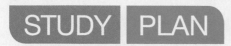

STUDY PLAN

Customize your study plan—and master your health!—in the Study Area of **MasteringHealth**.

ASSESS **YOURSELF**

Want to measure your muscular strength, flexibility, and cardiovascular endurance? Take the **How Physically Fit Are You?** assessment available on MasteringHealth.™

Need help creating a plan? Follow the strategies in the **Your Plan for Change** box for short- and long-term improvements to your health.

YOUR PLAN FOR **CHANGE**

The **ASSESS YOURSELF** activity mentioned above should help you determine your current level of physical fitness. Based on your results, you may decide that you should take steps to improve one or more components of your physical fitness.

TODAY, YOU CAN:

- ☐ Visit your campus fitness facility (or its website) and familiarize yourself with the equipment and resources. Find out what classes it offers, and take home (or print out) a copy of the schedule.
- ☐ Walk between your classes; make an extra effort to take the long way to get from building to building. Use the stairs instead of the elevator or escalator.
- ☐ Take an activity break. Spend 5 to 10 minutes between homework projects or just before bed doing some type of activity, such as abdominal crunches, push-ups, or yoga poses.

WITHIN THE NEXT 2 WEEKS, YOU CAN:

- ☐ Shop for comfortable workout clothes and appropriate athletic footwear.
- ☐ Look into group activities on your campus or in your community that you might enjoy.
- ☐ Ask a friend to join you in your workout once a week. Agree on a date and time in advance so you'll both be committed to following through.
- ☐ Plan for a physically active outing with a friend or date; perhaps you can go dancing, bowling, or shoot hoops. Use active transportation (e.g., walk or cycle) to get to a movie or go out for dinner.

BY THE END OF THE SEMESTER, YOU CAN:

- ☐ Establish a regular routine of engaging in physical activity or exercise at least three times a week. Mark your exercise times on your calendar and keep a log to track your progress.
- ☐ Take your workouts to the next level. If you are walking, try walking up hills, intermittent jogging, or sign up for a fitness event such as a charity 5K.

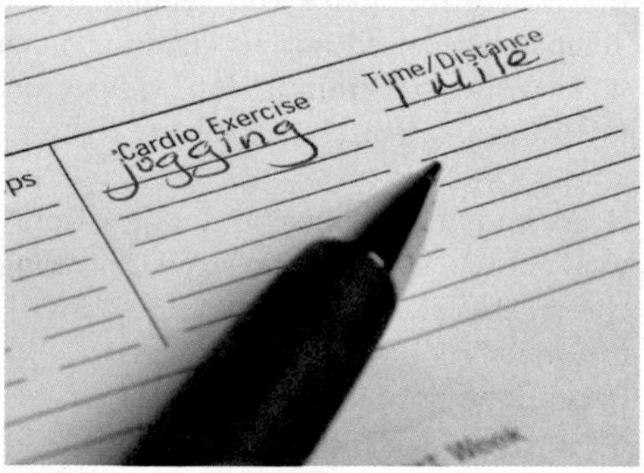

CHAPTER REVIEW

To hear an MP3 Tutor Session, scan here or visit the Study Area in **MasteringHealth.**

LO 1 Physical Activity for Health

- Health benefits of regular physical activity include reduced risk of heart attack, some cancers, hypertension, and type 2 diabetes and improved blood profile, bone mass, weight control, immunity to disease, mental health, and stress management.

LO 2 Physical Activity for Fitness and Performance

- Physical fitness involves achieving minimal levels in the health-related components of fitness: cardiorespiratory, muscular strength, muscular endurance, flexibility, and body composition. Skill-related components of fitness, such as agility, balance, reaction time, speed, coordination, and power, are essential for elite and recreational athletes to increase their performance.

LO 3 Committing to Physical Fitness

- Commit to physical activity by incorporating fitness activities into your life. If you are new to exercise, start slowly, keep your fitness program simple, and consider consulting your physician and/or a fitness instructor. Overcome obstacles to exercise by identifying them and then planning specific strategies to address them. Choose activities that are fun and convenient to increase your likelihood of sticking with them.

LO 4 Creating Your Own Fitness Program

- The FITT principle can be used to develop a progressive program of physical fitness. For general health benefits, every adult should participate in moderate-intensity activities for 30 minutes at least 5 days a week. To improve cardiorespiratory fitness, you should engage in vigorous, continuous, and rhythmic activities 3 to 5 days per week at an exercise intensity of 64 to 95 percent of your maximum heart rate for 20 to 30 minutes.
- Three key principles for developing muscular strength and endurance are overload, specificity of training, and reversibility. Muscular strength is improved by engaging in resistance-training exercises two to three times per week, using an intensity of greater than 60 percent of 1 RM, and completing two to four sets of 8 to 12 repetitions. Muscular endurance is improved by engaging in resistance-training exercises two to three times per week, using an intensity of less than 50 percent of 1 RM, and completing one to two sets of 15 to 25 repetitions.
- Flexibility is improved by engaging in two to four repetitions of static stretching exercises at least 2 to 3 days a week, where each stretch is held for 10 to 30 seconds.

LO 5 Implementing Your Fitness Program

- Planning to improve your physical fitness involves setting goals and designing a program to achieve these goals. A comprehensive workout repeated regularly will increase physical fitness and should include a warm-up with some light stretching, strength-development exercises, aerobic activities, and a cool-down period with a heavier emphasis on stretching exercises. Core strength training is important for mobility, stability, and preventing back injury.

LO 6 Taking in Proper Nutrition for Exercise

- Fueling properly for exercise involves eating a balance of healthy foods 3 to 4 hours before exercise. In exercise sessions lasting an hour or more, performance can benefit from some additional calories ingested during the exercise session. Hydrating properly for exercise is important for performance and injury prevention.

LO 7 Preventing and Treating Common Exercise Injuries

- Exercise injuries are generally caused by overuse or trauma; the most common are plantar fasciitis, shin splints, and runner's knee. Proper footwear and equipment can help prevent injuries. Exercising in the heat or cold requires taking special precautions. Minor exercise injuries should be treated with RICE (rest, ice, compression, and elevation).

POP QUIZ

Visit **MasteringHealth** to personalize your study plan with Chapter Review Quizzes and Dynamic Study Modules.

LO 1 Physical Activity for Health

1. What is physical fitness?
   a. The ability to respond to routine physical demands
   b. Having enough physical reserves to cope with a sudden challenge
   c. A balance of cardiorespiratory, muscle, and flexibility fitness
   d. All of the above
2. Which of the following is not associated with increased risk for type 2 diabetes?
   a. having type 1 diabetes
   b. obesity
   c. physical inactivity
   d. all of the above are risk factors for type 2 diabetes
3. Theresa wants increase the amount of weight she can bench press. She wants to work on her
   a. flexibility.
   b. muscular endurance.
   c. muscular strength.
   d. body composition.

LO 2 Physical Activity for Fitness and Performance

4. The volume of oxygen consumed by the muscles during maximal exercise defines
   a. fitness capacity.
   b. overall fitness.
   c. aerobic capacity.
   d. muscular endurance.
5. Muscular endurance is defined by your ability to
   a. contract muscles repeatedly over time.
   b. lift a heavy weight one time.
   c. hike for 8 hours.
   d. reach your toes during a muscle-stretching test.

LO 3 Committing to Physical Fitness

6. Miguel is thinking about becoming more active. Which of the following is *not* a good piece of advice to offer him?
   a. Incorporate physical activity into your daily life.
   b. Make multiple changes to diet and exercise routines simultaneously.
   c. Identify obstacles to being active.
   d. Set SMART goals.

LO 4 Creating Your Own Fitness Program

7. Exercise intensity can be assessed using
   a. the "talk test."
   b. perceived exertion.
   c. target heart rate range.
   d. any of the above.

LO 5 Implementing Your Fitness Program

8. At the start of an exercise session, you should always
   a. stretch.
   b. do 50 crunches to activate your core muscles.
   c. warm up with light cardiorespiratory activities.
   d. eat a meal to ensure that you are fueled for the activity.

LO 6 Taking in Proper Nutrition for Exercise

9. Chocolate milk is good for
   a. preworkout energy boost.
   b. postworkout recovery.
   c. slimming down.
   d. staying hydrated during exercise.

LO 7 Preventing and Treating Common Exercise Injuries

10. Overuse injuries can best be prevented by
    a. monitoring the quantity and quality of your workouts.
    b. engaging in only one type of aerobic training.
    c. working out daily.
    d. working out with a friend.

Answers to the Pop Quiz can be found on page A-1. If you answered a question incorrectly, review the section identified by the Learning Outcome. For even more study tools, visit MasteringHealth.

THINK ABOUT IT!

LO 1 Physical Activity for Health

1. How do you define *physical fitness*? Identify at least four physiological and psychological benefits of physical activity. How would you promote these benefits to nonexercisers?

LO 2 Physical Activity for Fitness and Performance

2. How are muscle strength and muscle endurance different? What are some ways you might work to increase muscle strength and muscle endurance?

LO 3 Committing to Physical Fitness

3. What do you do to motivate yourself to engage in physical activity on a regular basis?

LO 4 Creating Your Own Fitness Program

4. Describe the FITT prescription for cardiorespiratory fitness, muscular strength and endurance, and flexibility training.

LO 5 Implementing Your Fitness Program

5. Why is core strength important? What are some ways to increase your core strength every day?

LO 6 Taking in Proper Nutrition for Exercise

6. Why is when you eat as important as what you eat? How might your exercise preparation and routine differ in hot and cold climates?

LO 7 Preventing and Treating Common Exercise Injuries

7. Your roommate has decided to start running to improve cardiorespiratory fitness. What advice would you give to make sure he/she does not get injured and continues the program throughout the year?

ACCESS YOUR HEALTH ON THE INTERNET

Visit **MasteringHealth** for links to the websites and RSS feeds.

ACSM Online. This site is the link to the American College of Sports Medicine and all its resources. **www.acsm.org**

American Council on Exercise. Information is found here on exercise and disease prevention. **www.acefitness.org**

CDC Division of Nutrition, Physical Activity, and Obesity. This site is a great resource for current information on exercise and health. **www.cdc.gov/nccdphp/dnpao/index.html**

FOCUS ON Recognizing and Avoiding Addiction

Addiction isn't just for celebrities. Every day, people, young and old from all classes and backgrounds, struggle with many different types of addiction—some with far-reaching consequences.

LEARNING OUTCOMES

1 Define *addiction* and identify the signs of addiction.
2 Describe the impact of addiction on friends and family.
3 Discuss the addictive process, the physiology of addiction, and the biopsychosocial model of addiction.
4 Describe types of addictions, including disordered gambling, compulsive buying, compulsive Internet or technology use, work addiction, compulsive exercise, and sexual addiction.
5 Evaluate treatment and recovery options for addicts, including intervention, individual therapy, group therapy, family therapy, and 12-step programs.

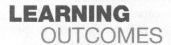

These days, it's easy to find high-profile cases of compulsive and destructive behavior. Stories of celebrities, athletes, and politicians struggling with addictions to alcohol, drugs, and sex are splashed in the headlines and profiled on TV news programs. But millions of people—young and old, rich and poor—from a wide range of socioeconomic conditions throughout the world are waging their own battles with addiction as well. People with addictions can sometimes be unaware that they have a problem because many potentially addictive activities may appear to enhance the lives of those who engage in them moderately. In addition to alcohol and drugs, the most commonly recognized addictions include food, sex, relationships, shopping, work, exercise, gambling, and using technology and the Internet.

LO 1 | WHAT IS ADDICTION?

Define *addiction* and identify the signs of addiction.

Addiction is a persistent, compulsive dependence on a behavior or substance, including mood-altering behaviors or

addiction Persistent, compulsive dependence on a behavior or substance, including mood-altering behaviors or activities, despite ongoing negative consequences.

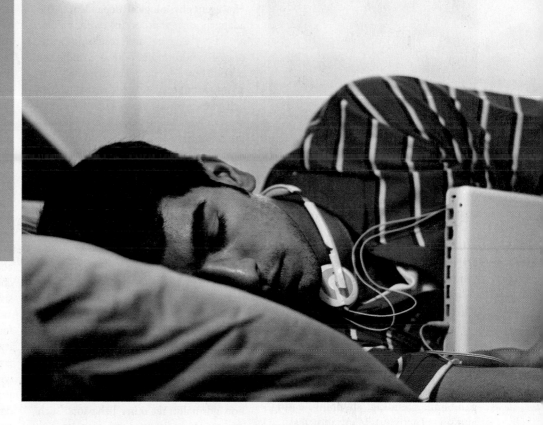

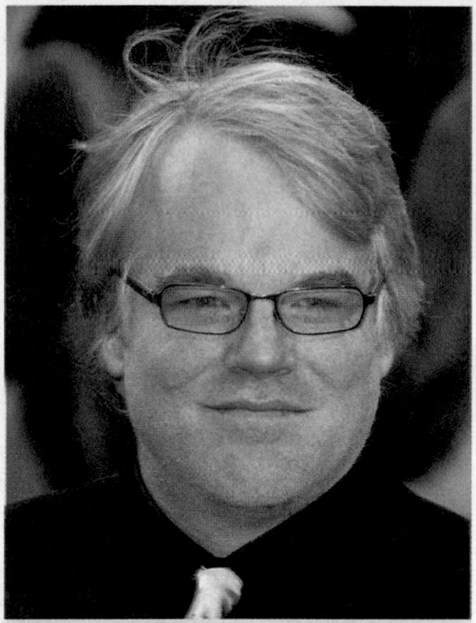

Addiction affects all kinds of people. Academy Award–winning actor Philip Seymour Hoffman, widely respected for his work, was found dead in his New York apartment with a needle in his arm. A mix of cocaine, heroin, and other drugs ultimately proved fatal.

activities, despite ongoing negative consequences. The American Society of Addiction describes addiction as a chronic disease that disrupts brain systems that regulate motivation and reward.[1] Some researchers speak of two types of addictions: *substance addictions* (e.g., alcoholism, drug abuse, and smoking) and *process addictions* (e.g., gambling, spending, shopping, eating, and sexual activity). Many addicts, such as *polydrug abusers*, are those addicted to more than one substance or process.

physiological dependence The adaptive state that occurs with regular addictive behavior and results in withdrawal syndrome.

compulsion Preoccupation with a behavior and an overwhelming need to perform it.

obsession Excessive preoccupation with an addictive object or behavior.

loss of control Inability to reliably predict whether a particular instance of involvement with the addictive substance or behavior will be healthy or damaging.

negative consequences Severe problems associated with addiction, such as physical damage, legal trouble, financial problems, academic failure, or family dissolution.

denial Inability to perceive or accurately interpret the self-destructive effects of the addictive behavior.

codependence A self-defeating relationship pattern in which a person is controlled by an addict's addictive behavior.

Regardless of the addictive behavior, the person experiencing it usually will feel a sense of pleasure or control that is beyond the addict's power to achieve in other ways. Eventually, the addicted person needs to do the behavior in order to feel like he or she is functioning normally.

In this text, *addiction* is used interchangeably with *physiological addiction.* However, **physiological dependence,** the adaptive state that occurs with regular addictive behavior and results in withdrawal syndrome, is only one indicator of addiction. Psychological dynamics play an important role too, which explains why behaviors not related to chemicals may also be addictive. To be addictive, a behavior must have the potential to produce a positive mood change. In many ways, addiction is a form of *operant conditioning* in which people do a drug or shop incessantly and it "feels good." Before they know it, they crave that pleasurable experience. Repeating the drug or the shopping reactivates the pleasure center in the brain. Before long, they lose control and would rather shop or do drugs to feel that pleasure than almost anything else in their lives. Chemicals are responsible for the most profound addictions because they produce dramatic mood changes and cause cellular changes to which the body adapts so well that it eventually requires the chemical in order to function normally. Yet other behaviors, such as gambling, working, and sex, also create changes at the cellular level along with positive mood changes.[2] A person with an intense, uncontrollable urge to continue engaging in a particular activity is said to have developed a psychological dependence. In fact, psychological and physiological dependence are so intertwined that it is not really possible to separate the two. Although the mechanism is not well understood, all forms of addiction probably reflect dysfunction of certain biochemical systems in the brain.[3]

Most drugs of abuse directly or indirectly target the brain's reward system by flooding the circuit with *dopamine.* Dopamine is a neurotransmitter present in regions of the brain that regulate movement, emotion, cognition, motivation, and feelings of pleasure. The overstimulation of this system, which rewards our natural behaviors, produces the euphoric effects sought by people who abuse drugs and teaches them to repeat the behavior.

Our brains are wired to ensure that we will repeat life-sustaining activities by associating those activities with reward or pleasure. Whenever the reward circuit is activated, the brain notes that something important is happening and needs to be remembered, and teaches us to do it again and again. Because drugs stimulate the same reward circuit as a satisfying meal or sexual encounter, we learn to abuse drugs.[4] We all engage in potentially addictive behaviors to some extent, because some are essential to our survival and are highly reinforcing, such as eating, drinking, and sex. At some point along the continuum, however, some individuals are not able to engage in these or other behaviors moderately—they become addicted and face a nearly uncontrollable urge to act on them 24/7.

Addiction has five common characteristics: (1) **compulsion,** which is characterized by **obsession,** or excessive preoccupation, with the behavior and an overwhelming need to perform it; (2) **loss of control,** the inability to reliably predict whether any isolated occurrence of the behavior will be healthy or damaging; (3) **negative consequences,** such as physical damage, legal trouble, financial problems, academic failure, and family dissolution, which do not occur with healthy involvement in any behavior; (4) **denial,** the inability to perceive that the behavior is self-destructive; and the (5) inability to abstain. These five components are present in all addictions, whether chemical or behavioral.[5]

LO 2 | ADDICTION AFFECTS FAMILY AND FRIENDS

Describe the impact of addiction on friends and family.

The family and friends of an addicted person can suffer many negative consequences. Often they struggle with **codependence,** a self-defeating relationship

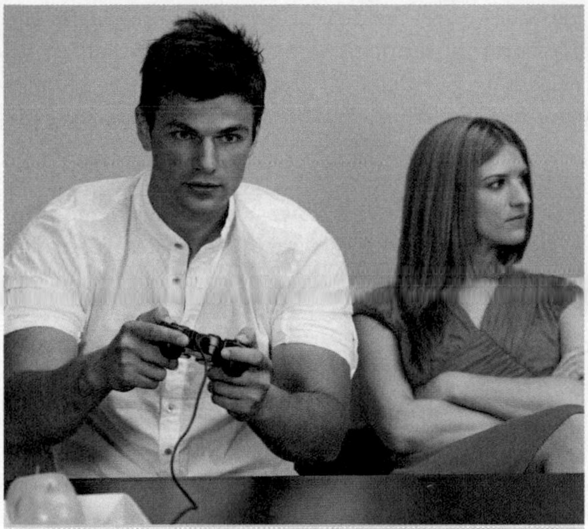

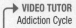

Addiction can be difficult to recognize or acknowledge. Symptoms to look for are an obsession or compulsion with a behavior or activity, a loss of control, and negative consequences as a result of the behavior. Another symptom, denial of a problem, may be easy to see in another person but difficult to recognize in yourself.

pattern in which a person is controlled by an addict's addictive behavior.

Codependence is often the result of growing up in an environment of addiction. Codependents find it hard to set healthy boundaries and often live in the chaotic, crisis-oriented mode that occurs around addicts. They assume responsibility for meeting others' needs to the point that they subordinate or even cease being aware of their own needs. They may be unable to perceive their needs because they have been taught that their needs are inappropriate or less important than someone else's. Although the word *codependent* is used less frequently today, treatment professionals still recognize the importance of helping addicts see how their behavior affects those around them and of working with family and friends to establish healthier relationships.

Family and friends can play an important role in getting an addict to seek treatment. They are most helpful when they refuse to be enablers. **Enablers** are people who knowingly or unknowingly protect addicts from the natural consequences of their behavior. If they don't have to deal with the consequences, addicts cannot see the self-destructive nature of their behavior and will therefore continue it. Codependents are the primary enablers of their addicted loved ones, although anyone who has contact with an addict can be an enabler and thus contribute to continuation of the addictive behavior. Enablers are generally unaware that their behavior has this effect. In fact, enabling is rarely conscious and certainly not intentional.

WHAT DO YOU THINK?

Why might friends and family members become enablers and codependents of people engaging in destructive behaviors?

- Have you ever confronted someone you were concerned about?
- If so, was the confrontation successful?
- What tips would you give someone who wants to address addiction with a loved one?

enablers People who knowingly or unknowingly protect addicts from the natural consequences of their behavior.

LO 3 | HOW ADDICTION DEVELOPS

Discuss the addictive process, the physiology of addiction, and the biopsychosocial model of addiction.

Addiction is a process that evolves over time. It begins when a person repeatedly seeks the illusion of relief to avoid unpleasant feelings or situations. This pattern is known as *nurturing through avoidance* and is a maladaptive way of taking care of emotional needs. As a person becomes increasingly dependent on the addictive behavior, there is a corresponding deterioration in relationships with family, friends, and coworkers; in performance at work or school; and in personal life. Eventually, addicts do not find the addictive behavior pleasurable but consider it preferable to the unhappy realities they are seeking to escape. **FIGURE 1** illustrates the cycle of psychological addiction.

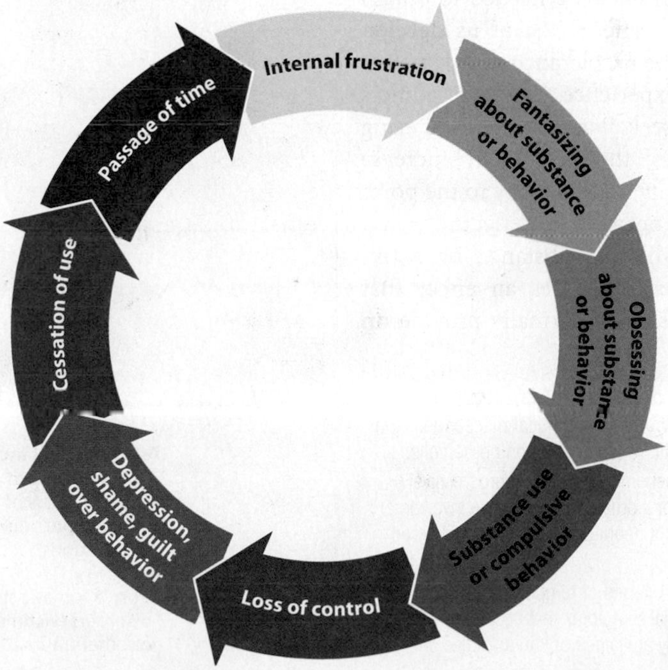

FIGURE 1 Cycle of Psychological Addiction

Source: Adapted from Recovery Connection, Cycle of Addiction, 2012, www.recoveryconnection.org/cycle-of-addiction.

VIDEO TUTOR Addiction Cycle

The Physiology of Addiction

Today, scientists view addiction as a chronic disease that involves disruption of the brain's system related to reward, motivation, and memory. Virtually all intellectual, emotional, and behavioral functions occur as a result of biochemical interactions between nerve cells in the body. Biochemical messengers, called **neurotransmitters,** exert their influence at specific receptor sites on nerve cells. Drug use and chronic stress can alter these receptor sites and cause the production and breakdown of neurotransmitters. Some people's bodies naturally produce insufficient quantities of these neurotransmitters, predisposing them to seek out chemicals, such as alcohol, as substitutes or pursue behaviors, such as exercise, that increase natural production. Thus, some people may be "wired" to look for substances or experiences that increase pleasure or reduce discomfort, making them more susceptible to addiction.

Mood-altering substances and experiences produce **tolerance,** a phenomenon in which progressively larger doses of a drug or more intense involvement in an experience are needed to obtain the desired effects. All of us develop some degree of tolerance to any mood-altering experience. Because addicts tend to seek intense mood-altering experiences, they eventually increase their amount and intensity to the point of causing negative side effects.

An addictive substance or activity replaces or causes an effect that the body should normally provide on its own. If the experience is repeated often enough, the body adjusts: It starts requiring the experience to obtain that effect. Stopping the behavior will cause **withdrawal,** because the body can no longer create the same effect naturally. Mood-altering chemicals, for example, fill up the receptor sites for the body's natural "feel-good" neurotransmitters (endorphins), and nerve cells shut down production of these substances temporarily. When the drug use stops, those receptor sites sit empty, resulting in uncomfortable feelings that remain until the body resumes normal neurotransmitter production or the person consumes more of the drug.

Withdrawal symptoms of chemical dependencies are generally the opposite of the effects of the drugs. For example, a cocaine addict who feels a high while using the drug will experience a characteristic "crash" (depression and lethargy) when he or she stops taking it. Conversely, a heroin addict experiences drowsiness, slowed speech and reactions, and uninhibited behavior while using the drug. When withdrawing from heroin, the addict experiences anxiety, elevated heart rate, trembling, irritability, insomnia, and convulsions. Withdrawal symptoms for addictive behaviors are usually less dramatic. They typically involve psychological discomfort such as anxiety, depression, irritability, guilt, anger, and frustration, with an underlying preoccupation with or craving for the behavior. Withdrawal syndromes range from mild to severe. The most severe form is delirium tremens (DTs), which can last from 1 day to 1 week and occur in approximately 5 to 10 percent of dependent individuals withdrawing from alcohol.[6] DTs can be life threatening; 1 to 2 percent of addicts die while withdrawing from alcohol.[7]

The Biopsychosocial Model of Addiction

The most effective treatment today is based on the **biopsychosocial model of addiction,** which proposes that addiction is caused by a variety of factors operating together. The biopsychosocial model was developed to explain the complex interaction between the biological, psychological, and social aspects of addiction. Although one factor may play a larger role than another in a specific individual, it is rarely sufficient to explain an addiction. **FIGURE 2** lists risk factors for addiction.

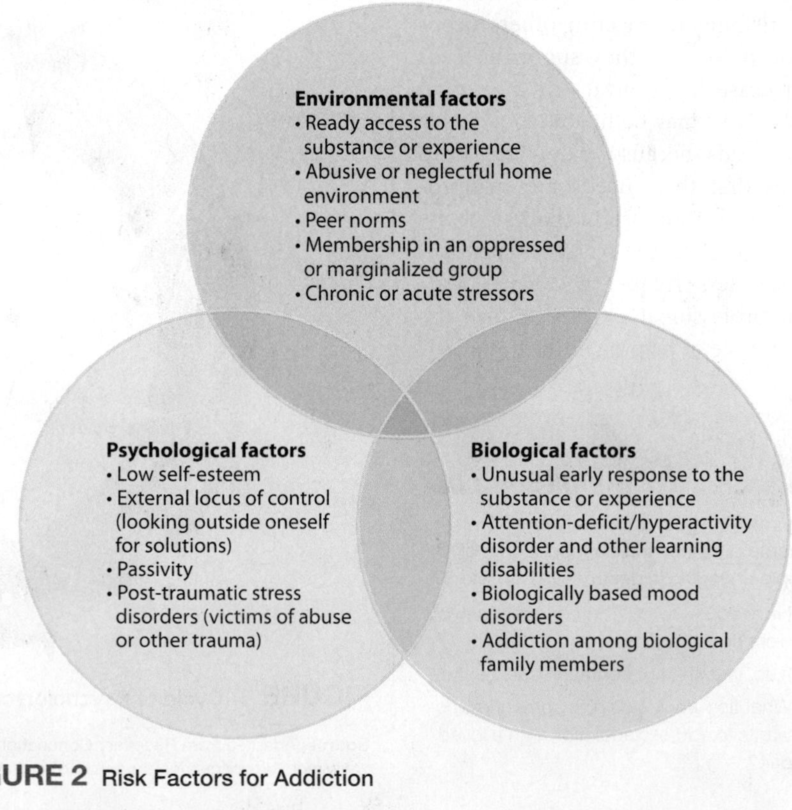

Environmental factors
• Ready access to the substance or experience
• Abusive or neglectful home environment
• Peer norms
• Membership in an oppressed or marginalized group
• Chronic or acute stressors
Psychological factors
• Low self-esteem
• External locus of control (looking outside oneself for solutions)
• Passivity
• Post-traumatic stress disorders (victims of abuse or other trauma)
Biological factors
• Unusual early response to the substance or experience
• Attention-deficit/hyperactivity disorder and other learning disabilities
• Biologically based mood disorders
• Addiction among biological family members

FIGURE 2 Risk Factors for Addiction

neurotransmitters Biochemical messengers that bind to specific receptor sites on nerve cells.

tolerance Phenomenon in which progressively larger doses of a drug or more intense involvement in a behavior is needed to produce the desired effects.

withdrawal A series of temporary physical and biopsychosocial symptoms that occurs when an addict abruptly abstains from an addictive chemical or behavior.

biopsychosocial model of addiction Theory of the relationship between an addict's biological (genetic) nature and psychological and environmental influences.

WHY SHOULD I CARE?

Addictions of any kind limit your ability to make good decisions and maintain your focus, making it hard for you to meet your full potential as a student and a member of the community. A seemingly harmless habit may actually be progressing into an addiction that prevents you from attending classes, meeting new people, or participating in other activities that you might find enjoyable.

Biological Influences

For many people, addiction is thought to be based in the brain and involves memory, motivation, and emotional state. The processes that control these aspects of brain function are thus logical subjects for genetic research into a biologically based risk for addiction, particularly to mood-altering substances. Studies show that drug addicts metabolize these substances differently than do nonaddicted people. Genes affecting the activity of the neurotransmitters serotonin and GABA (gamma-aminobutyric acid) are likely involved in the risk for alcoholism.[8]

Research also supports a genetic influence on addiction. It has been known for centuries that alcoholism runs in families. Studies have confirmed that identical twins, who share the same genes, are about twice as likely as fraternal twins, who share an average of 50 percent of their genes, to resemble each other in terms of the presence of alcoholism. Studies also show that half of the likelihood a person will develop an addiction is due to genetic factors.[9]

Psychological Factors

A person's psychological makeup also factors into the potential for addiction. People with low self-esteem, a tendency toward risk-taking behavior, or poor coping skills are more likely to develop addictive patterns. Individuals who consistently look outside themselves for solutions and explanations for life events (who have an external locus of control) are more likely to experience addiction.

Environmental Influences

Culture also plays a role in how an addiction begins. Social expectations and mores help determine whether people engage in certain behaviors. For example, although many Italians use alcohol abundantly, there is a low incidence of alcoholism in this culture. Low rates of alcoholism typically exist in countries and cultures where children are gradually introduced to alcohol in diluted amounts, on special occasions, and within a strong family group. There is deep disapproval of intoxication, which is not viewed as socially acceptable, stylish, or funny.[10] Such cultural traditions and values are less widespread in the United States, where the incidence of alcohol addiction and alcohol-related problems is very high.

Societal attitudes and messages also influence addictive behavior. The media's emphasis on appearance and the ideal body plays a significant role in exercise addiction. Societal glorification of money and material achievement can lead to work addiction, which is often admired. Societal changes, in turn, influence individual norms. People living in cities characterized by rapid social change or social disorganization often feel less connected to civic and religious institutions. The resulting disenfranchisement leads to increased destructive behaviors, including addiction.[11]

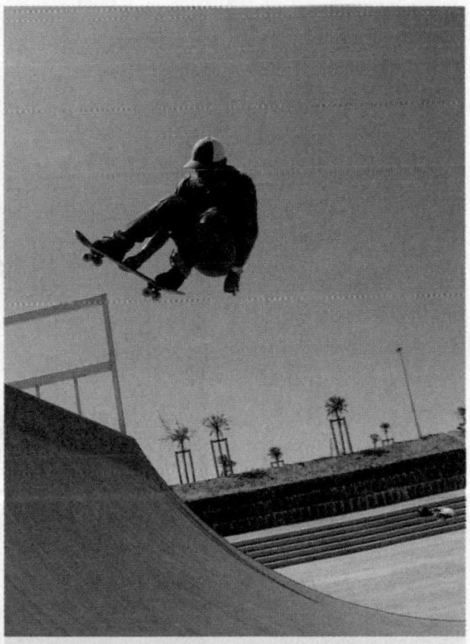

A tendency toward risk-taking behavior, as well as other psychological factors such as low self-esteem and poor coping skills, may put you at higher risk of developing an addiction than someone without these traits.

social learning theory Theory that people learn behaviors by watching role models—parents, caregivers, and significant others.

Social learning theory proposes that people learn behaviors by watching role models—parents, caregivers, and significant others. The effects of modeling, imitation, and identification with behavior from early childhood on are well documented.[12] Modeling is especially influential when it involves behavior that is mood altering.

On an individual level, major stressful life events—such as marriage, divorce, change in work status, or death of a loved one—may trigger addictive behaviors as traumatized people seek to medicate their pain. Addictive behaviors reliably alleviate personal pain for a short time. However, over the long term, addictive behaviors actually cause more pain than they relieve.

Family members whose needs for love, security, and affirmation are not consistently met; who are refused permission to express their feelings; and who frequently submerge their personalities to "keep the peace" are prone to addiction. Children whose parents are not consistently available to them (physically or emotionally); who are subjected to sexual abuse, physical abuse, neglect, or abandonment; or who receive inconsistent or disparaging messages about their self-worth may experience psychosocial or physical illness and addiction in adulthood.

LO 4 | ADDICTIVE BEHAVIORS

Describe types of addictions, including disordered gambling, compulsive buying, compulsive Internet or technology use, work addiction, compulsive exercise, and sexual addiction.

Thus far in this chapter, we have examined the fundamental concepts and processes of addiction and its associated problems. Clearly, tobacco, alcohol, and other drugs are addictive; they create multiple problems for addicted individuals and for their families and society. Later chapters will discuss these substance-related addictions.

Here we will look at **process addictions**—behaviors known to be addictive because they are mood altering. Traditionally, the word *addiction* has been used mainly with alcohol and other psychoactive substances. However, this is changing. New knowledge about the brain's reward system suggests that, as far as the brain is concerned, a reward is a reward, whether it is brought on by a chemical or a behavior.[13] Examples of process addictions include disordered gambling, compulsive buying, compulsive Internet or technology use, work addiction, compulsive exercise, and sexual addiction.

Gambling Disorder

Gambling is a form of recreation and entertainment for millions of Americans. Most people who gamble do so casually and moderately to experience the excitement of anticipating a win. However, more than 2 million Americans suffer from gambling disorder, and 6 million more are considered to be at risk for developing a gambling addiction.[14] The American Psychiatric Association (APA), which previously used the term *pathological gambling,* now uses the term **gambling disorder** and recognizes it as an addictive disorder. According to *the APA's Diagnostic and Statistical Manual of Mental Disorders,* 5th edition (*DSM-5*), characteristic behaviors associated with gambling disorder include a preoccupation with gambling, unsuccessful efforts to cut back or quit, gambling when feeling distressed, and lying to family members to conceal the extent of gambling.[15] Where casual gamblers can stop when they wish and are capable of seeing the necessity to do so, individuals with gambling disorder are unable to control the urge to gamble even in the face of devastating consequences like high debt or the loss of homes, families, jobs, health—even their lives.

There is strong evidence that disordered gambling has a biological component. A study of individuals with gambling disorder found the participants to have decreased blood flow to a key section of the brain's reward system. It is thought that individuals with gambling disorder, like people who abuse drugs, compensate for this deficiency in their brain's reward system by overdoing it and getting hooked.[16] Most individuals with a gambling disorder seek excitement even more than money. They place increasingly larger bets to obtain the desired level of excitement. Like drug addicts, they live from fix to fix. Their subjective cravings can be as intense as those of drug abusers; they show tolerance in their need to increase the amount of their bets; and they experience highs rivaling those brought on by drugs. Up to half of those with gambling disorder show withdrawal symptoms similar to a mild form of drug withdrawal, including sleep disturbance, sweating, irritability, and craving.

Who is at risk for getting hooked on the rush of gambling? Men are more likely to have gambling problems than are women. Women, however, tend to begin gambling later than do men, but they develop gambling problems more rapidly. Gambling prevalence is also higher among lower-income inividuals; those who are widowed, separated, or divorced; African Americans; individuals who begin gambling at a younger age; and older adults. Gambling disorder tends to run in families. If they are regularly exposed to gambling, family members of those with gambling disorder are more susceptible to developing gambling disorder themselves than are individuals with family members who don't have gambling disorder.

Individuals with gambling disorder are much more likely to have mental disorders and/or substance use disorders than are those without gambling disorder. It is not uncommon for gamblers to suffer from mood disorders such as depression, anxiety, or post-traumatic stress disorder. A significant number of those with gambling disorder are more likely to be alcoholics, drug use abusers, and/or smokers.[17]

Distorted thinking is one of the characteristics associated with gambling disorder. Similar to other addictions, denial is common. Gambling disorder differs from other addictions in the prevalence of superstitions, which serve to reinforce addictive behaviors. Another disordered thinking pattern is frequent and long-term chasing one's losses.

75%

OF COLLEGE STUDENTS **GAMBLED** DURING THE PAST YEAR.

process addictions Behaviors such as disordered gambling, compulsive buying, compulsive Internet or technology use, work addiction, compulsive exercise, and sexual addiction that are known to be addictive because they are mood altering.

gambling disorder Compulsive gambling that cannot be controlled.

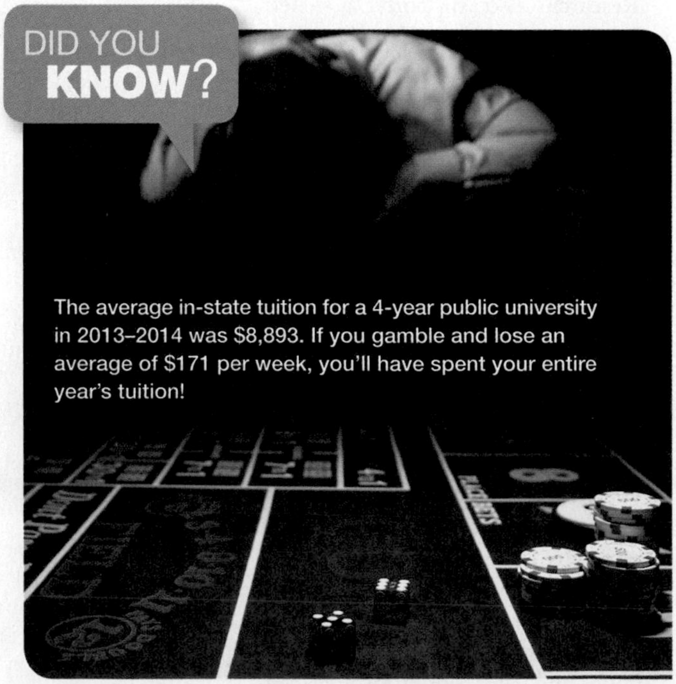
DID YOU KNOW?
The average in-state tuition for a 4-year public university in 2013–2014 was $8,893. If you gamble and lose an average of $171 per week, you'll have spent your entire year's tuition!

Source: The College Board, *Trends in College Pricing, 2013* (New York: The College Board, 2013), Available at https://trends.collegeboard.org/sites/default/files/college-pricing-2013-full-report-140108.pdf.

STUDENT HEALTH TODAY

GAMBLING AND COLLEGE STUDENTS

Although many people gamble occasionally without it ever becoming a problem, even model students can find themselv... dered gam... become a ...

A good ... campuses ... year during ... Collegiate A... lege basketl... $12 billion is ... during which ... more than is ... While over $... is from office ... these dollars ... of college stu... approximately ... reported they ... year, whether ... students give ... bling: risk, exc..., and the chance to make money. Consider the following:

I will be away on Tuesday, May 8th
R. Thebarge

- Almost 53 percent of college students have participated in most forms of gambling, including casino gambling, lottery tickets, racing, and sports betting, in the past month.
- At least 78 percent of youths have placed a bet by the age of 18.
- An estimated 6 percent of college students can be classified as problem...

...ege students who ... so without develop... signs of disordered ... llowing:

... gambling; encour... others to gamble ... or money on gam... can afford ... ing financial aid ... y, or committing ... nbling ... more gambling ... ng habits and ... confronted. ... paraphernalia ... or poker items ... r school, work, ... activities due to gambling

- Feeling sad, anxious, fearful, or angry about gambling losses

If any of these warning signs apply to you, consider talking with a counselor to get help.

Call, fold, or raise? For increasing numbers of college students, gambling and the debts it can incur are becoming serious problems

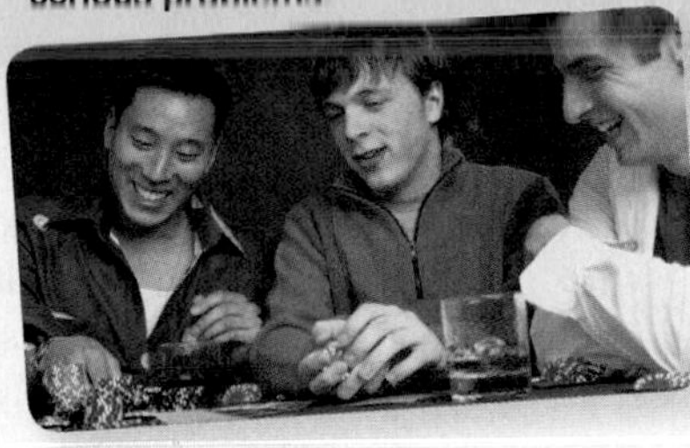

Sources: Task Force on College Gambling Policies, Division on Addictions at the Cambridge Health Alliance and the National Center for Responsible Gambling, *A Call to Action: Addressing College Gambling: Recommendations for Science-Based Policies and Programs* (Cambridge, MA: Cambridge Health Alliance and the National Center for Responsible Gambling, 2009), Available at www.ncrg.org/public_education/task force college gambling policies.cfm; N. Bhullar et al., "The Significance of Gender and Ethnicity in Collegiate Gambling and Drinking," *Addictive Disorders and Their Treatment* 11, no. 3 (2012): 154–64; National Council on Problem Gambling, "College Gambling Facts and Statistics," www.ncpgambling.org/files/NPGAWcollegefactsheet.pdf; N. Shead et al., "Characteristics of Internet Gamblers among a Sample of Students at a Large, Public University in the Southwestern United States," *Journal of College Student Development* 53, no. 1 (2012): 133–48; G. M. Barnes et al., "Comparisons of Gambling and Alcohol Use among College Students and Non-College Young People in the United States," *Journal of American College Health* 58, no. 5 (2010): 443–52; National Council on Problem Gambling, "March Madness Gambling Brings Out Warnings from NCAA to Tournament Players," 2011, Available at www.ncpgambling.org/i4a/headlines/headlinedetails.cfm?id=791&archive=1.

Although gambling is illegal for anyone under the age of 21, college students have easier access to gambling opportunities than ever before. The percentage of college students who gamble—about 75 percent (legally or illegally)—is consistent with these growing opportunities. About 18 percent of those students reported gambling once a week or more.[18] Regardless, with the advent of online gambling, televised poker tournaments, and a growing number of casinos, scratch tickets, lotteries, and sports-betting networks, there are many opportunities for college students to gamble. Students at most risk for problem gambling are males, African Americans, and those with lower socioeconomic status. It is estimated that 6 percent of college students in the United States have a serious gambling problem that can result in psychological difficulties, debt, and failing grades.[19] The **Student Health Today** box discusses student gambling in more detail.

Compulsive Buying Disorder

In the United States today, many people often use shopping as a way to make themselves feel better. However, **compulsive** buyers are preoccupied with shopping and spending and exercise little control over their impulses to buy. Shopping actually makes them feel worse, not better. Compulsive buying is estimated to afflict up to 5 percent of adults. The vast majority of compulsive buyers are women.[20]

Compulsive buying has many of the same characteristics as alcoholism, gambling, and other addictions. Symptoms that signal that a person has crossed the line into compulsive buying include preoccupation with shopping and spending, buying more than one of the same item, shopping for longer periods than intended, repeatedly buying much more than he or she needs or can afford, and buying to the point that it interferes with social activities or work and creates financial problems (e.g., indebtedness or bankruptcy). Compulsive buying frequently results in psychological distress, such as depression and

compulsive buying disorder People who are preoccupied with shopping and spending.

SEE IT! VIDEOS

How do you battle compulsive shopping? Watch **Woman's Shopping Addiction Revealed** available on MasteringHealth.™

feelings of guilt, as well as conflict with friends and between couples.[21]

Compulsive buying disorders are reported to begin in a person's late teens and early twenties, coinciding with the age that people first establish credit and independence from their parents. A recent study found approximately 3.5 percent of college students surveyed met the criteria for compulsive buying.[22] Access to student loans and financial aid may provide new financial resources not previously available.[23] In addition, the Internet makes it simple to access millions of items to purchase. Those who try to define who they are through material goods—especially young people—are most likely to show signs of compulsive buying and symptoms of Internet addiction.[24]

In addition to financial problems, college students experience personal distress, lower grade point averages, family and social problems, higher perceived stress, and poorer physical health. Students also report more depression, anxiety, and problems with impulse control disorders.[25]

Compulsive buying can be seasonal, such as shopping during the winter months to alleviate feelings of anxiety and depression. It can also occur when people feel depressed, lonely, or angry. Shopping and spending will not ensure more love, increase self-esteem, or heal the problems of daily living. It generally makes people feel worse because of increased debt. Like gambling disorder, compulsive buying can lead to compulsive borrowing to support the addiction. People may borrow money repeatedly from family, friends, or institutions in spite of the problems this causes.

$25,000

IS THE AVERAGE AMOUNT OF **DEBT** THAT A COMPULSIVE SHOPPER OWES.

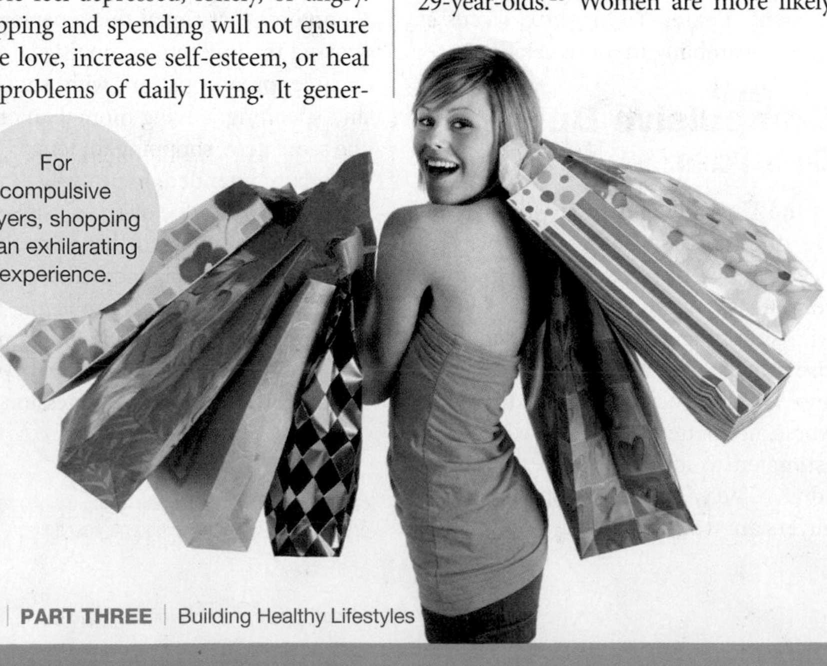

For compulsive buyers, shopping is an exhilarating experience.

Technology Addictions

Have you ever opened your Web browser to check something quickly, and an hour later found yourself still blogging or checking Facebook? Do you have friends who seem more concerned with texting or surfing the Internet than with eating, going out, studying, or having a face-to-face conversation? These behaviors are not unusual; many experts suggest that technology addiction is real and can present serious problems.

Recent data indicate that over 85 percent of adult Americans use the Internet, and 18- to 29-year-olds compose the largest users (with 98 percent using).[26] On average, Americans 18 years and older will spend 5.2 hours a day online, on non-voice mobile devices, or with other digital media.[27] Those most likely to use a social networking site are 18- to 29-year-olds.[28] Women are more likely than men to be on these sites.[29] This type of use does not come without risk: An estimated 1 in 8 Internet users will likely experience **Internet addiction.**[30] Younger people are more likely to be addicted to the Internet than are middle-aged users.[31] Approximately 12 percent of college students report that Internet use and computer games have interfered with their academic performance.[32] To read about the experiences of students taking part in an "unplug from technology day," see the **Tech & Health** box.

Internet addiction Compulsive use of the computer, personal digital device, cell phone, or other forms of technology to access the Internet for activities such as e-mail, games, shopping, social networking, or blogging.

So how important is technology to college students? A reported 91 percent of college students own at least one small mobile device.[33] Students own on average 6.9 electronic devices. Over 85 percent of students own laptops and rely on them for schoolwork; 70 percent use them for research and coursework, and 47 percent use them for note taking in a classroom.[34] However, these devices are also used frequently outside of schoolwork. The average time a day a college student spends texting on a cell phone is 3.5 hours, followed by over 5 hours on a laptop, 1.3 hours a day using a gaming console, roughly 1 hour per day with an e-reader or handheld gaming device, and approximately 3 hours per week watching TV.[35] Some online activities, such as gaming and cybersex, seem to be more potentially addictive than others.

Technology addicts typically exhibit symptoms such as general disregard for their health, sleep deprivation, depression, neglecting family and friends, lack of physical activity, euphoria when online, lower grades in school, and poor job performance. Internet addicts may feel moody or uncomfortable when they are not online. They may be using their behavior to compensate for loneliness, marital or work problems, a poor social life, or financial problems.

Work Addiction

To understand work addiction, we must first understand the concept of healthy work. Healthy work provides a sense of

TECH & HEALTH

MOBILE DEVICES, MEDIA, AND THE INTERNET *Could You Unplug?*

If someone asked you to give up your mobile devices, media, and the Internet for 24 hours, how hard would it be? Judging from the results of a study with participants hailing from 37 different countries on six continents—extremely hard. All students followed the same assignment: give up Internet, newspapers, magazines, TV, radio, phones, iPods/MP3 players, movies, Facebook, chat, Twitter, video games, and any other form of electronic or social media for 24 hours.

Students around the world repeatedly used the term *addiction* to speak about their dependence on media and likened their reactions to feelings of a drug withdrawal. "Media is my drug; without it I was lost," said one student from the UK. A student from the United States noted: "I was itching, like a crackhead, because I could not use my phone." A student from Argentina observed: "Sometimes I felt 'dead,'" and a student from Slovakia simply noted: "I felt sad, lonely, and depressed."

Students also reported that media—especially their mobile phones—have virtually become an extension of themselves. Going without media, therefore, made it seem like they had lost part of themselves.

Despite the withdrawal symptoms, many students found there were definite benefits to being unplugged for 24 hours. Some students found they had more time to talk, listen, and share with others. Students also reported feeling liberated. They took time to do things they normally would not do, such as visiting relatives, playing board games, or having face-to-face conversations.

How do you "unplug" from texting and Twitter for 24 hours (or more) without the anxiety of ignoring your friends online? Smartphone and computer apps can actually help! Available apps can post automatic status updates to Facebook and Twitter, send you reminders before scheduled technology breaks, or temporarily lock out your access to the Internet for a set interval. Here are a few suggested apps:

- **BRB.** (Free: iPhone) www.brbapp.com
- **Unplug and Reconnect.** (Free: Android) http://unplugreconnect.com
- **Freedom.** (Modest cost: Windows, Mac, Android) https://macfreedom.com

Source: The World Unplugged, Going 24 Hours Without Media, 2011, http://theworldunplugged.wordpress.com.

50%

OF AMERICANS WOULD GIVE UP CHOCOLATE, ALCOHOL, AND CAFFEINE FOR A WEEK BEFORE PARTING TEMPORARILY WITH THEIR **PHONES**.

identity; helps develop our strengths; and is a means of satisfaction, accomplishment, and mastery of problems. Healthy workers may work passionately for long hours. Although they have occasional projects that keep them away from family, friends, and personal interests for short periods of time, they generally maintain balance in their lives and full control of their schedules. Healthy work does not "consume" the worker.

Conversely, **work addiction** is the compulsive use of work and the work persona to fulfill needs of intimacy, power, and success. Work addicts usually set an intense work schedule, are unable to set boundaries regarding work, and feel driven to work even when they are away from work. Work addiction can be defined as a person's need for work becoming excessive to the point that it interferes with a person's physical health, personal happiness, interpersonal relationships, and the ability to maintain social relationships with others.[36] The disorder is characterized by excessive time spent working; difficulty disengaging from work; going above and beyond what the job calls for; a compulsive work style; high levels of stress; low life satisfaction; marital conflict; and work burnout.[37] Work addicts may feel too busy to take care of their health, and there is some evidence work addiction may cause physical symptoms such as sleep problems and exhaustion, high blood pressure, anxiety and depression, weight gain, ulcers and chest pain, or more chronic health conditions such as heart disease and asthmatic attacks.[38] **FIGURE 3** on the next page identifies other signs of work addiction.

Work addiction is found among all age, racial, and socioeconomic groups, but it typically develops in people in their forties and fifties. Male work addicts outnumber female work addicts, but this is changing as women gain equality in the workforce.[39] Most work addicts come from homes in which one or more parents were work addicts, rigid, violent, or otherwise dysfunctional.[40] While work addiction can bring admiration from society at large, as addicts often excel in their professions, the negative effects on individuals and those around them may be far-reaching.[41]

Exercise Addiction

Generally speaking, most Americans get too little physical activity, not too much. However, exercise, when taken to extremes, can become addictive due to its powerful mood-enhancing effects. **Exercise addicts** use exercise compulsively to try to meet needs—for nurturance, intimacy, self-esteem, and self-competency—that an object

work addiction The compulsive use of work and the work persona to fulfill needs for intimacy, power, and success.

exercise addicts People who exercise compulsively to try to meet needs of nurturance, intimacy, self-esteem, and self-competency.

FIGURE 3 Signs of Work Addiction

or activity cannot truly meet. Consequently, addictive or compulsive exercise results in negative consequences similar to those found in other addictions: alienation of family and friends, injuries from overdoing it, and a craving for more. Warning signs of exercise addiction include only exercising by yourself; adhering to a rigid workout plan; working out longer than 2 hours daily, repeatedly; exercising through illness or injury; becoming fixated on burning calories or losing weight; cancelling social plans, skipping work or missing class to exercise; or working out beyond the point of pain.[42]

Compulsive Sexual Behavior

Everyone needs love and intimacy, but the sexual practices of people addicted to sex involve neither. **Sexual addiction** is compulsive involvement in sexual activity.

Compulsive sexual behavior may involve a normally enjoyable sexual experience that becomes an obsession, or it may involve fantasies or activities outside the bounds of culturally, legally, or morally acceptable sexual behavior.[43] In fact, people with compulsive sexual behavior do not necessarily seek partners to obtain sexual arousal; they may be satisfied by masturbation, whether alone, during phone sex, or while reading or watching erotica. They may participate in a wide range of sexual activities, including affairs, sex with strangers, prostitution, voyeurism, exhibitionism, rape, incest, or pedophilia. People with compulsive sexual behavior frequently experience crushing episodes of depression and anxiety, fueled by the fear of discovery. The toll that compulsive sexual behavior exacts is most clearly seen in loss of intimacy with loved ones, which frequently leads to family disintegration and a host of health-related problems.

Compulsive sexual behaviors affect men and women of all ages, although it is more common in men, whether married or single, and it can affect anyone, regardless of sexual preference. Compulsive sexual behavior often occurs in people who experience other psychological conditions such as a mood disorder, impulse control disorders, or who have alcohol or drug abuse problems. Many may have a history of physical, emotional, and/or sexual abuse or a history of trauma.[44]

sexual addiction Compulsive involvement in sexual activity.

Multiple Addictions

Addicts often depend on more than one chemical or behavior. Although they tend to have a favorite drug or behavior—one that is most effective at meeting their needs—55 percent of people in treatment have problems with more than one addiction.[45] For example, alcohol addiction and eating disorders are commonly paired in women. Individuals trying to break a chemical dependency frequently resort to compulsive eating to keep themselves from taking drugs. Although multiple addictions complicate recovery, they do not make it impossible. As with single addictions, recovery begins with recognizing that there is a problem.

Costs of Addiction

Addiction affects approximately 16 percent of the United States population ages 12 and older (40.3 million), more than the share of the population with heart disease, diabetes, or cancer. Another 31.7 percent of the population (80.4 million), while not addicted, engages in risky use of substances in ways that threaten health and safety. Addiction and risky use constitute the largest preventable and most costly health problem facing the U.S. today. It is estimated that more than 20 percent of deaths in the U.S. are attributable to tobacco, alcohol, and other drug use. Addiction and risky use cause or contribute to more than 70 other conditions requiring medical care, including cancer, respiratory disease, cardiovascular disease, HIV/AIDS, pregnancy complications, cirrhosis, ulcers, and trauma. They also drive and contribute to a wide range of costly social consequences, including crime, accidents, suicide, child neglect and abuse, family dysfunction, unplanned pregnancies, and lost productivity. Costs of addiction and risky substance use to the government alone total at least $468 billion each year.[46]

WHAT DO YOU THINK?

Do you think any behavior can be addictive?

- Can one be a chocolate addict, a study addict, or a shoe addict? Why or why not?
- What dangers lie in using the word *addiction* too loosely?

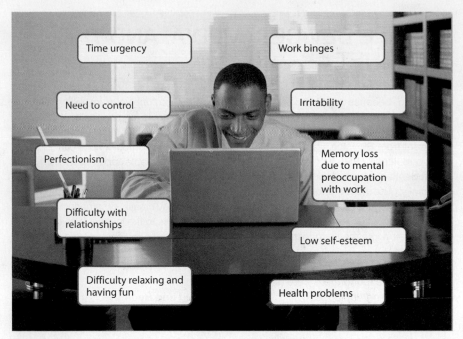

LO 5 | RECOVERING FROM ADDICTION

Evaluate treatment and recovery options for addicts, including intervention, individual therapy, group therapy, family therapy, and 12-step programs.

Recovery from addiction is a lifelong process. Before treatment can begin, the individual must recognize the addiction. This can be difficult because denial—the inability to see the truth—is the hallmark of addiction. Denial can be so powerful that intervention is sometimes necessary to break down the addict's defenses.

Intervention

Intervention is a planned process of confrontation by people who are important to the addict, including spouses, parents, children, bosses, and friends. Its purpose is to break down the denial compassionately so that the person can see the addiction's destructive nature. Getting addicts to admit they have a problem is not enough. They must perceive that the behavior is destructive and requires treatment.

Individual confrontation is difficult and often futile. However, an addict's defenses generally crumble when significant others collectively share their observations and concerns. Effective intervention includes (1) emphasizing care and concern for the addicted person; (2) describing the behavior that is the cause for concern; (3) expressing how the behavior affects the addict, each person taking part in the intervention, and others; and (4) outlining specifically what those participating in the intervention would like to see happen.

It is critical that those involved in the intervention clarify how they plan to end their enabling. In addition, persons contemplating interventions must choose consequences they are ready to stick to if the addict refuses treatment. Significant others must also be ready to give support if the addict is willing to begin a recovery program.

Intervention is a serious step that should be well planned and rehearsed. Most addiction treatment centers have specialists on staff who can help plan an intervention. In addition, books and Internet resources are available.

Treatment for Addiction

Treatment and recovery for any addiction generally begin with **abstinence**—refraining from the addictive behavior. For people addicted to behaviors such as work and sex, abstinence means restoring balance to their lives through noncompulsive engagement in the behaviors.

Detoxification refers to an early abstinence period during which an addict adjusts physically and cognitively to being free from the addiction's influence. It occurs in virtually every recovering addict. While it is uncomfortable for all addicts, it can be dangerous for some—primarily those addicted to chemicals—as early abstinence may involve profound withdrawal symptoms that require medical supervision. Therefore, most inpatient treatment programs provide a pretreatment component of supervised detoxification to achieve abstinence safely before treatment begins.

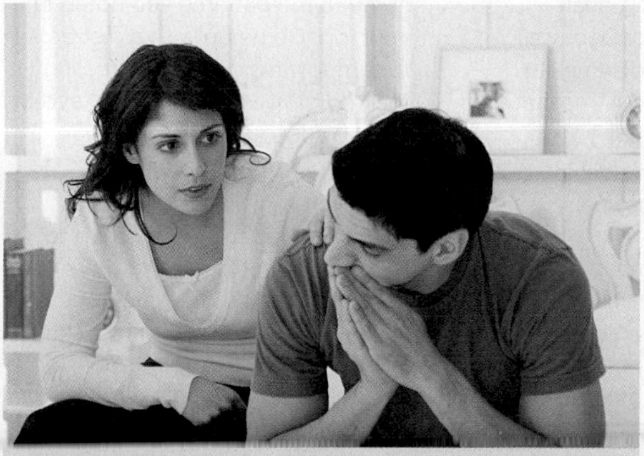

The process of acknowledging and overcoming an addiction is a long and difficult journey for everyone involved.

Abstinence alone does little to change the psychological, biological, and environmental dynamics that underlie the addictive behavior. Without treatment, an addict is apt to relapse repeatedly or simply change addictions. Treatment involves learning new ways of looking at oneself, others, and the world. It may require exploring a traumatic past so that psychological wounds can be healed. It also involves developing communication skills and new ways of having fun.

intervention A planned process of confronting an addict carried out by close family, friends, and significant others.

abstinence Refraining from a behavior.

detoxification The early abstinence period during which an addict adjusts physically and cognitively to being free from the influences of the addiction.

Finding a Quality Treatment Program

For a large number of addicts, recovery begins with a period of formal treatment. The best programs provide a combination of therapies (behavioral therapy, medications, or both) and other services to meet an addict's needs. A good treatment program includes the following:

- Professional staff familiar with the specific addictive disorder for which help is being sought
- A flexible schedule of inpatient and outpatient services
- Access to medical personnel who can assess the addict's health and treat all medical concerns as needed, including complicated detoxification
- Involvement of family members in the treatment process
- A coordinated team approach to treating addictive disorders (for example, medical staff, counselors, psychotherapists, social workers, clergy, educators, dietitians, and fitness counselors)
- Both group and individual therapy options
- Peer-led support groups that encourage the addict to continue involvement after treatment ends
- Structured aftercare and relapse-prevention programs
- Accreditation by the Joint Commission (a national organization that accredits and certifies health care organizations and programs) and a license from the state in which the program operates

WHAT DO YOU THINK?

Why might addicts resist seeking treatment, even when they may admit they have a problem?

- What factors need to be considered in helping prevent relapse?

Most programs apply a combination of family, individual, and group counseling, supplemented with attendance at a 12-step support group. Individuals may also wish to explore alternatives to 12-step groups. Organizations such as Rational Recovery and the Secular Organization for Sobriety provide support without the spiritual emphasis of 12-step groups such as Alcoholics Anonymous.

Relapse

Relapse is an isolated occurrence of or full return to addictive behavior. It is one of the defining characteristics of addiction. A person who does not relapse or have powerful urges to do so was probably not addicted in the first place. Addicts are set up to relapse long before they actually do so because of their tendency to meet change and stress with the same kind of denial they once used to justify their addictive behavior (for example, thinking, "I don't have a problem; I can handle this"). This sets off a series of events involving immediate or gradual abandonment of structured recovery plans. For example, the addict may quit attending support group meetings and slip into situations that previously triggered the addictive behavior.

relapse The tendency to return to the addictive behavior after a period of abstinence.

Because those who facilitate treatment programs recognize this strong tendency to relapse, they routinely teach clients and significant others to recognize the signs of imminent relapse and develop a plan for responding to these signs. Without such a plan, recovering addicts are likely to relapse more frequently, more completely, and perhaps permanently.

Relapse should not be interpreted as failure to change or lack of desire to stay well. The appropriate response to relapse is to remind addicts that they are addicted and to redirect them to the strategies that have previously worked for them. In addition to teaching skills, relapse prevention may involve aftercare planning such as connecting the recovering person with support groups, career counselors, or community services.

ASSESS YOURSELF

Are you affected by addiction? Want to find out? Take the **Are You Addicted?** assessment available on MasteringHealth.™

Need help creating a plan? Follow the strategies in the **Your Plan for Change** box for short- and long-term improvements to your health.

YOUR PLAN FOR CHANGE

The online **ASSESS YOURSELF** activity gave you a chance to evaluate signs of Internet, gambling, and shopping addictions. Depending on your results, you may need to take steps toward changing certain behaviors that could be detrimental to your health.

TODAY, YOU CAN:

- ☐ Identify any problem areas in which you may have an addiction. Be honest with yourself about your behaviors and commit to addressing the issue. The first step in beating an addiction is admitting you have a problem.
- ☐ Write a list of the things that contribute to the behavior you feel may be addictive. Include your reasons for engaging in the behavior and the things about it that are reinforcing. Why do you want to change it? Try to identify barriers that would make it hard to break away from the behavior or bring it under control. What would help you address these barriers?

WITHIN THE NEXT 2 WEEKS, YOU CAN:

- ☐ Look into support groups in your area that could possibly help you, such as Gamblers Anonymous or Debtors Anonymous. Visit your student health center to find out about programs that may be available on campus.
- ☐ Begin tracking your addictive behavior. Keep a log of dates, time spent engaging in the behavior, the way you are feeling, the amount of money spent (if pertinent), other people involved, and anything else you think is relevant. Look for patterns, such as particular times of day when you are most vulnerable to the addiction, a specific mood related to it, or certain people or places that trigger your compulsion.

BY THE END OF THE SEMESTER, YOU CAN:

- ☐ Take positive steps to address some of the patterns you noted in your log. Come up with a distraction to turn to when you begin feeling the addictive urge, and try to avoid settings or situations that trigger your addictive behavior.
- ☐ Establish new limits for your addictive behavior and strive to enforce them for several days at a time. For example, this could mean setting a time limit on Internet use. Enlist a trusted friend to help you enforce these limits—for example, by making plans to play Frisbee after your allotted half hour of Internet surfing.

10 Drinking Alcohol Responsibly

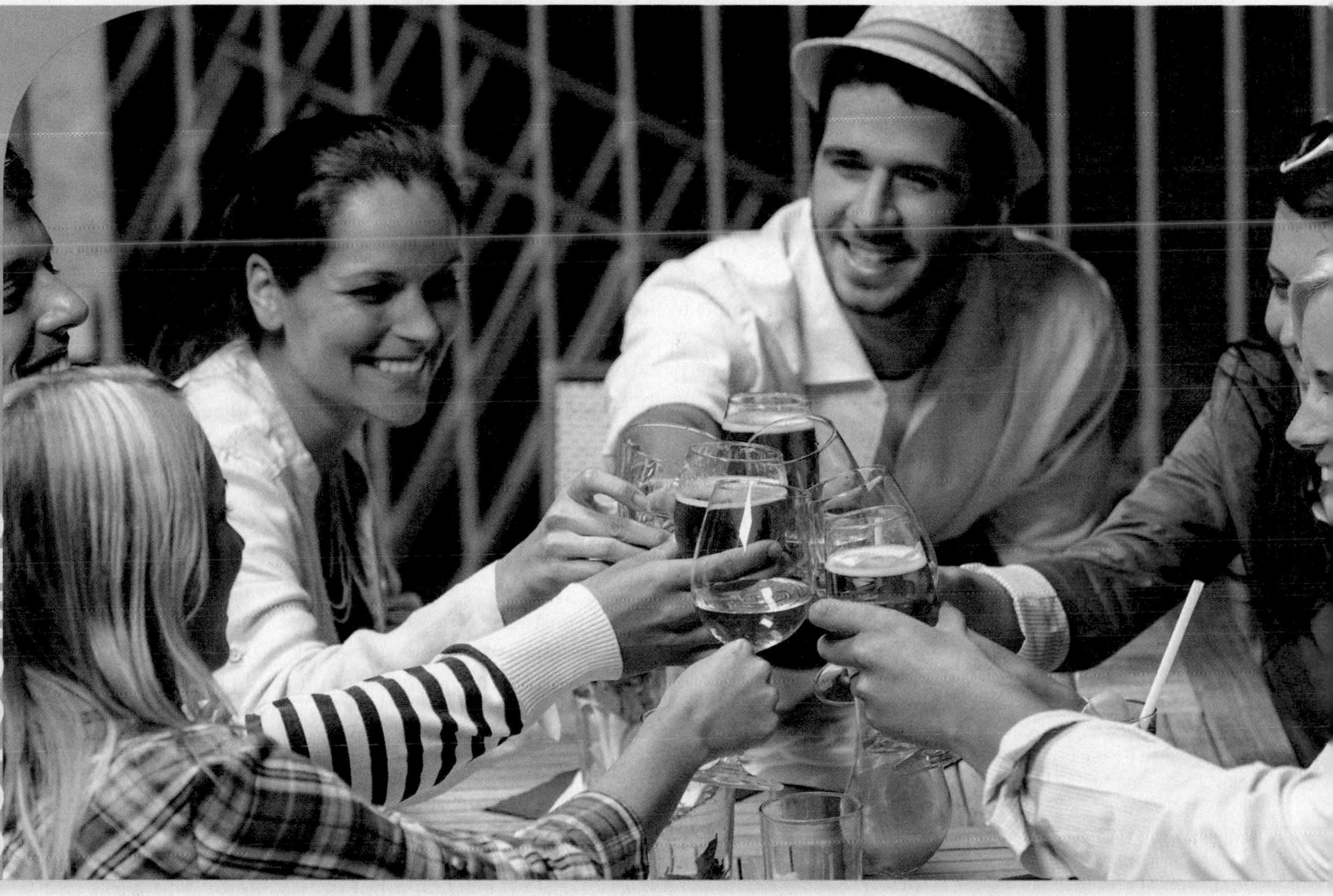

LEARNING OUTCOMES

1 Explain the physiological and behavioral effects of alcohol, including absorption, metabolism, and blood alcohol concentration.
2 Identify short- and long-term effects of alcohol consumption.
3 Describe alcohol use patterns of college students, practical strategies for drinking responsibly, and ways to cope with campus and societal pressures to drink.
4 Describe the impact of drinking and driving on society.
5 Compare the differences in alcohol consumption and abuse among various ethnic and racial minority groups.
6 Explain the risk factors associated with alcoholism, its symptoms, its costs to society, and its effects on family members.
7 Describe the various types of treatment programs for alcoholism and their effectiveness and explore the concepts of relapse, and recovery.

Throughout history, humans have used alcohol for everything from social gatherings to religious ceremonies. The consumption of alcoholic beverages is interwoven with many traditions, and moderate use of alcohol can enhance celebrations or special times. Research even shows that very low levels of alcohol consumption, particularly red wine, may actually lower some health risks in older adults.[1] Potential benefits include reduced risks of cardiovascular diseases and osteoporosis, though some critics of these studies argue that confounding factors, such as socioeconomic status, may account for the apparent benefits.[2] While alcohol can sometimes play a positive role in some people's lives, it is first and foremost a chemical substance that affects both physical and mental functions. Alcohol is a drug, and if it is not used responsibly, it can be dangerous.

It is estimated that half of Americans consume alcoholic beverages regularly, and about 21 percent abstain from drinking alcohol altogether.[3] Among those who drink, consumption patterns vary. More men are regular drinkers, and men typically drink more than women. White drinkers are more likely to drink daily or nearly daily than are nonwhites. Adults in poor families were twice as likely as adults in nonpoor families to be lifetime abstainers.[4]

New estimates also show that **binge drinking**—a pattern of drinking alcohol that brings blood alcohol concentration (BAC) to 0.08 gram-percent or above—is a bigger problem now than previously thought. More than 38 million U.S. adults binge drink (or approximately 1 in 6) about four times a month, and the largest number of drinks per binge is on average eight. Binge drinking prevalence (30%) and intensity of drinking (8.9 drinks) were highest among persons aged 18 to 24. Those households with incomes over $75,000 had the highest drinking prevalence (22.2%), but those with household incomes below $25,000 had the highest frequency (4.3 episodes per month) and intensity (7.1 drinks on occasion).[5]

In general, alcohol consumption among Americans declined steadily in the late 1970s until about 2000, when alcohol consumption began to increase slightly. Much of this increase can be linked to the downturn of the U.S. economy.[6] Since 2009 alcohol consumption has begun to decline. This downward trend has been tied to a stronger economy and a returned focus on personal health, weight management, and physical activity.[7]

binge drinking A pattern of drinking alcohol that brings BAC to 0.08 gram-percent or above; corresponds to consuming five or more drinks (adult male) or four or more drinks (adult female) in 2 hours.

ethyl alcohol (ethanol) Addictive drug produced by fermentation that is the intoxicating substance in alcoholic beverages.

fermentation Process in which yeast organisms break down plant sugars to yield ethanol.

distillation Process in which alcohol vapors are condensed and mixed with water to make hard liquor.

proof Measure of the percentage of alcohol in a beverage; the proof is double the percentage of alcohol in the drink.

standard drink Amount of any beverage that contains about 14 grams of pure alcohol.

LO 1 | ALCOHOL IN THE BODY

Explain the physiological and behavioral effects of alcohol, including absorption, metabolism, and blood alcohol concentration.

Learning about the metabolism and absorption of alcohol can help you understand how it affects each person differently and how it is possible to drink safely. It is also key to understanding how to avoid life-threatening alcohol-related circumstances such as alcohol poisoning.

The Chemistry and Potency of Alcohol

The intoxicating substance found in beer, wine, liquor, and liqueurs is **ethyl alcohol,** or **ethanol**. It is produced during a process called **fermentation,** in which yeast organisms break down plant sugars, yielding ethanol and carbon dioxide. For beers, ales, and wines, the process ends with fermentation. Hard liquor is produced through further processing called **distillation,** during which alcohol vapors are condensed and mixed with water to make the final product.

The **proof** of an alcoholic drink is a measure of the percentage of alcohol in the beverage and therefore the strength of the drink. Alcohol percentage is half of the given proof. For example, 80 proof whiskey or scotch is 40 percent alcohol by volume, and 100 proof vodka is 50 percent alcohol by volume. Lower-proof drinks will produce fewer alcohol effects than the same amount of higher-proof drinks. Most wines are between 12 and 15 percent alcohol, and most beers are between 2 and 8 percent, depending on state laws and the type of beer.

When discussing alcohol consumption, researchers usually talk in terms of "standard drinks." As defined by the National Institute on Alcohol Abuse and Alcoholism (NIAAA), a **standard drink** is any drink that contains about 14 grams of pure alcohol (about 0.6 fluid ounce or 1.2 tablespoons; see **FIGURE 10.1**). The actual size of a standard drink depends on the proof: A 12-ounce can of beer and a 1.5-ounce shot of vodka are both considered one standard drink because they contain the same amount of alcohol—about 0.6 fluid ounce. If you are estimating your blood alcohol concentration using standard drinks as a measure (see the following sections), you need to keep in mind the size of your drinks as well as their proof. For example, you may have bought only one beer while you were at the ballpark last weekend, but if that beer came in a 22-ounce cup, then you actually consumed two standard drinks.

Absorption and Metabolism

Unlike the molecules found in most foods and drugs, alcohol molecules are sufficiently small and fat soluble to be absorbed throughout the entire gastrointestinal system. Approximately 20 percent of ingested alcohol diffuses through the stomach lining into the bloodstream, and nearly 80 percent passes through the lining of the upper third of the small intestine. A negligible amount of alcohol is absorbed through the lining of the mouth.

Standard drink equivalent (and % alcohol)		Approximate number of standard drinks in:
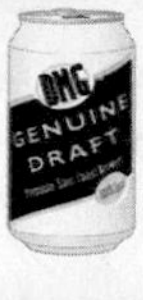	Beer = 12 oz (~5% alcohol)	12 oz = 1 16 oz = 1.3 22 oz = 2 40 oz = 3.3
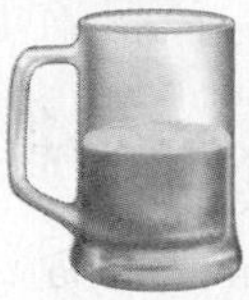	Malt liquor = 8.5 oz (~7% alcohol)	12 oz = 1.5 16 oz = 2 22 oz = 2.5 40 oz = 4.5
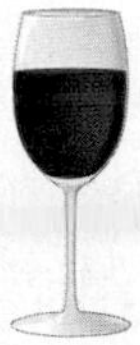	Table wine = 5 oz (~12% alcohol)	750-mL (25-oz) bottle = 5
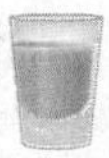	80 proof spirits (gin, vodka, etc.) = 1.5 oz (~40% alcohol)	mixed drink = 1 or more* pint (16 oz) = 11 fifth (25 oz) = 17 1.75 L (59 oz) = 39

FIGURE 10.1 What Is a Standard Drink?

*Note: It can be difficult to estimate the number of standard drinks in a single mixed drink made with hard liquor. Depending on factors such as the type of spirits and the recipe, a mixed drink can contain from one to three or more standard drinks. For example, a typical margarita may contain two shots (3-oz) of tequila, or two standard drinks.

Source: Adapted from National Institute on Alcohol Abuse and Alcoholism, *Rethinking Drinking: Alcohol and Your Health*, NIH Publication no. 10-3770 (Bethesda, MD: National Institutes of Health, 2010), http://pubs.niaaa.nih.gov/publications/Tips/tips.htm.

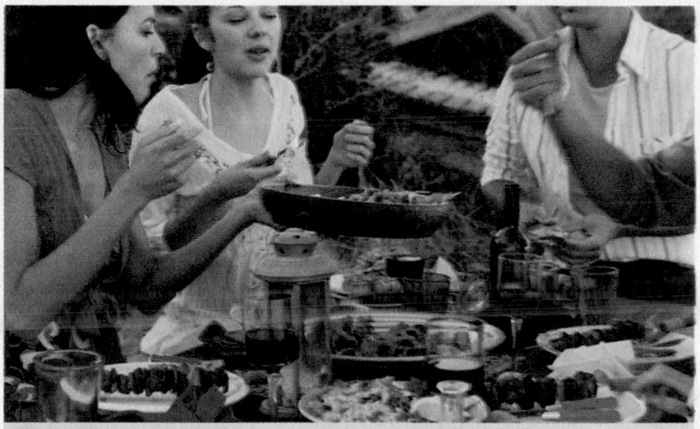

Eating while drinking slows the absorption of alcohol into your bloodstream. Other factors that influence how rapidly a person's body absorbs alcohol include gender, body weight, body composition, and mood.

Several factors influence how quickly your body will absorb alcohol: the alcohol concentration in your drink; the amount of alcohol you consume; the amount of food in your stomach; pylorospasm (spasm of the pyloric valve in the digestive system); your metabolism, weight, and body mass index; and your mood.

The higher the concentration of alcohol in your drink, the more rapidly it will be absorbed. As a rule, wine and beer are absorbed more slowly than distilled beverages. "Fizzy" alcoholic beverages—such as champagne and sparkling wines—are absorbed more rapidly than those containing no carbonation. Carbonated beverages and drinks served with mixers cause the pyloric valve to relax, thereby emptying the stomach's contents more rapidly into the small intestine. Because the small intestine is the site of the greatest absorption of alcohol, carbonated beverages increase the rate of absorption. The **Health Headlines** box on the next page discusses the effects of mixing energy drinks with alcohol.

The more alcohol you consume, the longer absorption takes. Alcohol can irritate the digestive system, which causes pylorospasm. When the pyloric valve is closed, nothing can move from the stomach to the upper third of the small intestine, which slows absorption. If the irritation continues, it can cause vomiting. Alcohol also takes longer to absorb if there is food in your stomach, because the surface area exposed to alcohol is smaller, and because a full stomach retards the emptying of alcoholic beverages into the small intestine.

Mood is another factor, because emotions affect how long it takes for the stomach's contents to empty into the intestine. Powerful moods like stress and tension are likely to cause the stomach to dump its contents into the small intestine more rapidly, meaning alcohol is absorbed much faster when people are tense than it is when they are relaxed.

Once it has been absorbed into the bloodstream, alcohol circulates throughout the body and is metabolized in the liver, where it is converted to *acetaldehyde*—a toxic chemical that can cause nausea and vomiting as well as long-term effects like liver damage—by the enzyme *alcohol dehydrogenase.* It is then rapidly oxidized to *acetate,* converted to carbon dioxide and water, and eventually excreted from the body. A very small portion of alcohol is excreted unchanged by the kidneys, lungs, and skin.

Alcohol contains 7 calories (kcal) per gram. This means that the average regular beer contains about 150 calories. Mixed drinks may contain more if they are combined with sugary soda or fruit juice. The body uses the calories in alcohol in the same manner it uses those found in carbohydrates: for immediate energy or for storage as fat if not immediately needed.

The breakdown of alcohol occurs at a fairly constant rate of 0.5 ounce per hour (slightly less than one standard

HEAR IT! PODCASTS

Want a study podcast for this chapter? Download the podcast on **Alcohol** available on MasteringHealth.™

HEALTH HEADLINES

ALCOHOL AND ENERGY DRINKS

A Dangerous Mix

Energy drinks are aggressively marketed on college campuses, with manufacturers often giving away samples to promote them. The success of these products is based on claims that they provide a burst of energy from caffeine and other plant-based stimulants and vitamins. Thirty-four percent of 18- to 24-year-olds are regular energy drink consumers.

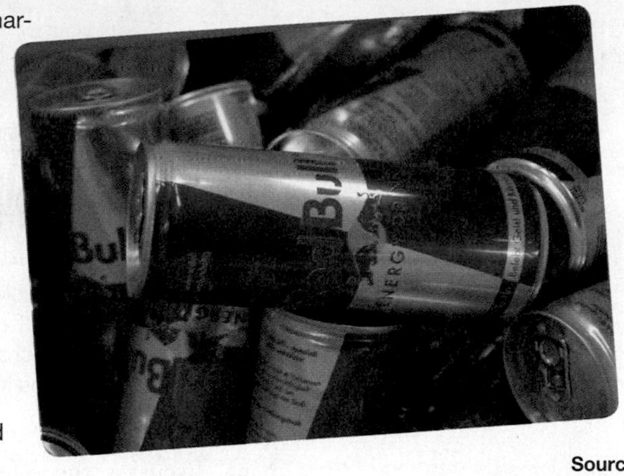

The alcohol industry has used the popularity of energy drinks to promote its own products, introducing premixed alcohol and energy drink products such as Sparks, Rockstar 21, and Tilt. In addition, energy drink companies promote mixing energy drinks with alcohol products. Red Bull, for example, promotes a top drinks list suggesting "Jaegerbombs" and "Tucker Death mix."

Students often mix energy drinks with alcohol, and these drinks can be particularly dangerous. College men who use alcohol-mixed energy drinks score more highly on risk taking measures. In a recent study, most college students had neutral or negative views of alcohol-mixed drinks. Those who most frequently consume alcohol-mixed drinks had positive expectations, such as being able to party longer.

Students also report not noticing the signs of intoxication (dizziness, fatigue, headache, or lack of coordination) when they had consumed alcohol-mixed energy drinks. Caffeine may delay the onset of normal sleepiness, increasing the amount of time a person would normally stay awake and drink. The caffeine in energy drinks also reduces the subjective feeling of drunkenness without actually reducing alcohol-related impairment.

Students who reported drinking alcohol-mixed energy drinks were more likely to consume large amounts of alcohol; have unprotected sex or sex under the influence of alcohol or drugs; be hurt or injured; and meet criteria for alcohol dependency.

Sources: D. L. Thombs et al., "Event-Level Analyses of Energy Drink Consumption and Alcohol Intoxication in Bar Patrons," *Addictive Behaviors* 35, no. 4 (2010): 325–30; A. Peacock et al., "Patterns of Use and Motivations for Consuming Alcohol Mixed with Energy Drinks," *Psychology of Addictive Behaviors* 27, no. 1 (2013): 202–206; J. Howland et al., Risks of Energy Drinks with Alcohol," *JAMA* 309, no. 3 (2013): 245–46; A. M. Arria et al., "Energy Drink Consumption and Increased Risk for Alcohol Dependence," *Alcoholism: Clinical and Experimental Research* 35, no. 2 (2011): 365–75; W. I. William et al., "Energy Drinks: Psychological Effects and Impact on Well-being and Quality of Life: A Literature Review," *Innovations in Clinical Neuroscience* 9, no. 1 (2012): 25–34.

drink). This amount of alcohol is approximately equivalent to 12 ounces of 5 percent beer, 5 ounces of 12 percent wine, or 1.5 ounces of 40 percent (80 proof) liquor. Unmetabolized alcohol circulates in the bloodstream until enough time passes for the body to break it down.

Blood Alcohol Concentration

Blood alcohol concentration (BAC) is the ratio of alcohol to total blood volume. It is the factor used to measure the physiological and behavioral effects of alcohol. Despite individual differences, alcohol produces some general behavioral effects, depending on BAC (see **FIGURE 10.2**).

blood alcohol concentration (BAC) The ratio of alcohol to total blood volume; the factor used to measure the physiological and behavioral effects of alcohol.

Blood Alcohol Concentration (BAC)	Psychological and Physical Effects
Not Impaired	
<0.01%	Negligible
Sometimes Impaired	
0.01–0.04%	Slight muscle relaxation, mild euphoria, slight body warmth, increased sociability and talkativeness
Usually Impaired	
0.05–0.07%	Lowered alertness, impaired judgment, lowered inhibitions, exaggerated behavior, loss of small muscle control
Always Impaired	
0.08–0.14%	Slowed reaction time, poor muscle coordination, short-term memory loss, judgment impaired, inability to focus
0.15–0.24%	Blurred vision, lack of motor skills, sedation, slowed reactions, difficulty standing and walking, passing out
0.25–0.34%	Impaired consciousness, disorientation, loss of motor function, severely impaired or no reflexes, impaired circulation and respiration, uncontrolled urination, slurred speech, possible death
0.35% and up	Unconsciousness, coma, extremely slow heartbeat and respiration, unresponsiveness, probable death

FIGURE 10.2 The Psychological and Physical Effects of Alcohol

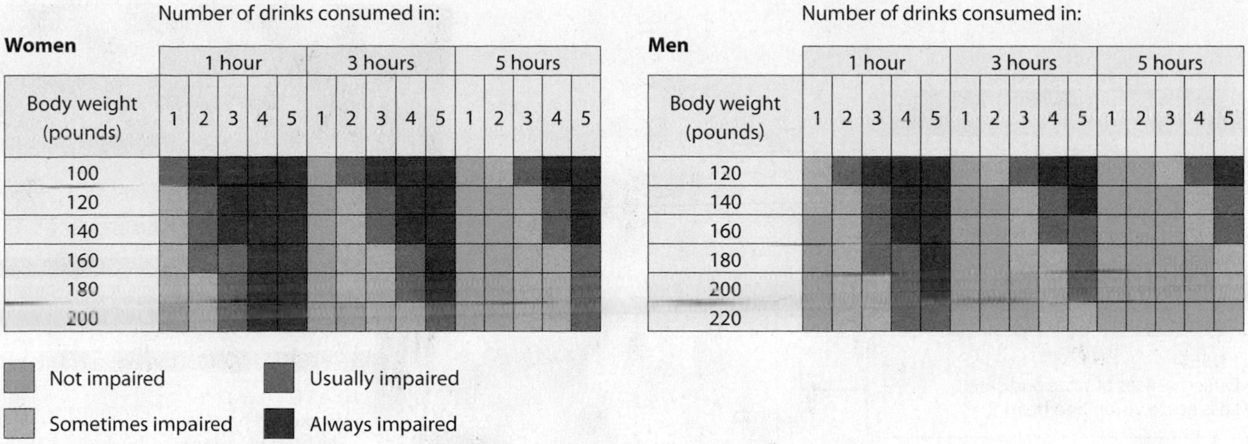

Women
Number of drinks consumed in:
1 hour
3 hours
5 hours
Body weight (pounds)
1 2 3 4 5 1 2 3 4 5 1 2 3 4 5
100
120
140
160
180
200
Men
Number of drinks consumed in:
1 hour
3 hours
5 hours
Body weight (pounds)
1 2 3 4 5 1 2 3 4 5 1 2 3 4 5
120
140
160
180
200
220
Not impaired
Sometimes impaired
Usually impaired
Always impaired

FIGURE 10.3 Approximate Blood Alcohol Concentration (BAC) and the Physiological and Behavioral Effects Remember that there are many variables that can affect BAC, so this is only an estimate of what your BAC would be.

At a BAC of 0.02 percent, a person feels slightly relaxed and in a good mood. At 0.05 percent, relaxation increases, there is some motor impairment, and a willingness to talk becomes apparent. At 0.08 percent, a person feels euphoric, and there is further motor impairment. The legal limit for driving a motor vehicle is a 0.08 percent BAC in all states and the District of Columbia. At 0.10 percent, the depressant effects of alcohol become apparent, drowsiness sets in, and motor skills are further impaired, followed by a loss of judgment. Thus, a driver may not be able to estimate distance or speed, and some drinkers may do things they would not do when sober. As BAC increases, the drinker suffers increasingly negative physiological and psychological effects.

A drinker's BAC depends on weight and percentage of body fat, the water content in body tissues, the concentration of alcohol in the beverage consumed, the rate of consumption, and the volume of alcohol consumed. Heavier people have larger body surfaces through which to diffuse alcohol; therefore, they have lower concentrations of alcohol in their blood than do thin people after drinking the same amount.

Blood Alcohol Concentration and Gender

Because alcohol does not diffuse as rapidly into body fat as it does into water, alcohol concentration is higher in a person with more body fat. Because women tend to have more body fat and less water in their tissues than men of the same weight, they will become more intoxicated after drinking the same amount of alcohol. Body fat is not the only contributor to the differences in alcohol's effects on men and women. Compared to men, women have half as much *alcohol dehydrogenase,* the enzyme that breaks down alcohol in the stomach before it reaches the bloodstream and the brain. So if a man and a woman drink the same amount of alcohol, the woman's BAC will be approximately 30 percent higher than the man's. Hormonal differences can also play a role: certain points in the menstrual cycle and the use of oral contraceptives are likely to contribute to longer periods of intoxication. This prolonged peak appears to be related to a woman's estrogen levels. **FIGURE 10.3** compares blood alcohol levels in men and women by weight and number of drinks consumed.

WHAT DO YOU THINK?

Why do some college students drink excessive amounts of alcohol?

- Are there particular traditions or norms related to when and why students drink on your campus?
- Have you ever had your sleep or studies interrupted or have you had to babysit a friend because he or she had been drinking?

Both breath analysis (breathalyzer test) and urinalysis are used to determine whether an individual is legally intoxicated, but blood tests are more accurate measures of BAC. An increasing number of states require blood tests for people suspected of driving under the influence of alcohol. In some states, refusal to take the breath, urine, or blood test results in immediate revocation of the person's driver's license.

People can develop physical and psychological tolerance of the effects of alcohol through regular use. The nervous system adapts over time, so greater amounts of alcohol are required to produce the same physiological and psychological effects. Though BAC may be quite high, the individual has learned to modify his or her behavior to appear sober. This ability is called **learned behavioral tolerance.**

learned behavioral tolerance The ability of heavy drinkers to modify behavior so they appear to be sober even when they have high BAC levels.

LO 2 | ALCOHOL AND YOUR HEALTH

Identify short- and long-term effects of alcohol consumption.

The immediate and long-term effects of alcohol consumption can vary greatly (**FIGURE 10.4**). Whether you experience any immediate or long-term consequences as a result of your

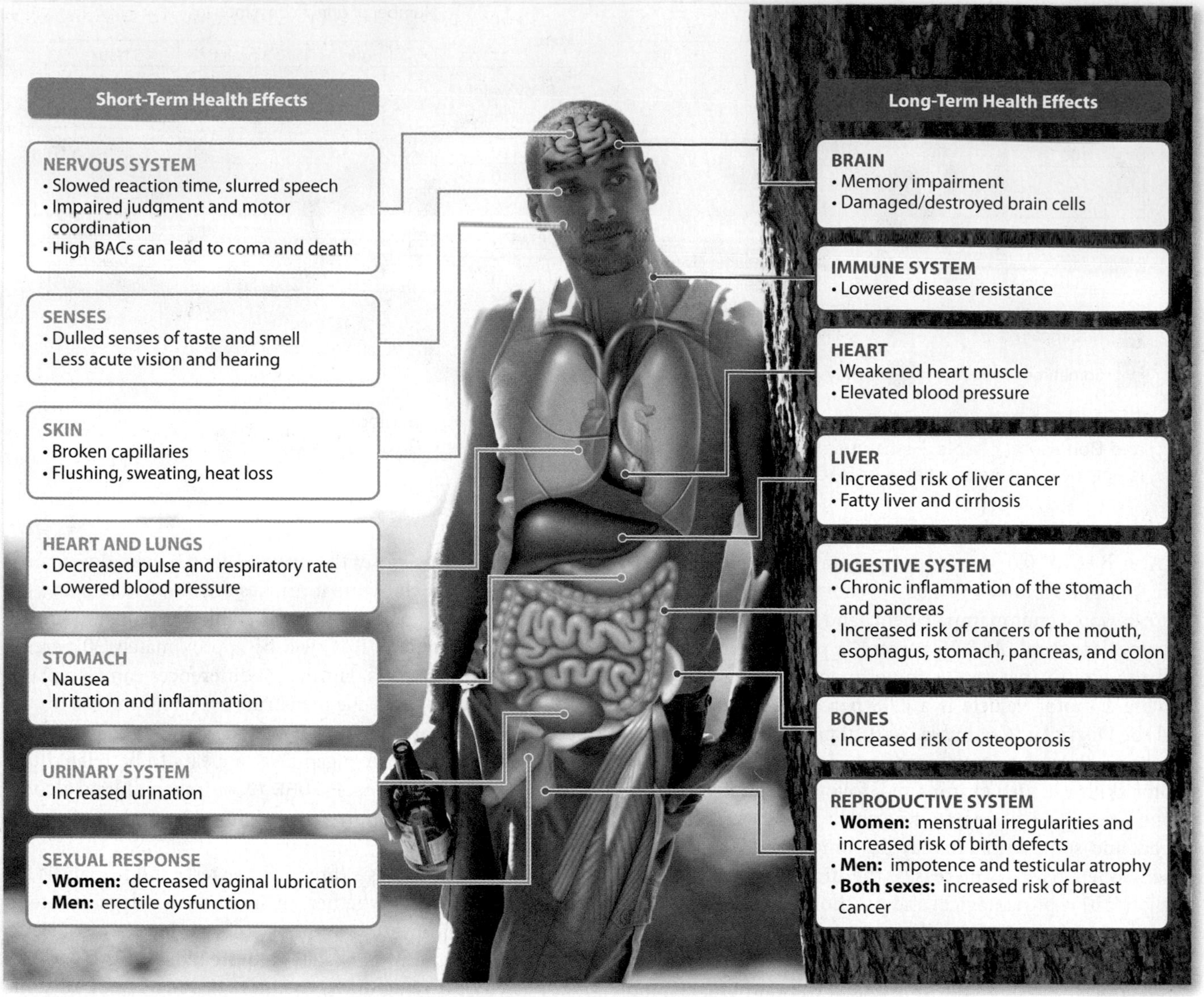
Short-Term Health Effects
NERVOUS SYSTEM
• Slowed reaction time, slurred speech
• Impaired judgment and motor coordination
• High BACs can lead to coma and death
SENSES
• Dulled senses of taste and smell
• Less acute vision and hearing
SKIN
• Broken capillaries
• Flushing, sweating, heat loss
HEART AND LUNGS
• Decreased pulse and respiratory rate
• Lowered blood pressure
STOMACH
• Nausea
• Irritation and inflammation
URINARY SYSTEM
• Increased urination
SEXUAL RESPONSE
• Women: decreased vaginal lubrication
• Men: erectile dysfunction
Long-Term Health Effects
BRAIN
• Memory impairment
• Damaged/destroyed brain cells
IMMUNE SYSTEM
• Lowered disease resistance
HEART
• Weakened heart muscle
• Elevated blood pressure
LIVER
• Increased risk of liver cancer
• Fatty liver and cirrhosis
DIGESTIVE SYSTEM
• Chronic inflammation of the stomach and pancreas
• Increased risk of cancers of the mouth, esophagus, stomach, pancreas, and colon
BONES
• Increased risk of osteoporosis
REPRODUCTIVE SYSTEM
• Women: menstrual irregularities and increased risk of birth defects
• Men: impotence and testicular atrophy
• Both sexes: increased risk of breast cancer

FIGURE 10.4 Effects of Alcohol on the Body and Health

VIDEO TUTOR
Long- and Short-Term Effects of Alcohol

alcohol use depends on you as an individual, the amount of alcohol you consume, and your circumstances.

Short-Term Effects of Alcohol

The most dramatic effects produced by ethanol occur within the central nervous system (CNS). Alcohol depresses CNS functions, which decreases respiratory rate, pulse rate, and blood pressure. As CNS depression deepens, vital functions become noticeably affected. In extreme cases, coma and death can result.

dehydration Loss of water from body tissues.

hangover Physiological reaction to excessive drinking, including headache, upset stomach, anxiety, depression, diarrhea, and thirst.

Alcohol is a diuretic that causes increased urinary output. Although this effect might be expected to lead to automatic **dehydration,** the body actually retains water, most of it in the muscles or in cerebral tissues. Because water is usually pulled out of the *cerebrospinal fluid* (fluid within the brain and spinal cord), drinkers may suffer symptoms that include "morning-after" effects.

Alcohol irritates the gastrointestinal system and may cause indigestion and heartburn if consumed on an empty stomach. In addition, people who engage in brief drinking sprees during which they consume unusually high amounts of alcohol put themselves at risk for irregular heartbeat or even total loss of heart rhythm, which can disrupt blood flow and damage the heart muscle.

Hangover

A **hangover** is often experienced the morning after a drinking spree. Its symptoms are familiar to most people who drink: headache, muscle aches, upset stomach, anxiety, depression, diarrhea, and thirst. Hangovers kick in for more than half of people after their blood alcohol content reaches 0.11. Approximately 20–25 percent of those who drink enough

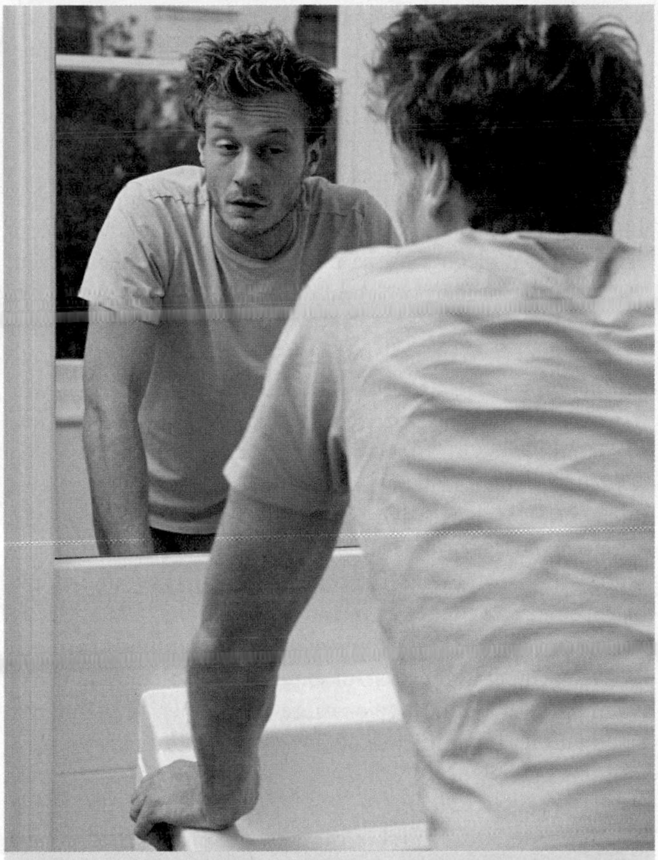

The only cure for a hangover is abstaining from excessive alcohol use in the first place.

to get a hangover do not experience them.[8] **Congeners,** forms of alcohol that are metabolized more slowly than ethanol and are more toxic, are thought to play a role in the development of a hangover. The body metabolizes the congeners after the ethanol is gone from the system, and their toxic by-products may contribute to the hangover. Alcohol also upsets the water balance in the body, which results in excess urination, dehydration, and thirst the next day. Increased production of hydrochloric acid can irritate the stomach lining and cause nausea. Recovery from a hangover usually takes 12 hours. Bed rest, solid food, plenty of water, and aspirin or ibuprofen may help relieve a hangover's discomforts, but the only sure way to avoid one is to abstain from excessive alcohol use in the first place.

Alcohol and Injuries Alcohol use plays a significant role in the types of injuries people experience. Hospitalizations from alcohol overdoses among 18- to 24-year-olds rose by 25 percent over the past 10 years, and about 30 percent of young adults hospitalized for overdoses involve excessive consumption of alcohol.[9] Alcohol use is involved in approximately 70 percent of fatal injuries during activities such as swimming and boating. A boat operator with a blood alcohol concentration (BAC) over 0.1 is 16 times more likely to be killed in a boating accident than an operator with zero BAC.[10] Alcohol is involved in 40 percent of fatal injuries due to house fires.[11]

Alcohol use is also a key risk factor for suicide—playing a role in approximately one-third of suicides in the United States. Alcohol may increase the risk for suicide by intensifying depressive thoughts or feelings of hopelessness, lowering inhibitions to hurt oneself, and interfering with the ability to assess future consequences of one's actions.[12]

Alcohol and Sexual Decision Making Because it lowers inhibitions, alcohol has a clear influence on one's ability to make good decisions about sex. People who are intoxicated are less likely to use safer sex practices and are more likely to engage in high-risk sexual activity. About 1 in 5 college students report engaging in sexual activity, including having sex with someone they just met, and having unprotected sex, after drinking.[13] The chance of acquiring a sexually transmitted infection or experiencing an unplanned pregnancy also increases among students who drink more heavily compared with those who drink moderately or not at all.

Alcohol and Rape, Sexual Assault, and Dating Violence Alcohol is a key factor in many rapes. More than 30 percent of rape victims reported that their assailant was under the influence of alcohol.[14] In a survey, almost 20 percent of undergraduate women reported experiencing some type of sexual assault since entering college—with most incidents involving alcohol or unknowingly consuming a drug placed in their drinks.[15] Perpetrators who drink before an assault are more likely to think their sex drive is increased by alcohol, and they are also more likely to think that drinking itself signals an interest in sex.[16]

Most college assault victims know their attacker, especially in incapacitated assaults, and assaults occur frequently at parties. One study found 58 percent of incapacitated rapes and 28 percent of forced rapes to occur at a party.[17] Students who have experienced recent sexual victimization are at higher risk of drinking—particularly binge drinking. Risky drinking, including binge drinking, in itself increases the risk of sexual victimization.[18]

congeners Forms of alcohol that are metabolized more slowly than ethanol and produce toxic by-products.

Another study of college students showed heavy drinking to be associated with dating violence by men in their freshman year. Among women, heavy drinking in their sophomore year predicted dating violence in their junior year.[19]

Alcohol and Weight Gain The "freshman 15" and other college-year weight gain may have more to do with alcohol consumption than the food served in the dining halls. Alcohol has 7 calories per gram—nearly as much as fat (9 calories per gram) and more than carbohydrates or protein (4 calories per gram)—and the calories from alcohol provide few nutrients. A standard drink contains 12 to 15 grams of alcohol, meaning a single drink can add about 100 empty calories to your daily intake. By drinking an extra 150 calories a day more than you need, you can gain 1 pound a month and up to 12 pounds a year.[20]

SKILLS FOR BEHAVIOR CHANGE

DEALING WITH AN ALCOHOL EMERGENCY

Heavy drinking can be life threatening. Anyone who has passed out from drinking should be watched very closely. Roll an unconscious drinker onto his or her side with knees bent to minimize the chance of vomit obstructing the airway. If the drinker vomits, you may need to reach into his or her mouth and clear the airway.

If you suspect that someone has alcohol poisoning, call 9-1-1 immediately to get help. For the safety of you and your friends, know the signs of acute alcohol intoxication:

- Confusion, stupor, or inability to be roused
- Vomiting and/or seizures
- Slow breathing (fewer than eight breaths per minute)
- Rapid or irregular pulse (100 beats or more per minute) or irregular breathing (10 seconds or more between breaths)
- Cool, clammy, skin; pale or bluish skin color; bluish lips or fingernails

Alcohol Poisoning **Alcohol poisoning** (also known as *acute alcohol intoxication*) occurs much more frequently than people realize, and all too often it can be fatal. Drinking large amounts of alcohol in a short period of time can cause the blood alcohol level to quickly reach the lethal range. Alcohol, used either alone or in combination with other drugs, is responsible for more toxic overdose deaths than any other substance.

The amount of alcohol that causes a person to lose consciousness, which for most people is 0.35% BAC (see Figure 10.3), is dangerously close to the lethal dose. Death from alcohol poisoning can be caused by CNS and respiratory depression or by the inhalation of vomit or fluid into the lungs. Alcohol depresses the nerves that control involuntary actions such as breathing and the gag reflex (which prevents choking). As BAC levels reach higher concentrations, eventually these functions can be completely suppressed. If a drinker becomes unconscious and vomits, there is a danger of asphyxiation through choking to death on the vomit. Blood alcohol concentration can continue rising even after a drinker becomes unconscious because alcohol in the stomach and intestine continues to empty into the bloodstream.

alcohol poisoning (acute alcohol intoxication) Potentially lethal BAC that inhibits the brain's ability to control consciousness, respiration, and heart rate; usually occurs as a result of drinking a large amount of alcohol in a short period of time.

The **Skills for Behavior Change** box describes the signs of alcohol poisoning. If you are with someone who has been drinking heavily and who exhibits these symptoms, or if you are unsure about the person's condition, call your local emergency number (9-1-1 in most areas) for immediate assistance.

Long-Term Effects

Alcohol is distributed throughout most of the body and may affect many organs and tissues. Problems associated with long-term, habitual alcohol abuse include diseases of the nervous system, cardiovascular system, and liver, as well as some cancers.

Effects on the Nervous System The nervous system is especially sensitive to alcohol. Even people who drink moderately experience shrinkage in brain size and weight and a loss of some degree of intellectual ability.

Research suggests that developing brains in adolescents are much more prone to damage than was previously thought. Alcohol appears to damage the frontal areas of the adolescent brain, which are crucial for controlling impulses and thinking through consequences of intended actions.[21] In addition, researchers suggest that people who begin drinking at an early age are at much higher risk of experiencing alcohol abuse or dependence, drinking five or more drinks per occasion, and driving under the influence of alcohol at least weekly.[22]

Cardiovascular Effects Alcohol affects the cardiovascular system in a number of ways. Numerous studies have associated light to moderate alcohol consumption (no more than two drinks a day) with a reduced risk of coronary artery disease.[23] Several mechanisms have been proposed to explain how this might happen. The strongest evidence points to an increase in high-density lipoprotein (HDL) cholesterol, which is known as "good" cholesterol. Studies have shown that moderate drinkers have higher levels of HDL.[24] Alcohol's effects on blood clotting, insulin sensitivity, and inflammation are also thought to play a role in protecting against heart disease. However, alcohol consumption is not a preventive measure against heart disease: It causes many more cardiovascular health hazards than benefits. Drinking too much alcohol contributes to high blood pressure and higher calorie intake, both of which are risk factors for cardiovascular disease.[25]

Liver Disease One result of heavy drinking is that the liver begins to store fat—a condition known as *fatty liver*. If there is insufficient time between drinking episodes, this fat cannot be transported to storage sites, and the fat-filled liver cells stop functioning. Continued drinking can cause a further stage of liver deterioration called *fibrosis*, in which the damaged

90%

OF PEOPLE WHO DRINK **ALCOHOL** ARE CLASSIFIED AS MODERATE, LIGHT, OR INFREQUENT DRINKERS.

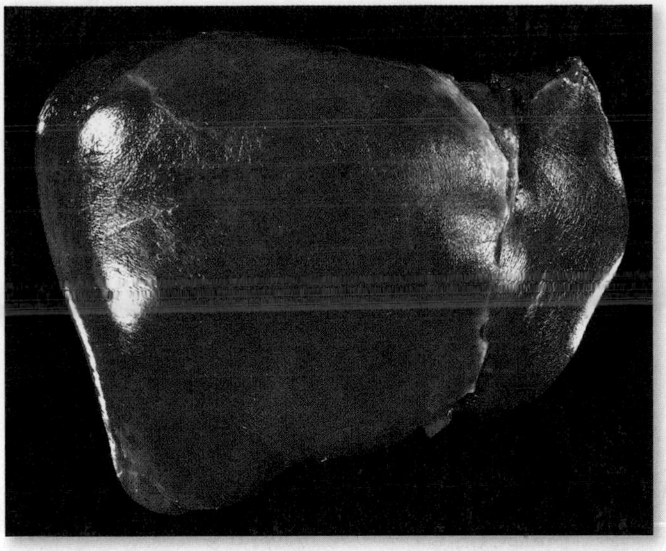

a A normal liver

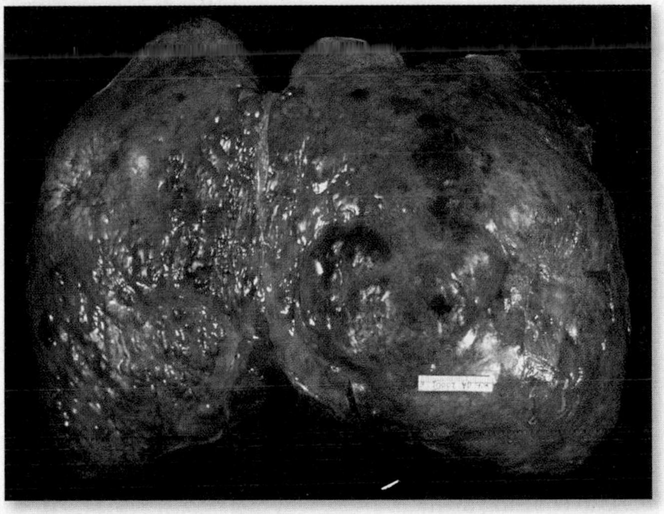

b A liver with cirrhosis

FIGURE 10.5 **Comparison of a Healthy Liver with a Cirrhotic Liver** In cirrhosis, healthy liver cells are replaced with scar tissue that interferes with the liver's ability to perform its many vital functions.

area of the liver develops fibrous scar tissue. Cell function can be partially restored at this stage with proper nutrition and abstinence from alcohol. However, if the person continues to drink, **cirrhosis** of the liver results (**FIGURE 10.5**). Among the top 10 causes of death in the United States, cirrhosis occurs as liver cells die and damage becomes permanent. **Alcoholic hepatitis** is another serious condition resulting from prolonged alcohol use. A chronic inflammation of the liver develops, which may be fatal in itself or progress to cirrhosis.

WHY SHOULD I CARE?

Going out drinking may be fun at the time, but excessive alcohol consumption can result in a hangover that ruins the day after you overindulge—leading you to skip class and to miss out on other activities.

Cancer Alcohol is considered a carcinogen. The repeated irritation caused by long-term alcohol use has been linked to cancers of the esophagus, stomach, mouth, tongue, and liver. In one study, NIAAA scientists discovered a possible link between acetaldehyde and DNA damage that could help explain the connection between drinking and certain types of cancer.[26]

There is substantial evidence that women who consume even low levels of alcohol (three to six drinks per week) have a higher risk of breast cancer compared with those who abstain, and the risk is even higher for women who consume more than two drinks per day.[27] Alcohol may make women more vulnerable to cancer by increasing estrogen levels. Health officials recommend women with a heightened risk of developing breast cancer due to factors like family history should only consume alcohol occasionally, or avoid it altogether.[28] Girls and young women who drink alcohol also increase their risk of benign (noncancerous) breast disease, which in turn increases the risk for developing breast cancer. In a recent study, girls and young women who drank 6 or 7 days a week were 5.5 times more likely to have benign breast disease than those who didn't drink or who had less than one drink per week.[29]

cirrhosis The last stage of liver disease associated with chronic heavy alcohol use, during which liver cells die and damage becomes permanent.

alcoholic hepatitis Condition resulting from prolonged use of alcohol in which the liver is inflamed; can be fatal.

Sleep People who suffer from insomnia are much more likely to develop drinking problems, and individuals with alcohol dependence are more likely to suffer from sleep problems. These sleep problems can persist for months or years after abstinence. A single drink has the potential to increase snoring and worsen sleep apnea. In young adults, binge drinking increases the frequency and severity of sleep problems.[30] For both young men and women, drinking alcohol significantly increases trouble with both falling asleep and staying asleep.

Other Effects Alcohol abuse is a major cause of chronic inflammation of the pancreas, the organ that produces digestive enzymes and insulin. Chronic alcohol abuse inhibits enzyme production, which further inhibits the absorption of nutrients. Drinking alcohol can block the absorption of calcium, a nutrient that strengthens bones. This should be of particular concern to women because of their risk for osteoporosis, as heavy consumption of alcohol worsens this condition. Evidence also suggests that alcohol impairs the body's ability to recognize and fight foreign bodies, such as bacteria and viruses.

Alcohol and Pregnancy

Teratogenic substances cause birth defects. Of the 30 known teratogens in the environment, alcohol is one of the most dangerous. If a woman ingests alcohol while pregnant, it will pass through the placenta and enter the growing fetus's bloodstream. A study found that more than 7.6 percent of children have been exposed to alcohol *in utero* and 1.4 percent of pregnant women reported binge drinking.[31] Consuming four or more drinks a day during pregnancy may significantly increase the risk of childhood mental health and learning problems. However, any use can result in varying degrees of effects, ranging from mild learning disabilities to major physical, mental, and intellectual impairment. Alcohol consumed during the first trimester poses the greatest threat to organ development; exposure during the last trimester, when the brain is developing rapidly, is most likely to affect CNS development.

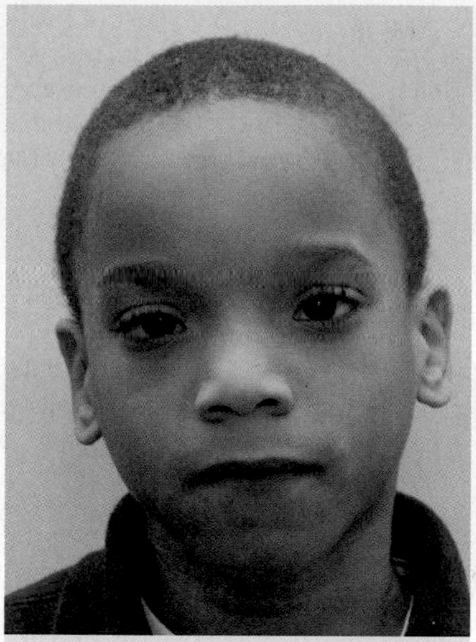

Characteristic facial features of FAS include a small, upturned nose with a low bridge and a thin upper lip.

A disorder called **fetal alcohol syndrome (FAS)** is associated with alcohol consumption during pregnancy. FAS is the third most common birth defect and the second leading cause of mental retardation in the United States, with an estimated incidence of 0.2 to 1.5 cases in every 1,000 live births.[32] It is the most common preventable cause of mental impairment in the Western world. Among the symptoms of FAS are mental retardation; small head size; tremors; and abnormalities of the face, limbs, heart, and brain. Children with FAS may experience problems such as poor memory and impaired learning, reduced attention span, impulsive behavior, and poor problem-solving abilities, among others.

fetal alcohol syndrome (FAS) Birth defect involving physical and mental impairment that results from the mother's alcohol consumption during pregnancy.

Some children may have fewer than the full physical or behavioral symptoms of FAS and may be diagnosed with disorders such as partial fetal alcohol syndrome (PFAS) or alcohol-related neurodevelopmental disorder (ARND); all of these disorders (including FAS) fall under the umbrella term *fetal alcohol spectrum disorder* (FASD). An estimated 40,000 infants in the United States are affected by FASD each year—more than those affected by spina bifida, Down syndrome, and muscular dystrophy combined.[33] Infants whose mothers habitually consumed more than 3 ounces of alcohol (approximately six drinks) in a short time period when pregnant are at high risk for FASD. Risk levels for babies whose mothers consume smaller amounts are uncertain. To avoid any chance of harming her fetus, any woman of childbearing age who is or may become pregnant is advised to refrain from consuming any amount of alcohol.

LO 3 | ALCOHOL USE IN COLLEGE

Describe alcohol use patterns of college students, practical strategies for drinking responsibly, and ways to cope with campus and societal pressures to drink.

Alcohol is the most popular drug on college campuses: Large numbers of students report having consumed alcoholic beverages in the past 30 days (**FIGURE 10.6**).[34] In a new trend on college campuses, women's consumption of alcohol has come close to equaling men's.

Approximately 40 percent of all college students engage in binge drinking.[35] For a typical adult, this means consuming five or more drinks (men), or four or more drinks (women),

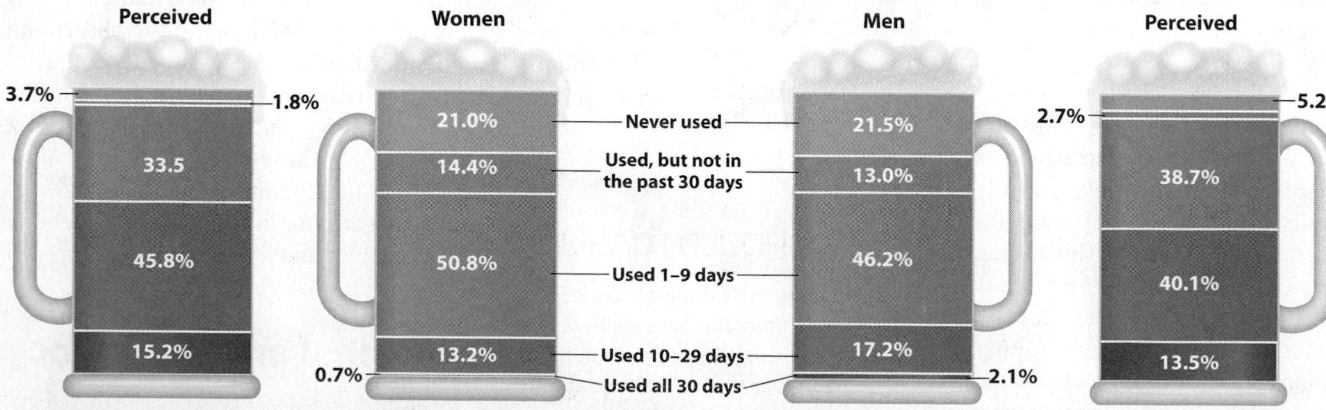

FIGURE 10.6 College Students' Patterns of Alcohol Use in the Past 30 Days

Source: Data from American College Health Association, *American College Health Association—National College Health Assessment II (ACHA-NCHA II) Reference Group Data Report Spring 2013* (Linthicum, MD: American College Health Association, 2013).

in about 2 hours.[36] Students who drink only once a week are considered binge drinkers if they consume these amounts within 2 hours. Binge drinking is especially dangerous because it can lead to extreme intoxication, unconsciousness, alcohol poisoning, and even death. Drinking competitions, celebrations, or games and hazing rituals encourage this type of drinking.

College is a critical time to become aware of and responsible for drinking. Many students are away from home, often for the first time, and are excited by their newfound independence. For some students, this independence and the rite of passage into the college culture are symbolized by alcohol use. Many students say they drink to have fun. "Having fun," which often means drinking simply to get drunk, may really be a way of coping with stress, boredom, anxiety, or pressures created by academic and social demands.

A significant number of students experience negative consequences as a result of their alcohol consumption (**FIGURE 10.7**). About 35 percent of college students who drank reported doing something they later regretted; 31 percent forgot where they were or what they did due to intoxication; approximately 14 percent accidentally injured themselves; and 20 percent had unprotected sex.[37] A recent study found students who played intramural sports, were in abusive relationships, had high stress levels, belonged to a fraternity or sorority, or were depressed reported higher levels of drinking and negative alcohol-related effects.[38]

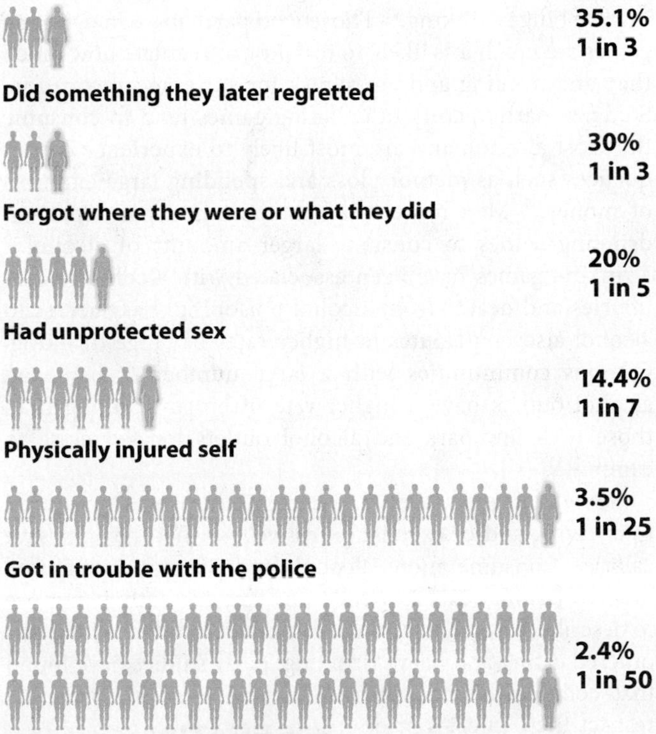

FIGURE 10.7 Prevalence of Negative Consequences of Drinking among College Students, Past Year

Source: Data from American College Health Association. *American College Health Association—National College Health Assessment II (ACHA-NCHA II) Reference Group Data Report Spring 2013* (Linthicum, MD: American College Health Association, 2013).

SKILLS FOR BEHAVIOR CHANGE

TIPS FOR DRINKING RESPONSIBLY

- Eat before and while you drink.
- Stay with the same group of friends for the entire time out.
- Don't drink before the party, or at all if you feel down or upset.
- Have no more than one alcoholic drink per hour.
- Alternate between alcoholic and nonalcoholic drinks.
- Set limits on how much to have before you start drinking.
- Avoid drinking games.
- Don't drink and drive.
- Avoid parties where you can expect heavy drinking.

Alcohol use among college students also has consequences related to academic performance. Alcohol consumption tends to disrupt sleep, particularly the second half of the night's sleep. These disruptive effects increase daytime sleepiness and decrease alertness, which negatively impacts students' academic performance.[39]

Fortunately, many college students report practicing protective behaviors when consuming alcohol to reduce the risk of negative consequences as a result of their alcohol use. Seventy-eight percent of students reported eating before or during drinking, about 84 percent said they usually or always stayed with the same group of friends the entire time they drank, 83 percent reported using a designated driver most or all of the time, and 65 percent always or usually kept track of how many drinks they consumed.[40] The **Skills for Behavior Change** box provides additional strategies for drinking responsibly.

High-Risk Drinking and College Students

According to one study, 1,825 college students die each year because of alcohol-related unintentional injuries, including car accidents.[41] Consumption of alcohol is the number one cause of preventable death among undergraduate college students in the United States today.

Who Drinks? It's likely that students who enter college will drink at some point, but there are groups of students who are more likely to drink more and more often. For example, students who believe that their parents approve of their drinking are more likely to drink.[42] Students who drank heavily in high school are also at risk for heavy drinking in college.[43] Most students have tried alcohol in high school.

By their senior year, 24 percent of high school students report engaging in binge drinking, 28 percent report having been drunk, and 42 percent report consuming some alcohol in the past month.[44]

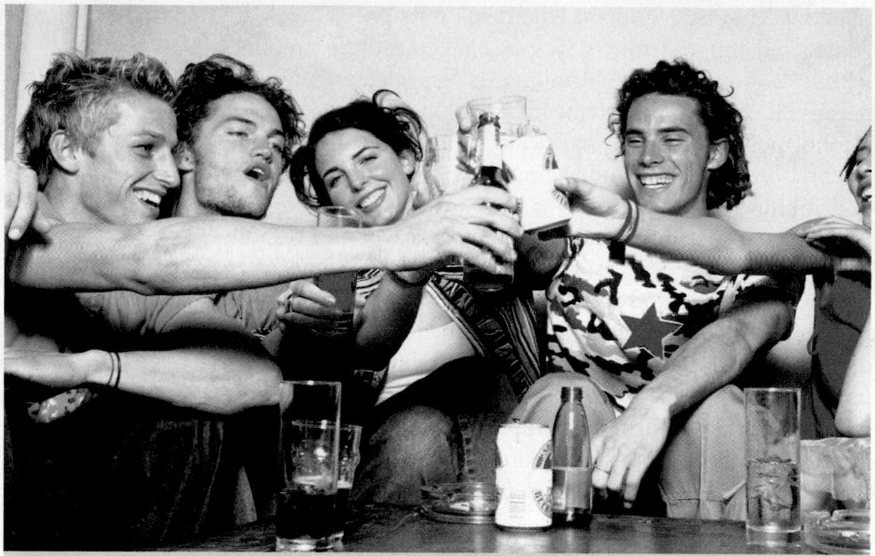

It may sometimes seem like your campus is crowded with heavy drinkers, but most college students—about 64 percent—drink only occasionally, and 21.3 percent don't drink at all. However, college students have high rates of binge drinking. Irresponsible consumption of alcohol can easily result in disaster, so it is important to take control of when you drink and how much.

Source: American College Health Association, *American College Health Association—National College Health Assessment II (ACHA-NCHA II) Reference Group Data Report Spring 2013* (Linthicum, MD: American College Health Association, 2013).

Why Do College Students Drink So Much? Although everyone who drinks is at some risk for alcohol-related problems, college students are particularly vulnerable for the following reasons:

- Alcohol exacerbates their already high risk for suicide, automobile crashes, and falls.
- Some university celebrations encourage certain dangerous practices and patterns of alcohol use.
- The alcoholic beverage industry heavily targets university campuses with promotions and ads.
- Drink specials enable students to consume large amounts of alcohol cheaply.
- College students are particularly vulnerable to peer influence.
- College administrators often deny that alcohol problems exist on their campuses.

College Student Drinking Behavior College students are more likely than their noncollegiate peers to drink recklessly, play drinking games, and engage in other dangerous practices. One such practice is **pre-gaming** (also called pre-loading or front-loading), which involves planned heavy drinking, usually in someone's home, apartment, or residence hall, prior to going out to a bar, nightclub, or sporting event. In a recent study, 75 percent of students reported pre-gaming in the past month. College men are more likely than women to pregame.[45] Some of the motivations for pre-gaming are to avoid paying for high-cost drinks, to socialize with friends, to reduce social anxiety, and to enhance male bonding. Pre-gamers have higher alcohol consumption during the evening and increase the risk for negative consequences such as blackouts, hangovers, passing out, and alcohol poisoning.

pre-gaming Drinking heavily at home before going out to an event or other location.

drunkorexia A colloquial term to describe the combination of disordered eating, excessive physical activity, and heavy alcohol consumption.

More than 80 percent of college students drink alcohol to celebrate their twenty-first birthday.[46] In a recent study, nearly half of students celebrating experienced at least one negative consequence of drinking alcohol (e.g., headache, feeling very sick to their stomach, etc.).[47]

Binge drinking is especially dangerous because it involves drinking a lot of alcohol in a very short period of time. Two-thirds of college students engage in drinking games that involve binge drinking.[48] Those who participate in drinking games are much less likely to monitor or regulate how much they are drinking and are at risk for extreme intoxication. Students participating in drinking games tend to consume the most alcohol, and are most likely to experience consequences such as memory loss and spending large amounts of money.[49] Men more often than women participate in drinking games to consume larger amounts of alcohol.[50] Drinking games have been associated with alcohol-related injuries and deaths from alcohol poisoning. Easy access to alcohol also contributes to higher rates of binge drinking. Campus communities with a large number of bars and alcohol outlets have a higher rate of binge drinking than those with few bars and alcohol outlets located close to campus.[51]

Some college students use extreme measures to control their eating and/or exercise excessively so that they can save calories, consume more alcohol, and become intoxicated faster.[52] **Drunkorexia** is a colloquialism currently being use to describe the combination of two dangerous behaviors: disordered eating and heavy drinking. Early studies have found that college students who restrict their calories prior to drinking are more likely to participate in binge drinking.[53] Similarly, another study found that highly physically active college students are more likely to binge drink than their non-active peers.[54]

SEE IT! VIDEOS

Heavy drinking during spring break can lead to bad decisions, or worse. Watch **Sloppy Spring Breaker** available on MasteringHealth.™

Motivations for drunkorexia include preventing weight gain, getting drunk faster, and saving money that would be spent on food to buy alcohol. Potential risks of drunkorexia include risk of blackouts, forced sexual activity, unintended sexual activity, and alcohol poisoning.

To see whether your alcohol consumption is a problem, complete the **Assess Yourself** online activity.

What Is the Impact of Student Drinking?

Unfortunately, recent studies confirm what students have been experiencing for a long time—drinking and binge drinkers cause problems not only for themselves, but also for those around them. One study indicated that more than 696,000 students between the ages of 18 and 24 were assaulted by another student who had been drinking.[55] There is significant evidence that campus rape is linked to binge drinking. Although exact numbers are hard to find, estimates are that more than 97,000 U.S. students between the ages of 18 and 24 experience alcohol-related sexual assault or date rape each year.[56] The laws regarding sexual consent are clear: A person who is drunk or passed out cannot consent to sex. Anyone who has sex with a person who is drunk or unconscious is committing rape. Claiming you were also drunk when you had sex with someone who was intoxicated or unconscious does not absolve you of your legal and moral responsibility for this crime.

Some students report sleep disruptions and academic problems related to alcohol. The more students drink, the more likely they are to miss class, do poorly on tests and papers, have lower grade point averages, and fall behind on assigned work. Some students even drop out of school as a result of their drinking.

DID YOU **KNOW?**

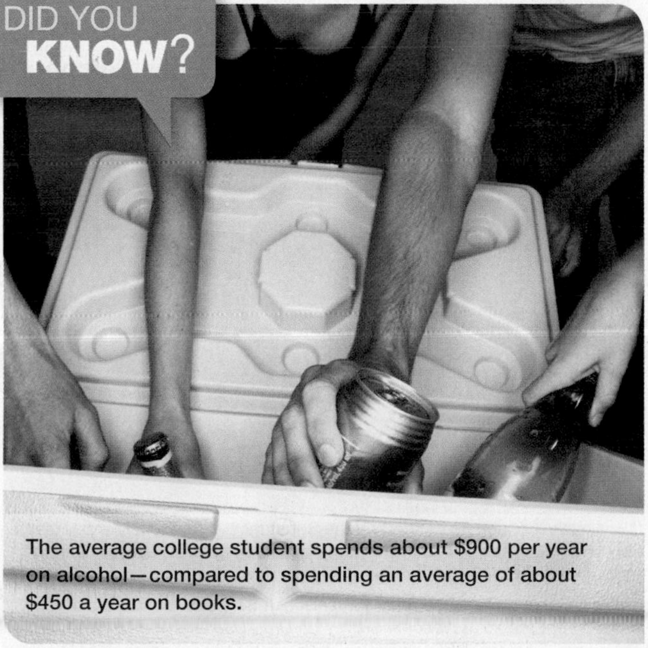

The average college student spends about $900 per year on alcohol—compared to spending an average of about $450 a year on books.

Source: Data from Facts on Tap, "School Daze?," Accessed May 2011, www.factsontap.org.

Efforts to Reduce Student Drinking

Some colleges are implementing strong policies against drinking to curb binge drinking and alcohol abuse. University policies include banning alcohol on campus or at university events, as well as banning advertising of alcohol in campus newspapers. Many fraternities have elected to have "dry" houses. At the same time, schools are making more help available to students with drinking problems. Today, most campuses offer both individual and group counseling and are directing more attention toward preventing alcohol abuse.

Programs that have proven particularly effective include cognitive-behavioral skills training with *motivational interviewing,* a nonjudgmental approach to working with students to change behavior. The NIAAA has recognized Brief Alcohol Screening and Intervention for College Students (BASICS) as an effective program for students who drink heavily and have experienced or are at risk for alcohol-related problems. A recent study found that both male and female students significantly decreased their alcohol consumption as a result of participating in this program.[57] E-interventions—electronically based alcohol education interventions using text messages, e-mails and podcasts—and Web interventions such as The Alcohol e-Check Up to Go (e-Chug) have shown promise in reducing alcohol-related problems among first year students.

Web-based education for first-year students, particularly those who are incoming, has become an increasingly important intervention. Because first-year students are at increased risk for alcohol-related problems, schools ensure that students are made aware of risks and effects of alcohol. Colleges and universities have been using a *social norms* approach to reducing alcohol consumption, sending a consistent message to students about actual drinking behavior on campus. Many students perceive that their peers drink more than they actually do, which may cause students to feel pressured to drink more themselves. This misperception includes inaccurately estimating the frequency and amount that students drink and the actual consequences of students' drinking. As a result of social norms campaigns, binge drinking has declined at campuses across the country. For example, Michigan State University, Florida State University, and the University of Arizona all reported 20 to 30 percent reductions in heavy episodic alcohol consumption within 3 years of implementing social norms campaigns, while Hobart and William Smith Colleges saw a 40 percent reduction in 5 years and Northern Illinois University saw a 44 percent reduction in 10 years.[58]

LO 4 | DRINKING AND DRIVING

Describe the impact of drinking and driving on society.

Traffic accidents are the leading cause of accidental death for all age groups from 1 to 44 years old.[59] In the United States, adults drank too much and got behind the wheel approximately 112 million times in a year.[60] Although the number of episodes of driving after drinking has gone down by 30 percent during the past 5 years, it remains a serious problem in the United States. Alcohol-impaired drivers are involved in about 1 in 3 crash deaths, resulting in nearly 11,000 deaths a year.[61] This number represents roughly one traffic fatality every 51 minutes.[62] Some groups are more likely to drink and drive than others. Men were responsible for 81 percent of the drinking and driving episodes, and 85 percent of people drinking and driving were reportedly binge drinking.[63] Unfortunately, college students are overrepresented in alcohol-related crashes. A recent survey reported that 23 percent of college students have driven after drinking, and about 3 percent said they had driven after drinking five or more drinks in the past 30 days.[64]

3 IN 10

AMERICANS WILL BE INVOLVED IN AN ALCOHOL-RELATED **ACCIDENT** AT SOME TIME IN THEIR LIVES.

Over the past 20 years, the percentage of intoxicated drivers involved in fatal crashes decreased for all age groups (**FIGURE 10.8**). Several factors probably contributed to these reductions in fatalities: laws that raised the drinking age to 21, stricter law enforcement, laws prohibiting anyone under 21 from driving with any detectable BAC, increased automobile safety, and educational programs designed to discourage drinking and driving. Furthermore, all states have zero-tolerance laws for driving while intoxicated, and the penalty is usually suspension of the driver's license.

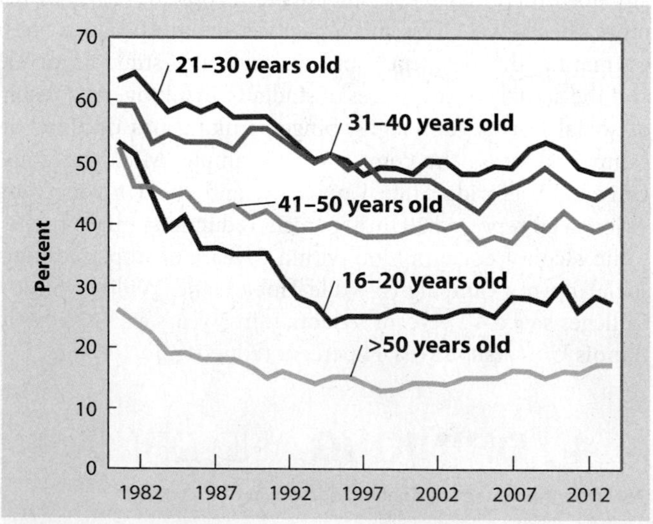

FIGURE 10.8 Percentage of Fatally Injured Drivers with BACs Greater Than 0.08 Percent, by Driver Age, 1982–2012

Source: Insurance Institute for Highway Safety, "Alcohol Impaired Driving 2012: Alcohol," Copyright 2014. Reprinted with permission.

Despite all these measures, the risk of being involved in an alcohol-related automobile crash remains substantial. Laboratory and test track research shows that the vast majority of drivers are impaired even at 0.08 BAC with regard to critical driving tasks. The likelihood of a driver being involved in a fatal crash rises significantly with a BAC of 0.05 percent and even more rapidly after 0.08 percent.[65]

Alcohol-related fatal car crashes occur more often at night than during the day, and the hours between 9:00 P.M. and 6:00 A.M. are the most dangerous. Sixty-seven percent of fatally injured drivers involved in nighttime single-vehicle crashes had BACs at or above 0.08 percent.[66] The risk of being involved in an alcohol-related crash increases not only with the time of day, but also with the day of the week; 24 percent of all fatal crashes during the week were alcohol related, compared with 46 percent on weekends.[67] For information on phone apps that claim to help you estimate your blood alcohol level, presumably so you can judge whether it is safe to drive after drinking, see the **Tech & Health** box.

LO 5 | **ETHNIC** DIFFERENCES IN ALCOHOL USE AND ABUSE

Compare the differences in alcohol consumption and abuse among various ethnic and racial minority groups.

Different ethnic and racial groups have their own patterns of alcohol consumption and abuse. Social or cultural factors, such as drinking norms and attitudes and, in some cases, genetic factors, may account for those differences. Better understanding of ethnic and racial differences in alcohol use patterns (**TABLE 10.1**) and factors that influence alcohol use can help guide the development of culturally appropriate prevention and treatment programs.

TABLE **10.1** | Prevalence of Heavy Alcohol Use* by Ethnicity

Ethnic Group	Percent of Total Population
Whites	7.6
African Americans	4.5
Latino	5.1
Native Americans/Alaska Natives	8.5
Asian Americans	1.7
Persons reporting two or more races	6.8

*"Heavy alcohol use" is defined by the Substance Abuse and Mental Health Services Administration as five or more drinks on at least 5 days within the past month.

Source: Substance Abuse and Mental Health Services Administration, *Results from the 2012 National Survey on Drug Use and Health: Summary of National Findings*, NSDUH Series H-46, HHS Publication no. (SMA) 13-4795 (Rockville, MD: Substance Abuse and Mental Health Services Administration, 2013).

TECH & HEALTH | SMARTPHONE BREATHALYZERS

Better Than BAC APPS?

Some smartphone applications can estimate a person's blood alcohol concentration (BAC) to help them decide if they should avoid driving after drinking. Enter how many drinks you've consumed along with weight, gender, and total number of hours spent drinking, and the apps estimate your BAC. Some even provide the phone number of a local taxi if a person has exceeded the legal BAC limit.

It is important to realize that these apps give general estimates, not your actual BAC. Many apps don't take into consideration elements such as food consumption, medication, general health, psychological conditions, and the time it takes for the body to fully absorb a drink. It can also be hard to accurately input how many drink servings you consume with a mixed drink, such as a margarita, which might contain two or three standard servings of alcohol.

Breathalyzer attachments for smartphones, which come with many of the same features as BAC apps, are perhaps a better indicator of your actual BAC. Like standard breathalyzers, these products work by measuring the amount of alcohol in your breath. They must be calibrated periodically to ensure accurate use.

While smartphone breathalyzer attachments cost more than BAC apps, they give more accurate information about your level of intoxication. Two smartphone breathalyzers are available:

- **Breathometer.** ($49: Android, iPhone) Small size, FDA-registered device that ensures accuracy to ±0.01 percent BAC. It hooks into the smartphone's audio jack and takes one AA battery, reading up to 75 BAC tests.
- **BACtrack Mobile Breathalyzer.** ($149.99: Android, iPhone). Small size, professional-grade device that senses BAC as low as 0.001 percent. Connects to the phone using Bluetooth technology, and the battery is rechargeable with a USB cord.

Remember, it isn't safe to rely on a BAC app or breathalyzer alone to decide if it's okay to drive after a night out. It's much better to arrange for a designated driver ahead of time or plan to take the bus or a taxi.

Sources: Join Together, "New Smartphone App Estimates Blood Alcohol Concentration," Accessed August 22, 2011, www.drugfree.org/join-together/alcohol/new-smartphone-app-estimates-blood-alcohol-concentration; Blood Alcohol Content Gauging Apps, "Apps Gone Free," http://appadvice.com/appguides/show/best-blood-alcohol-content-gauging-apps-for-the-iPhone; Breathometer, "Frequently Asked Questions," www.breathometer.com; BACtrack Mobile Breathalyzer, home page, www.bactrack.com/pages/bactrack-mobile-breathalyzers.

Among Native American populations, alcohol is the most widely used drug; the rate of alcoholism in this population is two to three times higher than the national average, and the death rate from alcohol-related causes is eight times higher than the national average.[68] When comparing other racial or ethnic groups, Native Americans have the highest alcohol-related motor vehicle crash and pedestrian fatalities, suicide, and falls.[69] Poor economic conditions and the cultural belief that alcoholism is a spiritual problem, not a physical disease, may partially account for high alcoholism rates.

African American and Latino populations also exhibit distinct patterns of abuse. On average, African Americans drink less than white Americans; however, those who do drink tend to be heavy drinkers, and twice as many African Americans die of cirrhosis of the liver.[70] Alcohol also contributes to high rates of hypertension, esophageal cancer, and homicide in African Americans. Among Latino populations, men have a higher than average rate of alcohol abuse and alcohol-related health problems. In contrast, many Latino cultures tend to discourage any drinking by women, and therefore many Latinas abstain; however, this cultural norm is changing. Recent evidence shows drinking rates among Latina women matching or surpassing those of young Latino men.[71] Many researchers agree that a major factor for alcohol problems in this ethnic group is the key role that drinking plays in Latino culture.[72]

Asian Americans have a very low rate of alcoholism.[73] When compared to other racial or ethnic groups, Asians have the lowest rates of alcohol-related injuries. Social and cultural influences, such as strong kinship ties, are thought to discourage heavy drinking in Asian American groups. Asians also have a genetic predisposition that might influence their low risk for alcohol abuse: Many possess a variant of the gene that codes for the enzyme aldehyde dehydrogenase, which plays a key role in the metabolism of alcohol.[74] People with this variant gene experience unpleasant side effects from consuming alcohol, making drinking a less pleasurable experience.

alcohol abuse Use of alcohol in a way that interferes with work, school, or personal relationships or that entails violations of the law.

alcoholism (alcohol dependence) Condition in which personal and health problems related to alcohol use are severe, and stopping alcohol use results in withdrawal symptoms.

The **Health in a Diverse World** box on the next page discusses global patterns of alcohol use and abuse.

LO 6 | ABUSE AND DEPENDENCE

Explain the risk factors associated with alcoholism, its symptoms, its costs to society, and its effects on family members.

Alcohol use becomes **alcohol abuse** when it interferes with work, school, or social and family relationships, or when it entails any violation of the law, including driving under the influence (DUI). **Alcoholism,** or **alcohol dependence,** results

HEALTH IN A DIVERSE WORLD

GLOBAL HEALTH AND ALCOHOL USE

Alcohol consumption comes with many serious social and developmental issues, including violence, child neglect and abuse, and absenteeism in the workplace. Throughout the world, alcohol is a factor in 60 types of diseases and injuries and a component cause in 200 others. Almost 4 percent of all deaths worldwide are attributed to alcohol, greater than deaths caused by HIV/AIDS, violence, or tuberculosis. Worldwide, the impact of alcohol use is as follows:

- Alcohol use results in 3.3 million deaths each year.
- 7.6% of male deaths and 4.0% of female deaths worldwide are attributable to alcohol consumption.
- Early alcohol use (before the age of 14) is positively correlated with harmful behaviors later in life, including alcohol addiction and drunk driving
- At the same level of alcohol consumption, men are more likely to become injured and women are more likely to experience negative health outcomes such as cancer (particularly breast cancer), cardiovascular disease, and gastrointestinal problems.

A large variation exists in adult per capita consumption. The highest consumption levels can be found in the developed world, including Europe and the Americas. Intermediate consumption levels can be found in regions of the Western Pacific and Africa. Low consumption levels can be found in Southeast Asia and the Eastern Mediterranean regions. Many factors, including culture, economic development, and socioeconomic status, contribute to these differences.

Sources: World Health Organization, "Global Status Report on Alcohol and Health," 2014, www.who.int/substance_abuse/publications/global_alcohol_report/en.

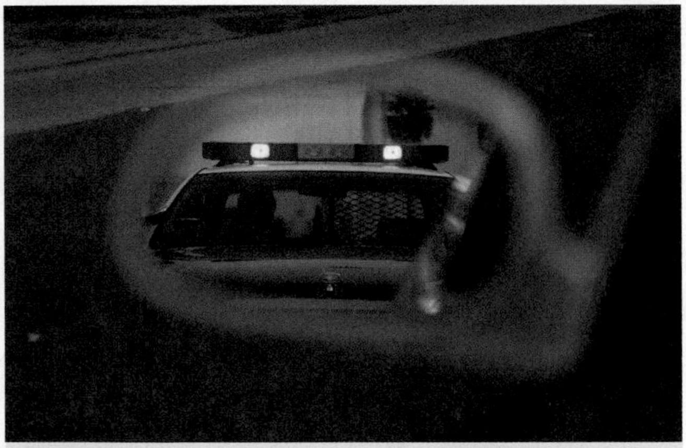

Getting behind the wheel after drinking alcohol is a dangerous choice, with serious legal consequences. Penalties for driving under the influence (DUI) include driving restrictions, fines, mandatory counseling, revoking your license, and jail time. In many states three DUI convictions make you a felon, meaning that you lose your right to vote and own a weapon, and you may also be permanently banned from driving. If you are involved in a drunk-driving accident in which someone dies, you may be charged with manslaughter or second-degree murder.

when personal and health problems related to alcohol use are severe and stopping alcohol use results in withdrawal symptoms.

Identifying an Alcoholic

As with other drug addictions, craving, loss of control, tolerance, psychological dependence, and withdrawal symptoms must be present to qualify a drinker as an addict (see **Focus On: Recognizing and Avoiding Addiction**). Irresponsible and problem drinkers, such as people who get into fights or embarrass themselves or others when they drink, are not necessarily alcoholics. Alcoholics can be found at all socioeconomic levels and in all professions, ethnic groups, geographical locations, religions, and races. Data indicate that about 15 percent of people in the United States are problem drinkers, and about 5 to 10 percent of male drinkers and 3 to 5 percent of females would be diagnosed as alcohol dependent.[75]

Recognizing and admitting the existence of an alcohol problem is often extremely difficult. Alcoholics often deny their problem, making statements such as, "I can stop any time I want to. I just don't want to right now." The fear of being labeled a "problem drinker" often prevents people from seeking help. People who recognize alcoholic behaviors in themselves may wish to seek professional help to determine whether alcohol has become a controlling factor in their lives.

Among full-time college students, 1 in 4 experienced alcohol abuse or dependence in the past year.[76] In a recent study, the progression to alcohol dependency based on college students' drinking patterns when they entered showed that 1.9 percent of nondrinkers, 4.3 percent of light drinkers, 12.8 percent of moderate drinkers, and 19 percent of heavy drinkers developed alcohol dependency.[77]

The Causes of Alcohol Abuse and Alcoholism

We know that alcoholism is a disease with biological and social/environmental components, but we do not yet know what role each component plays in the disease.

Biological and Family Factors Research into the hereditary and environmental causes of alcoholism has found higher rates of alcoholism among children of alcoholics than in the general population. The development of alcoholism among individuals with a family history of alcoholism is about four to eight times more common than it is among individuals with no such family history.[78]

Despite evidence of heredity's role in alcoholism, scientists do not yet understand the precise role of genes and increased risk for alcoholism, nor have they identified a specific "alcoholism" gene. Alcohol use disorders are between 50 and 60 percent heritable. Anxiety and depression, by comparison, are around 20 to 40 percent heritable, respectively.[79] Adoption studies demonstrate a strong link between biological parents' substance use and their children's risk for addiction. Recently, scientists have found a gene that, by controlling the way that alcohol stimulates the brain to release dopamine, can trigger feelings of reward. Alcohol gives individuals with the gene a stronger sense of reward from alcohol, making it more likely for them to be heavy drinkers.[80] However, there is nothing deterministic about the genetic basis for addiction. Although no single gene causes addiction, multiple genes can affect the ability to develop addiction.

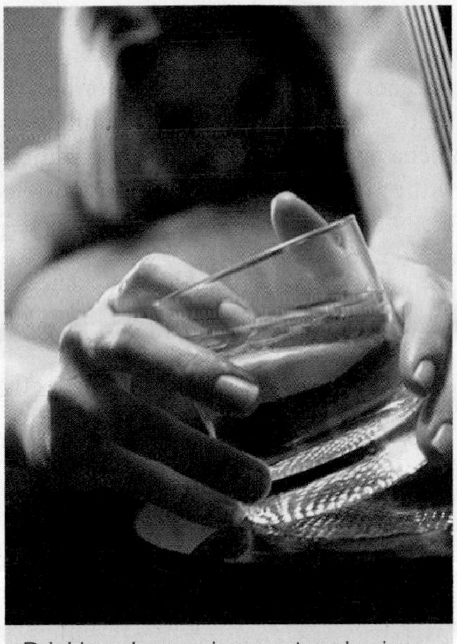

Drinking alone or in secret and using alcohol to cope with stress and emotional problems are all potential signs of alcohol dependency.

Social and Cultural Factors Some people begin drinking as a way to dull the pain of an acute loss or an emotional or social problem. Unfortunately, they become even sadder as the depressant effect of alcohol begins to take its toll, sometimes causing them to antagonize friends and other social supports. Eventually, the drinker becomes physically dependent on the drug.

Family attitudes toward alcohol also seem to influence whether a person will develop a drinking problem. It has been clearly demonstrated that people who are raised in cultures where drinking is a part of religious or ceremonial activities or part of the family meal are less prone to alcohol dependence. In contrast, societies where alcohol purchase is carefully controlled and drinking is regarded as a rite of passage to adulthood appear to have greater tendency for abuse.

The amount of alcohol a person consumes seems to be directly related to the drinking habits of that individual's social group. A recent study found that those whose friends and relatives drank heavily were 50 percent more likely to drink heavily themselves.[81] Even having friends of friends who drank heavily appeared to influence individual alcohol consumption. The opposite is also true, that people with abstinent friends or family members were less likely to drink themselves. This finding has increased importance for individuals who are in treatment or have been in treatment and their need to sever ties with heavy drinkers to successfully maintain their abstinence.

WHAT DO YOU THINK?

Why do you think women are drinking more heavily today than they did in the past?

- Does society look at men's and women's drinking habits in the same way?
- Can you think of ways to increase support for women in their recovery process?

Women and Alcoholism

Women tend to become alcoholics at later ages and after fewer years of heavy drinking than do men. Women also get addicted faster with less alcohol use. With greater risks for cirrhosis; excessive memory loss and shrinkage of the brain; heart disease; and cancers of the mouth, throat, esophagus, liver, and colon than male alcoholics, women suffer the consequences of alcoholism more profoundly.[82]

The highest risks for alcoholism occur among women who are unmarried but living with a partner, are in their twenties or early thirties, or have a husband or partner who drinks heavily. Other risks for women include a family history of drinking problems, pressure to drink from a peer or spouse, depression, and stress.

Alcohol and Prescription Drug Abuse

When alcohol and prescription drugs are taken together, severe medical problems can result, including alcohol poisoning, unconsciousness, respiratory depression, and death. The greatest risks from drug mixing occur when alcohol is mixed with prescription painkillers. Both drugs slow breathing rates in unique ways and inhibit the coughing reflex; when combined, they can stop breathing altogether. Alcohol also interacts with antianxiety medications, antipsychotics, antidepressants, sleep medications, and muscle relaxants, causing dizziness and drowsiness and making falls and unintentional injuries more likely. The prescription drugs that are most commonly combined with alcohol include opioids (e.g., Vicodin, OxyContin, Percocet); stimulants (e.g., Ritalin, Adderall, Concerta); sedative/anxiety medications (e.g., Ativan, Xanax); and sleeping medications (e.g., Ambien, Halcion).

Effects on Family and Friends

In addition to harming themselves, people who abuse alcohol cause tremendous harm to their family and friends. Everyone close to an addicted person—including family, friends, and roommates—suffers and becomes a part of the dynamics of addiction.

An estimated 7.5 million children in the United States live with a parent who has experienced an alcohol use disorder

delirium tremens (DTs) State of confusion, delusions, and agitation brought on by withdrawal from alcohol.

intervention A planned confrontation with an alcoholic led by a professional counselor in which family members and/or friends try to get the alcoholic to face the reality of his or her problem and to seek help.

in the past year. These children are at increased risk for a range of problems, including physical illness, emotional disturbances, behavioral problems, lower educational performance, and susceptibility to alcoholism or other addictions later in life.[83]

In dysfunctional families, children learn certain rules from an early age: Don't talk, don't trust, and don't feel. These unspoken rules allow the family to avoid dealing with real problems and issues as family members adapt to the alcoholic's behavior by adjusting their own behavior. Unfortunately, these behaviors enable the alcoholic to keep drinking. Children in such dysfunctional families generally assume at least one of the following roles:

- **Family hero.** Tries to divert attention from the problem by being too good to be true
- **Scapegoat.** Draws attention away from the family's primary problem through misbehavior
- **Lost child.** Becomes passive and quietly withdraws from upsetting situations
- **Mascot.** Disrupts tense situations by providing comic relief

For children in alcoholic homes, life is a struggle. They have to deal with constant stress, anxiety, and embarrassment. Because the alcoholic is the center of attention, the child's needs are often ignored. It is not uncommon for these children to be victims of violence, abuse, neglect, or incest.

Living with a family member (or friend or roommate) who is an alcoholic can be extremely stressful. People in close proximity to alcoholics can find themselves in codependent relationships that are often emotionally destructive or abusive and that enable the alcoholic's addiction. Codependents try to cover up for the addicted person: They may make excuses for the drinker's behavior or lie to others to cover for him or her. (For more information on how addiction can affect families and friends, see **Focus On: Recognizing and Avoiding Addiction**.)

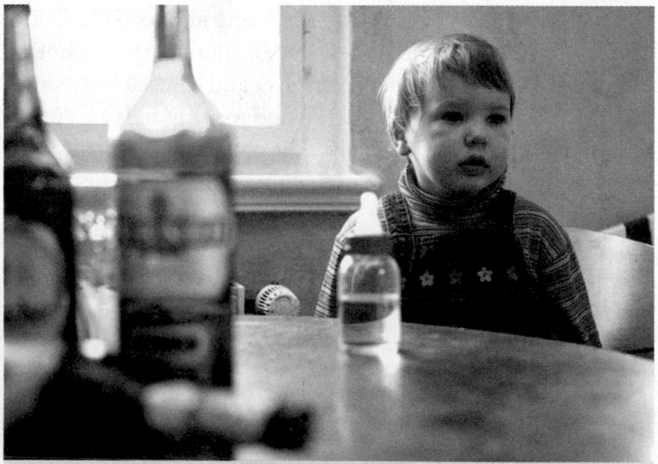

Adult children of alcoholics can have trouble developing social attachments and suffer low self-esteem and other problems from lack of parental nurturing. Fortunately, as they mature, many children of alcoholics can also develop resiliency in response to their families' problems.

Costs to Society

Alcohol related costs to society are estimated to be well over $223.5 billion when health insurance, criminal justice costs, treatment costs, and lost productivity are considered.[84] Alcoholism is directly or indirectly responsible for more than 25 percent of the nation's medical expenses and lost earnings.[85]

The Cost of Underage Drinking A recent study estimated that underage drinking costs society $62 billion annually.[86] The largest costs were related to violence ($35 billion) and drunk-driving accidents ($9.955 billion), followed by high-risk sex ($5 billion), property crime ($3 billion), and addiction treatment programs (nearly $2.5 billion). By dividing the cost of underage drinking by the estimated number of underage drinkers, the study estimated that every underage drinker costs society an average of $2,070 a year.[87]

LO 7 | TREATMENT AND RECOVERY

Describe the various types of treatment programs for alcoholism, and their effectiveness and explore the concepts of relapse and recovery.

Despite growing recognition of our national alcohol problem, only a very small percentage of alcoholics ever receive care in special treatment facilities. Numerous factors contribute to this low treatment utilization, including an inability or unwillingness to admit to an alcohol problem, the social stigma attached to alcoholism, potential loss of income, inability to pay for treatment, breakdowns in referral and delivery systems, and failure of the medical establishment to recognize and diagnose alcoholic symptoms among patients.[88] Most problem drinkers who seek help have experienced a turning point when the person recognizes that alcohol controls his or her life.

Alcoholics who quit drinking will experience *detoxification,* the process by which addicts end their dependence on a drug. Withdrawal symptoms include hyperexcitability, confusion, agitation, sleep disorders, convulsions, tremors, depression, headaches, and seizures. For a small percentage of people, alcohol withdrawal results in a severe syndrome known as **delirium tremens (DTs),** characterized by confusion, delusions, agitated behavior, and hallucinations.

The Family's Role in Recovery

Members of an alcoholic's family sometimes take action before the alcoholic does. An effective method of helping an alcoholic confront the disease is a process called **intervention** —a planned confrontation with the alcoholic that involves

SKILLS FOR BEHAVIOR CHANGE

THINKING AND TALKING ABOUT ALCOHOL USE

The following questions can help gauge whether you or a friend or relative could have an alcohol problem. The more questions you answer with a "yes," the more likely it is that there is a problem.

Does the person you are concerned about do any of the following?

- Lose time from classes, studying, or work because of drinking?
- Feel embarrassed about his or her behavior after sobering up?
- Drink to get drunk?
- Do dangerous things or get injured while drunk?
- Drink to cope with problems or stress?

Use these tips to talk to someone about alcohol abuse:

- Talk when he or she is sober. Avoid lecturing.
- Restrict comments to what you have experienced of the person's behavior.
- Use concrete examples: "You started a fight," or "You were hung over and failed an exam."
- Contrast sober and drunk behavior: "You have the most wonderful sense of humor, but when you drink it turns into cruel sarcasm."
- Distinguish between the person you like and the behavior you don't.
- Encourage him or her to consult a professional. Offer to go along for support.

family members and friends assisted by professional substance abuse counselors. (See **Focus On: Recognizing and Avoiding Addiction** for more on intervention.) See the **Skills for Behavior Change** box tips on confronting someone about alcohol abuse.

Treatment Programs

The alcoholic who is ready for help has several avenues of treatment: psychologists and psychiatrists specializing in the treatment of alcoholism, private treatment centers, hospitals specifically designed to treat alcoholics, community mental health facilities, and support groups.

Private Treatment Facilities Upon admission to a private treatment facility, the patient receives a complete physical exam to determine whether underlying medical problems will interfere with treatment. Shortly after detoxification, alcoholics begin their treatment for psychological addiction. Most treatment facilities keep their patients from 3 to 6 weeks.

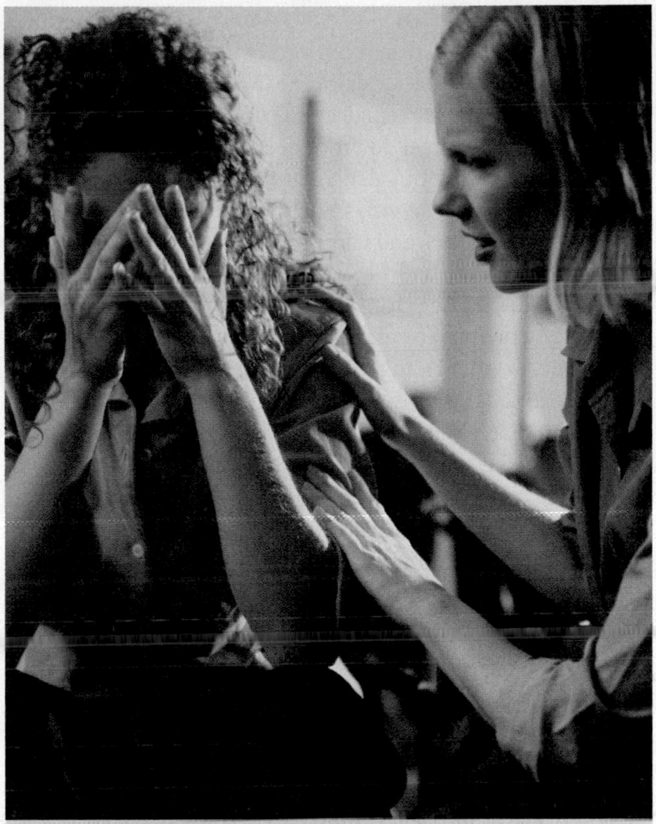

Most alcohol-dependent people need the help of others during their recovery, whether through support groups or individual, family, or group therapy.

Treatment at private facilities can cost several thousand dollars, but some insurance programs or employers will assume most of this expense.

Therapy Several types of therapy, including family therapy, individual therapy, and group therapy, are commonly used in alcoholism recovery programs. In family therapy, the person and family members examine the psychological reasons underlying the addiction and the environmental factors enabling it. In individual and group therapy, alcoholics learn positive coping skills for situations that have regularly caused them to turn to alcohol.

While there are many recovery management strategies for adults, understanding an appropriate recovery support system for college students has received less attention. In particular, there has been a lack of campus-based services for recovering students. The high prevalence of alcohol and other drug use on college campuses makes attending college a threat to sobriety. However, many campuses are beginning to recognize the need to create recovery-friendly space and supportive environments for students engaged in recovery. Common features of such programs include a designed campus meeting space, drug-free housing options, individual or group counseling, relapse prevention, and sober leisure activities; peer support and 12-step tenets are typically emphasized.[89]

Pharmacological Treatment Disulfiram (trade name Antabuse) is a drug commonly used for treating alcoholism. It is given to deter drinking, as it causes an individual to become acutely ill when he or she consumes alcohol. Disulfiram inhibits the breakdown of acetaldehyde from the liver. If individuals taking this drug drink alcohol or consume any foods with alcohol content, acetaldehyde will build up in the liver and cause nausea and vomiting. Other unpleasant effects, such as headache, bad breath, drowsiness, and temporary impotence discourage drinking. Because disulfiram does not reduce the cravings for alcohol, this treatment works best in conjunction with ongoing psychotherapy and support groups.

Naltrexone is used to reduce the craving for alcohol and decrease the pleasant reinforcing effects of alcohol without making the user ill. It also works most effectively with counseling and other forms of psychotherapy. Another pharmaceutical treatment for alcoholism approved by the U.S. Food and Drug Administration (FDA) is called acamprosate (Campral). Acamprosate helps people who have consumed large amounts of alcohol avoid drinking. Drinking large amounts of alcohol over a long period of time changes the way the brain works. Acamprosate helps stabilize the resulting chemical imbalance in the brain. It also helps to reduce the physical and emotional distress associated with the attempt to stay alcohol free. As with other pharmacological treatments, acamprosate should be used in conjunction with psychotherapy and support groups.

Support Groups The support gained from talking with others who have similar problems is one of the greatest benefits derived from self-help/support groups. **Alcoholics Anonymous (AA)** is a private, nonprofit, self-help organization founded in 1935. The organization, which relies on group support to help people stop drinking, currently has branches all over the world and more than 1 million members. At meetings, participants do not give their last names, and no one is forced to speak. Members are taught that alcoholism is a lifetime problem and that they can never drink alcohol again. They share their struggles and talk about the devastating effects alcoholism has had on their personal and professional lives. AA established the concept of the 12-step program for recovery from addiction, and its guiding principles are now used by other recovery organizations. The 12 steps ask members to address recovery one step at a time and to place their faith and control of their habit into the hands of a "Higher Power."

Alcoholics Anonymous (AA)
Organization whose goal is to help alcoholics stop drinking; includes auxiliary branches such as Al-Anon and Alateen.

Alcoholics Anonymous also has auxiliary groups to help spouses or partners, friends, and children of alcoholics. *Al-Anon* is the group dedicated to helping adult relatives and friends of alcoholics understand the disease and how they can contribute to the recovery process. *Alateen* helps adolescents living with alcoholic parents by teaching that they are not at fault for their parents' problems. They develop their self-esteem to overcome their guilt and function better socially.

Other self-help groups include Women for Sobriety and Secular Organizations for Sobriety (SOS). Women for Sobriety addresses the specific needs of female alcoholics, who often have more severe problems than do males. Unlike AA meetings, where attendance can be quite large, each group has no more than ten members. These meetings focus on behavioral changes through positive reinforcement, cognitive strategies, relaxation techniques, meditation, diet, exercise, and dynamic group involvement. SOS was founded to help people who are uncomfortable with AA's spiritual emphasis. It is a self-empowerment approach to recovery and maintains that sobriety is a separate issue from all else. Like AA, SOS holds confidential meetings, celebrates sobriety anniversaries, and views recovery as a one-day-at-a-time process.

Relapse

Success in recovery varies with the individual. Over half of alcoholics relapse (resume drinking) within the first 3 months of treatment. Treating an addiction requires more than getting the addict to stop using a substance; it also requires getting the person to break a pattern of behavior that has dominated his or her life. Many alcoholics refer to themselves as "recovering" throughout their lifetime rather than "cured."

People seeking to regain a healthy lifestyle must not only confront their addiction but also guard against the tendency to relapse. For alcoholics, it is important to identify situations that could trigger a relapse, such as becoming angry or frustrated and being around others who drink. During the initial recovery period, it can help to join a support group, maintain stability (resisting the urge to relocate, travel, take a new job, or make other drastic life changes), set aside time each day for reflection, and maintain a pattern of assuming responsibility for one's own actions. To be effective, recovery programs must offer alcoholics ways to increase self-esteem and resume personal growth.

STUDY PLAN

Customize your study plan—and master your health!—in the Study Area of **MasteringHealth**.

ASSESS YOURSELF

Are you at risk of alcohol abuse? Want to find out? Take the **What Is Your Risk of Alcohol Abuse?** assessment available on MasteringHealth.™

Need help creating a plan? Follow the strategies in the **Your Plan for Change** box for short- and long-term improvements to your health.

YOUR PLAN FOR CHANGE

If the results of your **ASSESS YOURSELF** exercise concern you, consider taking these steps to change your behavior.

TODAY, YOU CAN:

- ☐ Start a journal of your drinking habits to track how much alcohol you consume and what you spend on it.
- ☐ If you have a family history of alcohol abuse or addiction, consider whether your current use is healthy or is likely to create problems for you in the future.

WITHIN THE NEXT 2 WEEKS, YOU CAN:

- ☐ Make your first drink at a party something nonalcoholic.
- ☐ Intersperse alcoholic drinks with nonalcoholic beverages to help you pace yourself.

BY THE END OF THE SEMESTER, YOU CAN:

- ☐ Commit yourself to determining and limiting alcohol intake at every social function.
- ☐ Cultivate friendships and explore activities that do not center on alcohol. If your friends drink heavily you may need to step back from the group for a while or make an effort to meet new people who do not make drinking a major focus of their social activity.

CHAPTER REVIEW

To hear an MP3 Tutor Session, scan here or visit the Study Area in **MasteringHealth.**

LO 1 | Alcohol in the Body

- Alcohol is a central nervous system (CNS) depressant used by about half of all Americans. Alcohol's effect on the body is measured by the blood alcohol concentration (BAC). The higher the BAC, the greater the drowsiness and impaired judgment and motor function.

LO 2 | Alcohol and Your Health

- Excessive alcohol consumption can cause long-term damage to the nervous system and cardiovascular system, liver disease, and increased risk for cancer. Drinking during pregnancy can cause fetal alcohol spectrum disorders (FASD).

LO 3 | Alcohol Use in College

Large numbers of college students report drinking in the past 30 days. Negative consequences associated with alcohol use among college students include academic problems, traffic accidents, unplanned sex, hangovers, alcohol poisoning, injury to self or others, and dropping out of school.

LO 4 | Drinking and Driving

- Alcohol-impaired drivers are responsible for about 1 in 3 car crash deaths. College students have high rates of alcohol-related crashes.

LO 5 | Ethnic Differences in Alcohol Use and Abuse

- Rates of alcohol consumption and abuse vary among different racial and ethnic groups. African Americans, Latinos, and Native Americans have high rates of heavy alcohol use.

LO 6 | Abuse and Dependence

- Alcohol use becomes alcoholism when it interferes with school, work, or social and family relationships or entails violations of the law. Causes of alcoholism include biological, family, social, and cultural factors. Alcoholism has far-reaching effects on families and children, who may take those problems into adulthood.

LO 7 | Treatment and Recovery

- Most alcoholics do not admit to having a problem until reaching a major life crisis or until their families intervene. Treatment options include detoxification at private medical facilities, therapy (family, individual, or group), and self-help programs. Most recovering alcoholics relapse (over half within 3 months) because alcoholism is a behavioral addiction as well as a chemical addiction.

POP QUIZ

Visit **MasteringHealth** to personalize your study plan with Chapter Review Quizzes and Dynamic Study Modules.

LO 1 | Alcohol in the Body

1. If a man and a woman drink the same amount of alcohol, the woman's BAC will be approximately
   a. the same as the man's BAC.
   b. 60 percent higher than the man's BAC.
   c. 30 percent higher than the man's BAC.
   d. 30 percent lower than the man's BAC.
2. BAC is the
   a. concentration of plant sugars in the bloodstream.
   b. percentage of alcohol in a beverage.
   c. level of alcohol content in the blood.
   d. ratio of alcohol to the total blood volume.

LO 2 | Alcohol and Your Health

3. Drinking large amounts of alcohol in a short period of time that leads to passing out is known as
   a. learned behavioral tolerance.
   b. alcoholic unconsciousness.
   c. alcohol poisoning.
   d. acute metabolism syndrome.
4. Which of the following is typical of a child born with fetal alcohol syndrome?
   a. Deafness
   b. Impaired learning
   c. Cirrhosis
   d. Osteoporosis

LO 3 | Alcohol Use in College

5. When Amanda goes out with her friends on the weekends, she usually has four or five beers in a row. This type of high-risk drinking is called
   a. tolerance.
   b. alcoholic addiction.
   c. alcohol overconsumption.
   d. binge drinking.
6. Which is a strategy you could take to avoid drinking too much alcohol at a party?
   a. Pre-game before going out
   b. Drink only carbonated alcoholic beverages
   c. Don't eat before or during the party
   d. Alternate alcoholic and nonalcoholic drinks

LO 4 | Drinking and Driving

7. A BAC as low as ______ increases the likelihood of a driver being involved in a fatal car crash.
   a. 0.02
   b. 0.05
   c. 0.07
   d. 0.08

LO 5 **Ethnic Differences in Alcohol Use and Abuse**

8. Which of the following ethnic groups has the lowest rates of alcoholism?
   a. Asian Americans
   b. African Americans
   c. Latinos
   d. Native Americans

LO 6 **Abuse and Dependence**

9. Jake was raised in an alcoholic family. To adapt to his father's alcoholic behavior, he played the good, obedient son. Which role did Jake assume?
   a. Family hero
   b. Mascot
   c. Scapegoat
   d. Lost child

LO 7 **Treatment and Recovery**

10. The alcohol withdrawal syndrome that results in confusion, delusion, agitated behavior, and hallucination is known as
    a. automatic detoxification.
    b. delirium tremens.
    c. acute withdrawal.
    d. transient hyperirritability.

Answers to the Pop Quiz can be found on page A-1. If you answered a question incorrectly, review the section identified by the Learning Outcome. For even more study tools, visit MasteringHealth.

THINK ABOUT IT!

LO 1 **Alcohol in the Body and**
LO 2 **Alcohol and Your Health**

1. Would a person be more intoxicated after having four gin and tonics instead of four beers? Why or why not? At what point in your life should you start worrying about the long-term effects of alcohol abuse?

LO 3 **Alcohol Use in College**

2. What are some of the most common negative consequences college students experience as a result of drinking? Why do students tolerate the negative behaviors of students who have been drinking?

LO 4 **Drinking and Driving**

3. When it comes to drinking alcohol, how much is too much to drive? How can you avoid drinking amounts that will affect your judgment and impair your ability to safely operate a vehicle? If you see a friend having too many drinks at a party, what actions could you take to make sure he/she makes it home safely?

LO 5 **Ethnic Differences in Alcohol Use and Abuse**

4. In what ways do genetics influence ethnic differences in alcohol use and abuse? How much of the differences between ethnic groups in terms of alcohol use and abuse can be attributed to cultural or social differences?

LO 6 **Abuse and Dependence**

5. Describe the difference between a problem drinker and an alcoholic. What factors can cause someone to become an alcoholic? What effect does alcoholism have on an alcoholic's family?

LO 7 **Treatment and Recovery**

6. Does anyone ever permanently recover from alcoholism? Why or why not? Do you think society's views on drinking have changed over the years? Explain your answer.

ACCESS YOUR HEALTH ON THE INTERNET

Visit **MasteringHealth** for links to the websites and RSS feeds.

The following websites explore further topics and issues related to personal health.

Alcoholics Anonymous (AA). This website provides general information about AA and the 12-step program. **www.aa.org**

College Drinking: Changing the Culture. This resource center targets three audiences: the student population as a whole, the college and its surrounding environment, and the individual at risk or alcohol-dependent drinker. **www.collegedrinkingprevention.gov**

Students against Destructive Decisions. SADD is an organization of students dedicated to raising awareness about the dangers of underage drinking, drug use, and impaired driving, among other destructive decisions. **www.sadd.org**

11 Ending Tobacco Use

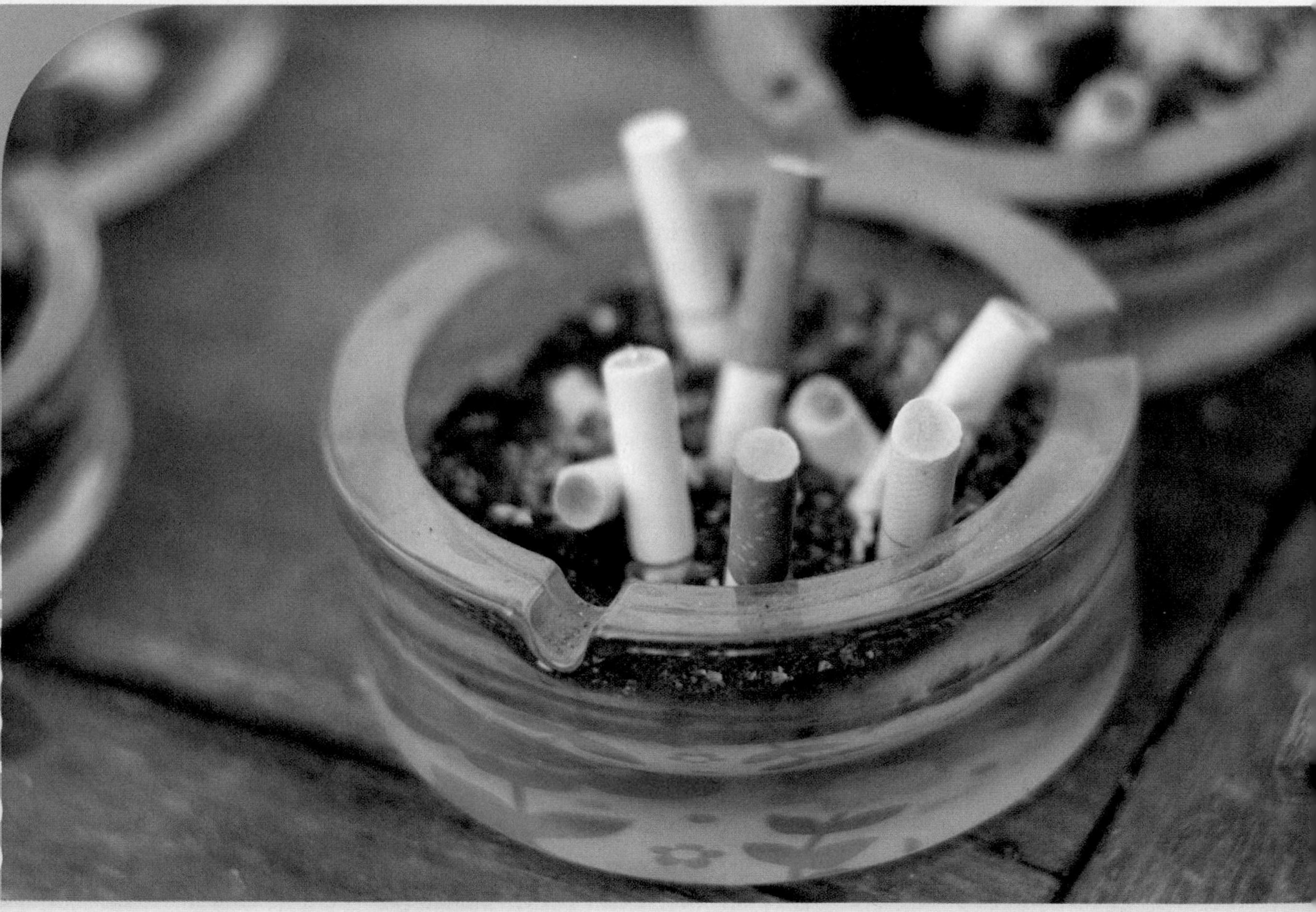

LEARNING OUTCOMES

1 Describe the rate of tobacco use in the United States, and explain the social and political issues involved in tobacco use.
2 Discuss the use of tobacco by college students, and identify some of the reasons college students smoke.
3 Describe how the chemicals in tobacco products affect the body.
4 Explain the health risks of smoking and using smokeless tobacco.
5 Explain the dangers created by environmental tobacco smoke.
6 Discuss prevention policies enacted by the U.S. government to curb tobacco use.
7 Describe various quitting strategies, including those aimed at ending the body's addiction to nicotine.

The prevalence of cigarette smoking among adults has declined significantly over the last 50 years.[1] However, tobacco use is still the single most preventable cause of death in the United States: Nearly 480,000 Americans die each year from tobacco-related diseases. Moreover, another 16 million people will suffer from health disorders caused by tobacco. To date, tobacco is known to cause more than 20 diseases, and about half of all regular smokers die of smoking-related causes. Smoking kills more Americans than alcohol, car accidents, suicide, AIDS, homicide, and illegal drugs combined.[2] Any contention by the tobacco industry that tobacco use is not dangerous completely ignores the overwhelming scientific evidence to the contrary.

LO 1 | UNITED STATES TOBACCO USE

Describe the rate of tobacco use in the United States, and explain the social and political issues involved in tobacco use.

Approximately 70 million Americans age 12 and older report using tobacco products (cigarettes, cigars, smokeless tobacco, and pipe tobacco) at least once in the past month.[3] Declines in cigarette smoking over the past two decades have slowed compared with earlier periods. In 2012, 20.5 percent of men and 15.8 percent of women were current cigarette smokers. Adults 25 to 44 years old had the highest percentage of current cigarette smoking (22 percent), and the percentage continues to decrease with age, with 19.5 percent of adults 45 to 64 years old and 9 percent of adults aged 65 years and older reported to be current smokers.[4]

The rate of past-month cigarette use among those 12 to 17 years old declined from 13 percent in 2002 to 8.6 percent in 2012. The rate of past-month smokeless tobacco use among those 12 to 17 years old increased from 2 percent in 2002 to 2.3 percent in 2012. In addition, every day over 3,000 teens under the age of 18 smoke their first cigarette, and approximately 1,000 of them become daily smokers.[5]

Cigarette use is closely linked to education: Adults with a bachelor's degree or higher education are two times *less* likely to smoke than are those with less than a high school education. Cigarette smoking also varies by ethnicity, with the highest rates of smoking found among American Indian and Alaska Natives, with a prevalence of 21.8 percent.[6] **TABLE 11.1** shows the percentage of Americans who smoke by demographic group.

50%

OF REGULAR SMOKERS EVENTUALLY **DIE** OF SMOKING-RELATED DISEASES.

TABLE 11.1 | Percentage of Population That Smokes (Age 18 and Older) among Select Groups in the United States

	Percentage
United States overall	18.1
Race	
Asian	10.7
Black, non-Hispanic	18.1
Hispanic	12.5
Native American	21.8
White, non-Hispanic	19.7
Age	
18–24	17.3
25–44	21.6
45–64	19.5
65+	8.9
Gender	
Male	20.5
Female	15.8
Education	
Undergraduate	9.1
High school	23.1
GED diploma	41.9
Less than 12 years (no diploma)	24.7
Postgraduate	5.9
Income Level	
Below poverty level	27.9
At or above poverty level	17

Source: Centers for Disease Control and Prevention, "Adult Cigarette Smoking in the United States: Current Estimate," February, 2014, www.cdc.gov/tobacco/data_statistics/fact_sheets/adult_data/cig_smoking.

More than 20 percent of Americans are former smokers, and about 60 percent have never smoked. The most commonly used tobacco product is cigarettes, more common among men (20.5%) than women (15.8%), followed by cigars (9.1% of men and 2.0% of women) and smokeless tobacco (3.5 percent of people 12 and older).[7]

Tobacco and Social Issues

The production and distribution of tobacco products involve many political and economic issues. Tobacco-growing states derive substantial income from tobacco production, and federal, state, and local governments benefit enormously from cigarette taxes.

Advertising The tobacco industry spends an estimated \$24 million per day on advertising and promotional material.[8]

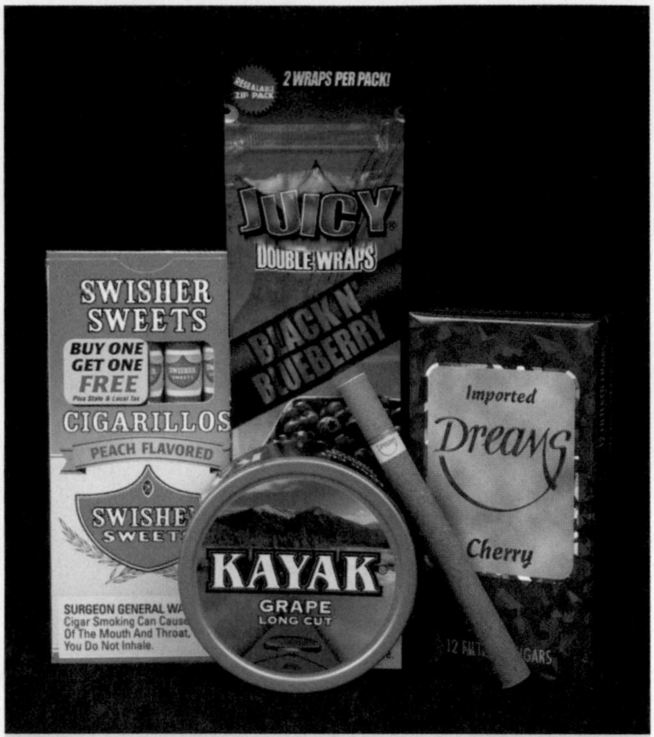

Tobacco companies know that once a person starts smoking, chances are good that he or she will get hooked, so they make a concerted effort to attract children and teens by using colorful images and flavored products that mask the harshness of tobacco.

With the number of smokers declining by about 1 million each year, the industry must actively recruit new smokers. Tobacco advertising encourages young people to begin smoking before they are old enough to understand the long-term health risks.[9] Of adult smokers, 90 percent started by age 21, and half became regular smokers by age 18. Tobacco companies target children and teens with tobacco products that are candy, fruit, or alcohol flavored, thus making them more palatable to young people.[10]

Advertisements in women's magazines imply that smoking is the key to financial success, thinness, independence, and social acceptance. These ads have apparently been working. From the mid-1970s through the early 2000s, cigarette sales to women increased dramatically. Not coincidentally, by 1987 cigarette-induced lung cancer had surpassed breast cancer as the leading cancer killer among women and has remained the leading cancer killer in every year since.[11]

Women are not the only targets of gender-based cigarette advertisements. Men are depicted in locker rooms, charging over rugged terrain in off-road vehicles, or riding stallions into the sunset in blatant appeals to a need to feel and appear masculine. Minorities are also often targeted. Tobacco advertising, particularly menthol cigarettes, is much more common in magazines aimed at African Americans, such as *Jet* and *Ebony*, than in similar magazines aimed at broader audiences, such as *Time* and *People*. Neighborhoods with large African American populations have a higher concentration of menthol advertisements and lower prices of menthol cigarettes compared to white neighborhoods.[12] Billboards and posters spreading the cigarette message have dotted the landscape in Hispanic communities for many years, especially in low-income areas. Recent innovations by tobacco companies have included sponsorship of community-based events such as festivals and annual fairs.

SEE IT! VIDEOS

What tools should you use to quit smoking? Watch **Do Nicotine Patches and Gum Work?** available on MasteringHealth.™

Financial Costs to Society

Estimates show annual costs attributed to smoking in the United States are between $289 and $333 billion. The economic burden of tobacco use totals more than $132–$176 billion in direct medical expenditures and $156 billion in lost productivity.[13] It is estimated that smoking-related health costs and productivity losses are $18.20 per pack of cigarettes sold.[14] These costs far exceed the tax revenues on the sale of tobacco products, even though the average cigarette tax in 2012 was $1.53 per pack and is rising in some states.[15]

LO 2 | COLLEGE STUDENTS AND TOBACCO USE

Discuss the use of tobacco by college students, and identify some of the reasons college students smoke.

College students are the targets of heavy tobacco marketing and advertising campaigns. The tobacco industry has set up aggressive marketing promotions at bars, music festivals, and other events specifically targeted at the 18- to 24-year-old age group. Being placed in a new, often stressful social and academic environment makes college students especially vulnerable to outside influences. Peer influence can prompt students to start or continue smoking, and many colleges and universities still sell tobacco products in campus stores. However, cigarette smoking among U.S. college students has decreased in recent years (see **FIGURE 11.1**). In a 2013 study, about 13.8 percent of college students reported having smoked cigarettes in the past 30 days.[16] College men have slight higher rates of smoking (17 percent) compared to women (12 percent).[17] Men also use more cigars and smokeless tobacco.[18]

Among those aged 18 to 22, full-time college students are less likely to smoke than their peers who are not enrolled full-time in college. In 2012, cigarette use in the past month was reported by 21.3 percent

WHAT DO YOU THINK?

Have you noticed a change in the number of your friends who smoke?

- How many smoked prior to college compared to now?
- What are their reasons for smoking?
- What keeps your friends from quitting?

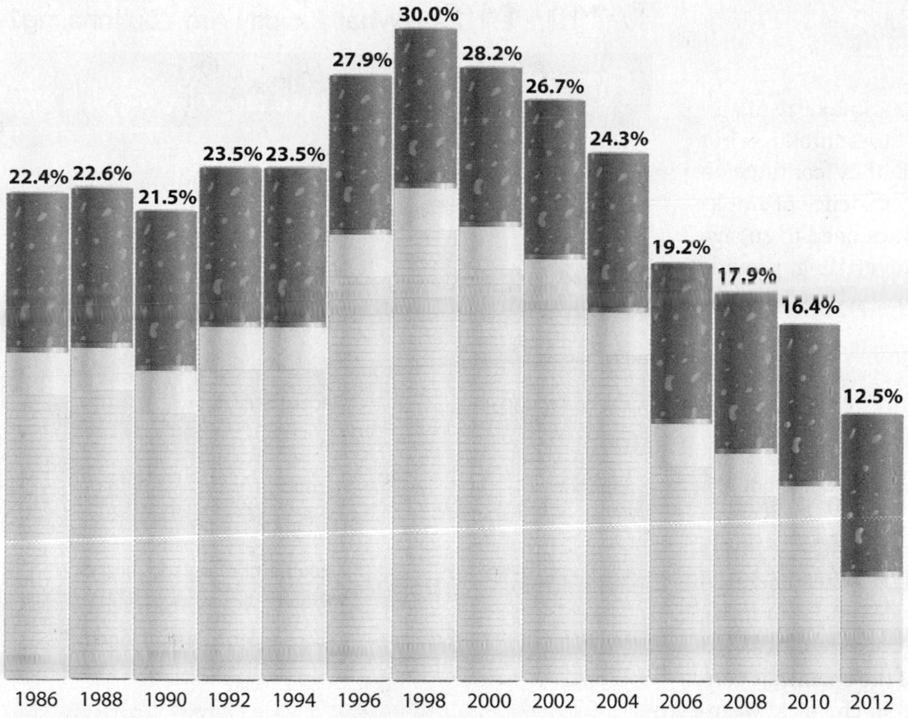

FIGURE 11.1 Trends in Prevalence of Cigarette Smoking in the Past Month among College Students

Source: Data from L. D. Johnston et al., "Monitoring the Future National Survey Results on Drug Use, 1975–2012, Volume II: College Students and Adults Ages 19–50" (Ann Arbor: Institute for Social Research, The University of Michigan, 2013).

of full-time college students, less than the rate of 37.2 percent for those not enrolled full time.[19] Among males age 18 to 22 who were full-time college students in 2012, cigarette use declined from 31.7 percent in 2009 to 24.5 percent.[20]

Why Do College Students Smoke?

Some of the reasons college students smoke are to relax or reduce stress (see **FIGURE 11.2**). Smokers are more likely to have higher levels of perceived stress than do nonsmokers. Other key reasons students smoke are to fit in or because they are addicted.

For some students, weight control is an important motivator, and fear of weight gain is a common reason for smoking relapse. Students diagnosed or treated for depression are much more likely to use tobacco compared to students who are not.[21]

Social Smoking

Many college-age smokers identify themselves as "social smokers"—those who smoke when they are with people, rather than alone. Up to half of college smokers deny being smokers, even though they reported smoking in the past 30 days. Many of these students smoke in social situations where they also drink alcohol.[22] Like regular smokers, social smokers engage in more alcohol use, illicit drug use, and higher sexual risk-taking behaviors than nonsmokers.[23] Even occasional smoking is not without risks of damaging health effects. Social smoking in college can lead to a complete dependence on nicotine and thus to all the same health risks as smoking regularly.

Smoking less than a pack of cigarettes a week has been shown to damage blood vessels and to increase the risk of heart disease and cancer.[24] Occasional or social smokers also experience an increased occurrence of colds, sore throats, shortness of breath, and fatigue.[25] In women taking birth control pills, even a few cigarettes a week can increase the likelihood of heart disease, blood clots, stroke, liver cancer, and gallbladder disease.[26] Pregnant women who smoke only occasionally still run a risk of giving birth to unhealthy babies.

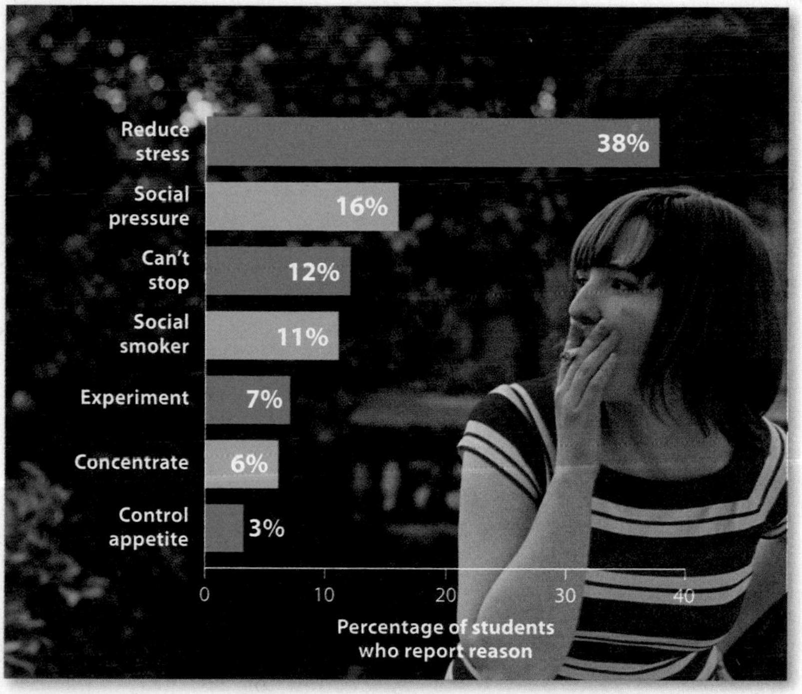

FIGURE 11.2 Reasons Why College Students Smoke

Source: National Center on Addiction and Substance Abuse at Columbia University, *Wasting the Best and the Brightest: Substance Abuse at America's Colleges and Universities* (New York: National Center on Addiction and Substance Abuse at Columbia University, March 2007), 48. Copyright © 2007. Used with permission.

Most Student Smokers Want to Quit

Unlike social smokers, most students who smoke regularly and are nicotine dependent do want to stop smoking, but in spite of their efforts or desire to quit, they continue to smoke throughout college. To reduce the incidence of smoking among students, colleges and universities need to engage in antismoking efforts, control tobacco advertising, provide smoke-free residence halls, and offer greater access to smoking-cessation programs.

LO 3 | EFFECTS OF TOBACCO

Describe how the chemicals in tobacco products affect the body.

Smoking, the most common form of tobacco use, delivers a strong dose of nicotine along with 7,000 other chemical substances, including arsenic, formaldehyde, and ammonia, directly to the lungs. Among these chemicals are at least 69 known or suspected carcinogens.[27] Some of the chemicals contained in tobacco smoke can also be found in chemical weapons, household cleaners, car exhaust, and embalming fluid (see **TABLE 11.2**). Inhaling toxic gases exposes sensitive mucous membranes to irritating chemicals that weaken the tissues and contribute to cancers of the mouth, larynx, and throat. The heat from tobacco smoke is also harmful to tissues.

TABLE 11.2 | What Exactly Are You Inhaling?

Chemical in Tobacco Smoke	Where Else Can You Find It?
Acetic acid	Vinegar
Acetone	Nail polish remover
Ammonia	Floor/toilet cleaner
Arsenic	Rat poison
Butane	Lighter fluid
Cadmium	Rechargeable batteries
Carbon monoxide	Car exhaust
DDT/dieldrin	Insecticides
Ethanol	Alcohol
Hexamine	Barbecue lighter
Hydrogen cyanide	Gas chamber poison, chemical weapons
Methane	Swamp gas, cow flatulence
Methanol	Rocket fuel
Naphthalene	Mothballs
Nicotine	Insecticide/addictive drug
Stearic acid	Candle wax
Toluene	Industrial solvent, paint thinner

Source: Utah Department of Health, TobaccoFreeUtah.org, "Chemicals Found in Tobacco Smoke," 2012, www.tobaccofreeutah.org/chemicals.html.

69 | OR MORE **CHEMICALS** IN SECONDHAND SMOKE ARE KNOWN TO CAUSE CANCER.

Nicotine

The highly addictive chemical stimulant **nicotine** is the major psychoactive substance in all tobacco products. In its natural form, nicotine is a colorless liquid that turns brown upon exposure to air. When tobacco leaves are burned in a cigarette, pipe, or cigar, nicotine is released and inhaled into the lungs. Sucking or chewing tobacco releases nicotine into the saliva, which is then absorbed through the mucous membranes in the mouth.

Nicotine is a powerful central nervous system stimulant that produces a variety of physiological effects. In the cerebral cortex, it produces an aroused, alert mental state. Nicotine stimulates the adrenal glands, which increases the production of adrenaline. It also increases heart and respiratory rates, constricts blood vessels, and, in turn, increases blood pressure because the heart must work harder to pump blood through the narrowed vessels.

nicotine Primary stimulant chemical in tobacco products that is highly addictive.

tar Thick, brownish sludge condensed from particulate matter in smoked tobacco.

carbon monoxide Gas found in cigarette smoke that reduces the ability of blood to carry oxygen.

Tar and Carbon Monoxide

Cigarette smoke is a complex mixture of chemicals and gases produced by the burning of tobacco and its additives. Particulate matter condenses in the lungs to form a thick, brownish sludge called **tar**, which contains various carcinogenic agents, such as benzopyrene, and chemical irritants, such as phenol. Phenol has the potential to combine with other chemicals that contribute to developing lung cancer.

In healthy lungs, millions of tiny hairlike projections (*cilia*) on the surfaces lining the upper respiratory passages sweep away foreign matter, which is expelled from the lungs by coughing. However, the cilia's cleansing function is impaired in smokers' lungs by nicotine, which paralyzes the cilia for up to 1 hour following a single cigarette. This allows tars and other solids in tobacco smoke to accumulate and irritate sensitive lung tissue. **FIGURE 11.3** illustrates how tobacco smoke damages the lungs.

Cigarette smoke also contains poisonous gases, the most dangerous of which is **carbon monoxide**, the deadly gas emitted in car exhaust. Carbon monoxide reduces the oxygen-carrying capacity of the red blood cells by binding

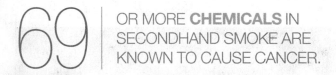

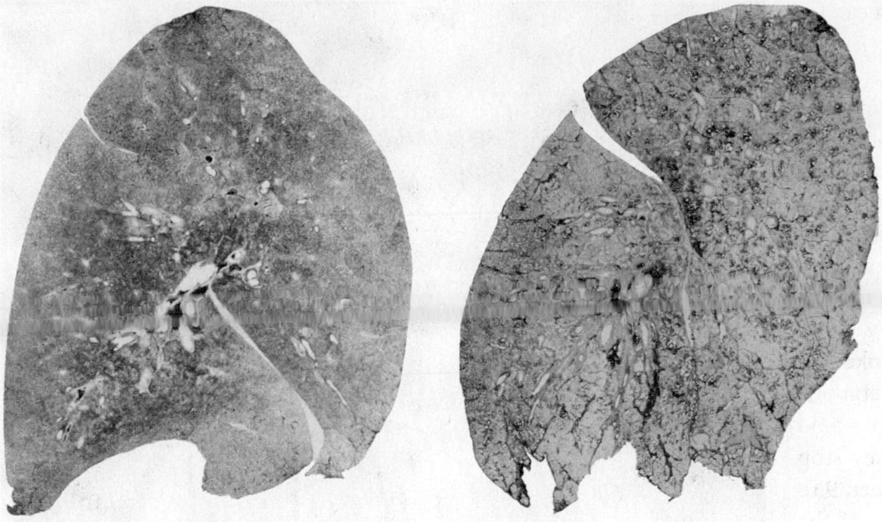
a A healthy lung
b A smoker's lung permeated with deposits of tar

FIGURE 11.3 Lung Damage from Chemicals in Tobacco Smoke Smoke particles irritate lung pathways, causing extra mucus production, and nicotine paralyzes the cilia that normally function to keep the lungs clear of excess mucus. The result is difficulty breathing, "smoker's cough," and chronic bronchitis. At the same time, tar collects within the alveoli (air sacs), ultimately causing their walls to break, leading to emphysema. Tar and other carcinogens in tobacco smoke also cause cellular mutations that lead to cancer.

with the receptor sites for oxygen, causing oxygen deprivation in many body tissues. It is at least partly responsible for the increased risk of heart attacks and strokes in smokers.

Tobacco Addiction

A recent study found that about half of high school students had experimented with smoking.[28] Why do some people walk away from cigarettes while others get hooked? This is a complicated question, but there are several possible reasons: Nicotine is a very addictive drug, people can become hooked on the behavior (inhalation) itself, weight control can be a motivating factor for either losing or maintaining weight, and U.S. residents are bombarded with cigarette advertising messages every day.

Nicotine Addiction Beginning smokers usually feel the effects of nicotine with their first puff. These symptoms, called **nicotine poisoning**, can include dizziness, lightheadedness, rapid and erratic pulse, clammy skin, nausea, vomiting, and diarrhea. These unpleasant effects cease as tolerance develops, which happens almost immediately in new users, perhaps after the second or third cigarette. In contrast, tolerance to most other drugs, such as alcohol, develops over a period of months or years. Regular smokers generally do not experience a "buzz" from smoking. They continue to smoke simply because quitting is so difficult.

Studies have found genetic factors to be significantly influential in smoking initiation and nicotine dependence. Specifically, one study found that teenagers carrying variants in two genes were three times more likely to become regular smokers in adolescence and twice as likely to be persistent smokers in adulthood compared to noncarriers.[29] These two specific genes may influence smoking behavior by affecting the action of the brain chemical dopamine.[30] Understanding the influence of genetics on nicotine addiction could be crucial to developing more effective smoking-cessation treatments.[31]

Behavioral Dependence People who smoke are not just physically dependent on nicotine, they are also psychologically dependent. Nicotine "tricks" the brain into creating pleasurable memory associations between sensory stimuli or environmental cues that may trigger the urge for a cigarette.[32] Even those who smoke only occasionally might find it hard to quit because of associations between smoking and a behavior such as having a drink or a morning cup of coffee.

Many smokers have a difficult time imagining not smoking. They often de-scribe their cigarette as their friend. For some smokers, simply holding a cigarette provides comfort and can have a calming effect. Some former smokers remain vulnerable to sensory and environmental

nicotine poisoning Symptoms often experienced by beginning smokers, including dizziness, diarrhea, lightheadedness, rapid and erratic pulse, clammy skin, nausea, and vomiting.

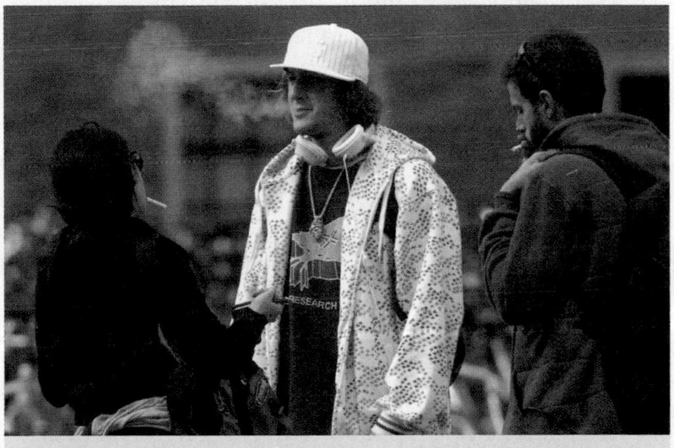
RESEARCH

An occasional puff once in a while when you are out with friends can't hurt, right? Wrong! There is no "safe" amount of tobacco use—any smoking or exposure to smoke increases your risks for negative health effects such as heart disease and lung cancer. And even if you smoke only once or twice a week and consider yourself a social smoker, chances are you're on the road to dependence and a more frequent smoking habit.

cues, such as the smell of tobacco or driving a car, for years after they quit.

Weight Control People who start smoking often lose weight. Nicotine is an appetite suppressant and slightly increases the smoker's *basal metabolic rate* (the rate of energy expended by the body at complete rest). After smoking, a smoker's metabolism increases right away and then returns to a normal level. Heavy smokers have surges in metabolism throughout the day. As a result, they experience less appetite than do those who smoke less or not at all. When a smoker quits, the metabolic rate slows down and appetite returns. People tend to eat more (sweets in particular) when they stop smoking, with an average weight gain between 9 to 11 pounds.[33] Fear of gaining weight is one of the biggest reasons smokers are reluctant to quit. Ways to avoid weight gain after quitting include avoiding crash diets, keeping low-calorie treats handy, and drinking plenty of water.

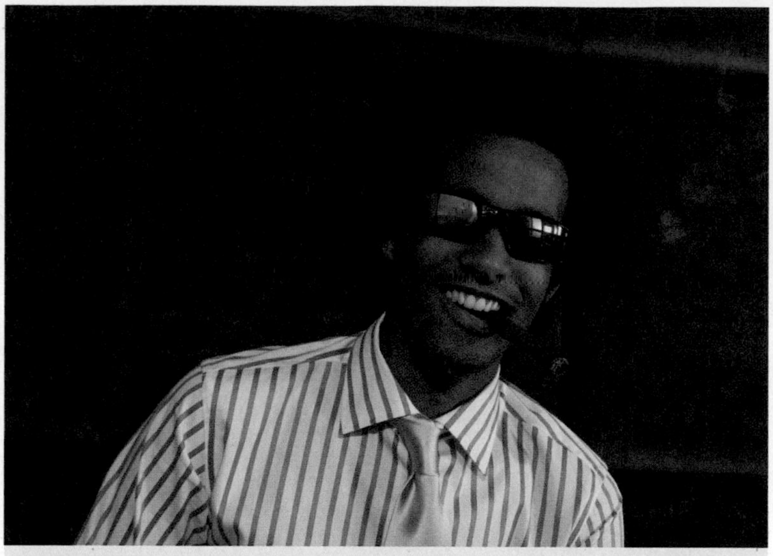

Cigars have two to three times the nicotine of a cigarette, and their smoke contains just as many toxic chemicals and carcinogens as cigarette smoke.

Tobacco Products

Tobacco comes in several forms. Cigarettes, cigars, pipes, and bidis are used for burning and inhaling tobacco. Smokeless tobacco is sniffed or placed in the mouth.

Cigarettes *Filtered cigarettes* are the most common form of tobacco available today. Almost all manufactured cigarettes have filters designed to reduce levels of gases such as hydrogen cyanide and carbon monoxide, but these products may actually deliver more hazardous gases to the user than nonfiltered brands. Some smokers use low-tar and low-nicotine products as an excuse to smoke more cigarettes, but wind up exposing themselves to more harmful substances than they would with a smaller number of regular-strength cigarettes.

Clove cigarettes contain about 40 percent ground cloves (a spice) and about 60 percent tobacco. Many users mistakenly believe that these products are made entirely of ground cloves and that smoking them eliminates the risks associated with tobacco. In fact, clove cigarettes contain higher levels of tar, nicotine, and carbon monoxide than do regular cigarettes—and the numbing effect of eugenol, an ingredient in cloves, allows smokers to inhale more deeply. The same effect is true of *menthol cigarettes:* The throat-numbing effect of the menthol allows for deeper inhalation. Menthol cigarettes also have higher carbon monoxide concentrations than regular cigarettes.

bidis Hand-rolled flavored cigarettes.

Cigars Many people believe that cigars are safer than cigarettes, when in fact the opposite is true. Cigar smoke contains 23 poisons and 43 carcinogens. Most cigars contain as much nicotine as several cigarettes, and when cigar smokers inhale, nicotine is absorbed as rapidly as it is with cigarettes. For those who don't inhale, nicotine is still absorbed through the mucous membranes in the mouth.

While cigar use has declined in recent years, the sale of little cigars has increased approximately 240 percent.[34] Little cigars are roughly the same size and shape as cigarettes; come in packs of 20, as do cigarettes; can be flavored; and cost much less than cigarettes. In a recent study, users of little cigars were more likely to be younger, male, black, and current cigarette, cigar, hookah, or marijuana smokers. Users also tended to have a lower perception of harm, greater sensation-seeking behaviors, and higher perceived levels of stress.[35]

Pipes and Hookahs Pipes have a long history of use throughout the world, including ritualistic and ceremonial use in many cultures. Often thought to be safer than cigarettes or cigars, pipes are not risk-free options. According to the National Cancer Institute and the American Cancer Society, pipe smoking carries risks similar to cigar smoking. Of concern in recent years is the increasing prevalence, particularly among college students, of the use of hookahs, or water pipes. Hookah smoking originated in the Middle East and involves burning flavored tobacco in a water pipe and inhaling the smoke through a long hose. Hookahs are marketed as a safe alternative to cigarettes because they reduce the risks from hazardous chemicals by filtering the smoke through water before it is inhaled. While water pipes may cool the smoke, they do not eliminate or filter out harmful substances.[36] In addition to the health risks associated with all tobacco products, risks associated with hookah use include the possibility of infectious disease transmission by sharing a pipe.

Bidis Generally made in India or Southeast Asia, **bidis** are small, hand-rolled cigarettes that come in a variety of flavors, such as vanilla, chocolate, and cherry. They have become

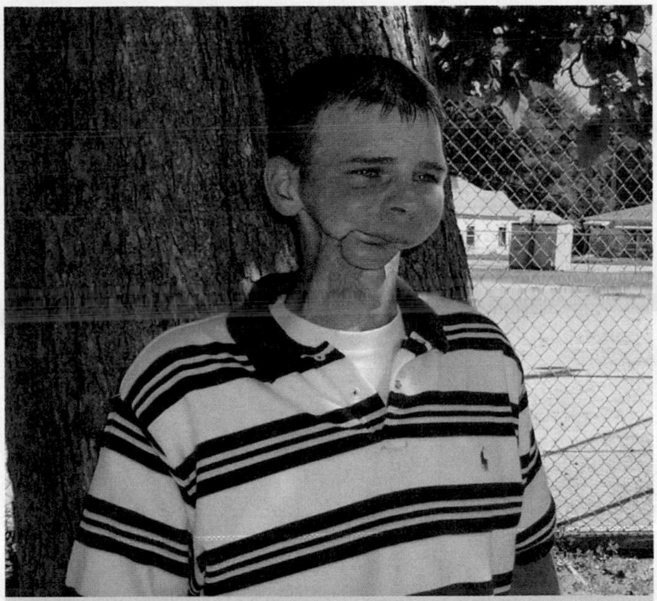

Any form of tobacco is hazardous to your health. This young cancer survivor began using smokeless tobacco at age 13; by age 17 he was diagnosed with squamous cell carcinoma and underwent surgery to remove neck muscles, lymph nodes, and his tongue.

increasingly popular with college students because they are viewed as safer and cheaper than cigarettes. However, they are far more toxic than cigarettes. Smoke from a bidi contains three times more carbon monoxide and nicotine and five times more tar than cigarettes.[37] The leaf wrappers are nonporous, which means that smokers must suck harder to inhale and must inhale more to keep the bidi lit. During testing, it took an average of 28 puffs to smoke a bidi, compared to only 9 puffs for a regular cigarette. This results in increased exposure to higher amounts of tar, nicotine, and carbon monoxide. Bidi smoking increases the risk for oral cancer, lung cancer, stomach cancer, and esophageal cancer and is also associated with emphysema and chronic bronchitis.[38]

Smokeless Tobacco There are two types of smokeless tobacco: chewing tobacco and snuff.

Chewing tobacco comes in three forms—loose leaf, plug, or in a pouch—and contains tobacco leaves treated with molasses and other flavorings. The user dips the tobacco by placing a small amount between the lower lip and teeth to stimulate the flow of saliva and release the nicotine. **Dipping** rapidly releases nicotine into the bloodstream. Use of chewing tobacco by teenagers, especially white males, has increased in recent years.[39]

WHAT DO YOU THINK?

Should nicotine be regulated as a controlled substance?

- Should more resources be used for research into nicotine addiction?
- Why or why not?

Snuff is a finely ground form of tobacco that can be inhaled, chewed, or placed against the gums. It comes in dry or moist powdered form or sachets (tea bag-like pouches). In 2009, "snus" became the latest form of smokeless tobacco to hit the market in the United States. Popular for more than 100 years in Sweden, these small sachets of tobacco are placed inside the cheek and sucked. Some people prefer snus to chewing tobacco because it doesn't require the user to spit frequently.

Smokeless tobacco is just as addictive as cigarettes and actually contains more nicotine—holding an average-sized dip or chew in the mouth for 30 minutes delivers as much nicotine as smoking four cigarettes. A two-can-a-week snuff user gets as much nicotine as a ten-pack-a-week smoker.

Dental problems are common among users of smokeless tobacco. Contact with tobacco juice causes receding gums, tooth decay, bad breath, and discolored teeth. Damage to both the teeth and jawbone can contribute to loss of teeth.

LO 4 | HEALTH HAZARDS OF TOBACCO PRODUCTS

Explain the health risks of smoking and using smokeless tobacco.

Each day, cigarettes contribute to approximately 1,200 deaths from cancer, cardiovascular disease, and respiratory disorders.[40] In addition, tobacco use can negatively affect the health of almost every system in your body. **FIGURE 11.4** on the next page summarizes some of the physiological and health effects of smoking.

Cancer

Lung cancer is the leading cause of cancer deaths in the United States. The American Cancer Society estimates that tobacco smoking causes 90 percent of all cases of lung cancer in men and 78 percent in women.[41] There were an estimated 242,550 *new* cases of lung cancer in the United States in 2013 alone, and an estimated 163,660 Americans died from the disease in 2013.[42] **FIGURE 11.5** on page 333 shows the association between tobacco consumption rates and lung cancer deaths.

Lung cancer can take 10 to 30 years to develop, and the outlook for its victims is poor. Most lung cancer is not diagnosed until it is fairly widespread in the body; at that point, the 5-year survival rate is only 17 percent. When a malignancy is diagnosed and recognized while still localized, the 5-year survival rate rises to 54 percent.[43]

If you are a smoker, your risk of developing lung cancer depends on several factors. First, the amount you smoke per day is important. Someone who smokes two packs a day is 15 to 25 times more likely to develop lung cancer than a nonsmoker. As little as one cigar per day can double the risk of several cancers, including cancer of the oral cavity (lip, tongue, mouth, and throat), esophagus, larynx, and lungs. A second factor is the age at which you started smoking; if you started in your teens, you

chewing tobacco Stringy form of tobacco that is placed in the mouth and then sucked or chewed.

dipping Placing a small amount of chewing tobacco between the lower lip and teeth for rapid nicotine absorption.

snuff Powdered form of tobacco that is sniffed or absorbed through the mucous membranes in the nose or placed inside the cheek and sucked.

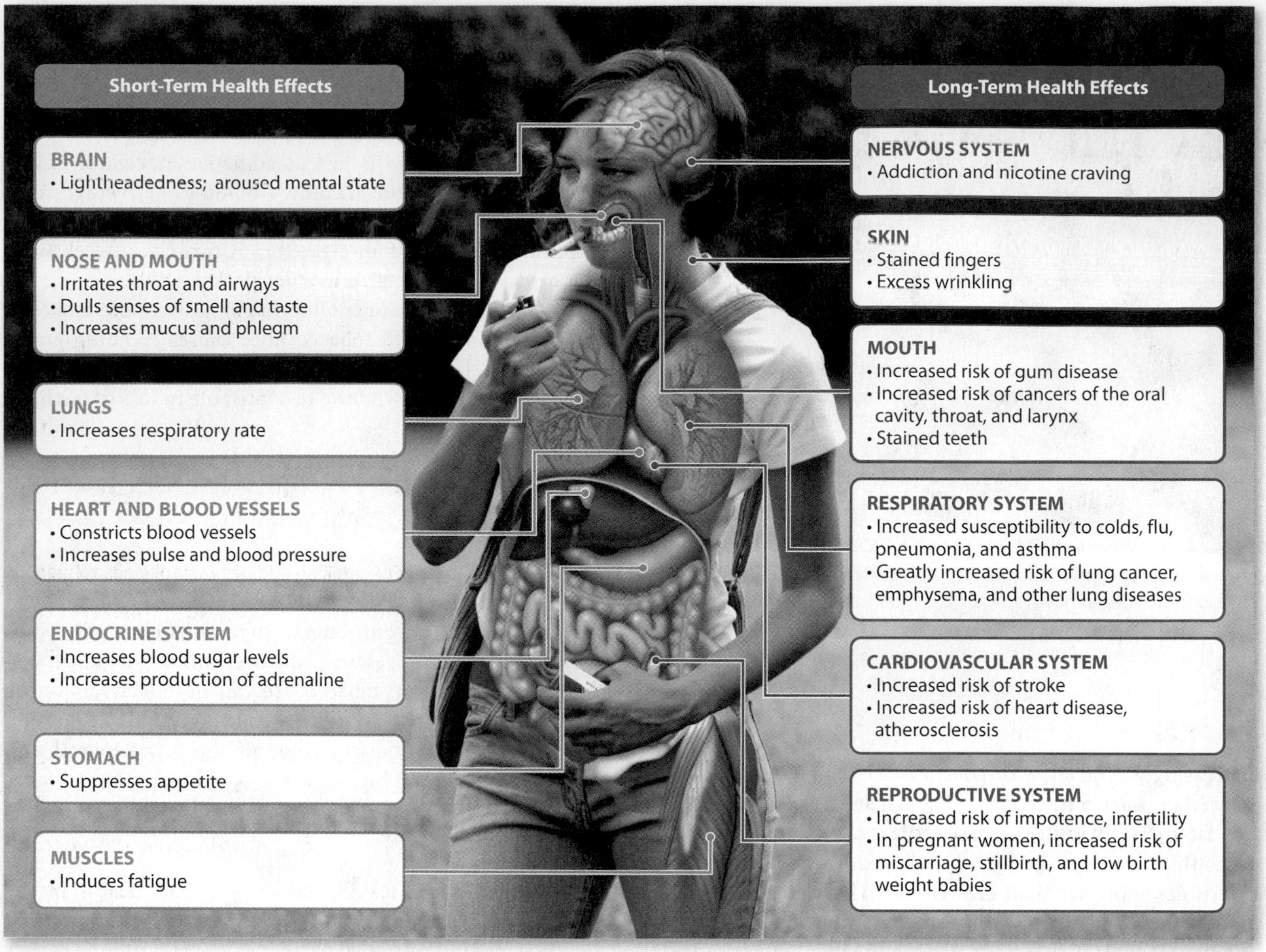
Short-Term Health Effects
BRAIN
• Lightheadedness; aroused mental state
NOSE AND MOUTH
• Irritates throat and airways
• Dulls senses of smell and taste
• Increases mucus and phlegm
LUNGS
• Increases respiratory rate
HEART AND BLOOD VESSELS
• Constricts blood vessels
• Increases pulse and blood pressure
ENDOCRINE SYSTEM
• Increases blood sugar levels
• Increases production of adrenaline
STOMACH
• Suppresses appetite
MUSCLES
• Induces fatigue
Long-Term Health Effects
NERVOUS SYSTEM
• Addiction and nicotine craving
SKIN
• Stained fingers
• Excess wrinkling
MOUTH
• Increased risk of gum disease
• Increased risk of cancers of the oral cavity, throat, and larynx
• Stained teeth
RESPIRATORY SYSTEM
• Increased susceptibility to colds, flu, pneumonia, and asthma
• Greatly increased risk of lung cancer, emphysema, and other lung diseases
CARDIOVASCULAR SYSTEM
• Increased risk of stroke
• Increased risk of heart disease, atherosclerosis
REPRODUCTIVE SYSTEM
• Increased risk of impotence, infertility
• In pregnant women, increased risk of miscarriage, stillbirth, and low birth weight babies

FIGURE 11.4 Effects of Smoking on the Body and Health

VIDEO TUTOR
Long- and Short-Term Effects of Tobacco

leukoplakia Condition characterized by leathery white patches inside the mouth, which is produced by contact with irritants in tobacco juice.

have a greater chance of developing lung cancer than do people who start later. And a third risk factor is whether you inhale deeply when you smoke. Smokers are also more susceptible to the cancer-causing effects of exposure to other irritants, such as asbestos and radon, than are nonsmokers.

A major risk of chewing tobacco is **leukoplakia**, a condition characterized by leathery white patches inside the mouth, produced by contact with irritants in tobacco juice. Approximately 1 out of 5 leukoplakias is either cancerous or precancerous on first sighting, eventually progressing to cancer if not treated.[44]

There were over 42,440 cases of oral cancer diagnosed in 2014—the vast majority of which were caused by smokeless tobacco or cigarettes.[45] Smokeless tobacco users have significantly higher rates of oral cancer than nonusers. Warning signs include lumps in the jaw or neck; color changes or lumps inside the lips; white, smooth, or scaly patches in the mouth or on the neck, lips, or tongue; a red spot or sore on the lips or gums or inside the mouth that does not heal in 2 weeks; repeated bleeding in the mouth; and difficulty or abnormality in speaking or swallowing.

The lag time between first use and contracting cancer is shorter for smokeless tobacco users than for smokers because

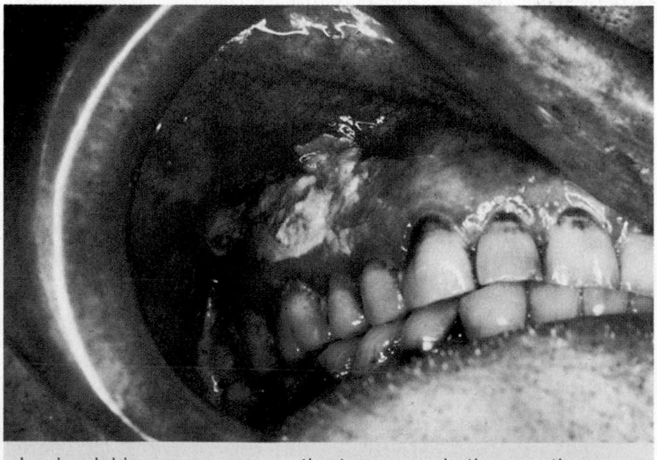

Leukoplakia can appear on the tongue or in the mouth, as shown here.

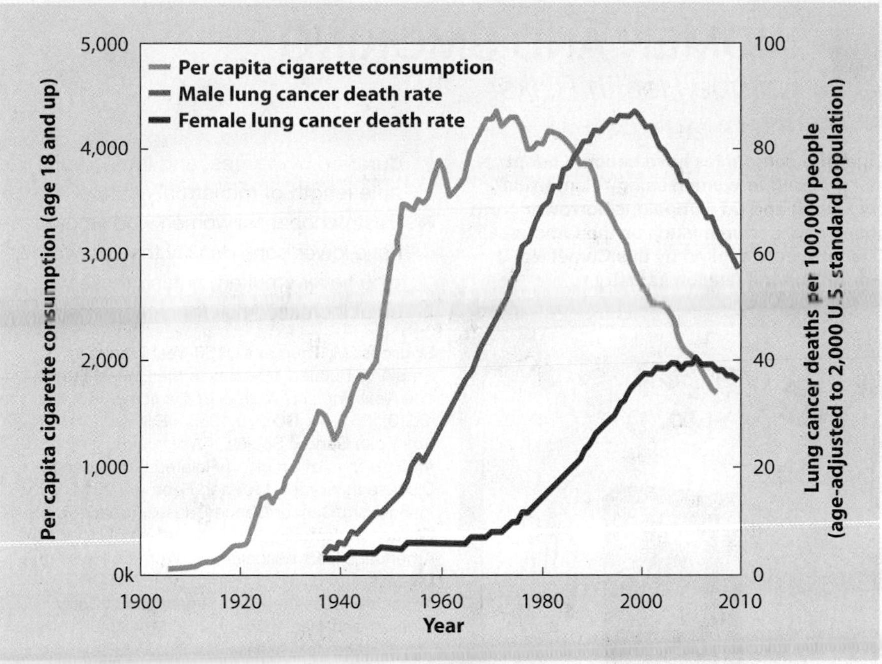

FIGURE 11.5 **Correlation between Tobacco Consumption and Lung Cancer Deaths in the United States** A dramatic rise in lung cancer death rates echoed the rise in popularity of cigarettes and other tobacco products in the last century. After tobacco use and smoking rates began to decline in the 1980s, the lung cancer death rates began to decline as well.

Sources: Death rates data from U.S. Mortality Files, National Center for Health Statistics, Centers for Disease Control and Prevention, 2010; E. Mendes, "The Study That Helped Spur the U.S. Stop-Smoking Movement," American Cancer Society, January 2014, www.cancer.org/research/acsresearchupdates/the-study-that-helped-spur-the-us-stop-smoking-movement.

absorption through the gums is the most efficient route of nicotine administration. Many smokeless tobacco users eventually "graduate" to cigarettes and increase their risk for developing additional problems.

Tobacco is linked to other cancers as well. The rate of pancreatic cancer is more than twice as high for smokers as for nonsmokers. Typically, the prognosis for people with pancreatic cancer is not good—the 5-year survival rate is 5 percent.[46] Smokers are at increased risk to develop cancers of the lip, tongue, salivary glands, and esophagus. A growing body of evidence suggests that long-term use of smokeless tobacco increases the risk of cancers of the larynx, esophagus, nasal cavity, pancreas, colon, kidney, and bladder.

Cardiovascular Disease

Over a third of all tobacco-related deaths occur from heart disease.[47] Smoking poses as great a risk for developing heart disease as high blood pressure and high cholesterol do. Daily cigar smoking, especially for people who inhale, also increases the risk of heart disease (cigar smokers double their risk of heart attack and stroke compared to nonsmokers).[48]

Smoking contributes to heart disease by aging the arteries.[49] This occurs because smoking and exposure to environmental tobacco smoke (ETS; see the definition on page 335), encourage and accelerate the buildup of fatty deposits (plaque) in the heart and major blood vessels (*atherosclerosis*). Smokers can experience a 50 percent increase in plaque accumulation in the arteries as compared with ex-smokers. Nonsmokers regularly exposed to ETS can have a 20 to 25 percent increase in plaque buildup.[50] For unknown reasons, smoking decreases blood levels of high-density lipoproteins (HDLs), the "good" cholesterol that helps protect against heart attacks.

Smoking also contributes to **platelet adhesiveness**, the sticking together of red blood cells associated with blood clots. The oxygen deprivation associated with smoking decreases the oxygen supplied to the heart and can weaken tissues. Smoking also contributes to irregular heart rhythms, which can trigger a heart attack. Both carbon monoxide and nicotine can precipitate angina attacks (chest pain due to the heart muscle not getting the blood supply it needs).

Smokers are two to four times as likely to suffer strokes as nonsmokers.[51] A stroke occurs when a small blood vessel in the brain bursts or is blocked by a blood clot, denying oxygen and nourishment to vital portions of the brain. Depending on the area of the brain affected, stroke can result in paralysis, loss of mental functioning, or death. Smoking contributes to strokes by raising blood pressure, which increases the stress on vessel walls. Platelet adhesiveness contributes to blood clot formation.

platelet adhesiveness Stickiness of red blood cells associated with blood clots.

If a person quits smoking, the risk of dying from a heart attack falls by half after only 1 year and declines steadily thereafter. After about 15 years without smoking, an ex-smoker's risk of coronary heart disease is similar to that of people who have never smoked.[52]

WHY SHOULD I CARE?

If the life-threatening health consequences aren't enough to make you give up smoking, consider the negative impact smoking can have on your social (and romantic!) life. Popular media may make smoking seem glamorous and sexy, but in reality, smoking makes your breath, hair, and clothing smell bad; it causes your skin to age prematurely; it yellows your teeth; and it can interfere with a man's ability to achieve and maintain an erection.

Respiratory Disorders

Smoking quickly impairs the respiratory system. Smokers can feel its impact in a relatively short period of time—they are more

HEALTH IN A DIVERSE WORLD

WOMEN AND SMOKING
Unique Health Risks

Today, 16.5 percent of women—slightly more than 1 in 6—smoke, compared with 21.6 percent of men. Women who smoke now are just as likely to die of cancer and other smoking-related diseases as men, and both active and passive smoking increase chances of breast cancer. Accordingly, women have assumed a much larger burden of smoking-related diseases than they did in the past, and the prevalence of tobacco-related disease continues to increase. Consider the following:

- Women are 25 times more likely to die from lung cancer than nonsmoking women compared to 30 years ago.
- Smoking reduces a woman's life expectancy on average by at least 10 years.
- Women who smoke are twice as likely to have a heart attack as nonsmoking women.
- Women who smoke (particularly those who also use oral contraceptives) are at increased risk for blood clots, as well as heavier menstrual bleeding, longer duration of cramps, and less predictable length of menstrual cycle.
- Postmenopausal women who smoke have lower bone density than do women who never smoked, putting these women at increased risk for osteoporosis.

Cigarette companies have become adept at marketing to women using "glamorous" packaging and ad campaigns borrowed from cosmetics, perfume (such as the famous Chanel scents evoked by this Camel No. 9 brand), and the fashion industry.

Sources: M. Thun et al., "50-Year Trends in Smoking-Related Mortality in the United States," *The New England Journal of Medicine* 368 (2013): 351–64, DOI: 10.1056/NEJMsa1211127; American Cancer Society, "Women and Smoking: An Epidemic of Smoking-Related Cancer and Disease in Women," revised February 2014, www.cancer.org/Cancer/CancerCauses/TobaccoCancer/WomenandSmoking/women-and-smoking-intro; American Heart Association, "Women, Heart Disease," 2012, www.heart.org/HEARTORG/Advocate/IssuesandCampaigns/QualityCare/Women-and-Heart-Disease_UCM_430484_Article.jsp; Centers for Disease Control and Prevention, "Cigarette Smoking among Adults and Trends in Smoking Cessation—United States 2009," *Morbidity and Mortality Weekly Report* 59, no. 35 (2010): 1135–40; P. Jha et al., "21st-Century Hazards of Smoking and Benefits of Cessation in the United States," *New England Journal of Medicine* 368, no. 4 (2013): 341–50; M. Thun et al. "50-Year Trends in Smoking-Related Mortality in the United States," *New England Journal of Medicine* 368, no. 4 (2013): 351–64.

prone to breathlessness, chronic cough, and excess phlegm production than are nonsmokers of the same age. Over time, cumulative lung damage can lead to chronic obstructive pulmonary disease (COPD), including chronic bronchitis and emphysema. Ultimately, smokers are up to 25 times more likely to die of lung disease than are nonsmokers.[53]

Chronic bronchitis may develop in smokers because their inflamed lungs produce more mucus, which they constantly try to expel along with foreign particles. This results in the persistent cough known as "smoker's hack." Smokers are also more prone to respiratory ailments such as influenza, pneumonia, and colds. Smokers tend to miss work one-third more often than nonsmokers, primarily because of respiratory conditions.

Emphysema is a chronic disease in which the alveoli (the tiny air sacs in the lungs) are destroyed, impairing the lungs' ability to obtain oxygen and remove carbon dioxide. As a result, breathing becomes difficult. While healthy people expend only about 5 percent of their energy in breathing, people with advanced emphysema expend nearly 80 percent. Because the heart has to work harder to do even the simplest tasks, it may become enlarged, and death from heart damage may result. There is no known cure for emphysema, and the damage is irreversible. Approximately 80 percent of all cases of emphysema are related to cigarette smoking.[54]

emphysema Chronic lung disease in which the tiny air sacs in the lungs are destroyed, making breathing difficult.

Sexual Dysfunction and Fertility Problems

Despite attempts by tobacco advertisers to make smoking appear sexy, research shows that it can actually cause impotence in men. Studies have found that male smokers are much more likely to experience erectile dysfunction than are nonsmokers.[55] Toxins in cigarette smoke damage blood vessels, reducing blood flow to the penis and leading to an inadequate erection. Impotence may indicate oncoming cardiovascular disease.

In women, smoking can lead to infertility and problems with pregnancy. Women who smoke increase their risk for infertility, ectopic pregnancy, miscarriage, and stillbirth. Smoking also increases the risk of sudden infant death syndrome and the chances of a baby being born with a cleft lip or cleft palate.[56] Smoking during pregnancy increases the

WHAT DO YOU THINK?

Should smokeless tobacco be banned wherever smoking is forbidden?

- Why do you think smokeless tobacco is popular with many athletes and young men?

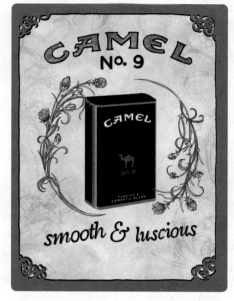

chance of premature birth and the risk of low birth weight (less than 5.5 pounds), which in turn increases the likelihood of illness or death of an infant.[57] For information on specific health risks faced by women smokers, see the **Health in a Diverse World** box on the previous page.

Other Health Effects

Studies have shown tobacco use to be a serious risk factor in the development of gum disease.[58] In addition, smoking increases the risk of macular degeneration, one of the most common causes of blindness in older adults. It also causes premature skin wrinkling, staining of the teeth, yellowing of the fingernails, and bad breath. Nicotine speeds up the process by which the body uses and eliminates drugs, making medications less effective. In addition, research suggests that smoking significantly increases the risk of Alzheimer's disease.[59]

LO 5 | ENVIRONMENTAL TOBACCO SMOKE

Explain the dangers created by environmental tobacco smoke.

Although fewer Americans smoke than in the past, air pollution from smoking in public places continues to be a problem. **Environmental tobacco smoke (ETS)** is divided into two categories: mainstream and sidestream smoke. **Mainstream smoke** refers to smoke drawn through tobacco while inhaling; **sidestream smoke** (commonly called *secondhand smoke*) refers to smoke from the burning end of a cigarette or smoke exhaled by a smoker. People who breathe smoke from someone else's smoking product are said to be *involuntary* or *passive* smokers.

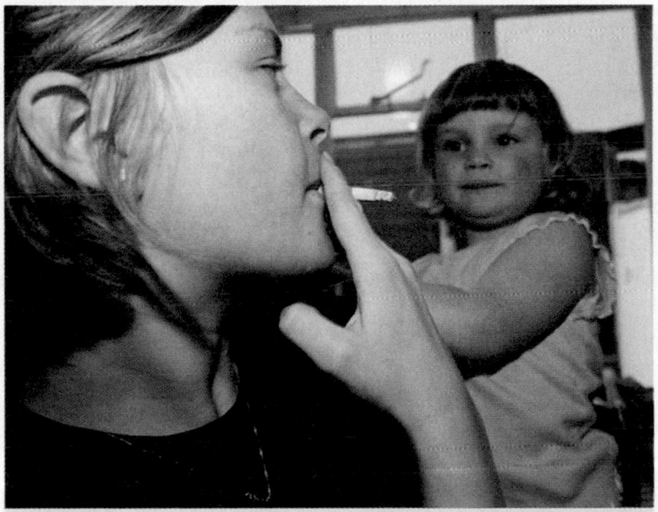

Every year, ETS is responsible for thousands of deaths from lung cancer and heart disease in nonsmoking adults, as well as hundreds of infant deaths from SIDS among babies who live with smokers. Because their bodies and brains are still developing, infants and children are particularly vulnerable to the toxins in secondhand smoke: It can cause respiratory problems, including lower respiratory infections and increased frequency and severity of asthma attacks, and other health concerns, such as greater risk of ear infections.

Between 1988 and 2008, detectable levels of nicotine exposure in nonsmoking Americans decreased from 87.9 percent to 40.1 percent.[60] The decrease in exposure to secondhand smoke is due to the growing number of laws that ban smoking in workplaces and other public areas. As of 2014, 39 states and the District of Columbia had laws in effect requiring workplaces, restaurants, and bars to be 100 percent smoke-free.[61] There are 22,487 municipalities—85 percent of the U.S. population—that are covered by either state, commonwealth, territorial, or local law.[62] Groups such as Action on Smoking and Health and Americans for Nonsmokers' Rights continue to push for policies and laws in support of smoke-free public places.[63]

WHAT DO YOU THINK?

Why do most smokers continue despite knowing long-term hazards?

- What strategies might be effective in reducing the number of people who begin smoking?

Risks from Environmental Tobacco Smoke

Although involuntary smokers breathe less tobacco than active smokers do, they still face risks from exposure. According to the American Lung Association, secondhand smoke has about 2 times more tar and nicotine, 5 times more carbon monoxide, and 50 times more ammonia than mainstream smoke. Every year, ETS is estimated to be responsible for approximately 3,400 lung cancer deaths in nonsmoking adults, 46,000 coronary and heart disease deaths in nonsmoking adults who live with smokers, and higher risk of death in newborns from sudden infant death syndrome.[64]

environmental tobacco smoke (ETS) Smoke from tobacco products, including secondhand and mainstream smoke.

mainstream smoke Smoke that is drawn through tobacco while inhaling.

sidestream smoke Smoke from the burning end of a cigarette, pipe, or cigar or exhaled by nonsmokers, commonly called *secondhand smoke*.

The Environmental Protection Agency has designated secondhand smoke as a known carcinogen. There are more than 69 cancer-causing agents found in secondhand smoke.[65] There is also strong evidence that secondhand smoke interferes with normal functioning of the heart, blood, and vascular systems, significantly increasing the risk for heart disease. Studies indicate that nonsmokers exposed to secondhand smoke were 20 to 30 percent more likely to have coronary heart disease than nonsmokers not exposed to smoke.[66]

Children and ETS Children are more heavily exposed to ETS than adults. More than 53 percent of U.S. children age 3 to 11 years—22 million children—are exposed to ETS. Exposure to ETS increases children's risk of lower respiratory tract infections. Consequently, there are an estimated 150,000 to 300,000 lower respiratory tract infections in children under 18 months of age and lung infections resulting in 7,500 to 15,000 hospitalizations each year.[67] Chemicals in tobacco smoke also show up in breast milk, and breast-feeding may pass more chemicals to the infant of a smoking mother than direct exposure to ETS. In addition, children exposed to secondhand smoke have a greater chance of developing other respiratory problems such as coughing, wheezing, asthma, and chest colds, along with a decrease in lung function. ETS is also linked to fluid buildup in the middle ear, a contributing factor in middle ear infections, a leading reason for childhood surgery. Children exposed to secondhand smoke daily in the home miss more school days and have more colds and acute respiratory infections than do those not exposed. Disparities in ETS also occur along ethnic, racial, and economic lines. African Americans have been found to have higher levels of exposure to ETS than whites and Latinos. ETS exposure is also higher among low-income persons.

Secondhand smoke affects not only children's physical health, but also their cognitive abilities and academic success. One study found that children exposed to high levels of secondhand smoke were twice as likely to develop learning disabilities, conduct disorders, and other behavioral disorders.[68] Boys were more likely to be at risk of developing learning disabilities than girls.[69]

ETS and Additional Health Problems ETS in enclosed areas presents other hazards; it can cause allergic reactions such as itchy eyes, difficulty in breathing, headaches, nausea, and dizziness. Environmental tobacco smoke may also increase the risk of breast cancer in women; cancer of the nasal sinus cavity and of the pharynx in adults; and leukemia, lymphoma, and brain tumors in children.[70] The level of carbon monoxide in cigarette smoke in enclosed spaces is 4,000 times higher than that allowed in the clean-air standard recommended by the EPA.

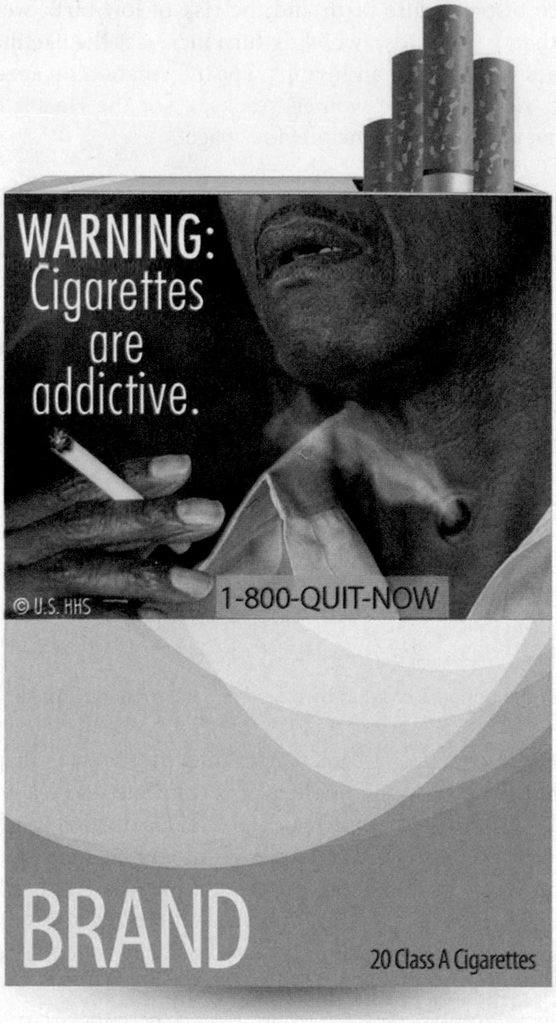

FIGURE 11.6 **Proposed New Cigarette Warning Labels**
The U.S. Food and Drug Administration proposed that graphic warning images such as this one be placed on all cigarette packages and advertisements. However, lawsuits prevented their implementation, and the FDA is now in the process of creating new warning labels.

Source: U.S. Food and Drug Administration, "Proposed Cigarette Product Warning Labels," accessed March 27, 2014, www.fda.gov/TobaccoProducts/Labeling/CigaretteWarningLabels/default.htm.

LO 6 | TOBACCO USE AND PREVENTION POLICIES

Discuss prevention policies enacted by the U.S. government to curb tobacco use.

It has been more than 40 years since the U.S. government began warning that tobacco use was hazardous to health. Despite all the education on the health hazards of tobacco use, health care spending and lost productivity associated with smoking costs between $289 and $333 billion each year.[71]

In 1998, the tobacco industry reached the Master Settlement Agreement with 46 states. The agreement requires tobacco companies to pay out more than $206 billion over 25 years. The agreement includes a variety of measures to support antismoking education and advertising and to fund research to determine effective smoking-cessation strategies. The agreement also curbs certain advertising and promotions directed at youth.

Unfortunately, most of the money designated for tobacco control and prevention at the state level has not been used for this purpose. Facing budget woes, many states have drastically cut spending on antismoking programs. In the few states that have spent the settlement money on smoking-cessation programs, there has been some success in decreasing cigarette use.[72] The Family Smoking Prevention and Tobacco Control Act of 2009 allows the U.S. Food and Drug Administration (FDA) to forbid advertising geared toward children, to lower the amount of nicotine in tobacco products, to ban sweetened cigarettes that appeal to young people, and to prohibit labels such as "light" and "low tar."[73] The FDA recently ordered four tobacco products (bidis) to be taken off the market when the company that created

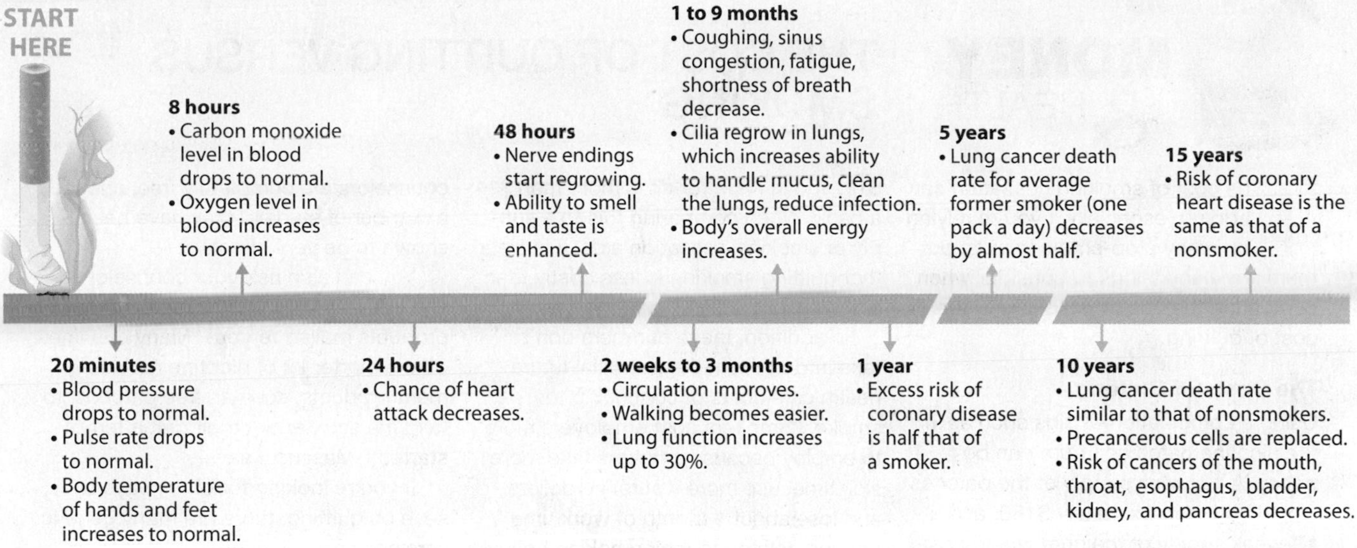

START HERE
8 hours
• Carbon monoxide level in blood drops to normal.
• Oxygen level in blood increases to normal.
48 hours
• Nerve endings start regrowing.
• Ability to smell and taste is enhanced.
1 to 9 months
• Coughing, sinus congestion, fatigue, shortness of breath decrease.
• Cilia regrow in lungs, which increases ability to handle mucus, clean the lungs, reduce infection.
• Body's overall energy increases.
5 years
• Lung cancer death rate for average former smoker (one pack a day) decreases by almost half.
15 years
• Risk of coronary heart disease is the same as that of a nonsmoker.
20 minutes
• Blood pressure drops to normal.
• Pulse rate drops to normal.
• Body temperature of hands and feet increases to normal.
24 hours
• Chance of heart attack decreases.
2 weeks to 3 months
• Circulation improves.
• Walking becomes easier.
• Lung function increases up to 30%.
1 year
• Excess risk of coronary disease is half that of a smoker.
10 years
• Lung cancer death rate similar to that of nonsmokers.
• Precancerous cells are replaced.
• Risk of cancers of the mouth, throat, esophagus, bladder, kidney, and pancreas decreases.

FIGURE 11.7 **When Smokers Quit** Within 20 minutes of smoking that last cigarette, the body begins a series of changes that continues for years. However, by smoking just one cigarette a day, the smoker loses all of these benefits of quitting smoking, according to the American Cancer Society.

Source: American Cancer Society, "When Smokers Quit—What Are the Benefits Over Time?," February 2014, www.cancer.org/healthy/stayawayfromtobacco/guidetoquittingsmoking/guide-to-quitting-smoking-benefits.

them was unwilling to provide ingredient information—the first time since being given the authority in 2009.

One of the most significant impacts of the law is that it requires more prominent health warnings on advertising of tobacco products. Smokeless tobacco ads must contain a warning that fills 20 percent of the advertising space. The FDA attempted to require cigarette packages and advertising to have larger, graphical warnings depicting the negative consequences of smoking (**FIGURE 11.6**), but a federal judge declared the requirement unconstitutional in 2012.

LO 7 | QUITTING

Describe various quitting strategies, including those aimed at ending the body's addiction to nicotine.

Smokers who want to quit must break both the physical addiction to nicotine and the psychological habit of lighting up at certain times or in certain situations. Approximately 70 percent of U.S. adult smokers want to quit smoking, and up to 44 percent make a serious attempt to quit each year. However, only 4 to 7 percent succeed.[74] Quitting is often a lengthy process involving several unsuccessful attempts before success is finally achieved. Even successful quitters suffer occasional slips. For those smokers unable to quit, they can expect to lose at least one decade of life compared to those who do not smoke.

Benefits of Quitting

Many body tissues damaged by smoking can repair themselves. As soon as smokers stop, the body begins the repair process. Within 8 hours, carbon monoxide and oxygen levels return to normal, and "smoker's breath" disappears. Often, within a month of quitting, the mucus that clogs airways is broken up and eliminated. Circulation and the senses of taste and smell improve within weeks. Many ex-smokers say that they have more energy, sleep better, and feel more alert.

After 1 year, the risk for lung cancer and stroke decreases. The risk of developing cancer of the mouth, throat, esophagus, larynx, pancreas, bladder, or cervix is considerably reduced, as is the risk of peripheral artery disease, COPD, coronary heart disease, and ulcers.[75] Women are less likely to bear babies of low birth weight. Within 2 years, the risk for heart attack drops to near normal. After 10 smoke-free years, ex-smokers can expect a normal life span. See **FIGURE 11.7** for a time line of how the body recuperates after a smoker quits.

Another significant benefit of quitting smoking is the money saved. A single pack of cigarettes ranges from about $5.00 (including tax) to as much as $11.00 to $14.50 in the most expensive states, so a pack-a-day smoker who lives in an area where cigarettes cost $8.00 per pack spends $56.00 per week, or $2,912 per year.[76] That is money that could have gone toward school expenses, a down payment on a car, or a vacation. See the **Money & Health** box on the next page for more on the cost of smoking versus quitting.

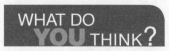

WHAT DO YOU THINK?

Do you know anyone who has tried to quit smoking?

- Why did they do so?
- What was their experience like?
- Were they successful?
- If not, what will they do differently the next time?

MONEY & HEALTH | THE COST OF QUITTING VERSUS SMOKING

The cost of smoking cessation can add up, especially if you're relying on many stop-smoking aids, but there are many things to consider when comparing the cost of smoking to the cost of quitting.

The Costs of Quitting

Using a combination of aids such as the nicotine patch and gum can be pricey. A 12-week supply of the patches would cost approximately $180, and a 12-week supply of the gum would cost about $240, according to Diane Massucci of the North Shore-LIJ Center for Tobacco Control in Great Neck, New York. The total for both aids would be estimated at $420 for less than 3 months of nicotine replacement treatment.

However, smoking-cessation experts state that it's important to keep these stop-smoking costs in perspective. "In Michigan, where I live, the average cost of a pack of cigarettes is over $6.50," says Amanda L. Holm, MPH, manager of Tobacco Treatment Services at the Henry Ford Health System in Detroit. "That means that over the span of a year, a pack-a-day smoker will pay more than $2,372. That's more than enough savings to buy 3 or 6 months' worth of nicotine replacement or other medications, or to pay for a class or a few counseling sessions."

In other states, the costs of smoking are even higher. In Rhode Island, Alaska, Illinois, and Hawaii, a pack of cigarettes costs anywhere from $9 to $12, and in New York it is more than $14 a pack. When comparing this to a supply of smoking-cessation aids, it is clear that quitting smoking is less costly than smoking.

In addition, these numbers don't take into account the potential future health care costs of continuing to smoke. "Smokers cost employers more to employ because smokers take more sick time, use more insurance dollars, and lose about 1 month of work time per year related to their smoking behaviors," Massucci says. "Quitting smoking or not smoking in the car or home can increase the resale value of the car or home. Nonsmokers have lower insurance premiums and increased wellness benefits, as some employers incentivize employees who do not smoke."

The Bottom Line

Add it all up, and the answer is evident. Even if you paid full price for all your smoking-cessation aids, it's still going to be less expensive in the long run than smoking. "Even if someone needed to take medications for longer than 6 months, the reduced health care costs down the road would likely result in substantial savings," Holm says.

Furthermore, people who want to quit smoking also have a number of resources at their disposal that can reduce the cost of quitting. The national smoking quit line, 1-800-QUIT-NOW, can transfer you to your local quit-smoking hotline. The therapy and counseling sessions offered by the over-the-phone counselors are completely free, and in a number of studies, they have been shown to be very effective.

You can also ask your counselor if you can get free nicotine replacement products mailed to you. "Many quit lines offer a starter kit of nicotine replacement products, such as free patches, to help the smoker get their quit attempt started," Massucci says.

If you're looking for other ways to save on quitting, there are many generic versions of medication or the generic or store versions of nicotine replacement products. Holm says that "generic drugs are usually as good as brand-name forms."

As a part of the Affordable Care Act, insurance companies now are required to cover tobacco cessation treatment with no cost to the smoker. This makes it clear: It doesn't pay to continue to smoke.

Sources: M. Kofman, "Implementation of Tobacco Cessation Coverage Under the Affordable Care Act: Understanding How Private Health Insurance Policies Cover Tobacco Cessation Treatments," *Health Policy Institute*, November 26, 2012, www.tobaccofreekids.org/pressoffice/2012/georgetown/coveragereport.pdf; Health Care.gov, "What Are My Preventive Care Benefits?" 2014, www.healthcare.gov/what-are-my-preventive-care-benefits/; L. Mahapatra, "The Price of Cigarettes: How Much Does a Pack Cost in Each US State?" *International Business Times*, February 5, 2014, www.ibtimes.com/price-cigarettes-how-much-does-pack-cost-each-us-state-map-1553445; W. Myers, "Is It Cheaper to Smoke or Quit?," 2011, *Everyday Health*, www.everydayhealth.com/stop-smoking/is-it-cheaper-to-smoke-or-quit.aspx; J. Kritz, "Quitting Smoking Makes Economic Sense," *LA Times*, 2011, http://articles.latimes.com/2011/jan/03/health/la-he-quit-smoking-20110103.

How Can You Quit?

A person who wishes to quit smoking has several options. Most people who are successful quit "cold turkey"—that is, they simply decide not to smoke again. Others focus on gradual reduction in smoking levels, which can reduce risks over time. Some rely on short-term programs, such as those offered by the American Cancer Society, which are based on behavior modification and a system of self-rewards. Still others turn to treatment centers, community outreach programs, or a telephone helpline. Finally, some people work privately with their physicians to reach their goal. Programs that combine several approaches have shown the most promise. Financial considerations, personality, and level of addiction are all factors to consider in deciding on a method.

nicotine withdrawal Symptoms including nausea, headaches, irritability, and intense tobacco cravings suffered by nicotine-addicted individuals who stop using tobacco.

Breaking the Nicotine Addiction

Nicotine addiction may be one of the toughest addictions to overcome. Symptoms of **nicotine withdrawal** include

TABLE 11.3 | Coping Strategies for Common Smoking Withdrawal Problems

Withdrawal Challenge	Estimated Length of Symptoms	Coping Strategies*
Anger, frustration, and irritability	Peaks in first week after quitting but can last 2–4 weeks.	Avoid caffeine, which can amp up an already agitated mood. Get a massage, try deep breathing or exercise.
Anxiety	Builds over the first 3 days and may last up to 2 weeks.	Same strategies as above. Also remind yourself that the symptoms usually pass by themselves over time.
Mild depression	One month or less.	Be with supportive friends, increase physical activity, make a list of things that are upsetting you and write down possible solutions. If depression lasts longer than a month, seek medical advice.
Weight gain	Usually begins in the early weeks and continues through the first year after quitting.	Studies show nicotine replacement products such as gum and lozenges can help counter weight gain. You may also ask your doctor about the drug bupropion (brand names Wellbutrin or Zyban), which has also been shown to counter weight gain.

*Asking your doctor for nicotine replacement products or other medications is a valid coping strategy for any of the withdrawal challenges listed here.

Source: Adapted from National Cancer Institute, National Institutes of Health, "Handling Withdrawal Symptoms When You Decide to Quit," National Cancer Institute Fact Sheet, 2010, www.cancer.gov/cancertopics/factsheet/Tobacco/symptoms-triggers-quitting.

irritability, restlessness, nausea, vomiting, and intense cravings for tobacco (see **TABLE 11.3**). The evidence is strong that consistent pharmacological treatments can help a smoker quit: An estimated 25 to 33 percent of people who have used nicotine replacement therapy or smoking-cessation medications continue to abstain from cigarettes for more than 6 months.[77]

Nicotine Replacement Products

Nontobacco products that replace depleted levels of nicotine in the bloodstream have helped some people stop using tobacco. The two most common are nicotine chewing gum and the nicotine patch, both of which are available over the counter. The FDA has also approved nicotine lozenges, a nicotine nasal spray, and a nicotine inhaler. Another product called the e-cigarette is also available, though it comes with its own health concerns. See the **Health Headlines** box on the next page for more information on e-cigarettes.

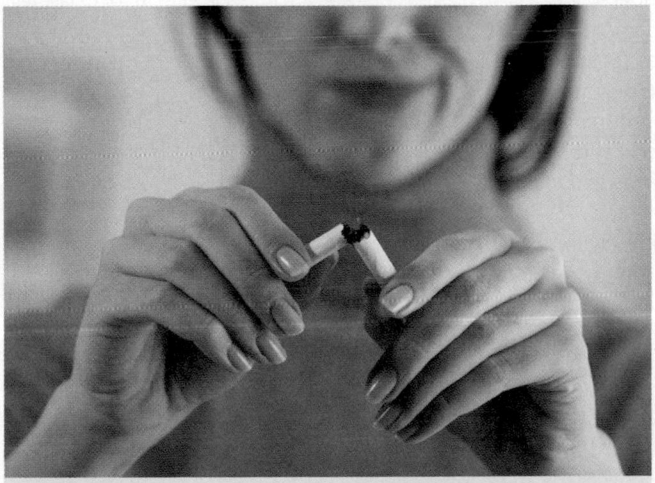

Tobacco causes serious injury to your heart and lungs, but when you quit, your body immediately starts to recover and repair the damage. Over time, the body's repair processes reduce a former smoker's risk of heart disease and cancer.

Nicotine gum is available without a prescription. The user chews up to 20 pieces of gum a day for 1 to 3 months. Nicotine gum delivers about the same amount of nicotine as a cigarette, but because it is absorbed through the mucous membrane of the mouth, it doesn't produce the same rush. Users experience no withdrawal symptoms and fewer cravings for nicotine as the dosage is reduced until they are completely weaned. Nicotine-containing lozenges are available in two strengths, and a 12-week program of use is recommended to allow users to taper off the drug.

The nicotine patch is generally used in conjunction with a comprehensive smoking-cessation program. A small, thin patch placed on the smoker's upper body delivers a continuous flow of nicotine through the skin, helping to relieve cravings. Patches can be bought with or without a prescription and are available in different dosages. The FDA recommends using the patch for 3 to 5 months. During this time, the dose of nicotine is gradually reduced until the smoker is fully weaned from the drug. The patch costs less than a pack of cigarettes—about $4—and some insurance plans will pay for it.[78]

The nasal spray, which requires a prescription, is much more powerful and delivers nicotine to the bloodstream faster than gum, lozenges, or the patch. Patients are warned to be careful not to overdose; as little as 40 mg of nicotine taken at once could be lethal. The FDA has advised that the spray should be used for no more than 3 months and never for more than 6 months so that smokers don't find themselves as dependent on nicotine in spray form as they were on cigarettes. The FDA also advises that no one who

HEALTH HEADLINES

E-CIGARETTES *Health Risks and Concerns*

Electronic cigarettes, also called e-cigarettes, are increasingly used worldwide, even though there is limited information on their health effects. In the United States, they are readily available in most states and on the Internet. A recent report from the Centers for Disease Control and Prevention (CDC) showed a sharp spike in e-cigarette experimentation among U.S. middle and high school students—from 4.7 percent to 10 percent.

Most e-cigarettes consist of a battery, a charger, an atomizer, and a cartridge containing nicotine and propylene glycol. When a smoker draws air through an e-cigarette, an airflow sensor activates the battery and heats the atomizer to vaporize the propylene glycol and nicotine. Upon inhalation, the aerosol vapor delivers a dose of nicotine into the lungs of the smoker, after which residual aerosol is exhaled into the environment. Nothing is known, however, about the chemicals present in the aerosolized vapors emanating from e-cigarettes.

Although manufacturers claim that electronic cigarettes are a safe alternative to conventional cigarettes, the U.S. Food and Drug Administration (FDA) analyzed samples of two popular brands and found variable amounts of nicotine and traces of toxic chemicals, including known cancer-causing substances (carcinogens). This prompted the FDA to issue a warning about potential health risks associated with electronic cigarettes. There is no quality control in the manufacturing of the product. Many of the e-cigarettes are manufactured in China under no controlled conditions.

Furthermore, New York City, Chicago, and Los Angeles have banned e-cigarette use in public places. Many employers are struggling with employees wanting to "vape" indoors on break. Some corporations such as Exxon allow vaping, while Starbucks Corp. and Wal-Mart Stores, Inc. do not. UPS charges nonunion e-cigarette and tobacco users a higher price for their insurance premiums.

Electronic cigarette, or e-cigarette.

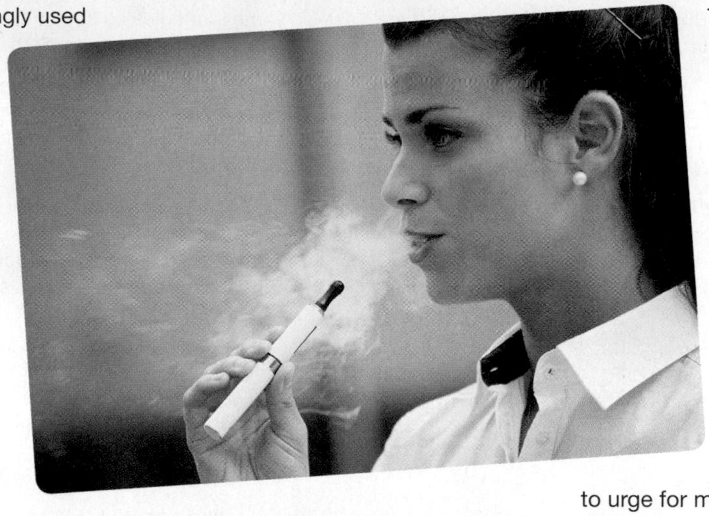

With various colors, fruity flavors, clever designs, and other options, e-cigarettes may hold too much appeal for young people, critics warn, offering an easy gateway to nicotine addiction.

Currently, e-cigarettes do not contain any health warnings comparable to FDA-approved nicotine replacement products or conventional cigarettes. They are often marketed as a method to quit smoking, but health professionals recommend using FDA-approved medications and aids that have been shown to be safe and effective for this purpose. A recent study found no merit to the claim that e-cigarettes are better in terms of helping people quit smoking over the nicotine patch.

As e-cigarettes have increased in popularity, a new health risk has emerged for those who do not smoke. The CDC has reported a dramatic increase in calls to poison control centers regarding e-cigarettes and liquid nicotine poisoning. Over 51 percent of these calls involved children under 5 years of age. The cartridges are not required to be childproof and feature flavors such as spearmint, banana, and bubble gum, making them appealing to children.

As a result, health professionals continue to urge for more action to regulate these products.

Sources: M. Hug, "Health-Related Effects Reported by Electronic Cigarette Users in Online Forums," *Journal of Medical Internet Research* 15, no. 4 (2014): e59; U.S. Food and Drug Administration, "FDA and Public Health Experts Warn About Electronic Cigarettes," 2010, www.fda.gov/newsevents/newsroom/pressannouncements/ucm173222.htm; L. Dale, Mayo Clinic, "Electronic Cigarettes: A Safe Way to Light Up?," 2011, www.mayoclinic.com/health/electronic-cigarettes/AN02025; E. Sohn, Discovery News, "How Safe are E-Cigarettes?," 2011, news.discovery.com/human/e-cigarettes-health-nicotine-tobacco-110127.html; A. Norton, "Are E-Cigarettes Bad for Health?," 2012, www.huffingtonpost.com/2012/01/05/study-finds-e-cigarettes-_n_1187166.html; L. M. Dutra and S. A. Glanz, "Electronic Cigarettes and Conventional Cigarette Use Among US Adolescents. A Cross-sectional Study," *JAMA Pediatrics,* (March 06, 2014), DOI:10.1001/jamapediatrics.2013.5488 (Epub ahead of print.); L. Weber et al., "E-Cigarette Rise Poses Quandary for Employers," *The Wall Street Journal,* January 16, 2014, 41–2; K. Chatham-Stephens et al., "Notes from the Field: Calls to Poison Centers for Exposures to Electronic Cigarettes—United States, September 2010–February 2014," *Morbidity and Mortality Weekly* 63, no. 13 (2014): 292–93; Centers for Disease Control and Prevention, "Youth and Tobacco Use," *Smoking and Tobacco Use,* February 2014, www.cdc.gov/tobacco/data_statistics/fact_sheets/youth_data/tobacco_use.

experiences nasal or sinus problems, allergies, or asthma should use it.

The nicotine inhaler, which also requires a prescription, consists of a mouthpiece and cartridge. By puffing on the mouthpiece, the smoker inhales air saturated with nicotine, which is absorbed through the lining of the mouth, not the lungs, entering the body much more slowly than does the nicotine in cigarettes. Using the inhaler mimics the hand-to-mouth actions used in smoking and causes the back of the throat to feel as it would when inhaling tobacco smoke.

STUDENT HEALTH TODAY

NONTRADITIONAL QUITTING METHODS *Are They Effective?*

In addition to nicotine-replacement products and smoking-cessation drugs, there are many complementary and alternative methods that claim to help you quit smoking. But while the system for evaluating traditional drug therapies automatically involves studying them for safety and effectiveness, alternative quit-smoking methods suffer from a lack of hard data. Furthermore, alternative therapies can be expensive, costing hundreds of dollars per session. And unlike drug therapies, insurance may not cover alternative methods. How is a smoker to judge if the cost is worth it?

In 2012 *The American Journal of Medicine* (AJM) published a study that is helpful for smokers hoping to evaluate these treatments. It conducted a meta-analysis of randomized controlled trials relating to alternative methods for quitting smoking. In meta-analysis, more than one study is examined to discover patterns in the overall data available.

Below is a description of popular nontraditional quitting methods, along with the AJM study's conclusion on effectiveness.

Acupuncture is one of several alternative therapies sometimes used to aid in smoking cessation.

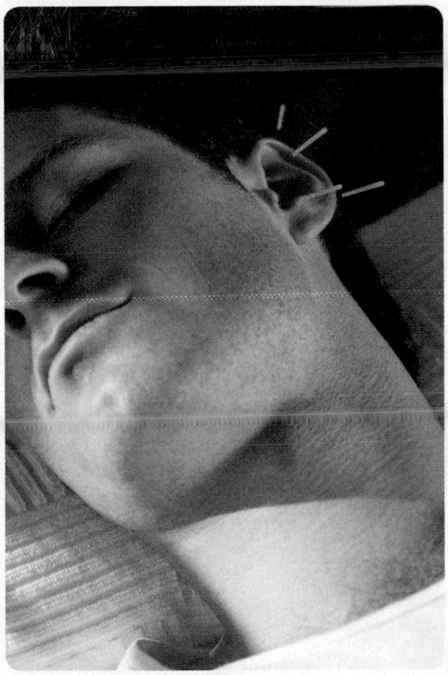

Acupuncture

For smoking cessation, acupuncture needles are generally placed along the ear. The AJM study found that people who used acupuncture were over 3.5 times more likely to quit smoking than those who quit "cold turkey." This is compared with current drug therapies, which are thought to increase smoking cessation by a factor of 2 to 2.5.

The study authors only used the best-quality studies in their analysis, but that meant the amount of data available was low, and they cautioned that this could throw results off. Still, study authors recommended that physicians promote acupuncture as a valid option for patients to use when quitting smoking.

Hypnosis

This deep-relaxation and mental suggestion technique was judged to increase odds of successfully quitting smoking by a factor of 4.26. Again, the lack of good studies available for the analysis made researchers caution the quality of these results. But there was enough evidence for the AJM study authors to suggest that doctors should bring this up as a viable quitting therapy for patients.

Smoking Aversion

In this technique, smokers rapidly take large numbers of puffs on a cigarette in a short period of time. This can make them feel sick—the goal being to remove the pleasure smokers feel when they light up, thereby making it easier for them to quit.

The AJM study found smoking aversion increased the success rate for quitting by a factor similar to hypnosis. However, there were very few recent studies on smoking aversion available, and that led the researchers to call for new and better research for this therapy, rather than endorsing it outright.

Sources: M. Tahiri, S. Mottillo, L. Joseph, and L. Pilote, "Alternative Smoking Cessation Aids: A Meta-Analysis of Randomized Controlled Trials," *American Journal of Medicine* 125, no. 6 (2012): 576–84; and M. J. Eisenberg, "Pharmacotherapies for Smoking Cessation: A Meta-Analysis of Randomized Controlled Trials," *Canadian Medical Association Journal* 179 (2008): 135–44.

Smoking-Cessation Medications Bupropion (brand name Zyban), an antidepressant, is FDA approved as a smoking-cessation aid. Varenicline (brand name Chantix) reduces nicotine cravings and the urge to smoke and blocks the effects of nicotine at nicotine receptor sites in the brain. Both drugs may cause changes in behavior such as hostility, agitation, depressed mood, and suicidal thoughts or actions. People taking one of these drugs who experience any unusual changes in mood are advised to stop taking the drug immediately and contact their health care professional.[79]

See **TABLE 11.4** for a summary of recommended smoking-cessation therapies. In addition to the medications and methods previously described, there are also a number of alternative or nontraditional methods promoted as helpful in quitting smoking. Unlike the strategies previously discussed, these methods have not been scientifically proven to be effective. However, because anything that may help a smoker quit is beneficial, some additional options are discussed in the **Student Health Today** box. Additionally, see the **Tech & Health** box on page 343 for information on smoking apps.

Breaking the Smoking Habit

For some smokers, the road to quitting includes antismoking therapy. Two common techniques are operant conditioning and self-control therapy. Pairing the act of smoking with an external stimulus is a typical example of an operant strategy.

TABLE 11.4 | Recommended Therapies for Smoking Cessation

Therapy	Duration
Buproprion (Zyban) A non–nicotine-based antidepressant that helps reduce nicotine withdrawal symptoms and the urge to smoke. Common side effects are dry mouth, difficulty sleeping, dizziness, and skin rash. Contraindicated if smoker has a history of seizures. *Availability:* Prescription only with a doctor consultation *Cost:* Approximately $2–$4 per day	7–12 weeks; maintenance up to 6 months; start 1–2 weeks before the quit date 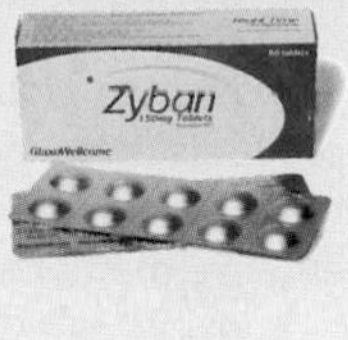
Varenicline (Chantix) A non–nicotine-based prescription medicine developed for the sole purpose of helping people stop smoking. Interferes with nicotine receptors in the brain to lessen the pleasurable physical effects from smoking and to reduce symptoms of nicotine withdrawal. Usually well tolerated, but reported side effects have included headaches, nausea, vomiting, difficulty sleeping, flatulence, changes in taste, and depressed mood. *Availability:* Prescription only with a doctor consultation *Cost:* Approximately $2–$4 per day	12 weeks; maintenance of 12 weeks after successfully quitting; start 1–2 weeks in advance 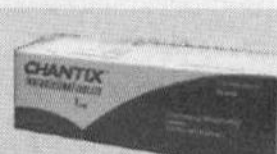
Nicotine Gum A chewing gum that releases nicotine into the bloodstream through the lining of the mouth; might not be appropriate for people with temporomandibular joint disease or those with dentures or other dental work. Up to 2 mg dose if less than 25 cigarettes/day; 4 mg dose if more than 25 cigarettes/day. *Availability:* Over the counter (OTC) *Cost:* Varies upon usage, ranging from $5 to $10 a day	Up to 12 weeks 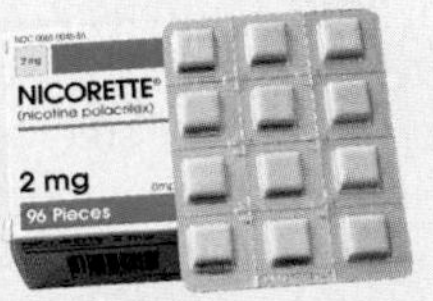
Nicotine Lozenges The lozenges are available in two strengths as part of a 12-week program. Doses can be regularly lowered as treatment progresses. Users should not eat or drink 15 minutes before using lozenges. *Availability:* OTC *Cost:* Depending on frequency of usage, ranges from $6 to $12 per day	The recommended dose is one lozenge every 1–2 hours for 6 weeks, then one lozenge every 2–4 hours for weeks 7–9, and one lozenge every 4–8 hours for weeks 10–12. 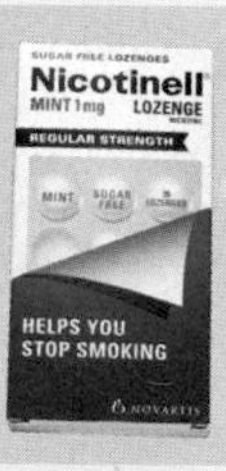
Nicotine Patch Patch supplies a steady amount of nicotine to the body through the skin. It is sold in varying strengths as an 8-week smoking-cessation treatment. Doses can be regularly lowered as treatment progresses or given as a steady dose during treatment. May not be a good choice for people with skin problems or allergies to adhesive tape. *Availability:* Either OTC or by prescription with a doctor consultation *Cost:* Approximately $4 per day.	4 weeks; then 2 weeks; then 2 weeks (8 weeks total) 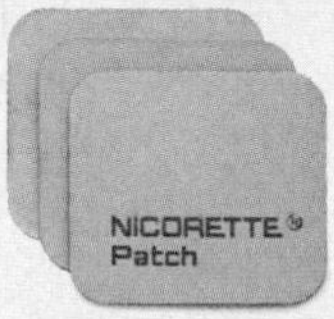
Nicotine Nasal Spray Comes in a pump bottle containing nicotine that tobacco users can inhale when they have an urge to smoke. Not recommended for people with nasal or sinus conditions, allergies, or asthma, or for young tobacco users. *Availability:* Prescription only with a doctor consultation *Cost:* Approximately $5–$15 per day, depending on frequency of use	3–6 months 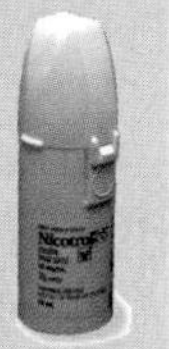
Nicotine Inhaler This device delivers a vaporized form of nicotine to the mouth through a mouthpiece attached to a plastic cartridge. Nicotine travels to the mouth and throat and is absorbed through the mucous membranes. Common side effects include throat and mouth irritation and coughing. Anyone with bronchial problems should use caution. *Availability:* Prescription only with a doctor consultation *Cost:* Ranges from $40 to $55 per package	Up to 6 months 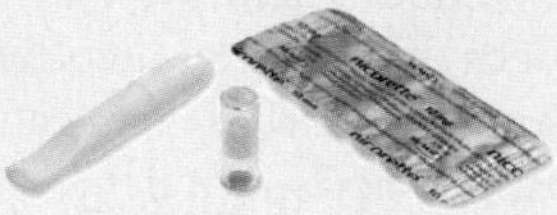

Sources: ShopWiki.com, Smoking Cessation, 2012, www.shopwiki.com/wiki/Smoking-Cessation-Products; QuitSmokingSupport.com, "Quit Smoking Using the Nicotrol Inhaler," 2012, www.quitsmokingsupport.com/inhaler.htm; *Everyday Health*, "Could Chantix or Zyban Help You to Stop Smoking?," 2011, www.everydayhealth.com/smoking-cessation/nicotine-free-smoking-cessation-aids.aspx.

TECH & HEALTH

CAN SMOKING APPS HELP YOU QUIT?

With the thousands of smart phone apps available for quitting smoking, it may seem like all you need to stop smoking is to start downloading. But users should proceed with caution: A recent study that examined popular smoking apps in 2012 found that most apps did not adhere to known cessation methods, meaning they may not be based on evidence or established behavior change strategies.

However, several research-based smoking apps available from reputable institutions may actually help you stop smoking:

- **QuitPal.** (Free: iPhone) http://smokefree.gov/apps-quitpal Developed by the National Cancer Institute, QuitPal allows users to track smoking habits, connect with social networks, chat online with an information service, and access other features to stay motivated.
- **QuitForLife.** (Free: iPhone, Android) www.quitforlifeapp.com The American Cancer Society developed this app with resources including a savings calculator, daily motivational tips, and a 24-hour coaching phone line and online community (for eligible individuals).
- **UCSF/SFGH Stop Smoking.** (Modest cost: iPhone) https://itunes.apple.com/us/app/ucsf-sfgh-stop-smoking/id393637213?mt=8 The University of California, San Francisco's app is a self-help tool that tracks your mood and triggers for smoking and helps you plan healthier activities.

Remember that these apps alone may not be enough to help you quit. Determining what works best for you is an individual process, and programs that combine multiple methods (behavior modification, telephone hotlines, etc.) are usually your best bet.

Source: Abroms et al., "A Content Analysis of Popular Smartphone Apps for Smoking Cessation," *American Journal of Preventive Medicine* 45, no. 6 (2013): 732–36; J. Choi et al., "Smoking Cessation Apps for Smartphones: Content Analysis with the Self-Determination Theory," *Journal of Medical Internet Research* 16, no.2 (2014): e44.

For example, one technique requires smokers to carry a timer that sounds a buzzer at various intervals. When the buzzer sounds, the patient is required to smoke a cigarette. Once the smoker is conditioned to associate the sound of the buzzer with smoking, the buzzer is eliminated, and, one hopes, so is the smoking.

Self-control strategies view smoking as a learned habit associated with specific situations. Therapy aims to identify these situations and teach smokers the skills necessary to resist smoking. The **Skills for Behavior Change** box presents one of the American Cancer Society's approaches to quitting.

SKILLS FOR BEHAVIOR CHANGE

TIPS FOR QUITTING SMOKING

Ready to quit tobacco? These strategies can help:

- Ask smokers who live with you to keep cigarettes out of sight and not offer you any.
- Use the four Ds: deep breaths, drink water, do something else, and delay (tell yourself you'll smoke in 10 minutes when the urge hits).
- Keep "mouth toys" handy: Hard candy, chewing gum, toothpicks, or carrot or celery sticks can help.
- Ask your doctor about nicotine gum, patches, nasal sprays, inhalers, or lozenges.
- Make an appointment with your dental hygienist to have your teeth cleaned.
- Examine those associations that trigger your urge to smoke.
- Spend your time in places that don't allow smoking.
- Take up a new sport, exercise program, hobby, or organizational commitment. This will help shake up your routine and distract you from smoking.

STUDY PLAN

Customize your study plan—and master your health!—in the Study Area of **MasteringHealth**.

ASSESS **YOURSELF**

Are you a smoker? Take the **Tobacco: Are Your Habits Placing You at Risk?** assessment available on MasteringHealth.™

Need help creating a plan? Follow the strategies in the **Your Plan for Change** box for short- and long-term improvements to your health.

YOUR PLAN FOR **CHANGE**

After completing the "Tobacco: Are Your Habits Placing You at Risk?" **ASSESS YOURSELF**, tobacco users can use these steps to help cut down on their smoking and quit.

TODAY, YOU CAN:

- ☐ Develop a plan to kick the tobacco habit. The first step is to identify why you want to quit. Write down your reasons and carry a copy with you. Every time you are tempted to smoke, go over your reasons for stopping.
- ☐ Think about the times and places you usually smoke. What could you do instead of smoking at those times? Make a list of positive alternatives.

WITHIN THE NEXT 2 WEEKS, YOU CAN:

- ☐ Pick a day to stop smoking, and tell a family member or friend to gain support and accountability.
- ☐ Throw away all your cigarettes, lighters, and ashtrays.

BY THE END OF THE SEMESTER, YOU CAN:

- ☐ Focus on the positives. Now that you have stopped smoking, your mind and body will begin to feel better. Make a list of the good things about not smoking. Carry a copy with you, and look at it whenever you have the urge to smoke.
- ☐ Reward yourself for stopping. Go to a movie, go out to dinner, or buy yourself a gift.
- ☐ If you are having difficulty quitting, consult with your campus health center or your doctor to discuss medications or other therapies that may help you quit.

CHAPTER REVIEW

To hear an MP3 Tutor Session, scan here or visit the Study Area in **MasteringHealth.**

LO 1 U.S. Tobacco Use

- Tobacco use involves many social and political issues, including advertising targeted at youth and women, the fastest-growing populations of smokers. Smoking costs the United States between $289 and $333 billion per year.

LO 2 College Students and Tobacco Use

- While smoking has decreased in college students in recent years, students are heavily targeted by tobacco marketing and advertising campaigns. College students smoke to reduce stress, to fit in socially, and because they are addicted.

LO 3 Effects of Tobacco

- Smoking delivers more than 7,000 chemicals to the lungs. Tobacco comes in smoking and smokeless forms; both contain nicotine, an addictive psychoactive substance.

LO 4 Health Hazards of Tobacco Products

- Health hazards include markedly higher rates of cancer, heart and circulatory disorders, respiratory diseases, sexual dysfunction, fertility problems, low birth weight babies, and gum diseases. Smokeless tobacco increases risks for oral cancer and other oral problems.

LO 5 Environmental Tobacco Smoke

- Environmental tobacco smoke puts nonsmokers at risk for cancer and heart disease.

LO 6 Tobacco Use and Prevention Policies

- The FDA requires prominent health warnings on tobacco products and enacts other policies to prevent young people from using tobacco products.

LO 7 Quitting

- To quit, smokers must kick a chemical addiction and a behavioral habit. Nicotine-replacement products or drugs such as Zyban and Chantix can help wean smokers off nicotine. Various types of psychotherapy and alternative methods can also help.

POP QUIZ

Visit **MasteringHealth** to personalize your study plan with Chapter Review Quizzes and Dynamic Study Modules.

LO 1 U.S. Tobacco Use

1. Smoking rates are highest among which of the following education levels?
   a. Undergraduate
   b. High school
   c. GED diploma
   d. Postgraduate

LO 2 College Students and Tobacco Use

2. Which age group is most targeted by tobacco advertisers?
   a. Teenagers age 14 to 17
   b. Young adults age 18 to 24
   c. Adults age 25 to 30
   d. Married men age 31 to 35

LO 3 Effects of Tobacco

3. What is the major psychoactive ingredient in tobacco products?
   a. Carbon monoxide
   b. Tar
   c. Formaldehyde
   d. Nicotine
4. What does nicotine do to cilia in the lungs?
   a. Instantly destroys them
   b. Thickens them
   c. Paralyzes them
   d. Accumulates on them
5. What effect does carbon monoxide have on a smoker's body?
   a. It accumulates on alveoli in lungs, making breathing difficult.
   b. It increases heart rate.
   c. It interferes with the ability of red blood cells to carry oxygen.
   d. It dulls taste and smell.
6. Which tobacco product contains eugenol, which allows smokers to inhale smoke more deeply?
   a. Bidis
   b. Cigars
   c. Snuff
   d. Clove cigarettes

LO 4 Health Hazards of Tobacco Products

7. A major health risk of chewing tobacco is
   a. lung cancer.
   b. leukoplakia.
   c. heart disease.
   d. emphysema.

LO 5 Environmental Tobacco Smoke

8. What is sidestream smoke?
   a. Smoke inhaled by a smoker
   b. Smoke released from the burning end of a cigarette
   c. Smoke from a low-tar cigarette
   d. Smoke from a pipe or hookah

LO 6 Tobacco Use and Prevention Policies

9. Which federal policy allows the FDA to regulate the amount of nicotine in tobacco products and to require health warnings on tobacco products?
   a. The Family Smoking Prevention and Tobacco Control Act
   b. The Master Settlement Agreement
   c. The Child Smoking Prevention and Anti-Tobacco Act
   d. The Environmental Assessment for Tobacco Products Act

LO 7 | Quitting

10. How quickly will an individual begin to see health benefits after quitting smoking?
    a. Within 8 hours
    b. Within a month
    c. Within a year
    d. Never

Answers to the Pop Quiz can be found on page A-1. If you answered a question incorrectly, review the section identified by the Learning Outcome. For even more study tools, visit MasteringHealth.

THINK ABOUT IT!

LO 1 | U.S. Tobacco Use

1. What tactics do tobacco companies use to target different groups of people?

LO 2 | College Students and Tobacco Use

2. What are some of the main reasons college students choose to use tobacco?

LO 3 | Effects of Tobacco

3. Discuss the various ways that tobacco is used. Is any method less addictive or less hazardous to health than another?

LO 4 | Health Hazards of Tobacco Products

4. Discuss the health hazards associated with tobacco. Who should be responsible for the medical expenses of smokers? Insurance companies? Smokers themselves?

LO 5 | Environmental Tobacco Smoke

5. How is sidestream smoke dangerous?

LO 6 | Tobacco Use and Prevention Policies

6. Do you think restrictions on smoking are fair? Why or why not?

LO 7 | Quitting

7. Describe the various methods of tobacco cessation. Which would be most effective for you? Why?

ACCESS YOUR HEALTH ON THE INTERNET

Visit **MasteringHealth** for links to the websites and RSS feeds.

Use the following websites to further explore topics and issues related to ending tobacco use.

For links to the websites below, visit **MasteringHealth.**

American Lung Association. This site offers a wealth of information regarding smoking trends, environmental smoke, and advice on smoking cessation. www.lungusa.org

Action on Smoking and Health (ASH). The nation's oldest and largest antismoking organization, ASH works to fight smoking and protect nonsmokers' rights. www.ash.org

Tobacco Information and Prevention Source (TIPS). This site provides information regarding tobacco use in the United States, with specific information for young people. www.cdc.gov/tobacco

The Tobacco Atlas. This book and website, produced by the World Lung Foundation and the American Cancer Society, cover a range of topics including the history of tobacco use, prevalence of use, youth smoking, secondhand smoke, quitting, and more. www.tobaccoatlas.com

Americans for Nonsmokers' Rights (ANR). This site provides information about smoke-free communities across the United States and tips for taking action to ban smoking in workplaces and other public areas. www.no-smoke.org

Tobacco-Free College Campus Initiative. Serves as a clearinghouse of key information to assist educational communities to establish their own tobacco-free environments. The site includes news updates, state-specific information, links to a wide range of external resources, and referrals to national experts. www.tobaccofreecampus.org

12 Avoiding Drug Misuse and Abuse

LEARNING OUTCOMES

1. Explain how drugs affect physical functions and activate the brain's pleasure circuit.
2. List and describe the six categories of drugs and their routes of administration.
3. Review problems relating to the misuse and abuse of prescription drugs, including the use of illicit drugs among college students.
4. Discuss the use and abuse of controlled substances, including cocaine, amphetamines, marijuana, opioids, hallucinogens, club drugs, inhalants, and steroids.
5. Provide examples of treatment and recovery options for addicts and their effectiveness.
6. Profile illicit drug use in the United States, including who uses illicit drugs, financial impact, and impact on college campuses and the workplace.

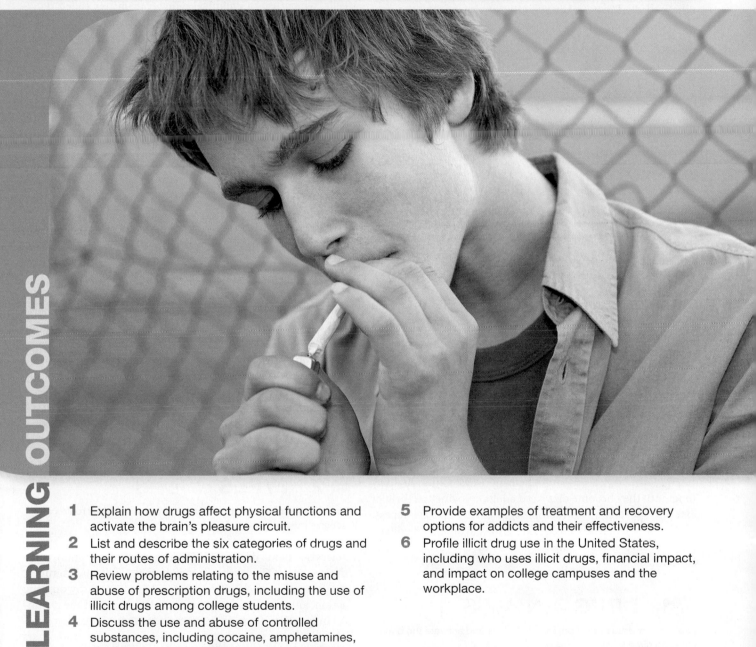

Drug misuse and abuse are enormous problems in our society. Whether it is the meth addict who has lost everything in a fall into dependence and crime or the high-functioning executive who gets hooked on prescription drugs such as OxyContin or Vicodin to ease excruciating back pain, drug addiction wreaks havoc on individuals, families, businesses, and society. The use and abuse of drugs occurs at all income levels, among all ethnic groups, and at all ages. Approximately 9 percent of Americans report using illicit drugs during the past month.[1] By late adolescence, 42 percent of Americans report having used illicit drugs in their lifetime.[2] Over 21 percent of high school students have taken prescription drugs without a doctor's permission.[3]

7.6%

OF COLLEGE STUDENTS REPORT HAVING ABUSED **PRESCRIPTION PAINKILLERS** SUCH AS CODEINE, VICODIN, AND OXYCONTIN IN THE PAST YEAR.

Recently, the overall rate of drug use in the United States rose to its highest level in almost a decade, mostly driven by an increase in the use of marijuana.[4] Drug abuse costs taxpayers more than $193 billion annually in health care costs, public costs related to crime, and lost productivity.[5] It's impossible to put a dollar amount on the pain, suffering, and dysfunction that drugs cause in our everyday lives.

Why do people use drugs? Human beings appear to have a need to alter their consciousness, or mental state. We like to feel good, escape, and feel different. Sometimes we like to reduce pain or dull our senses. Consciousness can be altered in many ways: Children spinning until they become dizzy and adults enjoying the thrill of extreme sports are two examples. To change our awareness, some of us listen to music, ski, read, daydream, meditate, pray, or have sexual relations. Others turn to drugs to alter consciousness.

neurotransmitter A chemical that relays messages between nerve cells or from nerve cells to other body cells.

psychoactive drugs Drugs that affect brain chemistry and have the potential to alter mood or behavior.

LO 1 | DRUG DYNAMICS

Explain how drugs affect physical functions and activate the brain's pleasure circuit.

Drugs work because they physically resemble chemicals produced naturally within the body. Most bodily processes result from chemical reactions or from changes in electrical charge. Because drugs possess an electrical charge and chemical structure similar to those of chemicals that occur naturally in the body, they can affect physical functions in many different ways.

How Drugs Affect the Brain

Pleasure, which scientists call *reward,* is a powerful biological force for survival. If you do something that feels pleasurable, the brain is wired in such a way that you tend to want to do it again. Life-sustaining activities, such as eating, activate a circuit of specialized nerve cells devoted to producing and regulating pleasure. One important set of these nerve cells, which uses a chemical **neurotransmitter** called *dopamine,* sits at the very top of the brain stem in the *ventral tegmental area* (*VTA*). These dopamine-containing neurons relay messages about pleasure through their nerve fibers to nerve cells in the limbic system, structures in the brain regulating emotions. Still other fibers connect to a related part of the frontal region of the cerebral cortex, the area of the brain that plays a key role in memory, perception, thought, and consciousness. Thus, this "pleasure circuit," known as the *mesolimbic dopamine* system, spans the survival-oriented brain stem, the emotional limbic system, and the thinking frontal cerebral cortex.

All drugs that are addicting can activate the brain's pleasure circuit. Drug addiction is a biological, pathological process that alters the way in which the pleasure center, as well as other parts of the brain, functions. Almost all **psychoactive drugs** (those that change the way the brain works) do so by affecting chemical neurotransmission, either enhancing it, suppressing it, or interfering with it. Some drugs, such as heroin and lysergic acid diethylamide (LSD), mimic the effects of a natural neurotransmitter. Others, such as phencyclidine (PCP), block receptors and thereby prevent neuronal messages from getting through. Still others, such as cocaine, block the *reuptake* of neurotransmitters by neurons, thus increasing the concentration of the neurotransmitters in the synaptic gap, the space between individual neurons (**FIGURE 12.1**). Finally, some drugs, such as methamphetamine, cause neurotransmitters to be released in greater amounts than is normal.

LO 2 | TYPES OF DRUGS

List and describe the six categories of drugs and their routes of administration.

Scientists divide drugs into six categories: prescription, over-the-counter (OTC), recreational, herbal, illicit, and commercial drugs. These classifications are based primarily on drug action, although some are based on the source of the chemical in question. Each category includes some drugs that stimulate the body, some that depress body functions, and others that produce hallucinations (sounds, images, or other sensations that are perceived but are not real). Each category also includes psychoactive drugs.

- **Prescription drugs.** These drugs can be obtained only with a prescription from a licensed health practitioner.

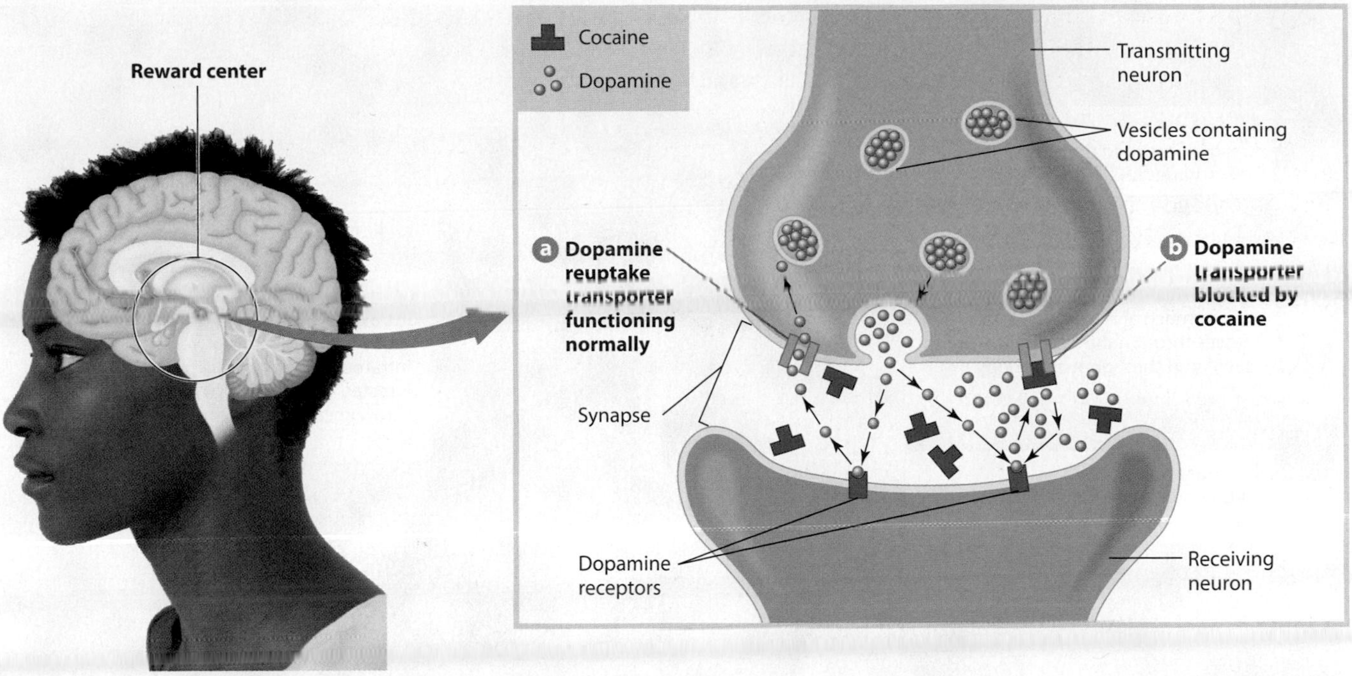

FIGURE 12.1 The Action of Cocaine at Dopamine Receptors in the Brain, an Example of Psychoactive Drug Action In normal neural communication, dopamine is released into the synapse between neurons. It binds temporarily to dopamine receptors on the receiving neuron and then is recycled back into the transmitting neuron by a transporter. When cocaine molecules are present, they attach to the dopamine transporter and block the recycling process. Excess dopamine remains active in the synaptic gaps between neurons, creating feelings of excitement and euphoria.

Source: Adapted from National Institute of Drug Research, *NIDA Research Report—Cocaine Abuse and Addiction*, NIH Publication no. 10-4166, May 1999, revised September 2010, www.drugabuse.gov.

VIDEO TUTOR
Psychoactive Drugs Acting on the Brain

Approximately 47 percent of Americans have reported using at least one prescription medication in the past month.[6]

- **Over-the-counter (OTC) drugs.** These can be purchased without a prescription in many locations such as grocery, drug, and convenience stores. OTC drugs, used to treat everything from headaches to pain, cold, stomach upsets, and athlete's foot, provide an important access to medicine. They create substantial savings for the health care system through decreased visits to health care providers and decreased use of prescription medications.[7] However, there is a risk of OTC drugs being used improperly or misused.[8] (See **Chapter 18** for more information on OTC drugs.)
- **Recreational drugs.** These belong to a somewhat vague category whose boundaries depend on how the term *recreation* is defined. Generally, recreational drugs contain chemicals used to help people relax or socialize. Most of them are legal even though they are psychoactive. Alcohol, tobacco, and caffeine products are included in this category.
- **Herbal preparations.** Herbals encompass approximately 750 substances, including herbal teas and other products of botanical (plant) origin that are believed to have medicinal properties. (See **Chapter 18** for more on herbal preparations.)
- **Illicit (illegal) drugs.** These are the most notorious type of drug. Although laws governing their use, possession, cultivation, manufacture, and sale differ from state to state, illicit drugs are generally recognized as harmful. All of them are psychoactive.
- **Commercial drugs.** These are drugs found in commercially sold products. More than 1,000 of them exist, including those used in seemingly benign items such as perfumes, cosmetics, household cleansers, paints, glues, inks, dyes, and pesticides.

oral ingestion Intake of drugs through the mouth.

Routes of Drug Administration

Route of administration refers to the way in which a drug is taken into the body. The route largely determines the rapidity of the drug's effect on the body (**FIGURE 12.2**). The most common route is **oral ingestion**—swallowing a tablet, capsule, or liquid. Drugs taken by mouth don't reach the bloodstream as quickly as do drugs introduced to the body by other means. A drug taken orally may not reach the bloodstream for 30 minutes.

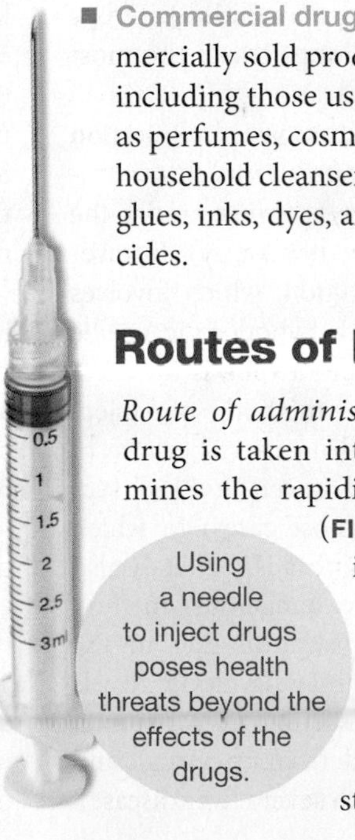

Using a needle to inject drugs poses health threats beyond the effects of the drugs.

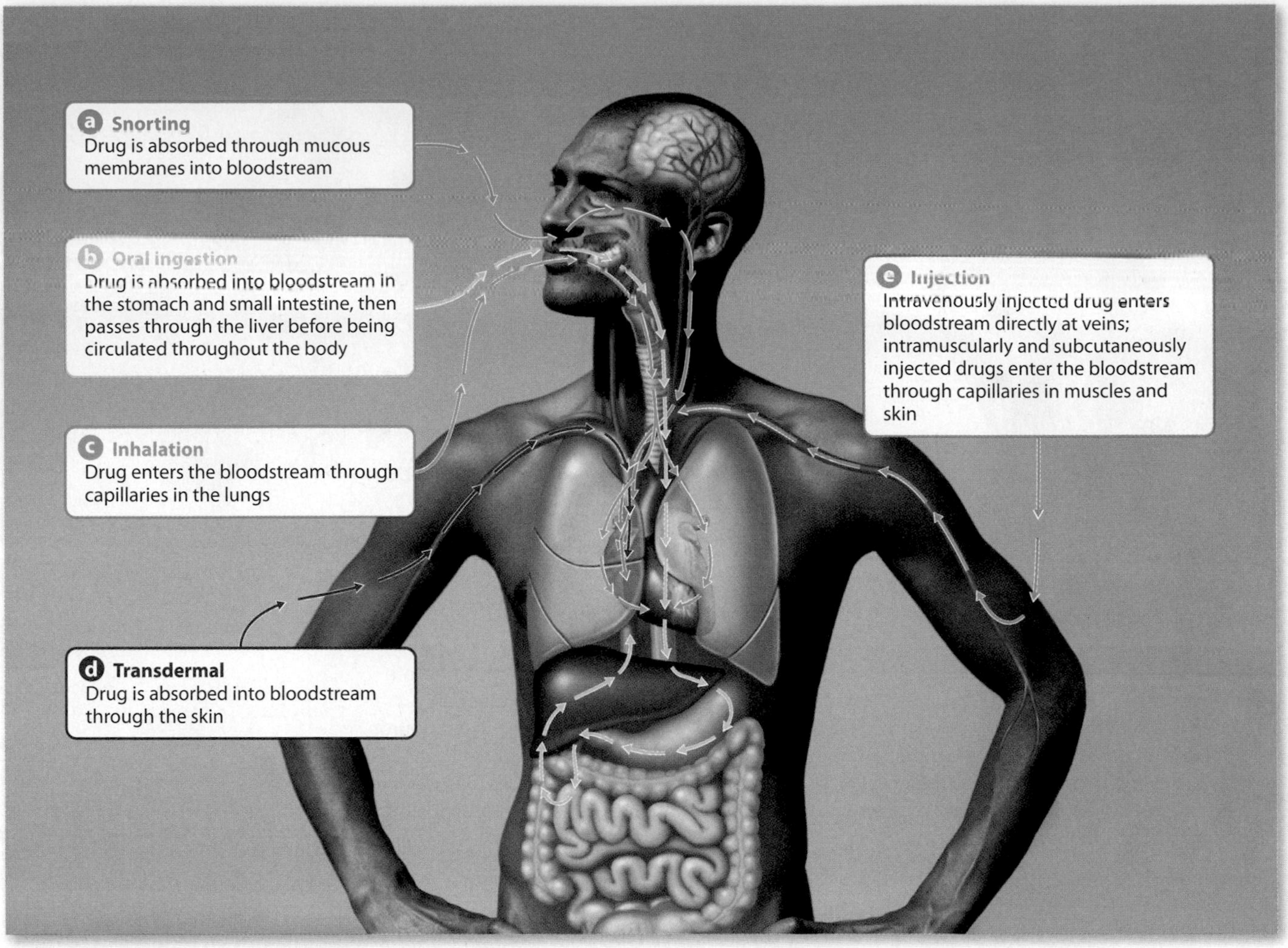

a Snorting
Drug is absorbed through mucous membranes into bloodstream
b Oral ingestion
Drug is absorbed into bloodstream in the stomach and small intestine, then passes through the liver before being circulated throughout the body
c Inhalation
Drug enters the bloodstream through capillaries in the lungs
d Transdermal
Drug is absorbed into bloodstream through the skin
e Injection
Intravenously injected drug enters bloodstream directly at veins; intramuscularly and subcutaneously injected drugs enter the bloodstream through capillaries in muscles and skin

FIGURE 12.2 Routes of Drug Administration Drugs are most commonly swallowed, inhaled, or injected. They can also be absorbed through the skin or mucous membranes (as in snorting) and suppository use (not shown here).

Drugs can also enter the body through the respiratory tract via sniffing, smoking, or inhaling (**inhalation**). Drugs that are inhaled and absorbed by the lungs travel the most rapidly of all the routes of drug administration.

Another rapid form of drug administration is by **injection** directly into the bloodstream (intravenously), muscles (intramuscularly), or just under the skin (subcutaneously). Intravenous injection, which involves inserting a hypodermic needle directly into a vein, is the most common method of injection for drug users because of the rapid speed (within seconds in most cases) in which a drug's effect is felt. It is also the most dangerous method of administration due to the risk of damaging blood vessels and contracting HIV (human immunodeficiency virus) and hepatitis (a severe liver disease).

inhalation The introduction of drugs through the respiratory tract via sniffing, smoking, or inhaling.

injection The introduction of drugs into the body via a hypodermic needle.

transdermal The introduction of drugs through the skin.

suppositories Mixtures of drugs and a waxy medium (designed to melt at body temperature) that are inserted into the anus or vagina.

receptor sites Specialized areas of cells and organs where chemicals, enzymes, and other substances interact.

Drugs can also be absorbed through the skin or tissue lining (**transdermal**)—the nicotine patch is a common example of a drug that is administered in this manner—or through the mucous membranes, such as those in the nose (snorting) or in the vagina or anus (**suppositories**). Suppositories are typically mixed with a waxy medium that melts at body temperature, releasing the drug into the bloodstream.

However the drug enters the system, it eventually finds its way to the bloodstream and circulates throughout the body to various **receptor sites** where chemicals, enzymes, and other substances interact. Psychoactive drugs are able to cross the blood–brain barrier to reach receptor sites in the brain, where they can affect cognition, emotions, and physiological functioning. Once a drug reaches receptor sites in the brain and other body organs, it may remain active for several hours before it dissipates and is carried by the blood to the liver where it is metabolized (broken down by enzymes). The products of enzymatic breakdown, called *metabolites*, are then excreted, primarily through the kidneys (in urine) or the bowels (in feces), but also through the skin (in sweat) or through the lungs (in expired air).

Drug Interactions

Polydrug use—taking several medications, vitamins, recreational drugs, or illegal drugs simultaneously—can lead to dangerous health problems. Alcohol in particular frequently has dangerous interactions with other drugs. The most hazardous interactions are synergism, antagonism, inhibition, intolerance, and cross-tolerance. Some drug interactions occur as a result of the foods we eat or drink or other environmental exposures that might seem harmless. For instance, consuming grapefruit or grapefruit juice while taking a statin, a medication used for lowering blood pressure, allows too much of the drug to enter the bloodstream and can cause liver damage, and exposure to the sun when taking sulfa-based antibiotics can cause a skin rash or a severe sunburn.

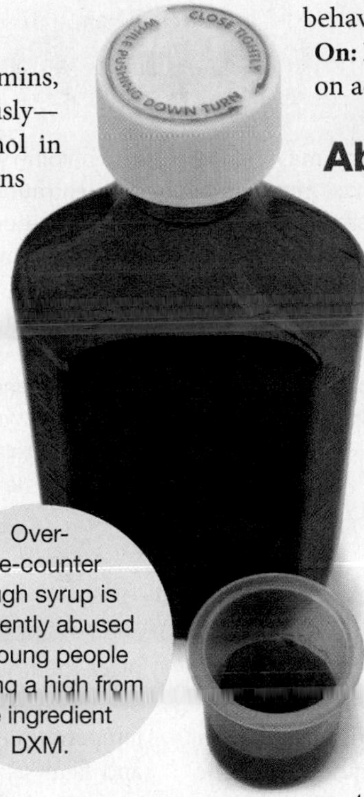

Over-the-counter cough syrup is frequently abused by young people seeking a high from the ingredient DXM.

Synergism, also called *potentiation*, is an interaction of two or more drugs in which the effects of the individual drugs are multiplied beyond what would normally be expected if they were taken alone. Think of synergism as 2 + 2 = 10. A synergistic reaction can be very dangerous and even deadly.

Antagonism, although usually less serious than synergism, can also produce unwanted and unpleasant effects. In an antagonistic reaction, drugs work at the same receptor site so that one drug blocks the action of the other. The blocking drug occupies the receptor site and prevents the other drug from attaching, thus altering its absorption and action.

With **inhibition**, the effects of one drug are eliminated or reduced by the presence of another drug at the receptor site.

Intolerance occurs when drugs combine in the body to produce extremely uncomfortable reactions. The drug Antabuse (disulfiram), used to help alcoholics give up alcohol, works by producing this type of interaction.

Cross-tolerance occurs when a person develops a physiological tolerance to one drug that also increases the body's tolerance to other substances that act similarly on the body.

LO 3 | USING, MISUSING, AND ABUSING DRUGS

Review problems relating to the misuse and abuse of prescription drugs, including the use of illicit drugs among college students.

Although drug abuse is usually referred to in connection with illicit drugs, many people misuse or abuse prescription, OTC, and recreational drugs. **Drug misuse** involves using a drug for a purpose for which it was not intended. For example, taking a friend's high-powered prescription painkiller for your headache is a misuse of that drug. This is not too far removed from **drug abuse**, or the excessive use of any drug, and may cause serious harm. The misuse and abuse of any drug may lead to addiction, the habitual reliance on a substance or a behavior to produce a desired mood. (See **Focus On: Recognizing and Avoiding Addiction** for more on addiction.)

Abuse of Over-the-Counter Drugs

OTC medications come in many different forms, including pills, liquids, nasal sprays, and topical creams. Although many people assume that no harm can come from legal nonprescription drugs, OTC medications can be abused, with resultant health complications and potential addiction. People who appear to be most vulnerable to abusing OTC drugs are teenagers, young adults, and people over age 65.

OTC drug abuse can involve taking more than the recommended dosage, combining it with other drugs, or taking it over a longer period of time than is recommended. Abuse of and addiction to OTC drugs can be accidental. A person may develop tolerance from continued use, creating an unintended dependence. However, teenagers and young adults sometimes intentionally abuse OTC medications in search of a cheap high—by drinking large amounts of cough medicine, for instance. The following are a few types of OTC drugs that are subject to misuse and abuse:

- **Sleep aids.** These drugs may be harmful in excess as they can cause problems with the sleep cycle, weaken areas of the body, or induce narcolepsy (a condition of excessive, intrusive sleepiness). Continued use can lead to tolerance and dependence.
- **Cold medicines (cough syrups and tablets).** There are many different ingredients in cough and cold medicines, but one of particular concern is dextromethorphan (DXM), which is present in many types of OTC medications. As many as 4 percent of high school seniors report taking drugs containing DXM to get high.[9] Large doses of products containing DXM can cause hallucinations, loss of motor control, and "out-of-body" (disassociative) sensations.

polydrug use Taking several medications, vitamins, recreational drugs, or illegal drugs simultaneously.

synergism The interaction of two or more drugs that produces more profound effects than would be expected if the drugs were taken separately; also called *potentiation*.

antagonism A drug interaction in which two drugs compete for the same available receptors, potentially blocking each other's actions.

inhibition A drug interaction in which the effects of one drug are eliminated or reduced by the presence of another drug at the same receptor site.

intolerance A drug interaction in which the combination of two or more drugs in the body produces extremely uncomfortable reactions.

cross-tolerance Development of a physiological tolerance to one drug that reduces the effects of another, similar drug.

drug misuse Use of a drug for a purpose for which it was not intended.

drug abuse Excessive use of a drug.

Other possible side effects of DXM abuse include confusion, impaired judgment, blurred vision, dizziness, paranoia, excessive sweating, slurred speech, nausea, vomiting, abdominal pain, irregular heartbeat, high blood pressure, headache, lethargy, numb fingers and toes, facial redness, and dry and itchy skin. In extreme cases, DXM abuse can lead to loss of consciousness, seizures, brain damage, and even death. Some states have passed laws limiting the amount of products containing DXM a person can purchase or prohibiting sale to individuals under age 18.[10]

Pseudoephedrine is another cold and allergy medication ingredient that is frequently abused, most commonly in the illegal manufacture of methamphetamine (discussed later). United States law limits the number of products containing this drug that an individual may purchase in a month and requires that it be sold "behind the counter" (i.e., without a prescription, but only through a pharmacist) and that photo identification be presented and recorded. Pharmacists are required to keep a record of purchasers for at least 2 years.[11]

- **Diet pills.** Some teens use diet pills as a way of getting high, whereas other people use these drugs in an attempt to lose weight. Diet pills often contain a stimulant such as caffeine (discussed later in the text) or an herbal ingredient claimed to promote weight loss, such as *Hoodia gordonii.* Many diet pills are marketed as "dietary supplements" and so are regulated by the U.S. Food and Drug Administration (FDA) as "food," not as "drugs."

WHY SHOULD I CARE?

You may think drugs are helping you relax, improving your concentration, or enhancing your social enjoyment, but those effects are transient—and often illusory—and they are nothing compared to the many negative effects those same drugs can have on your life and health. Sooner or later, drug misuse and abuse is likely to catch up with you and cause problems—be they academic, social, career, legal, financial, or health related. Are a few moments of excitement really worth a lifetime of trouble?

Nonmedical Use or Abuse of Prescription Drugs

In the United States today, the abuse of prescription medications is at an all-time high. Only marijuana is more widely abused.[12] Individuals abuse prescription medications because they are an easily accessible and inexpensive means of altering a user's mental and physical state. Women, in particular, are more likely to use prescription drugs as a method of self-medication for psychological distress.[13] Some people also have the mistaken idea that prescription drugs are a "safer high."

The latest data available indicate that approximately 6.1 million Americans age 12 and older used prescription drugs for nonmedical reasons in the past month.[14] Prescription drug abuse is particularly common among teenagers and young adults.

SEE IT! VIDEOS

Is illegal painkiller use spiraling out of control? Watch **Government Crackdown on Painkillers** available on MasteringHealth.™

Every day, a significantly large number of people begin misusing prescription drugs. In 2012, 3 percent of teenagers age 12 to 17 and 5 percent of people 18 to 25 reported abusing prescription drugs in the past month.[15] The problem may be getting worse, with nearly 15 percent of twelfth-graders reporting abuse of prescription drugs by the time they graduate from high school.[16]

The risks associated with prescription drug abuse vary depending on the drug. Abuse of opioids, narcotics, and pain relievers can result in life-threatening respiratory depression (reduced breathing). Overdoses involving prescription painkillers are at epidemic levels and now kill more Americans than heroin and cocaine combined.[17] Individuals who abuse depressants place themselves at risk of seizures, respiratory depression, and decreased heart rate. Stimulant abuse can cause elevated body temperature, irregular heart rate, cardiovascular system failure, and fatal seizures. It can also result in hostility or feelings of paranoia. Individuals who abuse prescription drugs by injecting them expose themselves to additional risks, including contracting HIV, hepatitis B and C, and other bloodborne viruses.

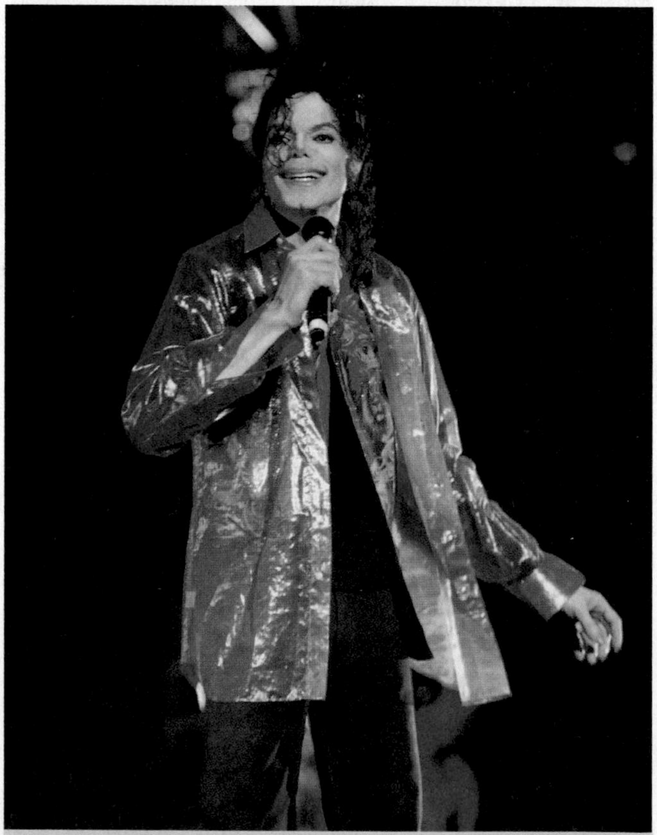

Abusing prescription drugs is no safer than abusing illicit drugs, as tragically demonstrated by the 2010 death of singer Michael Jackson, whose death ultimately stemmed from his abuse of numerous prescription medications.

STUDENT HEALTH TODAY

OXYCONTIN AND VICODIN ABUSE

Since the mid-1990s, there has been a sharp increase in prescription drug abuse among youth. The 2012 Monitoring the Future (MTF) study found that approximately 3.8 percent of college students had used Vicodin and 1.2 percent used OxyContin, both prescription painkillers, without a doctor's prescription in the past year.

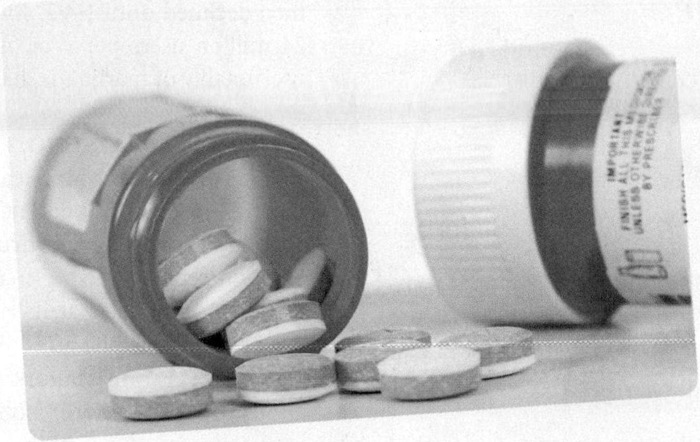

As with most other drugs, some of the reasons college students use OxyContin and Vicodin are that they feel young and often invincible; they need to express their new-found independence; they like the excitement of risk-taking; or they feel pressure from their peers. Often, there is the perception that prescription drugs are safer than illicit drugs.

However, painkillers such as OxyContin, Percocet, Percodan, Vicodin, and others are highly addictive; if they are taken daily for several weeks, that is enough time for addiction to develop. OxyContin, in particular, can be a highly addictive and dangerous narcotic when abused. The "rush" is similar to that of heroin. In fact, it's common for people who are addicted to OxyContin to turn to heroin when they can't afford to buy OxyContin. Chronic use can also result in increasing tolerance, and more of the drug is needed to achieve the desired effect.

Many people who abuse prescription medications are simultaneously abusing illegal drugs. According to the MTF study, students who obtained prescription painkillers from peers reported higher levels of binge drinking and marijuana abuse than nonabusers or those who received painkillers from family. This poses another set of problems, as alcohol in combination with any one of these medications can make a dangerous cocktail. If someone you know seems unusually drunk, drowsy, slurs speech, has trouble moving, or passes out, call for help immediately.

Sources: L. D. Johnston et al., *Monitoring the Future: National Survey Results on Drug Use, 1975–2012,* Volume 2, *College Students and Adults Ages 19–50* (Ann Arbor, MI: Institute for Social Research, The University of Michigan, 2013), Available at http://monitoringthefuture.org/new.html; Higher Education Center for Alcohol, Drug Abuse and Violence Prevention, "OxyContin & Oxycodone," 2010, www.higheredcenter.org/high-risk/drugs/prescription-drugs/oxycontin.

Unfortunately, prescription drugs are often easier to obtain than illegal ones. In some cases, unscrupulous pharmacists or other medical professionals either steal the drugs or sell fraudulent prescriptions. In a process called *doctor shopping,* abusers visit several doctors to obtain multiple prescriptions. Some may fake or exaggerate symptoms to persuade physicians to write prescriptions. Individuals may also call pharmacies with fraudulent prescriptions. Young people typically obtain prescription drugs from peers, friends, or family members. Some teenagers and college students who have legitimate prescriptions sell or give away their medications to other students or trade them for others. Some abusers order from Internet pharmacies where prescriptions are not always required.

College Students and Prescription Drug Abuse Prescription drug abuse among college students has increased dramatically over the past decade. Because prescription drugs are prescribed by doctors and approved by the FDA, many college students seem to perceive these drugs as safer or more socially acceptable than illicit drugs, or they believe prescription drugs will enhance their well-being or performance. However, nothing could be further from the truth when these drugs are misused.

According to the 2013 *American College Health Association–National College Health Assessment,* the illicit use of prescription drugs is a growing trend on campuses. The report shows 14.9 percent of surveyed students reported illegally using prescription drugs in the last year, compared to 13.5 percent in 2008.[18] Students who illegally use prescription drugs are also more likely to use other illegal drugs and binge drink.[19]

The most commonly abused prescription drugs on college campuses are painkillers (e.g., OxyContin and Vicodin). Approximately 7.6 percent of students report using painkillers that were not prescribed to them in the past 12 months. Of those reporting use, 8.3 percent were men and 7.2 percent women.[20] The **Student Health Today** box discusses OxyContin and Vicodin abuse.

Also of particular concern on college campuses is the increased abuse of stimulant drugs such as Adderall and Ritalin, which are intended to treat attention-deficit/hyperactivity disorder (ADHD). Students primarily report using ADHD drugs for academic gain. Approximately 8 percent of students report using stimulants that were not prescribed to them in the past 12 months.[21] According to a recent study, friends with prescriptions were the most commonly reported source of prescription stimulants, and most students obtained their drugs

TABLE 12.1 | 30-Day Drug Use Prevalence, Full-Time College Students vs. Respondents 1–4 Years beyond High School

	Full-Time College (%)	Others (%)
Any illicit drug	22.3	22.0
Any illicit drug other than marijuana	7.8	8.7
Marijuana	20.5	21.1
Inhalants	0.2	*
Hallucinogens	1.1	1.1
LSD	0.4	0.5
Hallucinogens other than LSD	0.7	1.1
Ecstasy (methylene-dioxymethamphetamine, MDMA)	1.4	1.6
Cocaine	1.1	1.0
Crack	*	0.1
Other cocaine	1.3	1.0
Heroin	*	0.5
Narcotics other than heroin	2.2	3.6
Amphetamines, adjusted	4.6	2.4
Crystal methamphetamine	0.3	0.2
Sedatives (barbiturates)	0.8	1.7
Tranquilizers	1.1	2.5
Alcohol	67.7	53.9
Been drunk	40.7	42.0
Flavored alcoholic beverage	31.3	26.8
Cigarettes	12.5	25.9
Approximate weighted N =	*1,150*	*750*

*Indicates prevalence less than 0.05%.

Source: L. D. Johnston et al., *Monitoring the Future National Survey Results on Drug Use, 1975–2012*, Volume 2, *College Students and Adults Ages 19–50* (Ann Arbor, MI: Institute for Social Research, The University of Michigan, 2013), Available at http://monitoringthefuture.org/new.html.

for free or at a cost of $1 to $5.[22] Users generally believed that the drugs were beneficial, despite frequent reports of adverse reactions. The most commonly reported adverse effects were sleeping difficulties, irritability, and reduced appetite.

Illicit Drugs

The problem of illicit drug use touches us all. We may use illicit substances ourselves, watch someone we love struggle with drug abuse, or become the victim of a drug-related crime. At the very least, we are forced to pay increasing taxes for law enforcement and drug rehabilitation. When our coworkers use drugs, the effectiveness of our own work is diminished. If the car we drive was assembled by drug-using workers at the plant, we are in danger. A drug-using bus driver, surgeon, or pilot jeopardizes our safety.

Illicit drug users span all age groups, genders, ethnicities, occupations, and socioeconomic groups. Illicit drug use has a devastating effect on users and their families in the United States and in many other countries.

The good news about illicit drugs in the United States is that it peaked at around 25 million users between 1979 and 1986, then declined until 1992, and has since remained stable around 24 million users per year. Among youth, however, illicit drug use, notably of marijuana, has been rising in recent years.[23]

Illicit Drug Use on Campus Illicit drug use has seen a resurgence on college campuses. Even so, it is not the norm. Close to 50 percent of college-aged students nationwide have tried an illicit drug at some point; the vast majority of them reported using marijuana (see TABLE 12.1).[24] Daily use of marijuana is at its highest point since 1989. Cocaine use is down sharply, but LSD use has more than doubled.[25]

College administrators, staff, and faculty are concerned about the link between substance abuse and poor academic performance, depression, anxiety, suicide, property damage, vandalism, fights, serious medical problems, and death. Students who use marijuana and/or other illicit drugs are at increased risk for disruptions in college attendance.[26] A longer-term consequence of illicit drug use among college students is a significantly increased chance of unemployment after college (FIGURE 12.3).

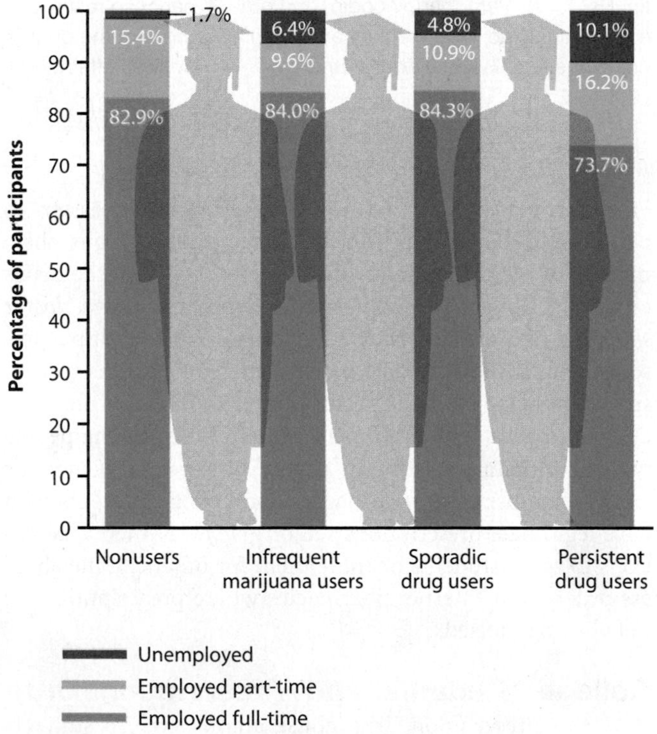

FIGURE 12.3 Employment Post-College Based on College Drug Use If you're inclined to think that drug use in college won't affect your life later, think again. Even periodically using drugs increases the chances of unemployment after college.

Source: A. M. Arria, "Drug Use Patterns in Young Adulthood and Post-College Employment," *Drug and Alcohol Dependence* 1, no. 127 (2013): 23–30, DOI: 10.1016/j.drugalcdep.2012.06.001.

Why Do Some College Students Use Drugs?

Research has identified the following factors in a student's life that increase the risk of substance abuse. The more factors there are, the greater the risk:

- **Positive expectations.** Some students take drugs such as Adderall and Ritalin believing that the drugs will help their ability to study. The vast majority of students say they take drugs to relax, reduce stress, or forget about problems.
- **Genetics and family history.** Genetics and family history play a significant role in the risk for developing an addiction.
- **Substance use in high school.** Two-thirds of college students who use illicit drugs began doing so in high school.[27]
- **Mental health problems.** Students who report being diagnosed with depression are more likely to have abused prescription drugs or to have used marijuana or other illicit drugs.
- **Sorority and fraternity membership.** Being a member of a sorority or fraternity increases the likelihood of using alcohol, marijuana, or cocaine and makes one twice as likely to abuse prescription drugs.
- **Stress.** For some students under academic and social stress, seemingly easy relief comes in the form of drugs or alcohol.

Why Don't Some College Students Use Drugs?

There can be many factors influencing a student to avoid drugs; some of the most commonly reported include the following:[28]

- **Parental attitudes and behavior.** Students who say they are more influenced by their parents' concerns or expectations drink, use marijuana, and smoke significantly less than students who are less influenced by parents.
- **Religion and spirituality.** The greater the students' level of religiosity (hours in prayer, attendance at services), the less likely they are to drink, smoke, or use other drugs.
- **Student engagement.** The more students are involved in learning and in extracurricular activities, the less likely they are to binge drink, use marijuana, or abuse prescription drugs.
- **College athletics.** College athletes drink at higher rates than nonathletes but are less likely to use illicit drugs.
- **Healthy social network.** Having a wide range of friends and supports to help cope with the challenges of life is a well-known protective factor for many negative behaviors, including drug use.

To prepare yourself for a possible offer of drugs on campus, and to be ready to make the decision that is best for *you*, see the **Skills for Behavior Change** box.

SKILLS FOR BEHAVIOR CHANGE

RESPONDING TO AN OFFER OF DRUGS

No matter what your experience has been up until now, it is likely that you will be invited to use drugs at some point in your life. Here are some questions to consider before you find yourself in a situation in which you are offered or feel pressure to use illicit drugs:

- Why am I considering trying drugs? Am I trying to fit in or impress my friends? What does this say about my friends if I need to take drugs to impress them? Are my friends really looking out for what is best for me?
- Am I using this drug to cope or feel different? Am I depressed?
- What could taking drugs cost me? Will this cost me my career if I am caught using? Could using drugs prevent me from getting a job?
- What are the long term consequences of using this drug?
- What will this cost me in terms of my friendships and family? How would my family and friends respond if they knew I was using drugs?

Even when you make the decision not to use drugs, it can be difficult to say no gracefully. Some good ways to turn down an offer:

- "Thanks, but I've got a big test (game, meeting) tomorrow morning."
- "I've already got a great buzz right now. I really don't need anything more."
- "I don't like how (insert drug name here) makes me feel."
- "I'm driving tonight. So I'm not using."
- "I want to go for a run in the morning."
- "No."

LO 4 | COMMON DRUGS OF ABUSE

Discuss the use and abuse of controlled substances, including cocaine, amphetamines, marijuana, opioids, hallucinogens, club drugs, inhalants, and steroids.

Hundreds of drugs are subject to abuse—some are legal, such as recreational drugs and prescription medications, while others are illegal and classified as "controlled substances." For general purposes, drugs can be divided into the following categories: *stimulants, cannabis products (cannabinoids) including marijuana, narcotics and depressants, hallucinogens, inhalants,* and *anabolic steroids.* These categories are discussed in subsequent sections; **TABLE 12.2** summarizes the categories, uses, and effects of various drugs of abuse, both legal and illicit.

TABLE 12.2 | Drugs of Abuse: Uses and Effects

Category	Drugs	Trade or Street Names	Dependence	Usual Method	Possible Effects	Overdose Effects	Withdrawal Syndrome
Stimulants	Cocaine	Coke, Flake, Snow, Crack, *Coca, Blanca, Perico*	*Physical:* Possible *Psychological:* High *Tolerance:* Yes	Snorted, smoked, injected	Increased alertness, excitation, euphoria, increased pulse rate and blood pressure, insomnia, loss of appetite	Agitation, increased body temperature, hallucinations, convulsions, possible death	Apathy, long periods of sleep, irritability, depression, disorientation
	Amphetamine, methamphetamine	Crank, Ice, Cristal, Crystal Meth, Speed, Adderall, Dexedrine	*Physical:* Possible *Psychological:* High *Tolerance:* Yes	Oral, injected, smoked			
	Methylphenidate	Ritalin (Illy's), Concerta, Focalin, Metadate	*Physical:* Possible *Psychological:* High *Tolerance:* Yes	Oral, injected, snorted, smoked			
Cannabis	Marijuana	Pot, Grass, Weed, Sinsemilla, Blunts, *Mota, Yerba*	*Physical:* Possible *Psychological:* High *Tolerance:* Yes	Oral, smoked	Euphoria, relaxed inhibitions, increased appetite, disorientation	Fatigue, paranoia, possible psychosis	Hyperactivity, decreased appetite, insomnia
	Hashish, hashish oil	Hash, Hash oil	*Physical:* Unknown *Psychological:* Moderate *Tolerance:* Yes	Smoked, oral			
Narcotics	Heroin	Diamorphine, Horse, Smack, Black tar, *Chiva*	*Physical:* High *Psychological:* High *Tolerance:* Yes	Injected, snorted, smoked	Euphoria, drowsiness, respiratory depression, constricted pupils, nausea	Slow and shallow breathing, clammy skin, convulsions, coma, possible death	Watery eyes, runny nose, yawning, loss of appetite, irritability, tremors, panic, cramps, nausea, chills and sweating
	Morphine	MS-Contin, Roxanol	*Physical:* High *Psychological:* High *Tolerance:* Yes	Oral, injected			
	Hydrocodone, oxycodone	Vicodin, OxyContin, Percocet, Percodan	*Physical:* High *Psychological:* High *Tolerance:* Yes	Oral			
	Codeine	Acetaminophen w/ Codeine, Tylenol w/ Codeine	*Physical:* Moderate *Psychological:* Moderate *Tolerance:* Yes	Oral, injected			
Depressants	Gamma-hydroxybutyrate	GHB, Liquid Ecstasy, Liquid X	*Physical:* Moderate *Psychological:* Moderate *Tolerance:* Yes	Oral	Slurred speech, disorientation, drunken behavior without odor of alcohol, impaired memory of events, interacts with alcohol	Shallow respiration, clammy skin, dilated pupils, weak and rapid pulse, coma, possible death	Anxiety, insomnia, tremors, delirium, convulsions, possible death
	Benzodiazepines	Valium, Xanax, Halcion, Ativan, Rohypnol (Roofies, R-2), Klonopin	*Physical:* Moderate *Psychological:* Moderate *Tolerance:* Yes	Oral, injected			
	Other depressants	Ambien, Sonata, Barbiturates, Methaqualone (Quaalude)	*Physical:* Moderate *Psychological:* Moderate *Tolerance:* Yes	Oral			
Hallucinogens	Methylenedioxymethamphetamine (MDMA), analogs	Ecstasy, XTC, Adam, MDA (Love Drug), MDEA (Eve)	*Physical:* None *Psychological:* Moderate *Tolerance:* Yes	Oral, snorted, smoked	Heightened senses, teeth grinding, dehydration	Increased body temperature, electrolyte imbalance, cardiac arrest	Muscle aches, drowsiness, depression, acne
	LSD	Acid, Microdot, Sunshine, Boomers	*Physical:* None *Psychological:* Unknown *Tolerance:* Yes	Oral	Hallucinations, altered perception of time and distance	Longer, more intense "trips"	None
	Phencyclidine, analogs	PCP, Angel Dust, Hog, Ketamine (Special K)	*Physical:* Possible *Psychological:* High *Tolerance:* Yes	Smoked, oral, injected, snorted		Unable to direct movement, feel pain, or remember	Drug-seeking behavior
	Other hallucinogens	Psilocybe mushrooms, Mescaline, Peyote, Dextromethorphan	*Physical:* None *Psychological:* None *Tolerance:* Possible	Oral			
Inhalants	Amyl and butyl nitrite	Pearls, Poppers, Rush, Locker Room	*Physical:* Unknown *Psychological:* Unknown *Tolerance:* No	Inhaled	Flushing, hypotension, headache	Methemoglobinemia	Agitation
	Nitrous oxide	Laughing gas, Balloons, Whippets	*Physical:* Unknown *Psychological:* Low *Tolerance:* No	Inhaled	Impaired memory, slurred speech, drunken behavior, slow-onset vitamin deficiency, organ damage	Vomiting, respiratory depression, loss of consciousness, possible death	Trembling, anxiety, insomnia, vitamin deficiency, confusion, hallucinations, convulsions
	Other inhalants	Adhesives, spray paint, hairspray, lighter fluid	*Physical:* Unknown *Psychological:* High *Tolerance:* No	Inhaled			
Anabolic Steroids	Testosterone	Depo Testosterone, Sustanon, Sten, Cypt	*Physical:* Unknown *Psychological:* Unknown *Tolerance:* Unknown	Injected	Virilization, edema, testicular atrophy, gynecomastia, acne, aggressive behavior	Unknown	Possible depression
	Other anabolic steroids	Parabolan, Winstrol, Equipose, Anadrol, Dianabol	*Physical:* Unknown *Psychological:* Yes *Tolerance:* Unknown	Oral, injected			

Source: Adapted from U.S. Department of Justice Drug Enforcement Administration, "DEA Drug Fact Sheets," 2011, www.justice.gov/dea/pubs/all_fact_sheets.pdf.

Stimulants

A **stimulant** is a drug that increases activity of the central nervous system. Its effects usually involve increased activity, anxiety, and agitation; users often seem jittery or nervous while high. Commonly used illegal stimulants include cocaine, amphetamines, and methamphetamine. Legal stimulants include caffeine and nicotine (see **Chapter 11** for a discussion of nicotine).

Cocaine

A white crystalline powder derived from the leaves of the South American coca shrub (not related to cocoa plants), *cocaine* ("coke") has been described as one of the most powerful naturally occurring stimulants.

Methods of Use and Physical Effects Cocaine can be taken in several ways, including snorting, smoking, and injecting. The powdered form is snorted through the nose, which can damage mucous membranes and cause sinusitis. It can destroy the user's sense of smell, and occasionally it even eats a hole through the septum. When snorted, the drug enters the bloodstream through the lungs in less than 1 minute and reaches the brain in less than 3 minutes. It binds at receptor sites in the central nervous system, producing an intense high that disappears quickly, leaving a powerful craving for more.

Cocaine alkaloid, or *freebase,* is obtained by removing the hydrochloride salt from cocaine powder. *Freebasing* refers to smoking freebase by placing it at the end of a pipe and holding a flame near it to produce a vapor, which is then inhaled. *Crack* is identical pharmacologically to freebase, but the hydrochloride salt is still present and is processed with baking soda and water. It is a cheap, widely available drug that is smokable and very potent. Crack is commonly smoked in the same manner as freebase. Because crack is such a pure drug, it takes little time to achieve the desired high, and a crack user can become addicted quickly.

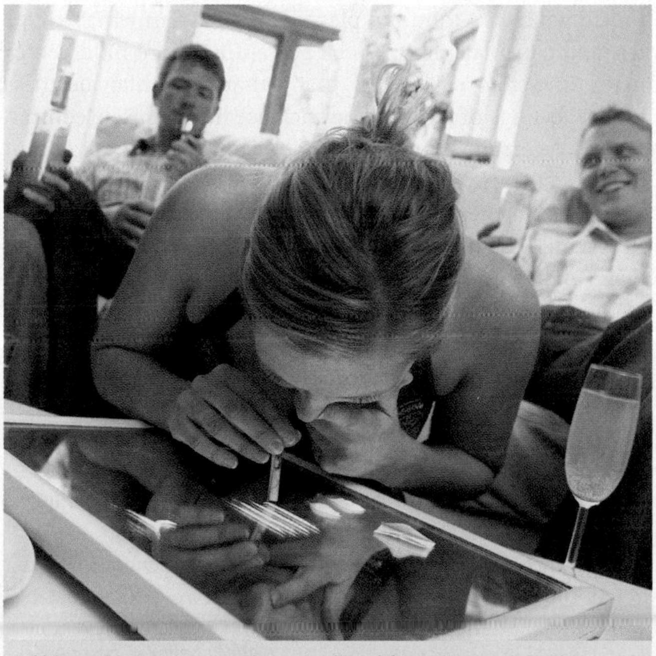

Although cocaine use has declined from its peak in the 1980s, it continues to be a commonly abused illicit drug.

stimulants Drugs that increase activity of the central nervous system.

amphetamines A large and varied group of synthetic agents that stimulate the central nervous system.

Some cocaine users inject the drug intravenously, which introduces large amounts into the body rapidly, creating a brief, intense high and subsequent crash. Injecting users place themselves at risk not only for contracting HIV and hepatitis (a serious liver disease) through shared needles, but also for skin infections, vein damage, inflamed arteries, and infection of the heart lining.

Cocaine is both an anesthetic and a central nervous system stimulant. In tiny doses, it can slow the heart rate. In larger doses, the physical effects are dramatic: increased heart rate and blood pressure, loss of appetite that can lead to dramatic weight loss, convulsions, muscle twitching, irregular heartbeat, and even death from overdose. Other effects of cocaine include temporary relief of depression, decreased fatigue, talkativeness, increased alertness, and heightened self-confidence. However, as the dose increases, users become irritable and apprehensive, and their behavior may turn paranoid or violent.

Amphetamines

The **amphetamines** include a large and varied group of synthetic agents that stimulate the central nervous system. Small doses of amphetamines improve alertness, lessen fatigue, and generally elevate mood. With repeated use, however, physical and psychological dependencies develop. Sleep patterns are affected (insomnia); heart rate, breathing rate, and blood pressure increase; and restlessness, anxiety, appetite suppression, and vision problems are common. High doses over long time periods can produce hallucinations, delusions, and disorganized behavior.

Certain types of amphetamines or amphetamine-like drugs are used for medicinal purposes. As discussed earlier, drugs prescribed to treat ADHD are stimulants, which are increasingly abused on campus.

Methamphetamine An increasingly common form of amphetamine, *methamphetamine* (commonly called "meth") is a potent, long-acting, addictive drug that strongly activates the brain's reward center by producing a sense of euphoria. Over 439,000 Americans are regular users of methamphetamine, and it is believed that more than 12 million Americans have tried it.[29] In 2012, about 2 percent of high school seniors reported using methamphetamine in their lifetime.[30] The rate of methamphetamine use may be increasing because it is relatively easy to make. Recipes often include common OTC ingredients such as ephedrine and pseudoephedrine.

In the short term, methamphetamine produces increased physical activity and body temperature, alertness, euphoria, rapid breathing, insomnia, tremors, anxiety, confusion, and decreased appetite.

Methamphetamine can be snorted, smoked, injected, or orally ingested. When snorted, the effects can be felt in 3 to 5 minutes; if orally ingested, effects occur within 15 to 20 minutes. The pleasurable effects of methamphetamine are typically an intense rush lasting only a few minutes when snorted;

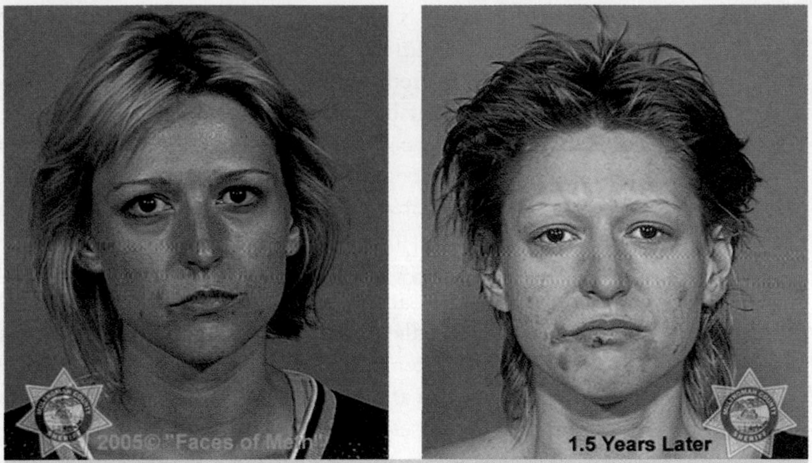

The physical consequences of methamphetamine use are often dramatic. The photos above show a person before and 1.5 years after methamphetamine use.

in contrast, smoking the drug can produce a high lasting more than 8 hours. Users often experience tolerance after the first use, making methamphetamine highly addictive.

Methamphetamine increases the release and blocks the reuptake of the neurotransmitter dopamine, leading to high levels of the chemical in the brain. This action occurs rapidly and produces the intense euphoria, or "rush," that many users feel. Over time, meth destroys dopamine receptors, making it impossible to feel pleasure. Researchers have now established that, due to the destruction of dopamine receptors, people who abuse methamphetamine (or cocaine) are at increased risk for developing Parkinson's disease later in life.[31]

Other long-term effects of methamphetamine can include severe weight loss, cardiovascular damage, increased risk of heart attack and stroke, hallucinations, extensive tooth decay and tooth loss ("meth mouth"), violence, paranoia, psychotic behavior, and even death. Recent studies of chronic methamphetamine abusers have revealed severe structural and functional changes in areas of the brain associated with emotion and memory, which may account for the emotional and cognitive problems observed in chronic methamphetamine abusers. Some of these changes persist after the methamphetamine abuse has stopped. Other changes reverse after sustained periods of abstinence from methamphetamine, lasting typically longer than a year, but problems often remain.

caffeine A stimulant drug that is legal in the United States and found in many coffees, teas, chocolates, energy drinks, and certain medications.

Bath Salts "Bath salts" is the latest addition to the growing list of items people are using to get high. The new designer drug is synthetic powder sold legally online and in corner stores and truck stops. The powder substance is sold in a packet with a disclaimer "not for human consumption." It is not subject to FDA regulation; however, some of the substances used in making bath salts were made illegal in 2012. These packages contain various amphetamine or cocaine-like substances such as methylenedioxypyrovalerone (MPDV), mephedrone, and pyrovalerone. The powder can be smoked, snorted, injected, and wrapped in pieces of paper and ingested or "bombed." These chemicals cannot be detected by routine drug screening, making them attractive for misuse.[32]

Effects include intense stimulation, alertness, euphoria, elevated mood, and pleasurable "rush." Users may describe feelings of closeness, sociability, and moderate sexual arousal. Other symptoms can include tremor, shortness of breath, and loss of appetite. Changes in body temperature regulation are accompanied by hot flashes and sweating, with bleeding from the nose and throat from ulcerations when snorted.[33]

This drug also can have significant effects on the cardiovascular system, resulting in rapid heart rate, increased blood pressure, and chest pain. Psychiatric effects at higher doses consist of anxiety, agitation, hallucinations, paranoia, and erratic behavior. Depression and suicide have also been reported as a result of use. While withdrawal symptoms are reported as minimal, users often have described a strong craving for the drug.[34]

Caffeine Unlike cocaine and methamphetamine, **caffeine** is a legal stimulant.

More than half of all Americans drink coffee every day, and many others consume caffeine in some other form, making it the most popular and widely consumed drug in the United States.[35] Coffee, tea, soft drinks, chocolate, and other caffeine-containing products are loved for their wake-up effects. Caffeine may be commonplace, but excessive consumption is associated with addiction and certain health problems.

Caffeine is derived from the chemical family called *xanthines,* which are found in plant products from which coffee, tea, and chocolate are made. The xanthines are mild central nervous system stimulants that enhance mental alertness, reduce feelings of fatigue, and increase heart muscle contractions, oxygen consumption, metabolism, and urinary output. Side effects of the xanthines include wakefulness, insomnia, irregular heartbeat, dizziness, nausea, indigestion, and sometimes mild delirium. Some people also experience heartburn. A person feels these effects within 15 to 45 minutes of ingesting a caffeinated product. It takes 4 to 6 hours for the body to metabolize half of the caffeine ingested, so, depending on the amount of caffeine taken in, it may continue to exert effects for a day or longer. **FIGURE 12.4** compares the caffeine content of various products.

As the effects of caffeine wear off, frequent users may feel let down—mentally or physically depressed, tired,

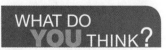

WHAT DO YOU THINK?

How much caffeine do you consume regularly, and why?

- What is your pattern of caffeine consumption?
- Have you ever experienced any ill effects after going without caffeine for a period of time?

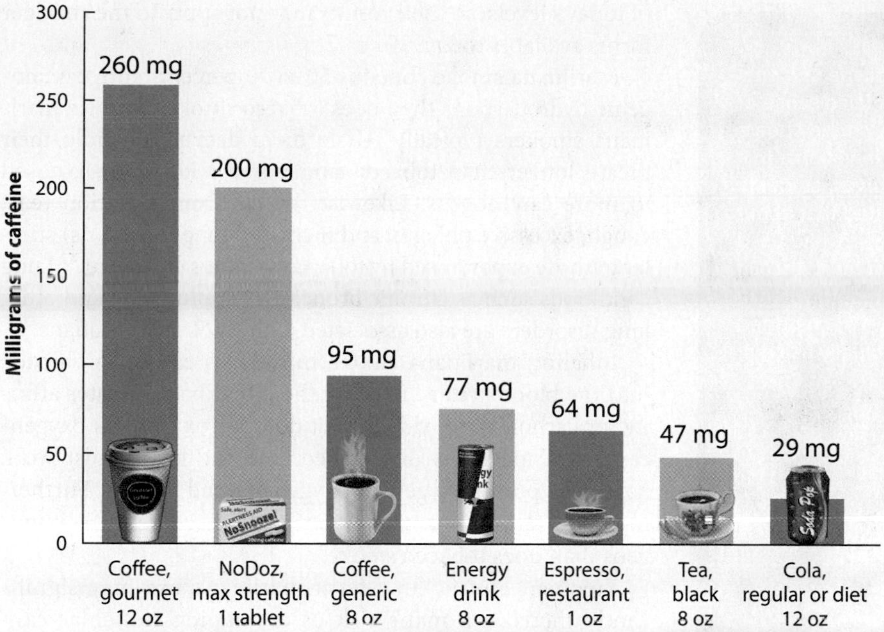

FIGURE 12.4 Caffeine Content Comparison

Source: Data are from *USDA National Nutrient Database for Standard reference*, Release 25 (2012), www.ars.usda.gov.

and weak. To counteract this, they commonly choose to drink another cup of coffee, tea, or soda. Habitually engaging in this practice leads to tolerance and psychological dependence. Symptoms of excessive caffeine consumption include chronic insomnia, jitters, irritability, nervousness, anxiety, and involuntary muscle twitches. Withdrawing from caffeine may compound the effects and produce headaches, fatigue, and nausea. Because caffeine meets the requirements for addiction—tolerance, psychological dependence, and withdrawal symptoms—it can be classified as addictive.

Long-term caffeine use has been suspected of being linked to several serious health problems. However, no strong evidence exists to suggest that moderate caffeine use (less than 300 mg daily, approximately 3 cups of regular coffee) produces harmful effects in healthy, nonpregnant people. For most people, caffeine poses few health risks and may actually have some benefits. Drinking coffee has been associated with lower prostate cancer rates in men, lower depression rates among women, and a lower risk of lower risk of stroke in general. Caffeine may also protect against Alzheimer's disease, Parkinson's disease, liver disease, and some types of cancer.[36]

Marijuana and Other Cannabinoids

Although archaeological evidence documents the use of **marijuana** ("grass," "weed," "pot") as far back as 6,000 years, the drug did not become popular in the United States until the 1960s. Today, marijuana is the most commonly used illicit drug in the United States. Approximately 43 percent of Americans over the age of 12 have tried marijuana at least once.[37] Some 32 million Americans have reported using marijuana in the past year, and more than 19 million have reported using marijuana within the past month. More than 1 million Americans over the age of 12 reported receiving treatment for marijuana use, more than any other illicit drug. Marijuana use is also on the rise on college campuses, following the trend of increased use in the general population.[38]

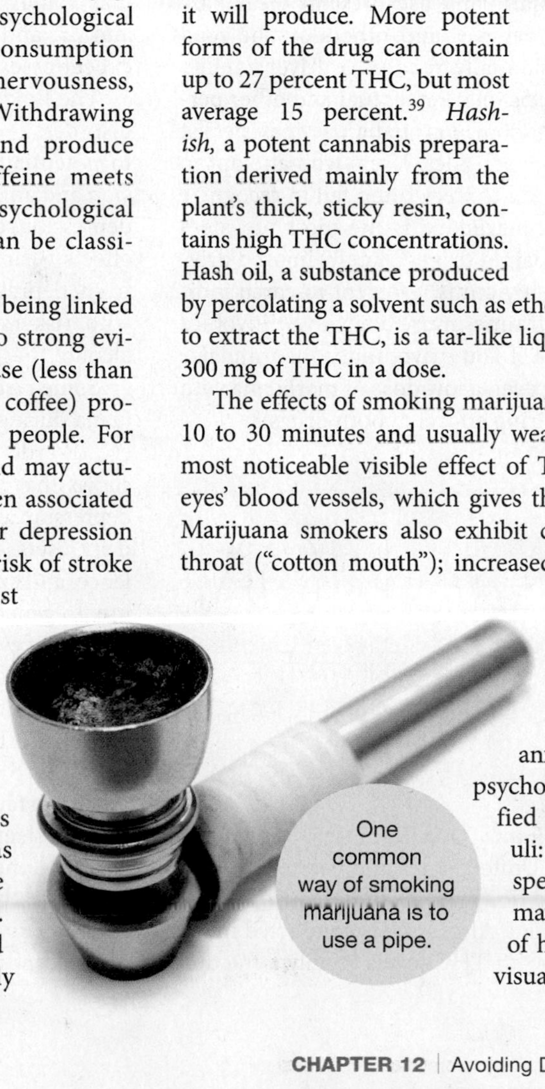

One common way of smoking marijuana is to use a pipe.

Methods of Use and Physical Effects

Marijuana is derived from either the *Cannabis sativa* or *Cannabis indica* (hemp) plant. Most of the time, marijuana is smoked, although it can also be ingested, as in brownies baked with marijuana in them. When marijuana is smoked, it is usually rolled into cigarettes (joints) or placed in a pipe or water pipe (bong).

Tetrahydrocannabinol (THC) is the psychoactive substance in marijuana and the key to determining how powerful a high it will produce. More potent forms of the drug can contain up to 27 percent THC, but most average 15 percent.[39] *Hashish,* a potent cannabis preparation derived mainly from the plant's thick, sticky resin, contains high THC concentrations. Hash oil, a substance produced by percolating a solvent such as ether through dried marijuana to extract the THC, is a tar-like liquid that may contain up to 300 mg of THC in a dose.

marijuana Chopped leaves and flowers of *Cannabis indica* or *Cannabis sativa* plants (hemp); a psychoactive stimulant.

tetrahydrocannabinol (THC) The chemical name for the active ingredient in marijuana.

The effects of smoking marijuana are generally felt within 10 to 30 minutes and usually wear off within 3 hours. The most noticeable visible effect of THC is the dilation of the eyes' blood vessels, which gives the smoker bloodshot eyes. Marijuana smokers also exhibit coughing; dry mouth and throat ("cotton mouth"); increased thirst and appetite; lowered blood pressure; and mild muscular weakness, primarily exhibited in drooping eyelids. Users can also experience severe anxiety, panic, paranoia, and psychosis, and may have intensified reactions to various stimuli: Colors, sounds, and the speed at which things move may seem altered. High doses of hashish may produce vivid visual hallucinations.

DID YOU **KNOW?**

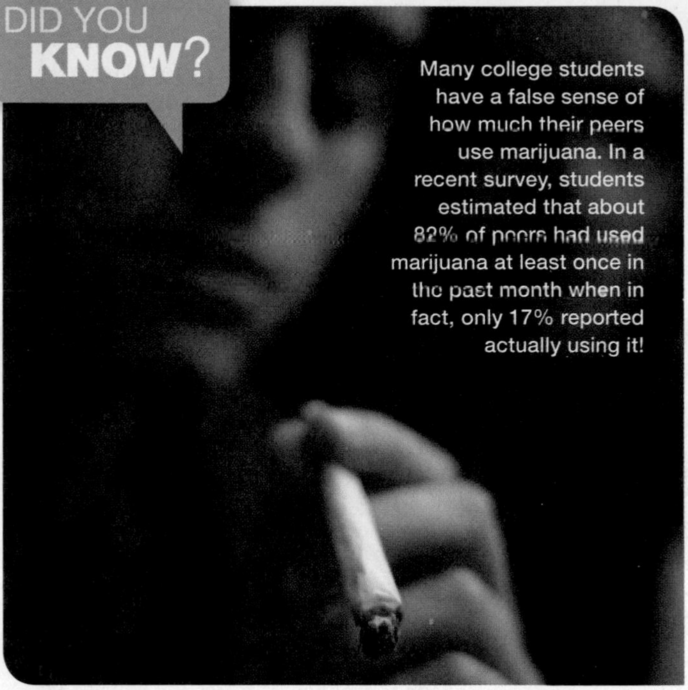

Many college students have a false sense of how much their peers use marijuana. In a recent survey, students estimated that about 82% of peers had used marijuana at least once in the past month when in fact, only 17% reported actually using it!

Source: Data are from American College Health Association, *American College Health Association—National College Health Assessment II (ACHA-NCHA II): Reference Group Data Report, Spring 2013* (Baltimore, MD: American College Health Association, 2013).

Marijuana and Driving Marijuana use presents clear hazards for drivers of motor vehicles and others on the road with them. The drug substantially reduces a driver's ability to react and make quick decisions. Perceptual and other performance deficits resulting from marijuana use may persist for some time after the high subsides. Users who attempt to drive, fly, or operate heavy machinery often fail to recognize their impairment. Overall, marijuana is the most prevalent illegal drug detected in impaired drivers, fatally injured drivers, and motor vehicle crash victims.[40] Recent research indicates you are two and a half times more likely to be involved in a motor vehicle accident if you drive under the influence of marijuana.[41] Combining even a low dose of marijuana with alcohol enhances the impairing effects of both drugs.

10.3 MILLION

PEOPLE REPORTED DRIVING UNDER THE **INFLUENCE** OF ILLICIT DRUGS IN THE PAST YEAR.

Effects of Chronic Marijuana Use Because marijuana is illegal in most parts of the United States and has been widely used only since the 1960s, long-term studies of its effects have been difficult to conduct. Also, studies conducted in the 1960s involved marijuana with THC levels at only a fraction of today's levels, so their results may not apply to the stronger forms available today.

Marijuana smoke contains 50 to 70 percent more carcinogenic hydrocarbons than does tobacco smoke. Because marijuana smokers typically inhale more deeply and hold their breath longer than tobacco smokers, the lungs are exposed to more carcinogens. Likewise, effects from irritation (e.g., cough, excessive phlegm, and increased lung infections) similar to those experienced by tobacco smokers can occur.[42] Lung conditions such as chronic bronchitis, emphysema, and other lung disorders are also associated with smoking marijuana.

Inhaling marijuana smoke introduces carbon monoxide into the bloodstream. Because the blood has a greater affinity for carbon monoxide than it does for oxygen, its oxygen-carrying capacity is diminished, and the heart must work harder to pump oxygen to oxygen-starved tissues. Furthermore, the tar from cannabis contains higher levels of carcinogens than does tobacco smoke.

Frequent and/or long-term marijuana use may significantly increase a man's risk of developing testicular cancer. The risk was particularly elevated (about twice that of those who never smoked marijuana) for those who used marijuana at least weekly or who had long-term exposure to the substance beginning in adolescence. The results also suggested that the association with marijuana use might be limited to *nonseminoma,* an aggressive, fast-growing testicular malignancy that tends to strike early, between ages 20 and 35, and accounts for about 40 percent of all testicular cancer cases.[43]

The link between marijuana and common mental health disorders is somewhat conflicting, because marijuana is said to potentially cause as well as relieve symptoms of depression and anxiety. While marijuana may ease the symptoms of depression, depression may actually worsen once the positive effects wear off.[44] Marijuana users are more likely to suffer from depression and depressive symptoms than nonusers, with risk increasing for people using both marijuana and alcohol.[45]

Some research suggests that frequent or heavy use of marijuana during adolescence may be associated developing anxiety disorders in young adulthood.[46] Additionally, research shows that frequent cannabis use in teenagers predicts both depression and anxiety later in life, with the highest risk among daily users. Certain personality disorders, interpersonal violence, and suicidal ideation are also correlated with marijuana use. In general, the younger marijuana use started, the greater the risk of eventually developing a mental health disorder.[47]

Chronic use of marijuana can decrease the quality of sleep. Studies have found that chronic users of marijuana experience less rapid eye movement (REM) and slow-wave sleep (SWS), often referred to as deep sleep, both of which are important for the consolidation of memories. Not getting enough sleep interferes with the ability to think and remember, challenging students' ability to learn and perform well academically.[48]

Other risks associated with marijuana include suppression of the immune system, blood pressure changes, and impaired memory. Recent studies suggest that pregnant women who smoke marijuana may have children who have subtle brain changes that can cause difficulties with problem-solving skills, memory, and attention, and can more than double the risk of women giving birth prematurely.[49]

Legalization of Marijuana and Medicinal Uses

Although recognized as a dangerous drug by the U.S. government, marijuana has been legalized for medicinal uses in 21 states and the District of Columbia. While marijuana's legal status for medicinal purposes continues to be hotly debated, marijuana has several medical purposes. Marijuana also reduces the muscle pain and spasticity caused by diseases such as multiple sclerosis.

Two FDA-approved medications based on the scientific study of cannabinoids—the active chemicals in marijuana—that harness therapeutic benefits of cannabinoids while reducing or eliminating side effects have been developed. *Dronabinol* (Marinol) and *nabilone* (Cesamet®) both contain THC and are used to lessen the chemotherapy-induced nausea, as well as the effects of wasting disease (extreme weight loss) caused by AIDS. A drug called *Sativex* is already authorized for use in treating symptoms of multiple sclerosis in the United Kingdom and several European countries. It is currently moving through Phase III clinical trials in the United States as an option for treating cancer pain.

A cannabidiol-based drug called *Epidiolex* has also been developed for the treatment of different types of childhood epilepsy. Although the drug is not yet FDA tested or approved, some parents of children with Dravet syndrome—a severe form of epilepsy—initially report success controlling seizures in their children.[50]

Voters in Washington and Colorado recently passed ballot initiatives to legalize marijuana for recreational use. Many arguments have been made for legalization, including the revenue boost to state and local governments (Colorado will receive an estimated $99 million in tax revenues from marijuana), more effective law enforcement and criminal justice since police officers will have more time and money to pursue criminals for other crimes, decrease in the violence associated with selling marijuana as a result of cutting off revenue streams to organized crime, and safety controls that help eliminate the risk of smoking marijuana potentially laced with toxic substances.[51]

On the other side of the coin, people have argued that marijuana is addictive—with research suggesting that as many as 10 percent of users will develop dependence over time. Additionally, others have suggested marijuana alters the way users perceive things while under the influence, can be a gateway drug with the potential to introduce users to more serious illegal substances, and has negative health impacts as a result of high levels of carcinogens, ability to raise heart rate, and links to mental health issues such as depression, anxiety, and suicidal ideation.[52]

Synthetic Marijuana

Also known as K2 or "Spice," synthetic marijuana is used to describe a diverse family of herbal blends marketed under many names, including K2, fake marijuana, Yucatan Fire, Skunk, Moon Rocks, and others. These products contain dried, shredded plant material and one or more synthetic cannabinoids, with results that mimic marijuana intoxication but with longer duration and poor detection on urine drug screens. K2 is sold legally as herbal blend incense. However, K2 is smoked by people to gain effects similar to marijuana, hashish, and other forms of cannabis.[53]

K2 is used by nearly 1 in 10 college students and is more commonly used by males and first- and second-year college students. Students who reported using K2 were more likely to have smoked cigarettes, marijuana, and hookahs. It is also gaining more attention among high school seniors, with reports that 1 in every 9, or 11.3 percent, of high school seniors are using this drug.[54]

The most common way of smoking K2 is in a "joint," followed by hookah use. People smoking K2 may experience several adverse health effects such as hallucinations, severe agitation, extremely elevated heart rate and blood pressure, coma, suicide attempts, and drug dependence, which is not common among cannabis users. Emergency departments are also reporting a significant increase in the numbers of people being treated for K2 use.[55]

Depressants and Narcotics

Whereas central nervous system stimulants increase muscular and nervous system activity, **depressants** have the opposite effect. These drugs slow down neuromuscular activity and cause sleepiness or calmness. If the dose is high enough, brain function can stop, causing death. Alcohol is the most widely used central nervous system depressant. (For details on alcohol's effect on the body, see **Chapter 10**.) Other forms include benzodiazepines, barbiturates, and opioids.

depressants Drugs that slow down the activity of the central nervous and muscular systems and cause sleepiness or calmness.

benzodiazepines A class of central nervous system depressant drugs with sedative, hypnotic, and muscle relaxant effects.

barbiturates Drugs that depress the central nervous system and have sedating, hypnotic, and anesthetic effects.

Benzodiazepines and Barbiturates

A *sedative* drug promotes mental calmness and reduces anxiety, whereas a *hypnotic* drug promotes sleep or drowsiness. The most common sedative-hypnotic drugs are **benzodiazepines**, more commonly known as *tranquilizers*. These include prescription drugs such as Valium, Ativan, and Xanax. Benzodiazepines are most commonly prescribed for tension, muscular strain, sleep problems, anxiety, panic attacks, and alcohol withdrawal. **Barbiturates** are sedative-hypnotic drugs such as Amytal and Seconal. Today, benzodiazepines have largely replaced barbiturates, which were used medically in the past for relieving tension and inducing relaxation and sleep.

Sedative-hypnotics have a synergistic effect when combined with alcohol, another central nervous system depressant.

opioids Drugs that induce sleep, relieve pain, and produce euphoria, including derivatives of opium and synthetics with similar chemical properties; also called *narcotics.*

opium The parent drug of the opioids; made from the seedpod resin of the opium poppy.

endorphins Opioid-like hormones that are manufactured in the human body and contribute to natural feelings of well-being.

Taken together, these drugs can lead to respiratory failure and death. All sedative or hypnotic drugs can produce physical and psychological dependence in several weeks. A complication specific to sedatives is cross-tolerance, which occurs when users develop tolerance for one sedative or become dependent on it and develop tolerance for others as well. Withdrawal from sedative or hypnotic drugs may range from mild discomfort to severe symptoms, depending on the degree of dependence.

Rohypnol One benzodiazepine of concern is Rohypnol, a potent tranquilizer similar in nature to Valium but many times stronger. The drug produces a sedative effect, amnesia, muscle relaxation, and slowed psychomotor responses. The most publicized "date rape" drug, Rohypnol has gained notoriety as a growing problem on college campuses. The drug has been added to punch and other drinks at parties, where it is reportedly given to women in hopes of lowering their inhibitions and facilitating potential sexual conquests. (See **Chapter 19** for more information about rape.)

GHB *Gamma-hydroxybutyrate (GHB)* is a central nervous system depressant known to have euphoric, sedative, and anabolic (bodybuilding) effects. The FDA banned OTC sales of GHB in 1992, and it is now a Schedule I controlled substance.[56] Gamma-hydroxybutyrate is an odorless, tasteless fluid that can be made easily at home or in a chemistry lab. Like Rohypnol, GHB has been slipped into drinks without being detected, resulting in loss of memory, unconsciousness, amnesia, and even death. Other dangerous side effects include nausea, vomiting, seizures, hallucinations, coma, and respiratory distress.

Opioids (Narcotics)

Opioids cause drowsiness, relieve pain, and produce euphoria. Also called *narcotics,* opioids are derived from the parent drug **opium**, a dark, resinous substance made from the milky juice of the opium poppy seedpod, and they are all highly addictive. Opium and heroin are both illegal in the United States, but some opioids are available by prescription for medical purposes: Morphine is sometimes prescribed for severe pain, and codeine is found in prescription cough syrups and other painkillers. Several prescription drugs, including Vicodin, Percodan, OxyContin, Demerol, and Dilaudid, contain synthetic opioids.

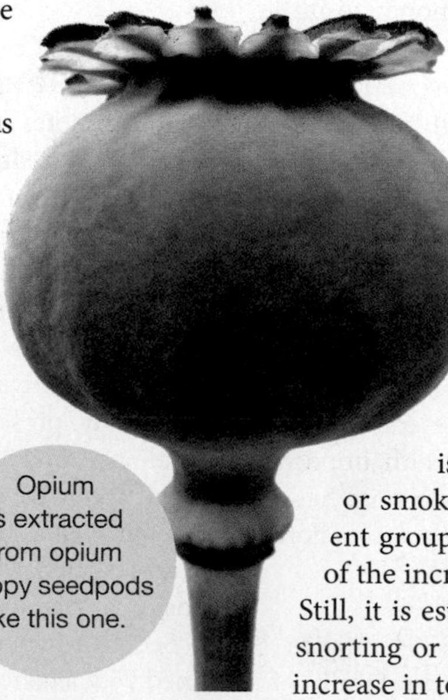

Opium is extracted from opium poppy seedpods like this one.

Physical Effects of Opioids Opioids are powerful depressants of the central nervous system. In addition to relieving pain, these drugs lower heart rate, respiration, and blood pressure. Side effects include weakness, dizziness, nausea, vomiting, euphoria, decreased sex drive, visual disturbances, and lack of coordination.

54%

OF PEOPLE WHO USE PAIN RELIEVERS **NONMEDICALLY** GET THE DRUG FROM A FRIEND OR RELATIVE.

The human body's physiology could be said to encourage opioid addiction. Opioid-like hormones called **endorphins** are manufactured in the body and have multiple receptor sites, particularly in the central nervous system. When endorphins attach themselves at these points, they create feelings of painless well-being; medical researchers refer to them as "the body's own opioids." When endorphin levels are high, people feel euphoric. The same euphoria occurs when opioids or related chemicals are active at the endorphin receptor sites. While the following section discusses heroin addiction, addiction to any opioid follows a similar path.

Heroin Use *Heroin* is a white powder derived from morphine. *Black tar heroin* is a sticky, dark brown, foul-smelling form of heroin that is relatively pure and inexpensive. Once considered a cure for morphine dependence, heroin was later discovered to be even more addictive and potent than morphine. Today, heroin has no medical use.

Heroin is a depressant that produces drowsiness and a dreamy, mentally slow feeling. It can cause drastic mood swings, with euphoric highs followed by depressive lows. Heroin slows respiration and urinary output and constricts the pupils of the eyes. Symptoms of tolerance and withdrawal can appear within 3 weeks of first use.

In 2012, 669,000 Americans reported using heroin in the past year, a considerable increase since 2002.[57] This trend appears to be driven largely by 18- to 25-year-olds, among whom there have been the largest increases. This younger age group may be more likely to purchase heroin since it is both cheaper and generally easier to obtain than prescription opioids.

While heroin is usually injected ("mainlined"), the contemporary version of heroin is so potent that users can get high by snorting or smoking the drug. This has attracted a more affluent group of users who may not want to inject because of the increased risk of contracting diseases such as HIV. Still, it is estimated that within 2 to 3 weeks of beginning snorting or smoking, the majority of users experience an increase in tolerance and begin injecting their heroin.

Many users describe the "rush" they feel when injecting themselves as intensely pleasurable, whereas others report unpredictable and unpleasant side effects. The temporary nature of the rush contributes to the drug's high potential for addiction—many addicts shoot up four or five times a day. Mainlining can cause veins to scar and eventually collapse. Once a vein has collapsed, it can no longer be used to introduce heroin into the bloodstream. Addicts become expert at locating new veins to use: in the feet, the legs, the temples, under the tongue, or in the groin.

Heroin addicts experience a distinct pattern of withdrawal. Symptoms include intense desire for the drug, sleep disturbance, dilated pupils, loss of appetite, irritability, goose bumps, and muscle tremors. The most difficult time in the withdrawal process occurs 24 to 72 hours following last use. All of the preceding symptoms continue, along with nausea, abdominal cramps, restlessness, insomnia, vomiting, diarrhea, extreme anxiety, hot and cold flashes, elevated blood pressure, and rapid heartbeat and respiration. Once the peak of withdrawal has passed, symptoms begin to subside.

Hallucinogens

Hallucinogens, or *psychedelics,* are substances that are capable of creating auditory or visual hallucinations and unusual changes in mood, thoughts, and feelings. The major receptor sites for most of these drugs are in the reticular formation (located in the brain stem at the upper end of the spinal cord), which is responsible for interpreting outside stimuli before allowing these signals to travel to other parts of the brain. When a hallucinogen is present at a reticular formation site, messages become scrambled, and the user may see wavy walls instead of straight ones or may "smell" colors and "hear" tastes. This mixing of sensory messages is known as *synesthesia.* Users may also become less inhibited or recall events long buried in the subconscious mind. The most widely recognized hallucinogens are LSD, Ecstasy, mescaline, psilocybin, PCP, and ketamine. All are illegal and carry severe penalties for manufacture, possession, transportation, or sale.

LSD First synthesized in the late 1930s by Swiss chemist Albert Hoffman, *lysergic acid diethylamide* (*LSD*) received media attention in the 1960s when young people used the drug to "turn on and tune out." In 1970, federal authorities placed LSD on the list of controlled substances (Schedule I). Today, this dangerous psychedelic drug, known alternately as "acid," has been making a comeback. It is estimated that 6 percent of Americans aged 18 to 25 have used LSD at least once in their lifetime.[58] A national survey of college students showed that 3 percent had used the drug in their lives.[59]

hallucinogens Substances capable of creating auditory or visual distortions and unusual changes in mood, thoughts, and feelings.

The most common and popular form of LSD is blotter acid—small squares of blotter-like paper that have been impregnated with a liquid LSD mixture. The blotter is swallowed or chewed briefly. LSD also comes in tiny thin squares of gelatin called *windowpane* and in tablets called *microdots,* which are less than an eighth of an inch across (it would take ten or more to equal the size of an aspirin tablet).

One of the most powerful drugs known to science, LSD can produce strong effects in doses as low as 20 micrograms (μg). (To give you an idea of how small a dose this is, the average postage stamp weighs approximately 60,000 μg.) The potency of a typical dose currently ranges from 20 to 80 μg, compared to 150 to 300 μg commonly used in the 1960s.

Depending on the quantity users have eaten, LSD usually takes 20 to 60 minutes to take effect, and can last 6 to 8 hours. For many people there is also a period (2 to 6 hours) where it becomes difficult to sleep, and everyday reality is noticeably different. The psychological effects of LSD vary. Euphoria is the common psychological state produced by the drug, but dysphoria (a sense of evil and foreboding) may also be experienced. LSD also distorts ordinary perceptions, such as the movement of stationary objects, as well as auditory or visual hallucinations. In addition, the drug shortens attention span, causing the mind to wander. Thoughts may be interposed and juxtaposed, so the user experiences several different thoughts simultaneously. Users become introspective, and suppressed memories may surface, often taking on bizarre symbolism. Many more effects are possible, including decreased aggressiveness and enhanced sensory experiences.

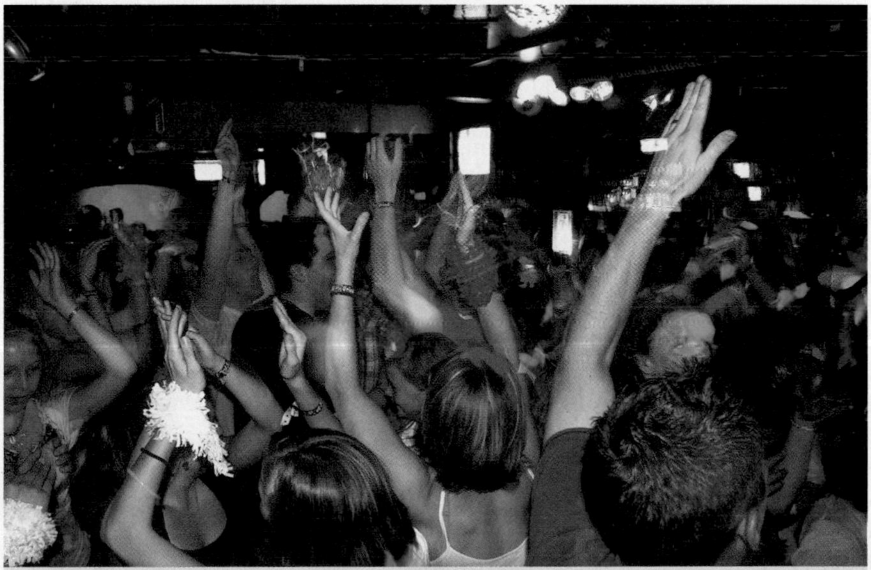

Although users may think so-called "club drugs" (such as Ecstasy, GHB, and ketamine) are harmless, research has shown that they can produce hallucinations, paranoia, amnesia, dangerous increases in heart rate and blood pressure, coma, and, in some cases, death.

In addition to its psychedelic effects, LSD produces several physical effects, including increased heart rate, elevated blood pressure and temperature, gooseflesh (roughened skin), increased reflex speeds, muscle tremors and twitches, perspiration, increased salivation, chills, headaches, and mild nausea. Because the drug also stimulates uterine muscle contractions, it can lead to premature labor and miscarriage in pregnant women. Research into long-term effects has been inconclusive.

Although there is no evidence that LSD creates physical dependency, it may well create psychological dependence. Many LSD users become depressed for 1 or 2 days following a trip and turn to the drug to relieve this depression. The result is a cycle of LSD use to relieve post-LSD depression, which can lead to psychological addiction.

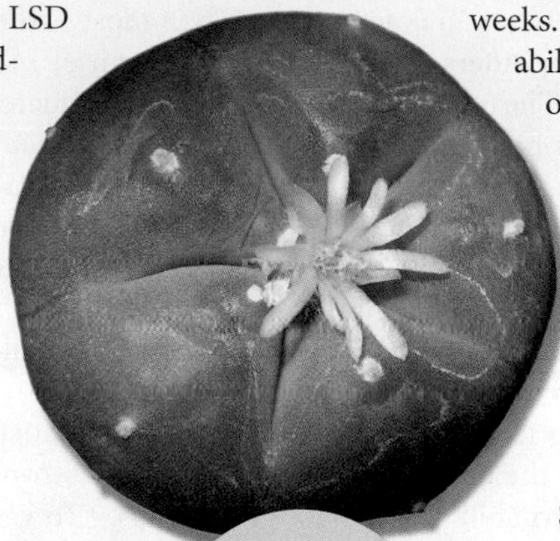

Mescaline comes from "buttons" of the peyote cactus, like this one.

Ecstasy *Ecstasy* is the most common street name for the drug *methylene-dioxymethamphetamine* (*MDMA*), a synthetic compound with both stimulant and mildly hallucinogenic effects. It is one of the most well-known **club drugs** or "designer drugs," terms applied to synthetic analogs of existing illicit drugs popular at nightclubs and all-night parties. Ecstasy creates feelings of extreme euphoria, openness, and warmth; an increased willingness to communicate; feelings of love and empathy; increased awareness; and heightened appreciation for music. Ecstasy can enhance the sensory experience and distort perceptions, but it does not create visual hallucinations. Effects begin within 20 to 90 minutes and can last for 3 to 5 hours.

club drugs Synthetic analogs (drugs that produce similar effects) of existing illicit drugs.

Some of the risks associated with Ecstasy use are similar to those of other stimulants. Because of the nature of the drug, Ecstasy users are at greater risk of inappropriate or unintended emotional bonding and have a tendency to say things they might feel uncomfortable about later. More physical consequences of Ecstasy use may include mild to extreme jaw clenching, tongue and cheek chewing, short-term memory loss or confusion, increased body temperature, and increased heart rate and blood pressure. Combined with alcohol, Ecstasy can be extremely dangerous and sometimes fatal. As the effects of Ecstasy wear off, the user can experience mild depression, fatigue, and a hangover that can last from days to weeks. Chronic use appears to damage the brain's ability to think and to regulate emotion, memory, sleep, and pain. Some studies indicate that the drug may cause long-lasting neurotoxic effects by damaging brain cells that produce serotonin.[60]

MDMA in powder or crystal form—called "Molly," short for molecule—has become a popular festival drug. Unlike Ecstasy, which tends to be laced with ingredients like caffeine or methamphetamine, Molly is considered pure MDMA. Still, many powders sold as Molly contain zero actual MDMA. Some typical side effects of using Molly include grinding one's teeth, becoming dehydrated, feeling anxious, having trouble sleeping, fever, and losing one's appetite, as well as uncontrollable seizures, elevated blood pressure, high body temperature, and depression.[61]

Mescaline *Mescaline* is one of hundreds of chemicals derived from the peyote cactus, a small, button-like plant that grows in the southwestern United States and in Latin America. Natives of these regions have long used the dried peyote "buttons" for religious purposes. It is both a powerful hallucinogen and a central nervous system stimulant.

Products sold on the street as mescaline are likely to be synthetic chemical relatives of the true drug. Street names of these products include DOM, STP, TMA, and MMDA. Any of these can be toxic in small quantities.

Users typically swallow 10 to 12 buttons. They taste bitter and generally induce immediate nausea or vomiting. Longtime users claim that the nausea becomes less noticeable with frequent use. Those who are able to keep the drug down begin to feel the effects within 30 to 90 minutes, when mescaline reaches maximum concentration in the brain. Effects may persist for 9 or 10 hours.

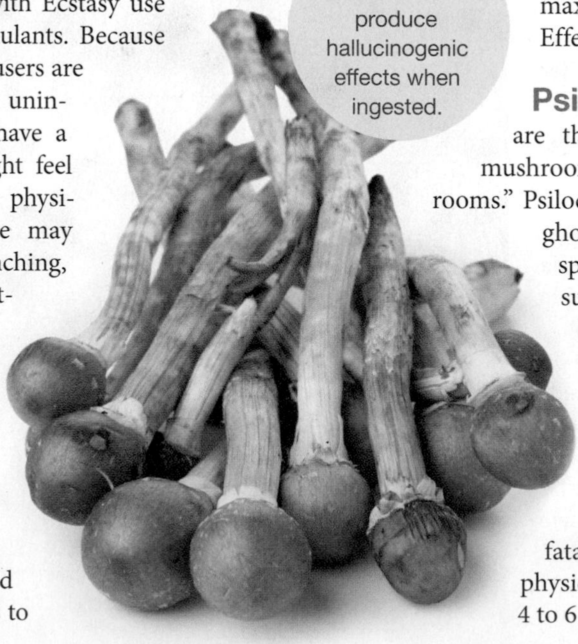

Psilocybe mushrooms produce hallucinogenic effects when ingested.

Psilocybin *Psilocybin* and *psilocin* are the active chemicals in a group of mushrooms sometimes called "magic mushrooms." Psilocybe mushrooms, which grow throughout the world, can be cultivated from spores or harvested wild. When consumed, these mushrooms can cause hallucinations. Because many mushrooms resemble the psilocybe variety, people who harvest wild mushrooms for any purpose should be certain of what they are doing. Mushroom varieties can be easily misidentified, and mistakes can be fatal. Psilocybin is similar to LSD in its physical effects, which generally wear off in 4 to 6 hours.

PCP The synthetic substance *phencyclidine* (*PCP*) was originally developed as a dissociative anesthetic—patients administered this drug could keep their eyes open, apparently remain conscious, and feel no pain during a medical procedure. Afterward, they would experience amnesia for the time that the drug was in their system. Such a drug had obvious advantages as an anesthetic, but its unpredictability and drastic effects (postoperative delirium, confusion, and agitation) caused it to be withdrawn from the legal market.

On the illegal market, PCP is a white, crystalline powder that users often sprinkle onto marijuana cigarettes. It is dangerous and unpredictable regardless of the method of administration. The effects of PCP depend on the dosage. A dose as small as 5 mg will produce effects similar to those of strong central nervous system depressants—slurred speech, impaired coordination, reduced sensitivity to pain, and reduced heart and respiratory rate. Doses between 5 and 10 mg cause fever, salivation, nausea, vomiting, and total loss of sensitivity to pain. Doses greater than 10 mg result in a drastic drop in blood pressure, coma, muscular rigidity, violent outbursts, and possible convulsions and death.

Psychologically, PCP may produce either euphoria or dysphoria. It is also known to produce hallucinations as well as delusions and overall delirium. Some users experience a prolonged state of "nothingness." The long-term effects of PCP use are unknown.

Ketamine The liquid form of *ketamine* ("Special K") is used as an anesthetic in some hospital and veterinary clinics. After stealing it from hospitals or medical suppliers, dealers typically dry the liquid (usually by cooking it) and grind the residue into powder. Special K causes hallucinations, as it inhibits the relay of sensory input; the brain fills the resulting void with visions, dreams, memories, and sensory distortions. The effects of ketamine are similar to those of PCP—confusion, agitation, aggression, and lack of coordination—but even less predictable. The aftereffects of Special K are less severe than those of Ecstasy, so it has grown in popularity as a club drug.

Inhalants

Inhalants are chemicals whose vapors, when inhaled, can cause hallucinations and create intoxicating and euphoric effects. Not commonly recognized as drugs, inhalants are legal to purchase and widely available, but dangerous. They generally appeal to young people who can't afford or obtain illicit substances. Some misused products include rubber cement, model glue, paint thinner, aerosol sprays, lighter fluid, varnish, wax, spot removers, and gasoline. Most of these substances are sniffed or "huffed" by users in search of a quick, cheap high.

inhalants Chemical vapors that are sniffed or inhaled in order to produce highs.

anabolic steroids Artificial forms of the hormone testosterone that promote muscle growth and strength.

ergogenic drug Substance believed to enhance athletic performance.

Because they are inhaled, the volatile chemicals in these products reach the bloodstream and then the brain within seconds. This characteristic, along with the fact that dosages are extremely difficult to control because everyone has unique lung and breathing capacities, makes inhalants particularly dangerous. The effects of inhalants usually last for fewer than 15 minutes and resemble those of central nervous system depressants: dizziness, disorientation, impaired coordination, reduced judgment, and slowed reaction times. Combining inhalants with alcohol produces a synergistic effect and can cause severe and sometimes fatal liver damage. An overdose of fumes from inhalants can cause unconsciousness. If the user's oxygen intake is reduced during the inhaling process, death can result within 5 minutes. *Sudden sniffing death* syndrome can be a fatal consequence, whether it's the user's first time or not. This syndrome can occur if a user inhales deeply and then participates in physical activity or is startled.

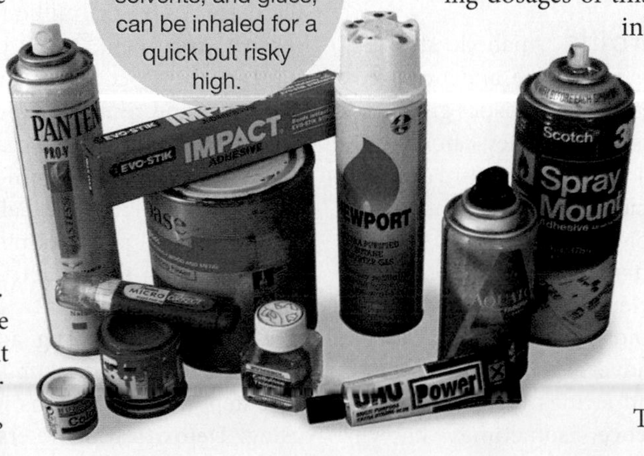

Common household products, such as aerosol sprays, solvents, and glues, can be inhaled for a quick but risky high.

Amyl Nitrite Sometimes called "poppers" or "rush," *amyl nitrite* is packaged in small, cloth-covered glass capsules that can be crushed to release the active chemical for the user to inhale. The drug is often prescribed to alleviate chest pain in heart patients because it dilates small blood vessels and reduces blood pressure. Dilation of blood vessels in the genital area is thought to enhance sensations or perceptions of orgasm. It also produces fainting, dizziness, warmth, and skin flushing.

Nitrous Oxide *Nitrous oxide* is sometimes used as dental or minor surgical anesthesia. It is also a propellant chemical in aerosol products such as whipped toppings. Users who inhale nitrous oxide experience a state of euphoria, floating sensations, and illusions. Effects also include pain relief and a silly feeling (hence its nickname "laughing gas"). Regulating dosages of this drug can be difficult. Sustained inhalation can lead to unconsciousness, coma, and death.

Anabolic Steroids

Anabolic steroids are artificial forms of the male hormone testosterone that promote muscle growth and strength. Steroids are available in two forms: injectable solutions and pills. These **ergogenic drugs** are used

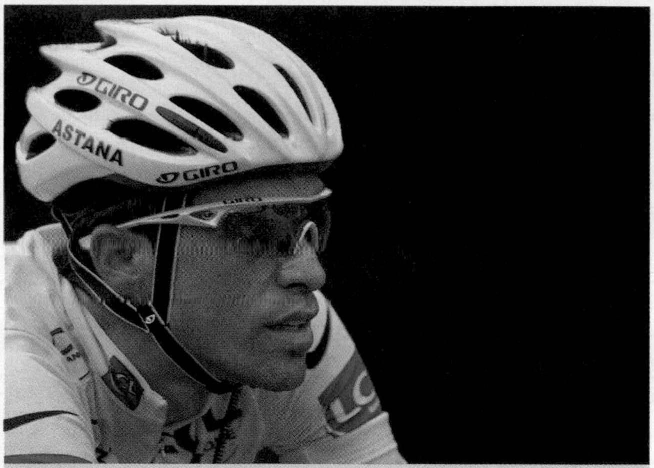

Cyclist Alberto Contador was suspended from the Tour de France for 2 years and stripped of 2010 victory after testing positive for performance-enhancing drug use.

primarily by people who believe the drugs will increase their strength, power, bulk (weight), speed, and athletic performance.

It was once estimated that up to 20 percent of college athletes used steroids. Now that stricter drug-testing policies have been instituted by the National Collegiate Athletic Association (NCAA), reported use of anabolic steroids among intercollegiate athletes has decreased. Currently, less than half of 1 percent of college athletes surveyed report use of anabolic steroids within the past 12 months. Those who report using anabolic steroids use them less than once per week. Of those, half reported their first experience with anabolic steroids occurred after the age of 18.[62] The use of anabolic steroids on the college campus is very low; approximately 1 percent report using them within the past 30 days. However, the perception of anabolic steroid use on the college campus is much higher, with 31 percent of students perceiving their classmates had used anabolic steroids in the past 30 days.[63] It has been estimated that approximately 1 million adults have used anabolic steroids.[64] Among both adolescents and adults, steroid abuse is higher among men than it is among women. However, steroid abuse is growing most rapidly among young women.[65]

Physical Effects of Steroids Anabolic steroids produce a state of euphoria, diminished fatigue, and increased bulk and power in both sexes. These characteristics give steroids an addictive quality. When users stop, they can experience psychological withdrawal and sometimes severe depression, in some cases leading to suicide attempts. If untreated, depression associated with steroid withdrawal has been known to last for a year or more after steroid use stops.

detoxification The early abstinence period during which an addict adjusts physically and cognitively to being free from the substance's influence.

Men and women who use steroids experience a variety of adverse effects, including mood swings (aggression and violence, sometimes known as "roid rage"); acne; liver tumors; elevated cholesterol levels; hypertension; kidney disease; and immune system disturbances. There is also a danger of transmitting HIV and hepatitis through shared needles. In women, large doses of anabolic steroids may trigger the development of masculine attributes such as deeper voice, increased facial and body hair, and male pattern baldness; they may also result in an enlarged clitoris, smaller breasts, and changes in or absence of menstruation. When taken by healthy males, anabolic steroids shut down the body's production of testosterone, causing men's breasts to grow and testicles to atrophy.

WHAT DO YOU THINK?

Do you believe an athlete's admission of steroid use invalidates his or her athletic achievements?

- How do you think professional athletes who have used steroids or other performance enhancers should be disciplined?
- If you are an athlete, have you ever considered using some type of ergogenic aid to improve your performance?

Steroid Use and Society The Anabolic Steroids Control Act (ASCA) of 1990 makes it a crime to possess, prescribe, or distribute anabolic steroids for any use other than the treatment of specific diseases. Penalties for their illegal use include up to 5 years' imprisonment and a $250,000 fine for the first offense and up to 10 years' imprisonment and a $500,000 fine for subsequent offenses.

In recent years, high-profile athletes in sports such as cycling, track and field, swimming, and baseball have garnered media attention for suspected use of steroids or other banned performance-enhancing drugs. Six athletes were barred from the 2014 Winter Olympic Games for illegal drug use.

LO 5 | TREATMENT AND RECOVERY

Provide examples of drug treatment and recovery options for addicts and their effectiveness.

An estimated 23.1 million Americans age 12 or older needed treatment for an illicit drug or alcohol use problem in 2012. Of these, only 2.5 million—approximately 10.8 percent—received treatment.[66] This gap between needing and receiving treatment occurs because the most difficult step in the treatment and recovery process is for the substance abuser to admit that he or she is an addict. Admitting to addiction is difficult because of the power of *denial*—the inability to see the truth. Denial is the hallmark of addiction. It can be so powerful that a planned intervention is sometimes necessary to break down the addict's defenses against recognizing the problem.

Recovery from drug addiction is a long-term process and frequently requires multiple episodes of treatment. The first step generally begins with abstinence—refraining from using. **Detoxification** refers to the early abstinence period during which an addict adjusts physically and cognitively to

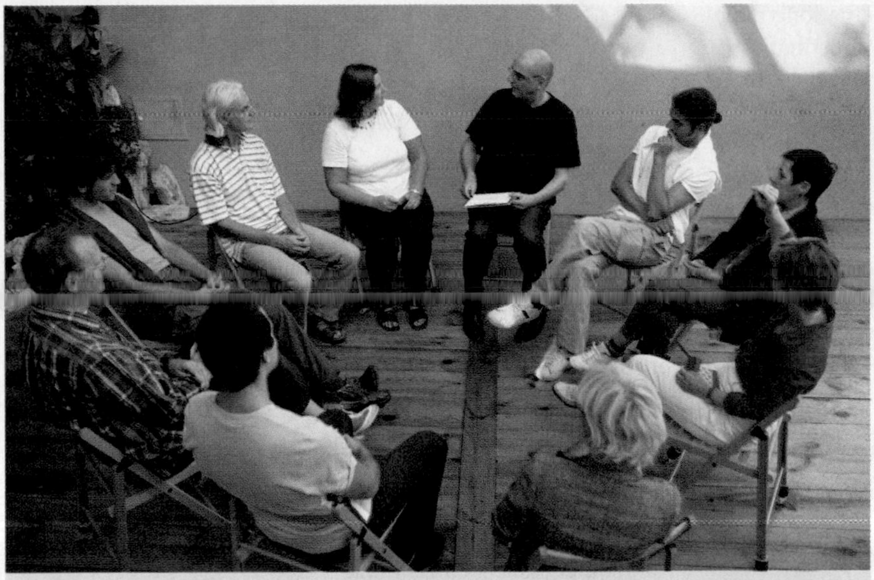

For most addicts, recovery is a long, difficult progress—for some people it can be a lifelong journey. Therapy often takes the form of group meetings, such as those held by 12-step programs, for example Narcotics Anonymous.

being free from the substance's influence. It occurs in virtually every recovering addict. Detoxification is uncomfortable and can be dangerous. For some addicts, early abstinence may involve profound withdrawal that requires medical supervision.

Treatment Approaches

Outpatient behavioral treatment encompasses a variety of programs for addicts who visit a clinic at regular intervals. Most of the programs involve individual or group drug counseling. *Residential treatment programs* can also be very effective, especially for those with more severe problems. Therapeutic communities (TCs) are highly structured programs in which addicts remain at a residence, typically for 6 to 12 months, with a focus on resocializing the addict to a drug-free lifestyle.

12-Step Programs The first 12-step program was Alcoholics Anonymous (AA), begun in 1935 in Akron, Ohio. The 12-step program has since become the most widely used approach to dealing not only with alcoholism, but also with drug abuse and other dysfunctional behaviors. There are more than 200 different recovery programs based on the concept, including Narcotics Anonymous, Cocaine Anonymous, Crystal Meth Anonymous, Gamblers Anonymous, and Pills Anonymous.

The 12-step program is nonjudgmental and based on the idea that a program's only purpose is to work on personal recovery. Working the 12 steps involves admitting to having a serious problem, recognizing there is an outside power that could help, consciously relying on that power, admitting and listing character defects, seeking deliverance from defects, apologizing to those individuals one has harmed in the past, and helping others with the same problem. There is no membership cost, and meetings are open to anyone who wishes to attend.

Vaccines against Addictive Drugs A promising new cocaine vaccine is in development. The vaccine does not eliminate the desire for cocaine; instead, it keeps the user from getting high by stimulating the immune system to attack the drug when it's taken. Clinical human trials are expected to begin soon.

Vaccines against nicotine and methamphetamine are also in development.

Other Treatments Methadone maintenance is one treatment available for people addicted to heroin or other opioids. Methadone is chemically similar enough to opioids to control the tremors, chills, vomiting, diarrhea, and severe

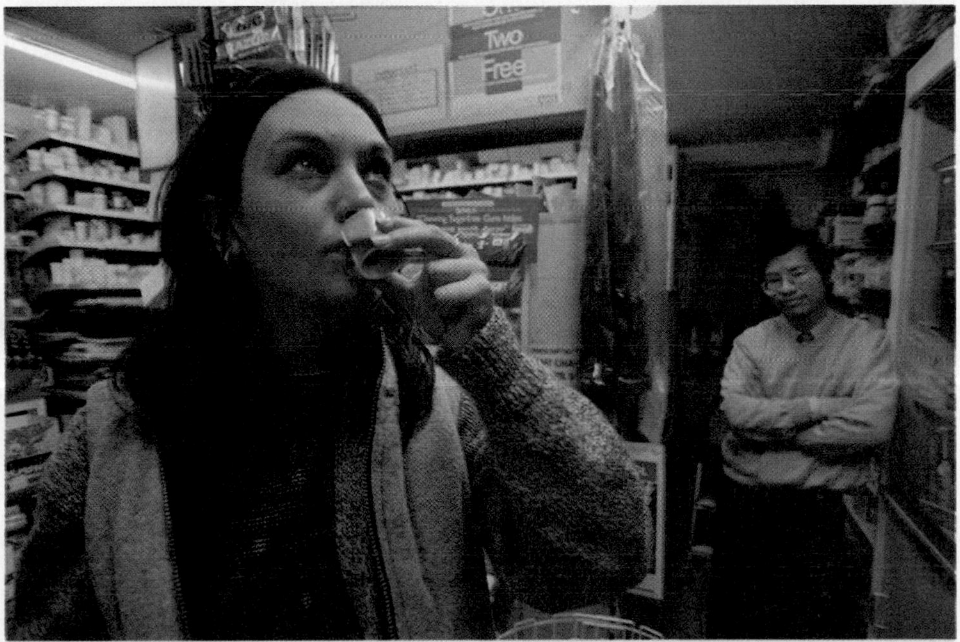

Methadone is a synthetic narcotic that blocks the effects of heroin withdrawal. Although it is still a narcotic and must be administered under the supervision of clinic or pharmacy staff, methadone allows many heroin addicts to lead somewhat normal lives.

abdominal pains of withdrawal. Critics of methadone maintenance contend that the program merely substitutes one addiction for another. Proponents argue that people on methadone maintenance are less likely to engage in criminal activities to support their habits than heroin addicts are. For this reason, many methadone maintenance programs are financed by state or federal government and are available free of charge or at reduced cost.

A number of new drug therapies for opioid dependence are emerging. Naltrexone (Trexan), an opioid antagonist, has been approved as a treatment. While on naltrexone, recovering addicts do not have the compulsion to use heroin, and if they do use it, they don't get high, so there is no point in using the drug. More recently, researchers have reported promising results with buprenorphine (Temgesic), a mild, nonaddicting synthetic opioid that, like heroin and methadone, bonds to certain receptors in the brain, blocks pain messages, and persuades the brain that its craving for heroin has been satisfied.

College Students' Treatment and Recovery

For college students who have developed substance or behavioral addictions, early intervention increases the likelihood of successful treatment. The needs of college students seeking drug treatment in rehab do not differ greatly from other adult recovering addicts, but for best results, the community of addicts should include others of a similar age and educational background. Private therapy, group therapy, cognitive training, nutrition counseling, and health therapies can all help with recovery.

A growing number of colleges and universities offer "recovery communities" to students who are recovering from addiction and want to stay in school without being exposed to excessive drinking or drug use. Students can get specialized counseling and support that is not typically provided on a college campus.

For instance, at Kennesaw State's 4-year-old program, students first enter the Center for Young Adult Addiction and Recovery, where addiction specialists use clinical techniques to support the social and academic success of students while they abstain from substance use. After students have been sober for 6 months, they enter the center's Collegiate Recovery Community, which includes weekly meetings and seminars on relapse prevention and community building and meetings with academic advisers.

A scholarship may be available for students who have a 3.0 grade point average and participate in the "peer community." Recovering students are trained to go back into the classroom and educate their peers who are most at risk of developing substance abuse problems, such as fraternity and sorority members and incoming first-year students.[67]

Another campus, Texas Tech University, received a federal grant to create a national model of its students-in-recovery program. The program offers scholarships to students in recovery, as well as on-campus 12-step meetings and academic support.[68]

LO 6 | ADDRESSING DRUG MISUSE AND ABUSE IN THE UNITED STATES

Profile illicit drug use in the United States, including who uses illicit drugs, financial impact, and impact on college campuses and the workplace.

While stories of people who have tried illegal drugs may tempt you to try them yourself, the risks associated with drug use extend beyond the personal. The decision to try any illicit substance supports illicit drug manufacture and transport, thus contributing to the national drug problem.

Illegal drug use in the United States costs about $193 billion per year.[69] This estimate includes $11 billion in the cost of health care, $120 billion in lost productivity, and $61 billion in the cost of criminal investigation, prosecution, incarceration, and other associated criminal justice costs.[70]

Drugs in the Workplace

According to the National Survey on Drug Use and Health, 50 percent of all U.S. workers who use illicit drugs are employed full time.[71] Many companies have instituted drug testing for their employees. Mandatory drug urinalysis is controversial. Critics argue that such testing violates Fourth Amendment rights of protection from unreasonable search and seizure. Proponents believe the

WHAT DO YOU THINK?

What do you believe are the moral and ethical issues surrounding drug testing of employees?

- Are you in favor of drug testing?
- Should employers have the right to conduct drug testing at the worksite?

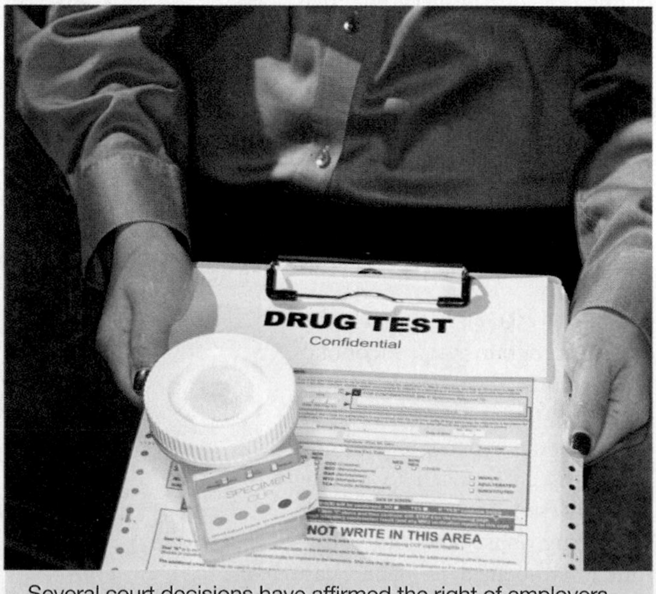

Several court decisions have affirmed the right of employers to test their employees for drug use. Most Americans apparently support drug testing for certain types of jobs.

TECH & HEALTH | TYPES OF DRUG TESTS

Linn State Technical College, a 2-year public institution, made the news in 2011 when it implemented a mandatory drug-testing program for all students. The policy was later ruled to be a violation of students' right to privacy. But beyond the campus, drug testing is an ever-more-common condition of many employers.

There are many types of drug tests.

Urine Tests

Urine tests are the least expensive test method, with costs varying between $7 and $50 for the home versions. They can be conducted anywhere, but labs must verify results. Urine tests are best at detecting drug use within the past week, although if someone uses a drug over a long period of time the ability of urine tests to detect it outside that effective window increases. There are some problems with this test: Many find giving a urine sample to be embarrassing and intrusive, and if drug users know the date of an upcoming urine test they can abstain for a short period of time to get a clean result and then go back to using afterward.

Saliva Tests

At $15 to $75 per test, saliva tests are cost effective, easy to administer, and they are not seen by sample givers to be as much of a violation of privacy as urine tests often are. Like urine tests, they can be done at any location, but results must be verified by a lab. Saliva tests are growing in popularity and can detect more recent drug use than other testing methods, especially use in the past few days. They are good at detecting methamphetamine and opiates, but less reliable for THC and cannabinoids found in marijuana.

Hair Tests

Hair and follicle tests cost about $100 to $150 to perform. They can give information on a person's drug use for the past 90 days rather than for just a few days or weeks, as with saliva or urine tests. These tests have a positive result a little more than twice as often as urine tests. Hair tests also do not have as many false positives for certain substances, such as poppy seed ingestion versus opiate abuse. The tests are also difficult to "game," since shampoos and other follicle-cleansing products have not been shown to reliably remove drug metabolites from hair.

Opiates (codeine, morphine, heroin) lay down on the hair shaft very tightly and are shown not to migrate along the shaft; thus, if a long segment of hair is available, one can draw some "relative" conclusions about when the use occurred. However, cocaine, although very easy to detect, is able to migrate along the shaft, making it very difficult to determine when the drug was used and for how long.

A drawback of hair tests is that they are not good at detecting very recent use, such as in the past week. While hair tests are not considered to be as much of an intrusion of privacy as urine tests, the amount of hair required for a sample is about the diameter of a pencil and 1.5 inches long.

Blood Tests

Blood tests are the most expensive type of testing, and they are therefore the type least frequently used. They are considered the most intrusive method of testing, but also the most accurate. The detection period is small—just hours or days, depending on the substance.

Sources: N. Koppel, "Suit Claims Public College's Drug Testing Policy is Unconstitutional," *The Wall Street Journal*, September 15, 2011, http://blogs.wsj.com/law/2011/09/15/suit-claims-public-colleges-drug-testing-policy-is-unconstitutional/; The Vaults of EROWID, "Drug Testing Basics," www.erowid.org/psychoactives/testing/testing_info1.shtml.

personal inconvenience entailed in testing pales in comparison to the problems caused by drug use in the workplace.

Drug testing is expensive, with costs running as high as $100 per test. Moreover, some critics question the accuracy and reliability of the results. Both false positives and false negatives can occur. Despite the controversy, drug testing is becoming more common in the work environment. For more information on drug testing, see the **Tech & Health** box.

Preventing Drug Use and Abuse on Campus

Strategies that universities should consider to reduce the number of students who become involved in substance use include:

- Changing student expectations that college is a time to party and experiment with drugs
- Engaging parents about substance use on campus and encouraging them to continue open communication with their children
- Identifying high-risk students through early detection screening programs
- Providing services such as treatment programs specifically tailored for students

The pressure to take drugs is often tremendous, and the reasons for using them are complex. People who develop drug problems generally believe they can control their drug use when they start out. Initially, they view taking drugs as a fun and manageable pastime. However, since most illegal drugs and many prescription drugs produce physical and psychological dependency, it is unrealistic to think that a person can use them regularly without becoming addicted. Peer influence is also a strong motivator, especially among adolescents, who fear not being accepted as part of the group.

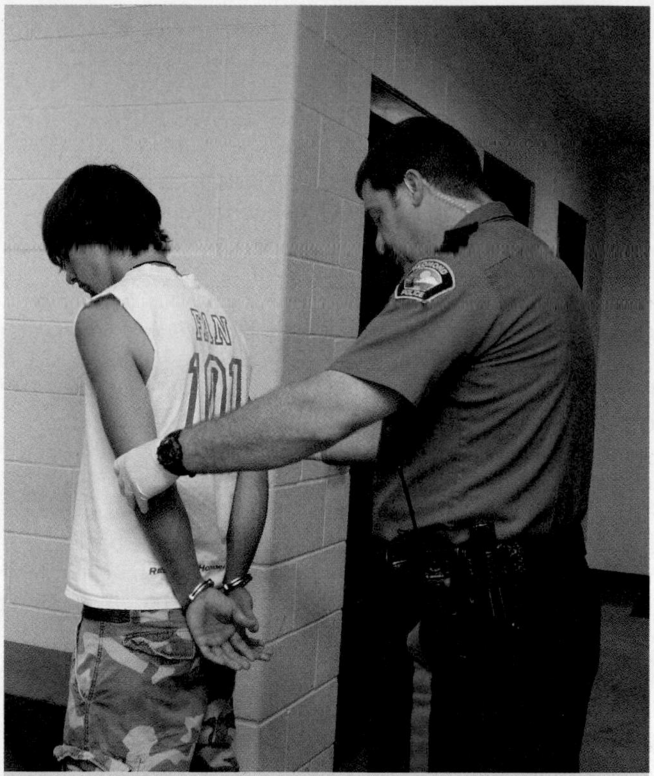

A high percentage of violent and nonviolent crime is linked to drug abuse, affecting not only the abuser, but also entire communities.

Possible Solutions to the Drug Problem

Americans are alarmed by the increasing use of illegal drugs. Respondents in public opinion polls feel that the most important strategy for fighting drug abuse is educating young people. They also endorse strategies such as:

- Stricter border surveillance to reduce drug trafficking
- Longer prison sentences for drug dealers
- Increased government spending on prevention
- Enforcing antidrug laws
- Greater cooperation between government agencies and private groups and individuals providing treatment assistance

All of these approaches will probably help, but they do not offer a total solution to the problem. Drug abuse has been a part of human behavior for thousands of years, and it is not likely to disappear in the near future. For this reason, it is necessary to educate ourselves and develop the self-discipline necessary to avoid dangerous drug dependence.

For many years, the most popular antidrug strategy has been total prohibition. This approach has proved to be ineffective. Prohibition of alcohol during the 1920s created more problems than it solved, as did prohibition of opioids in 1914. A more recent campaign is commonly referred to as the "War on Drugs," undertaken by the U.S. government and other countries. This campaign includes laws and policies that are intended to discourage the production, distribution, and consumption of illicit substances.

In general, researchers in the field of drug education agree that a multimodal approach is best. Students should be taught the difference between drug use, misuse, and abuse. Factual information must be presented without scare tactics; lecturing and moralizing have proven ineffective.

Harm Reduction Strategies Harm reduction is a set of practical approaches to reducing negative consequences of drug use, incorporating a spectrum of strategies from safer use to abstinence. For example, needle exchange programs for injection drug users provide clean needles and syringes and bleach for cleaning needles; these efforts help reduce the number of cases of HIV and hepatitis B. Harm reduction may involve changing the legal sanctions associated with drug use, increasing the availability of treatment services to drug abusers, making use safer through programs like needle exchange, and attempting to change drug users' behavior through education. Harm reduction strategies meet drug users "where they're at," addressing conditions of use along with the use itself. This strategy recognizes that people always have and always will use drugs and, therefore, attempts to minimize the potential hazards associated with drug use rather than the use itself.

WHAT DO YOU THINK?

What is the attitude toward drug use on your campus?

- Are some substances considered more acceptable than others?
- Is drug use considered acceptable at certain times or on occasions?

STUDY PLAN

Customize your study plan—and master your health!—in the Study Area of **MasteringHealth.**

ASSESS YOURSELF

Is your relationship with drugs unhealthy? Take the **Learn to Recognize Drug Use and Potential Abuse** assessment available on MasteringHealth.™

Need help creating a plan? Follow the strategies in the **Your Plan for Change** box for short- and long-term improvements to your health.

YOUR PLAN FOR CHANGE

The **ASSESS YOURSELF** activity describes signs of being controlled by drugs or by a drug user. Depending on your results, you may need to change certain behaviors that may be detrimental to your health.

TODAY, YOU CAN:

- ☐ Imagine a situation in which someone offers you a drug and think of several different ways of refusing. Rehearse these scenarios in your head.
- ☐ Think about the drug use patterns among your social group. Are you ever uncomfortable with these people because of their drug use? Is it difficult to avoid using drugs when you are with them? If you answered yes, begin exploring ways to expand your social circle.

WITHIN THE NEXT 2 WEEKS, YOU CAN:

- ☐ Stop by your campus health center to find out about drug treatment programs or support groups they may have.
- ☐ If you are concerned about your own drug use or the drug use of a close friend, make an appointment with a counselor to talk about the issue.

BY THE END OF THE SEMESTER, YOU CAN:

- ☐ Participate in clubs, activities, and social groups that do not rely on substance abuse for their amusement.
- ☐ If you have a drug problem, make a commitment to enter a treatment program. Acknowledge that you have a problem and that you need the assistance of others to help you overcome it.

CHAPTER REVIEW

To hear an MP3 Tutor Session, scan here or visit the Study Area in **MasteringHealth.**

LO 1 | Drug Dynamics

- Mood-altering substances and experiences produce biochemical reactions that make the body feel good; when absent, the person feels the effects of withdrawal.

LO 2 | Types of Drugs

- The six categories of drugs are prescription drugs, over-the-counter (OTC) drugs, recreational drugs, herbal preparations, illicit drugs, and commercial preparations. Routes of administration include oral ingestion, inhalation, injection (intravenous, intramuscular, and subcutaneous), transdermal, and insertion of suppositories.

LO 3 | Using, Misusing, and Abusing Drugs

- Over-the-counter medications do not require a prescription. Some OTC medications, including sleep aids, cold medicines, and diet pills, can be addictive.
- Prescription drug abuse is at an all-time high, particularly among college students. Only marijuana is more commonly abused. The most commonly abused prescription drugs are opioids/narcotics, depressants, and stimulants.
- People from all walks of life use illicit drugs, although college students report higher usage rates than do the general population. Drug use declined from the mid-1980s to the early 1990s but has remained steady since then. However, among young people, use of drugs has been rising in recent years.

LO 4 | Common Drugs of Abuse

- Drugs of abuse (both legal and illegal) include stimulants; cannabis products, including marijuana; narcotics/depressants; hallucinogens; inhalants; and anabolic steroids. Each has its own set of risks and effects.

LO 5 | Treatment and Recovery

- Treatment begins with abstinence from the drug or addictive behavior, usually instituted through intervention by close family, friends, or other loved ones. Treatment programs may include individual, group, or family therapy, as well as 12-step programs.

LO 6 | Addressing Drug Misuse and Abuse in the United States

- The drug problem reaches everyone through crime and elevated health care costs. Public health and governmental approaches to the problem involve regulation, enforcement, education, and harm reduction.

POP QUIZ

Visit **MasteringHealth** to personalize your study plan with Chapter Review Quizzes and Dynamic Study Modules.

LO 1 | Drug Dynamics

1. Drugs that have the potential to alter mood or behavior are called
   a. recreational drugs.
   b. psychoactive drugs.
   c. psychotic drugs.
   d. dopamine reactor drugs.

LO 2 | Types of Drugs

2. Cross-tolerance occurs when
   a. drugs work at the same receptor site so that one blocks the action of the other.
   b. the effects of one drug are eliminated or reduced by the presence of another drug at the receptor site.
   c. a person develops a physiological tolerance to one drug and shows a similar tolerance to select other drugs as a result.
   d. two or more drugs interact and the effects of the individual drugs are multiplied beyond what normally would be expected if they were taken alone.
3. Rebecca takes a number of medications for various conditions, including Prinivil (for high blood pressure), insulin (a diabetic medication), and Claritin (an antihistamine). This is an example of
   a. synergism.
   b. illegal drug use.
   c. polydrug use.
   d. antagonism.
4. The most common method for taking drugs is
   a. injection.
   b. inhalation.
   c. oral ingestion.
   d. transdermal.

LO 3 | Using, Misusing, and Abusing Drugs

5. The most commonly reported illicit drug used on college campuses is
   a. Adderall.
   b. marijuana.
   c. Ecstasy.
   d. tranquilizers.

LO 4 | Common Drugs of Abuse

6. Which of the following is classified as a stimulant drug?
   a. Amphetamines
   b. Alcohol
   c. Marijuana
   d. LSD
7. *Freebasing* is
   a. mixing cocaine with heroin.
   b. burning heroin and inhaling the vapor.
   c. injecting a drug into the veins.
   d. burning cocaine and inhaling the vapor.

8. The psychoactive drug mescaline is found in what plant?
   a. Mushrooms
   b. Peyote cactus
   c. Marijuana
   d. Belladonna

LO 5 Treatment and Recovery

9. Generally, the first step in a drug treatment program is
   a. cognitive therapy.
   b. behavioral therapy.
   c. resocialization.
   d. detoxification.

LO 6 Addressing Drug Misuse and Abuse in the United States

10. Which of the following is an example of a *harm reduction strategy*?
    a. Providing clean needles and syringes to a heroin user
    b. Using scare tactics to show the negative consequences of drug use
    c. Enforcing antidrug laws
    d. Favoring longer prison sentences for drug dealers

Answers to the Pop Quiz can be found on page A-1. If you answered a question incorrectly, review the section identified by the Learning Outcome. For even more study tools, visit MasteringHealth.

THINK ABOUT IT!

LO 1 Drug Dynamics

1. Why and how do drugs work? What are some of the different ways that different types of drugs interact with brain chemistry?

LO 2 Types of Drugs

2. Explain the terms *synergism, antagonism,* and *inhibition.*

LO 3 Using, Misusing, and Abusing Drugs

3. Do you think there is such a thing as responsible use of illicit drugs? Would you change any of the current laws governing drugs? How would you determine what is legitimate and illegitimate use?
4. Why do you think so many young people today are abusing prescription drugs? Do you perceive prescription drug abuse as being less dangerous or illegal than illicit drug use? Why? Do you think this is an accurate or biased perception?

LO 4 Common Drugs of Abuse

5. What accounts for the fact that some drugs are more addictive than others, chemically, culturally, and psychologically?

LO 5 Treatment and Recovery

6. What could you do to help a friend who is fighting a substance abuse problem? What resources on your campus could help you?

LO 6 Addressing Drug Misuse and Abuse in the United States

7. What are the arguments for and against drug testing in the workplace? Would you apply for a job that had drug testing as an interview requirement? Why or why not?
8. What types of programs do you think would be effective in preventing drug abuse among high school and college students? How might programs for high school students differ from those for college students?

ACCESS YOUR HEALTH ON THE INTERNET

Visit **MasteringHealth** for links to the websites and RSS feeds.

The following websites explore further topics and issues related to personal health.

Club Drugs. The website provides science-based information about club drugs. **www.drugabuse.gov/drugs-abuse/club-drugs**

Join Together. This excellent site has the most current information related to substance abuse. It also includes information on alcohol and drug policy and provides advice on organizing and taking political action. **www.drugfree.org/join-together**

National Institute on Drug Abuse (NIDA). The home page of this U.S. government agency has information on the latest statistics and findings in drug research. **www.nida.nih.gov**

Substance Abuse and Mental Health Services Administration (SAMHSA). This website is an outstanding resource for information about national surveys, ongoing research, and national drug interventions. **www.samhsa.gov**

13 Protecting against Infectious Diseases

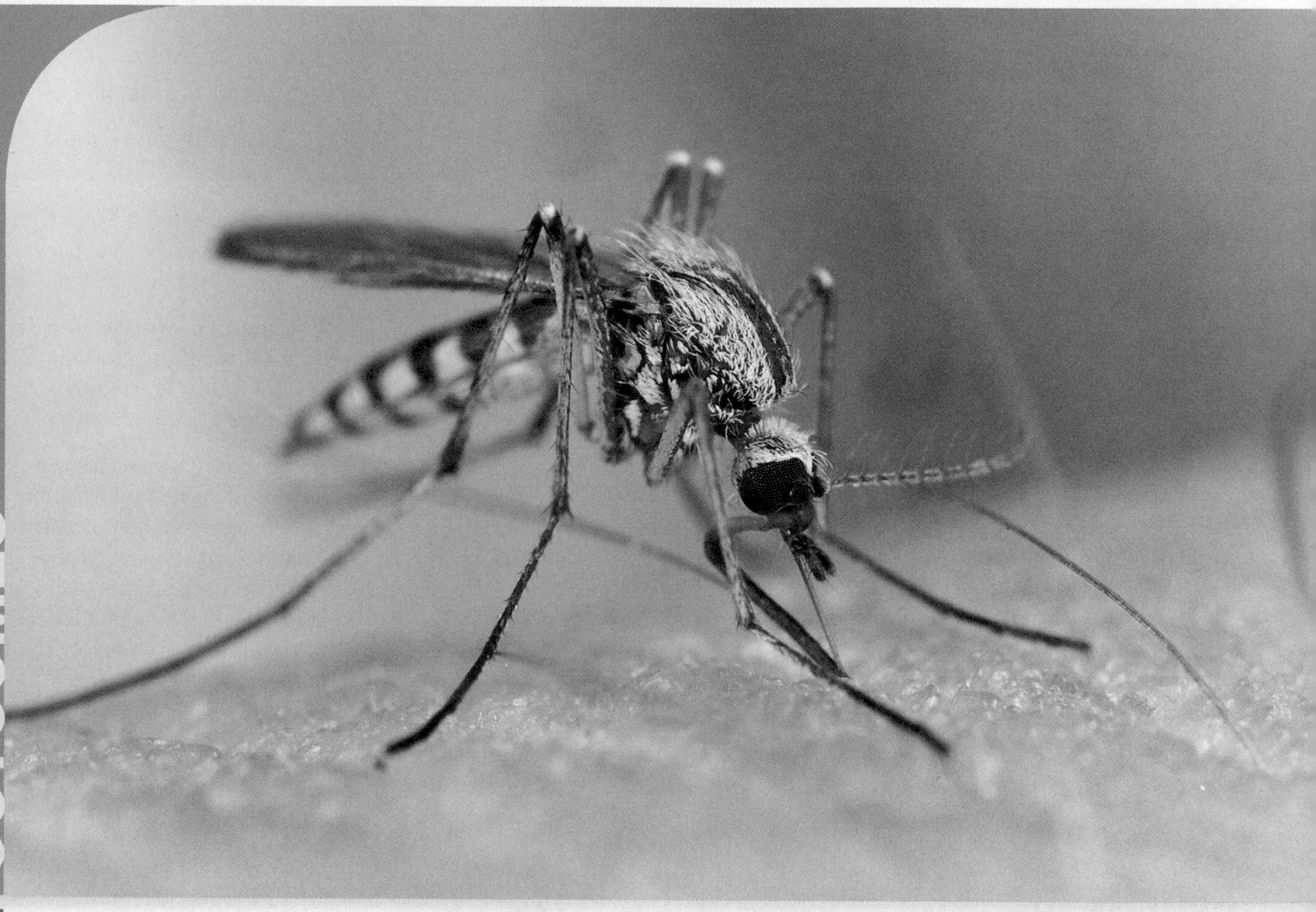

LEARNING OUTCOMES

1. Describe the process of infection and the risk factors for infectious diseases.
2. Explain how your immune system protects you, factors that diminish its effectiveness, and what you can do to boost its effectiveness.
3. Describe the most common pathogens infecting humans today, key diseases caused by each, and the threat of growing antimicrobial resistance as well as individual- and community-based strategies to reduce the threat of infectious diseases.

Throughout history, humans have faced wave after wave of infectious diseases, wiping out civilizations, killing the most vulnerable, and leaving their mark on survivors. Particularly powerful strains of *influenza* have emerged several times in our history, the most notable of which was the "Spanish Flu" of 1918–1919, affecting between 20 and 40 percent of the world's population and killing over 50 million people—675,000 of whom died in the United States.[1] Vaccines and other preventive strategies have kept large-scale deaths from influenza strains in check for decades; however, several new strains have emerged that could pose an ominous threat. *H1N1,* also known as *swine flu,* became a global threat in 2009. This new version—"novel *H1N1*"—was notably different from past strains in that it was reported to have killed over 500,000 people globally—mainly young, otherwise healthy adults.[2] Schools were closed, churches canceled services, and people feared the slightest cough or sneeze from others.

In 2013–2014, a new variant known as *pH1N1* struck in several regions of the world. Although fears of mutations that would allow an Armageddon-like jump of deadly new viruses swirl, so far these newer forms have remained primarily carried by their nonhuman hosts, often in isolated areas. One of the most recent threats, Middle Eastern Respiratory Syndrome (MERS), a potent respiratory disease that has spread primarily on the Arabian Peninsula, sickened two people in the United States and has migrated to other international locations. The virus causes severe coughing and congestion, and has killed over 30 percent of those infected in the Middle East. Health officials are monitoring this one closely.

With the advent of antibiotics, antivirals, and vaccinations, many envisioned a world where infectious diseases could become eradicated. However, in spite of massive educational campaigns, changes in sanitation and infection control, and major investments in vaccinations, infectious diseases continue to be among the leading causes of death globally. Fueled by media attention, worry over getting infected from others has prompted precautions such as elementary teachers wiping their students' hands after recess and grocery stores putting sanitary wipes next to their shopping carts. Sales of masks and antimicrobial wipes, soaps, and cleansers have soared. Is all of this anxiety over germs really necessary? Is the next great killer lurking, ready to kill millions and disrupt life as we know it? What are the most ominous threats that we currently face? Who is at greatest risk? How can we protect ourselves and our loved ones? What policies, agencies, and programs are currently in place to protect us? The old adage is probably the best advice: "To be *forewarned* (knowledgeable) is to be *forearmed* (prepared)."

Disease-causing agents, called **pathogens**, are everywhere—on every inch of our bodies, on everything we touch, smell, and taste. We inhale them, swallow them, rub them in our eyes, and are constantly in a hidden, high-stakes battle with them. Although many pathogens have existed as long as there has been life on the planet, new varieties of pathogens seem to be emerging daily. Some infectious diseases, like the common cold, are **endemic**, meaning that they are present at expected prevalence rates in virtually all populations on Earth, with rates that rise and fall predictably each season. When the number of cases of a disease increases, often suddenly, with higher than projected endemic numbers in a population area, it becomes an **epidemic**. Epidemics such as the Black Death, or bubonic plague, which killed up to one-third of the population of Europe in the 1300s, have been well documented. **Pandemics**, or global epidemics that occur in several continents at once, have been particularly devastating, striking again and again in different regions of the world. HIV, malaria, tuberculosis, and other pandemics continue to be major threats to human health today.

pathogen A disease-causing agent.

endemic Present at expected prevalence rates in a given population or area.

epidemic Disease outbreak that affects many people in a community or region at the same time.

pandemic Global epidemic of a disease that occurs in several countries at the same time.

virulent Strong enough to overcome host resistance and cause disease.

multifactorial disease Disease caused by interactions of several factors.

immunocompromised Having an immune system that is impaired.

Fortunately for us, despite constant bombardment by pathogens, our immune systems are remarkably adept at protecting us. Exposure to invading microorganisms actually helps us build resistance to various pathogens and teaches our immune systems to be more efficient. Millions of *endogenous microorganisms* live in and on our bodies all the time, usually in a symbiotic, peaceful coexistence. These are generally harmless to someone in good health, but can cause serious health problems for sick people or those with weakened immune systems.

Exogenous microorganisms are those that do not normally inhabit the body. When they do, they are apt to produce an infection or illness. The more easily these pathogens can gain a foothold in the body and sustain themselves, the more **virulent**, or aggressive, they may be in causing disease. By keeping your immune system strong, you increase your ability to resist and fight off even the most virulent pathogen.

LO 1 | THE PROCESS OF INFECTION

Describe the process of infection and the risk factors for infectious diseases.

Most diseases are **multifactorial**: They are caused by the interaction of several factors inside and outside the person. For a disease to occur, the person, or *host,* must be *susceptible,* which means that the immune system must be in a weakened condition (**immunocompromised**); an *agent* capable of *transmitting* a disease must be present; and the *environment*

HEAR IT! PODCASTS

Want a study podcast for this chapter? Download **Infectious and Noninfectious Conditions** available on MasteringHealth.™

autoinoculate Transmit a pathogen from one part of your body to another part.

zoonotic diseases Diseases of animals that may be transmitted to humans.

must be *hospitable* to the pathogen in terms of temperature, light, moisture, and other requirements. If, for example, you cut your arm, virulent pathogens breech the protective skin layer that normally keeps them out, and your immune system is weakened—that cut may become infected.

Routes of Transmission

Pathogens enter the body in several ways. They may be transmitted by *direct contact* between infected persons or by *indirect contact,* such as touching an object the infected person has had contact with. (**TABLE 13.1** lists common routes of transmission.) You may also **autoinoculate** yourself, or transmit a pathogen from one part of your body to another. For example, if you touch a herpes sore on your lip, you may transmit the virus to your eye when you scratch your itchy eyelid.

In addition to person-to-person transmission, your furry and feathered friends may also be sources of **zoonotic diseases** or diseases of animals that may be transmitted to humans. Dogs, cats, livestock, and wild animals can spread numerous diseases through their body fluids, bites, or feces or by carrying infected insects or pathogens into living areas and transmitting diseases either directly or indirectly. Although *interspecies transmission* of diseases (diseases passed from humans to animals and vice versa) is rare, it does occur. The Centers for Disease Control and Prevention's (CDC's) National Center for Emerging and Zoonotic Infectious Diseases (www.cdc.gov/ncezid) provides an excellent up-to-date overview of these diseases.

Risk Factors You Can Control

With all these pathogens floating around, how can you be sure you don't get sick? Fortunately, there are some things you can do to stay healthy. Too much stress, overuse of antibiotics, inadequate nutrition, a low fitness level, lack of sleep, drug misuse or abuse, poor personal hygiene, unsafe food handling, and other high-risk behaviors significantly increase the risk for many diseases. College students, in particular, often are at higher risk because of many of the above factors, in addition to the fact that alcohol and other drugs, increasing numbers of sexual experiences, and close living conditions all create higher risk for exposure to pathogens. The **Skills for Behavior Change** box lists some actions you can take to eliminate, reduce, or change your susceptibility to infections. There are also changes you can make in your community to clean up toxins; increase food safety; establish policies on contaminant levels in foods, water, and other household items; and reduce the likelihood of exposure to harmful pathogens or toxins. The chain of infection between pathogen, environment, and host presents multiple opportunities for individuals and communities to intercede and "break the chain," preventing and controlling disease transmission (see **FIGURE 13.1**).

TABLE **13.1** | Routes of Disease Transmission

Mode of Transmission	Aspects of Transmission
Contact	Either *direct* (e.g., skin or sexual contact) or *indirect* (e.g., infected blood or body fluid)
Foodborne or waterborne	Eating or coming in contact with contaminated food or water, or products passed through them
Airborne	Inhalation; droplet-spread as through sneezing, coughing, or talking
Vector-borne	Vector-transmitted via secretions, biting, egg laying, as done by mosquitoes, ticks, snails, or birds
Perinatal	Similar to contact infection; happens in the uterus or as the baby passes through the birth canal, or through breast-feeding

SKILLS FOR BEHAVIOR CHANGE

REDUCE YOUR RISK OF INFECTIOUS DISEASE

- **Limit exposure to pathogens.** Don't drag yourself to classes or work and infect others when you are seriously ill. Also, don't share towels, utensils, or drinking glasses, and keep your toothbrush away from those of others. Wash your hands often, and keep them away from your mouth, nose, and eyes. Keep purses and backpacks off of kitchen counters and restroom floors.
- **Exercise regularly.** Regular exercise raises core body temperature, strengthens the immune system, and kills pathogens. Sweat and oil make the skin a hostile environment for many bacteria.
- **Get enough sleep.** Sleep allows the body time to refresh itself, produce necessary cells, and reduce inflammation. Even a single night without sleep can increase inflammatory processes and delay wound healing.
- **Stress less.** Rest and relaxation, stress management practices, laughter, and calming music have all been shown to promote healthy cellular activity and bolster immune functioning.
- **Optimize eating.** Enjoy a balanced, healthy diet, including adequate amounts of water, protein, and complex carbohydrates. Eat more omega-3 fatty acids to reduce inflammation, and replace saturated fats with good fats such as olive oil. Antioxidants are believed to be important in immune functioning, so make sure you get your daily fruits and vegetables. Avoid excess alcohol, and use caution with over-the-counter remedies for boosting the immune system.

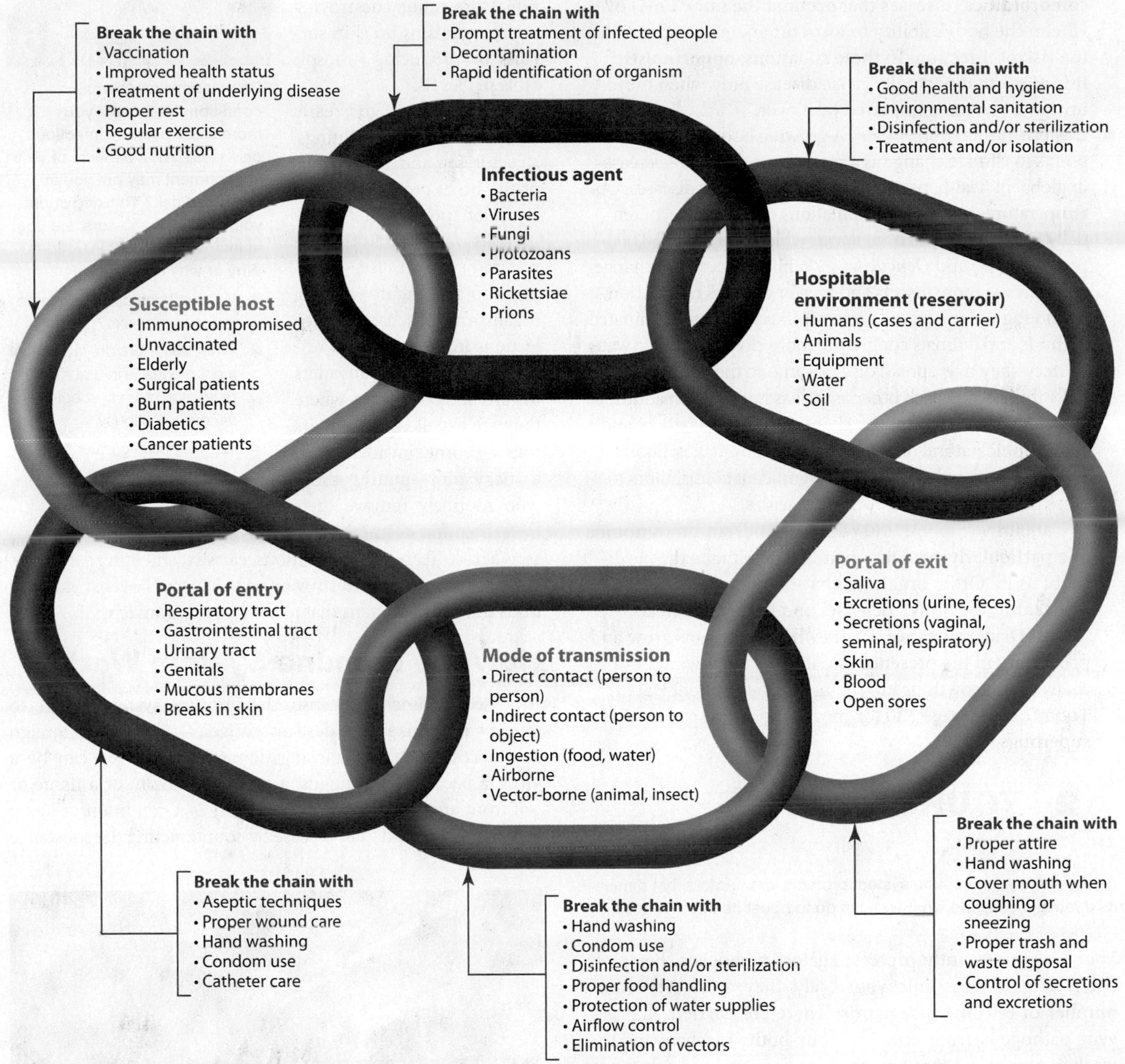

FIGURE 13.1 **The Chain of Infection** The three key factors in transmission of an infectious disease are a *susceptible host*, an *infectious agent*, and a *hospitable environment*. Connecting these three factors are the portal of entry, mode of transmission, and portal of exit. Interfering with any of the links in the chain can prevent the transmission of infectious disease.

VIDEO TUTOR
Chain of Infection

Risk Factors You Typically Cannot Control

Some of the factors that make you susceptible to a certain disease are either hard or impossible to control. The following are the most common:

- **Heredity.** One of the key factors influencing disease risk is genetics. It is often unclear whether hereditary diseases are due to inherited genetic traits or to inherited insufficiencies in the immune system. Some believe that we may inherit the quality of our immune system, making some people more resistant to disease and infection.
- **Age.** People under age 5 and over age 65 are often more vulnerable to infectious diseases because body defenses that we take for granted are either not fully developed or not as effective as they once were. Thinning of the skin, reduced sweating and oil gland secretions, and other physical changes can make the elderly more vulnerable to disease. In addition, as people age, certain

comorbidities (diseases that occur at the same time) overwhelm the body's ability to ward off enemies and increase the risk of infection. In these situations, **opportunistic infections** that normally cause disease only when the immune system is impaired take over.

- **Environmental conditions.** A growing body of research points to climate change as a major contributor to increases in global ill health, particularly from infectious diseases.[3] As temperatures rise, insect populations may increase, potentially increasing cases of *malaria* (which kills over 650,000 people a year) and *Dengue fever*. While temperature change often means more insects and greater chances of infection, dwindling water supplies are more likely to be contaminated. As birds and animals congregate more closely at scarce water sources, they may spread diseases among themselves, potentially threatening each other as well as humans.[4] In addition, long-term exposure to toxic chemicals, poor nutrition, and catastrophic natural disasters such as earthquakes, floods, and tsunamis are believed to be significant contributors to increasing numbers of infectious diseases.[5]
- **Organism virulence and resistance.** Even tiny amounts of a particularly virulent organism may make the hardiest of us ill. Other organisms have mutated and become resistant to the body's defenses and to medical treatments. **Drug resistance** occurs when pathogens grow and proliferate in the presence of chemicals that would normally slow growth or kill them. See the **Student Health Today** box on page 380 for more on drug resistance and superbugs.

LO 2 | YOUR BODY'S DEFENSES AGAINST INFECTION

Explain how your immune system protects you, factors that diminish its effectiveness, and what you can do to boost its effectiveness.

Your body constantly protects against pathogens. For pathogens to gain entry into your body, they must overcome a number of effective safeguards: There are barriers that prevent pathogens from entering your body, mechanisms that weaken organisms that breach these barriers, and substances that counteract the threat that pathogens pose. **FIGURE 13.2** summarizes some of the body's defenses.

comorbidities The presence of one or more diseases at the same time.

opportunistic infections Infections that occur when the immune system is weakened or compromised.

drug resistance That which occurs when microbes, such as bacteria, viruses, or other pathogens grow and proliferate in the presence of chemicals that would normally kill them or slow their growth.

antigen Substance capable of triggering an immune response.

Physical and Chemical Defenses

Our first line of defense is also the largest organ in the body: the skin. Structured to provide an intricate web of physical and chemical barriers, the skin allows few pathogens to enter. When they do breech this barrier, *enzymes* in body secretions such as sweat provide additional protection, destroying microorganisms on skin surfaces by producing inhospitable pH levels.

In addition to early defenses, internal linings, structures, and secretions of the body provide another layer of protection. Sticky mucous membranes in the respiratory tract, for example, trap and engulf invading organisms. Cilia, hairlike projections in the lungs and respiratory tract, sweep invaders toward body openings, where they are expelled. Nose hairs trap airborne invaders with a sticky film—putting those who routinely remove their nose hair for cosmetic reasons at risk. Tears, nasal secretions, earwax, and other secretions contain enzymes that destroy or neutralize pathogens. Stomach acids destroy pathogens that make it to the stomach.

WHAT DO YOU THINK?

Do you have any chronic conditions that make you more susceptible to infectious diseases? What aspects of your environment may put you at increased risk? Thinking about your lifestyle behaviors, are you at increased risk for infections? Why or why not?

- What actions can you take to reduce your risks?
- What behaviors do you or your friends engage in that might make you more susceptible to various infections?
- Are your risks greater today than before you entered college? Why or why not?

How the Immune System Works

As a second line of defense, the immune system is able to quickly recognize and destroy **antigens**—outside or foreign substances capable of causing disease. An antigen can be a virus, a bacterium, a fungus, a parasite, a toxin, or a tissue or cell from another organism. *Immunity* is a condition of being able to resist a particular disease by counteracting the substance

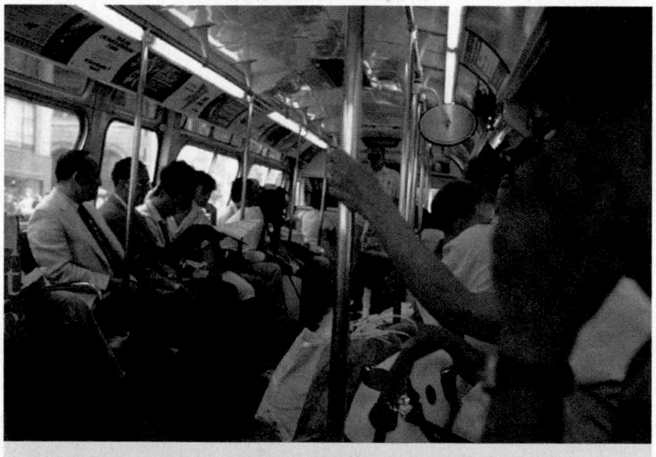

Vaccinations are key in protecting us from infectious diseases, yet many people "opt out" of recommended vaccines for religious or philosophical reasons. College students and those who live or routinely hang out in crowded areas, ride on public transportation, travel internationally, attend major sporting events or concerts, or spend time in hospitals where sick people congregate are more likely to come in contact with those who are sick. Keeping up-to-date on your vaccines is a big part of being responsible and protecting yourself and others.

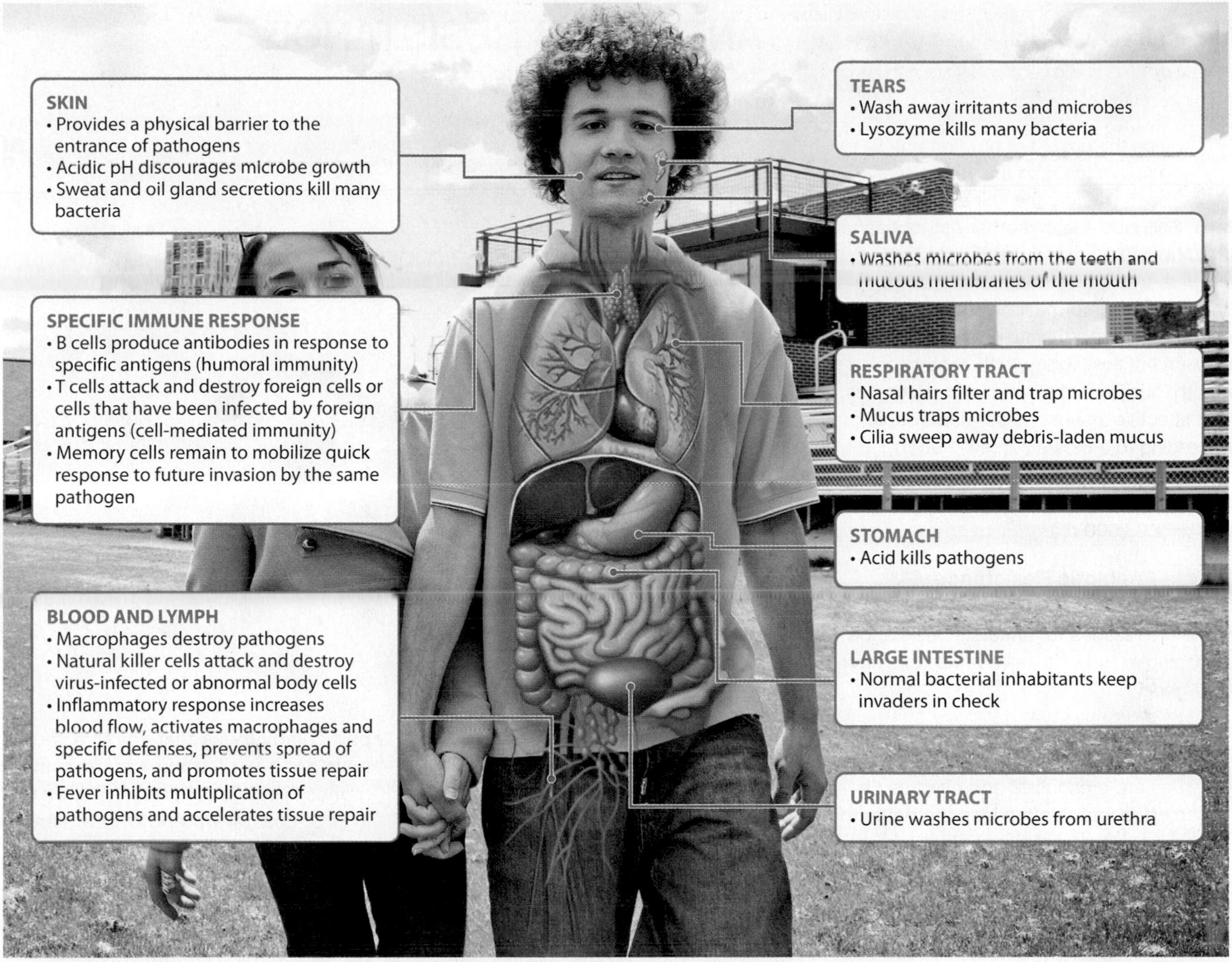
SKIN
• Provides a physical barrier to the entrance of pathogens
• Acidic pH discourages microbe growth
• Sweat and oil gland secretions kill many bacteria
SPECIFIC IMMUNE RESPONSE
• B cells produce antibodies in response to specific antigens (humoral immunity)
• T cells attack and destroy foreign cells or cells that have been infected by foreign antigens (cell-mediated immunity)
• Memory cells remain to mobilize quick response to future invasion by the same pathogen
BLOOD AND LYMPH
• Macrophages destroy pathogens
• Natural killer cells attack and destroy virus-infected or abnormal body cells
• Inflammatory response increases blood flow, activates macrophages and specific defenses, prevents spread of pathogens, and promotes tissue repair
• Fever inhibits multiplication of pathogens and accelerates tissue repair
TEARS
• Wash away irritants and microbes
• Lysozyme kills many bacteria
SALIVA
• Washes microbes from the teeth and mucous membranes of the mouth
RESPIRATORY TRACT
• Nasal hairs filter and trap microbes
• Mucus traps microbes
• Cilia sweep away debris-laden mucus
STOMACH
• Acid kills pathogens
LARGE INTESTINE
• Normal bacterial inhabitants keep invaders in check
URINARY TRACT
• Urine washes microbes from urethra

FIGURE 13.2 **The Body's Defenses against Disease-Causing Pathogens** In addition to the defenses listed, many of the body's defensive secretions and fluids, such as earwax, tears, mucus, and blood, contain enzymes and other proteins that can kill some invading pathogens or prevent or slow their reproduction.

that produces the disease. The immune system has elaborate mechanisms for protecting you from invading microbes.

As soon as an antigen breaches the body's initial defenses, the body responds by forming substances called **antibodies** that are matched to that specific antigen, much as a key is matched to a lock. The body analyzes the antigen, considers the size and shape of the invader, verifies that the antigen is not part of the body itself, and then produces a specific antibody to destroy or weaken the antigen. This process is part of a complex system called *humoral immune responses.* **Humoral immunity** is the body's major defense against many bacteria and the toxins—poisonous substances—they produce.

In **cell-mediated immunity**, specialized white blood cells called **lymphocytes** attack and destroy the foreign invader. Lymphocytes constitute the body's main defense against viruses, fungi, parasites, and some bacteria, and they are found in the blood, lymph nodes, bone marrow, and certain glands. Other key players in this immune response are **macrophages** (a type of phagocytic, or cell-eating, white blood cell).

Two forms of lymphocytes in particular, the *B lymphocytes* (B cells) and *T lymphocytes* (T cells), are involved in the immune response. *Helper T cells* are essential for activating B cells to produce antibodies. They also activate other T cells and macrophages. Another form of T cell, known as the *killer T cell,* directly attacks infected or malignant cells. *Suppressor T cells* turn off or suppress the activity of B cells, killer T cells, and macrophages. After a successful attack on a pathogen, some of the attacker T and B cells are preserved as *memory T and B cells,* enabling the body to recognize and respond quickly to subsequent attacks by the same kind of organism.

antibodies Substances produced by the body that are individually matched to specific antigens.

humoral immunity Aspect of immunity that is mediated by antibodies secreted by white blood cells.

cell-mediated immunity Aspect of immunity that is mediated by specialized white blood cells that attack pathogens and antigens directly.

lymphocyte A type of white blood cell involved in the immune response.

macrophage A type of white blood cell that ingests foreign material.

STUDENT HEALTH TODAY

ANTIBIOTIC RESISTANCE

Bugs Versus Drugs

Since the advent of our first antibiotic, penicillin, in the 1920s, we've been winning the war against bacteria. Still, bacteria and other pathogens learn how to outmaneuver the drugs we throw at them; they adapt and change, share genetic information with other bacteria, and morph into stronger, more resilient entities. Today, with each passing month, our arsenal of antibiotics becomes less effective against these "superbugs." According to a recent "Threat Report," over 2 million people in the United States are infected with super-bugs each year, and over 23,000 die.

To prevent the spread of infectious disease, wash your hands and keep your hands away from your eyes, nose, and mouth!

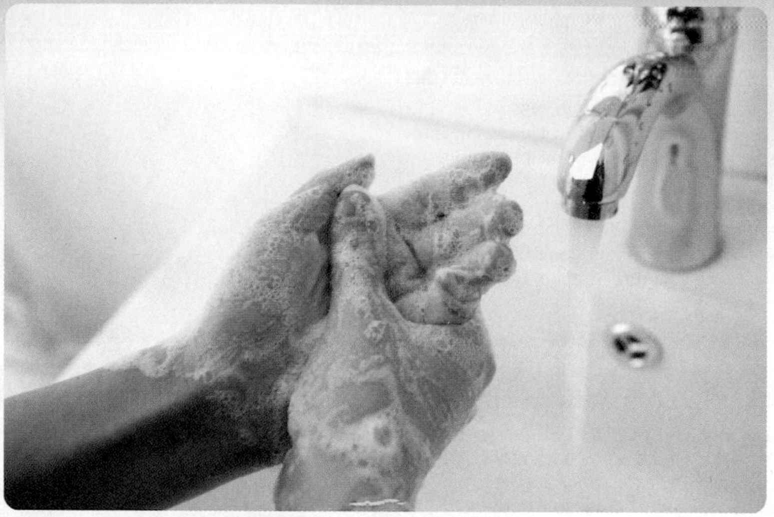

Why Is Antibiotic Resistance on the Rise?

While the reasons for antibiotic resistance are complex, several key contributors have emerged:

- **Improper use of antibiotics and resulting growth of superbugs.** When drugs are prescribed and used as directed, bacteria often lose the battle to survive. However, prescription misuse can speed the natural evolution of resistance. Quitting your prescription as soon as you feel better can result in killing off weaker bacteria, but allowing tougher, more drug-resistant ones to survive. Doctors who overprescribe antibiotics or give them for virally caused diseases also contribute to antibiotic resistance.
- **Overuse of antibiotics in food production.** About 70 percent of antibiotic production today is used to treat sick animals and to encourage growth in livestock, poultry, and even farmed fish. Many believe that ingesting animal products full of antibiotics may contribute to resistance in humans. In addition, water runoff and sewage from feedlots can contaminate rivers and streams with antibiotics. A growing problem is the use of antibiotics to treat household pets. Many of these prescriptions go unused and are dumped in toilets and garbage, posing a threat to community water systems.
- **Misuse and overuse of antibacterial soaps and other cleaning products.** Preying on the public's fear of germs and disease, the cleaning industry adds antibacterial ingredients to many of its dish soaps, hand cleaners, shower scrubs, surface scrubs, and most household products. Just how much these products contribute to overall resistance is difficult to assess; as with antibiotics, the germs these products do not kill may become stronger than before.

What Can You Do?

- **Get regular vaccinations.** If someone in your house has a resistant bacterial infection, be careful about hand washing and general hygiene. Don't share towels or personal items.
- **Be responsible with medications.** Take medications as prescribed and finish the full course. Talk to your local pharmacist or waste disposal company about how to dispose of unused drugs.
- **Use regular soap—not antibacterial soap—when washing your hands.** Research suggests that antibacterial agents contained in soaps actually may kill normal bacteria, thus creating an environment for resistant, mutated bacteria impervious to antibacterial cleaners and antibiotics.
- **Avoid food treated with antibiotics.** Buy organic meat and poultry, particularly those that say that they have not been fed antibiotics or hormones. Look for farmed fish grown in U.S. coastal waters, where there is less likelihood of questionable fish feeding practice, contaminated waters, and antibiotics or growth hormones.
- **Be Safe in the Kitchen.** Wash hands after handling uncooked meats and keep hands away from your eyes, nose, and mouth. Cook meats thoroughly.

Sources: CDC, "Antibiotic Resistance Threats in the United States, 2013," September 2013, www.cdc.gov/features/antibioticresistancethreats/; D. Meeker et al., "Nudging Guideline-Concordant Antibiotic Prescribing: A Randomized Clinical Trial," *JAMA Internal Medicine* (January 2014), 174 (3): 425–31; Association for Professionals in Infection Control and Epidemiology, "Responsible Use of Antibiotics," 2013, www.apic.org; Association for Professionals in Infection Control and Epidemiology, "Antibiotics, Preserving Them for the Future," 2012, www.apic.org; Centers for Disease Control and Prevention, National Center for Emerging and Zoonotic Infectious Diseases, Division of Healthcare Quality Promotion, "Diseases/Pathogens Associated with Antimicrobial Resistance," Updated January, 2013, www.cdc.gov/drugresistance/diseasesconnectedar.html; Centers for Disease Control and Prevention, National Center for Immunization and Respiratory Diseases, Division of Bacterial Diseases, "Antibiotic Resistance Questions & Answers," Updated November 2011, www.cdc.gov/getsmart/antibiotic-use/anitbiotic-resistance-faqs.html.

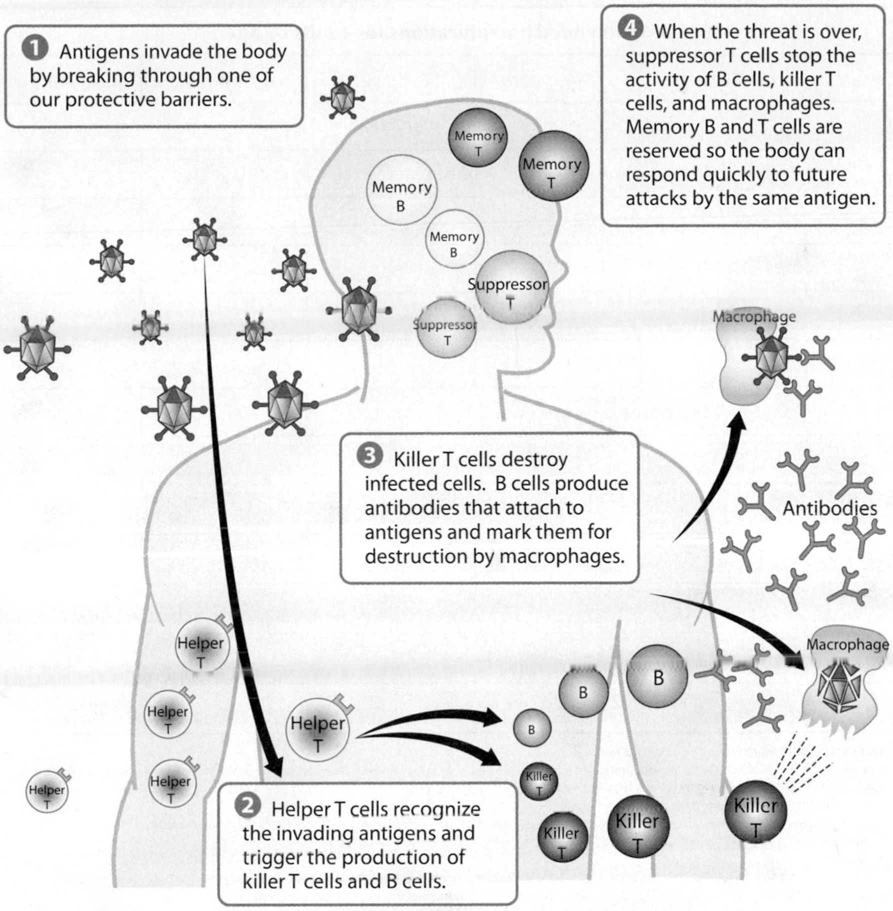

1 Antigens invade the body by breaking through one of our protective barriers.
4 When the threat is over, suppressor T cells stop the activity of B cells, killer T cells, and macrophages. Memory B and T cells are reserved so the body can respond quickly to future attacks by the same antigen.
Memory T
Memory T
Memory B
Memory B
Suppressor T
Suppressor T
Macrophage
3 Killer T cells destroy infected cells. B cells produce antibodies that attach to antigens and mark them for destruction by macrophages.
Antibodies
Macrophage
Helper T
Helper T
Helper T
Helper T
Helper T
B
B
B
Killer T
Killer T
Killer T
Killer T
2 Helper T cells recognize the invading antigens and trigger the production of killer T cells and B cells.

FIGURE 13.3 Overview of the Cell-Mediated Immune Response

Once people have survived certain infectious diseases, they become immune to those diseases, meaning they will likely not develop them again. Upon subsequent attack by the same disease-causing microorganisms, their memory T and B cells are quickly activated to come to their defense. **FIGURE 13.3** provides a summary of the cell-mediated immune response.

When the Immune System Misfires: Autoimmune Diseases Although the immune response generally works in our favor, the body sometimes makes a mistake and targets its own tissue as the enemy. This is known as **autoimmune disease** (*auto* means "self"). The National Institutes of Health estimates that over 32 million Americans have *autoantibodies*, which are proteins made by the immune system that target the body's tissues. Their presence can indicate autoimmunity, in many cases well before the symptoms of autoimmune diseases actually begin.[6] Researchers estimate that there are between 80 and 140 different types of autoimmune disease, many of which are chronic, debilitating, and life threatening. They can affect virtually any part of the body and cause disability and death. Some of the most common autoimmune diseases include type 1 Diabetes (see **Focus On: Minimizing Your Risk for Diabetes** for more on this disease), rheumatoid arthritis, psoriasis, Graves disease, multiple sclerosis, Guillain-Barré syndrome, lupus, celiac disease, Crohn disease, and irritable bowel syndrome. Many people do not realize that autoimmune diseases are among the leading causes of death in female children and women under the age of 65 in the United States.[7] (See **Chapter 17**.)

WHY SHOULD I CARE?

An increasing number of chronic diseases are being linked to the inflammation that occurs when certain pathogens invade. Avoiding infections and their inflammatory side effects now has the added benefit that it may help you avoid certain chronic diseases later.

Inflammatory Response, Pain, and Fever If an infection is localized, pus formation, redness, swelling, and inflammation often occur. These symptoms, part of the body's inflammatory response, indicate that the invading organisms are being fought systemically. The four cardinal signs of inflammation are *redness, swelling, pain,* and *heat*.

Pain is often one of the earliest signs that an injury or infection has occurred. Pathogens can kill or injure tissue at the site of infection, causing swelling that puts pressure on nerve endings in the area, causing pain. Pain plays a valuable, protective role in the body's response to injury or invasion by signaling to you that something is wrong and causing you to reduce or avoid activities that can aggravate the injury or site of infection.

In addition to *inflammation*, another frequent indicator of infection is *fever*, or a body temperature above the average norm of 98.6°F. Fever is frequently caused by toxins secreted by pathogens that interfere with the control of body temperature. Although extremely elevated temperatures are harmful to the body, a mild fever is protective: Raising body temperature by 1 or 2 degrees provides an environment that destroys some disease-causing organisms. A fever also stimulates the body to produce more white blood cells, which destroy more invaders. As fevers increase beyond 101 or 102°F, risks to the patient outweigh any fever benefits, and medical treatment should be obtained.

autoimmune disease Disease caused by an overactive immune response against the body's own cells.

vaccination Inoculation with killed or weakened pathogens or similar, less dangerous antigens to prevent or lessen the effects of some disease.

Vaccines Bolster Immunity

Recall that once people have been exposed to a specific pathogen, subsequent attacks will activate their memory T and B cells, thus giving them immunity. This is the principle on which **vaccination** is based.

<table>
<tr><th></th><th colspan="6">2014 recommended immunizations for adults by age</th></tr>
<tr><th>Vaccine</th><th>19–21 years</th><th>22–26 years</th><th>27–49 years</th><th>50–59 years</th><th>60–64 years</th><th>65+ years</th></tr>
<tr><td>Influenza (Flu)[1]</td><td colspan="6">Get a flu vaccine every year</td></tr>
<tr><td>Tetanus, diphtheria, pertussis (Td/Tdap)2</td><td colspan="6">Get a Tdap vaccine once, then a Td booster vaccine every 10 years</td></tr>
<tr><td>Varicella (Chickenpox)[3]</td><td colspan="6">2 doses</td></tr>
<tr><td>HPV Vaccine for Women[3,4]</td><td colspan="2">3 doses</td><td></td><td></td><td></td><td></td></tr>
<tr><td>HPV Vaccine for Men[3,4]</td><td>3 doses</td><td>3 doses</td><td></td><td></td><td></td><td></td></tr>
<tr><td>Zoster (Shingles)[5]</td><td></td><td></td><td></td><td></td><td colspan="2">1 dose</td></tr>
<tr><td>Measles, mumps, rubella (MMR)[3]</td><td colspan="4">1 or 2 doses</td><td></td><td></td></tr>
<tr><td>Pneumococcal (PCV13)[7]</td><td colspan="6">1 dose</td></tr>
<tr><td>Pneumococcal (PPSV23)[7]</td><td colspan="5">1 or 2 doses</td><td>1 dose</td></tr>
<tr><td>Meningococcal</td><td colspan="6">1 or more doses</td></tr>
<tr><td>Hepatitis A[3]</td><td colspan="6">2 doses</td></tr>
<tr><td>Hepatitis B[3]</td><td colspan="6">3 doses</td></tr>
<tr><td>Haemophilus influenzae type b (Hib)</td><td colspan="6">1 or 3 doses</td></tr>
</table>

1. Influenza vaccine: There are several flu vaccines available—talk to your healthcare professional about which flu vaccine is right for you.
2. Td/Tdap vaccine: Pregnant women are recommended to get tdap vaccine with each pregnancy in the third trimester to increase protection for infants who are too young for vaccination, but at highest risk for severe illness and death from pertussis (whooping cough). People who have not had Tdap vaccine since age 11 should get a dose of Tdap followed by TD booster doses every 10 years.
3. Varicella, HPV, MMR, Hepatitis A, Hepatitis B vaccine: These vaccines are needed for adults who didn't get these vaccines when they were children.
4. HPV vaccine: There are two HPV vaccines, but only one, HPV (Gardasilr), should be given to men. Gay men or men who have sex with men who are 22 through 26 years old should get HPV vaccine if they haven't already started or completed the series.
5. Zoster vaccine: You should get the zoster vaccine even if you've had shingles before.
6. MMR vaccine: If you were born in 1957 or after, and don't have a record of being vaccinated or having had these infections, talk to your healthcare professional about how many doses you may need.
7. Pneumococcal vaccine: There are two different types of pneumococcal vaccines: PCV13 and PPSV23. Talk with your healthcare professional to find out if one or both pneumococcal vaccines are recommneded for you.

If you travel outside of the United States, you may need additional vaccines. Ask your healthcare professional which vaccines you may need.
For more information, call toll free 1-800-CDC-INFO (1-800-232-4636) or visit http://www.cdc.gov/vaccines

Boxes this color show that the vaccine is recommended for all adults who have not been vaccinated, unless your healthcare professional tells you that you cannot safely receive the vaccine or that you do not need it.

Boxes this color show when the vaccine is recommended for adults with certain risks related to their health, job or lifestyle that put them at higher risk for serious diseases. Talk to your halthcare professional to see if you are at higher risk.

No recommendation

FIGURE 13.4 **Recommended Adult Immunization Schedule, by Vaccine and Age Group, 2014** Note there are important explanations and additions to these recommendations that should be consulted by checking the latest schedule at www.cdc.gov/vaccines/recs/schedules/adult-schedule.htm.

Source: Centers for Disease Control and Prevention, "Recommended Adult Immunization Schedule, by Vaccine and Age Group, United States, 2014," Updated February 2014, www.cdc.gov/vaccines/schedules/hcp/imz/adult.html.

A vaccine consists of killed or weakened versions of a disease-causing microorganism or an antigen that is similar to but less dangerous than the disease antigen. It is administered to stimulate the person's immune system to produce antibodies against future attacks—without actually causing the disease (or by causing a very minor case of it). Vaccines typically are given orally or by injection, and this form of immunity is termed *artificially acquired active immunity,* in contrast to *naturally acquired active immunity* (which is obtained by exposure to antigens in the normal course of daily life) or *naturally acquired passive immunity* (as occurs when a mother passes immunity to her fetus via their shared blood supply or to an infant via breast milk).

Specific vaccination schedules have been established for various population groups. See **FIGURE 13.4** for the recommended vaccination schedule for the general adult population. Childhood vaccine schedules are available at the CDC website. Concern about the safety of vaccines and religious opposition have caused an increase in the number of parents who refuse to vaccinate their children (see the **Health Headlines** box).

@ HEALTH HEADLINES

VACCINE CONTROVERSY *Should Parents Be Allowed to Opt Out?*

Immunizations against widespread infectious diseases are one of the greatest public health success stories of all time—so successful, in fact, that most people have never seen or heard of anyone having diseases such as smallpox that once wiped out entire populations. Today, fear of the old "killer" diseases has waned and been replaced with distrust of the vaccines themselves, leading to a growing trend for parents to "opt out" of vaccinations for their children, even though failure to vaccinate puts children and communities at risk.

Why opt out? Typical reasons for vaccine exemptions include religious beliefs, personal beliefs, and medical reasons, while others consider vaccinations to be a government intrusion into their individual rights. In some states, exemptions have been as easy to get as checking a box on a form. With the proliferation of misleading information about supposed dangers of vaccination, many mistakenly believe that they are doing the right thing by avoiding some or all vaccines.

Undervaccination rates are particularly high in non-Hispanic, college-educated white families with incomes above $75,000 a year. In recent years, exemption rates in states like California and Oregon have increased significantly, with corresponding increases in childhood diseases. In 2009, when exemption rates skyrocketed to nearly 8 percent, Washington State passed a law requiring a doctor's signature to opt out of vaccinations. Today, Washington has one of the highest vaccine rates in the country, along with Vermont, Massachusetts, Florida, and New Hampshire, as these states make exemptions more difficult to obtain.

Some parents have expressed concern over the safety of vaccinations; however, the vast majority of public health professionals believe they are essential.

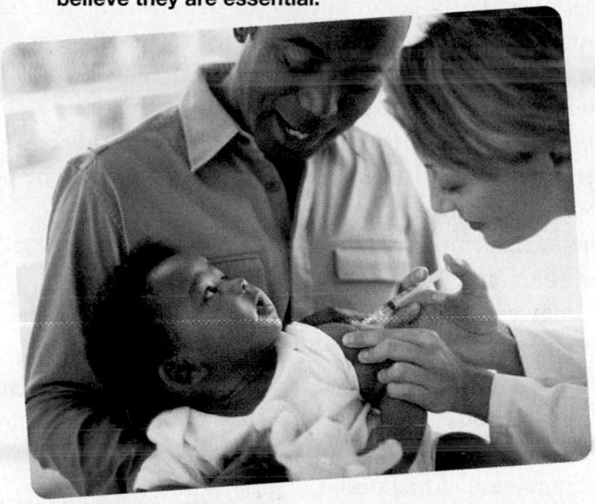

Much initial anxiety was fueled by an article in the medical journal *Lancet* in 1998, linking the MMR vaccine to increased risk of autism and bowel disease. The article prompted many to refuse the vaccine in the United States and elsewhere, and the resulting drop-off in immunizations led to increased cases of measles in many parts of the world. Over 10 years later, after a thorough investigation of ethical and factual issues with the research, *Lancet* retracted the article as being false. The lead author of the paper was later fired from his research position and had his license to practice revoked.

While research is ongoing, the Centers for Disease Control and Prevention (CDC) has found no evidence to substantiate claims that vaccines lead to conditions like autism, multiple sclerosis, or sudden infant death syndrome. Virtually all medical and public health organizations support vaccinations, pointing to stringent safety controls in the manufacturing and testing of vaccines, as well as ongoing safety monitoring and the long history of vaccines in wiping out killer diseases across the globe. If large numbers of people were to avoid vaccinations, old killers would be likely to reemerge, and those people who were already sick or weak from other conditions would be extremely vulnerable.

Today, the CDC's Immunization Safety Office monitors complaints and investigates potential problems with vaccines as they occur. Still, the danger of major complications from getting vaccinations is extremely low, and generally pales in comparison to the effects of contracting the diseases that the vaccinations protect against.

Sources: S. Omer et al., "Legislative Challenges to School Immunization Mandates, 2009–2012," *JAMA* 3111, no. 6 (2014): 620–21; Centers for Disease Control and Prevention, "Vaccine Safety: Concerns about Autism," Modified March 2012, www.cdc.gov/vaccinesafety/Concerns/Autism/Index.html; The Editors of the *Lancet*, "Retraction—Ileal-lymphoid-nodular hyperplasia, non-specific colitis, and pervasive development disorder in Children," *Lancet* 375, no. 9713 (2010): 445; Centers for Disease Control and Prevention, National Immunization Survey, 2010–2011, Accessed May 2014, www.cdc.gov/nchs/nis.htm; S. Robinson, H. Groom, and C. Young, "Frequency of Alternative Immunization Schedule Use in a Metropolitan Area," *Pediatrics*, 130(32:32–138) (2012); S. Bean, "Vaccine Beliefs of Complementary and Alternative Medical (CAM) Providers in Oregon, Doctoral Dissertation, Oregon State University, May 2014; V. Martinez-Sernandez, and A. Figueiras, "Central Nervous System Demyelinating disease and recombinant hepatitis B. Vaccinations: A critical systematic review of scientific production," *Journal of Neurology* 260 (1951–1959) (2013).

Because of their close living quarters and frequent interactions with people, college students face a higher than average risk of infection from diseases that are largely preventable. If you aren't up to date on your vaccines or never had them, catch-up vaccines that should be a priority among 20-somethings include *tetanus-diphtheria-pertussis vaccine (Tdap); meningococcal conjugate vaccine (MCV4); human papillomavirus (HPV)*; the *influenza vaccine; hepatitis A and B; measles, mumps, and rubella (MMR); polio; and Varicella.*[8]

Allergies: The Immune System Overreacts

An **allergy** occurs as part of the body's attempt to defend itself against a specific *antigen* or **allergen** by producing specific *antibodies*. The production of antibodies is usually

allergy Hypersensitive reaction to a specific antigen in which the body produces antibodies to a normally harmless substance.

allergen An antigen that induces a hypersensitive immune response.

histamine Chemical substance that dilates blood vessels, increases mucous secretions, and produces other symptoms of allergies.

immunotherapy Treatment strategies based on the concept of regulating the immune system by administering antibodies or desensitizing shots of allergens.

allergist Medical doctor specialty focusing on the diagnosis and treatment of allergies.

bacteria (singular: *bacterium*) Simple, single-celled microscopic organisms; about 100 known species of bacteria cause disease in humans.

antibiotics Medicines used to kill microorganisms, such as bacteria.

antibiotic resistance The ability of bacteria or other microbes to withstand the effects of an antibiotic.

a positive part of the body's defense system. However, in some people, the body overreacts by developing an overly protective mechanism against relatively harmless substances. The resulting *hypersensitivity reaction* is fairly common, as anyone who has awakened with a runny nose or itchy eyes will testify. Most commonly, these hypersensitivity, or allergic, reactions occur as a response to environmental antigens such as molds, animal dander (hair and dead skin), pollen, ragweed, or dust. Some people are also allergic to certain foods. (See **Chapter 7** for more about food allergies.) Once excessive antibodies to allergens are produced, they trigger the release of **histamine**, a chemical that dilates blood vessels, increases mucous secretions, causes tissues to swell, and produces rashes, difficulty breathing, and other allergy symptoms. Many people have found that **immunotherapy** treatment, or "allergy shots," somewhat reduce the severity of their symptoms. In most cases, once the offending antigen has disappeared, allergy-prone people suffer few symptoms. One of the more common allergic reactions affecting humans is hay fever. See **Chapter 17** on chronic conditions for other allergy-related chronic problems.

Hay Fever Hay fever, or *seasonal allergic rhinitis,* occurs throughout the world and is one of the most common chronic diseases in the United States, affecting nearly 17.6 million adults and nearly 7 million children every year.[9] It is most prevalent when pollen levels are high from ragweed, flowers, and grasses. Hay fever attacks are characterized by sneezing and itchy, watery eyes and nose. You are more likely to have hay fever if you have a family history of allergies or asthma, are male, were exposed to cigarette smoke during your first year of life, or live or work in environments where allergens are constantly present.

Typical over-the-counter treatment consists of antihistamines. These work well for mild cases, but may become less effective over time. Air-conditioning, whole house air filters, air purifiers, and other options can also help relieve symptoms. To determine if you have pollen allergy, the best bet is to get tested by an **allergist**—a doctor specializing in allergies. Typical treatments include prescription medications and/or allergy shots. While allergy shots are one of the most effective ways of treatment, side effects are possible and doctors recommend them for limited time periods.[10]

LO 3 | TYPES OF PATHOGENS AND THE DISEASES THEY CAUSE

Describe the most common pathogens infecting humans today, key diseases caused by each, and the threat of growing antimicrobial resistance as well as individual- and community-based strategies to reduce the threat of infectious diseases.

We can categorize pathogens into six major types: bacteria, viruses, fungi, protozoans, parasitic worms, and prions. Each has a particular route of transmission and unique characteristic elements. **FIGURE 13.5** shows examples of several of these pathogens.

Bacteria

Bacteria (singular: *bacterium*) are simple, single-celled organisms. There are three major types of bacteria, which are classified by their shape: *cocci, bacilli,* and *spirilla.* Although there are several thousand known species of bacteria (and many thousands more that are unknown), just over 100 cause disease in humans. In many cases, it is not the bacteria themselves that cause disease but rather the toxins that they produce.

Antibiotics are among the potent groups of drugs designed to fight and kill specific bacteria. However, overuse and misuse of antibiotics has led to **antibiotic resistance**, in which successive generations of bacteria change or adapt so that

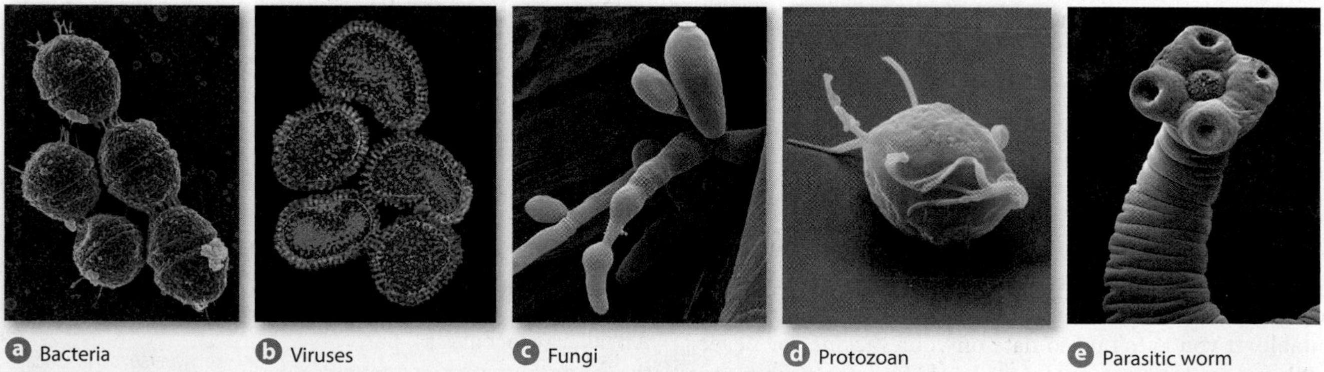

(a) Bacteria (b) Viruses (c) Fungi (d) Protozoan (e) Parasitic worm

FIGURE 13.5 Examples of Five Major Types of Pathogens (a) Color-enhanced scanning electron micrograph (SEM) of *Streptococcus* bacteria, magnified 40,000×. (b) Colored transmission electron micrograph (TEM) of influenza (flu) viruses, magnified 32,000×. (c) Color SEM of *Candida albicans,* a yeast fungus, magnified 50,000×. (d) Color TEM of *Trichomonas vaginalis,* a protozoan, magnified 9,000×. (e) Color-enhanced SEM of a tapeworm, magnified 50×.

SEE IT! VIDEOS

How can you protect yourself from a staph infection? Watch **Toxic Staph Outbreak** available on MasteringHealth.™

antibiotics are less effective in killing them. Many believe that antibiotic resistance is one of the world's greatest problems and that we may lose our ability to fight bacteria at rates faster than our ability to develop more powerful antibiotics. Even as antibiotic use has declined in the United States in the last decade, the percentage of bacteria that are resistant continues to increase. Each year, over 2 million people contract antibiotic-resistant infections, and 23,000 die as a direct result.[11] Many more die as a result of other health problems that become more complicated as a result of these infections, such as hip replacements that become infected and lead to slow or no recovery.[12]

Staphylococcal Infections

Staphylococci are among the most common bacterial pathogens causing diseases in humans. They are normally present on the skin or in the nostrils of most people at any given time and usually present no problems for otherwise healthy persons. The presence of bacteria on or in a person without infection is called **colonization**. A colonized person can be a carrier, spreading infection to others, yet never develop the disease. Additionally, when the pathogen is present and there is a cut or break in the *epidermis,* or outer layer of the skin, staphylococci may enter the system and cause an **infection**. If you have ever suffered from acne, boils, sties (infections of the eyelids), or infected wounds, you have probably had a "staph" infection.

Although most of these pathogens are handily nixed by the immune system, resistant forms are on the rise. One of these resistant forms of staph, **methicillin-resistant *Staphylococcus aureus*** **(MRSA)**, has come under intense international scrutiny as numerous cases have arisen around the world, especially in the United States.[13] There were over 80,000 cases of MRSA in the United States in 2013, with nearly 11,300 deaths.[14] Symptoms of MRSA infection often start with a rash or pimple-like skin irritation. Within hours, early symptoms may progress to redness, inflammation, pain, and deeper wounds. If untreated, MRSA may invade the blood, bones, joints, surgical wounds, heart valves, and lungs, and can be fatal.[15]

In the past, most cases of MRSA were contracted in health care facilities such as hospitals, nursing homes, or clinics; these are known as *health care–associated MRSA (HA-MRSA).* However, growing numbers of cases are appearing among people who have not sought medical treatment. Known as *community-acquired MRSA (CA-MRSA),* this form of MRSA is a growing concern. Finally, linezolid-resistant *Staphylococcus aureus,* or LRSA, is a particularly potent bacterium that has evolved among patients using one of the last effective antibiotics, linezolid, as treatment for MRSA. Reports of deaths from LRSA in many regions of the world are on the rise. Questions about what happens when linezolid no longer works and the antibiotic "well" runs dry have raised red flags for health professionals everywhere. People recovering from surgery, those with weakened immune systems, and those with underlying respiratory problems may be at tremendous risk if this resistant form of MRSA remains unchecked.

Three Urgent Resistant Bacterial Threats

Clostridium difficile (C. difficile) is a highly resistant bacteria that affects the intestinal tract, causing diarrhea and serious complications. It is responsible for over 250,000 hospitalizations and 14,000 deaths per year.[16] In most infections, patients had been on long-term antibiotic treatment that eventually led to resistance. Stopping antibiotic treatment is a key part of treatment for many victims; however, in some cases, other antibiotic regimens are necessary.

Although Enterobacteriaceae have been effectively treated for years, a newer strain, known as **carbapenem-resistant Enterobacteriaceae (CRE),** has proven to be highly resistant to nearly all conventional antibiotics. CRE was responsible for over 9,000 hospitalizations and 600 deaths in 2013.[17] **Drug-resistant *Neisseria gonorrhoeae*** is the third urgent resistant bacterial threat in the United States, affecting nearly 250,000 people each year.[18]

Streptococcal Infections

At least five types of the ***Streptococcus*** microorganism are known to cause infections. Group A streptococci (GAS) cause the most common diseases, such as streptococcal pharyngitis ("strep throat") and scarlet fever.[19] One particularly virulent group of GAS can lead to rare but serious diseases such as *toxic shock syndrome,* which can cause dramatic drops in blood pressure and death, or *necrotizing fasciitis* (often referred to as "flesh-eating strep").[20] Group B streptococci can cause illness in newborn babies, pregnant women, older adults, and adults with illnesses like diabetes or liver disease. A form of resistant *Streptococcus pneumoniae* is a leading cause of bacterial pneumonia, as well as ear infections, sinus infections, and bloodstream infections or "*sepsis.*"

Meningitis

Meningitis is an infection and inflammation of the *meninges,* the membranes that surround the brain and spinal cord. Some forms of bacterial meningitis are contagious and can be spread through contact with saliva, nasal discharge, feces, or respiratory and throat secretions. *Pneumococcal meningitis,* the most common form of the disease, is also the most dangerous. *Meningococcal meningitis,* a virulent form of meningitis, remains prevalent on college campuses.[21] Although meningitis can

staphylococci A group of round bacteria, usually found in clusters, that cause a variety of diseases in humans and other animals.

colonization The process of bacteria or some other infectious organisms establishing themselves in a host without causing infection.

infection The state of pathogens being established in or on a host and causing disease.

methicillin-resistant *Staphylococcus aureus* (MRSA) Highly resistant form of staph infection that is growing in international prevalence.

Clostridium difficile (C. difficile) A highly resistant bacteria that affects the intestinal tract.

carbapenem-resistant Enterobacteriaceae (CRE) A form of Enterobacteriaceae resistant to nearly all conventional antibiotics.

drug-resistant *Neisseria gonorrhoeae* Drug-resistant form of *Neisseria gonorrhoeae.*

Streptococcus A round bacterium, usually found in chain formation.

meningitis An infection of the meninges, the membranes that surround the brain and spinal cord.

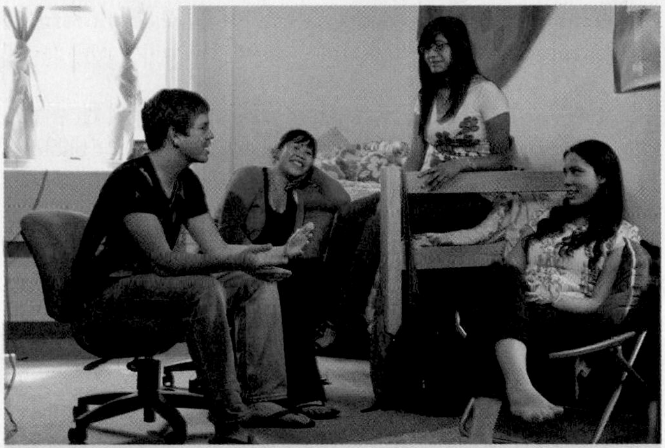

Close quarters, such as college dorms, are prime breeding grounds for contagious diseases such as the flu, colds, and meningitis.

occur at any age, adolescents ages 16 to 21 have the highest rates, particularly those living in close quarters such as dormitories. The other vaccine-preventable form of bacterial meningitis is *Haemophilus influenzae* type b (Hib).

Typical signs of meningitis are sudden fever, severe headache, and a stiff neck, particularly causing difficulty touching your chin to your chest. Persons who are suspected of having meningitis should receive immediate, aggressive medical treatment. Talk to the medical or health education staff at your local student health center to see if they have the vaccine most likely to protect you in your area.

pneumonia Inflammatory disease of the lungs characterized by chronic cough, chest pain, chills, high fever, and fluid accumulation; may be caused by bacteria, viruses, fungi, chemicals, or other substances.

tuberculosis (TB) A disease caused by bacterial infiltration of the respiratory system.

multidrug-resistant TB (MDR-TB) Form of TB that is resistant to at least two of the best antibiotics available.

extensively drug-resistant TB (XDR-TB) Form of TB that is resistant to nearly all existing antibiotics.

Pneumonia A wide range of conditions can result in inflammation of the lungs and difficulty breathing. These are generally referred to as **pneumonia**. Pneumonia is characterized by chronic cough, chest pain, chills, high fever, fluid accumulation, and eventual respiratory failure. Although bacterial and viral pathogens are the most common causes, pneumonia can also be caused by fungi, occupational exposure, or trauma.

Bacterial pneumonia responds readily to antibiotic treatment in the early stages, but it can be deadly in more advanced stages. Other forms of pneumonia caused by viruses, fungi, chemicals, or other substances in the lungs are more difficult to treat. Although medical advances have reduced the overall incidence of pneumonia, it continues to be a major threat in the United States and throughout the world. Vulnerable populations include children; the poor; those displaced by war, famine, and natural disasters; older adults; those who have been occupationally exposed to chemicals and particulates that damage the lungs; and those already suffering from other illnesses.

Tuberculosis With an astounding one-third of the world's population infected, and over 1.3 million deaths each year, only HIV/AIDS is a greater global infectious agent killer than **tuberculosis (TB)**.[22] Historically, people used the term "consumption" to refer to a bacterial disease with symptoms that include wasting/weight loss, fever, chronic cough and blood streaked sputum, fluid- and blood-filled lungs, and eventual spread throughout the body. While the term is still used in some parts of the world, TB is now widely recognized for these symptoms. Coughing is the most common mode of transmitting TB, and infected people can be contagious without showing symptoms. Those at highest risk for TB include the poor, especially children, and the chronically ill. People residing in poorly ventilated crowded prisons and homeless shelters who continuously inhale the same contaminated air are at higher risk. Persons with compromised immune systems are also at high risk, as are comorbid individuals (people suffering from more than one disease).

Many health professionals assumed that TB was conquered in the United States, and though rates have declined in the United States and globally in the last two decades, there were still nearly 10,000 cases of TB documented in the United States in 2012.[23] During the past 20 years, overcrowding and poor sanitation in some developing nations kept the disease alive. Failure to isolate active cases of TB and fully treat them, plus a migration of TB to the United States through immigration and international travel, as well as a weakened public health infrastructure that funded less screening, kept the disease from disappearing in North America.

Most tuberculosis-related deaths occur in developing countries, where it accounts for 26 percent of all preventable deaths.[24] Most TB cases and deaths occur in men; however, TB is among the top three killers of women globally, as well as the leading cause of death among HIV-positive patients.[25]

The current recommended treatment for TB involves taking four drugs for 6 to 9 months, though a new 12-dose regimen is available for high-risk populations.[26] Medications may cause side effects ranging from minor stomach irritation to liver failure.[27] The lengthy, difficult treatment, along with barriers to obtaining drugs and care in many developing areas, leads to missed doses and treatments that end before the cure and breed drug-resistant bacteria.

Multidrug-resistant TB (MDR-TB) is currently resistant to at least two of the best anti-TB drugs in use today, and an even more dangerous form, **extensively drug-resistant TB (XDR-TB)**, is resistant to nearly all first- and second-line drug defenses and is extremely difficult to treat. These newer

THERE ARE

8.6 MILLION

NEW CASES EACH YEAR OF **TB** AND 1.3 MILLION DEATHS.

strains are reaching epidemic proportions in many regions of the world, particularly among those whose immune systems are already compromised by HIV and other diseases.[28]

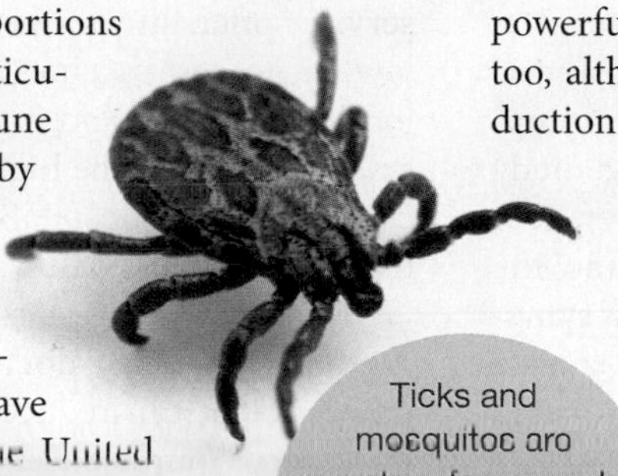

Ticks and mosquitoes are vectors for several devastating diseases in the United States and around the globe.

Tick-Borne Bacterial Diseases

In the past few decades, certain tick-borne diseases have become major health threats in the United States. The most noteworthy include two bacterially caused diseases that spike in the summer months in many states. *Lyme disease* is present in many regions of the United States, particularly the upper Midwest. Symptoms range from none, to a rash or bull's eye lesion and flu-like symptoms, to chronic arthritis, blindness, and long-term disability. *Ehrlichiosis* has flu-like symptoms that may progress quickly to respiratory difficulties and even death. Fortunately, antibiotics given early in the disease course are effective in preventing any serious threats.

Once believed to be closely related to viruses, **rickettsia** are now considered a small form of bacteria. They produce toxins and multiply within small blood vessels, causing vascular blockage and tissue death. Rickettsias require an insect vector (carrier) for transmission to humans. Two common forms are *Rocky Mountain spotted fever* (*RMSF*), carried by a tick, and *typhus,* carried by a louse, flea, or tick. These diseases produce similar symptoms, including high fever, weakness, rash, and coma. Both can be life threatening.

For all insect-borne diseases, the best protection is to stay indoors at dusk and early morning to avoid hours of high insect activity. If you must go out, wear protective clothing or use bug sprays containing natural oils, pyrethrins, or DEET (diethyltoluamide), all products regarded as generally safe. If you are traveling in areas where insect-borne diseases are prevalent, bed nets, routine "tick checks," and other protective measures may be necessary. Lastly, if you have flu-like symptoms during typically "non-flu" seasons, get checked out.

Viruses

Viruses are the smallest known pathogens, approximately 1/500th the size of bacteria. Essentially, a virus consists of a protein structure that contains either *ribonucleic acid* (*RNA*) or *deoxyribonucleic acid* (*DNA*). To reproduce, they must invade and inject their own DNA or RNA into a host cell and force it to make copies. The new viruses then erupt out of the host cell and seek other cells to invade. While viruses are incapable of carrying out any life processes on their own, hundreds of viruses are known to cause diseases in humans.

Viral diseases can be difficult to treat because many viruses can withstand heat, formaldehyde, and large doses of radiation. Some viruses have **incubation periods** (the length of time required to develop fully and cause symptoms in their hosts) that last for years, which delays diagnosis. Drug treatment for viral infections is also limited. Drugs powerful enough to kill viruses generally kill the host cells, too, although some medications block stages in viral reproduction without damaging the host cells.

The Common Cold

Some experts believe there are at least 200 different viruses responsible for colds. Any given cold's most likely cause is the rhinovirus, which causes 30–50 percent of all colds, followed by the coronavirus, responsible for another 10–15 percent.[29] Colds are **endemic** (always present to some degree) throughout the world, with increasing prevalence in colder weather as people spend more time indoors. Otherwise healthy people carry cold viruses in their noses and throats most of the time, held in check until defenses are weakened. It is possible to "catch" a cold from airborne transmission and skin-to-skin or mucous membrane contact, though the hands are the greatest avenue for transmitting cold viruses and other pathogens. Covering your nose and mouth with a tissue, handkerchief, or even the crook of your elbow when sneezing is better than using your bare hand.

Several common sense strategies for preventing a cold include bolstering your immune system with healthy diet, exercise, stress reduction, sleep, and other behaviors. Washing your hands with regular soap and water and keeping your hands away from your eyes, nose, and mouth are also key. If you have a cold, keep away from others; if others have a cold, avoid close contact and wash your hands often. Remember that many cold viruses can last for hours on the skin or other objects. Throw used tissues in the trash, and disinfect TV remotes and other objects that you have been touching. Contrary to popular belief, you cannot catch a cold from getting a chill, but the chill may lower your immune system's resistance to a pathogenic virus if one is present.

rickettsia A small form of bacteria that live inside other living cells.

viruses Pathogens that invade and inject their own DNA or RNA into a host cell, take it over, and force it to make copies of the pathogen.

incubation period The time between exposure to a disease and the appearance of symptoms.

endemic Describes a disease that is always present to some degree.

influenza A common viral disease of the respiratory tract.

While many products are touted as cold remedies, the evidence that *Echinacea* can prevent or shorten the duration of colds is inconclusive according to summaries of several studies.[30] Although it may come as a surprise, there is also scant evidence that mega-doses of vitamin C can cure or even reduce symptoms of the cold.[31]

Influenza

In otherwise healthy people, **influenza**, or flu, is usually not life threatening. However, for certain vulnerable populations, such as individuals with respiratory problems or heart disease, older adults (over age 65), or young children (under age 5), the flu can be very serious. Approximately 200,000 Americans will need hospitalization each year for influenza treatment.[32] Once a person gets the flu, treatment is *palliative*—focused on relief of symptoms, rather than cure.

mononucleosis A viral disease that causes pervasive fatigue and other long-lasting symptoms.

hepatitis A viral disease in which the liver becomes inflamed, producing symptoms such as fever, headache, and possibly jaundice.

Determining whether you have a cold or the flu is a matter of assessing your symptoms: If you have bad body aches, fatigue, and fever, it is likely that you have the flu. In the absence of these symptoms, but the presence of a stuffy or runny nose, sneezing, a sore throat, and often a cough, over-the-counter medicines targeting symptoms of the common cold may help.[33]

To date, three major varieties of flu virus have been discovered, with many different strains existing within each variety. The *A form* of the virus is generally the most virulent, followed by the *B* and the very mild *C varieties*. If you contract one form of influenza, you may develop immunity to it, but you will not necessarily be immune to other forms.

Strains of influenza are constantly changing, so flu vaccines are formulated each year that combine three types of killed flu viruses from the A and B varieties (called trivalent vaccines).[34] The viruses are selected based on forecasting of the strains likely to emerge in various regions of the world. If researchers correctly predict strains, vaccines are between 70 and 90 percent effective in healthy adults for about a year; if the prediction is off, a shot may not totally protect you from the flu; however, symptoms may be less severe.[35] If you have had a severe reaction to past flu shots, have a severe allergy to chicken eggs, are running a fever, or have other issues, consult with your doctor before having a shot. An optional nasal spray flu vaccine is available for healthy people age 1 to 49 who are not pregnant. Flu shots take 2 to 3 weeks to become effective, so people at risk should get these shots in the fall before the flu season begins. Most campus health services offer flu vaccines for $20 or less. Other options for low- or no-cost vaccines are local public health departments, local pharmacies and big box stores, and community centers. Compared to the high cost of lost days of work or missed classes, possible hospitalization, and expensive medicines to treat symptoms, the flu vaccine is a sound investment.

If you feel you've been exposed to the flu or have early symptoms, see your doctor, as antiviral sprays, capsules, and powders that can reduce symptoms, prevent complications, and speed your recovery are available. For more information about antiviral drugs, see www.cdc.gov/flu/antivirals/whatyoushould.htm.

DID YOU **KNOW?**

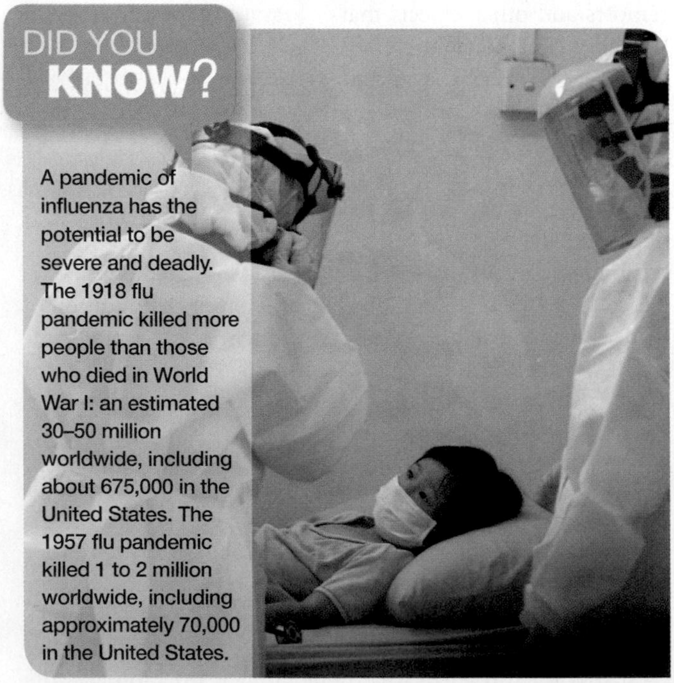

A pandemic of influenza has the potential to be severe and deadly. The 1918 flu pandemic killed more people than those who died in World War I: an estimated 30–50 million worldwide, including about 675,000 in the United States. The 1957 flu pandemic killed 1 to 2 million worldwide, including approximately 70,000 in the United States.

Source: Flu.gov, "Pandemic Flu History," Accessed April 2014, www.flu.gov/pandemic/history.

3,000–49,000

IS THE RANGE IN YEARLY **DEATHS** ATTRIBUTABLE TO THE FLU IN THE UNITED STATES

Infectious Mononucleosis Caused primarily by the Epstein-Barr virus, **mononucleosis** is most widespread among people between the ages of 15 and 24, with college students or those living in close quarters among those at highest risk. By adulthood, 90 to 95 percent of people have been infected, many without ever showing symptoms.[36] Because saliva seems to be a key route of transmission, "mono" has often referred to as the "kissing disease." However, sharing eating utensils, drinking vessels, towels, or cosmetics such as lipstick, or even coughing, can spread the virus. Body fluids, including blood, genital secretions, and mucus, can also spread the disease. Common symptoms include bone-crushing fatigue, headache, fever, aches and pains, sore throat, rashes, and swollen lymph nodes. Pain in the area of the spleen may indicate spleen enlargement, a potentially dangerous risk for those involved in exercise or athletics where contact with the ground or others is common. Anything that weakens the immune system, such as high stress, lack of sleep, poor diet, or too much alcohol or drug use, can increase risk. A simple blood test can determine whether you have mono. Rest, balanced nutrition, stress management, and healthy lifestyle are the best treatments.

Hepatitis One of the most highly publicized viral diseases is **hepatitis**, an inflammation of the liver that is a leading cause of liver cancer and liver transplantation internationally. Currently, nearly 4.5 million Americans have one of several forms of hepatitis (A, B, C, D, and E), with hepatitis A, B, and C having the highest rates of incidence.[37]

Hepatitis A (HAV) is contracted by eating food or drinking water contaminated with human feces. Since vaccinations became available, HAV rates have declined dramatically, yet an estimated 2,700 new cases are diagnosed and treated annually.[38] Food handlers, children at day care centers, those who have sexual contact with HAV-positive individuals, those who travel to regions where HAV is endemic, and those who use contaminated needles are at higher risk. Ingesting shellfish from sewage-infested waters is a major cause of infection in U.S. coastal areas. Fortunately, individuals infected with hepatitis A do not become chronic carriers, and vaccines for the disease are available.

Hepatitis B (HBV) is spread through body fluid exchange during unprotected sex; sharing needles or accidental needlesticks; or, in the case of a baby, from an infected mother. Hepatitis B can lead to chronic liver disease or liver cancer. Since vaccines became available in 1981, numbers of HBV cases have declined rapidly, and needle exchange programs have helped reduce risks of HBV infection in many populations in the last decade. Still, nearly 40,000 cases are reported each year in the United States, and over 1.4 million are chronic carriers. The highest rates of infection are among males ages 30–39 and Black non-Hispanics. The lowest rates are among Asian Pacific Islanders and Hispanics.[39] Globally, HBV infections are on the decline, but over 240 million are chronically infected.[40] Because the hepatitis B virus is particularly virulent, efforts to increase global vaccination rates have become a major priority.

Hepatitis C (HCV) infections are on an epidemic rise in many regions of the world as resistant forms emerge. Some cases can be traced to blood transfusions or organ transplants. Currently, an estimated 17,000 new cases of HCV are diagnosed in the United States each year, with over 3.2 million people chronically infected.[41] Of those infected, 75–85 percent develop chronic infections; if the infection is left untreated, the person may develop cirrhosis of the liver, liver cancer, or liver failure.[42] Although there is no vaccine for HCV, there are new drugs that have been successful in treating the disease. The problem is that millions of people, primarily "baby boomers," do not know that they are infected and are not seeking these treatments. Educating these individuals about potential risks and getting them tested and treated is a top priority.

To prevent the spread of HBV and HCV, follow these precautions: use latex condoms correctly every time you have sex; don't share personal-care items that might have blood on them, such as razors or toothbrushes; get a blood test for HBV so you know your status; never share needles; and if you are having body art done, go only to reputable artists or piercers who follow established sterilization and infection-control protocols.

Mumps With vaccine introduction, reported cases of **mumps** declined from 80 per 100,000 people in 1968 to less than 2 per 100,000 in 1984. However, in the last decade, several outbreaks of the mumps have occurred in the United States and globally, largely attributed to parents' unsubstantiated fears of vaccine complications keeping many school-aged children from being vaccinated.

Approximately one-half of all mumps infections produce only minor symptoms, with about one-third of infected people never showing any. The most common symptom is the swelling of the parotid (salivary) glands. One of the greatest dangers associated with mumps is the potential for sterility in men who contract the disease in young adulthood. Some victims also suffer hearing loss.

mumps A once common viral disease that is controllable by vaccination.

chickenpox A highly infectious disease caused by the herpes varicella zoster virus.

shingles A disease characterized by a painful rash that occurs when the chickenpox virus is reactivated.

herpes gladiatorum A skin infection caused by the herpes simplex type 1 virus and seen among athletes participating in contact sports.

Herpes Viruses: Chickenpox, Shingles, and Herpes Gladiatorum

From the cold sores to chickenpox, herpes-caused diseases are known for painful, blistering rashes and are easily transmitted via physical contact. They can become chronic problems for the person infected. (Genital herpes is covered in **Chapter 14**.)

Caused by the *herpes varicella zoster virus* (*HVZV*), **chickenpox** produces characteristic symptoms of fever and fatigue 13 to 17 days after exposure, followed by skin eruptions that itch, blister, and produce a clear fluid. The virus is present in these blisters for approximately 1 week. Although a vaccine for chickenpox is available, many parents incorrectly assume that the vaccine is not necessary and that contracting the disease will ensure lifelong immunity.

For a small segment of the population, the chickenpox virus reactivates later in life during times of high stress or when the immune system is taxed by other diseases. This painful, blistering rash, extreme pain, and other possible complications is called **shingles.** The disease shingles affects over 1 million people in the United States, most of whom are over the age of 60.[43] The best way to prevent shingles is to get vaccinated.[44]

Another form of herpes-caused disease that is increasing on college campuses is **herpes gladiatorum** (**FIGURE 13.6**), which shows itself as a blistered rash on the face, neck, or torso. Caused by the herpes simplex type 1 virus, herpes gladiatorum is also referred to as "mat pox" or "wrestler's herpes," as it's highly contagious via mats used in a yoga studio or gym, or through body-to-body contact.

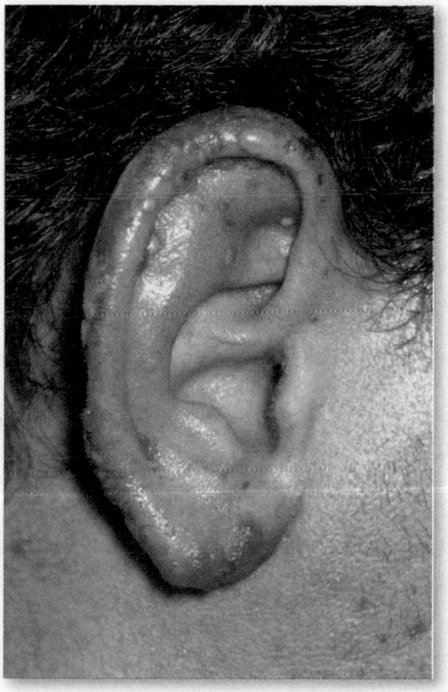

FIGURE 13.6 Herpes Gladiatorum
A series of fluid-filled blisters on the face, neck, or torso can be a sign of this form of herpes, which is easily spread, especially among athletes.

Measles and Rubella **Measles** is a highly contagious viral disorder that often affects young children, but it is increasing among young adults today, particularly on college campuses. Many young adults may not have been fully vaccinated in their youth, as their parents may have thought the disease was no longer a problem in the United States. During the first 2 months of 2014, there were nearly as many cases (54) of confirmed measles in the United States as usually occur in a full year (64), and numbers may surpass record high cases in 2013, when unvaccinated international travelers and large numbers of children whose parents objected to vaccinations on religious or philosophical reasons created a perfect storm of illnesses.[45] Those who refuse vaccination put the immunocompromised and others at risk, as babies are typically not vaccinated until after 1 year of age. Although vaccination rates are fairly high for these diseases in the United States, many regions of the world have large numbers of unvaccinated individuals.[46] Today, with outbreaks on several U.S. campuses, increased numbers of colleges and universities require verification of immunization with the measles, mumps, rubella (MMR) vaccination or a blood test that indicates immunity prior to admission.

measles A viral disease that produces symptoms such as an itchy rash and a high fever.

rubella (German measles) A milder form of measles that causes a rash and mild fever in children and may damage a fetus or a newborn baby.

rabies A viral disease of the central nervous system; often transmitted through animal bites.

fungi A group of multicellular and unicellular organisms that obtain their food by infiltrating the bodies of other organisms, both living and dead; several microscopic varieties are pathogenic.

Coccidioidomycosis (Valley Fever) An infection that occurs when humans or pets inhale soil-dwelling fungal spores.

protozoans Microscopic single-celled organisms that can be pathogenic.

Symptoms, appearing about 10 days after exposure, include an itchy rash and a high fever. Many people don't realize that measles can be life threatening, causing high fever, pneumonia, encephalitis, and other complications. Symptoms tend to be worse for those under 5 and those 20 and over. In 2011, nearly 40 percent of children under the age of 5 with measles had to be hospitalized.[47]

Rubella (German measles) is a milder viral infection that causes rashes, usually on upper extremities, and is believed to be spread by inhalation. Mild in most adults, rubella is a threat to the very young and unborn, as it is known to cause blindness, deafness, heart defects, and cognitive impairments in fetuses and newborns. Immunization has reduced the incidence of both measles and rubella. Infections in children not immunized against measles can lead to fever-induced problems such as rheumatic heart disease, kidney damage, and neurological disorders.

Rabies The **rabies** virus infects many warm-blooded animals. Bats are believed to be asymptomatic carriers. Their urine, which they spray when flying, contains the virus, so even the air of densely populated bat caves may be infectious. In most other hosts, the disease is extremely virulent and usually fatal. The most obvious symptoms of the disease are extreme activity in the cerebral region of the brain, rage, increased salivation, spasms in the throat muscles, extreme drive to find water, and the inability to swallow. Rabid animals may attempt to bite other animals and people. Not only does this behavior cause injury, but it also spreads the virus through saliva.

The incubation period for rabies is usually 1 to 3 months. The disease may be fatal if not treated immediately with the rabies vaccine. Anyone bitten by an animal that might be carrying rabies should seek immediate medical attention and try to bring the animal along for testing. If you are wondering whether you should spring for the cost of rabies shots for your pets, do it. Pets that bite and are not current on their rabies vaccinations are routinely euthanized.

Bats and other small mammals infected with rabies do not exhibit symptoms of the disease and easily spread it.

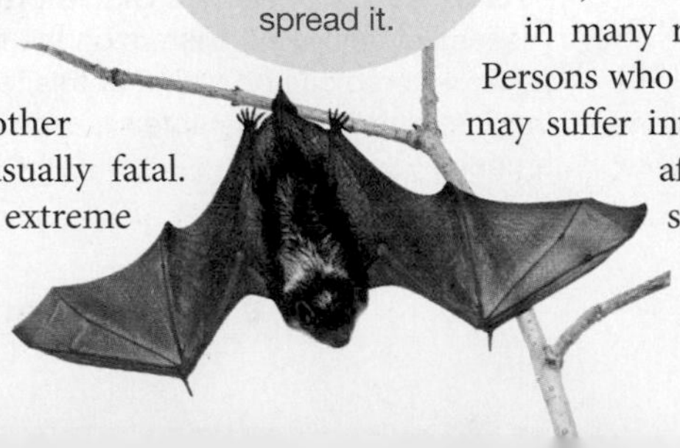

Other Pathogens

While bacteria and viruses account for many common diseases in both adults and children, other organisms can also infect and cause disease symptoms in a host. Among these are fungi, protozoans, parasitic worms, and prions.

Fungi Hundreds of species of **fungi** exist. While many of these multi- or unicellular organisms are beneficial—such as edible mushrooms, penicillin, and the yeast used in making bread—*candidiasis* (as in a vaginal yeast infection; see **Chapter 14**), athlete's foot, ringworm, jock itch, and toenail fungus are examples of some of the most common fungal diseases. With most fungal diseases, keeping the affected area clean and dry and treating it promptly with appropriate medications (often available over the counter) will generally bring relief. Fungal diseases typically transmit via physical contact, so avoid going barefoot in public showers, hotel rooms, and other areas where fungus may be present.

Coccidioidomycosis, also known as **Valley Fever**, is an infection that occurs when humans or pets inhale soil-dwelling fungal spores. In the last decade, rates have soared in desert regions of Mexico, Central and South America, and the southwestern United States.[48] Because early symptoms of headache, aches, fever, etc. are common, cases often go unreported. Unfortunately, these symptoms can quickly progress to pneumonia, meningitis, or other life-threatening complications. As many as 40 percent of cases require hospitalization and have symptoms lasting weeks or months.[49] The best means of prevention is to avoid actions that stir the soil and cause spores to be aerosolized. Staying indoors during dust storms may also help reduce risks.

Protozoans **Protozoans** are single-celled organisms that cause diseases such as African sleeping sickness and malaria. Although prevalent in nonindustrialized countries, they are largely controlled in the United States. The most common protozoan disease in the United States is *trichomoniasis* (discussed in **Chapter 14**). A common waterborne protozoan disease in many regions of the country is *giardiasis*. Persons who are exposed to the *giardia* pathogen may suffer intestinal pain and discomfort weeks after infection. Protection of water supplies is the key to prevention.

parasitic worms The largest of the pathogens, most of which are more a nuisance than a threat.

prion A recently identified self-replicating protein-based pathogen.

Parasitic Worms

Parasitic worms are the largest pathogens. Ranging in size from small pinworms typically found in children to large tapeworms that can take up large portions of the human intestines, they are more nuisance than threat. Of special note are worm infestations associated with eating raw fish such as sushi. You can prevent worm infestations by cooking fish and other foods to temperatures sufficient to kill the worms and their eggs. Other preventive measures include getting your pets checked and wearing shoes in parks or public places where animal feces are present.

Prions

A **prion** is a self-replicating, protein-based agent that can infect humans and animals. One such prion is believed to be the underlying cause of spongiform diseases such as *bovine spongiform encephalopathy (BSE)* or "mad cow disease" found in beef cattle in various regions of the world. If humans eat contaminated meat from cattle with BSE, they may develop a mad cow-like disease known as *variant Creutzfeldt-Jakob disease (vCJD)*. Symptoms of vCJD include loss of memory, tremors, and muscle spasms or "ticks." Within a fairly short time period, depression, difficulty walking, seizures, and severe dementia can ultimately lead to death in both cows and humans.[50] An increasing number of infected cattle have been found in the United States and globally. To date, there have been three cases of vCJD in the United States.[51] Improved surveillance and reporting is necessary to determine if more cases exist. In the meantime, because infected brain and spinal tissue of cattle have been implicated in global infections, these animal parts from high-risk older cattle are prohibited from the human food chain.[52]

Emerging and Resurgent Diseases

Within the past decade, rates for infectious diseases have rapidly increased. This trend can be attributed to a combination of overpopulation, inadequate health care systems, increasing poverty, extreme environmental degradation, and drug resistance.[53] At the same time, world travel and trade of goods has become increasingly fast and easy, giving many pathogens ample opportunity to hitch a ride to new locations.

Ebola Virus Disease

Ebola virus disease (EVD), formerly called *Ebola Hemorrhagic Fever*, is a rare, often fatal, disease that is ravaging parts of Central and West Africa, with over 8,000 cases reported in September 2014 and death rates of 50 to 90 percent. Fruit bats, chimps, and other animals are natural hosts and spread the disease to humans, who spread it to others via contact with infected body fluids or surfaces such as sheets and clothing. Once infected, blood clotting ability diminishes, leading to internal and external bleeding. Without rehydration, organ failure and death can occur. Body rash, vomiting, diarrhea, fever, pain, and headache are early symptoms. Currently no vaccines are available, although two are being tested. At the time of this book's publication, international efforts to improve treatment centers and train hundreds of community workers in infection control and population education were underway. Until vaccines are available, prevention of infection, quarantine of those infected, and symptom relief are the best means of slowing Ebola's spread.[54]

West Nile Virus

Spread by infected mosquitoes, there are several thousand active cases of West Nile virus in the United States every year. Although most people infected have minor flu-like symptoms and fully recover, approximately 1 percent of those infected have neurological symptoms, indicative of a more serious form of *West Nile encephalitis* (inflammation of the brain).[55] Symptoms can include severe neurological complications, including respiratory failure, paralysis, seizures, and death.[56] Survivors often face years of intensive rehabilitation. Those with compromised immune systems or other health problems are more likely to have complications.[57] Today, only Alaska and Hawaii remain free of the disease, and avoiding mosquito bites is the best way to prevent it.[58]

Avian (Bird) Flu

Avian influenza is an infectious disease of birds, with strains capable of crossing the species barrier to cause severe illness in humans who come in contact with bird droppings or fluids. Bird flu appears to have originated in Asia and spread via migrating bird populations.[59] Although the virus has yet to mutate into a form highly infectious to humans, outbreaks in which people contract the disease from birds in rural areas of the world (where people often live in close proximity to poultry and other animals) have occurred. As of March 2013, the World Health Organization (WHO) had recorded 650 cases of bird flu in humans, with 386 deaths.[60]

Many health experts suggest that if this virus becomes transmissible between humans, it is virulent enough to surpass the lethality of the influenza epidemics of 1918 and 1919, which caused millions of deaths. This type of pandemic flu or global epidemic could decimate the world's population.

Escherichia coli O157:H7

Escherichia coli O157:H7 is one of over 170 types of *E. coli* bacteria that can infect humans. Most *E. coli* organisms are harmless and live in the intestines of healthy animals and humans. *E. coli* O157:H7, however, produces a lethal toxin and can cause severe illness or death. It can live in the intestines of healthy cattle and then contaminate food products at slaughterhouses. Eating ground beef that is rare or undercooked, drinking unpasteurized milk or juice, or swimming in sewage-contaminated water or public pools can also cause infection.

A symptom of infection is nonbloody diarrhea, usually 2 to 8 days after exposure; however, asymptomatic cases have been noted. Children, older adults, and people with weakened immune systems are particularly vulnerable to serious side effects such as kidney failure, intestinal damage, or death.

Listeriosis

Luncheon meats or deli foods are particularly susceptible to transmitting the bacterium responsible for listeriosis, a disease that has proved fatal in many cases in recent years. Early symptoms begin with mild fever and progress to headache and inflammation of the brain. Those who are immunocompromised and pregnant women are at greatest risk. New regulations that require strict monitoring of food-processing plants should help reduce the risk of listeria infection.

Malaria Today, approximately 50 percent of the world's population, mostly those living in the poorest countries, are at risk for malaria. The disease is transmitted by mosquitoes carrying a parasite. There were 207 million cases of malaria and an estimated 627,000 deaths in 2012, even though mortality rates have dropped significantly in the last decade.[61] Most deaths occur among poor and vulnerable children and pregnant women in sub-Saharan Africa.[62]

Travelers from malaria-free regions entering areas where there is malaria transmission are highly vulnerable, as they have little or no immunity and often receive a delayed or wrong malaria diagnosis when they return home.[63] Mosquito nets and use of insect repellents are particularly important to prevention, as is removal of standing water in yards. Natural disasters that leave standing water in which mosquitoes can flourish pose increased risks. Resistance to chloroquine, once a widely used and highly effective treatment, is now found in most regions of the world, and other treatments are losing their effectiveness at alarming rates.

STUDY PLAN

Customize your study plan—and master your health!—in the Study Area of **MasteringHealth.**

ASSESS YOURSELF

How much do you really know about infectious diseases? Take the **Myth or Fact? Test Your Infectious Diseases IQ** assessment available on MasteringHealth.™

Need help creating a plan? Follow the strategies in the **Your Plan for Change** box for short- and long-term improvements to your health.

YOUR PLAN FOR **CHANGE**

After completing the "Are You Protecting Yourself against Infectious Diseases?" **ASSESS YOURSELF**, you can begin to change behaviors that may be putting you at risk for infection.

TODAY, YOU CAN:

- ☐ Get in the habit of washing your hands regularly. After you cough, sneeze, blow your nose, use the bathroom, or prepare food, find a sink, wet your hands with warm water, and lather up with soap. Scrub your hands for about 20 seconds (count to 20 or recite the alphabet), rinse well, and dry your hands.
- ☐ Make sure to cook and store food properly. Meats and fish should be well done and never rare, and luncheon meats should be refrigerated until you're ready to put them on your sandwich. Always drink pasteurized milk and juice. These same guidelines apply for eating out at restaurants or in the dining hall.

WITHIN THE NEXT 2 WEEKS, YOU CAN:

- ☐ Take action to keep your immune system strong: Exercise regularly and eat lots of fruits and vegetables.
- ☐ Adjust your sleep schedule so that you're getting an adequate amount of rest every night. Being well rested is one key aspect of maintaining a healthy immune system.

BY THE END OF THE SEMESTER, YOU CAN:

- ☐ Check your immunization schedule and make sure you're current with all recommended vaccinations. Make an appointment with your health care provider if you need a booster or vaccine. If flu season is coming up, get a flu shot.
- ☐ Make an appointment with your health care provider if you're planning a trip abroad to determine what vaccinations, if any, you'll need for the trip. Once you're traveling, avoid mosquito bites by using insect repellents, and stay away from standing water (unless it's chlorinated).

CHAPTER REVIEW

To hear an MP3 Tutor Session, scan here or visit the Study Area in **MasteringHealth.**

LO 1 The Process of Infection

- For a person to become infected with a disease, the immune system must be weakened, an agent capable of transmitting the disease must be present, and the environment must be hospitable to the pathogen.
- Getting enough sleep and exercise, having adequate nutrition, and avoiding alcohol and drugs are some of the controllable risk factors for infectious diseases. Heredity, age, environmental conditions, and organism resistance are uncontrollable risk factors.

LO 2 Your Body's Defenses against Infection

- Your body uses several defense systems to keep pathogens from invading. The skin is the body's major protection, helped by enzymes and body chemistry. The immune system creates antibodies to destroy antigens. Fever and pain play a role in defending the body. Vaccines bolster the body's immune system against specific diseases. If you are immunocompromised, your risk for disease increases. Allergies are an overreaction of the immune system.

LO 3 Types of Pathogens and the Diseases They Cause

- The major classes of pathogens are bacteria, viruses, fungi, protozoans, parasitic worms, and prions. Bacterial infections include staphylococcal infections, streptococcal infections, meningitis, pneumonia, tuberculosis, and tick-borne diseases. Major viral infections include the common cold; influenza; mononucleosis; hepatitis; mumps; the herpes viruses, including chickenpox, shingles, and herpes gladiatorum; measles and rubella; and rabies.
- Emerging and resurgent diseases such as avian flu or West Nile virus pose significant threats for future generations. Many factors contribute to these risks. Possible solutions focus on a public health approach to prevention.
- Antibiotic resistance for several pathogens continues to be a major threat to United States and global health. Several strategies for prevention at the individual and community level are key to reducing risks.

POP QUIZ

Visit **MasteringHealth** to personalize your study plan with Chapter Review Quizzes and Dynamic Study Modules.

LO 1 The Process of Infection

1. Fernando catches a cold after his roommate Jason sneezes and coughs near Fernando in their shared dorm room. The likely mode of transition for Fernando's cold was
   a. waterborne.
   b. airborne.
   c. vector-borne.
   d. perinatal.
2. Jennifer touched her viral herpes sore on her lip and then touched her eye. She ended up with the herpes virus in her eye as well. This is an example of
   a. acquired immunity.
   b. passive spread.
   c. autoinoculation.
   d. self-vaccination.
3. Which of the following would put a 70-year-old person at a greater risk for infectious diseases?
   a. Vaccinations from birth wearing off or not as effective
   b. Thickening of the skin
   c. Losing sense of smell
   d. Getting "chilled" from a drafty room.

LO 2 Your Body's Defenses against Infection

4. Which of the following do not assist the body in fighting disease?
   a. Antigens
   b. Antibodies
   c. Lymphocytes
   d. Macrophages
5. An example of passive immunity is
   a. inoculation with a vaccine containing weakened antigens.
   b. when the body makes its own antibodies to a pathogen.
   c. the antibody-containing part of the vaccine that came from someone else.
   d. when lymphocytes attack and destroy a foreign invader.
6. A hypersensitive reaction that occurs when the body attempts to defend itself against an antigen by producing antibodies to a normally harmless substance is known as a(n)
   a. allergy.
   b. opportunistic infection.
   c. autoimmune disease.
   d. vaccination.

LO 3 Types of Pathogens and the Diseases They Cause

7. Which of the following diseases is caused by a prion?
   a. Shingles
   b. Listeria
   c. Mad cow disease
   d. Trichomoniasis
8. Which of the following is a *viral* disease?
   a. Pneumonia
   b. Measles
   c. Malaria
   d. Streptococcal infection
9. Because colds are always present to some degree throughout the world, they are said to be
   a. globally acquired.
   b. vector-borne.
   c. endemic.
   d. resistant to antibiotics.

10. For which of the following diseases can you reduce your risk by using mosquito repellent when outdoors?
    a. Candidiasis
    b. West Nile virus
    c. Rubella
    d. *E. coli* O157:H7

Answers to the Pop Quiz can be found on page A-1. If you answered a question incorrectly, review the section identified by the Learning Outcome. For even more study tools, visit MasteringHealth.

THINK ABOUT IT!

LO 1 The Process of Infection

1. What are three lifestyle changes you could make right now that would reduce your risk of developing an infectious disease? What could you do to help protect your friends, partner, and family members? Discuss uncontrollable and controllable risk factors that can make you more or less susceptible to infectious pathogens.

LO 2 Your Body's Defenses against Infection

2. What is a pathogen? What does it mean if someone says a pathogen is particularly *virulent*? What is the difference between *antigens* and *antibodies*?
3. What is the difference between active and passive immunity? How do they compare to natural and acquired immunity? What type of immunity do vaccines provide?

LO 3 Types of Pathogens and the Diseases They Cause

4. What are some of the differences between bacteria and viruses? How do certain pathogens develop drug resistance? What are the implications for growing numbers of drug-resistant pathogens?

ACCESS YOUR HEALTH ON THE INTERNET

Visit **MasteringHealth** for links to the websites and RSS feeds.

The following websites explore further topics and issues related to personal health.

Centers for Disease Control and Prevention (CDC). This is the home page for the government agency dedicated to disease intervention and prevention, with links to all the latest data and publications put out by the CDC—including the *Morbidity and Mortality Weekly Report* (*MMWR*) and the *Journal of Emerging Infectious Diseases*—and access to the CDC research database, Wonder. www.cdc.gov

Specialized CDC sites. These sites focus on infectious diseases:

- National Center for Immunization and Respiratory Diseases. www.cdc.gov/ncird/index.html
- National Center for Emerging and Zoonotic Infectious Diseases. www.cdc.gov/ncezid
- ArboNET. ArboNET is a national surveillance system for arboviral (arthropod-caused) diseases in the United States, monitoring West Nile disease, eastern equine encephalitis, dengue, and other mosquito and tick-borne diseases. www.cdc.gov/westnile/resourcepages/survResources.html

World Health Organization (WHO). You'll gain access to the latest information on world health issues and direct access to publications and fact sheets at WHO's site. www.who.int

Association for Professionals in Infection Control and Epidemiology (APIC). Excellent resource for health professionals and consumers, covering a wide range of infectious disease issues in health care, workplaces, schools, and in one's personal environment. www.apic.org

14 Protecting against Sexually Transmitted Infections

LEARNING OUTCOMES

1. Explain the risk factors for sexually transmitted infections and actions that can prevent their spread.
2. Describe common types of sexually transmitted infections, including their symptoms and treatment methods.
3. Discuss human immunodeficiency virus (HIV) and acquired immunodeficiency syndrome (AIDS), trends in infection and treatment, and the impact of HIV/AIDS on special populations.

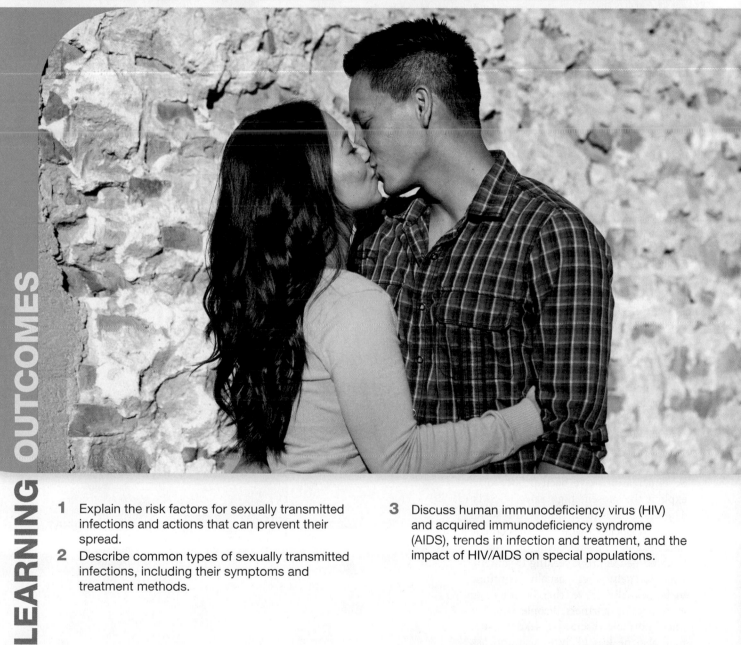

Every year, there are at least 20 million new cases of **sexually transmitted infections (STIs)**, only some of which are curable. Often used as being synonymous with sexually transmitted diseases (STDs), the term *STI* is more appropriate since, medically, the term "disease" is used only with conditions that cause visible symptoms. While some people with STIs may eventually show symptoms, and all STDs begin as STIs, it is possible for a person to be infected without having the infection exhibit visible symptoms or develop into a full-blown disease.[1] Almost half of the newly diagnosed cases of STIs are in people ages 15–24.[2] Sexually transmitted infections affect people of all backgrounds and socioeconomic levels. However, they disproportionately affect women, minorities, and infants, and are most prevalent in teens and young adults.[3]

sexually transmitted infections (STIs) Infections transmitted through some form of intimate, usually sexual, contact.

There are more than 20 known types of STIs. More virulent strains and antibiotic resistant forms indicate the potential for ominous threats to those who engage in risky behaviors in the days ahead.

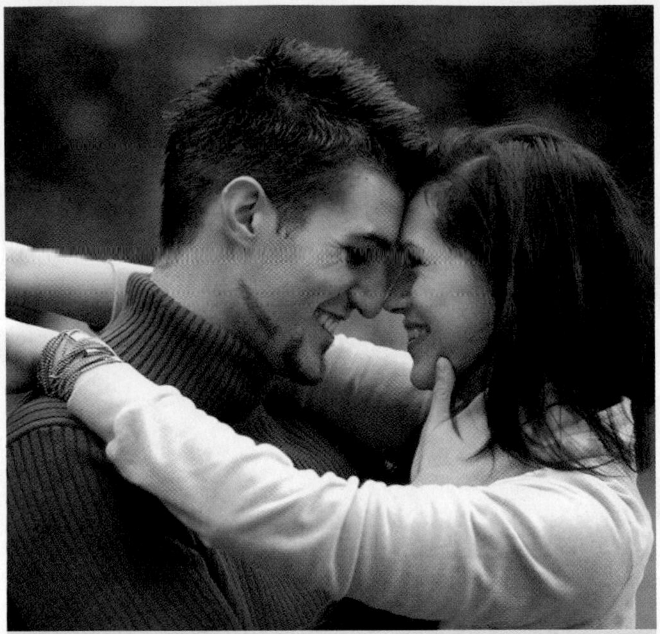

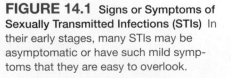

You can't tell if someone has an STI just by looking at them. The only way to know for sure is to go to a clinic and get tested.

LO 1 | SEXUALLY TRANSMITTED INFECTIONS

Explain the risk factors for sexually transmitted infections and actions that can prevent their spread.

Early symptoms of an STI are often mild and unrecognizable (see **FIGURE 14.1**). Left untreated, some of these infections can have grave consequences, such as sterility, blindness, central nervous system destruction, disfigurement, and even death. Infants born to mothers carrying the organisms for these infections are at risk for a variety of health problems.

What's Your Risk?

Several reasons have been proposed to explain the present high rates of STIs. The first relates to the moral and social stigmas associated with these infections. Shame and embarrassment often keep infected people from seeking treatment. Unfortunately, they usually continue to be sexually active, thereby infecting unsuspecting partners. People who are uncomfortable discussing sexual issues may also be less likely to use and ask their partners to use condoms to protect against STIs and pregnancy.

Another reason proposed for the STI epidemic is our casual attitude about sex. Bombarded by media that glamorizes sex, many people consider sex to be without consequences. Some are pressured into sexual relationships that they don't want, or before they are really ready. Generally, the more sexual partners a person has, the greater the risk for contracting an STI.

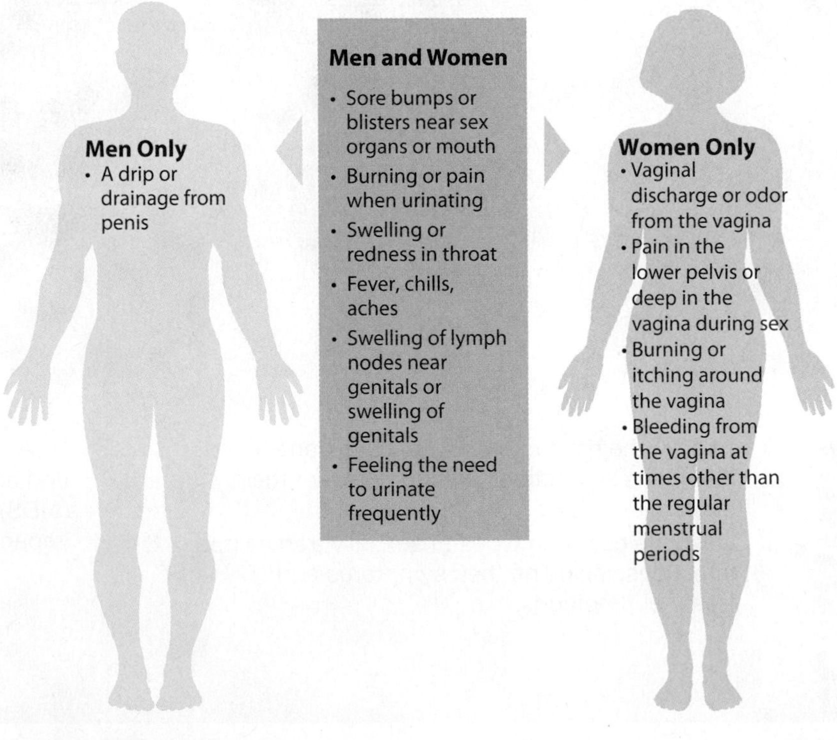

Men Only
• A drip or drainage from penis
Men and Women
• Sore bumps or blisters near sex organs or mouth
• Burning or pain when urinating
• Swelling or redness in throat
• Fever, chills, aches
• Swelling of lymph nodes near genitals or swelling of genitals
• Feeling the need to urinate frequently
Women Only
• Vaginal discharge or odor from the vagina
• Pain in the lower pelvis or deep in the vagina during sex
• Burning or itching around the vagina
• Bleeding from the vagina at times other than the regular menstrual periods

FIGURE 14.1 Signs or Symptoms of Sexually Transmitted Infections (STIs) In their early stages, many STIs may be asymptomatic or have such mild symptoms that they are easy to overlook.

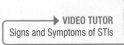

VIDEO TUTOR
Signs and Symptoms of STIs

STUDENT HEALTH TODAY

MAKING ORAL SEX SAFE *Condoms, Dental Dams, and Abstinence*

Oral sex refers to orally stimulating the penis (*fellatio*), vagina and clitoris (*cunnilingus*), and/or anus (*analingus*). Many young people tend to believe that oral sex is safe, and while the risks of contracting an STI are lower with oral sex than with vaginal or anal intercourse, the risk is still not zero. It is entirely possible to contract HIV from oral sex, as well as herpes, gonorrhea, syphilis, genital warts, and other diseases. Beyond common STIs, it's also possible to spread or contract intestinal parasites, as well as hepatitis A and B. That being the case, here are a couple things you can do to minimize your risk:

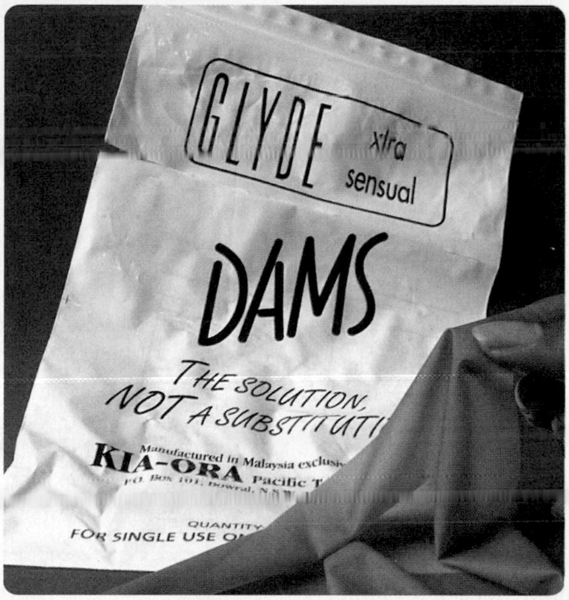

- **Use a Condom Correctly:** Condom use during oral sex is especially important for HIV prevention. When performing or receiving fellatio, use a new latex condom each time. Check it for holes before using, and discard it after use. Never reuse a condom.
- **Use a Dental Dam:** A dental dam is essentially a small square of latex. While they were originally developed to be used during dental procedures, they are now commonly used as barriers when performing cunnilingus or analingus. Before using a dental dam, visually check it for holes, and be sure to use a new one every time. Discard it after use, and never reuse a dental dam.

Lastly, keep in mind that condoms and dental dams provide less protection against STIs spread through contact with exposed sores, like HPV or herpes, than for other STIs. Abstinence is the only way to be 100 percent sure you don't transmit or contract an STI.

Sources: Centers for Disease Control and Prevention, "Oral Sex and HIV Risk," January 2014, www.cdc.gov/hiv/risk/behavior/oralsex.html; Centers for Disease Control and Prevention, "HIV Prevention," March 2014, www.cdc.gov/hiv/basics/prevention.html; U.S. Department of Veterans Affairs, "Tips for Using Condoms and Dental Dams," www.hiv.va.gov/patient/daily/sex/condomtips.asp; Mayo Clinic, "Sexually Transmitted Diseases (STDs): Prevention," February 2013, www.mayoclinic.org/diseases-conditions/sexually-transmitted-diseases-stds/basics/prevention/con-20034128.

Ignorance—about the infections, their symptoms, and the fact that someone can be asymptomatic but still infected—is also a factor. A person who is infected but asymptomatic can unknowingly spread an STI to others who also ignore or misinterpret symptoms. By the time either partner seeks medical help, he or she may have infected several others. In addition, many people mistakenly believe that certain sexual practices—oral sex, for example—carry no risk for STIs. In fact, oral sex practices among young adults may be responsible for increases in herpes and other STIs (see the **Student Health Today** box on making oral sex safe). **FIGURE 14.2** shows the continuum of risk for various sexual behaviors, and the **Skills for Behavior Change** box on the next page offers tips for ways to practice safer sex.

High-risk behaviors	Moderate-risk behaviors	Low-risk behaviors	No-risk behaviors
Unprotected vaginal, anal, and oral sex—any activity that involves direct contact with bodily fluids, such as ejaculate, vaginal secretions, or blood—are high-risk behaviors.	Vaginal, anal, or oral sex with a latex or polyurethane condom and a water-based lubricant used properly and consistently can greatly reduce the risk of STI transmission. Dental dams used during oral sex can also greatly reduce the risk of STI transmission.	Mutual masturbation, if there are no cuts on the hand, penis, or vagina, is very low risk. Rubbing, kissing, and massaging carry low risk, but herpes can be spread by skin-to-skin contact from an infected partner.	Abstinence, phone sex, talking, and fantasy are all no-risk behaviors.

FIGURE 14.2 Continuum of Risk for Various Sexual Behaviors There are different levels of risk for various behaviors and various sexually transmitted infections (STIs); however, no matter what, any sexual activity involving direct contact with blood, semen, or vaginal secretions is high risk.

Routes of Transmission

Sexually transmitted infections are generally spread through some form of intimate sexual contact. Vaginal intercourse, oral–genital contact, hand–genital contact, and anal inter-course are the most common modes of transmission. Less likely modes of transmission include mouth-to-mouth contact or contact with fluids from body sores that may be spread by the hands. Although each STI is a different infection caused by a different pathogen, all STI pathogens prefer dark, warm, moist places, especially the mucous membranes lining the reproductive organs. Most of them are susceptible to light and excess heat, cold, and dryness, and many die quickly on exposure to air. Like other communicable infections, STIs have both pathogen-specific *incubation periods* (time between introduction of the pathogen and infection/disease) and periods of *communicability*—times during which transmission is most likely.

WHY SHOULD I CARE?

Getting an STI can be painful, and you can infect your current partner with it. In the long term it could affect your health, the health of your children, and even your ability to have children.

LO 2 | COMMON TYPES OF SEXUALLY TRANSMITTED INFECTIONS

Describe common types of sexually transmitted infections, including their symptoms and treatment methods.

Almost half of all college students report having vaginal sex with at least one partner over the past 30 days, and yet only half of those students used a condom or other protective barrier.[4] In addition to other risky behaviors, sex without a condom—whether it's with a well-known lover or someone whom you just met—puts you at significantly higher risk for STIs. It pays to know about the different types of STIs, including the signs and symptoms to watch out for, so you can protect yourself and your partners.

Chlamydia

Chlamydia, an infection caused by the bacterium *Chlamydia trachomatis* that is often asymptomatic, is the most commonly reported STI in the United States. Chlamydia infects an estimated 2.8 million Americans annually, the majority of them women.[5] Public health officials believe that this estimate could be higher, because many cases go unreported.

chlamydia Bacterially caused STI of the urogenital tract; most commonly reported STI in the United States.

Signs and Symptoms In men, early symptoms may include painful and difficult urination; frequent urination; and a watery, pus-like discharge from the penis. Symptoms in women may include a yellowish discharge, spotting between periods, and occasional spotting after intercourse. However, many chlamydia victims display no symptoms and therefore do not seek help until the disease has done secondary damage. Women are especially likely to be asymptomatic; many do not realize they have the disease, which can put them at risk for secondary damage.

SKILLS FOR BEHAVIOR CHANGE — SAFE IS SEXY

Practicing the following behaviors will help you reduce your risk of contracting a sexually transmitted infection (STI):

- Avoid casual sexual partners. All sexually active adults who are not in a lifelong monogamous relationship should practice safer sex.
- Always use a condom or a dental dam (a sensitive latex sheet, about the size of a tissue, that can be placed over the female genitals to form a protective layer) during vaginal, oral, or anal sex. Remember that condoms do not provide 100 percent protection against all STIs.
- Postpone sexual involvement until you are assured that your partner is not infected; discuss past sexual history and, if necessary, get tested for any potential STIs.
- Avoid injury to body tissue during sexual activity. Some pathogens can enter the bloodstream through microscopic tears in anal or vaginal tissues.
- Avoid unprotected oral, anal, or vaginal sexual activity in which semen, blood, or vaginal secretions could penetrate mucous membranes or enter through breaks in the skin.
- Avoid using drugs and alcohol, which can dull your senses and affect your ability to take responsible precautions with potential sex partners.
- Wash your hands before and after sexual encounters. Urinate after sexual relations and, if possible, wash your genitals.
- Total abstinence is the only absolute way to prevent the transmission of STIs, but abstinence can be a difficult choice to make. If you have any doubt about the potential risks of having sex, consider other means of intimacy (at least until you can assure your safety)—massage, dry kissing, hugging, holding and touching, and masturbation (alone or with a partner).
- Think about situations ahead of time to avoid risky behaviors, including settings with alcohol and drug use.
- If you are worried about your own HIV or STI status, get tested. Don't risk infecting others.
- If you contract an STI, ask your health care provider for advice on notifying past or potential partners.

Sources: American College of Obstetricians and Gynecologists, *How to Prevent Sexually Transmitted Diseases,* ACOG Education Pamphlet AP009 (Washington, DC: American College of Obstetricians and Gynecologists, 2013), Available at www.acog.org/~/media/For%20 Patients/faq009.pdf?dmc=1&ts=20120215T1334311398; American Social Health Association, "Sexual Health: Reduce Your Risk,"2014, www.ashastd.org/std-sti/reduce-your-risk.html.

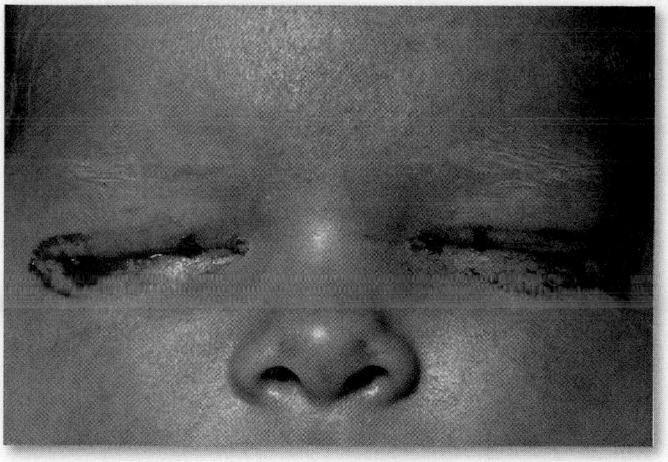

FIGURE 14.3 Conjunctivitis in a Newborn's Eyes Untreated chlamydia and gonorrhea in a pregnant woman can be passed to her child during delivery, causing the eye infection conjunctivitis.

Complications

Men can suffer injury to the prostate gland, seminal vesicles, and bulbourethral glands, as well as arthritis-like symptoms and inflammatory damage to the blood vessels and heart. Men can also experience *epididymitis*, inflammation of the area near the testicles.

In women, chlamydia-related inflammation can injure the cervix or fallopian tubes, causing sterility, and it can damage the inner pelvic structure, leading to **pelvic inflammatory disease (PID)**. If an infected woman becomes pregnant, she has a high risk for miscarriage and stillbirth. Symptoms of PID vary, but generally include lower abdominal pain, fever, unusual vaginal discharge, painful intercourse, painful urination, and irregular menstrual bleeding. The vague symptoms associated with PID can cause women to delay seeking medical care, thereby increasing the risk of permanent damage and scarring that can lead to infertility and ectopic pregnancy.

Women with chlamydia and those who are sexually active with multiple partners are also at greater risk for **urinary tract infections (UTIs)**. Women are disproportionately affected by UTIs because a woman's urethra is much shorter than a man's, making it easier for bacteria to enter the bladder. In addition, a woman's urethra is closer to her anus than is a man's, allowing bacteria to spread into her urethra and cause an infection. Symptoms of a UTI in women include a burning sensation during urination and lower abdominal pain. A UTI can be diagnosed through a urine test and treated by antibiotics. If left untreated, UTIs can cause kidney damage.

Men can also get UTIs, although they are rarer than UTIs in women. One form most commonly caused by *Chlamydia trachomatis* is *nongonococcal urethritis*. Infections should be taken seriously—if you have a milky penile discharge and/or burning during urination, contact your health care provider.[6]

Chlamydia may also be responsible for one type of *conjunctivitis*, an eye infection that affects not only adults but also infants, who can contract the disease from an infected mother during delivery (**FIGURE 14.3**). Untreated conjunctivitis can cause blindness.[7]

Diagnosis and Treatment

A sample of urine or fluid from the vagina or penis is collected and tested to identify the presence of the bacteria. Unfortunately, chlamydia tests are not a routine part of many health clinics' testing procedures and must be specifically requested. If detected early, chlamydia is easily treatable with antibiotics such as tetracycline, doxycycline, or erythromycin.

110 MILLION

PEOPLE ARE LIVING WITH AN **STI** IN THE UNITED STATES.

Gonorrhea

Gonorrhea is one of the most common STIs in the United States, surpassed only by chlamydia in number of cases. The Centers for Disease Control and Prevention (CDC) estimates that there are over 820,000 cases per year, plus many more cases that go unreported.[8] Caused by the bacterial pathogen *Neisseria gonorrhoeae*, gonorrhea primarily infects the linings of the urethra, genital tract, pharynx, and rectum. It may spread to the eyes or other body regions by the hands or through body fluids, typically during vaginal, oral, or anal sex. Most cases occur in individuals between the ages of 15 and 24.[9]

pelvic inflammatory disease (PID) Term used to describe various infections of the female reproductive tract; can be caused by chlamydia or gonorrhea.

urinary tract infection (UTI) Infection, more common among women than men, of the urinary tract; causes include untreated STIs.

gonorrhea Second most common bacterial STI in the United States; if untreated, may cause sterility.

Signs and Symptoms

In men, a typical symptom is a white, milky discharge from the penis accompanied by painful, burning urination 2 to 9 days after contact (**FIGURE 14.4**).

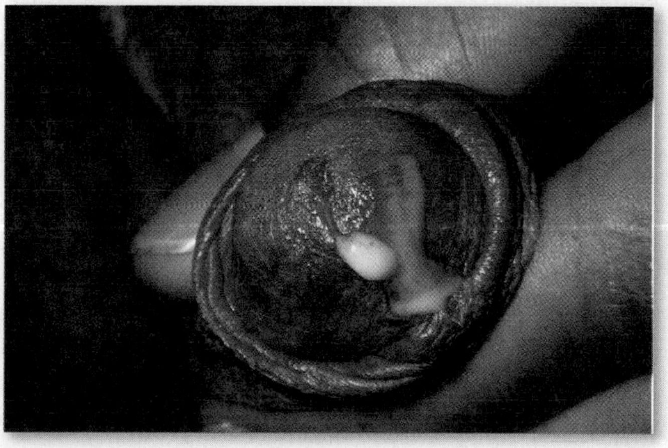

FIGURE 14.4 Gonorrhea One common symptom of gonorrhea in men is a milky discharge from the penis, accompanied by burning sensations during urination. Whereas these symptoms will cause most men to seek diagnosis and treatment, women with gonorrhea are often asymptomatic, so they may not be aware they are infected.

Epididymitis can also occur as a symptom of infection. However, some men with gonorrhea are asymptomatic.

When women contract gonorrhea, the situation is just the opposite: Most do not experience any symptoms; however, if a woman does experience symptoms, they can include vaginal discharge or a burning sensation on urinating.[10] The organism can remain in the woman's vagina, cervix, uterus, or fallopian tubes for long periods with no apparent symptoms other than an occasional slight fever. Thus a woman can be unaware that she has been infected and that she is infecting her sexual partners.

Complications In a man, untreated gonorrhea may spread to the prostate, testicles, urinary tract, kidney, and bladder, and blockage of the vasa deferentia caused by scar tissue may cause sterility. In some cases, the penis develops a painful curvature during erection. If the infection goes undetected in a woman, it can spread to the fallopian tubes and ovaries, causing sterility or, at the very least, severe inflammation and PID. The bacteria can also spread up the reproductive tract or, more rarely, through the blood and infect the joints, heart valves, or brain. If an infected woman becomes pregnant, the infection can be transmitted to her baby during delivery, potentially causing blindness, joint infection, or a life-threatening blood infection.

Diagnosis and Treatment Diagnosis of gonorrhea is similar to that of chlamydia, requiring a sample of either urine or fluid from the vagina or penis to detect the presence of the bacteria. If detected early, gonorrhea is treatable with antibiotics, but the *Neisseria gonorrhoeae* bacterium has begun to develop resistance to some antibiotics. It is also important to recognize that chlamydia and gonorrhea often occur at the same time, but different treatment plans are needed to treat each infection separately. The new guidelines for gonorrhea treatment recommend dual therapy to address the issue of antibiotic-resistant strains.[11]

Syphilis

Syphilis is caused by a bacterium, the spirochete called *Treponema pallidum.* The incidence of syphilis is highest in adults aged 20 to 39, and it is particularly high among African Americans and men who have sex with men. Because it is extremely delicate and dies readily on exposure to air, dryness, or cold, the organism is generally transferred only through direct sexual contact or from mother to fetus. The incidence of syphilis in newborns has continued to increase in the United States.[12]

syphilis One of the most widespread bacterial STIs; characterized by distinct phases and potentially serious results.
chancre Sore often found at the site of syphilis infection.

Signs and Symptoms Syphilis is known as the "great imitator," because its symptoms resemble those of several other infections. It should be noted, however, that some people experience no symptoms at all. Syphilis can occur in four distinct stages:[13]

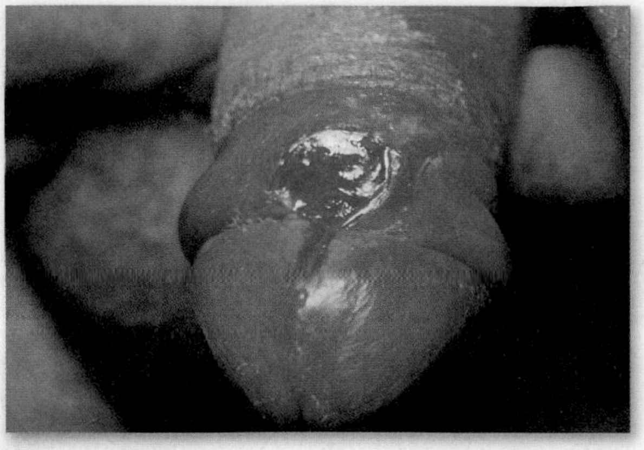

(a) Primary syphilis

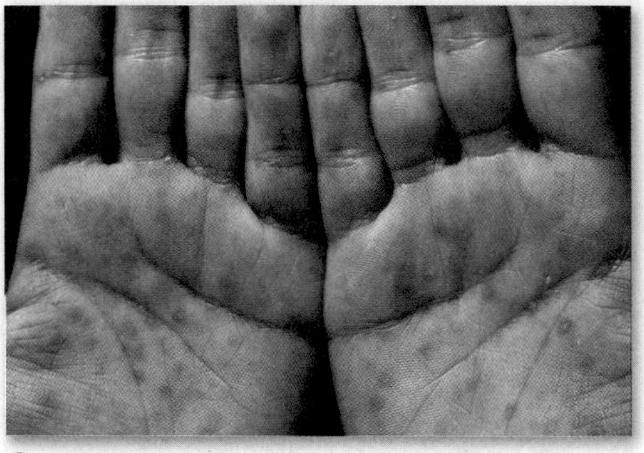

(b) Secondary syphilis

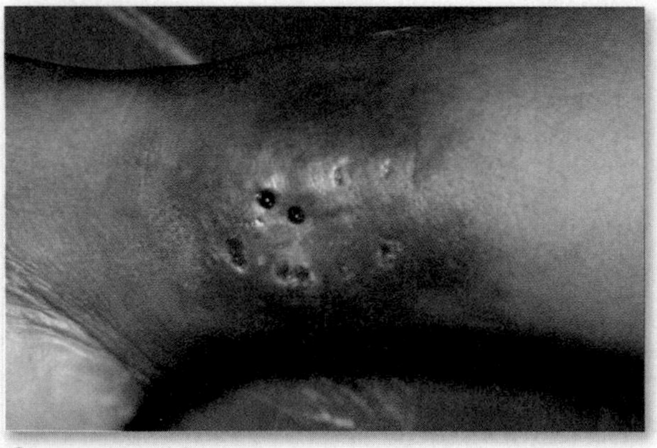

(c) Latent syphilis

FIGURE 14.5 Syphilis A chancre on the site of the initial infection is a symptom of primary syphilis **(a)**. A rash is characteristic of secondary syphilis **(b)**. Lesions called "gummas" are often present in latent syphilis **(c)**.

- **Primary syphilis.** The first stage of syphilis, particularly for men, is often characterized by the development of a **chancre** (pronounced "shank-er"), a sore located most frequently at the infection site that usually appears about a month after initial infection (see **FIGURE 14.5**). In men, the site of the chancre tends to be the penis or scrotum; in women, the site of infection is often internal, on the vaginal wall or high on the cervix where the chancre is not readily apparent and the likelihood of detection is not great. Detected or not, the chancre oozes with bacteria, ready to infect an unsuspecting partner. In both men and women, the chancre will disappear in 3 to 6 weeks.

- **Secondary syphilis.** If the infection is left untreated, a month to a year after the chancre disappears secondary symptoms may appear, including a rash or white patches on the skin or on the mucous membranes of the mouth, throat, or genitals. Hair loss may occur, lymph nodes may enlarge, and the victim may develop a slight fever or headache. In rare cases, sores develop around the mouth or genitals. As during the active chancre phase, these sores contain infectious bacteria, and contact with them can spread the infection.
- **Latent syphilis.** After the secondary stage, if the infection is left untreated, the syphilis spirochetes begin to invade body organs, causing lesions called *gummas.* The infection now is rarely transmitted to others, except during pregnancy, when it can be passed to the fetus.
- **Tertiary/late syphilis.** Years after syphilis has entered the body, its effects become all too evident if still untreated. Late-stage syphilis indications include heart and central nervous system damage, blindness, deafness, paralysis, premature senility, and, ultimately, dementia.

Complications Pregnant women with syphilis can experience complications, including premature births, miscarriages, and stillbirths. An infected pregnant woman may transmit the syphilis to her unborn child. The infant will then be born with *congenital syphilis,* which can cause death; severe birth defects such as blindness, deafness, or disfigurement; developmental delays; seizures; and other health problems. Because in most cases the fetus does not become infected until after the first trimester, treatment of the mother during this time will usually prevent infection of the fetus.

Diagnosis and Treatment

There are two methods that can be used to diagnose syphilis. In the primary stage, a sample from the chancre is collected to identify the bacteria. Another method of diagnosing syphilis is through a blood test. Syphilis can easily be treated with antibiotics, usually penicillin, for all stages except the late stage.

Herpes

As mentioned previously in this chapter text, herpes is a general term for a family of infections characterized by sores or eruptions on the skin and caused by the herpes simplex virus. The herpes family of diseases is not transmitted exclusively by sexual contact. Kissing or sharing eating utensils can also exchange saliva and transmit the infection. Herpes infections range from mildly uncomfortable to extremely serious. **Genital herpes** affects approximately 16.2 percent of the population aged 14 to 49 in the United States.[14]

genital herpes STI caused by the herpes simplex virus.

There are two types of herpes simplex virus. Only about 1 in 6 Americans currently has HSV-2; however, about half of adults have HSV-1, usually appearing as cold sores on their mouths.[15] Both herpes simplex types 1 and 2 can infect any area of the body, producing lesions (sores) in and around the vaginal area; on the penis; and around the anal opening, buttocks, thighs, or mouth (see **FIGURE 14.6**). Whether you contract HSV-1 or HSV-2 on your genitals, the net results may be just as painful, just as long term, and just as infectious for future partners. Herpes simplex virus remains in certain nerve cells for life and can flare up when the body's ability to maintain itself is weakened.

People may contract genital herpes from sexual contact with others who may not realize they are infected, or with those who do know they are infected but may be having outbreaks of herpes without any sores. Genital herpes can also be transferred during oral sex. Herpes is spread very rarely by touching shared objects like toilet seats.

Signs and Symptoms The precursor phase of a herpes infection is characterized by a burning sensation and redness at the site of infection. This phase of the disease is quickly followed by the second phase, in which a blister filled with a clear fluid containing the virus forms. If you pick at this blister or otherwise touch the site and spread this fluid with fingers, lipstick, lip balm, or other products, you can autoinoculate other body parts. Particularly dangerous is the

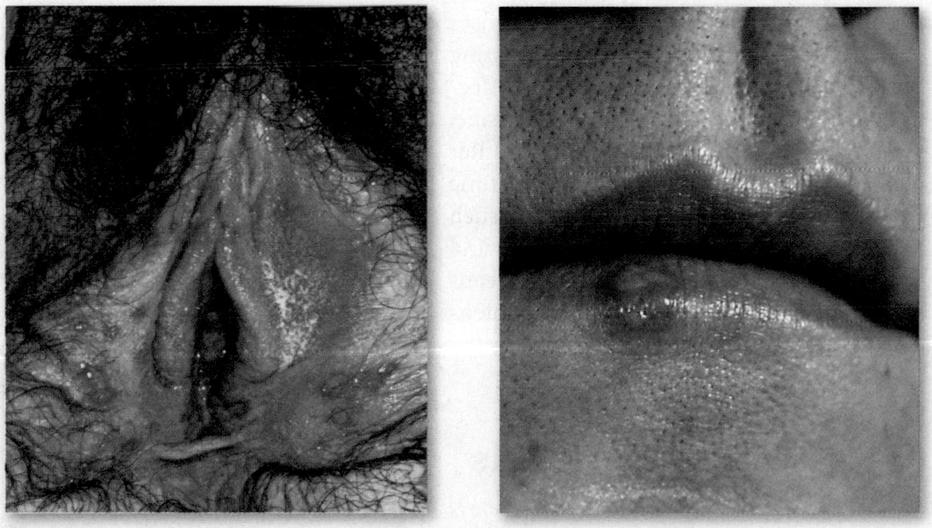

(a) Genital herpes is a highly contagious and incurable STI. It is characterized by recurring cycles of painful blisters on the genitalia.

(b) Oral herpes, caused by the same virus as genital herpes, is extremely contagious and can cause painful sores and blisters around the mouth.

FIGURE 14.6 **Herpes** Both genital and oral herpes can be caused by either herpes simplex virus type 1 or 2. Genital herpes is highly contagious and incurable **(a)**. Oral herpes is the same virus as genital herpes, but occurs in and around the mouth **(b)**.

possibility of spreading the infection to your eyes, since a herpes lesion on the eye can cause blindness.

Over a period of days, the unsightly blister will crust over, dry up, and disappear, and the virus will travel to the base of an affected nerve supplying the area and become dormant. Only when the victim becomes overly stressed, when diet and sleep are inadequate, when the immune system is overworked, or when excessive exposure to sunlight or other stressors occur will the virus become reactivated (at the same site every time) and begin the blistering cycle all over again. Each time a sore develops, it casts off (sheds) viruses that can be highly infectious. However, it is important to note that a herpes site can shed the virus even when no overt sore is present, particularly during the interval between the earliest symptoms and blistering.

genital warts Warts that appear in the genital area or the anus; caused by the human papillomavirus (HPV).

human papillomavirus (HPV) A group of viruses, many of which are transmitted sexually; some types of HPV can cause genital warts or cervical cancer.

Complications Genital herpes is especially serious in pregnant women because the baby can be infected as it passes through the vagina during birth. Many physicians recommend cesarean deliveries for infected women. Additionally, women with a history of genital herpes appear to have a greater risk of developing cervical cancer.

Diagnosis and Treatment Diagnosis of herpes can be determined by collecting a sample from the suspected sore or by performing a blood test to identify an HSV-1 or HSV-2 infection. Although there is no cure for herpes at present, certain drugs can be used to treat symptoms. During the precursor phase, prescription medicines such as acyclovir and over-the-counter medications such as Abreva will often keep the disease from spreading. However, most drugs only seem to work if the infection is confirmed during the first few hours after contact. The effectiveness of other treatments, such as L-lysine, is largely unsubstantiated. Over-the-counter medications may reduce the length of time you have sores/symptoms. Other drugs, such as famciclovir (FAMVIR), may reduce viral shedding between outbreaks. This means that if you have outbreaks, you may potentially reduce risks to your sexual partners.[16]

Human Papillomavirus (HPV) and Genital Warts

Genital warts (also known as *venereal warts* or *condylomas*) are caused by a group of viruses known as **human papillomavirus (HPV)**. There are over 100 different types of HPV; more than 40 types are sexually transmitted and are classified as either low risk or high risk. A person becomes infected when certain types of HPV penetrate the skin and mucous membranes of the genitals or anus. This is among the most common forms of STI, with 79 million Americans currently infected with genital HPV and approximately 14 million new cases each year.[17]

Signs and Symptoms Genital HPV appears to be relatively easy to catch. The typical incubation period is 6 to 8 weeks after contact. People infected with low risk types of HPV may develop genital warts, a series of bumps or growths on the genitals, ranging in size from small pinheads to large cauliflower-like growths (see **FIGURE 14.7**).

Complications HPV poses a significant risk for cervical cancer in women. High-risk types of HPV (16 and 18) are responsible for an estimated 70 percent of cervical cancer cases.[18] Exactly how high-risk HPV infection leads to cervical cancer is uncertain, though it may lead to *dysplasia*, or changes in cells that may lead to a precancerous condition. It is known that a pap test done as routine screening for women aged 21 to 65 years old can help prevent cervical cancer.[19]

Of those cases that become precancerous and are left untreated, 70 percent will eventually result in actual cancer. In addition, HPV may also pose a threat to a fetus that is exposed to the virus during birth. Cesarean deliveries may be considered in serious cases. HPV can cause cancers—called "oropharyngeal cancers"—in the back of the throat, often around the tonsils or the base of the tongue. Each year, approximately 8,400 Americans are diagnosed with HPV-caused cancers of the oropharynx.[20] Men are about three times more likely to develop cancers of the oropharynx than are women.[21]

Diagnosis and Treatment Diagnosis of genital warts from low-risk types of HPV is determined through a visual examination by a health care provider. High-risk types

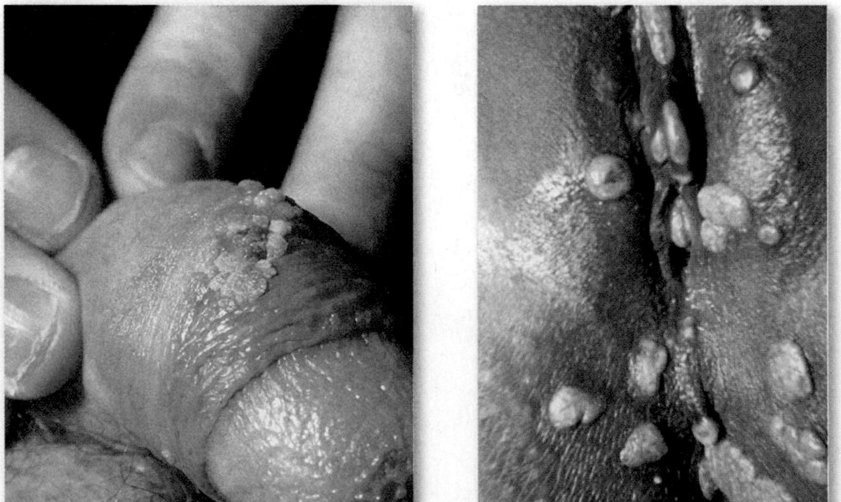

FIGURE 14.7 Genital Warts Genital warts are caused by certain types of the human papillomavirus.

STUDENT HEALTH TODAY

Q&A ON HPV VACCINES

Most sexually active people will contract some form of human papillomavirus (HPV) at some time in their lives, though they may never even know it. There are about 40 types of sexually transmitted HPV, most of which cause no symptoms and go away on their own. Low-risk types can cause genital warts, but some high-risk types can cause cervical and other cancers. Every year in the United States, about 12,000 women are diagnosed with cervical cancer, and almost 4,000 die from this disease. There are currently two HPV vaccines that can help prevent women from becoming infected with HPV and subsequently developing cervical cancer.

- **Who should get the HPV vaccine?** There are two vaccines currently available—Cervarix and Gardasil. HPV vaccines are recommended for 11- and 12-year-old girls, but can be given to girls as young as 9 years old. It is also recommended for girls and women ages 13 through 26 who have not yet been vaccinated or completed the vaccine series. Ideally, females should get a vaccine before they become sexually active. Females who are sexually active may get less benefit from it because they may have already contracted an HPV type targeted by the vaccines.

  One of the HPV vaccines, Gardasil, is also licensed, safe, and effective for males ages 9 through 26 years. The CDC recommends Gardasil for all boys 11 or 12 years old and for males ages 13 through 21 years who did not get any or all of the three recommended doses when they were younger. All men may receive the vaccine through the age of 26, but it is recommended that they should speak with their doctor to find out if getting vaccinated is right for them.

- **How are the two HPV vaccines, Cervarix and Gardasil, similar and different?** Both vaccines are very effective against high-risk HPV types 16 and 18, which cause 70 percent of cervical cancer cases. Both vaccines are given as shots and require three doses, but only Gardasil protects against low-risk HPV types 6 and 11. These HPV types cause 90 percent of cases of genital warts in females and males, so Gardasil is approved for use with males as well as females.

- **What do the two vaccines not protect against?** The vaccines do not protect against all types of HPV, so about 30 percent of cervical cancers will not be prevented by the vaccines. It will be important for women to continue getting screened for cervical cancer through regular Pap tests. Also, the vaccines do not prevent other sexually transmitted infections (STIs).

- **How safe are the HPV vaccines?** The vaccines are licensed by the FDA and approved by the CDC as safe and effective. They have been studied in thousands of females (ages 9 through 26) around the world, and their safety continues to be monitored by the CDC and the FDA. Studies have found no serious side effects.

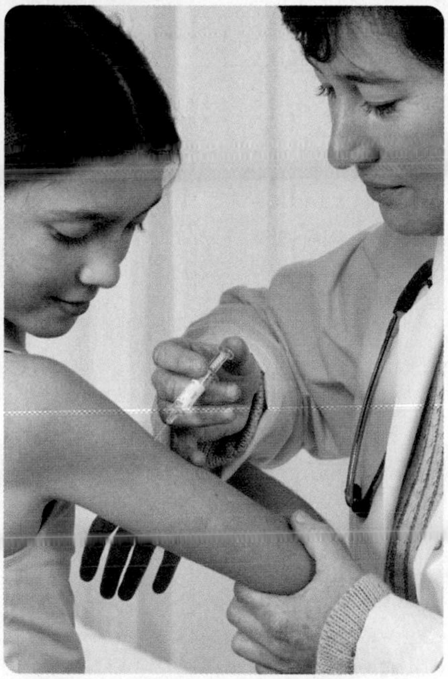

Many state health departments and college campuses offer free or low-cost vaccines for those whose insurance does not cover the cost.

Sources: Centers for Disease Control and Prevention, "Vaccines and Preventable Diseases: HPV Vaccine—Questions & Answers," Reviewed July 2012, www.cdc.gov/vaccines/vpd-vac/hpv/vac-faqs.htm; American Cancer Society, 2014, "Human Papillomavirus (HPV), Cancer and HPV Vaccines—Frequently Asked Questions," Revised 2014, www.cancer.org/cancer/cancercauses/othercarcinogens/infectiousagents/hpv/humanpapillomavirusandhpvvaccinesfaq/index.

can be diagnosed in women through microscopic analysis of cells from a Pap smear or by collecting a sample from the cervix to test for HPV DNA. There is currently no HPV DNA test for men.

Treatment is available only for the low-risk forms of HPV that cause genital warts. The warts can be treated with topical medication or can be frozen with liquid nitrogen and then removed. Large warts may require surgical removal. There are currently two HPV vaccines that are licensed by the U.S. Food and Drug Administration (FDA) and recommended by the CDC. See the **Student Health Today** box for more information about these vaccines.

Candidiasis (Moniliasis)

Most STIs are caused by pathogens that come from outside the body; however, the yeast-like fungus *Candida albicans* is a normal inhabitant of the vaginal tract in most women. (See Figure 13.5c in **Chapter 13** for a micrograph of this fungus.) Only when the normal chemical balance of the vagina is disturbed will these organisms multiply and cause the fungal disease **candidiasis**, also sometimes called *moniliasis* or a *yeast infection.*

candidiasis Yeast-like fungal infection often transmitted sexually; also called *moniliasis* or *yeast infection.*

Signs and Symptoms Symptoms of candidiasis include severe itching and burning of the vagina and vulva and a white, cottage cheese–like vaginal discharge.[22] When this microbe infects the mouth, whitish patches form, and the condition is referred to as *thrush*. Thrush infection can also occur in men and is easily transmitted between sexual partners. Symptoms of candidiasis can be aggravated by contact with soaps, douches, perfumed toilet paper, chlorinated water, and spermicides.

Diagnosis and Treatment Diagnosis of candidiasis is usually made by collecting a vaginal sample and analyzing it to identify the pathogen. Antifungal drugs applied on the surface or by suppository usually cure candidiasis in just a few days.

Trichomoniasis

Unlike many STIs, **trichomoniasis** is caused by a protozoan, *Trichomonas vaginalis*. (See Figure 13.5d in **Chapter 13** for a micrograph of this organism.) An estimated 3.7 million Americans have the infection, but only about one-third of those who contract it experience symptoms.[23] Although usually transmitted by sexual contact, the "trich" organism can also be spread by toilet seats, wet towels, or other items that have discharged fluids on them.

Signs and Symptoms Symptoms among women include a foamy, yellowish, unpleasant-smelling discharge accompanied by a burning sensation, itching, and painful urination. Most men with trichomoniasis do not have any symptoms, though some men experience irritation inside the penis, mild discharge, and a slight burning after urinating.[24]

Diagnosis and Treatment Diagnosis of trichomoniasis is determined by collecting and testing fluid samples from the penis or vagina to test for the presence of the protozoan. Treatment includes oral metronidazole, usually given to both sexual partners to avoid the "ping-pong" effect of repeated cross-infection.

trichomoniasis Protozoan STI characterized by foamy, yellowish discharge and unpleasant odor.

pubic lice Parasitic insects that can inhabit various body areas, especially the genitals.

acquired immunodeficiency syndrome (AIDS) A disease caused by a retrovirus, the human immunodeficiency virus (HIV), that attacks the immune system, reducing the number of helper T cells and leaving the victim vulnerable to infections, malignancies, and neurological disorders.

human immunodeficiency virus (HIV) The virus that causes AIDS by infecting helper T cells.

Pubic Lice

Pubic lice, often called "crabs," are small parasitic insects that are usually transmitted during sexual contact (see **FIGURE 14.8**). More annoying than dangerous, they move easily from partner to partner during sex. Lice have an affinity for pubic hair and attach themselves to the base of these hairs, where they deposit their eggs (nits). One to 2 weeks later, these nits develop into adults that lay eggs and migrate to other body parts, thus perpetuating the cycle.

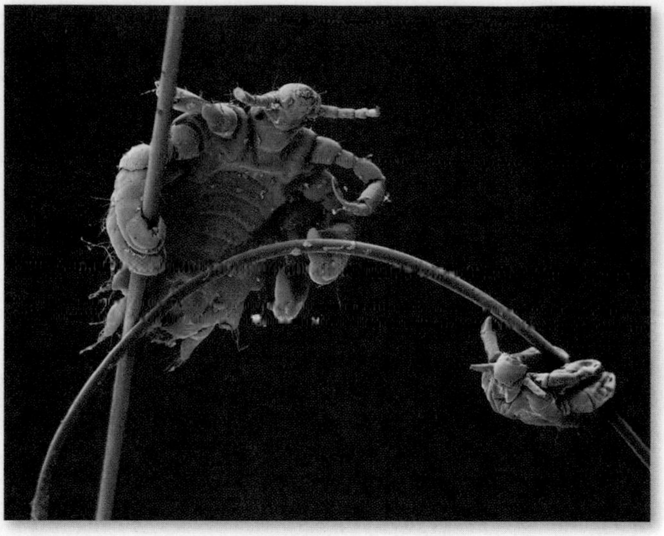

FIGURE 14.8 Pubic Lice Pubic lice, also known as "crabs," are small, parasitic insects that attach themselves to pubic hair.

Signs and Symptoms Symptoms of pubic lice infestation include itchiness in the area covered by pubic hair, bluish-gray skin color in the pubic region, and sores in the genital area.

Diagnosis and Treatment Diagnosis of pubic lice involves an examination by a health care provider to identify the eggs in the genital area. Treatment includes washing clothing, furniture, and linens that may harbor the eggs. Over-the-counter lotions containing permethrin can kill lice and eggs in affected areas.[25] It usually takes 2 to 3 weeks to kill all larval forms. Although sexual contact is the most common mode of transmission, you can "catch" pubic lice from lying on sheets or sitting on a toilet seat that an infected person has used.

LO 3 | HIV/AIDS

Discuss human immunodeficiency virus (HIV) and acquired immunodeficiency syndrome (AIDS), trends in infection and treatment, and the impact of HIV/AIDS on special populations.

Acquired immunodeficiency syndrome (AIDS) is a significant global health threat. Since 1981, when AIDS was first recognized, approximately 75 million people in the world have become infected with **human immunodeficiency virus (HIV)**, the virus that causes AIDS. About 35.3 million people worldwide are living with HIV.[26] The vast majority of HIV-infected individuals (approximately 70%) are in sub-Saharan Africa. Globally, the numbers of people living with HIV have increased, even though the numbers of new infections have decreased in the last decade.[27] In the United

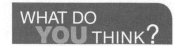

WHAT DO YOU THINK?

Do you think we have grown too apathetic about HIV/AIDS in the United States?

- Is HIV/AIDS prevention discussed on your campus?
- Are people as concerned with HIV as they are with other STIs?

States, there are over 1 million people infected with HIV. About 15,000 people die from HIV/AIDS each year.[28]

Initially, people with HIV were diagnosed as having AIDS only when they developed blood infections, the cancer known as Kaposi's sarcoma, or any of 21 other indicator diseases, most of which were common in male AIDS patients. The CDC has expanded the indicator list to include pulmonary tuberculosis, recurrent pneumonia, and invasive cervical cancer. Perhaps the most significant indicator today is a drop in the level of the body's master immune cells, CD4 cells (also called helper T cells), to one-fifth the level in a healthy person.

AIDS cases have been reported state by state throughout the United States since the early 1980s. Today, the CDC recommends that all states report HIV infections as well as AIDS. Because of medical advances in treatment and increasing numbers of HIV-infected persons who do not progress to AIDS, it is believed that AIDS incidence statistics may not provide a true picture of the epidemic, the long-term costs of treating HIV-infected individuals, whether we continue to make progress on prevention, and other key information.

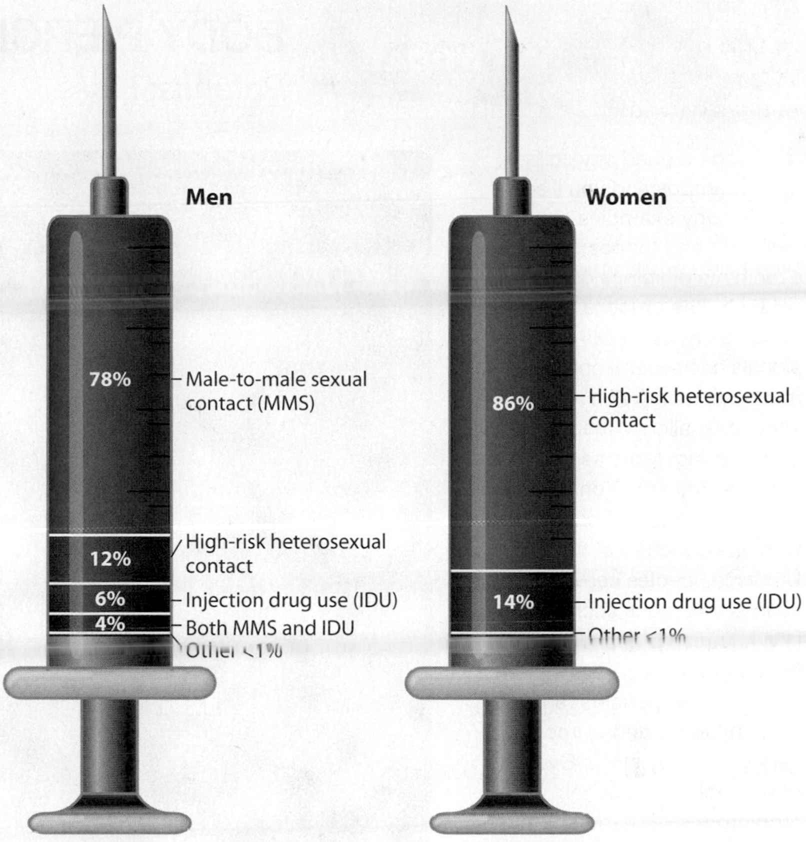

FIGURE 14.9 **Sources of HIV Infection among Adults and Adolescents in the United States, 2011**

Source: Data are from the Centers for Disease Control and Prevention, *HIV Surveillance: Epidemiology of HIV Infection (through 2011)*, Updated 2013, www.cdc.gov/hiv/library/reports/surveillance.

How HIV Is Transmitted

HIV typically enters one person's body when another person's infected body fluids (e.g., semen, vaginal secretions, blood) gain entry through a breach in body defenses. Mucous membranes of the genital organs and the anus provide the easiest route of entry. If there is a break in the mucous membranes (as can occur during sexual intercourse, particularly anal intercourse), the virus enters and begins to multiply. After initial infection, HIV multiplies rapidly, invading the bloodstream and cerebrospinal fluid. It progressively destroys helper T cells (recall that these cells call the rest of the immune response to action), weakening the body's resistance to disease.

ONLY 34%

OF THOSE WITH HIV IN LOW- AND MIDDLE-INCOME COUNTRIES RECEIVE **TREATMENT**.

It is important to know that HIV is transmitted in very specific ways. It cannot reproduce outside a living host, except in a controlled laboratory environment, and does not survive well in open air. As a result, HIV cannot be transmitted through casual contact, including sharing glasses, utensils, or musical instruments. Transmission also cannot occur through swimming pools, showers, or by sharing washing facilities or toilet seats.[29] Research also provides overwhelming evidence that insect bites do not transmit HIV.[30]

Engaging in High-Risk Behaviors AIDS is not a disease of gay people or minority groups. Although during the early days of the epidemic it appeared that HIV infected only homosexuals, it quickly became apparent that the disease was not confined to groups of people, but rather was related to high-risk behaviors such as having unprotected sexual intercourse and sharing needles. People who engage in high-risk behaviors increase their risk for the disease; people who do not engage in these behaviors have minimal risk. **FIGURE 14.9** shows the breakdown of sources of HIV infection among U.S. men and women.

The majority of HIV infections arise from the following high-risk behaviors:

- **Exchange of body fluids.** The greatest risk factor is the exchange of HIV-infected body fluids during vaginal or anal intercourse. Substantial research indicates that blood, semen, and vaginal secretions are the major fluids of concern. In rare instances, the virus has been found in saliva, but most health officials state that saliva is a less significant risk than other shared body fluids.

STUDENT HEALTH TODAY

BODY PIERCING AND TATTOOING

Potential Risks

Look around any college campus and you'll see many examples of body piercings and tattoos; you may even have piercings or tattoos yourself. The practice can be done safely, but health professionals cite several concerns, most commonly skin reactions, infections, allergic reactions, and scarring. More serious is the potential transmission of dangerous pathogens that can occur with any puncture of the skin. Unsterile needles can spread serious infections such as staph, HIV, hepatitis B and C, and tetanus.

Laws and policies regulating body piercing and tattooing vary greatly by state. Because of the lack of universal regulatory standards and the potential for transmission of dangerous pathogens, anyone who receives a tattoo, body piercing, or permanent makeup tattoo cannot donate blood for 1 year. Finding a safe and reputable body artist for a tattoo or piercing should be the priority. The following tips can help reduce risks:

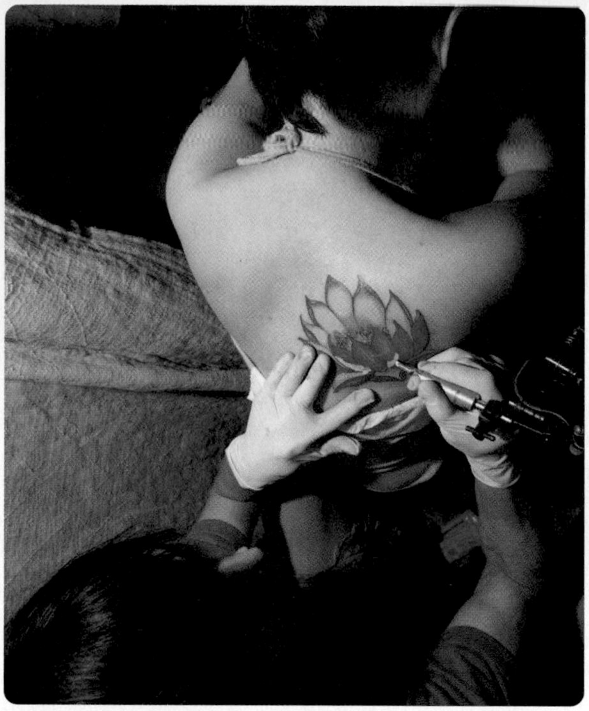

Like any activity that involves bodily fluids, tattooing carries some risk of disease transmission.

- Look for clean, well-lighted work areas, and inquire about sterilization procedures. Be wary of establishments that won't answer questions or show you their sterilization equipment.
- Packaged, sterilized needles should be used only once and then discarded. A piercing gun should not be used, because it cannot be sterilized properly. Watch that the artist uses new needles and tubes from a sterile package before your procedure begins. Ask to see the sterile confirmation logo on the bag itself.
- Immediately before piercing or tattooing, the body area should be carefully sterilized. The artist should wash his or her hands and put on new latex gloves for each procedure. Make sure the artist changes gloves if he or she touches anything else, such as the telephone, while working.
- Leftover tattoo ink should be discarded after each procedure. Do not allow the artist to reuse ink that has been used for other customers. Used needles should be disposed of in a "sharps" container, a plastic container with the biohazard symbol clearly marked on it.

Source: Mayo Clinic Staff, "Tattoos: Understand Risks and Precautions," March 2012, www.mayoclinic.com/health/tattoos-and-piercings/MC00020.

- **Contaminated needles.** A significant percentage of AIDS cases in the United States result from sharing or using HIV-contaminated needles and syringes. Although users of illegal drugs are commonly considered the only members of this category, others may also share needles—for example, people with diabetes who inject insulin or athletes who inject steroids. People who share needles and also engage in sexual activities with members of high-risk groups, such as those who exchange sex for drugs, increase their risks dramatically. Tattooing and piercing can also be risky (see the **Student Health Today** box).

Mother-to-Child (Perinatal) Transmission

Mother-to-child transmission occurs when an HIV-positive woman passes the virus to her baby. This can occur during pregnancy, during labor and delivery, or through breast-feeding. Without antiretroviral treatment, approximately 15 to 45 percent of HIV-positive pregnant women will transmit the virus to their infant.[31]

Signs and Symptoms of HIV/AIDS

A person may go for months or years after infection by HIV before any significant symptoms appear. The incubation time varies greatly from person to person. For adults who receive no medical treatment, it takes an average of 8 to 10 years for the virus to cause the slow, degenerative changes in the immune system that are characteristic of AIDS. During this time, the person may experience *opportunistic infections* (infections that gain a foothold when the immune system is not functioning effectively). Colds, sore throats, fever, tiredness, nausea, night sweats, and other generally non–life-threatening conditions commonly appear and are described

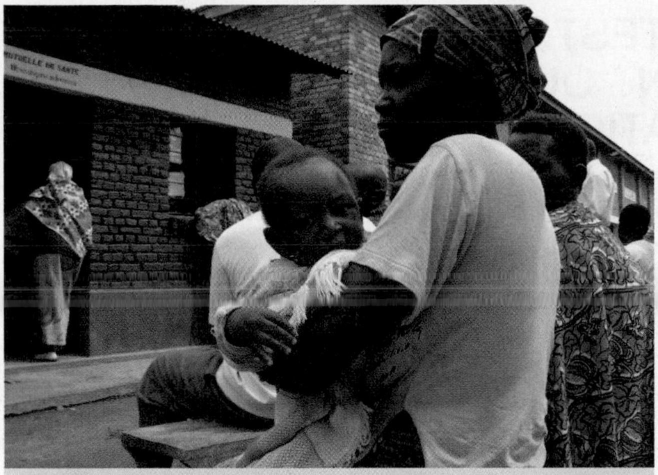

In North America, 1.4 million people are living with HIV, and HIV and AIDS are still at epidemic levels all over the world, especially in developing nations. Sub-Saharan Africa has been hit hardest by HIV/AIDS, with nearly 1 in every 20 adults living with HIV.

Sources: Joint United Nations Programme on HIV/AIDS (UNAIDS) and World Health Organization (WHO), *2013 UNAIDS Report on the Global AIDS Epidemic* (Geneva: UNAIDS, 2013), Available at www.unaids.org/en/resources/publications/2013/name,85053,en.asp; Care.org, "HIV/AIDS," 2013, www.care.org/work/health/hiv-aids/hiv-aids-facts.

as pre-AIDS symptoms. Other symptoms of progressing HIV infection include wasting syndrome, swollen lymph nodes, and neurological problems. As the immune system continues to decline, the body becomes more vulnerable to infection. A diagnosis of AIDS, the final stage of HIV infection, is made when the infected person has either a dangerously low CD4 (helper T) cell count (below 200 cells per cubic milliliter of blood) or has contracted one or more opportunistic infections characteristic of the disease (such as Kaposi's sarcoma or *Pneumocystis carinii* pneumonia).

Testing for HIV Antibodies

Once antibodies have formed in reaction to HIV, a blood test known as the *ELISA* (enzyme-linked immunosorbent assay) may detect their presence. It can take 3 to 6 months after initial infection for sufficient antibodies to develop in the body to show a positive test result. Therefore, individuals with negative test results should be retested within 6 months. If sufficient antibodies are present, the test will be positive. When a person who previously tested *negative* (no HIV antibodies present) has a subsequent test that is *positive,* seroconversion is said to have occurred. In such a situation, the person would typically take another ELISA test, followed by a more precise test known as the *Western blot,* to confirm the presence of HIV antibodies.

A polymerase chain reaction (PCR) test detects the genetic material of HIV instead of the antibodies to the virus and can identify HIV within the first few weeks of infection. It is often performed on babies born to mothers who are HIV positive. Rapid HIV tests using blood or oral fluids are also available and can produce results in 20 minutes. However, they require a confirmatory test with positive results, which may take up to several weeks. Home kits are also available, allowing a person to take a blood or saliva sample and anonymously send it to a laboratory. The person then calls a number to find out their results, with professional counselors available to provide support.[32]

It should be noted that these tests are not AIDS tests per se. Rather, they detect antibodies for HIV, indicating the presence of the virus in the person's system. Whether the person will develop AIDS depends to some extent on the strength of the immune system.

Health officials distinguish between *reported* and *actual* cases of HIV infection because it is believed that many HIV-positive people avoid being tested. One reason is fear of knowing the truth. Another is the fear of recrimination from employers, insurance companies, and medical staff. However, early detection and reporting are important because immediate treatment for someone in the early stages of HIV disease is critical.

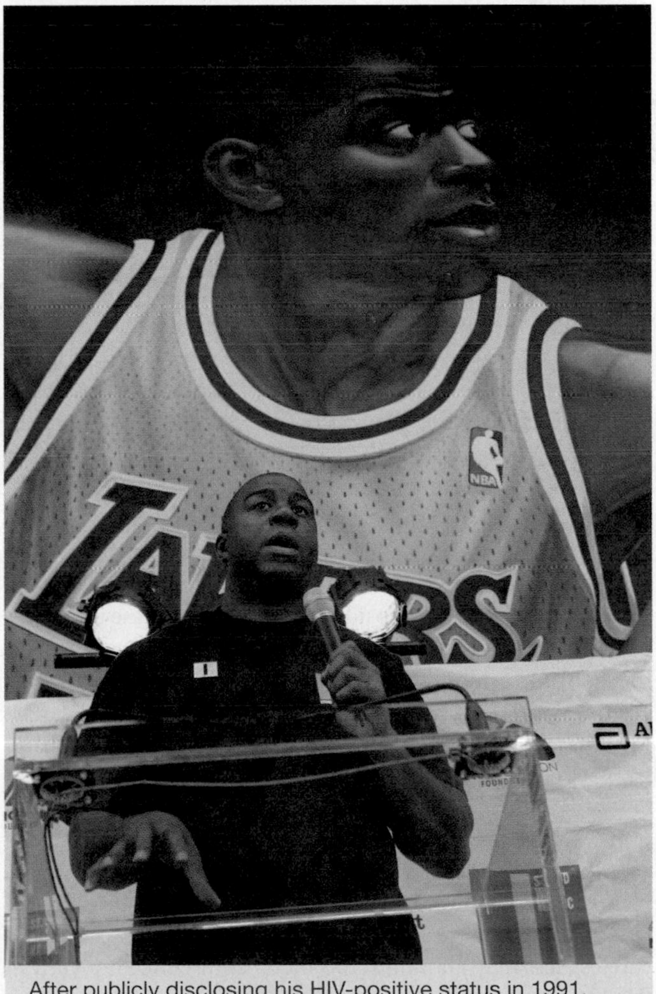

After publicly disclosing his HIV-positive status in 1991, former L.A. Laker star Earvin "Magic" Johnson became the first openly HIV-positive basketball player in the NBA.

TECH & HEALTH

SIMPLER TESTS CAN IMPROVE TREATMENT OUTCOMES FOR HIV AND TB PATIENTS

One of the side effects of AIDS antiviral therapy and tuberculosis treatment is liver failure due to the toxicity of the medication used to treat those diseases. In Africa that's been especially difficult to combat, as the tests routinely used to monitor liver function for signs of trouble require tubes of blood, laboratory facilities, and time for processing results, as well as money for all of the above. In a place where poverty is widespread and patients are many, but skilled health care workers and equipment are scarce, liver function often goes unmonitored in those who are at greatest risk. It is estimated that in resource-poor countries, approximately 25 percent of HIV/AIDS patients lack access to diagnostic tools and die as a result of liver complications related to treatment. But a new cheap and simple test that determines liver function could change that.

The new test is a piece of specially treated paper the size of a stamp that costs around 10 cents. A small amount of blood or urine is applied, and then chemicals in the paper change color to show the result. As with diabetes or pregnancy home-testing kits, the test is designed to be simple enough so the person reading it doesn't need to be a trained medical professional to understand the results, and it doesn't need any external power or equipment. This test improves the odds for patients with tuberculosis or HIV/AIDS to able to withstand the side effects of their treatments successfully.

Source: Diagnostics for All, "Liver Function Test," 2012, www.dfa.org/projects/liver-function.php; D. McNeil, "Far from Any Lab, Paper Bits Find Illness," September 27, 2011, *The New York Times*; A. Maloney, "AlterNet's Top 20 Big Ideas that Don't Cost the Earth," 2011, www.trust.org/alertnet/news/alertnets-top-20-big-ideas-that-dont-cost-the-earth.

New Hope and Treatments

Drugs have slowed the progression from HIV to AIDS and have prolonged life expectancies for most AIDS patients. Evidence is increasing that treating HIV-positive babies within a few hours of birth can dramatically restrict—and perhaps eliminate—infection, as indicated in two recent cases of babies who were born with HIV and who are now HIV negative. A clinical trial is being conducted to study this treatment and to further investigate implications.[33] Antiretroviral therapy (ART), the current treatment method, combines selected drugs, especially protease inhibitors and reverse transcriptase inhibitors. *Protease inhibitors* (e.g., amprenavir, ritonavir, and saquinavir) act to prevent the production of the virus in chronically infected cells that HIV has already invaded. Other drugs, such as azidothymidine (AZT), rilpivirine (RPV), ddI, ddC, d4T, and 3TC, inhibit the HIV enzyme *reverse transcriptase* before the virus has invaded the cell, thereby preventing the virus from infecting new cells. These drugs are categorized as either non-nucleoside reverse transcriptase inhibitors or nucleoside reverse transcriptase inhibitors, based on their mechanism to inhibit the enzyme. All of the protease drugs seem to work best in combination with other therapies. The FDA has approved several fixed-dose combinations of drugs from two or more classes, most recently, *Complera*, which combines nucleoside reverse transcriptase inhibitors with non-nucleoside reverse transcriptase inhibitors.[34]

Although these drugs provide new hope and longer survival rates for people living with HIV, it is important to maintain caution. We are still a long way from a cure. Apathy and carelessness may abound if too much confidence is placed in these treatments. Newer drugs that held much promise are becoming less effective as HIV develops resistance to them. Costs of taking multiple drugs are prohibitive, and they can cause serious damage to the liver if they are not carefully monitored (see the **Tech & Health** box for more on efforts to make these drug regimens safer). Furthermore, the number of people becoming HIV infected each year has increased in some communities, meaning that we are still a long way from beating this disease.

Preventing HIV Infection

Although scientists have been working on a variety of HIV vaccine trials, none is currently available. The only way to prevent HIV infection is through the choices you make in sexual behaviors and drug use and by taking responsibility for your own health and the health of your loved ones. You can't determine the presence of HIV by looking at a person; you can't tell by questioning the person, unless he or she has been tested recently and is giving an honest answer. So what should you do?

Of course, the simplest answer is abstinence. If you don't exchange body fluids, you won't get the disease. As a second line of defense, if you decide to be intimate, the next best option is to use a condom. However, in spite of all the educational campaigns, surveys consistently indicate that most college students throw caution to the wind if they think they "know" someone—and they have unprotected sex.

Where to Go for Help If you are concerned about your own risk or that of a close friend, arrange a confidential meeting with the health educator or other health professional at your college health service. He or she will provide you with the information that you need to decide whether you should be tested for HIV antibodies. If the student health service is not an option for you, seek assistance through your local public health department or community STI clinic.

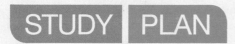

STUDY PLAN

Customize your study plan—and master your health!—in the Study Area of **MasteringHealth**.

ASSESS **YOURSELF**

Is misinformation about STIs putting your health at risk? Take the **STIs: Do You Really Know What You Think You Know?** assessment available on MasteringHealth.

Need help creating a plan? Follow the strategies in the **Your Plan for Change** box for short- and long-term improvements to your health.

YOUR PLAN FOR **CHANGE**

After completing the "STIs: Do You Really Know What You Think You Know?" **ASSESS YOURSELF**, you can begin to change behaviors that may be putting you at risk for STIs.

TODAY, YOU CAN:

- ☐ Put together an "emergency" supply of protection including condoms and possibly dental dams, and remember to use them. Outside of abstinence, condoms are your best protection against an STI. Both men and women are responsible for preventing the transmission of STIs.
- ☐ Avoid mixing alcohol, drugs, and sex. Alcohol can lower your inhibitions, increasing the risk of STIs, and drugs can affect your judgment, increasing risk-taking behaviors.

WITHIN THE NEXT 2 WEEKS, YOU CAN:

- ☐ Talk with your significant other or sexual partner(s) honestly about your sexual history. Make appointments to get tested if either of you think you may have been exposed to an STI.
- ☐ If you engage in high-risk sexual behaviors, think of ways to substitute those behaviors with ones that carry low to no risk. For example, rather than having sex with someone you just met, don't get more intimate than kissing or massage—until you know you're both disease-free.

BY THE END OF THE SEMESTER, YOU CAN:

- ☐ Get vaccinated for HPV if you're age 26 years or younger, and make sure you're up-to-date on all your other vaccinations.
- ☐ If you are due for a pelvic exam, make an appointment. Ask your partner if he or she has had an exam recently and encourage him or her to make an appointment if not.

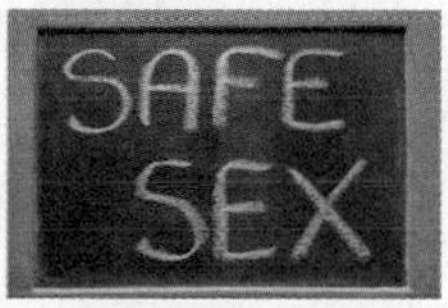

CHAPTER **REVIEW**

LO 1 Sexually Transmitted Infections

- Sexually transmitted infections (STIs) are spread through sexual intercourse, oral–genital contact, anal sex, hand–genital contact, and sometimes through mouth-to-mouth contact.

LO 2 Common Types of Sexually Transmitted Infections

- Major STIs include chlamydia, gonorrhea, syphilis, herpes, human papillomavirus (HPV) and genital warts, candidiasis, trichomoniasis, and pubic lice.

LO 3 HIV/AIDS

- Acquired immunodeficiency syndrome (AIDS) is caused by the human immunodeficiency virus (HIV). Globally, HIV/AIDS has become a major threat to the world's population. Anyone can get HIV by engaging in high-risk sexual activities that include exchange of body fluids or by injecting drugs (or by having sex with someone who does). You can reduce your risk for contracting HIV significantly by not engaging in risky sexual activities or IV drug use.

POP **QUIZ**

Visit **MasteringHealth** to personalize your study plan with Chapter Review Quizzes and Dynamic Study Modules.

LO 1 Sexually Transmitted Infections

1. Which behavior from the following list is considered the riskiest behavior for a sexually transmitted infection?
   a. Anal sex with a condom
   b. Mutual masturbation
   c. Massage
   d. Unprotected oral sex
2. What types of environments do STI pathogens prefer?
   a. Any environment, whether it's dark, light, cold, hot, dry, or moist
   b. Dark, moist places
   c. Light, dry places
   d. Excessively hot and humid places

LO 2 Common Types of Sexually Transmitted Infections

3. Which of the following is a common sign of gonorrhea in men?
   a. Whitish patches in the mouth
   b. Itchiness in the pubic hair region
   c. A milky discharge from the penis
   d. Gummas appearing near the penis
4. Which of the following STIs cannot be treated with antibiotics?
   a. Chlamydia
   b. Gonorrhea
   c. Syphilis
   d. Herpes
5. The most widespread sexually transmitted bacterium is
   a. gonorrhea.
   b. chlamydia.
   c. syphilis.
   d. chancroid.

LO 3 HIV/AIDS

6. Which of the following is a true statement about HIV?
   a. Drugs can provide longer survival rates for HIV.
   b. An infected mother cannot pass the virus to her baby.
   c. You can get HIV from a public restroom toilet seat.
   d. HIV symptoms usually appear immediately after initial infection.

Answers to the Pop Quiz can be found on page A-1. If you answered a question incorrectly, review the section identified by the Learning Outcome. For even more study tools, visit MasteringHealth.

THINK ABOUT IT!

LO 1 Sexually Transmitted Infections

1. What kind of behaviors should you avoid to prevent contracting a sexually transmitted infection? What kind of behaviors put people at increased risk? What might you tell a friend who is being sexually irresponsible?

LO 2 Common Types of Sexually Transmitted Infections

2. Identify five STIs and their symptoms. How do they develop? What are their potential long-term effects?

LO 3 HIV/AIDS

3. Why are women more susceptible to HIV infection than men? What implication does this have for prevention, treatment, and research?

ACCESS YOUR HEALTH ON THE INTERNET

Visit **MasteringHealth** for links to the websites and RSS feeds.

The following websites explore further topics and issues related to personal health.

American Social Health Association. This site provides facts, support, resources, and referrals about sexually transmitted infections and diseases. **www.ashastd.org**

San Francisco AIDS Foundation. This community-based AIDS service organization focuses on ending the HIV/AIDS pandemic through education, services for AIDS patients, advocacy and public policy efforts, and global programs. **www.sfaf.org**

HIV/AIDS and STIs Prevention. Learn more about sexual health through news, topics, publications, and reports at this CDC website. **www.cdc.gov/nchhstp**

AVERT. This is an international site with information on HIV/AIDS, global STI statistics, interactive quizzes, and graphics displaying current statistics for vulnerable populations. **www.avert.org**

FOCUS ON

Understanding Your Health Inheritance

Your family influences everything that defines you, from the foods you like to eat to the way you interact with others. Through the genes you inherit, your family also plays a significant role in your present and future health.

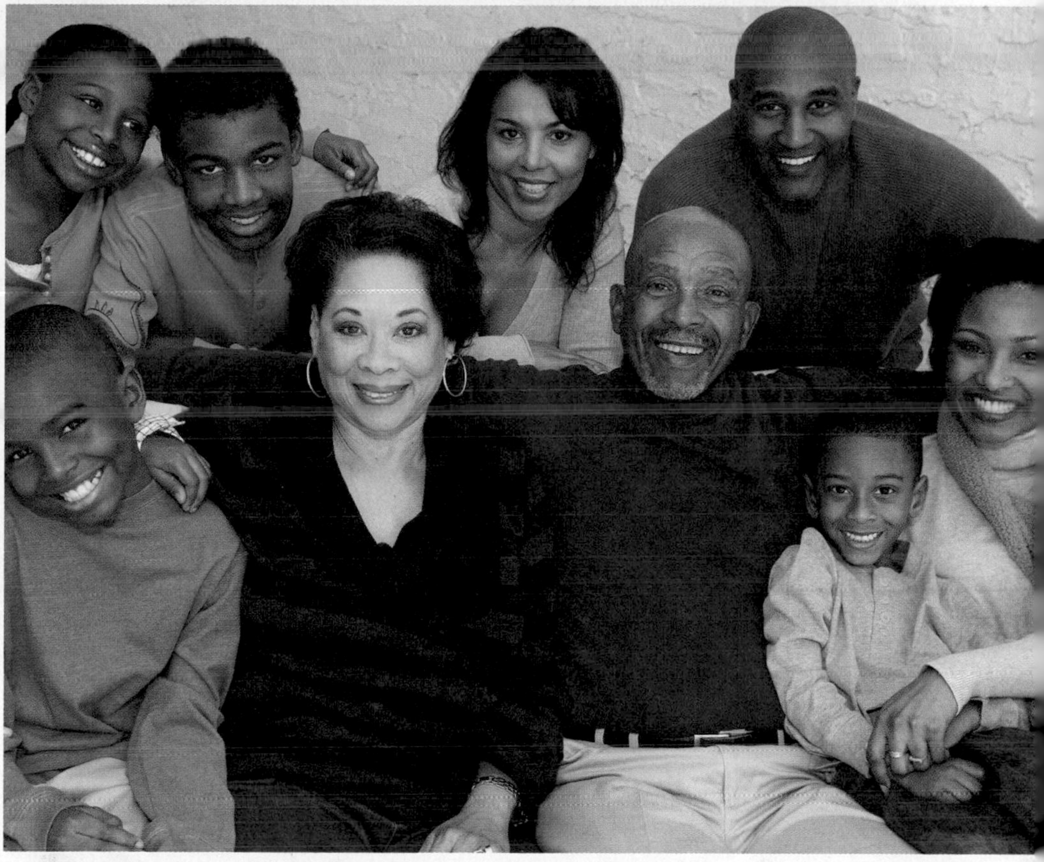

LEARNING OUTCOMES

1 Describe the relationship between chromosomes, DNA, and genes, and explain the role genes play in inheritance.

2 Discuss the inheritance of genetic disorders, including the ways genes interact with the environment.

3 Discuss genetic factors that contribute to various behaviors.

We seldom think of young adults dying of heart disease or other chronic illnesses, and statistically such situations are rare. However, research points to a clear hereditary risk for certain conditions in certain families. Not only do we inherit our tendency to be short or tall or have blue or brown eyes, we also inherit a tendency for an increased or decreased risk for some forms of cardiovascular disease, type 2 diabetes, early-onset Alzheimer disease, and even certain types of cancer. Are we "doomed" by our genes?

Although inheritance can play a significant role in determining your health, your behaviors—from what you eat and how much you exercise to whether you smoke or misuse alcohol—also affect your quality of life and your risk of disease and disability. If that's the case, then why should you bother to find out your family health history? There are three reasons. First, if you know that certain diseases run in your family, you can change your behaviors to reduce your risk. Second, you can share your family health portrait with your health care providers so that they can provide better care, for instance, by looking for early warning signs of a condition in your family. Third, compiling a family health history is important if you are planning to have children. A handful of disorders—known collectively as *genetic disorders*—are determined by inheritance, and we'll discuss them later in this chapter. If your research were to reveal a family history of any of these genetic disorders, you could then talk to your health care provider about genetic testing and counseling.

If you're adopted or your parents and grandparents are already deceased, then it may be more challenging for you to determine your family health history. But undertaking the investigation is important because it has become increasingly evident that your genetic background plays a role in your future health. Before you set out to gather your family health history, you need to understand the basic substances, structures, and processes involved in human inheritance.

inheritance Process by which physical and biological characteristics—called traits—are transmitted from parents to their offspring.

DNA (deoxyribonucleic acid) Compound residing in the nucleus of body cells that stores in its sequence of chemical subunits the instructions for assembling body proteins.

chromosome Discrete bundle of DNA, 46 of which are present in the nucleus of almost all cells of the human body.

WHY SHOULD I CARE?

You may have inherited traits or characteristics that affect your health every day, such as color blindness or a tendency toward depression. Knowing your family's health history, and sharing it with your health care provider, may help you treat symptoms or head off conditions that you might otherwise overlook or ignore.

LO 1 | WHAT ROLE DO GENES PLAY IN INHERITANCE?

Describe the relationship between chromosomes, DNA, and genes, and explain the role genes play in inheritance.

Inheritance is the process by which physical and biological characteristics—called *traits*—are transmitted from parents to their offspring. For instance, you may have inherited your dad's curly hair, but your mom's blood type. To appreciate how transmission of traits occurs, let's look at the key players in the process.

Genes Are Coding Regions of DNA

You probably know that all of the structures of your body—from your skin to your bones—are composed of functional units called *cells*. Within each cell is a small, dark sac called the *nucleus*. It's dark because it's densely packed with **DNA (deoxyribonucleic acid)**, a complex molecule that stores all of the programming code that your body uses for its initial assembly, growth from infancy to adulthood, and functioning throughout life. DNA is an extraordinarily long molecule that's shaped like a twisted rope ladder (commonly known as a *double helix*) with two long-side strands connected by short "rungs." For much of the life of a cell, its DNA exists as tangled masses dispersed within the nucleus. But when a cell gets ready to divide, its DNA becomes organized into 46 distinct bundles called **chromosomes** (see **FIGURE 1**). These 46 chromosomes exist as two sets of 23; you get one full set of 23 chromosomes from each parent.

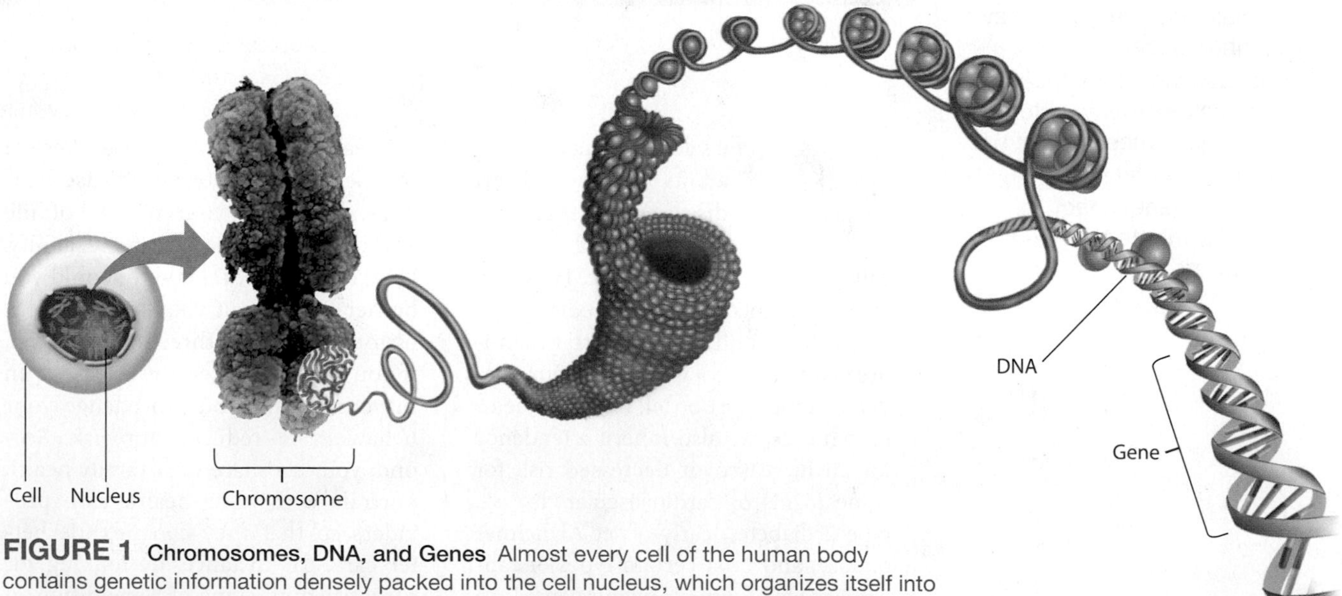

FIGURE 1 Chromosomes, DNA, and Genes Almost every cell of the human body contains genetic information densely packed into the cell nucleus, which organizes itself into 46 chromosomes when the cell is preparing to divide. Chromosomes are bundles composed of DNA, a weak acid that forms long strands of a characteristic double-helix shape. DNA consists of noncoding regions as well as regions called *genes* that code for the assembly of body proteins.

Source: Adapted from Michael D. Johnson, *Human Biology: Concepts and Current Issues,* 5th ed., © 2010. Printed and electronically reproduced by permission of Pearson Education, Inc., Upper Saddle River, New Jersey.

DID YOU KNOW?

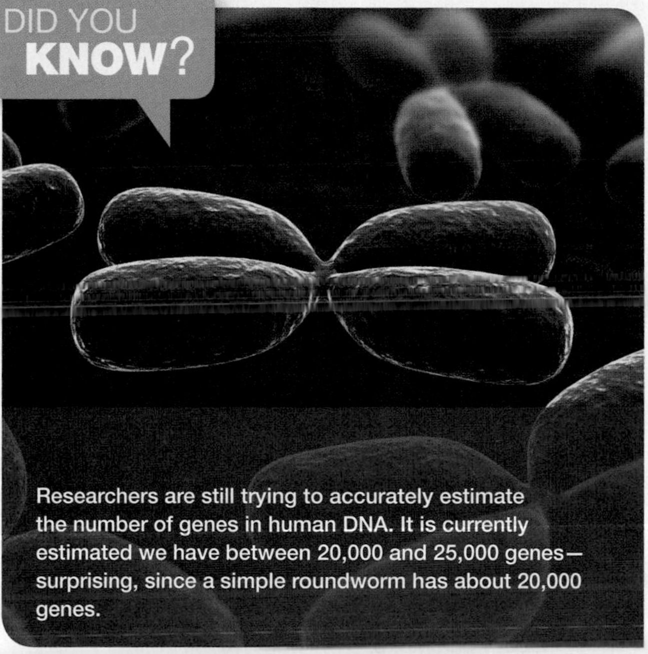

Researchers are still trying to accurately estimate the number of genes in human DNA. It is currently estimated we have between 20,000 and 25,000 genes—surprising, since a simple roundworm has about 20,000 genes.

Source: Genetics Home Reference, "What Is a Gene?" March 2014, http://ghr.nlm.nih.gov/handbook/basics/gene.

The long rope ladder of DNA that makes up each chromosome contains unique regions called **genes,** which store the code for assembling particular body proteins. Genes occupy about 1 percent of the total DNA in human chromosomes.[1] Most chromosomes have several hundred genes, but a few have over 1,000.[2] The rest of your DNA has noncoding functions, such as assisting in regulating the quantity of proteins made or maintaining the structure of the chromosome.[3] Your full complement of DNA—including genes and noncoding regions—is your **genome.** The branch of human biology that studies the human genome, genetic variation, and inheritance is known as *genetics.*

Genes Are Expressed as Proteins

Genes can be likened to particular "pages" in the code book of DNA, in that they contain the instructions for assembling—or *expressing*—specific body proteins. But what makes proteins so important? First, all cells and tissues of the human body are composed of proteins. Second, proteins include a vast array of molecules such as enzymes, antibodies, and hormones that participate in processes that enable you to function. By controlling the expression of proteins, genes control your body's appearance and structure as well as its functioning.

To understand how genes express proteins, it's important to recall that proteins are made up of subunits called *amino acids.* Just as a vast quantity of 20 different Lego parts could be assembled in various combinations into thousands of different shapes, a vast quantity of the 20 amino acids in your body can be assembled into an estimated 10,000 to 50,000 unique body proteins.[4] For the instructions indicating how to make each of these proteins, the cell turns to DNA: Each gene on the DNA is a sequence of chemical instructions for combining amino acids into a specific protein.

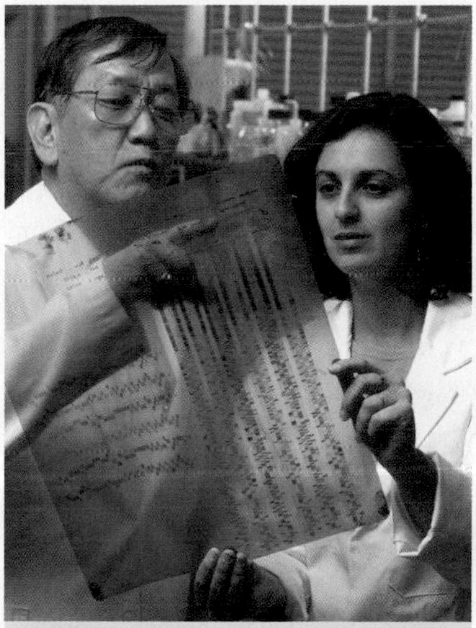

Genes contain the code for assembling proteins necessary for your body's structures and functions. The way these proteins are put together can affect whether you are more at risk for certain conditions or have particular traits that can influence your health.

gene Discrete segment of DNA in a chromosome that stores the code for assembling one or more body proteins.

genome All of the genetic information an organism possesses.

MORE THAN 99% OF THE DNA SEQUENCE IN HUMANS IS IDENTICAL; THE REMAINING FRACTION IS WHAT MAKES EACH PERSON **UNIQUE**.

Proteins Express Traits

Minute differences in proteins from one person to another result in the unique physical and physiological characteristics each of us possesses. For instance, pigments are proteins, and they account for variations in the color of people's skin, hair, and eyes. But proteins also account for traits that are not visible. For example, certain proteins contribute to three different types of cone cells in the eye. Cone cells allow us to distinguish colors, and if we don't have the genes to code for all three types of cone cells, we will have some form of color blindness.

LO 2 | HOW ARE TRAITS INHERITED?

Discuss the inheritance of genetic disorders, including the ways genes interact with the environment.

You may have inherited your father's height or your mother's hazel eyes, or even a grandparent's jawline or big nose. Just as people can inherit aspects of their

allele One of potentially several variants of the same gene.

dominant Term describing an allele that is expressed even if there is only one copy in the pair.

recessive Term describing an allele that is expressed only in the absence of a dominant allele; that is, if both alleles are recessive or if the recessive gene is on the X chromosome of the twenty-third pair.

single-gene disorder A disorder characterized by structural and/or functional impairments resulting from a defect involving only one gene.

appearance from family members, people can also inherit genetic disorders or susceptibility to chronic diseases experienced by others in their family. But precisely how are such traits passed down?

Traits Are Inherited via Chromosomes

We said earlier that your body cells have two sets of 23 chromosomes, one set from each parent. In other words, chromosomes exist as pairs that are alike in size and appearance. Geneticists can arrange chromosomes by pair in a configuration called a *karyotype* (**FIGURE 2**), with pair 1 being the largest and pair 22 the smallest. These are the 22 pairs of body chromosomes, called *autosomes.*

Pair 23 is your solitary pair of *sex chromosomes,* called XX or XY, which determines whether you are female or male, respectively. That is, every female gets one X chromosome from each parent to make up her twenty-third pair. The one she gets from her mother is one of the two Xs that make up her mother's twenty-third pair. The one she gets from her father is the only X he has to give—because the other chromosome in his twenty-third pair is a Y. Every male gets his father's only Y chromosome, but he could get either one of his mother's two Xs. For this reason, it is the father's genetic contribution that determines the baby's sex.

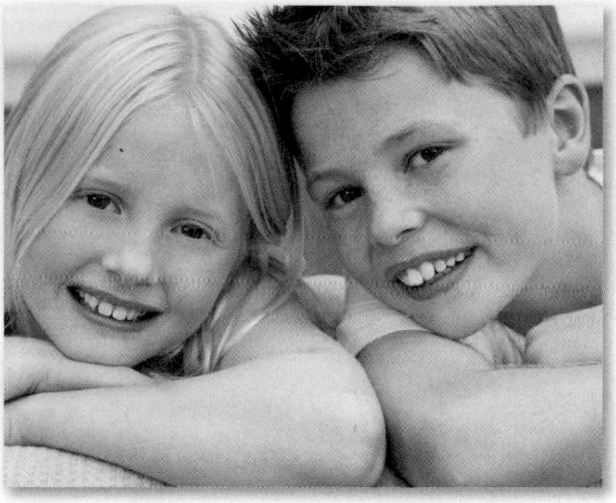

FIGURE 3 Effect of Dominant versus Recessive Alleles Freckles are coded for by a single gene with two forms, or alleles. The allele that codes for freckles is dominant, whereas the allele that results in absence of freckles is recessive. If you inherit the dominant allele from both parents, or even from just one parent, you'll have freckles (right). If you inherit the recessive gene from both parents, you won't have freckles (left).

Because you have two copies of each chromosome, you have two copies of each gene. Again, one copy comes from your father, and one from your mother. Your two gene copies may be similar, or they may be different. Different forms of the same gene are known as **alleles.**

For example, do you have freckles? Researchers believe that, in most people, the presence or absence of freckles is coded by just one gene, the *MC1R* gene on chromosome 16.[5] However, that gene has two alleles—two forms. If you have freckles, you may have inherited the allele for freckles from both of your parents. But even if you inherited the freckle allele from just one parent, you'll still have freckles! Why? Because the allele for freckles is **dominant,** whereas the allele for absence of freckles is **recessive.** A dominant allele always expresses the trait it codes for—it "dominates." In contrast, a recessive allele "recedes" in the presence of a dominant allele. When there is no dominant allele around and you inherit two recessive alleles, then you express that recessive trait (**FIGURE 3**).

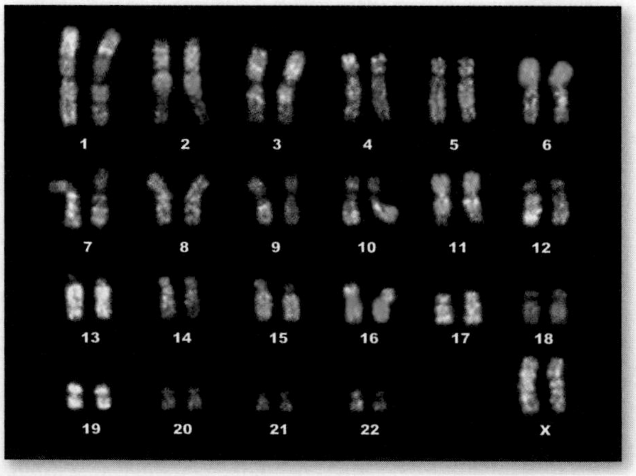

FIGURE 2 Human Karyotype A karyotype is a complete set of chromosomes arranged into pairs by size. This karyotype is from a female. You can tell because the chromosomes making up the last pair (pair 23) look almost identical (XX). In contrast, the male's XY chromosomes look different (the Y chromosome is shorter).

So if you *don't* have freckles, you must have inherited the recessive allele from both of your parents. Is it possible for you to have freckle-free skin even if both of your parents have freckles? The answer is yes. If both parents have one dominant and one recessive allele, they will both have freckles. Yet they could both have transmitted to you their recessive allele, in which case you would not have freckles.

Just as humans can pass on physical traits—like freckles—that are the expressions of proteins, they can also pass on genetic disorders. That's because any genetic defect, at its most fundamental level, is either the production of a defective form of a body protein or a failure to produce a body protein at all. *Geneticists*—scientists who specialize in genetics—recognize three types of genetic disease: single-gene disorders, multifactorial disorders, and chromosome disorders.

Single-Gene Disorders

Single-gene disorders occur as a result of a defect, called a *mutation,* involving just one gene. For example, the

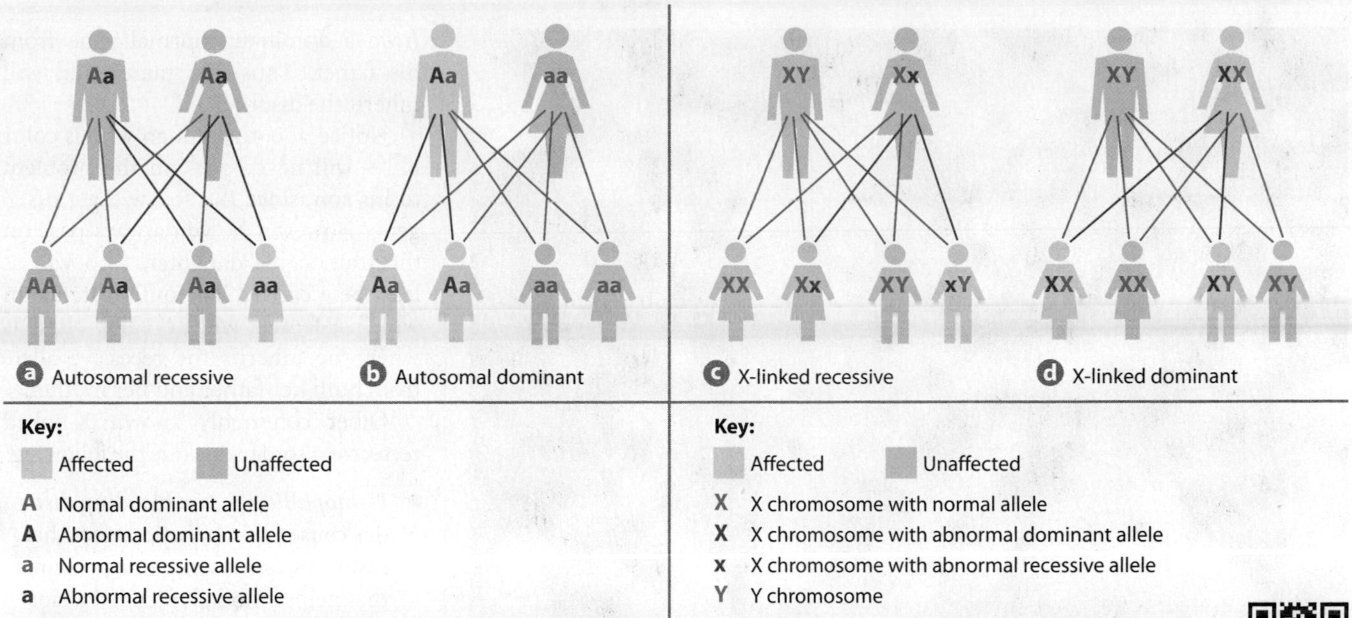

FIGURE 4 Inheritance Patterns of Single-Gene Disorders

VIDEO TUTOR
Inheritance Pattern of Single-Gene Disorders

disease *cystic fibrosis* occurs because of a defect on the *CFTR* gene on chromosome 7. Without the protein normally coded by this gene, a person with cystic fibrosis develops thick, sticky mucus that clogs his or her airways and gastrointestinal tract, interfering with breathing and digestion and absorption of food. Although many single-gene disorders, like cystic fibrosis, show up in childhood, a few manifest only in adulthood.

There are four common types of single-gene disorders (**FIGURE 4**). These are classified according to the type of chromosome affected (autosome or sex chromosome) and type of allele (recessive or dominant).

Autosomal Recessive Disorders

Cystic fibrosis is classified as an **autosomal recessive disorder** because it occurs on an autosome (recall that all body chromosomes, 1 through 22, are autosomes) and the allele responsible is recessive. Autosomal recessive disorders are rare because very few people inherit the recessive allele for the disorder from both parents. However, many more people are "silent carriers" of the responsible recessive gene. A **carrier** is a person who has one dominant normal allele and one recessive abnormal allele. Carriers thus do not develop the disorder and may have no idea that they carry the recessive gene.

In addition to cystic fibrosis, common autosomal recessive disorders include the following:

- *Albinism*—a partial or complete lack of pigmentation of the skin, hair, and eyes.
- *Sickle-cell disease*—a group of disorders in which various genetic mutations change the structure of hemoglobin, the oxygen-carrying protein in red blood cells. In sickle-cell anemia, normally disc-shaped red blood cells distort into an S-shape. These inflexible, sticky sickled cells can accumulate within small blood vessels, blocking blood flow and causing severe pain and organ damage. Sickled cells also break down prematurely, causing anemia.
- *Tay-Sachs disease*—a neurological disorder that causes a progressive deterioration of mental and physical abilities. It results from a defect in a gene coding for a protein that helps clear nerve-cell "debris." As a result, toxic deposits build up in the brain and spinal cord. Signs of Tay-Sachs typically begin to appear around 3 to 6 months of age. It is typically fatal before age 4.

Autosomal Dominant Disorders

An **autosomal dominant disorder** will occur even if an individual inherits just one defective allele because the defective allele is dominant (see Figure 4b). This is the case, for example, with *Huntington disease,* in which a defective *HTT* gene on chromosome 4 causes cells to synthesize a flawed protein. This flaw eventually causes nerve cells in the brain and spinal cord to deteriorate, triggering involuntary movements, memory loss, and changes in personality. Although the disease can develop in childhood, it typically begins to manifest around middle age. Its progression varies according to the extent of the genetic defect, but most patients die within 15 years of initial symptoms.[6]

With autosomal recessive disorders, it's entirely possible for both parents to

autosomal recessive disorder Single-gene disorder that occurs in individuals who have inherited two copies of an autosome with the affected recessive allele.

carrier Individual who has one copy of an autosome with a recessive allele for a particular trait, but is unaffected by it.

autosomal dominant disorder Single-gene disorder that occurs in individuals who have inherited at least one copy of an autosome with the affected dominant allele.

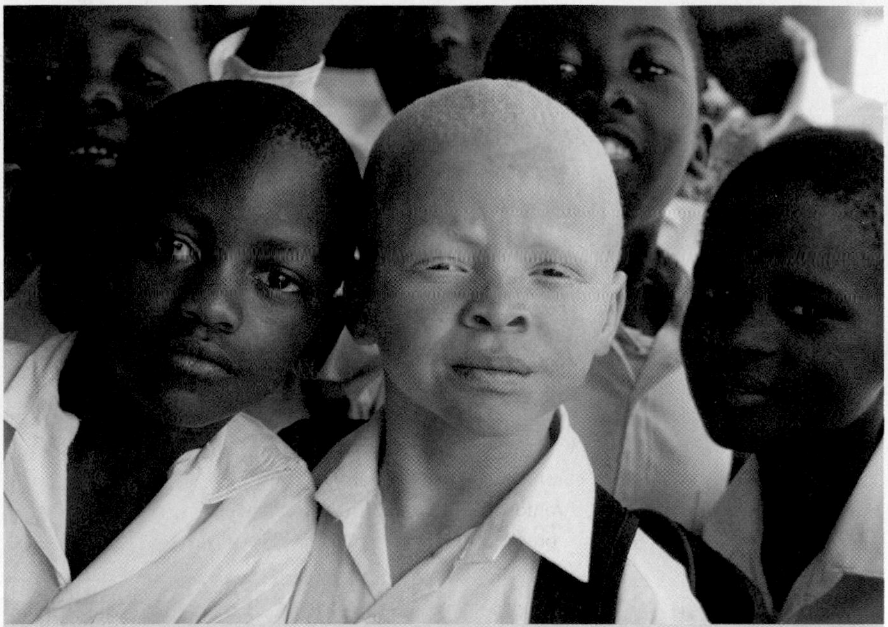

Albinism—a partial or total lack of pigmentation of the skin, hair, and eyes—is an autosomal recessive disorder: It occurs only if the defective allele is passed on from both parents.

X-linked recessive disorder Single-gene disorder that occurs in males who have inherited one copy of an X chromosome with the affected recessive allele and in females who have inherited two copies.

X-linked dominant disorder Single-gene disorder that occurs in individuals who have inherited at least one copy of an X chromosome with the affected dominant allele.

be unaware they are "silent carriers" of the same recessive gene. In contrast, in autosomal dominant disorders, a parent has the disease; still, if the effects manifest only in middle age, that parent may not have been aware of his or her condition and thus may not have sought genetic counseling before conception.

X-Linked Recessive Disorders

Some single-gene disorders are carried on the twenty-third chromosome pair—the sex chromosomes. The most common are **X-linked recessive disorders.** An example of X-linked inheritance is color blindness. This condition is coded by a recessive allele, so if a dominant, normal gene is present, the child will not be color blind. However, it is carried on the X chromosome of pair 23—the sex chromosomes, which determine gender. Recall that, whereas females inherit an X chromosome each from their father and their mother, males inherit an X chromosome from their mother but a Y chromosome from their father. The Y chromosome has fewer genes than the X chromosome, and most of them code for aspects of male reproductive function. So if the X chromosome a male inherits from his mother has a defective gene, even if it's recessive, it won't have any competition from a dominant, normal gene from his father. Thus, the male child will inherit the disorder.

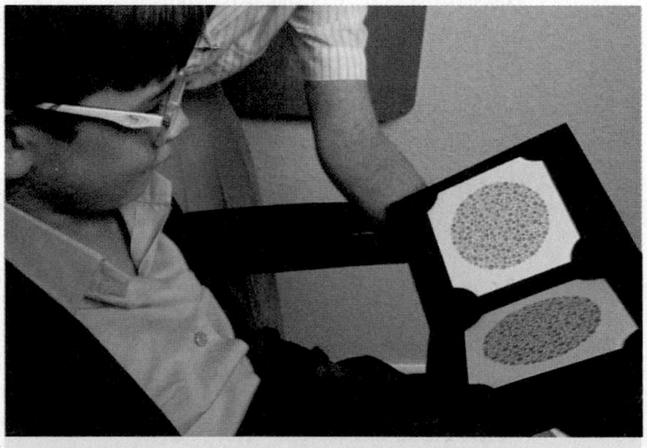

One out of every 10 American males is color blind. The most common color blindness is the inability to distinguish between red and green. It is more common in males because the trait is carried by a gene on the X chromosome.

Notice, too, that a man who is color blind will never pass on the problem to his son, since the son will get his Y gene. However, he will always pass on the trait to his daughter, who will at least be a carrier. The only instance in which a female will be color blind is when she inherits the recessive allele from both her father and her mother.

Other commonly known X-linked recessive disorders include the following:

- *Hemophilia*—a rare bleeding disorder caused by a genetic defect that results in the absence of a protein that helps blood clot (called a clotting factor). Fortunately, the missing clotting factor is now produced in laboratories and can be injected into the bloodstream.
- *Duchenne muscular dystrophy*—an X-linked disorder that causes muscle weakness that progresses throughout childhood until, by about age 12, the child is usually unable to walk. It is caused by a defective gene for dystrophin, a muscle protein.

X-Linked Dominant Disorders

X-linked dominant disorders are extremely rare (see Figure 4d). The most common affect the bones or the kidneys, and in males they are often fatal. Even though the responsible allele is dominant, when females inherit it, the single copy of the recessive, normal allele can mitigate somewhat the disorder's effects.

In Multifactorial Disorders, Genes Interact with Other Factors

Genes operate in a complex network, interacting and overlapping with one another in ways that can promote health or lead to disease. Moreover, our genes interact with the genes of the bacteria residing in our body, as well as with compounds in our diet, cigarette smoke and other toxins, disease-causing microbes, radiation, and many other factors. These can act like a switch, turning on or off genes so that the proteins they code for are, or are not, assembled. For this reason, certain health-related choices, such as what to eat and whether or not to smoke, influence our risk for disease.

Chemicals that don't affect the structure of our genes, but instead alter their activity, are collectively known as our **epigenome**. Epigenetic chemicals attach to DNA, turning on or off certain genes and influencing how and how much of a given protein they produce. Errors in the epigenetic process, such as altering the wrong gene or altering a gene in the wrong way, can cause an assembly of abnormal proteins. These epigenetic errors are now known to play a role in a wide range of disorders, including cancers, metabolic disorders, and degenerative diseases.[7]

Moreover, it is becoming clear that aspects of an individual's epigenome can be passed down to offspring, and even grandchildren! Several recent studies have yielded evidence supporting the theory that, during pregnancy, aspects of a woman's health—such as obesity or consumption of a high-fat diet—contribute significantly to metabolic diseases such as type 2 diabetes in her offspring.[8] Moreover, geneticists studying dietary patterns over two centuries in Sweden have found a link between food shortages in boys between the ages of 9 and 12—when cells that produce sperm are forming—and a longer life span in their grandchildren. In contrast, abundant food during the same growth period increased the risk for cardiovascular disease, type 2 diabetes, and an earlier death in grandchildren.[9]

Disorders in which genes and epigenetics play a role—but not the only role—are called **multifactorial disorders** (**FIGURE 5**). They are known to include obesity, heart disease, type 2 diabetes, Alzheimer disease, and certain types of cancer; however, some researchers contend that nearly all conditions and diseases have a genetic component.[10]

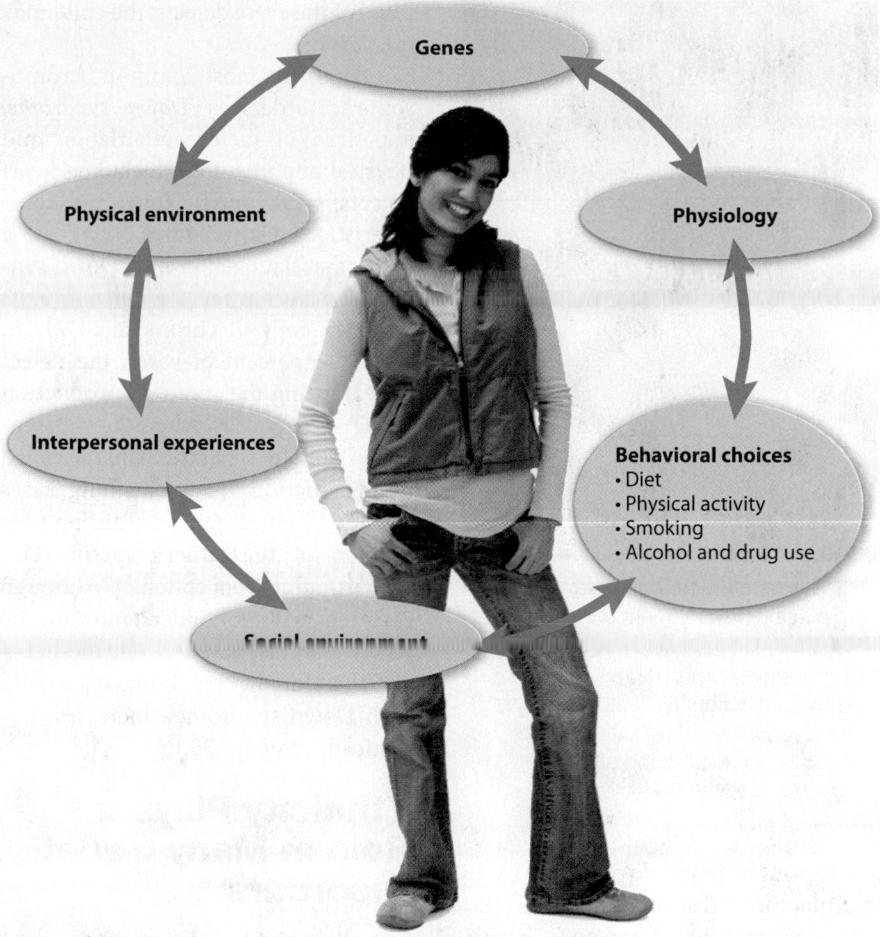

FIGURE 5 **Multifactorial Disorders** Whereas single-gene disorders are determined entirely by genes, multifactorial disorders result from the influence of multiple genes and epigenetic chemicals on a vast number of physiological processes, all interacting with behavioral choices, interpersonal experiences, and a variety of factors in the social and physical environment.

In addition, genes are known to play at least some role in certain psychiatric disorders, including the following:

- *Schizophrenia*—a complex disorder in which the person interprets reality abnormally. Researchers have now identified a number of genes accounting for at least 32 percent of the variance in risk. In addition, exposure to malnutrition or infection during fetal development is linked to schizophrenia, as are stress, the use of certain psychoactive drugs, and other metabolic factors.[11]
- *Bipolar disorder*—formerly known as manic-depression. Bipolar disorder is characterized by periods of excitability and exuberance alternating with periods of depression. Twin and family studies have shown that bipolar disorder has a strong genetic component: An estimated 80 percent of people diagnosed as bipolar have a close relative with the disorder. Despite considerable efforts, genetic researchers have not been able to identify specific genes involved.[12]
- *Clinical depression* (also called *major depressive disorder*)—a condition characterized by persistent feelings of sadness, hopelessness, and/or irritability. Like bipolar disorder, it tends to run in families, but no specific "depression" genes have yet been identified, and many other factors are also thought to be involved.[13]

epigenome The sum total of chemical compounds that influence the activity of an individual's genes.

multifactorial disorder A disorder attributable to more than one of a variety of factors.

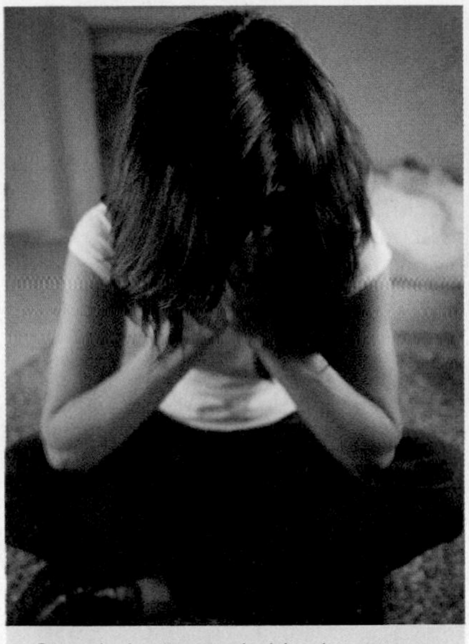

Genetic factors probably play some role in the development of psychiatric disorders such as depression, schizophrenia, and bipolar disorder. However, factors such as stress, use of psychoactive drugs, imbalances in body chemicals, and others also contribute to the risk.

Although genes do play a role in multifactorial disorders, they are just one determinant of anyone's health. If a multifactorial disorder runs in your family, you should learn about the other factors influencing development of the disorder and make healthy choices to reduce your risk.

Some Disorders Involve Missing, Extra, or Damaged Chromosomes

Chromosome disorders are caused by errors in an entire chromosome or part of a chromosome, rather than in one or a few genes. For example, an entire chromosome may be missing, or an extra chromosome may be present; a chromosome may be broken, or a portion of one chromosome may transfer to another. The altered genetic code can be expressed as a wide range of abnormalities, including heart defects, kidney disorders, and mental retardation. With severe defects, the child may not survive.

One of the most common chromosome disorders is *Down syndrome,* a pattern of mental retardation and physical abnormalities, including heart defects, weak muscle tone, and characteristic facial features such as a somewhat flattened profile. Down syndrome occurs when the child inherits an extra copy of chromosome 21. In about 90 percent of cases, the defect arises during the mother's production of mature egg cells, when the chromosomes fail to separate. This is called nondisjunction. The remaining cases are due to nondisjunction during production of the father's sperm cells, or just after conception.[14] Although researchers do not understand why, the risk of nondisjunction in the mother—and therefore her risk of having a child with Down syndrome—increases dramatically after age 35.[15]

chromosome disorder A disorder arising from a damaged, missing, or extra chromosome or transfer of one portion of a chromosome to another.

Ethnicity Plays a Role in Many Genetic Disorders

Some genetic disorders tend to occur more frequently among people who trace their ancestry to a particular geographic area.[16] People in an ethnic group often share certain versions of their genes, which have been passed down from common ancestors. If one of these genes contains a disease-causing mutation, the disease may be more frequent in this group.

For example, Tay-Sachs disease, mentioned earlier, is more common among Jewish people of eastern and central Europe, French Canadians, and Cajuns. About 1 in 27 American Jews carries the recessive allele for Tay-Sachs disease, whereas only about 1 in 250 are carriers in the population at large.[17] In addition, both cystic fibrosis and Huntington disease are more common among Americans of European descent.[18]

Ethnicity is also believed to play at least some role in many multifactorial diseases. For example, hypertension, heart attack, and stroke are all more common among African Americans. Type 2 diabetes is more common among African Americans, Hispanic Americans, Native Americans, and Asian Americans than among Caucasian Americans. Although it's not clear why, African Americans are also more likely to develop and die from cancer than any other ethnic group.[19] Asian

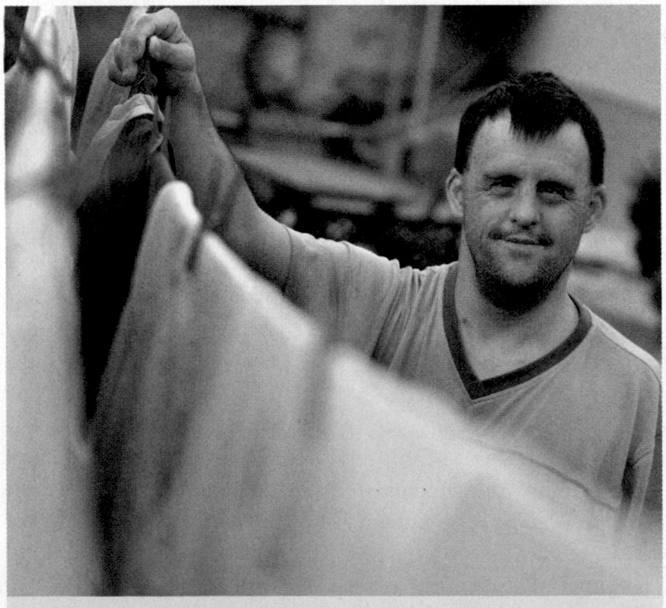

Some children born with Down syndrome have severe health problems, though the majority have mild to moderate mental retardation and physical challenges, as well as unique gifts and talents.

TECH & HEALTH

AT-HOME GENETIC TESTING

Dubious at Best

Do Alzheimer disease, depression, cancer, or alcoholism "run in your family"? If you saw an ad promoting a test you could take at home to find out whether or not you have "the gene" associated with such disorders, would you be tempted? As more Americans seek genetic testing, many are purchasing tests they can conduct without anyone—including their physician—getting involved.

Typically, so-called direct-to-consumer (DTC) tests are purchased online or in drugstores, and cost upwards of several hundred dollars. The consumer mails a swab from inside the cheek or a very small blood sample to a laboratory for analysis. Results are sent back via mail or posted online with a confidential code.

It sounds simple, but the tests raise a number of ethical concerns, including the following:

- **Validity.** The U.S. Food and Drug Administration (FDA) reports that some of these tests lack scientific validity, and others provide results that are meaningful only in the context of a full medical evaluation. In November 2013, for example, the FDA ordered the genetic testing company 23andMe to immediately discontinue marketing their "personal genome service" until it had been reviewed and approved for marketing. Genetic experts warn that until genomic tests have been validated, their results can be misleading or entirely false and could cause patients more harm than good.
- **Ambiguity.** Even for disorders known to be linked to specific genes, the results of most genetic tests are not black-and-white. They require evaluation and interpretation by a qualified health care provider.
- **Fraud.** As mentioned, these tests are costly. Some companies profit not only from the tests themselves, but also by selling products they claim will reduce the consumer's genetic vulnerability to specific disorders. A company might offer, for example, an "oxidative stress supplement" for clients with a genetic profile suggestive of cancer.
- **Privacy.** Consumers sending a DNA sample to a testing company may be opening the door for that company to use their genetic profile without their authorization—for example, to sell their information to insurance companies, manufacturers of dubious health care products or services, and so on.
- **Potential for harm.** Without genetic counseling, consumers are left on their own to respond to the results of a DTC test. When genetic tests are conducted by qualified health care providers, results are interpreted and explained by a clinician with training in genetics, and follow-up support is offered, not only from a professional counselor, but also from others who have faced similar diagnoses.

Although all states have laws protecting consumers from false advertising, none has laws specific to genetic testing. In the meantime, the FDA, the U.S. Centers for Disease Control, and the National Society of Genetic Counselors advise that all genetic tests be performed in a registered laboratory certified to handle DNA specimens and that results be interpreted by a physician or trained genetic counselor who understands the value of genetic testing for the particular situation. The bottom line? If you're considering genetic testing, see your doctor.

Sources: Federal Trade Commission, "Direct-to-Consumer Genetic Tests," January 2014, www.consumer.ftc.gov/articles/0166-direct-consumer-genetic-tests; G. J. Annas and S.L. Elias, "23andMe and the FDA," *New England Journal of Medicine* 370 (2014): 985–88, DOI: 10.1056/NEJMp1316367; The National Society of Genetic Counselors, "Position Statement: Direct-to-Consumer Genetic Testing," June 2011, www.nsgc.org/Media/PositionStatements/tabid/330/Default.aspx#DTC.

Americans and Pacific Islanders are the least likely to develop or die from cancer.[20] Still to be determined is how large a role genetics play in these trends and how much is a result of diet, access to health care, stress, exposure to pollution and infection, and other factors shared by people of a certain ethnicity.

Genetic Counseling Helps Families Evaluate Options

If you were to discover a family history of a genetic or multifactorial disease, one smart response would be to see a genetic counselor. Most genetic counselors have graduate degrees, experience in medical genetics, and work within health care organizations to provide information and support to families. They can help couples identify their risk for giving birth to a baby with a genetic disorder, investigate disorders already present within a family, review available options, and provide supportive counseling.[21]

Some people who consult a genetic counselor decide to undergo testing. A DNA sample can be obtained from any tissue. Gene tests can tell you whether or not you are a carrier of a genetic disorder, as well as give a prenatal diagnosis; provide newborn screening; or predict the presence of an adult-onset genetic disorder prior to symptom development. Testing is also available to estimate the risk of certain rare cancers associated with specific genes, as well as a particularly severe form of Alzheimer disease linked to certain genes. Genetic testing can also confirm or rule out a preliminary diagnosis. There are significant ethical issues connected with genetic testing, especially with direct-to-consumer testing; see the **Tech & Health** box.

LO 3 | DO GENES INFLUENCE BEHAVIORAL TRAITS?

Discuss genetic factors that contribute to various behaviors.

Animal breeders have long recognized that certain species of domestic and farm animals have a higher prevalence of certain desirable behavioral traits than others. For instance, border collies are famous for their herding instincts, and belted Galloways (a Scottish breed of cattle) are known for their docility. The field of **behavioral genetics** explores how genetic factors might contribute to these kinds of variations in humans as well. Studies in behavioral genetics are typically *twin studies* involving identical twins. Because identical twins have the same DNA, differences between them are assigned to variations in their epigenome and environment—whether during fetal life, growing up in the same family, or growing up apart.

Even in studies involving twins, determining the role of genetics is challenging for several reasons.[22] First, in order to study a behavior, researchers have to be able to define and measure it precisely. It's easy to define and measure, say, short stature in a child. But what would constitute a valid scientific definition of shyness? And how would you measure it? Researchers are also limited by the fact that epigenetic chemicals potentially relevant to behavioral traits cannot be studied since cells in the living brain manufacture them. Moreover, the pace at which studies in molecular biology yield new information about genetics and epigenetics has become so rapid that studies in behavioral genetics can become outdated even while they're still underway. Finally, any claim researchers make about the hereditary nature of a behavior applies only to the precise group studied. We can't readily extrapolate from any study cohort to the general population.

behavioral genetics The science that studies the role of inheritance in human behavior.

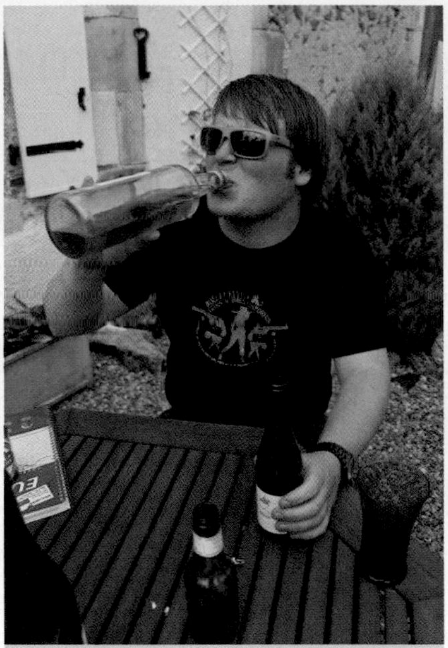

No one is destined to engage in addictive behaviors. Genes only affect body processes that interact with one another and with your life experiences to influence your susceptibility.

With these limitations in mind, let's look at what the research has to say about the heritability of the following behavioral traits:

- **Personality.** Human personality traits that can be reliably measured by rating scales do show a considerable heritable component.[23] Researchers have asserted claims for a genetic basis of impulsivity, novelty seeking, and aggression, as well as positive traits such as autonomy, sociability, sense of purpose, and self-control. However, environmental factors modify gene effects.
- **Intelligence.** Research evidence suggests that an adult's general cognitive ability is 25 to 50 percent attributable to variations in individual genes, and that their influence is further increased by interactions within networks of functionally linked genes.[24] Nongenetic factors contributing to intelligence are thought to include nutrition, socioeconomic status, stress level, and aspects of the fetal environment such as exposure to alcohol.
- **Substance abuse and addiction.** Over the past 75 years, genetic researchers have identified a diverse range of genetic variations that influence addiction and substance abuse.[25] This literature overwhelmingly suggests that, although they are multifactorial, genes explain up to 60 percent of these traits. Still, genes, epigenetics, and environmental factors interact with one another and with an individual's life experiences to influence this risk.

ASSESS YOURSELF

What is your health inheritance? Want to find out? Take the **What's Your Family History?** assessment available on MasteringHealth.™

Need help creating a plan? Follow the strategies in the **Your Plan for Change** box for short- and long-term improvements to your health.

YOUR PLAN FOR CHANGE

The **ASSESS YOURSELF** activity gave you the chance to create your own family health history and identify the health risks present in your family. Now you can take steps to help you take charge of your destiny!

TODAY, YOU CAN:

- ☐ List the disorders that occur within your family. Identify the environmental factors and/or lifestyle choices most strongly associated with development of each disorder.
- ☐ Jot down one small step you can take to positively influence your risk. For example, let's say that two close relatives have experienced lung cancer. You identify smoking as a lifestyle factor in each case. Maybe you don't smoke—but your roommate does. Today, you can share with your roommate your family history of lung cancer and ask your roommate to smoke away from you.

WITHIN THE NEXT 2 WEEKS, YOU CAN:

- ☐ Share your health history—and the patterns it reveals—with other members of your family. Invite them to fill in any gaps, and talk to them about the healthy choices you're making.

BY THE END OF THE SEMESTER, YOU CAN:

- ☐ Share your health history with your primary health care provider. Ask him or her for more advice about choices you can make to take charge of your health.
- ☐ If there is a multifactorial disorder in your family history, commit to behavior changes that reduce your risk of developing the disorder, such as getting your cholesterol checked or beginning an exercise program.

15 Preventing Cardiovascular Disease

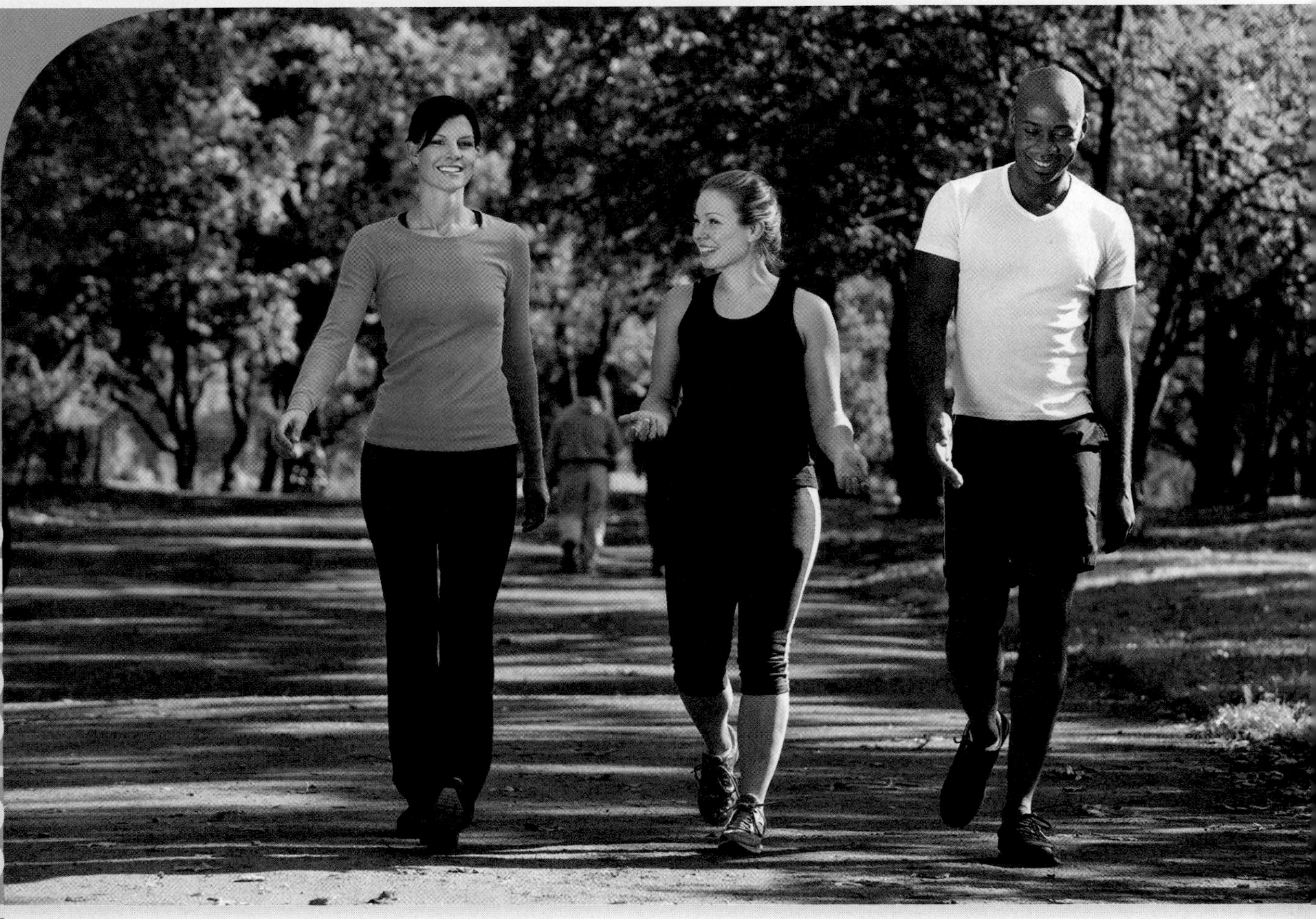

LEARNING OUTCOMES

1 Describe the anatomy and physiology of the heart and circulatory system and the importance of healthy heart function.

2 Explain the incidence, prevalence, and outcomes of cardiovascular disease in the United States, including its impact on society.

3 Review major types of cardiovascular disease and their symptoms.

4 Describe the modifiable and nonmodifiable risk factors for cardiovascular disease and methods of prevention.

5 Examine current strategies for diagnosis and treatment of cardiovascular disease.

Early in 2013, the American Heart Association (AHA) reported that death rates from cardiovascular disease had declined by nearly 33 percent in the last decade.[1] Sounds great, doesn't it? In spite of this promising decline, nearly 84 million Americans—more than 1 out of every 3 adults—suffer from one or more types of **cardiovascular disease (CVD)**, the broad term used to describe diseases of the heart and blood vessels.[2] Much of the improvement in death rates is due to improved diagnosis, early intervention and treatment, and a multibillion dollar market in pharmaceuticals designed to keep the heart and circulatory system ticking along. We've also made improvements in knowledge about risks and selected behavioral areas, yet CVD continues to be a threat regardless of age, socioeconomic status, or gender.[3] In fact, it has been the leading killer of U.S. adults every year since 1900, except in 1918, when a pandemic flu killed more people. Each day, as you are sitting in classes or studying in your room, over 2,150 Americans die of CVD.[4] Put into perspective, that would be the equivalent of ten Boeing 737 crashes. Even though the sheer magnitude of deaths and disability attributable to these diseases is sobering, CVD deaths often go unnoticed. The greatest barriers to change appear to be growing increases in obesity and diabetes.

2,150

IS THE NUMBER OF AMERICANS WHO **DIE** EVERY DAY OF CVD.

Americans are more obese and spending more on treatment of cardiovascular disease than ever before. Current direct and indirect costs of CVD are approximately 315 billion dollars.[5] By 2030, costs are projected to exceed $918 billion![6] Recognizing that selected risk factors are key to changing the course of CVD, the American Heart Association is aiming, by 2020, to improve Americans' cardiovascular health by 20 percent and to reduce death from CVDs and stroke by 20 percent. Achieving these goals will take a concerted effort and the collective will of policymakers, legislators, community leaders and community groups, and individuals.[7] As part of this strategy, the AHA has begun to focus more on **ideal cardiovascular health (ICH)** rather than mortality rates and the disease process. ICH is defined as the absence of clinical indicators of CVD and the simultaneous presence of the following seven behavioral and health factor metrics:[8]

Behaviors:

- Not smoking
- Sufficient physical activity
- A healthy diet
- An appropriate energy balance and normal body weight

Health factors:

- Having optimal total cholesterol without medication
- Having optimal blood pressure without medication
- Having optimal fasting blood glucose without medication

How are we doing with respect to measures? Not so hot. Less than 1 percent of the total population meets all of the ideal heart health measures, whereas just over 17 percent meet two to three of the indicators.[9] Nearly 83 percent had poor ICH.[10] The young in America tend to be most likely to meet the above measures.[11]

Clearly, the best defense against CVD is to prevent it from developing in the first place. Knowing how your cardiovascular system works, the factors that put your system at risk, and what happens when various diseases occur will help you understand your risk and how to reduce it.

cardiovascular disease (CVD) Diseases of the heart and blood vessels.

ideal cardiovascular health (ICH) The absence of clinical indicators of CVD and the presence of certain behavioral and health factor metrics.

cardiovascular system Organ system, consisting of the heart and blood vessels, that transports nutrients, oxygen, hormones, metabolic wastes, and enzymes throughout the body.

LO 1 | UNDERSTANDING THE CARDIOVASCULAR SYSTEM

Describe the anatomy and physiology of the heart and circulatory system and the importance of healthy heart function.

The **cardiovascular system** is the network of organs and vessels through which blood flows as it carries oxygen and nutrients to all parts of the body. It includes the heart, arteries, arterioles (small arteries), veins, venules (small veins), and capillaries (minute blood vessels).

The Heart: A Mighty Machine

The heart is a muscular, four-chambered pump, roughly the size of your fist. It is a highly efficient, extremely flexible organ that contracts 100,000 times each day and pumps the equivalent of 2,000 gallons of blood through the body. In a 70-year lifetime, an average human heart beats 2.5 billion times.

Under normal circumstances, the human body contains approximately 6 quarts of blood, which transports nutrients, oxygen, waste products, hormones, and enzymes throughout the body. Blood also aids in regulating body temperature, cellular water levels, and acidity levels of body components, and it helps defend the body against toxins and harmful microorganisms. An adequate blood supply is essential to health and well-being.

The heart's four chambers work together to circulate blood constantly throughout the body. The two upper

HEAR IT! PODCASTS

Want a study podcast for this chapter? Download **Cardiovascular Disease: Reducing Your Risk** available on MasteringHealth.™

atria (singular: *atrium*) The heart's two upper chambers, which receive blood.

ventricles The heart's two lower chambers, which pump blood through the blood vessels.

arteries Vessels that carry blood away from the heart to other regions of the body.

arterioles Branches of the arteries.

capillaries Minute blood vessels that branch out from the arterioles and venules; their thin walls permit exchange of oxygen, carbon dioxide, nutrients, and waste products among body cells.

veins Vessels that transport waste and carry blood back to the heart from other regions of the body.

venules Branches of the veins.

sinoatrial node (SA node) Cluster of electric pulse-generating cells that serves as a natural pacemaker for the heart.

chambers of the heart, called **atria**, are collecting chambers that receive blood from the rest of the body. The two lower chambers, known as **ventricles**, pump the blood out again. Small valves regulate the steady, rhythmic flow of blood between chambers and prevent leakage or backflow between them.

Heart Function

Heart activity depends on a complex interaction of biochemical, physical, and neurological signals. FIGURE 15.1 shows blood flow through the heart:

1. Deoxygenated blood enters the right atrium after having been circulated through the body.
2. From the right atrium, blood moves to the right ventricle and is pumped through the pulmonary artery to the lungs, where it receives oxygen.
3. Oxygenated blood from the lungs then returns to the left atrium of the heart.
4. Blood from the left atrium moves into the left ventricle. The left ventricle pumps blood through the aorta to all body parts.

Various types of blood vessels are required for different parts of this process. **Arteries** carry blood away from the heart; all arteries carry oxygenated blood, *except* for pulmonary arteries, which carry deoxygenated blood to the lungs, where the blood picks up oxygen and gives up carbon dioxide. After the arteries branch off from the heart, they branch into smaller blood vessels called **arterioles**, and then branch into even smaller blood vessels known as **capillaries.** Capillaries have thin walls that permit the exchange of oxygen, carbon dioxide, nutrients, and waste products with body cells. Carbon dioxide and other waste products are transported to the lungs and kidneys through **veins** and **venules** (small veins).

For the heart to function properly, the four chambers must beat in an organized manner. Your heartbeat is governed by an electrical impulse that directs the heart muscle to move when the impulse travels across it, resulting in a sequential contraction of the chambers. This signal starts in a small bundle of highly specialized cells in the right atrium, called the **sinoatrial node (SA node)**. The SA node serves as a natural pacemaker for the heart. People with a damaged SA node must often have a mechanical pacemaker implanted to make the heart beat.

At rest, the average adult heart beats 70 to 80 times per minute, although a well-conditioned heart may beat only 50 to 60 times per minute to achieve the same results. If your resting heart rate is routinely in the high 80s or 90s, it may indicate that you are out of shape, carrying too much weight, or suffering from some underlying illness. When overly stressed, a heart may beat more than 200 times per minute.

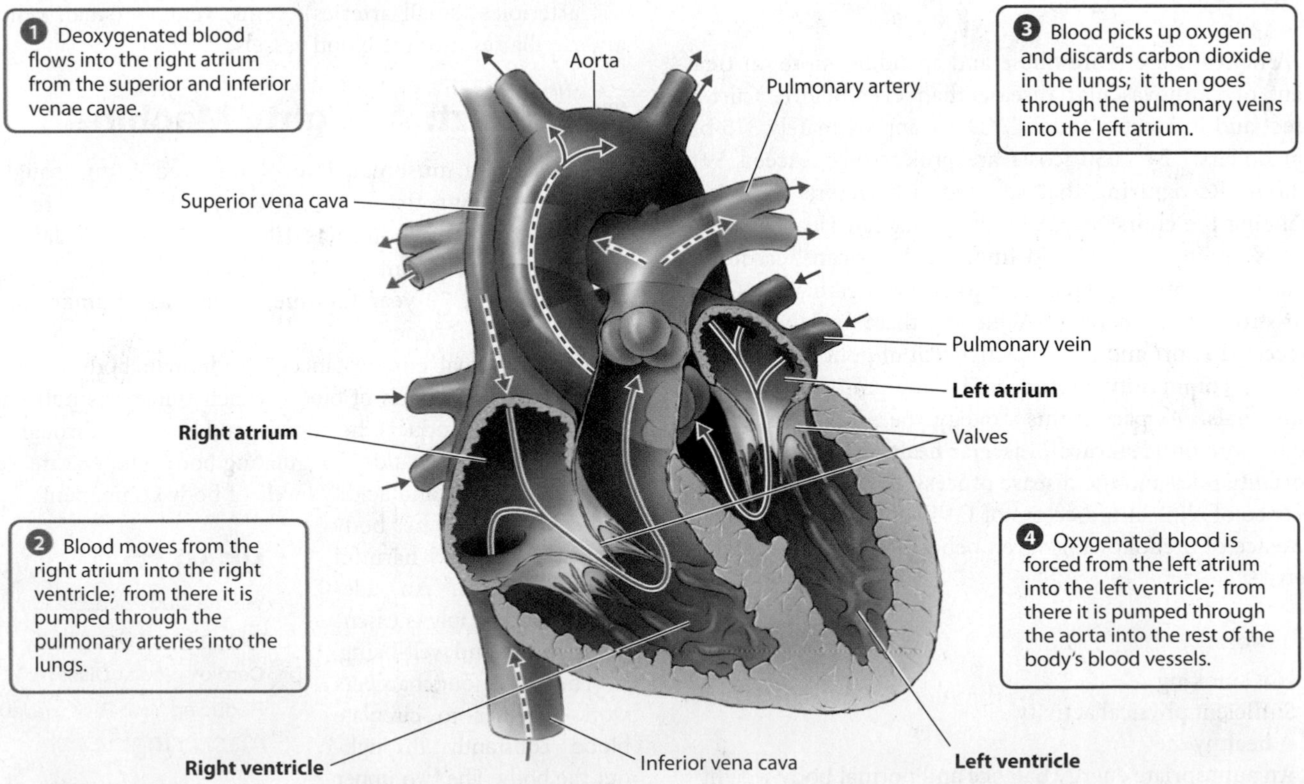
1 Deoxygenated blood flows into the right atrium from the superior and inferior venae cavae.
Aorta
Pulmonary artery
3 Blood picks up oxygen and discards carbon dioxide in the lungs; it then goes through the pulmonary veins into the left atrium.
Superior vena cava
Pulmonary vein
Left atrium
Right atrium
Valves
2 Blood moves from the right atrium into the right ventricle; from there it is pumped through the pulmonary arteries into the lungs.
4 Oxygenated blood is forced from the left atrium into the left ventricle; from there it is pumped through the aorta into the rest of the body's blood vessels.
Right ventricle
Inferior vena cava
Left ventricle

FIGURE 15.1 Blood Flow within the Heart

A healthy heart functions more efficiently and is less likely to suffer damage when overworked by stress or physical activity.

LO 2 | CARDIOVASCULAR DISEASE: AN EPIDEMIOLOGICAL OVERVIEW

Explain the incidence, prevalence, and outcomes of cardiovascular disease in the United States, including its impact on society.

Every year about 620,000 Americans have a first coronary attack, and 295,000 have a recurrent attack (**FIGURE 15.2**).[12] Cardiovascular disease claims more lives each year than the next three leading causes of death combined (cancer, chronic lower respiratory diseases, and accidents), accounting for nearly 33 percent of all deaths in the United States.[13]

33% IS THE PERCENTAGE OF **DECLINE** IN DEATH RATES FROM CVD IN THE LAST DECADE.

Consider the following facts:[14]

- Many CVD related fatalities are **sudden cardiac deaths**, meaning an abrupt, profound loss of heart function (cardiac arrest) that causes death either instantly or shortly after symptoms occur. Fifty percent of men and 64 percent of women who die suddenly have had no previous symptoms.[15]
- CVD has claimed the lives of more women than men every year since 1984. Only among those people ages 20 to 39 is CVD significantly more prevalent among men than it is among women (**FIGURE 15.3**).[16] Women also have a higher lifetime prevalence of stroke.[17]
- African American and Asian/Pacific Islander women (particularly South Asians) have the highest percentages of CVD deaths at 34 and 33 percent, respectively.
- Asian/Pacific Islander and African American males also have the highest percentages of death from CVD at 32.8 percent and 31.7 percent, respectively. In contrast, American Indian and Alaska Natives have the lowest percentages of deaths from CVD.[18]
- Among those aged 20 to 39, 20.3 percent have metabolic syndrome (MetS), a dangerous grouping of key risk factors for CVD. Among those aged 40 to 59, rates jumped to a whopping 40.8 percent, and for those 60 and over, the rates of MetS soared to nearly 52 percent.[19]

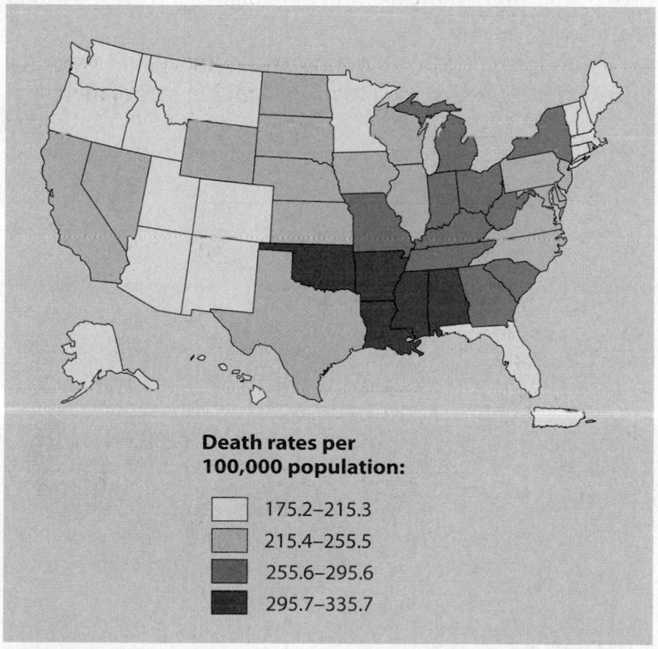

FIGURE 15.2 Major Cardiovascular Disease Age-Adjusted Death Rates by State

Source: Data from A. S. Go et al., "Heart Disease and Stroke Statistics—2014 Update: A Report from the American Heart Association," *Circulation* 129 (2014): e28–e292.

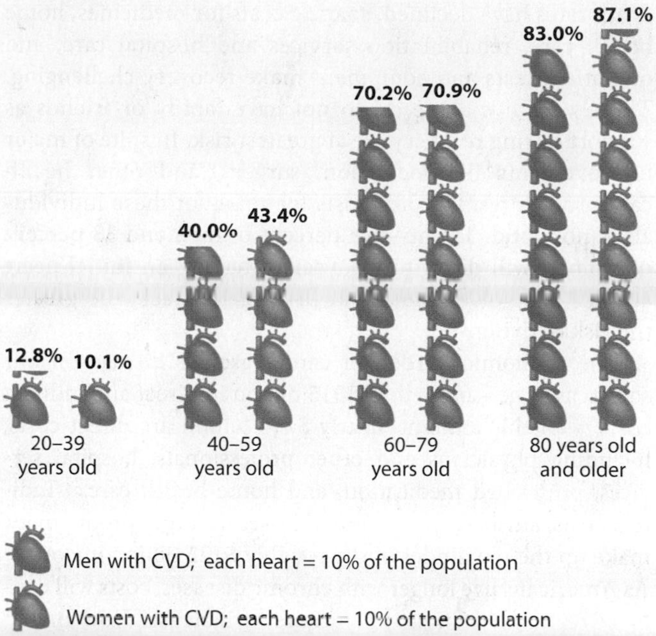

FIGURE 15.3 Prevalence of Cardiovascular Disease (CVD) in U.S. Adults Aged 20 and Older by Age and Sex

Source: Data from A. S. Go et al., "Heart Disease and Stroke Statistics—2014 Update: A Report from the American Heart Association," *Circulation* 129 (2014): e28–e292.

Although millions of Americans are living longer with CVD problems, many lack adequate health insurance and fail to obtain screenings and treatments early enough. Large numbers of CVD survivors suffer from physical and emotional disability in the form of fear, depression, and/or inability to perform activities of daily living. While actual

sudden cardiac death Death that occurs as a result of abrupt, profound loss of heart function.

death rates have declined, soaring costs for medicines, home health care, rehabilitation services and hospital care, and outpatient tests and equipment make recovery challenging. Those who live alone or do not have family or friends as support during recovery are at greatest risk. In spite of major improvements in medication, surgery, and other health care procedures, the prognosis for many of these individuals is not good: Twenty-five percent of men and 38 percent of women will die within 1 year of having an initial heart attack.[20] The older the age at first heart attack, the greater the risk of dying.[21]

The economic burden of cardiovascular disease on our society is huge—more than $315 billion in direct and indirect costs.[22] Of this amount, nearly $194 billion are direct costs, including physicians and other professionals, hospital services, prescribed medication, and home health care.[23] Indirect costs, attributed to projected losses in future productivity, make up the remainder of the roughly $122 billion in costs.[24] As Americans live longer with chronic diseases, costs will continue to increase. How much? Based on current trends, projections of total direct and indirect costs of CVD will surpass $918 billion, almost triple current costs, by 2030![25] While economic concerns are huge, the effects of CVD on patients, families, communities, and society may be even greater.

hypertension Sustained elevated blood pressure.

Cardiovascular disease is not a uniquely American health problem. With an international trend toward obesity, more and more countries face epidemic CVD rates. In fact, according to the most recent World Health Organization (WHO) estimates, CVD accounts for 30 percent of all deaths globally.[26] Many have the mistaken idea that CVD is only a developed nation problem. Unfortunately, over 80 percent of the world's deaths from CVD occur in low- and middle-income countries, places where people have more risks and fewer options for prevention and treatment.[27] People with CVD in these countries die at younger ages, often during their most productive years.[28]

$918 BILLION

IS THE PROJECTED TOTAL DIRECT MEDICAL **COST** OF CVD BY 2030.

LO 3 | KEY CARDIOVASCULAR DISEASES

Review major types of cardiovascular disease and their symptoms.

There are several types of cardiovascular disease, including hypertension, atherosclerosis, coronary heart disease (CHD), stroke, angina pectoris, arrhythmia, congestive heart failure (CHF), and congenital cardiovascular defects. **FIGURE 15.4** presents a breakdown of deaths from common diseases in the United States.

Although death rates are relatively easy to calculate, the short- and long-term psychological problems that occur after a person has a heart attack are harder to measure. Imagine the anxiety caused by wondering if your heart will fail each time you exercise or fearing that sexual activity might cause another heart attack. Knowing more about your specific CVD risks, your limitations, and what you can do about them is key to taking healthy action.

Hypertension

Hypertension refers to sustained high blood pressure. It is known as the "silent killer" because it often has few overt symptoms. Untreated hypertension damages blood vessels and increases your chance of angina, heart failure, peripheral artery disease, stroke, and heart attack. Hypertension can also cause kidney damage and contribute to vision loss, erectile dysfunction, and memory problems.[29]

The prevalence of hypertension in the United States continues to increase in spite of significant efforts aimed at treatment and control. Today, more than 1 in 3 American adults have high blood pressure. At nearly 47 percent, African Americans have the highest rate of high blood pressure in the United States, or even worldwide.[30] Rates are also much higher among the elderly, men, and those who don't have a high school education.[31] Although awareness of hypertension has increased and most diagnosed individuals are using hypertension medications, only 47 percent of those on meds have their hypertension under control.[32] Women who take oral contraceptives are two to three times more likely to have high blood pressure than women who do not.[33]

Blood pressure is measured by two numbers, for example, 110/80 mm Hg, stated as "110 over 80 millimeters of mercury."

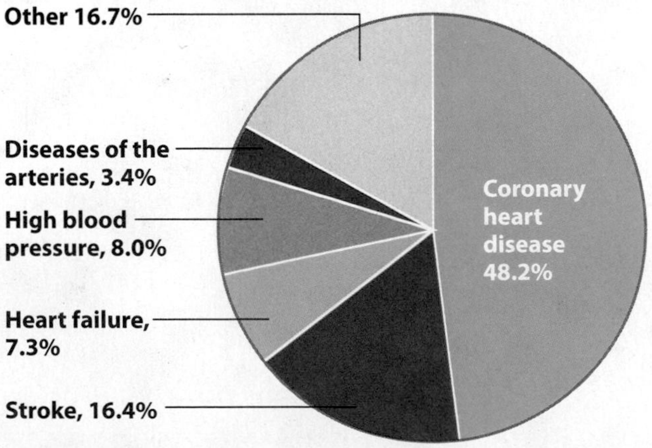

FIGURE 15.4 Percentage Breakdown of Deaths Attributable to Cardiovascular Disease

Source: Data from A. S. Go et al., "Heart Disease and Stroke Statistics—2014 Update: A Report from the American Heart Association," *Circulation* 129 (2014): e28–e292.

WHAT DO **YOU** THINK?

Why are certain populations within the United States especially at risk for CVD?

- Why are developing regions of the world experiencing major increases in CVD rates?
- With all of the media focus on reducing risks for CVD, why do you think we aren't seeing more dramatic reductions in CVD deaths?

The top number, **systolic blood pressure**, refers to the pressure of blood in the arteries when the heart muscle contracts, sending blood to the rest of the body. The bottom number, **diastolic blood pressure**, refers to the pressure of blood on the arteries when the heart muscle relaxes, as blood is reentering the heart chambers. Normal blood pressure varies depending on age, weight, and physical condition. High blood pressure is usually diagnosed when systolic pressure is 140 or above. When only systolic pressure is high, the condition is known as *isolated systolic hypertension* (*ISH*), the most common form of high blood pressure in older Americans. See **TABLE 15.1** for a summary of blood pressure guidelines.

Systolic blood pressure tends to increase with age, whereas diastolic blood pressure typically increases until age 55 and then declines. Men under the age of 45 are at nearly twice the risk of becoming hypertensive as their female counterparts; however, women tend to have higher rates of hypertension after age 65.[34] A key indicator of a growing threat from hypertension is the fact that more and more people (over 30 percent of the population) are considered to be **prehypertensive**, meaning that their blood pressure is above normal, but not yet in the hypertensive range. These individuals have a significantly greater risk of becoming hypertensive.[35]

In a society increasingly medicated for chronic conditions, the committee charged with setting new guidelines for blood pressure came out with a controversial new plan. Essentially, they relaxed blood pressure goals for adults over the age of 60 from 140/90 to 150/90, and eased recommendations for higher risk adults who have diabetes and kidney diseases. Effectively, their recommendations mean that nearly 14 million adults over the age of 60 would be considered to have their BP under control and could be taken off blood pressure medications or have their dosage reduced, while others might not be given them to begin with.[36] Not surprisingly, these recommendations are being viewed with caution by the American Heart Association and the American College of Cardiology.

TABLE **15.1** | Blood Pressure Classifications

Classification	Systolic Reading (mm Hg)		Diastolic Reading (mm Hg)
Normal	Less than 120	and	Less than 80
Prehypertension	120–139	or	80–89
Hypertension			
Stage 1	140–159	or	90–99
Stage 2	Greater than or equal to 160	or	Greater than or equal to 100

Note: If systolic and diastolic readings fall into different categories, treatment is determined by the highest category. Readings are based on the average of two or more properly measured, seated readings on each of two or more health care provider visits.

Source: National Heart, Lung, and Blood Institute, *The Seventh Report of the Joint National Committee on Prevention, Detection, Evaluation, and Treatment of High Blood Pressure,* NIH Publication no. 03-5233 (Bethesda, MD: National Institutes of Health, 2003).

Atherosclerosis and Coronary Artery Disease

Atherosclerosis comes from the Greek words *athero* (meaning gruel or paste) and *sclerosis* (hardness). In this condition, fatty substances, cholesterol, cellular waste products, calcium, and fibrin (a clotting material in the blood) build up in the inner lining of an artery. *Hyperlipidemia* (an abnormally high blood lipid level) is a key factor in this process, and the resulting buildup is called **plaque**. Atherosclerosis underlies many cardiovascular health problems and is believed to be the biggest contributor to disease burden globally.

As plaque accumulates, vessel walls become narrow and may eventually block blood flow or cause vessels to rupture (**FIGURE 15.5**). The pressure buildup is similar to putting your thumb over the end of a hose while water is on. Pressure builds within arteries just as pressure builds in the hose. If vessels are weakened and pressure persists, they may burst or the plaque itself may break away from the walls of the vessels and obstruct blood flow. In addition, fluctuation in the blood pressure levels within arteries can damage their internal walls, making it even more likely that plaque will stick to injured wall surfaces and accumulate.

Atherosclerosis is often called **coronary artery disease (CAD)** because of the damage to the body's main coronary arteries on the outer surface of the heart. These are the arteries that provide blood supply to the heart muscle itself. Most heart attacks result from blockage of these arteries. Atherosclerosis and other circulatory impairments also often reduce blood flow and limit the heart's blood and oxygen supply, a condition known as **ischemia**.

systolic blood pressure The upper number in the fraction that measures blood pressure, indicating pressure on the walls of the arteries when the heart contracts.

diastolic blood pressure The lower number in the fraction that measures blood pressure, indicating pressure on the walls of the arteries during the relaxation phase of heart activity.

prehypertensive Blood pressure is above normal, but not yet in the hypertensive range.

atherosclerosis Condition characterized by deposits of fatty substances (plaque) on the inner lining of an artery.

plaque Buildup of deposits in the arteries.

coronary artery disease (CAD) A narrowing or blockage of coronary arteries, usually caused by atherosclerotic plaque buildup.

ischemia Reduced oxygen supply to a body part or organ.

Peripheral Artery Disease

When atherosclerosis occurs in the upper or lower extremities, such as in the arms, feet, calves, or legs, and causes narrowing or complete blockage of arteries, it is often called

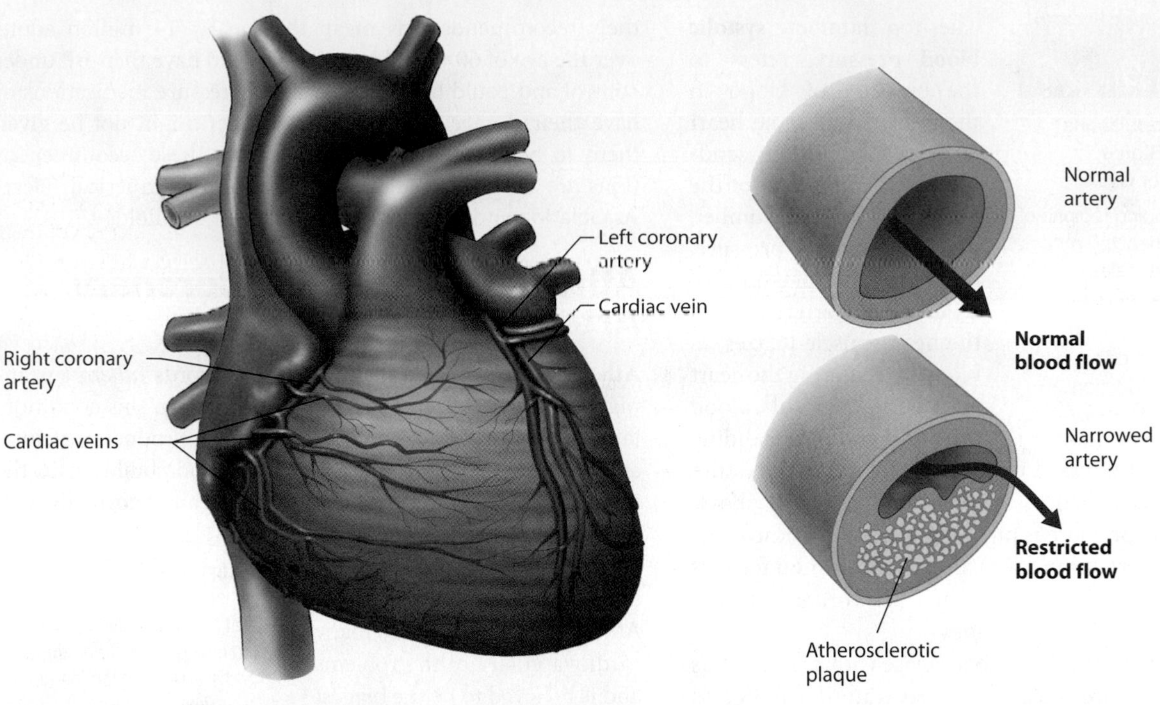

FIGURE 15.5 **Atherosclerosis and Coronary Artery Disease** The coronary arteries are located on the exterior of the heart and supply blood and oxygen to the heart muscle itself. In atherosclerosis, arteries become clogged by a buildup of plaque. When atherosclerosis occurs in coronary arteries, blood flow to the heart muscle is restricted and a heart attack may occur.

Sources: Adapted from Joan Salge Blake, *Nutrition & You,* 2nd ed., MyPlate edition, and Michael D. Johnson, *Human Biology: Concepts and Current Issues*, 6th ed., both copyright © 2012 Pearson Education, Inc. Reprinted by permission.

VIDEO TUTOR
Atherosclerosis and Coronary Artery Disease

peripheral artery disease (PAD). In the United States, over 8.5 million people—particularly those over 65, non-Hispanic blacks, and women—have PAD, and many are not receiving treatment because they are asymptomatic or don't recognize subtle symptoms.[37] Most often characterized by pain and aching in the legs, calves, or feet upon walking or exercise (known as *intermittent claudication*), PAD is a leading cause of disability in people over the age of 50. While it strikes both men and women, men, smokers, and diabetics tend to develop it more frequently.[38] In recent years, increased attention has been drawn to PAD's role in subsequent blood clots and resultant heart attacks, particularly among people who sit in cramped airplanes for long distances without getting up and moving. Sometimes PAD in the arms can be caused by trauma, certain diseases, radiation therapy, surgery, repetitive motion syndrome, or a combination of

peripheral artery disease (PAD) Atherosclerosis occurring in the lower extremities, such as in the feet, calves, or legs, or in the arms.

coronary heart disease (CHD) A narrowing of the small blood vessels that supply blood to the heart.

myocardial infarction (MI) or **heart attack** A blockage of normal blood supply to an area in the heart.

coronary thrombosis A blood clot occurring in a coronary artery.

thrombus A blood clot attached to a blood vessel's wall.

embolus A blood clot that becomes dislodged from a blood vessel wall and moves through the circulatory system.

collateral circulation Adaptation of the heart to partial damage accomplished by rerouting needed blood through unused or underused blood vessels while the damaged heart muscle heals.

TABLE 15.2 | Common Heart Attack Symptoms and Signs

Sign or Symptom	Gender That Most Commonly Experiences It
Crushing or squeezing chest pain	More common in men
Pain radiating down arm, neck, or jaw	More common in men
Chest discomfort or pressure with shortness of breath, nausea/vomiting, or lightheadedness	Women more likely to feel pressure than pain. Shortness of breath and nausea, and lightheadedness common in both women and men
Shortness of breath without chest pain, discomfort in back, neck, or jaw or in one or both arms	More common in women
Unusual weakness	More common in women
Unusual fatigue	More common in women
Sleep disturbances	More common in women
Indigestion, flulike symptoms	More common in women

Sources: American Heart Association, "Symptoms of Heart Attack in Women," 2014, http://www.heart.org/HEARTORG/Conditions/HeartAttack/WarningSignsofaHeartAttack/Heart-Attack-Symptoms-in-Women_UCM_436448_Article.jsp.

HEALTH IN A DIVERSE WORLD

WOMEN AND HEART ATTACKS

"Having a heart attack" usually brings to mind an older man gasping for breath, clutching his chest, and toppling over in the middle of a workout. So the story of comedian and former talk show host Rosie O'Donnell's heart attack doesn't seem to fit the mold: O'Donnell, 50, didn't even know she'd had one at first. She reported on her blog that "my body hurt, I had an ache in my chest, both my arms were sore; everything felt bruised." At first, she wondered if she might have strained a muscle. Later she felt hot, clammy, and vomited. Fortunately, she took an aspirin and eventually went to the doctor, despite initially doubting a serious problem. It turned out O'Donnell had an almost complete blockage of a heart artery that required a stent.

Rosie isn't alone. According to a recent study, women who suffer heart attacks under the age of 55 are not only less likely to have classic chest pain or pressure, but also they tend to delay going to the doctor. When they do seek medical attention, they often report more atypical symptoms, such as shortness of breath or pain in the neck, shoulder, arms, and stomach. Many women chalk up heart symptoms to stress, flu, or lack of exercise. Because of treatment delays, women are more likely to have heart damage and to die from a heart attack than are men of the same age.

So how can a woman tell if she is having a heart attack? In addition to the symptoms already mentioned, women may experience chest pressure or pain; radiating pains in the arms, shoulder, neck, jaw, or back; dizziness; abdominal pain; and unexplained feelings of fatigue, anxiety, or weakness—especially during exertion. But the real answer to the question of how to tell if a woman is having a heart attack is this: *let a doctor* determine that. If you or someone you know has even a few of these symptoms, don't delay. Crush or chew a full strength aspirin and swallow it with water. In addition to being a pain killer, aspirin has blood-thinning properties, so taking one can prevent fatal blood clots from forming. Then have someone drive you to a health care facility for evaluation, or call 9-1-1 to get an ambulance.

Sources: J. Cant, et al., "Association of Age and Sex with Myocardial Infarction Symptom Presentation and in Hospital Mortality," *Journal of the American Medical Association* 307, no. 8 (2012,): 813–22; National Coalition for Women with Heart Disease, Women Heart, "Are You Having a Heart Attack?," 2012, www.womenheart.org.

factors. Damage to vessels and threats to health can be severe, with a two- to three-times greater risk of stroke and heart attack among those who have PAD.[39]

Coronary Heart Disease

Of all the major cardiovascular diseases, **coronary heart disease (CHD)** is the greatest killer, accounting for nearly 1 in 6 deaths in the United States. Nearly 1 million new and recurrent heart attacks occur in the United States each year.[40] A **myocardial infarction (MI),** or **heart attack**, involves an area of the heart that suffers permanent damage because its normal blood supply has been blocked. This condition is often brought on by a **coronary thrombosis** (clot) or an atherosclerotic narrowing that blocks a coronary artery (an artery supplying the heart muscle with blood; refer to Figure 15.5). When a clot, or **thrombus**, becomes dislodged and moves through the circulatory system, it is called an **embolus**. Whenever blood does not flow readily, there is a corresponding decrease in oxygen flow to tissue below the blockage. If the blockage is extremely minor, an otherwise healthy heart will adapt over time by enlarging existing blood vessels and growing new ones to reroute needed blood through other areas. This system, called **collateral circulation**, is a form of self-preservation that allows an affected heart muscle to cope with damage.

When a heart blockage is more severe, however, the body is unable to adapt on its own, and outside lifesaving support is critical. The events of the first hour after an attack are critical to survival. See the **Health in a Diverse World** box, the **Skills for Behavior Change** box, and **TABLE 15.2** to learn common signs and symptoms, as well as what to do in case of a heart attack.

SKILLS FOR BEHAVIOR CHANGE

WHAT TO DO WHEN A HEART ATTACK HITS

People often miss the signs of a heart attack, or they wait too long to seek help, which can have deadly consequences. Knowing what to do in an emergency could save your life or somebody else's. (See Table 15.2 for information on signs and symptoms.)

- Keep a list of emergency rescue service numbers next to your telephone and in your pocket, wallet, or purse. Be aware of whether your local area has a 9-1-1 emergency service.
- Expect the person to deny the possibility of anything as serious as a heart attack, particularly if that person is young and appears to be in good health. If you're with someone who appears to be having a heart attack, don't take no for an answer; insist on taking prompt action.
- If you are with someone who suddenly collapses, perform cardiopulmonary resuscitation (CPR). See www.heart.org for information on the new chest-compression-only techniques recommended by the American Heart Association. If you're trained and willing, use conventional CPR methods.

Sources: Adapted from American Heart Association, "Warning Signs of Heart Attack, Stroke, and Cardiac Arrest," 2014, http://www.heart.org/HEARTORG/Conditions/911-Warnings-Signs-of-a-Heart-Attack_UCM_305346_SubHomePage.jsp.

Stroke

Brain cells must have a continuous and adequate supply of oxygen in order to survive. A **stroke** (also called a *cerebrovascular accident*) occurs when the blood supply to the brain is interrupted. Strokes may be either *ischemic,* caused by plaque formation or a clot that reduces blood flow, or *hemorrhagic,* meaning a blood vessel weakens and either bulges or ruptures. FIGURE 15.6 illustrates some of the blood vessel disorders that can lead to a stroke. An **aneurysm** is the most well-known and life-threatening of the hemorrhagic strokes. When any of these events occur, oxygen deprivation kills brain cells.

stroke A condition occurring when the brain is damaged by disrupted blood supply; also called *cerebrovascular accident.*

aneurysm A weakened blood vessel that may bulge under pressure and, in severe cases, burst.

transient ischemic attack (TIA) Brief interruption of the blood supply to the brain that causes only temporary impairment; often an indicator of impending major stroke.

Some strokes are mild and cause only temporary dizziness or slight weakness or numbness. More serious interruptions in blood flow may impair speech, memory, or motor control. Other strokes affect the parts of the brain that regulate heart and lung function and kill within minutes. According to the American Heart Association's latest statistics, nearly 7 million Americans suffer a stroke every year, and almost 129,000 die as a result. Strokes account for 1 in 19 deaths each year, surpassed only by CHD, cancer, and chronic lower respiratory diseases.[41] Even scarier, it is thought that more young people are having strokes than ever before, possibly due to increased obesity and hypertension.[42]

Although stroke survivors at any age often face significant disability, nearly one third of young and middle-age adult stroke survivors have difficulty living independently without assistance.[43] Whether due to the severity of the stroke, depression, or a combination of variables, the long-term costs for individuals, families, and the health care system are significant.

Many strokes are preceded days, weeks, or months earlier by **transient ischemic attacks (TIAs)**, brief interruptions

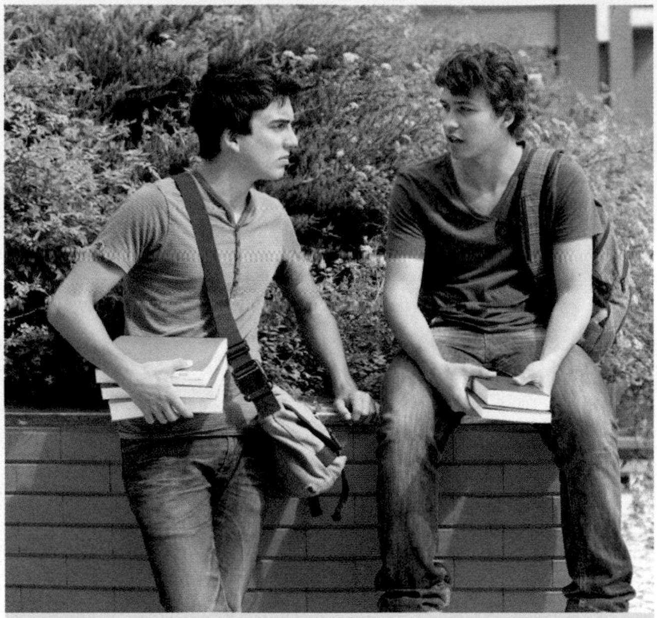

Strokes aren't just diseases that older people have. In increasing numbers, hypertension and strokes affect younger adults, with young men having the greatest risk of stroke in persons under age 50.

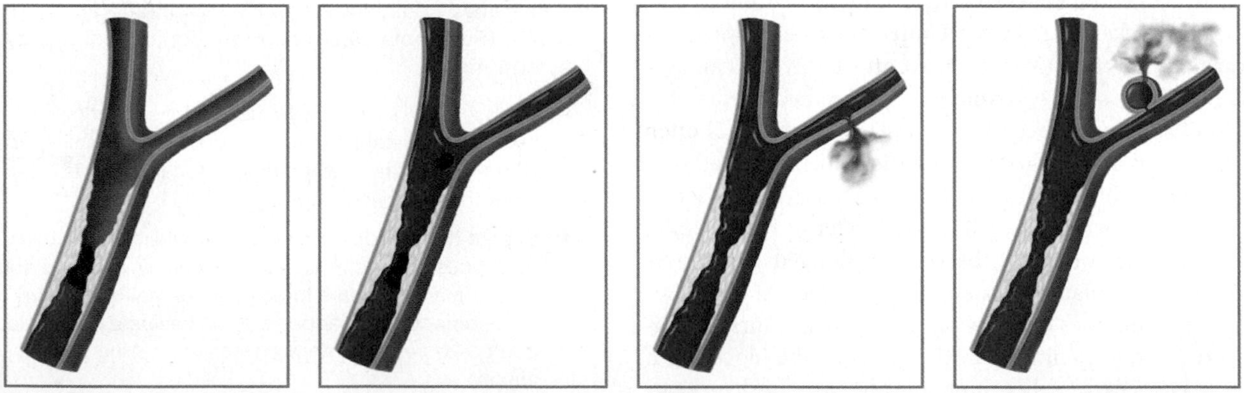

ⓐ A thrombus is a blood clot that forms inside a blood vessel and blocks the flow of blood at its origin. A thrombus in a cerebral artery can lead to an ischemic stroke.

ⓑ An embolus is a blood clot that breaks off from its point of formation and travels in the bloodstream until it lodges in a narrowed vessel and blocks blood flow. Emboli in brain blood vessels can cause ischemic strokes.

ⓒ A hemorrhage occurs when a blood vessel bursts, allowing blood to flow into the surrounding tissue or between tissues. There are two types of hemorrhagic strokes: subarachnoid, in which a vessel on the brain's surface bursts, and intracerebral, in which a vessel within the brain bursts.

ⓓ An aneurysm is the bulging of a weakened blood vessel wall. Aneurysms in the brain can cause hemorrhagic strokes if they burst.

FIGURE 15.6 Blood Vessel Disorders That Can Lead to Stroke

SEE IT! VIDEOS

See how two young women have regained their lives after experiencing a stroke. Watch **Stroke in Young Adults** available on MasteringHealth.™

of the blood supply to the brain that cause temporary impairment.[44] Symptoms of TIAs include dizziness, particularly when first rising in the morning, weakness, temporary paralysis or numbness in the face or other regions, temporary memory loss, blurred vision, nausea, headache, slurred speech or difficulty in speaking, or other unusual physiological reactions. Some people may actually experience unexpected falls or have blackouts; others may have no obvious symptoms. Transient ischemic attacks often indicate an impending major stroke. The earlier a stroke is recognized and treatment started, the more effective that treatment will be. See the **Skills for Behavior Change** box for tips on recognizing a stroke.

One of the great medical successes in recent years has been the decline in the death rate from strokes, which has dropped by over one-third in the United States since the 1980s and continues to fall.[45] Greater awareness of stroke symptoms, improvements in emergency medicine protocols and medicines, and a greater emphasis on fast rehabilitation and therapy after a stroke have helped many survive. Unfortunately, stroke survivors do not always make a full recovery. Problems with speech, memory, swallowing, activities of daily living, and other consequences can persist, even with physical therapy and medications. Depression is also an issue for many poststroke survivors.

SKILLS FOR BEHAVIOR CHANGE

A SIMPLE TEST FOR STROKE

People often ignore, minimize, or misunderstand stroke symptoms. Starting treatment within just a few hours is crucial for the best recovery outcomes. So if you suspect someone is having a stroke, use the tool many emergency teams use to assess what is happening. Think FAST.

- **F**acial droop: Ask the person to smile. It is normal for both sides of the face to move equally, and it is abnormal if one side moves less easily.
- **A**rm weakness: Ask the person to raise both arms. It is normal if both arms move equally (or not at all). It is abnormal if one arm drifts or cannot be raised as high as the other.
- **S**peech difficulty: Have the patient restate a sentence such as, "You can't teach an old dog new tricks." It is normal if they can say the sentence correctly, and it is abnormal if they use inappropriate words, slur, or cannot speak.
- **T**ime to ACT and call 9-1-1. Don't delay if you note 1–3 above. Time is of the essence.

Source: "Cincinnati Prehospital Stroke Scale," adapted from the Uniform Document for Georgia EMS Providers, Department of Public Health, State of Georgia. 2011, http://dph.georgia.gov/sites/dph.georgia.gov/files/Georgia%20Stroke%20Assessment%20Form%20-%20v.1%20-%2011-02-2011.pdf.

Angina Pectoris

Angina pectoris occurs when there is not enough oxygen to supply the heart muscle, resulting in chest pain or pressure. Nearly 8 million people in the United States suffer from mild-to-severe symptoms of angina—from indigestion or heartburn-like sensations to crushing chest pain.[46] Generally, the more serious the oxygen deprivation, the more severe the pain. Although angina pectoris is not a heart attack, it does indicate underlying heart disease.

Mild cases of angina may be treated simply with rest. Drugs such as *nitroglycerin* can dilate veins and provide pain relief. Other medications, such as *calcium channel blockers*, can relieve cardiac spasms and arrhythmias, lower blood pressure, and slow heart rate. *Beta-blockers* control potential overactivity of the heart muscle.

Arrhythmias

Over the course of a lifetime, most people experience some type of **arrhythmia**, an irregularity in heart rhythm that occurs when the electrical impulses in your heart that coordinate heartbeat don't work properly. A person with a racing heart in the absence of exercise or anxiety may be experiencing *tachycardia*, the medical term for abnormally fast heartbeat. On the other end of the continuum is *bradycardia*, or abnormally slow heartbeat. When a heart goes into **fibrillation**, it beats in a sporadic, quivering pattern, resulting in extreme inefficiency in moving blood through the cardiovascular system. If untreated, fibrillation may be fatal.

Not all arrhythmias are life-threatening. In many instances, excessive caffeine or nicotine consumption can trigger an arrhythmia episode. However, severe cases may require drug therapy or external electrical stimulus to prevent serious complications. When in doubt, it is always best to check with your doctor.

angina pectoris Chest pain occurring as a result of reduced oxygen flow to the heart.

arrhythmia An irregularity in heartbeat.

fibrillation A sporadic, quivering pattern of heartbeat that results in extreme inefficiency in moving blood through the cardiovascular system.

WHY SHOULD I CARE?

Hypertension is becoming more common among college students. You can't tell whether you have it by how you feel or how you look in the mirror, but it poses a major potential threat to your quality of life. Get your blood pressure checked. It's easy to do, and it could save your life!

Heart Failure

When the heart muscle is damaged and can't pump enough blood to supply body tissues, fluids may begin to accumulate in various

heart failure (HF) or congestive heart failure (CHF) An abnormal cardiovascular condition that reflects impaired cardiac pumping and blood flow; pooling blood leads to congestion in body tissues.

cardiomyopathy Damage to heart muscle due to enlargement, atrophy, and/or rigidity that results in decreased heart function.

congenital cardiovascular defect Cardiovascular problem that is present at birth.

rheumatic heart disease A heart disease caused by untreated streptococcal infection of the throat.

parts of the body, most notably, the lungs, feet, ankles, and legs. Acute shortness of breath and fatigue are often key symptoms of **heart failure (HF)** or **congestive heart failure (CHF)**. This condition is increasingly common, particularly among those with a history of other heart problems. Currently in the United States, nearly 6.6 million adults age 20 and over have HF, with cases estimated to rise to nearly 10 million by 2030.[47]

Underlying causes of HF may include heart injury that results in damage to heart muscle (**cardiomyopathy**), affects heart valves, or causes problems with heart rhythms. Infectious diseases, such as rheumatic fever, can damage heart valves. Bacteria and viruses can inflame blood vessels, increasing atherosclerotic plaque formation. Uncontrolled high blood pressure, coronary artery disease, diabetes, and other chronic conditions can all lead to heart failure. Certain prescription drugs such as NSAIDS and diabetes medications also increase risks, as do chronic drug and alcohol abuse. In some cases, damage is due to cancer radiation or chemotherapy treatments. Untreated, HF can be fatal. However, most cases respond well to treatment that includes *diuretics* ("water pills") to relieve fluid accumulation; drugs, such as *digitalis*, that increase the pumping action of the heart; and drugs called *vasodilators*, which expand blood vessels, allowing blood to flow more freely and making the heart's work easier. Prevention of underlying CVD risks, such as reducing sodium intake and following a heart-smart diet, are the best ways to reduce your risks of HF.

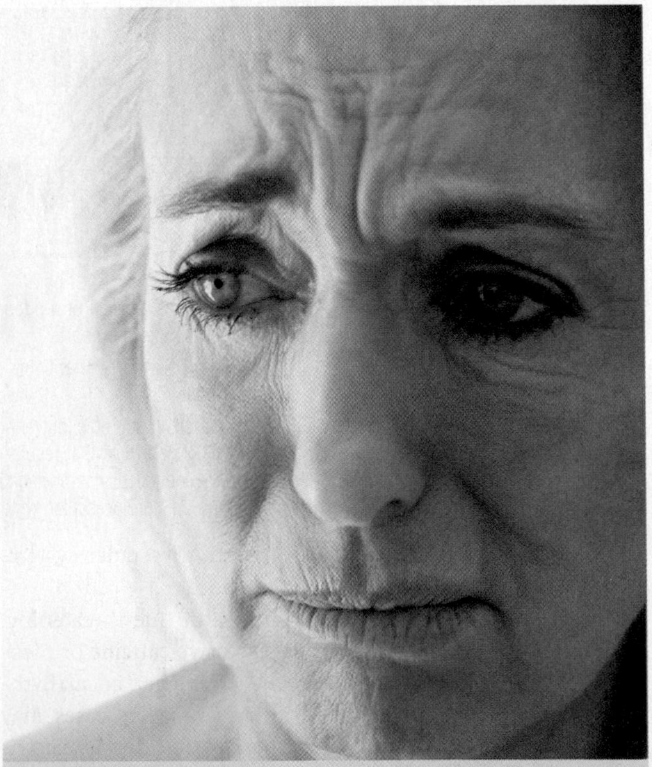

Research shows evidence of "broken heart syndrome," also known as *stress cardiomyopathy*, where traumatic emotional events trigger a "concussion," a type of heart attack caused by overwhelming grief. The first 24 hours after a loved one dies pose the biggest risk for a heart attack, particularly among those with CVD risks.

Source: E. Mostosfsky et al., "Risk of Acute Myocardial Infarction After Death of a Significant Person in One's Life: The Determinants of MI Onset Study," *Circulation* 125 (2012): 491–96.

Congenital and Rheumatic Heart Disease

Approximately 32,000 infants are expected to be born in the United States each year with some form of **congenital cardiovascular defect** (*congenital* means the problem is present at birth).[48] These forms may be relatively minor, such as slight *murmurs* (low-pitched sounds caused by turbulent blood flow through the heart) caused by valve irregularities that some children outgrow. About 25 percent of those born with congenital heart defects must undergo invasive procedures to correct problems within the first year of life.[49] The underlying causes of these defects are unknown, but may be related to hereditary factors; maternal diseases, such as rubella, that occurred during fetal development; or the mother's chemical intake (particularly alcohol or methamphetamine) during pregnancy. Because of advances in pediatric cardiology, the prognosis for children with congenital heart defects is better than ever before.

Rheumatic heart disease is attributed to rheumatic fever, an inflammatory disease caused by an unresolved *streptococcal infection* of the throat (strep throat). Over time, this strep infection can affect many connective tissues of the body, especially those of the heart, joints, brain, or skin. In some cases, this infection can lead to an immune response in which antibodies attack the heart as well as the bacteria. Many of the thousands of operations on heart valves performed per year in the United States are related to rheumatic heart disease.

LO 4 | REDUCING YOUR RISKS

Describe the modifiable and nonmodifiable risk factors for cardiovascular disease and methods of prevention.

CVD takes a tremendous toll in terms of mortality and morbidity in the United States. Recently, the *U.S. Burden of Disease Collaborators* determined that greatest contributor to overall CVD burden was *suboptimal diet*, followed by *tobacco smoking, high body mass index, high blood pressure, high fasting plasma glucose,* and *physical inactivity*.[50] A growing body of research has implicated selected CVD risks and conditions such as obesity and hypertension, with an increased risk for impaired cognitive function and an increased risk for Alzheimer's disease.[51]

TABLE 15.3 | Prevalence of Major CVD Risks in United States by Gender and Race

Women	Men
Overweight/Obesity (overall: 63.7%)	**Overweight/Obesity (overall: 72.9%)**
White 60.2%	White 73.3%
Black 79.9%	Black 68.7%
Mexican American 78.2%	Mexican American 81.3%
Total Cholesterol > 200 mg/dl (overall: 44.9%)	**Total Cholesterol > 200 mg/dl (overall: 41.3%)**
White 45.8%	White 40.5%
Black 40.7%	Black 38.6%
Mexican American 44.7%	Mexican American 48.1%
High Blood Pressure (overall: 32.2%)	**High Blood Pressure (overall: 33.6%)**
White 30.7%	White 33.4%
Black 47.0%	Black 42.6%
Mexican American 28.8%	Mexican American 30.1%
Diagnosed Type 2 Diabetes (overall: 7.9%)	**Diagnosed Type 2 Diabetes (overall: 8.7%)**
White 6.2%	White 7.7%
Black 15.4%	Black 13.5%
Mexican American 12.0%	Mexican American 11.4%

Source: Data taken from Tables 25.1 and 25.2 found in A. S. Go et al., "Heart Disease and Stroke Statistics—2014 Update: A Report from the American Heart Association," *Circulation* 129 (2014): e28–e292, www.heart.org/idc/groups/ahamah-public/@wcm/@sop/@smd/documents/downloadable/ucm_459072.pdf.

Cardiometabolic risks are the combined risks, which indicate physical and biochemical changes that can lead to diseases. Some risks result from choices and behaviors and are modifiable, whereas others are inherited or are intrinsic (such as your age and gender) and cannot be changed. See **TABLE 15.3** for a breakdown of CVD risk factors by race and gender.

Metabolic Syndrome: Quick Risk Profile

Over the past decade, different health professionals have attempted to establish diagnostic cutoff points for a cluster of combined cardiometabolic risks, variably labeled as *syndrome X*, *insulin resistance syndrome*, and most recently, **metabolic syndrome (MetS)**. Historically, metabolic syndrome is believed to increase the risk for atherosclerotic heart disease by as much as three times the normal rates. It has captured international attention because over 20 percent of people age 20 to 39, 41 percent of people age 40 to 59, and nearly 52 percent of those over the age of 60 meet the criteria for MetS.[52] Although different professional organizations have slightly different criteria for MetS, that of the National Cholesterol Education Program's Adult Treatment Panel (NCEP/ATPIII) is most commonly used. According to these criteria, for a diagnosis of metabolic syndrome a person would have three or more of the following risks (**FIGURE 15.7**):[53]

cardiometabolic risks Physical and biochemical changes that are risk factors for the development of cardiovascular disease and type 2 diabetes.

metabolic syndrome (MetS) A group of metabolic conditions occurring together that increase a person's risk of heart disease, stroke, and diabetes.

- Abdominal obesity (waist measurement of more than 40 inches in men or 35 inches in women)
- Elevated blood fat (triglycerides greater than 150)
- Low levels of HDL ("good") cholesterol (less than 40 in men and less than 50 in women)
- Elevated blood pressure greater than 135/85 mm Hg

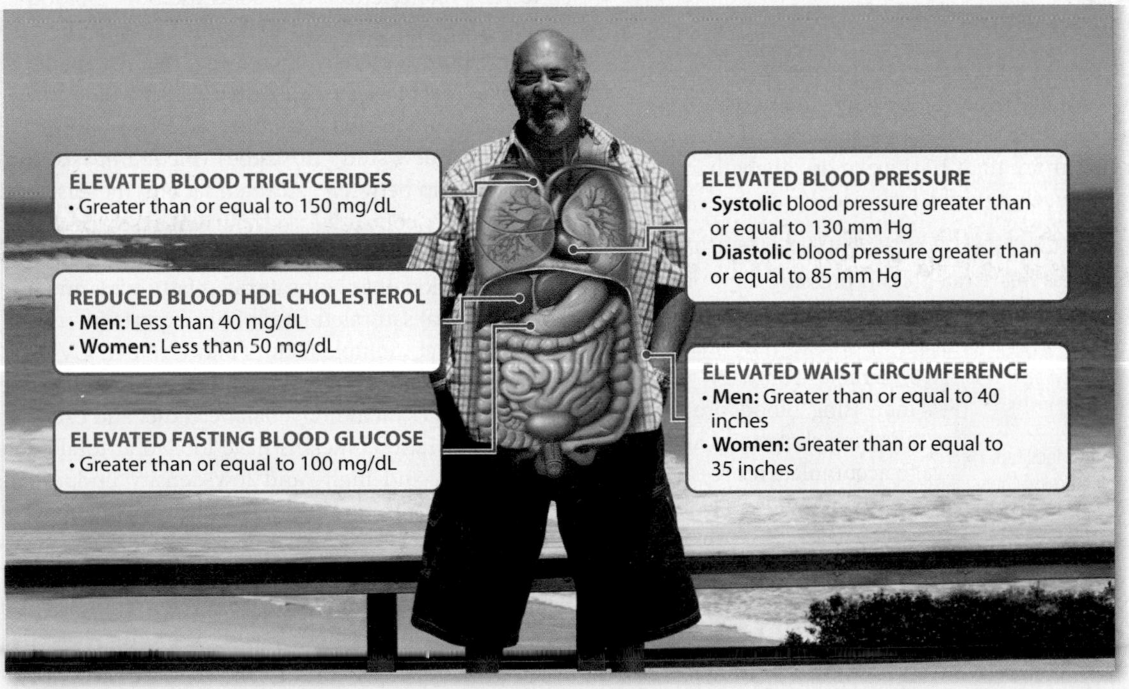

ELEVATED BLOOD TRIGLYCERIDES
• Greater than or equal to 150 mg/dL
REDUCED BLOOD HDL CHOLESTEROL
• Men: Less than 40 mg/dL
• Women: Less than 50 mg/dL
ELEVATED FASTING BLOOD GLUCOSE
• Greater than or equal to 100 mg/dL
ELEVATED BLOOD PRESSURE
• Systolic blood pressure greater than or equal to 130 mm Hg
• Diastolic blood pressure greater than or equal to 85 mm Hg
ELEVATED WAIST CIRCUMFERENCE
• Men: Greater than or equal to 40 inches
• Women: Greater than or equal to 35 inches

FIGURE 15.7 Risk Factors Associated with Metabolic Syndrome

- Elevated fasting glucose greater than 100 mg/dL (a sign of insulin resistance or glucose intolerance)

The use of the metabolic syndrome classification and other, similar terms has been important in highlighting the relationship between the number of risks a person possesses and that person's likelihood of developing CVD and diabetes. Groups such as the AHA and others are giving increased attention to multiple risks and emphasizing cardiovascular health in lifestyle interventions.

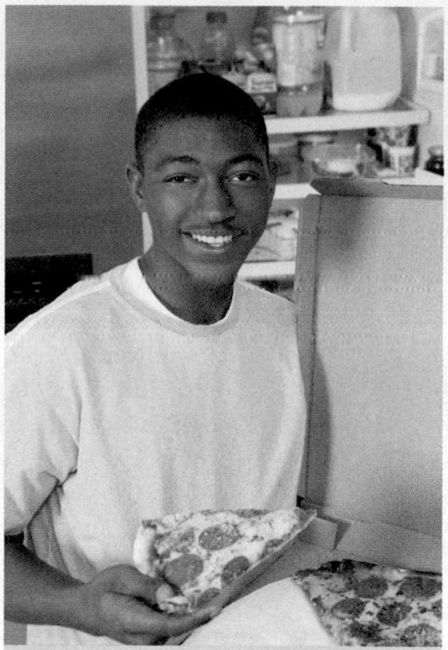
About 25 percent of your blood cholesterol level comes from foods you eat, and this is where you can make real improvements.

Modifiable Risks

Younger adults are not invulnerable to CVD risks. From the first moments of your life, you begin to accumulate risks. Your past and current lifestyle choices may haunt you as you enter your middle and later years of life. Behaviors you choose today and over the coming decades can actively reduce or promote your risk for CVD.

Avoid Tobacco Although smoking rates declined by over 50 percent between 1965 and 2007, about 21 percent of U.S. adults age 18 and over are still regular smokers.[54] Tobacco use remains the leading cause of preventable death in the United States, accounting for around 1 of every 5 deaths.[55] Likewise, nonsmokers regularly exposed to secondhand smoke have a 25 to 30 percent increased risk of heart disease, with over 35,000 deaths per year.[56]

Just how great a risk is smoking when it comes to CVD? Consider these statistics:[57]

- Cigarette smokers are two to four times more likely to develop coronary heart disease than are nonsmokers.
- Cigarette smoking doubles a person's risk of stroke.
- Smokers are more than 10 times more likely than nonsmokers to develop peripheral vascular diseases.

Smoking is thought to damage the heart in several ways. Nicotine increases heart rate, blood pressure, and oxygen use by heart muscles, which over time forces the organ to work harder. Additionally, chemicals in smoke may damage and inflame coronary arteries, increasing blood pressure and allowing cholesterol and plaque to accumulate more easily.

low-density lipoproteins (LDLs) Compounds that facilitate the transport of cholesterol in the blood to the body's cells and cause the cholesterol to build up on artery walls.

high-density lipoproteins (HDLs) Compounds that facilitate the transport of cholesterol in the blood to the liver for metabolism and elimination from the body.

The good news is that if you stop smoking, your heart begins to mend itself. A former smoker's risk of heart disease drops by 50 percent 1 year after quitting. Between 5 and 15 years after quitting, the risk of stroke and CHD becomes similar to that of nonsmokers. College-age students, take note: Studies show quitting by age 30 reduces chances of dying prematurely from tobacco-related diseases by more than 90 percent.[58] Numerous studies have shown that smoking increases the risk of respiratory diseases, lung cancer, and other problems that ultimately affect the heart and circulatory system.[59] Newer research points to the fact that stopping smoking may have a significant positive effect on stress levels, overall mood, depression, and anxiety; all factors that can affect diet, weight, motivation to exercise, and ultimately risk for CVD.[60] In short, when you are mentally healthy, you're more likely to engage in behaviors that reduce risks from CVD.

Cut Back on Saturated Fat and Cholesterol *Cholesterol* is a type of soft, waxy, fat-like substance found in your bloodstream and in your body cells. Cholesterol plays an important role in the production of cell membranes and hormones (estrogen and testosterone), it protects nerves, and it helps with digestion as well as processing vitamin D. However, when levels of cholesterol in the blood get too high, your risk for CVD increases. Much of your blood cholesterol level is predetermined: About 75 percent of it is produced by your body, and the rest comes from foods in your diet. The good news is that changing your diet can make real improvements in your overall cholesterol level, even if yours is naturally high.

Diets high in saturated fat and *trans* fats are widely believed to raise cholesterol levels, send the body's blood-clotting system into high gear, and make the blood more viscous in just a few hours, thereby increasing the risk of heart attack or stroke. High levels of cholesterol in the blood have long been thought to contribute to atherosclerosis. However, during an extensive new study of studies (*meta-analysis*) looking at the relationship between saturated fat and increased risk of CVD, researchers concluded that current research evidence doesn't clearly support cardiovascular guidelines that encourage high consumption of polyunsaturated fatty acids and low consumption of total saturated fats.[61] Still, experts increasingly point to the fact that multiple factors play a role in CVD risk and continue to recommend reduction of saturated fats as part of lifestyle changes including a balanced diet and exercising.

Historically, clinicians have looked at total cholesterol, triglycerides, and high- and low-density lipoproteins as being key to determining CVD risks. **Low-density lipoprotein (LDL)**, often referred to as "bad" cholesterol, is believed to build up on artery walls. In contrast, **high-density lipoprotein (HDL)**, or "good" cholesterol, appears to remove cholesterol from artery walls. In theory, if LDL levels get too high or HDL levels get too low, cholesterol will accumulate inside arteries and lead to cardiovascular problems. **Triglycerides** are also gaining increasing attention as a key factor in CVD risk. When you

TABLE 15.4 | Recommended Cholesterol Levels for Lower/Moderate-Risk Adults

Total Cholesterol Level (lower numbers are better)	
Less than 200 mg/dL	Desirable
200–239 mg/dL	Borderline high
240 mg/dL and above	High
HDL Cholesterol Level (higher numbers are better)	
Less than 40 mg/dL (for men)	Low
60 mg/dL and above	Desirable
LDL Cholesterol Level (lower numbers are better)	
Less than 100 mg/dL	Optimal
100–129 mg/dL	Near or above optimal
130–159 mg/dL	Borderline high
160–189 mg/dL	High
190 mg/dL and above	Very high
Triglyceride Level (lower numbers are better)	
Less than 150 mg/dL	Normal
150–199 mg/dL	Borderline high
200–499 mg/dL	High
500 mg/dL and above	Very high

Source: Adapted from *ATP III Guidelines At-a-Glance Quick Desk Reference*, National Heart, Lung, and Blood Institute, National Institutes of Health. Update on Cholesterol Guidelines, 2004, http://www.nhlbi.nih.gov/guidelines/cholesterol/atp3upd04.htm.

consume extra calories, the body converts the extra to triglycerides, which are stored in fat cells. Hormones release triglycerides throughout the day to provide energy. High counts of blood triglycerides are often found in people who are obese and overweight and have high cholesterol levels, heart problems, or diabetes. As they age, particularly if they gain weight, people's triglyceride and cholesterol levels tend to rise. It is recommended that a baseline cholesterol test (known as a lipid panel or lipid profile) be taken at age 20, with follow-ups every 5 years. Men over the age of 35 and women over the age of 45 should have their lipid profile checked annually, with more frequent tests for those at high risk. See **TABLE 15.4** for recommended levels of cholesterol and triglycerides.

Until recently, there has been general agreement that the higher the level of LDL cholesterol, the greater is the risk of a heart attack or stroke. Cutting *trans* fats and reducing saturated fats has been the standard recommendation for reducing risks. The goal has been to keep LDL levels between 100 and 129 mg/dL, ideally, and to maintain HDL levels higher than 60 dL to keep cardiovascular risk low.[62] However, new research indicates that raising HDL to prevent negative CVD outcomes may not be as beneficial as once thought.[63] Drugs that were effective in raising HDL levels had little or no effect on CVD risks or mortality.

SEE IT! VIDEOS

Can a way of eating reduce your risk of heart disease? Watch **Mediterranean Diet Could Help Reduce Heart Disease** available on MasteringHealth.™

triglycerides The most common form of lipid in the body; excess calories are converted into triglycerides and stored as body fat.

plant sterols Essential components of plant membranes that, when consumed in the diet, appear to help lower cholesterol levels.

In 2013, the American College of Cardiology and the American Heart Association developed guidelines to identify those who might benefit from cholesterol lowering lifestyle changes and/or drug therapy. These guidelines essentially go beyond lowering cholesterol and aiming for ideal LDL and HDL levels to a more aggressive drug treatment regimen for those likely to benefit. They include assessment of stroke risk and provide new gender and ethnicity specific methods for determining risk. Four lifestyle areas (exercise, healthy diet, weight control, and avoidance of tobacco) are key elements of individual assessments and treatment plans. LDL and other measures will be assessed to determine whether patients are following recommended treatment regimens, including whether drug treatments are working for them. Adjustments in dosage will be made to achieve optimum results over a 10-year period.[64]

In spite of all of the education on the dangers of high cholesterol, Americans continue to have higher-than-recommended levels. Nearly 44 percent of adults age 20 and older have cholesterol levels at or above 200 mg/dL, and another 14 percent have levels in excess of 240 mg/dL.[65] Millions of Americans are on cholesterol-lowering drugs, with numbers increasing yearly.

Strive for a Heart-Healthy Diet Research continues into other dietary modifications that may affect heart health. An overall approach, such as the DASH (Dietary Approaches to Stop Hypertension) eating plan from the National Heart, Lung, and Blood Institute (**FIGURE 15.8**), has strong evidence to back up its recommendations. DASH guidelines include the following:

- Consume 5 to 10 milligrams per day of soluble fiber from sources such as oat bran, fruits, vegetables, legumes, and psyllium seeds. Even this small dietary modification may result in a 5 percent drop in LDL levels.
- Consume about 2 grams per day of **plant sterols**, which are naturally present in small quantities in many fruits, vegetables, nuts, seeds, and other plant sources. Intake of plant sterols can reduce LDL by another 5 percent.
- Eat less sodium. Excess sodium has been linked to high blood pressure, which can in turn affect CVD risk.

See the **Health Headlines** box for more information on foods that may be heart protective.

Maintain a Healthy Weight No question about it—body weight plays a role in CVD. Researchers are not sure whether high-fat, high-sugar, high-calorie diets are a direct risk for CVD or whether such diets invite risk by causing obesity, which strains the heart, forcing it to push blood through the many miles of capillaries that supply each pound of fat. A heart

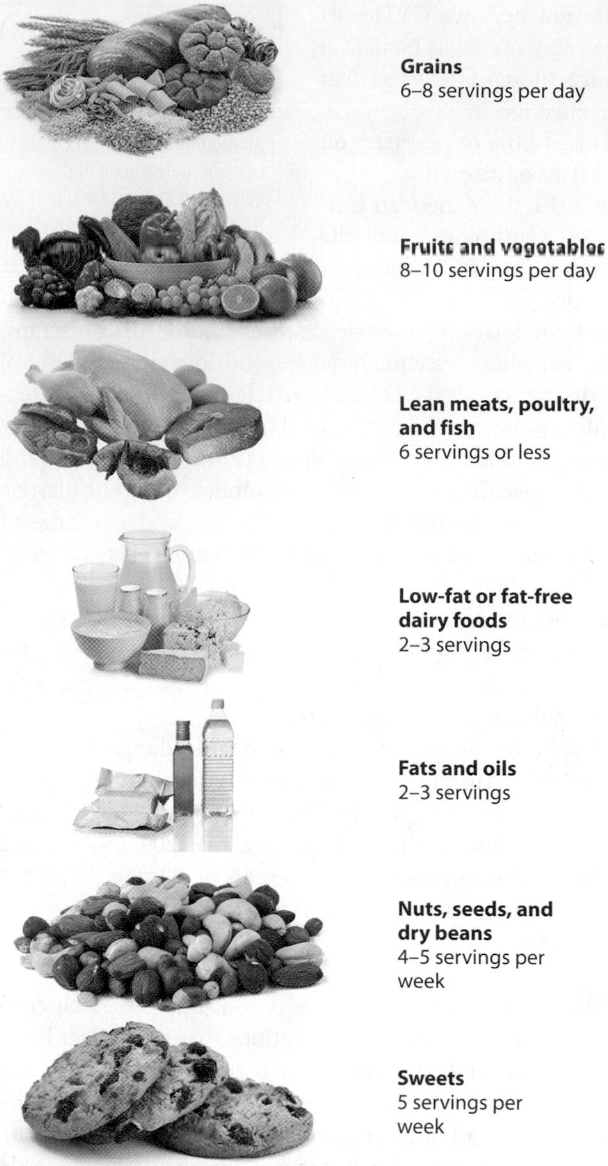
Grains
6–8 servings per day
Fruits and vegetables
8–10 servings per day
Lean meats, poultry, and fish
6 servings or less
Low-fat or fat-free dairy foods
2–3 servings
Fats and oils
2–3 servings
Nuts, seeds, and dry beans
4–5 servings per week
Sweets
5 servings per week

FIGURE 15.8 The DASH Eating Plan Based on a 2,000 calorie/day diet. All serving suggestions are per day unless otherwise noted.

Source: National Heart, Lung, and Blood Institute, "Following the DASH Eating Plan," July 2012, www.nhlbi.nih.gov/health/health-topics/topics/dash/followdash.html.

that has to continuously move blood through an overabundance of vessels may become damaged. Overweight people are more likely to develop heart disease and stroke even if they have no other risk factors. If you're heavy, losing even 5 to 10 pounds can make a significant difference.[66] This is especially true if you're an "apple" (thicker around your upper body and waist) rather than a "pear" (thicker around your hips and thighs).

Exercise Regularly Inactivity is a definite risk factor for CVD.[67] The good news is that you do not have to be an exercise fanatic to reduce your risk. Even modest levels of low-intensity physical activity—walking, gardening, housework, dancing—are beneficial if done regularly and over the long term. Exercise can increase HDL, lower triglycerides, and reduce coronary risks.

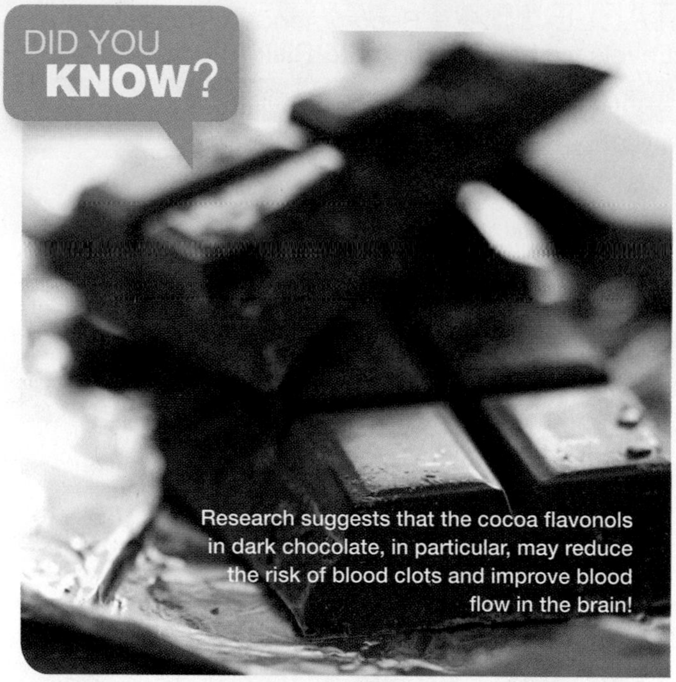
DID YOU KNOW?
Research suggests that the cocoa flavonols in dark chocolate, in particular, may reduce the risk of blood clots and improve blood flow in the brain!

Control Diabetes Heart disease death rates among adults with diabetes are two to four times higher than the rates for adults without diabetes. At least 68 percent of people with diabetes die of some form of heart disease or stroke.[68] (See **Focus On: Minimizing Your Risk for Diabetes** starting on page 444 for more on preventing and controlling diabetes.)

Control Your Blood Pressure Although blood pressure typically creeps up with age, lifestyle changes can dramatically reduce risks. Among the most beneficial actions you can take are losing weight, cutting back sodium in your diet, exercising more, reducing alcohol intake, quitting smoking, getting enough sleep, and reducing your caffeine intake.

Manage Stress People under stress may suffer from a variety of health-related problems. They may smoke or suffer extreme anxiety reactions. They may also anger more easily, have difficulty sleeping, experience gastrointestinal difficulties, have spikes in blood sugar, and have a host of negative health outcomes.[69] In recent years, scientists have shown compelling evidence that both acute and chronic stress may trigger acute cardiac events or even sudden cardiac death, as well as increase risks of hypertension, stroke, and elevated cholesterol levels. Newer research indicates that everyday, chronic stressors can lead to increased risk of coronary events, high blood pressure, strokes, and sudden cardiac death in much the same way that acute stress caused by natural disasters does. Financial stressors, pressure to succeed in college and get a great job, pressure to find a partner, and pressure to please significant others can have a tsunami-like effect on people young and old.[70]

Nonmodifiable Risks

Unfortunately, not all risk factors for CVD can be prevented or controlled. The most important are the following:

@ HEALTH HEADLINES

HEART-HEALTHY SUPER FOODS

The foods you eat play a major role in your CVD risk. While many foods can increase your risk, several have been shown to reduce the chances that cholesterol will be absorbed in the cells, reduce levels of LDL cholesterol, or enhance the protective effects of HDL cholesterol. To protect your heart, include the following in your diet:

- **Dark chocolate.** Dark chocolate contains 70 percent or more of flavonoid-rich cocoa, and much less sugar than milk chocolate. If you must indulge, buy the highest percent cocoa you can find, and savor the 1 to 2 ounces a bit at a time.
- **Fish high in omega-3 fatty acids.** Consumption of fish such as salmon, sardines, and herring helps reduce blood pressure and the risk associated with blood clots and helps lower cholesterol.
- **Olive oil.** Using monounsaturated fats in cooking, particularly extra virgin olive oil, helps lower total cholesterol and raise your HDL levels. Canola oil; margarine labeled "*trans* fat free"; and cholesterol-lowering margarines such as Benecol, Promise Activ, or Smart Balance are also excellent choices.
- **Whole grains and fiber.** Getting enough fiber each day in the form of 100 percent whole wheat, steel cut oats, oat bran, flaxseed, fruits, and vegetables helps lower LDL or "bad" cholesterol. Soluble fiber, in particular, seems to keep cholesterol from being absorbed in the intestines.
- **Plant sterols and stanols.** These essential components of plant membranes are found naturally in vegetables, fruits, and legumes. In addition, many food products, including juices and yogurt, are now fortified with them. These compounds are believed to benefit your heart health by blocking cholesterol absorption in the bloodstream, thus reducing LDL levels.
- **Nuts.** Long maligned for being high in calories, walnuts, almonds, and other nuts are naturally high in omega-3 fatty acids, which are important in lowering cholesterol and good for the blood vessels themselves.
- **Green tea.** Several studies have indicated that green tea may reduce LDL cholesterol. The flavonoids in it act as powerful antioxidants that protect the cells of the heart and blood vessels.
- **Red wine.** In recent years, many observational studies have indicated that one glass of red wine per day may be protective and reduce your risk of CHD. Although the research is promising, the American Heart Association is slow to endorse drinking alcohol to reduce CVD risk and instead recommends dietary modification, exercise, and stress reduction, while supporting additional research. While one drink of red wine might be protective, adding additional "doses" of wine won't help and, in fact, is likely to be harmful.

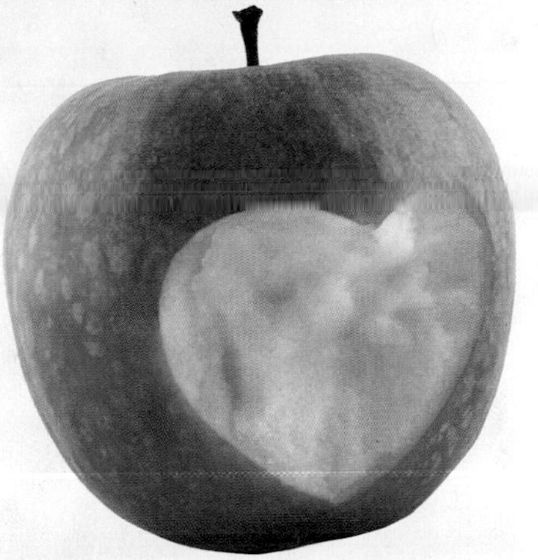

Sources: L. Hooper et al., "Effects of Chocolate, Cocoa, and Flavanols on Cardiovascular Health: A Systematic Review and Meta-Analysis of Randomized Trials," *American Journal of Clinical Nutrition* 95, no. 3 (2012): 740–51; American Heart Association, "Alcoholic Beverages and Cardiovascular Disease," 2014, http://www.heart.org/HEARTORG/GettingHealthy/NutritionCenter/HealthyEating/Alcohol-and-Heart-Health_UCM_305173_Article.jsp; P. Ronksley et al., "Association of Alcohol Consumption with Selected Cardiovascular Disease Outcomes: A Systematic Review and Meta-Analysis," *British Medical Journal* 342 (2011): 671–81; S. Kalesi et al., "Green Tea Catechins and Blood Pressure: A Systematic Review and Meta Analysis of Randomized Controlled Trials," *European J. Nut.*, May, 2014. doi. 10.1007/s00394-014-0720-1.

- **Race and ethnicity.** African Americans tend to have the highest overall rates of CVD and hypertension and the lowest rates of physical activity (**FIGURE 15.9**). The rate of high blood pressure in African Americans is among the highest in the world. Mexican Americans have the highest percentage of adults with cholesterol levels exceeding 200 mg/dL and the highest rates of obesity and overweight.[71]
- **Heredity.** A family history of heart disease increases risk of CVD significantly. The amount of cholesterol you produce, tendencies to form plaque, and a host of other factors seem to have genetic links. The difficulty comes in sorting out genetic influences from the modifiable factors shared by family members, such as environment, stress, dietary habits, and so on. Newer research has focused on studying the interactions between nutrition and genes (*nutrigenetics*) and the role that diet may play in increasing or decreasing risks among certain genetic profiles.[72]
- **Age.** Although cardiovascular disease can affect all ages, 82 percent of heart attacks occur in people over age 65.[73] Increasing age ups the risk for CVD for all.
- **Gender.** Men are at greater risk for CVD until about age 60, when women catch up and then surpass them. Otherwise healthy women under age 35 have a fairly low risk, although oral contraceptive use and smoking increase the risk. After menopause, or after estrogen levels are otherwise reduced (for example, because of a hysterectomy), women's LDL levels tend to go up, which increases the chance for CVD. Women also have poorer health outcomes and higher death rates than men when they have a heart attack.[74]

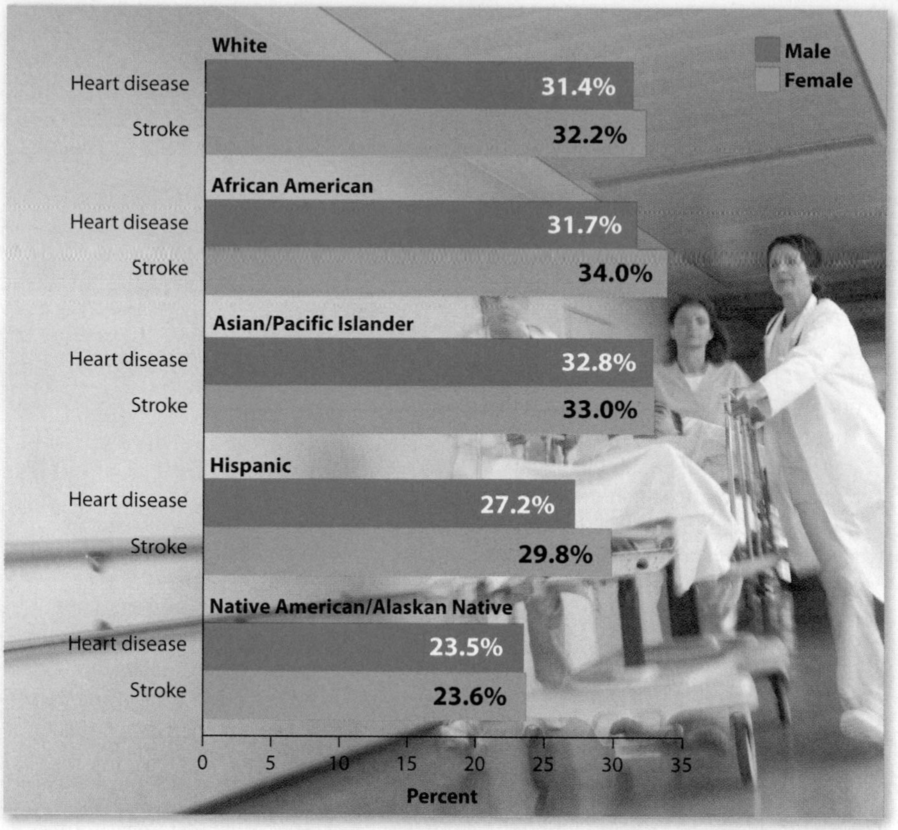

FIGURE 15.9 Percent CVD Deaths by Race and Gender

Sources: AHA, Statistics at a Glance—2014. Population Fact Sheets, 2014, also, Chart 13.8; A. S. Go et al., "Heart Disease and Stroke Statistics—2014 Update: A Report from the American Heart Association," *Circulation* 129 (2014): e28–e292, http://circ.ahajournals.org/content/129/3/e28.full.

Other Risk Factors

Several other factors and indicators have been linked to CVD risk, including inflammation and homocysteine levels.

Inflammation and C-Reactive Protein Many experts believe inflammation plays a major role in atherosclerosis development. It occurs when bacteria, trauma, toxins, or heat injure blood vessel walls, making them more prone to plaque formation. Cigarette smoke, high blood pressure, high LDL cholesterol, diabetes, certain forms of arthritis, and exposure to toxins have all been linked to increased risk of inflammation. However, the greatest risk appears to be from certain infectious disease pathogens, most notably *Chlamydia pneumoniae,* a common cause of respiratory infections; *Helicobacter pylori,* a bacterium that causes ulcers; herpes simplex virus; and *Cytomegalovirus,* another herpes virus infecting most Americans before the age of 40. During an inflammatory reaction, C-reactive proteins (CRPs) tend to be present at high levels. A recent meta-analysis shows a strong association between CRPs in the blood and increased risks for atherosclerosis and CVD.[75] Blood tests can test these proteins using a highly sensitive assay called *hs-CRP* (high-sensitivity C-reactive protein); if levels are high, action could be taken to reduce inflammation.

Fish oil, flax, and other foods high in omega-3 have been recommended by the AHA and other groups for their anti-inflammatory properties.[76] While some studies have cast doubt on omega-3's benefits, the bulk of research has shown beneficial effects of omega-3, leading to AHA recommendations for obtaining it in diet or supplement form.[77] More research is necessary to determine the actual role that inflammation plays in increased risk of CVD or if there is something unique about inflammation that omega-3 may work to counter.[78]

Homocysteine Over the last decade, there was mounting evidence that homocysteine, an amino acid normally present in the blood, increased the risk of CVD. Early studies indicated that at high levels homocysteine was a prelude to coronary heart disease, peripheral artery disease, and increased risk of stroke. Scientists hypothesized that homocysteine worked to inflame the inner lining of the arterial walls and promote fat deposits on the damaged walls, as well as to encourage the development of blood clots.[79] When

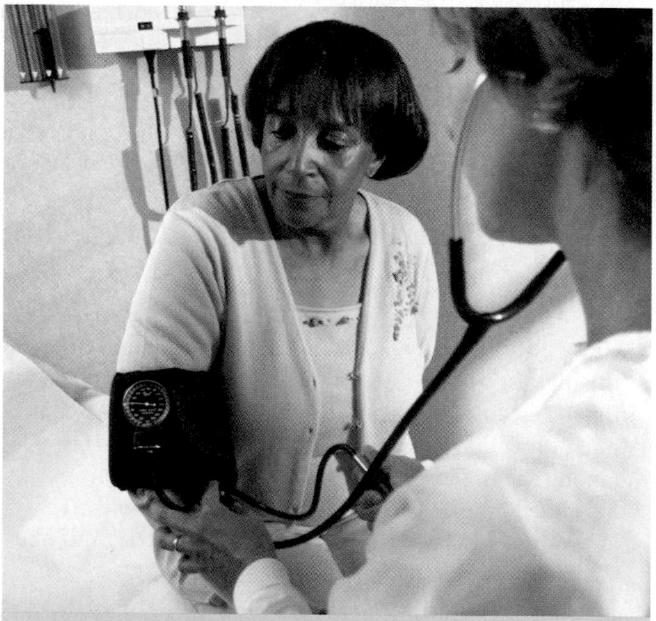

If there is a history of CVD in your family or your racial or ethnic background indicates a propensity for CVD, it is all the more important for you to have regular blood pressure and blood cholesterol screenings and for you to avoid lifestyle risks, including tobacco use, physical inactivity, and poor nutrition.

SEE IT! VIDEOS

What habits can you change now to improve your heart health? Watch **Importance of Heart Health in Your Youth** available on MasteringHealth.™

early studies indicated that folic acid and other B vitamins may help break down homocysteine in the body, food manufacturers responded by adding folic acids to a number of foods and touting the CVD benefits. Professional groups such as the American Heart Association do not currently recommend taking folic acid supplements to lower homocysteine levels and prevent CVD.[80] Instead, they recommend a healthy diet as the best way to reduce risk. Newer research has shown a positive association between taking vitamin B to reduce homocysteine and subsequent reductions in strokes.[81]

Lipoprotein Scientists now believe that there are other blood lipid factors that may also increase CVD risk, such as *lipoprotein-associated phospholipase A2* ($Lp\text{-}PLA_2$), an enzyme that circulates in the blood and attaches to LDL. $Lp\text{-}PLA_2$ plays an important role in plaque accumulation and increased risk for stroke and coronary events, particularly in men. Studies suggest that the higher the $Lp\text{-}PLA_2$ level, the higher the risk of a large artery stroke; however, the evidence is less clear that $Lp\text{-}PLA_2$ increases risk for other coronary events.[82] Another relatively new consideration is the presence of *apolipoprotein B* (apo B), a primary component of LDL that is essential for cholesterol delivery to cells. Although the mechanism is unclear, a growing body of research has shown that apo B levels may be as important as LDL levels in predicting risk of CHD.[83]

LO 5 | DIAGNOSING AND TREATING CARDIOVASCULAR DISEASE

Examine current strategies for diagnosis and treatment of cardiovascular disease.

There are many diagnostic, treatment, prevention, and rehabilitation options for cardiovascular disease. Medications can strengthen heartbeat, control arrhythmias, remove fluids, reduce blood pressure, and improve heart function. *Statins* can lower blood cholesterol levels, *ACE inhibitors* can lower blood pressure by causing the muscles surrounding blood vessels to contract, and *beta-blockers* can reduce blood pressure by blocking the effects of the hormone epinephrine. Long-standing methods of cardiopulmonary resuscitation (CPR) have also changed to focus primarily on chest compressions rather than mouth-to-mouth procedures. The thinking behind this is that people will be more likely to do CPR if the risk for exchange of body fluids is reduced, and any effort to save a person in trouble is better than inaction.

Electrocardiogram, angiography, and positron emission tomography scans are some techniques for diagnosing CVD. An **electrocardiogram (ECG)** is a record of the heart's electrical activity. Patients may undergo a *stress test*—standard exercise on a stationary bike or treadmill with an electrocardiogram and no injections—or a *nuclear stress test,* which involves injecting a radioactive dye and taking images of the heart to reveal problems with blood flow. Although these tests provide a good indicator of potential heart blockage or blood flow abnormalities, a more accurate method of testing for heart disease is **angiography** (also referred to as *cardiac catheterization*), in which a needle-thin tube called a *catheter* is threaded through heart arteries, a dye is injected, and an X-ray is taken to discover which areas are blocked in arteries or veins supplying the heart, lungs, head and neck, brain, and arms and legs.

A more recent and even more effective method of measuring heart activity is a *positron emission tomography (PET) scan,* which produces 3D images of the heart as blood flows through it. Other common tests include the following:

- **Magnetic resonance imaging** (MRI) involves using powerful magnets to look inside the body. Computer-generated pictures can show the heart muscle and help physicians identify damage from a heart attack, diagnose congenital heart defects, and evaluate disease of larger blood vessels such as the aorta.
- **Ultrafast computed tomography** (CT), an especially fast form of heart X-ray, can be used to evaluate bypass grafts, diagnose ventricular function, and identify other heart irregularities.
- **Coronary calcium score** is derived from another type of ultrafast CT used to diagnose levels of calcium in heart vessels. Calcium accumulations on vessel walls provide an indication of plaque formation and heart attack risks; however, most people will show some level of calcium accumulation.

electrocardiogram (ECG) A record of the electrical activity of the heart; may be measured during a stress test.

angiography A technique for examining blockages in arteries or veins supplying the heart, lungs, head and neck, or limbs, utilizing a small camera on a catheter and dye passed through key vessels.

magnetic resonance imaging (MRI) Precise diagnostic technique for identifying heart damage, diagnosing heart defects, and evaluation of blood vessel problems through the use of powerful magnetic, radiation free imaging.

ultrafast computed tomography (CT) A newer, faster form of heart X-ray used to evaluate bypass grafts, diagnose ventricular function, and identify other heart irregularities.

coronary calcium score A type of ultrafast CT used to diagnose levels of calcium in heart vessels or plaque formation and heart attack risk (involves radiation exposure).

coronary bypass surgery A surgical technique whereby a blood vessel taken from another part of the body is implanted to bypass a clogged coronary artery.

Surgical Options: Bypass Surgery, Angioplasty, and Stents

Coronary bypass surgery has helped many patients who suffered coronary blockages or heart attacks. In a coronary artery bypass graft (CABG, referred to as a "cabbage"), a blood vessel is taken from another site in

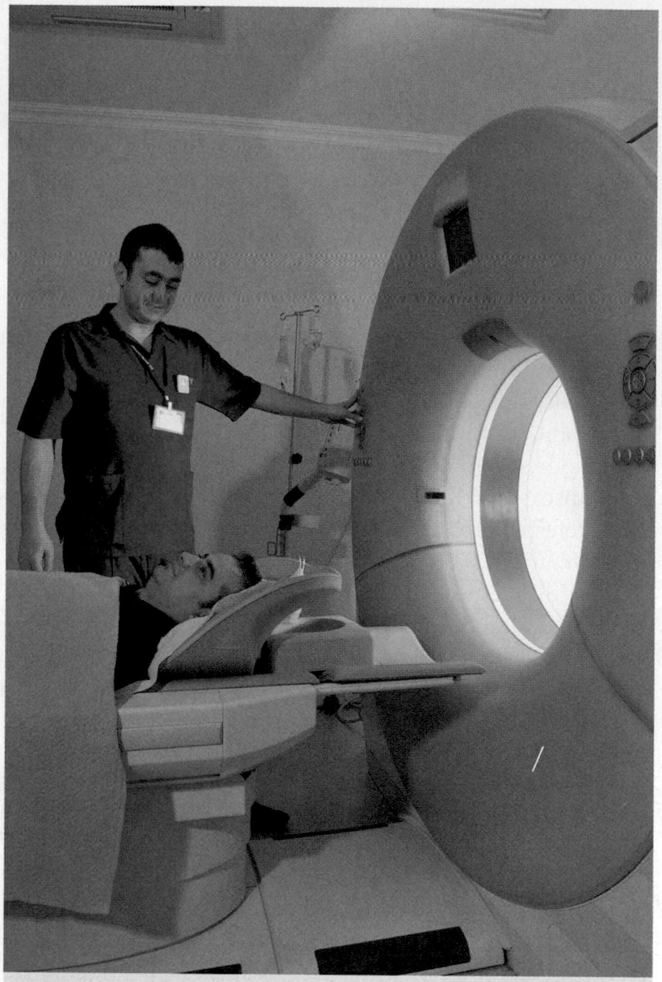

Magnetic resonance imaging is one of several methods used to detect heart damage, abnormalities, or defects.

the patient's body (usually the saphenous vein in the leg or the internal thoracic artery in the chest) and implanted to "bypass" blocked coronary arteries and transport blood to heart tissue. Increasing numbers of heart surgeries are done using a minimally invasive bypass surgery in which the chest is not cracked; the surgeon enters the body through a series of ports and performs the surgery with cameras.

Another procedure, **angioplasty** (sometimes called *balloon angioplasty*), carries fewer risks and may be more effective than bypass surgery in selected cases. As in angiography, a thin catheter is threaded through blocked heart arteries. The catheter has a balloon at the tip, which is inflated to flatten fatty deposits against the arterial walls, allowing blood to flow more freely. Today, many people with heart blockage undergo angioplasty and have a **stent** inserted to hold the vessel open after the procedure. A stent is a stainless steel mesh-like tube that is inserted to prop open the artery. Although stents are highly effective, inflammation and tissue growth in the area may actually increase after the procedure, leading to another blockage. In about 30 percent of patients, the treated arteries become clogged again within 6 months. Newer stents are usually medicated to reduce this risk. Nonetheless, some surgeons argue that given this high rate of recurrence, bypass may be a more effective treatment. Today, newer forms of laser angioplasty and *atherectomy*, a procedure that removes plaque, are being done in several clinics.

angioplasty A technique in which a catheter with a balloon at the tip is inserted into a clogged artery; the balloon is inflated to flatten fatty deposits against artery walls, and a stent is typically inserted to keep the artery open.

stent A stainless steel, mesh-like tube that is inserted to prop open the artery.

thrombolysis Injection of an agent to dissolve clots and restore some blood flow, thereby reducing the amount of tissue that dies from ischemia.

Aspirin and Other Drug Therapies

Although aspirin has been touted as possibly reducing risks for future heart attacks among those who already have had MI events, the benefits of an aspirin regimen for otherwise healthy adults remains in question. New research seems to indicate an increased risk of gastrointestinal bleeding and stroke in those who take it daily.[84] Furthermore, once a patient has taken aspirin regularly for possible protection against CHD, stopping this regimen may, in fact, increase his or her risk.[85]

When a coronary artery is blocked, the heart muscle doesn't die immediately. If a victim reaches an emergency room and is diagnosed fast enough, a form of clot-busting therapy called **thrombolysis** can be performed. Thrombolysis involves injecting an agent such as *tissue plasminogen activator (tPA)* to dissolve the clot and restore some blood flow to the heart, thereby reducing the amount of tissue that dies from ischemia.[86] These drugs must be administered within 1 to 3 hours after a heart attack for best results.

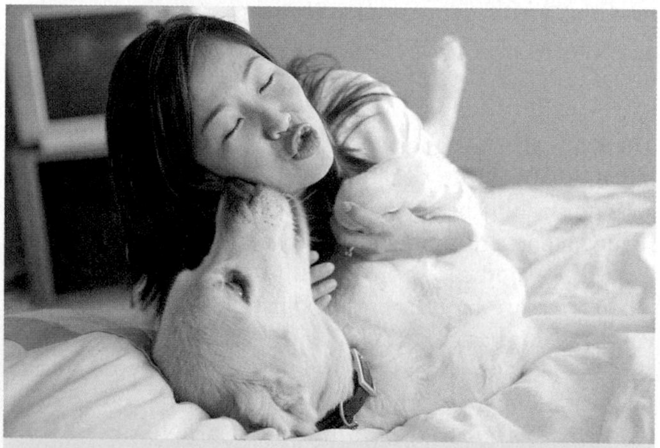

The path to recovery after a heart attack, stroke, or other cardiac problem can be a challenging one, possibly involving medication, physical therapy, and diet modifications. Another important element is stress reduction. Having a pet is one way to focus on something other than your medical condition.

Cardiac Rehabilitation and Recovery

Every year, more than 1 million Americans survive heart attacks. Millions more have a number of medical interventions to help them survive and thrive. In spite of our best diagnostic and treatment options, many cardiac patients find recovery difficult and live in fear of subsequent attacks. Others are disabled, have difficulty breathing and need supportive oxygen, retain fluid due to congestive heart failure, and have difficulties with activities of daily living. Those with friends and family for support and the financial ability to purchase necessary medication and travel for follow-up care can live out their lives with minimal dysfunction.

Perhaps the biggest deterrent is fear of having another attack due to exercise. The benefits of cardiac rehabilitation (including increased stamina and strength and faster recovery), however, far outweigh the risks when these programs are run by certified health professionals.

STUDY PLAN

Customize your study plan—and master your health!—in the Study Area of **MasteringHealth**.

ASSESS YOURSELF

What do your behaviors and family history tell you about your CVD risk? Want to find out? Take the **What's Your Personal CVD Risk?** assessment available on MasteringHealth.™

Need help creating a plan? Follow the strategies in the **Your Plan for Change** box for short- and long-term improvements to your health.

YOUR PLAN FOR **CHANGE**

An **ASSESS YOURSELF** activity for evaluating your risk of heart disease is found at **MasteringHealth**. Based on your results and the advice of your physician, you may need to take steps to reduce your risk of CVD.

TODAY, YOU CAN:

- ☐ Get up and move! Take a walk in the evening, use the stairs instead of the escalator, or ride your bike to class. Start thinking of ways you can incorporate more physical activity into your daily routine.
- ☐ Begin improving your dietary habits by reading labels and making healthier choices with low sodium foods, low fat foods, and nutrient dense fruits and vegetables. Replace the meat and processed foods you might normally eat with a serving of fresh fruit or soy-based protein and green leafy vegetables several times per week. Eat more monounsaturated fat and foods with lower cholesterol counts, and watch your total calorie consumption.

WITHIN THE NEXT 2 WEEKS, YOU CAN:

- ☐ Begin a regular exercise program, even if you start slowly. Set small goals and try to meet them. (See **Chapter 9** for ideas.)
- ☐ Practice a new stress management technique. For example, learn how to meditate. (See **Chapter 3** for other ideas for managing stress.)
- ☐ Get enough rest. Make sure you get at least 8 hours of sleep per night.

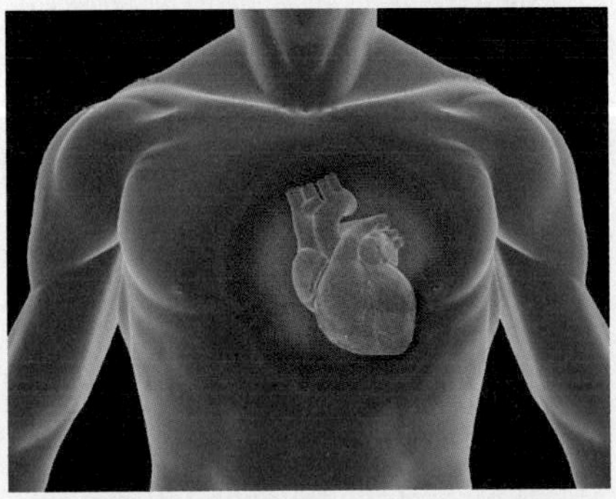

BY THE END OF THE SEMESTER, YOU CAN:

- ☐ Find out your hereditary risk for CVD. Call your parents and find out if your grandparents or aunts or uncles developed CVD. Ask if they know their latest cholesterol LDL/HDL levels. Do you have a family history of diabetes?
- ☐ Get a full lipid panel for yourself and have your blood pressure checked. Once you know your levels, you'll have a better sense of what risk factors to address. If your levels are high, talk to your doctor about how to reduce them.

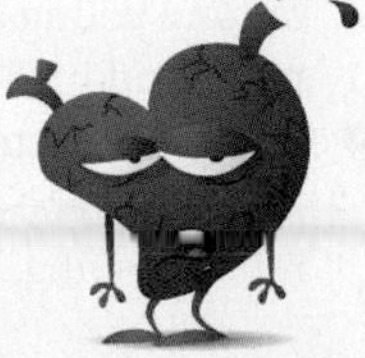

CHAPTER REVIEW

To hear an MP3 Tutor Session, scan here or visit the Study Area in **MasteringHealth**.

LO 1 Understanding the Cardiovascular System

- The cardiovascular system consists of the heart and circulatory system and is a carefully regulated, integrated network of vessels that supplies the body with the nutrients and oxygen necessary to perform daily functions.

LO 2 Cardiovascular Disease: An Epidemiological Overview

- Cardiovascular disease is the leading cause of death in the United States, and it puts a huge economic burden on our society. African Americans have the highest rates of CVD deaths out of any group in the United States. CVD is also a leading cause of death globally and is an increasing threat in the developing world.

LO 3 Key Cardiovascular Diseases

- Cardiovascular diseases include atherosclerosis, coronary artery disease, peripheral artery disease, coronary heart disease, stroke, hypertension, angina pectoris, arrhythmias, congestive heart failure, and congenital and rheumatic heart disease.

LO 4 Reducing Your Risks

- *Cardiometabolic risks* refer to combined factors that increase a person's chances of CVD and diabetes. A person who possesses three or more cardiometabolic risk factors may have metabolic syndrome. Metabolic syndrome is increasing at all levels—among young and old, rich and poor, and in all ethnicities.
- Many risk factors for cardiovascular disease can be modified, such as cigarette smoking, high blood cholesterol and triglyceride levels, hypertension, lack of exercise, a diet high in saturated fat, obesity, diabetes, and emotional stress. Some risk factors, such as age, gender, and heredity, cannot be modified. The more risks you have, the greater your chances of developing CVD at an early age.

LO 5 Diagnosing and Treating Cardiovascular Disease

- Coronary bypass surgery is an established treatment for heart blockage; however, increasing numbers of angioplasty procedures and stents are being used with great success. Increasing numbers of pharmacological interventions such as statins are being used to reduce risk and prevent problems. Drug therapies can be used to prevent and treat CVD.

POP QUIZ

Visit **MasteringHealth** to personalize your study plan with Chapter Review Quizzes and Dynamic Study Modules.

LO 1 Understanding the Cardiovascular System

1. The heart's upper chambers are called the
   a. Valves.
   b. Ventricles.
   c. Atria.
   d. Sinoatrial node.
2. Which type of blood vessels carry oxygenated blood away from the heart?
   a. Ventricles
   b. Arteries
   c. Pulmonary arteries
   d. Venules

LO 2 Cardiovascular Disease: An Epidemiological Overview

3. Which of the following is true about CVD?
   a. It's only a problem in developed nations.
   b. It claims the lives of more men than women every year.
   c. Risk factors are only an issue starting at age 50.
   d. It's the leading cause of death in America.

LO 3 Key Cardiovascular Diseases

4. A stroke results
   a. when a heart stops beating.
   b. when cardiopulmonary resuscitation has failed to revive the stopped heart.
   c. when blood flow in the brain has been compromised, either due to blockage or hemorrhage.
   d. when blood pressure rises above 120/80 mm Hg.
5. An irregularity in the heartbeat is called a(n)
   a. fibrillation.
   b. bradycardia.
   c. tachycardia.
   d. arrhythmia.
6. Severe chest pain due to reduced oxygen flow to the heart is called
   a. angina pectoris.
   b. arrhythmias.
   c. myocardial infarction.
   d. congestive heart failure.

LO 4 Reducing Your Risks

7. What does a person's cholesterol level indicate?
   a. The formation of fatty substances, called *plaque,* which can clog the arteries
   b. The level of triglycerides in the blood, which can increase risk of coronary disease
   c. Hypertension, which leads to thickening and hardening of the arteries
   d. The level of *C-reactive proteins* in the blood, indicating inflammation

8. The "bad" type of cholesterol found in the bloodstream is known as
   a. high-density lipoprotein (HDL).
   b. low-density lipoprotein (LDL).
   c. total cholesterol.
   d. triglyceride.
9. Which of the following is *correct* about metabolic syndrome?
   a. It is decreasing among the general population both in the United States and globally.
   b. It lowers your risk of cardiovascular disease.
   c. It includes high fasting blood glucose, obesity, high triglyceride levels, hypertension, and other risks.
   d. It is a nonmodifiable risk factor for CVD.

LO 5 Diagnosing and Treating Cardiovascular Disease

10. The surgery in which a blood vessel is taken from another site in the patient's body and implanted to bypass the blocked artery and transport blood to the heart is called
    a. atherosclerosis surgery.
    b. thrombolysis.
    c. coronary bypass surgery.
    d. angioplasty.

Answers to the Pop Quiz can be found on page A-1. If you answered a question incorrectly, review the section identified by the Learning Outcome. For even more study tools, visit MasteringHealth.

THINK ABOUT IT!

LO 1 Understanding the Cardiovascular System

1. What can your resting heart rate tell you about your overall health? What are some reasons a person's resting heart rate might be higher or lower than the median?

LO 2 Cardiovascular Disease: An Epidemiological Overview

2. Why do you think hypertension rates are rising among today's college students?

LO 3 Key Cardiovascular Diseases

3. List the different types of CVD. Compare and contrast their symptoms, risk factors, prevention, and treatment.

LO 4 Reducing Your Risks

4. Discuss the role that exercise, stress management, dietary changes, medical checkups, sodium reduction, and other factors can play in reducing risk for CVD. What role might infectious diseases play in CVD risk?
5. Discuss why age is an important factor in women's risk for CVD. Do men face the same age-related risks? Why or why not? What can be done to decrease women's risk in later life?

LO 5 Diagnosing and Treating Cardiovascular Disease

6. Describe some of the diagnostic, preventive, and treatment alternatives for CVD. If you had a heart attack today, which treatment would you prefer? Explain why.

ACCESS YOUR HEALTH ON THE INTERNET

Visit **MasteringHealth** for links to the websites and RSS feeds.

The following websites explore further topics and issues related to personal health.

American Heart Association. This is the home page of the leading private organization dedicated to heart health. This site provides information, statistics, and resources regarding cardiovascular care, including an opportunity to test your risk for CVD. **www.heart.org**

National Heart, Lung, and Blood Institute. This valuable resource provides information on all aspects of cardiovascular health and wellness. **www.nhlbi.nih.gov**

Global Cardiovascular Infobase. This site contains epidemiological data and statistics for cardiovascular diseases for countries throughout the world, with a focus on developing nations. **www.cvdinfobase.ca**

FOCUS ON Minimizing Your Risk for Diabetes

The behaviors you take up in college could lead you on a path toward diabetes. Do you know whether your lifestyle or family history put you at risk?

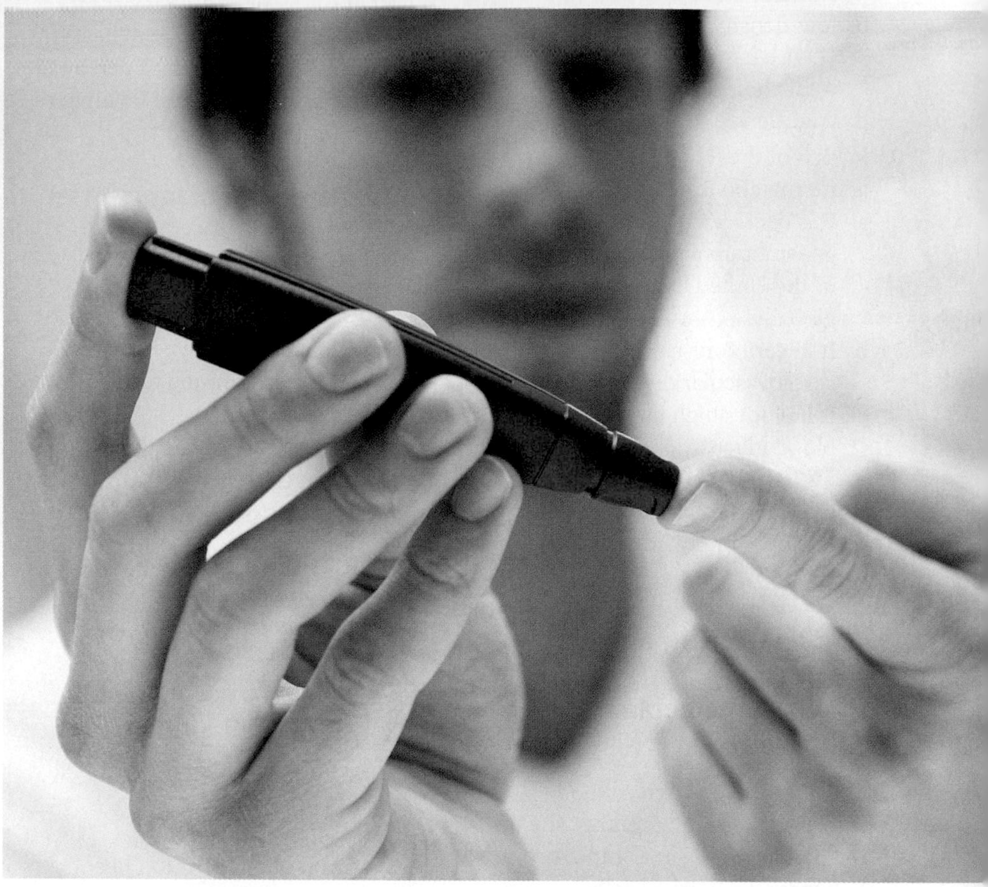

LEARNING OUTCOMES

1. Explain trends in diabetes in the United States and globally, describe the effect of diabetes on the body, and differentiate among types of diabetes and their risk factors.
2. Describe the main tests for, symptoms of, and complications associated with diabetes.
3. Explain how diabetes can be prevented and treated.

Nora is overweight. She used to figure it was no big deal; she'd go on a strict diet and exercise program as soon as she graduated and started to live "a normal life." But last week, her mom called with some bad news. She told Nora that she'd just been diagnosed with type 2 diabetes. Her voice sounded shaky as she reminded Nora about her own mother's death from kidney failure—a complication of diabetes—at age 52, a few months before Nora was born. Later, Nora searched online for information about her risk for diabetes. Her Hispanic ethnicity, family history, high stress level and lack of sleep, excessive weight, and sedentary lifestyle made her a prime candidate.

Nora made an appointment for a diabetes screening. She was instructed to fast the night before and was scheduled for an appointment first thing in the morning. At her visit, the nurse practitioner took a blood sample. A few days later, she called to tell Nora that her blood glucose was elevated, and although she wasn't diabetic yet, she needed to make changes to her diet and lifestyle to reduce her risk for developing type 2 diabetes like her mom.

Diabetes is one of the fastest growing health threats in the world today, with over 382 million people classified as diabetic in 2013 and cases expected to rise to 592 million by 2035.[1] While the number of people with diabetes has increased in virtually all countries of

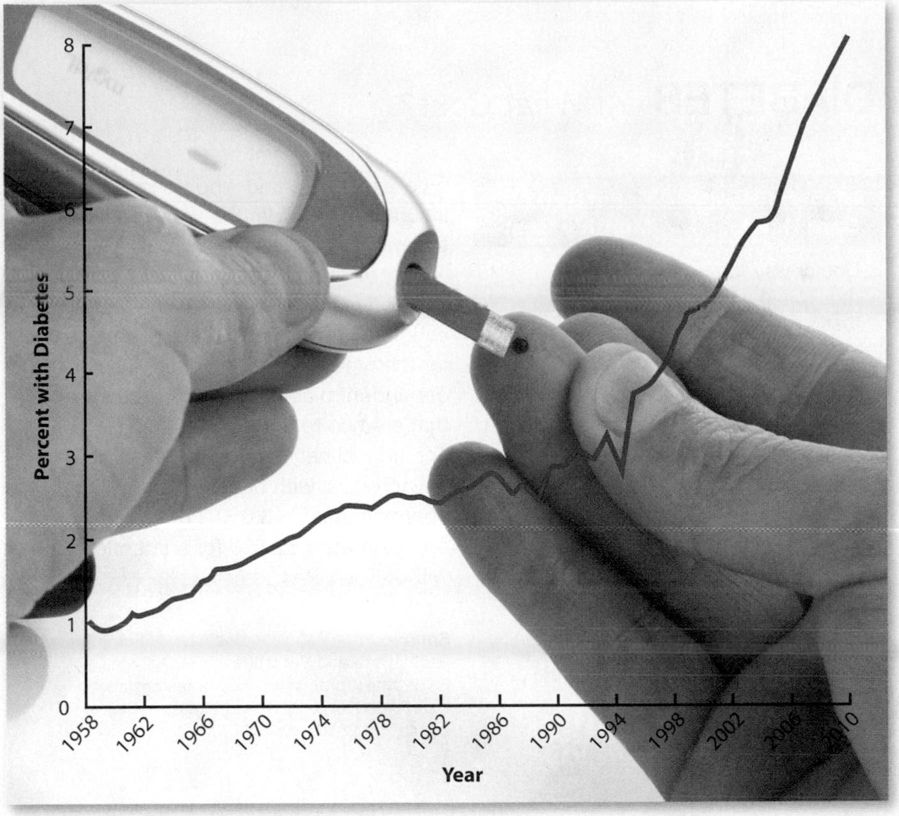

FIGURE 1 Percentage of U.S. Population with Diagnosed Diabetes, 1958–2010

Source: Data from Centers for Disease Control and Prevention, "Increasing Prevalence of Diagnosed Diabetes—United States and Puerto Rico, 1995–2010," 2012, www.cdc.gov.

the world, 80 percent of those with diabetes live in low- and middle-income countries where access to prevention and treatment may be lacking. Globally, the most people with diabetes are between 40 and 59 years of age.[2]

The United States isn't immune to epidemic rates of diabetes. Over the past two decades, diabetes rates have increased dramatically.[3] The Centers for Disease Control and Prevention (CDC) estimates that over 29.1 million people—almost 10 percent of the U.S. population—have diabetes.[4] Experts predict more than 1 in 3 Americans will have diabetes by 2050. Diabetes kills more Americans each year than breast cancer and AIDS, and millions suffer the physical and emotional burdens of dealing with this difficult disease[5] (see **FIGURE 1**).

Diabetes rates climb with age. While they aren't as high for college-age adults, overall rates have increased, even among the youngest populations. Among persons aged 20–44 years, approximately 4.1 percent have diabetes, compared to roughly 16.2 percent of those aged 45–64 and over 25.9 percent of those aged 65–74.[6] Diabetes is the primary cause of death each year for over 69,000.[7] All told, diabetes is listed as an underlying cause of death for over 234,000 Americans, ravaging the immune system, contributing to cardiovascular disease (CVD) and kidney, respiratory, liver, and a host of other problems.[8] Additionally, the costs of diagnosing and treating diabetes are staggering. The younger a person is when he/she develops the disease, the greater the long-term costs.

For an explanation of the financial toll that goes along with the damage to the body with diabetes, read the **Money & Health** box on the next page.

1 IN 3

THE NUMBER OF PEOPLE IN THE U.S. WHO WILL HAVE **DIABETES** BY 2050 BASED ON CURRENT TRENDS.

diabetes mellitus A group of diseases characterized by elevated blood glucose levels.

LO 1 | WHAT IS DIABETES?

Explain trends in diabetes in the United States and globally, describe the effect of diabetes on the body, and differentiate among types of diabetes and their risk factors.

Diabetes mellitus is actually a group of diseases, each with its own mechanism, but all are characterized by a persistently high level of glucose, a type of sugar, in the blood. One sign of diabetes is the production of an unusually

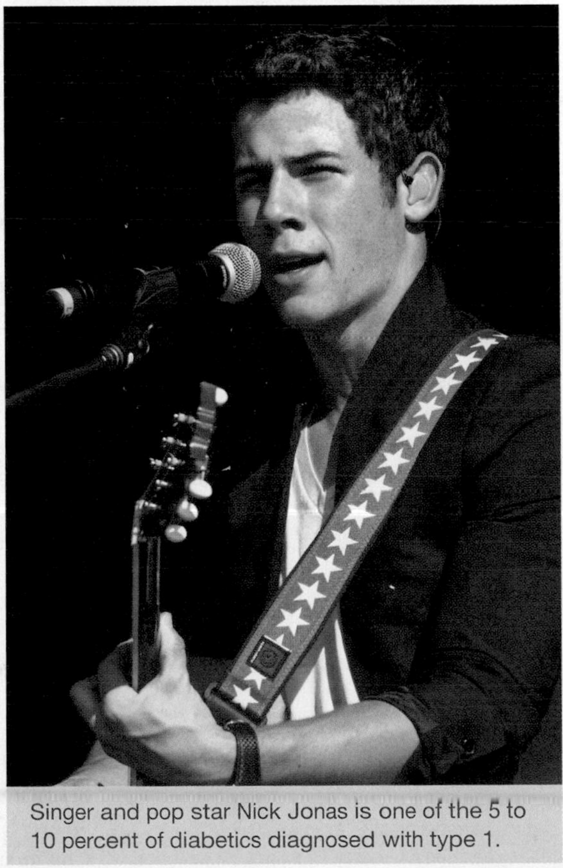

Singer and pop star Nick Jonas is one of the 5 to 10 percent of diabetics diagnosed with type 1.

MONEY & HEALTH

DIABETES *At What Cost?*

One in every 5 health care dollars is spent on diabetes care today. Fees for doctor visits, testing supplies, laboratory results, and other necessities are often only partially covered, even for those with insurance. If you are underinsured or uninsured, the *diabetes drain* on your bank account could be major. Diabetes is estimated to cost over $245 billion annually in direct and indirect costs. Those diagnosed with diabetes have health care costs that are nearly 2.5 times higher than those without diabetes in comparable age groups. The more years a person has diabetes, the greater the economic burden on the health care system and on society as a whole.

To give you an idea of what it might cost someone who is diagnosed with type 2 diabetes and who doesn't have insurance, consider the very conservative monthly estimates listed to the left.

Diabetic Health Care Need	Estimated Monthly Cost
Doctor visit for monitoring and testing	$200
Lab tests: A1C glucose tolerance	$35–$75
Glucose meter test strips	$100
Lancets and lancing devices, alcohol wipes	$5–$10
Oral medications (metformin)	$13–$15 (less for some generics, more for newer medications)

These numbers are consistent with American Diabetes Association estimates of $350–$900 per month for the typical type 2 diabetic. Insulin-dependent diabetics may have costs that are two to three times higher. The annual health care costs for an individual with diabetes are approximately $13,000, compared to approximately $2,600 for someone without diabetes.

Source: American Diabetes Association. "Fast Facts: Data and Statistics about Diabetes," 2013, http://professional.diabetes.org/admin/UserFiles/0%20-%20Sean/FastFacts%20March%202013.pdf.

high volume of glucose-laden urine, a fact reflected in its name: *Diabetes* derives from a Greek word meaning "to flow through," and *mellitus* is the Latin word for "sweet." The high blood glucose levels—or **hyperglycemia**—seen in diabetes can lead to many serious health problems and even premature death.

Before we describe what causes the different types of diabetes, let's look at how the body regulates blood glucose in a healthy person. The digestive system breaks down the carbohydrates we eat into glucose, which it releases into the bloodstream for use by all body cells. Glucose is one of our main sources of energy. Our red blood cells can only use glucose to fuel functioning, and brain and other nerve cells prefer glucose over other fuels. When glucose levels drop below normal, you may feel unable to concentrate, and certain mental functions may be impaired. When there is more glucose available than required to meet your body's immediate needs, the excess is stored as glycogen in the liver and muscles for later use. The average adult has about 5 to 6 grams of glucose in the blood at any given time, enough to provide energy for about 15 minutes under normal activity levels. Once that circulating glucose is used, the body begins to draw upon its glycogen reserves.

Glucose can't simply cross cell membranes on its own. Instead, cells have structures that transport glucose across in response to a signal that is generated by the **pancreas**, an organ located just beneath the stomach. Whenever a surge of glucose enters the bloodstream, the pancreas secretes a hormone called **insulin**. Insulin stimulates cells to take up glucose from the bloodstream and carry it into the cell, where it's used for immediate energy. Conversion of glucose to glycogen for storage in the liver and muscles is also assisted by insulin. These actions lower the blood level of glucose, and in response, the pancreas stops secreting insulin—until the next influx of glucose arrives.

hyperglycemia Elevated blood glucose level.

pancreas Organ that secretes digestive enzymes into the small intestine and hormones, including insulin, into the bloodstream.

insulin Hormone secreted by the pancreas and required by body cells for the uptake and storage of glucose.

type 1 diabetes Form of diabetes mellitus in which the pancreas is not able to make insulin, and therefore blood glucose cannot enter the cells to be used for energy.

Type 1 Diabetes Is an Immune Disorder

The more serious and less prevalent form of diabetes, called **type 1 diabetes** (or insulin-dependent diabetes), is an autoimmune disease in which the individual's immune system attacks and destroys the insulin-making cells in the pancreas. Destruction of these cells causes a dramatic reduction, or total cessation, of insulin production. Without insulin, cells cannot take up glucose, and blood glucose levels become permanently elevated. Too much glucose in the bloodstream can wreak havoc with tissues and organs in the body, damaging the kidneys and the nerves in the hands and feet and causing a wide range of other serious health consequences. The higher and longer sustained the blood glucose level, the greater the risk.

This form of diabetes used to be called *juvenile diabetes* because it most often appears during childhood or adolescence; however, it can begin at any age. Only about 5 percent of diabetic cases are type 1.[9] European ancestry, a genetic predisposition, and certain viral infections all increase the risk.[10]

People with type 1 diabetes require daily insulin injections or infusions and must carefully monitor their diet and exercise levels. Often they face unique challenges as the "lesser known" diabetic type, with fewer funds available for research and fewer options for treatment.

Type 2 Diabetes Is a Metabolic Disorder

Type 2 diabetes (non-insulin-dependent diabetes) accounts for 90 to 95 percent of all cases.[11] In type 2, either the pancreas does not make sufficient insulin, or body cells are resistant to its effects and don't use it efficiently (**FIGURE 2**). This latter condition is generally referred to as **insulin resistance.**

Development of the Disease

Unlike type 1 diabetes, which can appear suddenly, type 2 usually develops slowly. In early stages, cells throughout the body begin to resist the effects of insulin. An overabundance of free fatty acids concentrated in a person's fat cells (as may be the case in an obese individual) inhibit glucose uptake by body cells and suppress the liver's sensitivity to insulin. As a result, the liver's ability to self-regulate its conversion of glucose into glycogen begins to fail, and blood levels of glucose gradually rise. The pancreas attempts to compensate by producing more insulin, but it cannot maintain its hyperproduction of insulin indefinitely. As the progression to type 2 diabetes continues, more and more pancreatic insulin-producing cells sustain physical damage and become nonfunctional. Insulin output declines, and blood glucose levels rise high enough to warrant a diagnosis of type 2 diabetes.

Nonmodifiable Risk Factors

Type 2 diabetes is associated with a cluster of nonmodifiable risk factors, that is, factors over which you have no control. These include increased age, certain ethnicities, genetic factors, and biological factors.

One in 4 adults over age 65 has type 2 diabetes.[12] In fact, it used to be referred to as *adult-onset diabetes*, but it is now being diagnosed at younger ages, even among children and teens.

type 2 diabetes Form of diabetes mellitus in which the pancreas does not make enough insulin or the body is unable to use insulin correctly.

insulin resistance State in which body cells fail to respond to the effects of insulin; obesity increases the risk that cells will become insulin resistant.

WHAT DO YOU THINK?

Why do you think type 2 diabetes is increasing in the United States?

- Why is it increasing among young people?
- Do you think young people are generally aware of what diabetes is and their own susceptibility for it?

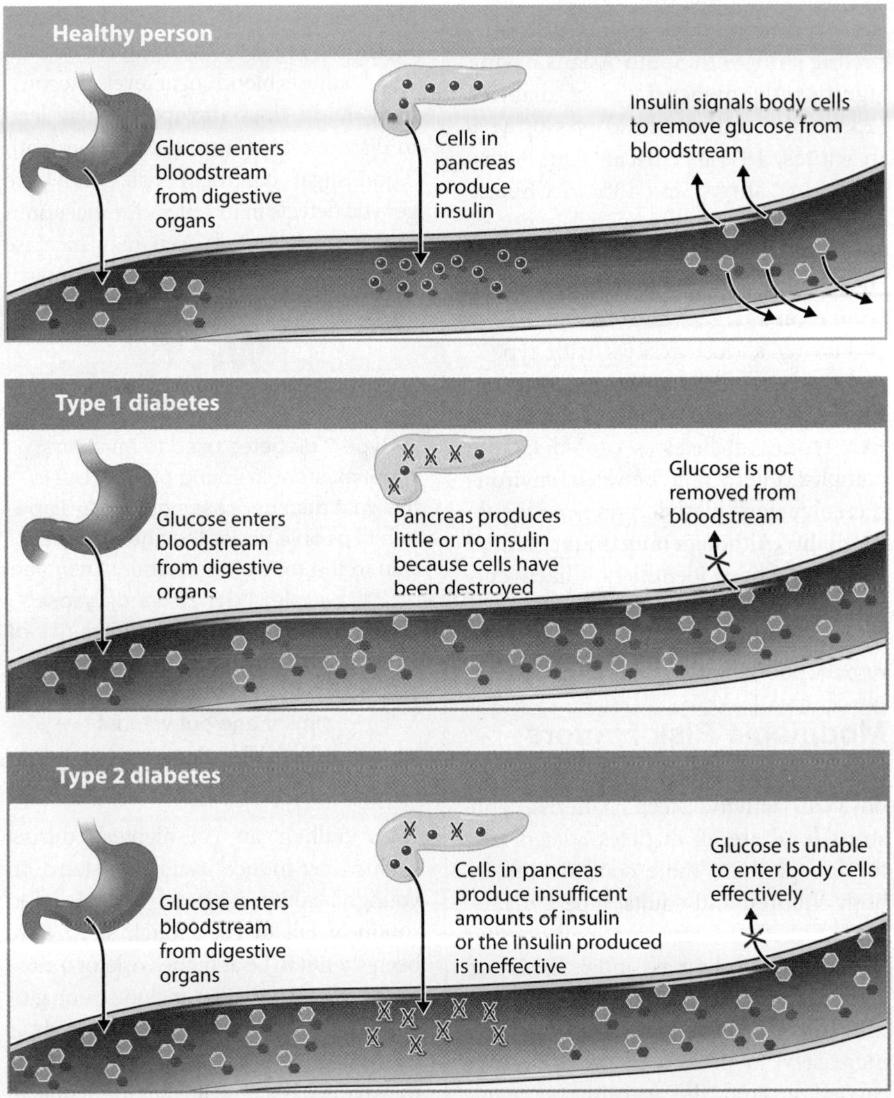

FIGURE 2 Diabetes: What It Is and How It Develops In a healthy person, a sufficient amount of insulin is produced and released by the pancreas and used efficiently by the cells. In type 1 diabetes, the pancreas makes little or no insulin. In type 2 diabetes, either the pancreas does not make sufficient insulin, or cells are resistant to insulin and are not able to use it efficiently.

VIDEO TUTOR How Diabetes Develops

SEE IT! VIDEOS

Are diabetes patients getting even younger? Watch **Young Adults and Diabetes** available on MasteringHealth.™

According to the most recent data, type 2 diabetes rates are soaring among U.S. teens—up from 9 percent in 2000 to 23 percent 2009.[13] Rates of youth diabetes have historically increased with age, with females having higher rates than males.[14] Non-Hispanic whites, Native Americans, and black youth have the highest rates while Asian/Pacific Islanders have the lowest rates.[15] However, recent research points to a surprising shift, with South Asians having significantly higher rates of diabetes (23%) than other ethnic groups (6% in whites, 18% in African Americans, 12.7% in Latinos, and 13% in Chinese Americans).[16] More research is necessary to determine if this is an isolated study group, or if the results will be similar on a larger scale.

Having a close relative with type 2 diabetes is another significant risk factor. In fact, most experts support the theory that type 2 diabetes is caused by the complex interaction between environmental factors, lifestyle, and genetic susceptibility. Although numerous potential genes have been identified as likely culprits in increased risk, the mechanisms by which inherited diabetes develops remain poorly understood.[17]

Modifiable Risk Factors

Body weight, dietary choices, level of physical activity, sleep patterns, and stress level are all diabetes-related factors people have more control over. In both children and adults, type 2 diabetes is linked to overweight and obesity. In adults, a body mass index (BMI) of 25 or greater increases the risk, with significantly higher risks for each 5 kg/m^2 increase.[18] In particular, excess weight carried around the waistline—a condition called *central adiposity*—and measured by waist circumference is a significant risk factor for older women.[19] People with type 2 diabetes who lose weight and increase their physical activity can significantly improve their blood glucose levels.

Inadequate sleep may contribute to the development of both obesity and type 2 diabetes, possibly due to the fact that sleep-deprived people tend to engage in less physical activity.[20] There also seems to be a link between the body clock hormone *melatonin* and type 2 diabetes. Melatonin regulates the release of insulin, which adjusts blood sugar levels. Accordingly, body clock disruptions may lead to disruptions in insulin and issues with blood sugar control. People who have genetic defects in receptors for melatonin and have disrupted sleep may increase their risk of type 2 diabetes by six times.[21]

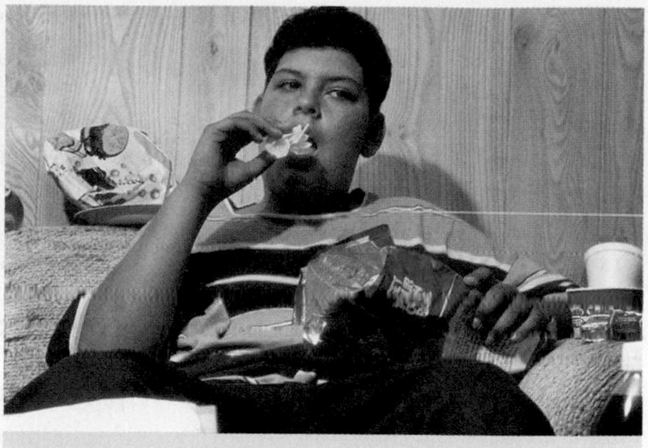

Unhealthy eating habits and a sedentary lifestyle can lead to type 2 diabetes, even among children.

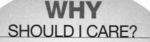

WHY SHOULD I CARE?

Type 2 diabetes used to be almost nonexistent in young people, but in the past decade, cases of type 2 diabetes in people under the age of 20 have risen to the tens of thousands. Each year, 3,700 people under 20 are diagnosed with type 2 diabetes. Overall, the risk of death among people with diabetes is about twice that of people of similar age but without diabetes.

Even pulling an "all-nighter" during exams may induce insulin resistance in young, healthy subjects.[22] People who routinely fail to get enough sleep have been shown to be at higher risk for a cluster of risk factors that include poor glucose metabolism.[23] A large meta-analysis has shown that melatonin supplements may reduce the time it takes for people to get to sleep and improve overall quality of sleep and amount of actual sleep time.[24] If melatonin helps sleep, and lack of sleep increases risk of diabetes, it is possible that behaviors that increase sleep may also reduce type 2 diabetes risks.

Recent data from large epidemiological studies provide evidence of a link between diabetes and psychological or physical stress; however, a recent analysis of studies focused on the role of work-related stress on type 2 diabetes development has shown mixed results, with sleep being more important than stress. Shift workers, in particular, appear to have a greater risk of diabetes, even when BMI and other risks are considered.[25]

A recent study of young adults with impaired fasting glucose experiencing significant financial stressors showed that physical activity played a key role in reducing stress and blood sugar levels.[26] Research on the effect of chronic stress and lack of sleep on insulin production and diabetes development is in its infancy. The best rule of thumb appears to be to manage stress, exercise, and sleep more if you want to reduce your risks.[27]

Prediabetes Can Lead to Type 2 Diabetes

An estimated 86 million Americans age 20 or older—37 percent of the population over 20, and 51 percent of those over 65—have an ominous set of symptoms known as **prediabetes**, a condition in which blood glucose levels are higher than normal, but not high enough to be classified as diabetes.[28] Having a fasting blood glucose level between 100 and 125 mg/dL is the typical guideline for diagnosing

prediabetes Condition in which blood glucose levels are higher than normal, but not high enough to be classified as diabetes.

prediabetes. Current rates of prediabetes in college students are unknown; however, based on increased rates of obesity and the fact that 37 percent of people 20 and older are already prediabetic, college students are likely not immune.[29]

Although prediabetes doesn't cause overt symptoms, the condition is like a ticking time bomb: If it's not "defused," diabetes eventually strikes. On the upside, a diagnosis of prediabetes represents a tremendous opportunity to take actions that could prevent diabetes or at least delay its onset.

Often, prediabetes is one of the risk factors linked to overweight and obesity that together constitute a dangerous health risk known as **metabolic syndrome**. You would be labeled as having metabolic syndrome if you have three of the following factors:

- Abdominal obesity
- Triglyceride level of 150 milligrams per deciliter (mg/dL) of blood or greater
- HDL cholesterol of less than 40 mg/ dL in men or less than 50 mg/ dL in women
- Systolic blood pressure (top number) of 130 millimeters of mercury (mm Hg) or greater
- Diastolic blood pressure (bottom number) of 85 mm Hg or greater
- Fasting glucose of 100 mg/dL or greater
- Insulin resistance or glucose intolerance (the body can't properly use insulin or blood sugar)

Of the seven conditions, prediabetes and central adiposity appear to be the dominant factors for metabolic syndrome.[30] A person who has metabolic syndrome is five times more likely to develop type 2 diabetes than is a person without it.[31] Overall, Mexican Americans have the highest rates of metabolic syndrome, with white Americans and African Americans not far behind.[32] Women who have uterine fibroids or ovarian cysts also are at increased risk.[33]

If you have already been diagnosed with prediabetes or type 2 diabetes, you can follow the tips in the **Skills for Behavior Change** box to halt or slow the progression of your condition. Even if you've never had your blood glucose tested, these steps could reduce your risk.

SKILLS FOR BEHAVIOR CHANGE

Key Steps to Begin Reducing Your Risk for Diabetes

- Maintain a healthy weight, and lose weight if you need to.
- Eat smaller portions and choose foods with less fat, salt, and added sugars. Keep calories equal to energy expended. Eat more fruits, vegetables, and complex carbohydrates, and make sure you consume lean protein.
- Get your body moving. At least 30 minutes of moderate activity 5 days a week is a minimum recommendation.
- Quit smoking. In addition to cancer and heart disease, smoking increases blood glucose levels.
- Reduce or eliminate alcohol consumption. It's high in calories and can interfere with blood glucose regulation.
- Get enough sleep. Inadequate sleep may contribute to the development of type 2 diabetes.
- Inoculate yourself against stress. Learn to take yourself less seriously, find time for fun, develop a strong support network, and use relaxation skills.
- If you have a family history, or several risk factors, get regular checkups.
- Check out this website and get involved in this program: www.cdc.gov/diabetes/prevention/recognition/curriculum.htm

Sources: Centers for Disease Control and Prevention, "National Diabetes Prevention Program," 2014, www.cdc.gov/diabetes/prevention/recognition/curriculum.htm.

metabolic syndrome: Cluster of risks for CVD and diabetes; persons with more than three of these risks greatly increase their risks of CVD and type 2 diabetes.

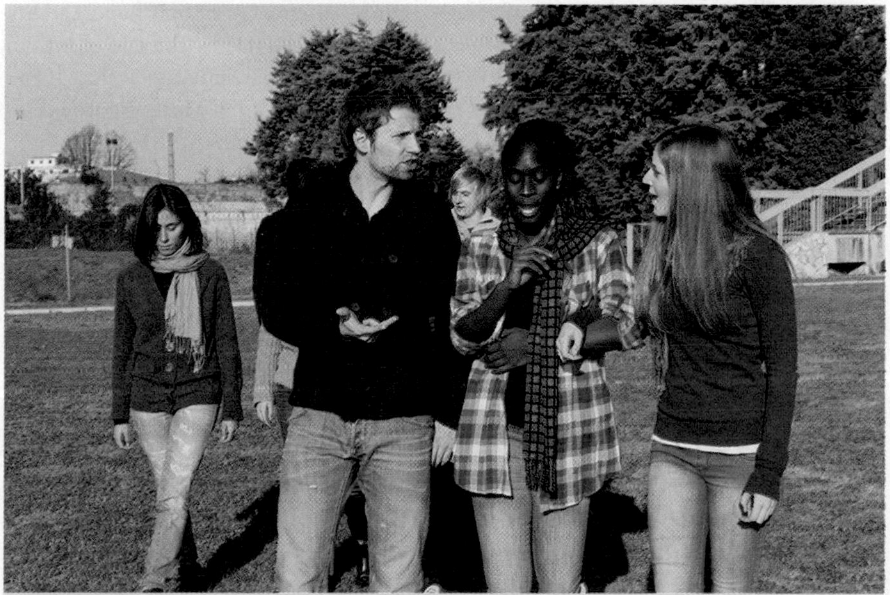

About 215,000 people younger than age 20 have type 1 or type 2 diabetes, with thousands more estimated to have prediabetes.

Source: American Diabetes Association. "Fast Facts: Data and Statistics about Diabetes," 2013, http://professional.diabetes.org/admin/UserFiles/0%20-%20Sean/FastFacts%20March%202013.pdf.

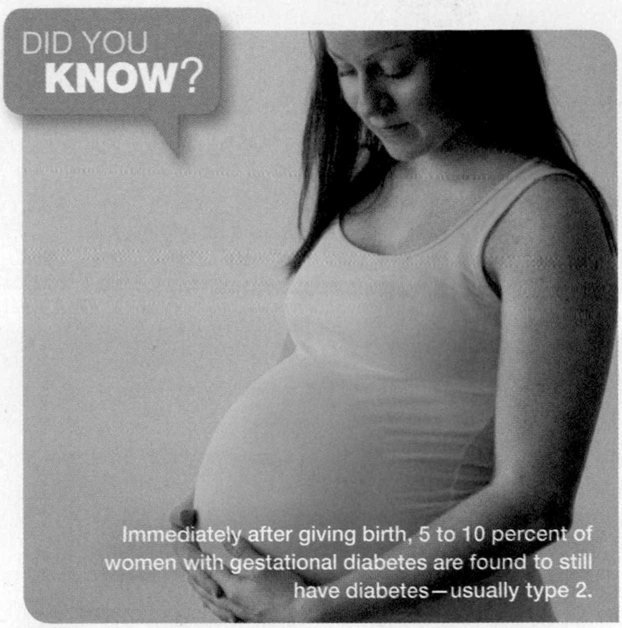

Immediately after giving birth, 5 to 10 percent of women with gestational diabetes are found to still have diabetes—usually type 2.

Source: Data from Centers for Disease Control and Prevention, "National Diabetes Statistics Report, 2014," June 2014, http://www.cdc.gov/diabeteS/pubs/statsreport14.htm; Centers for Disease Control and Prevention, "National Diabetes Fact Sheet: National Estimates and General Information on Diabetes and Pre-diabetes in the United States, 2011" (Atlanta, GA: U.S. Department of Health and Human Services, Centers for Disease Control and Prevention, 2011).

Gestational Diabetes

A third type of diabetes, **gestational diabetes**, is a state of high blood glucose level during pregnancy. It is thought to be associated with metabolic stresses that occur in response to changing hormonal levels. As many as 18 percent of pregnancies are affected by gestational diabetes, posing added risks for the mother and developing fetus.[34] Studies show that between 40 and 50 percent of gestational diabetics may develop type 2 diabetes within a decade of their initial diagnosis if they don't incorporate risk-reducing behaviors such as weight control, improved diet, and physical exercise.[35] If a woman enters pregnancy prediabetic and develops gestational diabetes, she has a 71 percent chance of developing type 2 diabetes if she doesn't make significant lifestyle changes.[36]

Women who are overweight and have high blood sugar or those with gestational diabetes have been shown to have increased risks of birth-related complications such as difficult labor, high blood pressure, high blood acidity, increased infections, and death. One of the adverse outcomes for these women is to give birth to large babies, a result of excess fat accumulation that is often a hallmark of gestational diabetes. The large size of these babies increases the risk of injury during normal delivery and often results in caesarean sections, which increase risks to both mother and infant. High blood sugar and excess weight in a pregnant woman can trigger higher insulin levels and blood sugar fluctuations in the newborn. In addition to increased risk of obesity and diabetes, babies born to women with gestational diabetes are also at risk for malformations of the heart, nervous system, and bones; respiratory distress; and fetal death.[37]

Results from a small, preliminary investigation raise the specter of a new threat. Children raised by mothers with gestational diabetes were shown to have twice the risk of developing attention deficit/hyperactivity disorder (ADHD) by the age of 6 than their peers, particularly among low-income families.[38] More rigorous research is necessary.

gestational diabetes Form of diabetes mellitus in which women who have never had diabetes have high blood sugar (glucose) levels during pregnancy.

LO 2 | WHAT ARE THE SYMPTOMS OF DIABETES?

Describe the main tests for, symptoms of, and complications associated with diabetes.

The symptoms of diabetes are similar for both type 1 and type 2. The following are among the most common:

- **Thirst.** Kidneys filter excessive glucose by diluting it with water. This can pull too much water from the body and result in dehydration.
- **Excessive urination.** For the same reason, increased need to urinate occurs.
- **Weight loss.** Because so many calories are lost in the glucose that passes into urine, a person with diabetes often feels hungry. Despite eating more, he or she typically loses weight.
- **Fatigue.** When glucose cannot enter cells, fatigue and weakness occur.
- **Nerve damage.** A high glucose concentration damages the smallest blood vessels of the body, including those supplying nerves in the hands and feet. This can cause numbness and tingling.
- **Blurred vision.** Too much glucose causes body tissues to dry out. This can be particularly damaging to the eyes.
- **Poor wound healing and increased infections.** High levels of glucose can affect the body's ability to ward off infections and may affect overall immune system functioning.

Complications of Diabetes

The main complications of poorly controlled diabetes include:[39]

- **Diabetic coma.** A coma from high blood acidity known as *diabetic ketoacidosis* can occur when, in the absence of glucose, body cells break down stored fat for energy. The process produces acidic molecules called *ketones*. Although essential to provide fuel to the brain in the absence of glucose, too many ketones can raise blood acid level dangerously high. The diabetic person slips into a coma and, without medical intervention, will die.
- **Cardiovascular disease.** More than 70 percent of diabetics have one or more forms of cardiovascular disease, including hypertension, increasing risk of heart attack and stroke significantly. Blood vessels become damaged as glucose-laden blood flows sluggishly and essential nutrients and other substances are not transported as effectively.
- **Kidney disease.** Diabetes is the leading cause of kidney failure. The kidneys become scarred by overwork and the high blood pressure in their vessels. More than 229,000 Americans are currently living with kidney failure caused by diabetes.

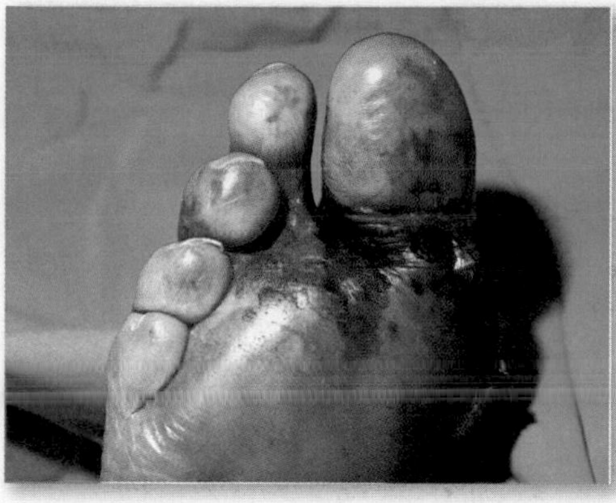

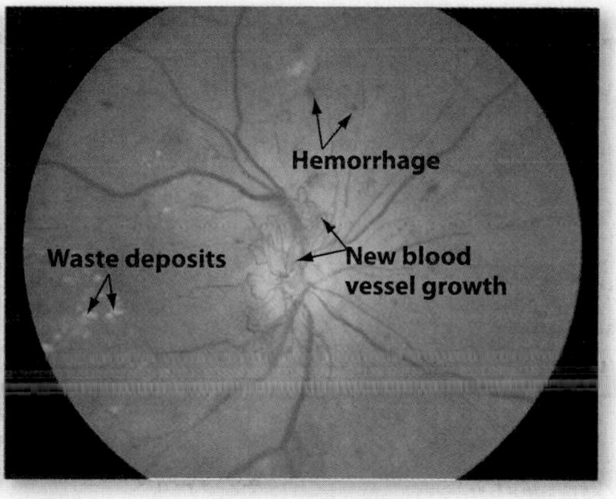

ⓐ Diabetics are prone to wounds that don't heal on the feet as nerves may be damaged, healing impaired and sensation diminished. Blisters, infections and other irritants can easily progress to more serious problems.

ⓑ Uncontrolled diabetes can damage the eye, causing swelling, leaking, and rupture of blood vessels; growth of new blood vessels; deposits of wastes; and scarring. All of these can progress to blindness.

FIGURE 3 Complications of Uncontrolled Diabetes: Amputation and Eye Disease

Many of these people are on dialysis or waiting for a kidney transplant that may never come.[40]

- **Amputations.** More than 73 percent of nontraumatic amputations of legs, feet, and toes are due to diabetes (see **FIGURE 3a**). In fact, each year nearly 66,000 nontraumatic lower-limb amputations are performed on people with diabetes (180/day).[41]
- **Eye disease and blindness.** Diabetes is the leading cause of new blindness in the United States. Nearly 7.7 million people over the age of 40 have early-stage retinopathy, which could lead to blindness without treatment (**FIGURE 3b**).[42]
- **Infectious diseases.** Persons with diabetes have increased risk of poor wound healing and greater susceptibility to infectious diseases, particularly influenza and pneumonia. Once infection occurs, it is more difficult to treat.
- **Other complications.** Diabetics may have gum and tooth disease, foot neuropathy, and chronic pain that makes walking, driving, and simple tasks more difficult. A recent study of persons with diabetes showed that *periodontitis*—an inflammation of the gums that can lead to decay, tooth loss and a variety of other health risks—was present to varying degrees in the majority of all diabetics. In addition, persons with diabetes are more likely to suffer from depression, making intervention and treatment more difficult. Those who are depressed are 60 percent more likely to develop type 2 diabetes.

Blood Tests Diagnose and Monitor Diabetes

Diabetes and prediabetes are diagnosed when a blood test reveals elevated blood glucose levels. Generally, a physician orders one of the following blood tests:

- The *fasting plasma glucose (FPG) test* requires the patient to fast for 8 to 10 hours prior to the test. Then, a small sample of blood is tested for glucose concentration. As you can see in **FIGURE 4**, an FPG level greater than or equal to 100 mg/dL indicates prediabetes, and a level greater than or equal to 126 mg/dL indicates diabetes.
- The *oral glucose tolerance test (OGTT)* requires the patient to drink concentrated glucose. A sample of blood is drawn for testing 2 hours after the patient drinks the solution. A reading greater than or equal to 140 mg/dL indicates prediabetes, whereas a reading greater than or equal to 200 mg/dL indicates diabetes.
- A third test, *A1C* or *glycosylated hemoglobin test (HbA1C)*, gives the average value of a patient's blood glucose over the past 2 to 3 months,

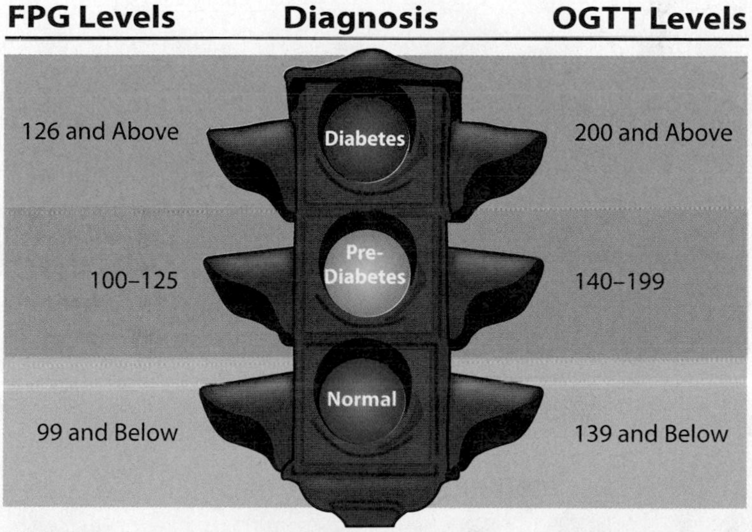

FIGURE 4 Blood Glucose Levels in Prediabetes and Untreated Diabetes The fasting plasma glucose (FPG) test measures levels of blood glucose after a person fasts overnight. The oral glucose tolerance test (OGTT) measures levels of blood glucose after a person consumes a concentrated amount of glucose.

Source: Data for FPG and OGTT levels taken from Table 1 (FPG Test) and Table 2 (OGTT) of "Diagnosis of Diabetes," National Diabetes Information Clearinghouse (NDIC), a service of the National Institute of Diabetes and Digestive and Kidney Diseases (NIDDK), National Institutes of Health (NIH), http://diabetes.niddk.nih.gov/dm/pubs/diagnosis.

instead of at one moment in time. It doesn't require fasting, which makes it more convenient for most. In general, an A1C of 5.7 to 6.4 means that you are at high risk for diabetes or are prediabetic. If your A1C is 6.5 or higher, diabetes may be diagnosed.[43] **Estimated average glucose (eAG)** shows how A1C numbers correspond to the blood glucose numbers people are used to seeing. For example, someone with an A1C value of 6.1 would be able to look at a chart and see that his or her average blood glucose was around 128—a high level that should encourage healthy lifestyle modifications.

People with diabetes also need to check their blood glucose level several times throughout each day to make sure they stay within their target range. To check blood glucose, diabetics must prick their finger to obtain a drop of blood. A handheld glucose meter is then used to evaluate the blood sample.

estimated average glucose (eAG) A method for reporting A1C test results that gives the average blood glucose levels for the testing period using the same units (milligrams per deciliter, or mg/dL) that patients are used to seeing in self-administered glucose tests.

LO 3 | TREATING DIABETES

Explain how diabetes can be prevented and treated.

Treatment options for people with prediabetes and type 1 and type 2 diabetes vary according to type and how far the disease has progressed. In addition to pharmaceutical options, several lifestyle changes can help reduce the risks of diabetes complications.

Lifestyle Changes

For people with prediabetes, it's important to initiate lifestyle changes to prevent progression of the condition. Studies have shown that lifestyle changes can prevent or delay the development of type 2 diabetes by up to 58 percent.[44] Even for people with type 2 diabetes, lifestyle changes can sometimes prevent or delay the need for medication or insulin injections. Weight loss, exercise, and a high-quality diet are all parts of the lifestyle formula.

Weight Loss

The key to preventing type 2 diabetes in people with prediabetes is weight loss. Results of a landmark clinical trial, the *Diabetes Prevention Program (DPP)*, show that a loss of as little as 5 to 7 percent of current body weight and regular physical activity significantly lowered the risk of progressing to diabetes.[45]

5%–7%

OF BODY WEIGHT LOSS. THE AMOUNT NEEDED TO CAUSE SIGNIFICANT REDUCTIONS IN **BLOOD GLUCOSE LEVELS** AND HELP PREVENT DIABETES.

Adopting a Healthy Diet

The DPP recommends losing weight by adopting a low-fat, reduced-calorie eating plan. In addition, diabetes researchers have studied a variety of specific foods for their effect on blood glucose levels. Here is a brief summary of some intriguing findings:

- **Whole grains.** A recent review of studies over many years suggests that a diet high in whole grains reduces a person's risk of developing type 2 diabetes.[46]
- **High-fiber foods.** The American Diabetes Association (ADA) indicates that evidence is inconclusive that cutting refined carbohydrates alone may reduce your risk of type 2 diabetes. However, recent research seems to indicate that eating high fiber foods may reduce diabetes risk.[47] Eating low-carbohydrate diets appear to reduce overall CVD risks and may have a significant effect on preventing and controlling type 2 diabetes.
- **Fatty fish.** An impressive body of evidence has linked the consumption of fish high in omega-3 fatty acids with decreased progression of insulin resistance.[48] Newer research has called omega-3's beneficial effects into question (see **Chapter 15**). More research is necessary to determine whether omega 3 and omega 6 fatty acids play a role in diabetes risk reduction.[49]

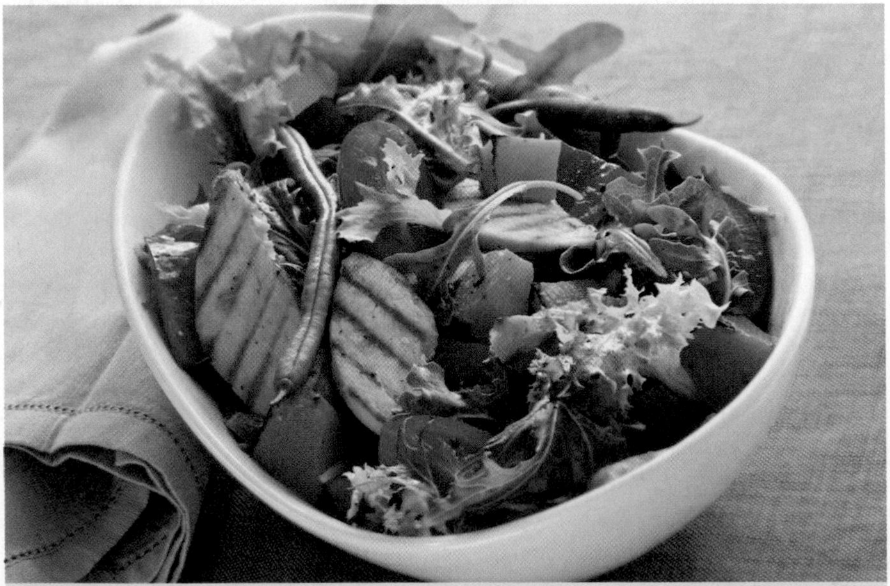

People with diabetes can occasionally indulge in sweets in moderation, particularly if they balance carbohydrates with protein. However, meals low in saturated and *trans* fats and high in fiber, like this salad of salmon and fresh vegetables, are recommended for helping to control blood glucose and body weight.

It is also important for people with diabetes to prevent surges in blood sugar after they eat. The **glycemic index** (GI) compares foods with the same amount of carbohydrates and determines how quickly and how much each raises blood glucose levels. Foods low on the GI have far less effect on blood glucose than do those that are high on the GI. **Glycemic load** is a measure of how much of a given carbohydrate (in grams) is in a serving of food. The concept of glycemic load was developed by scientists to simultaneously describe the quality (glycemic index) and quantity of carbohydrate in a meal.[50] By learning to combine high- and low-glycemic index foods to avoid surges in blood glucose, diabetics can help control their average blood glucose levels throughout the day. Eating smaller amounts, several times a day, from low GI sources is an important part of glucose control.

Increasing Physical Fitness

The DPP and other organizations recommend at least 30 minutes of physical activity 5 days a week to reduce your risk of type 2 diabetes.[51] Exercise increases sensitivity to insulin. The more muscle mass you have and the more you use your muscles, the more efficiently cells use glucose for fuel, meaning there will be less glucose circulating in the bloodstream. For most people, activity of moderate intensity can help keep blood glucose levels under control.

Oral Medications and Weight Loss Surgery

When lifestyle changes fail to control type 2 diabetes, oral medications may be prescribed. With new medications being developed constantly, diabetics have an increasing number of choices. Some medications reduce glucose production by the liver, whereas others slow the absorption of carbohydrates from the small intestine. Other medications increase insulin production by the pancreas, whereas still others work to increase the insulin sensitivity of cells.

The newest class of diabetes drugs are known as SGLT2 inhibitors. These drugs cause the kidneys to actually excrete more glucose, which lowers the levels of glucose circulating in the body. All diabetic drugs have side effects and contraindications; however, each person must balance risks of medications with risks of elevated blood glucose.

Some people use their diabetes meds as a form of crutch without altering lifestyle, thinking that the drugs are taking care of the problem. With time, meds become less effective and options for treatment become increasingly scarce. It is best to follow ADA recommendations on diet, exercise, and lifestyle in general.

When lifestyle changes prove challenging and risks are high and increasing, surgery is another option. People who undergo gastric/bariatric surgery for weight loss have shown remarkable reductions in blood glucose and diabetes symptoms for 2 to 3 years after surgery.[52] Those who combined gastric bypass or sleeve gastrectomy (a surgery where about 80 percent of the stomach is removed, leaving a small sleeve of stomach tissue connected to the intestines) with intensive medical therapy had similar outcomes.[53] In many cases, former diabetics can stop taking medications for some of their CVD risks, and stop diabetes symptoms altogether. Many professional groups are pushing for wider use of these more drastic weight loss methods.[54] Gastric bypass surgeries are not without risks, however, and can include death and serious complications. (See **Chapter 8** for more on gastric bypass surgeries.)

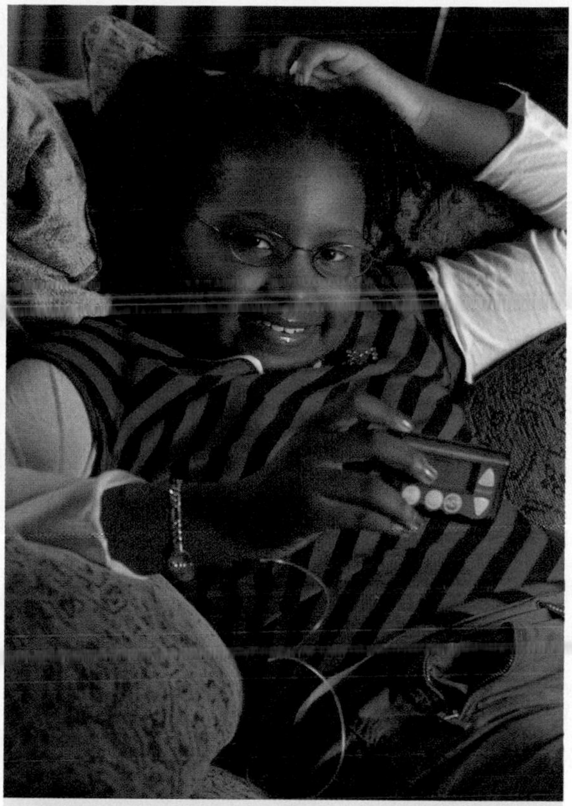

Some type 2 diabetics can control their condition with changes in diet and lifestyle habits or with oral medications. However, some type 2 diabetics and all type 1 diabetics require insulin injections or infusions.

Insulin Injections May Be Necessary

Since the pancreas can no longer produce adequate amounts of insulin with type 1 diabetes, insulin injections are absolutely essential for daily functioning. In addition, people with type 2 diabetes whose blood glucose levels cannot be adequately controlled with other treatment options require insulin injections. Since insulin is a protein and would be digested in the gastrointestinal tract in pill form, it must be injected into the fat layer under the skin, from which it is absorbed into the bloodstream.

People with diabetes used to need two or more insulin injections each day. Now, many diabetics use an *insulin infusion pump*. The external portion is only about the size of an MP3 player and can easily be hidden by clothes. It delivers insulin in minute amounts throughout the day through a thin

glycemic index (GI) Compares foods with the same amount of carbohydrates and determines how much each raises blood glucose levels.

glycemic load (GL) A means of assessing the likely rise in blood glucose based on dietary quality and quantity of food. Determined by consumption of carbohydrates in grams times glycemic index divided by 100.

tube and catheter inserted under the patient's skin. This infusion is less painful and more effective than delivering a few larger doses of insulin. To overcome the limitations of current insulin therapy, researchers are currently working to link glucose monitoring and insulin delivery by developing an artificial pancreas. An artificial pancreas would be a system that would mimic, as closely as possible, the way a healthy pancreas detects changes in blood glucose levels and responds automatically to secrete appropriate amounts of insulin. Although the first prototype devices received FDA approval, they cannot yet do the job of a fully functional pancreas. However, they have great potential to help those with insulin-dependent diabetes better control the highs and lows of blood glucose.[55]

ASSESS **YOURSELF**

Could you have diabetes? Want to find out what behaviors and symptoms to look out for? Take the **Are You at Risk for Diabetes?** assessment available on MasteringHealth.™

Need help creating a plan? Follow the strategies in the **Your Plan for Change** box for short- and long-term improvements to your health.

YOUR PLAN FOR **CHANGE**

If the results of the **ASSESS YOURSELF** activity, "Are You at Risk for Diabetes?," indicate you need to take further steps to decrease your risks, then follow this plan.

TODAY, YOU CAN:

- ☐ Talk to your parents and ask them if there is a history of prediabetes or diabetes mellitus in your family. If there is, find out who had it, when they developed it, and what type they had.
- ☐ Take stock of other risk factors you may have for diabetes—do you exercise regularly and watch your weight? Do you eat healthfully? Have you ever had your blood glucose measured? Make a list of small steps you can take right now to address any of your potential risk factors.

WITHIN THE NEXT 2 WEEKS, YOU CAN:

- ☐ Make an appointment with your health care provider to have your blood glucose levels tested.
- ☐ If you smoke, begin devising a plan to quit. **Chapter 11** can give you some ideas.

BY THE END OF THE SEMESTER, YOU CAN:

- ☐ Pay attention to what you eat; increase your intake of whole grains, fruits, and vegetables; and decrease your consumption of saturated fats, *trans* fats, and sugar.
- ☐ Make physical activity and exercise part of your daily routine, aiming for at least 30 minutes 5 days a week.

16 Reducing Your Cancer Risk

LEARNING OUTCOMES

1 Describe the impact of cancer on people in the United States and compare it to other major health problems in terms of morbidity/mortality, costs, and overall effectiveness of prevention and control.

2 Describe cancer and how it develops, as well as key risk factors.

3 Explain the suspected causes of cancer, and describe your own risks based on genetics and your lifestyle.

4 Describe the different types of cancer and the risks they pose to people at different ages and stages of life, as well as key actions to prevent cancer development.

5 Discuss cancer diagnosis and treatment, including radiotherapy and chemotherapy and other common methods of detection and treatment, indicating where we've made progress in recent decades.

6 Discuss what it really means to be a "cancer survivor" and how it means more than living cancer free for 5 years after diagnosis.

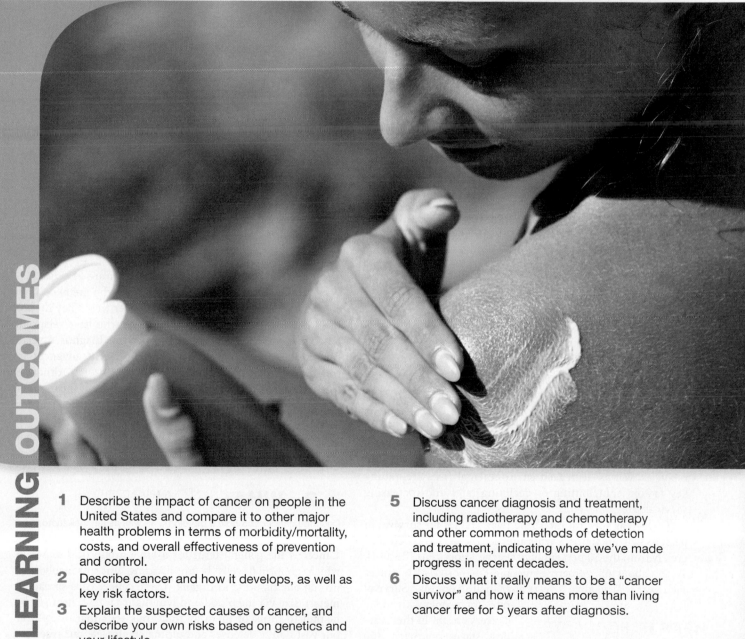

As recently as 50 years ago, a cancer diagnosis was typically a death sentence. Health professionals could only guess at the cause, and treatments were often as deadly as the disease itself. Because we didn't understand the disease process, fears about "catching cancer" from those who had it led to ostracism and bigotry. Fortunately, we've come a long way in our understanding of cancer, our willingness to talk about the disease openly, and our ability to treat it.

Knowledge of risks and symptoms, early detection, and significant developments in technology and treatment have dramatically improved the prognosis for most cancer patients, particularly those diagnosed in early stages. There are also many actions we can take individually and as a society to prevent cancer. Understanding the facts about cancer, recognizing your own risk, and taking action to reduce your risk are important steps in the battle.

LO 1 | AN OVERVIEW OF CANCER

Describe the impact of cancer on people in the United States and compare it to other major health problems in terms of morbidity/mortality, costs, and overall effectiveness of prevention and control.

Cancer is the second most common cause of death in the United States, exceeded only by heart disease.[1] Although there were nearly 1.7 million *new* cancer diagnoses and over 585,000 deaths in 2014, the good news is that cancer death rates have been declining by over 2 percent per year in the last decades. Increased emphasis on education and awareness, greater emphasis on prevention and early intervention, advancements in diagnosis and treatment, and policies and programs designed to decrease disparities in early access and treatment, as well as decreased environmental risks are among key factors contributing to declining rates and increasing survival rates.[2]

5-year survival rates The percentage of people in a study or treatment group who are alive 5 years after they were diagnosed with or treated for a disease, such as cancer.

cancer A large group of diseases characterized by the uncontrolled growth and spread of abnormal cells.

metastasize Process by which cancer spreads from one area to different areas of the body.

The **5-year survival rates** (the relative rates for survival in persons who are living 5 years after diagnosis) have increased greatly from the 50 percent of past generations (**FIGURE 16.1**). Today, about 68 percent of people diagnosed with cancer each year will be alive 5 years after their diagnosis.[3] Survival rates for people with many cancers caught in their earliest stages approach 100 percent; of those treated for cancer, many will be considered "cured," meaning that they have no new cancer in their bodies 5 years after their original diagnosis. These rates are *relative survival* rates, meaning they represent those who are alive after 5 years compared to those who are cancer free. They do not include those still in treatment or those who have relapsed. Since they are calculated based on patients diagnosed years earlier, they may not reflect the most recent advances in treatment and should be viewed with caution.[4] Although treatments and survival statistics have improved, nearly half of all American males and one-third of American females will still develop cancer at some point in their life.[5] In the following sections, we provide an overview of factors that increase risk of cancer and discuss ways to reduce those risks.

HEAR IT! PODCASTS

Want a study podcast of this chapter? Download **Cancer: Reducing Your Risk** available on MasteringHealth.™

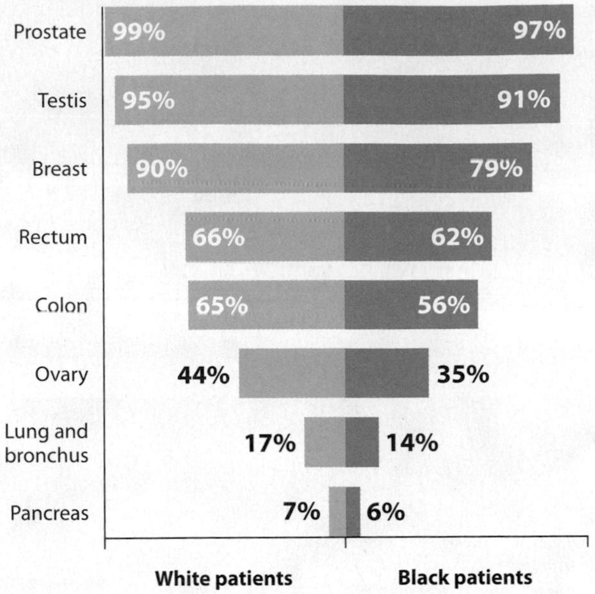

FIGURE 16.1 Five-Year Survival Cancer Rates by Site

Since the 1970s, survival rates have increased steadily for nearly all types of cancer. The exception to this trend has been lung cancer survivorship. Its survival rates remain both relatively steady and low, most likely due to the late stage at which most lung cancer cases are detected.

Source: N. Howlader et al., National Cancer Institute, "SEER Cancer Statistics Review, 1975–2011," based on November 2013 SEER data submission, April 2014, http://seer.cancer.gov/csr/1975_2011.

LO 2 | WHAT IS CANCER?

Describe cancer and how it develops, as well as key risk factors.

Cancer is the general term for a large group of diseases in which abnormal cells begin dividing uncontrollably and invade our tissues and organs. These cancer cells spread or **metastasize** via the blood and lymphatic system. It might be helpful to think of them as traitorous cells that overpower our vast bodily defenses and ultimately deplete our reserves. If we are already weakened by virtue of age, other "comorbidities," immune system breakdown, chronic stress, exposure to toxins, or other health risks, cancers have a better chance of successfully invading. When cancer cells invade and ramp up their growth, they interrupt normal cell programming and

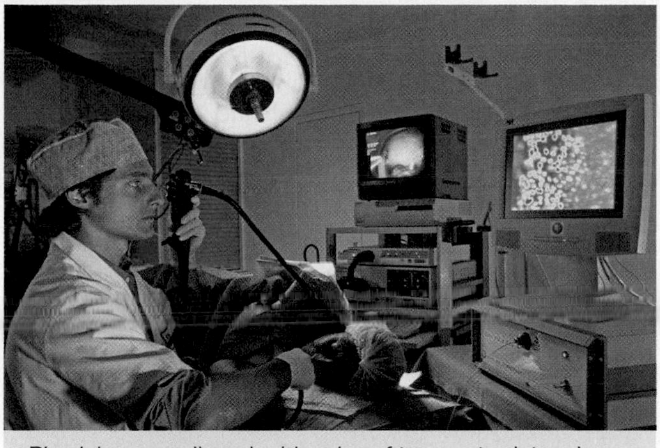

Physicians usually order biopsies of tumors to determine whether they are cancerous. Newer techniques, such as the minimally invasive "optical biopsy" shown here, allow microscopic examination of tissue without doing a physical biopsy.

develop into a **neoplasm**, a new growth of tissue serving no physiological function. This neoplasmic mass often forms a clump of cells known as a **tumor.** Tumors can grow rapidly or take months or years for them to cause noticeable symptoms.

Not all tumors are **malignant** (cancerous). In fact, most are **benign** (noncancerous). Benign tumors are generally harmless unless they grow to obstruct or crowd out normal tissues. A benign tumor of the brain, for instance, becomes life threatening when it grows enough to restrict blood flow and cause a stroke. The only way to determine whether a tumor is malignant is through **biopsy**, the removal and microscopic examination of a sample of cells.

Benign tumors generally consist of ordinary-looking cells enclosed in a fibrous shell or capsule that prevents their spreading to other body areas. Malignant tumors are usually not enclosed in a protective capsule and can therefore spread to other organs (**FIGURE 16.2**). This *metastatic* spread makes some forms of cancer particularly aggressive. By the time they are diagnosed, malignant tumors have frequently metastasized throughout the body, making treatment extremely difficult. Malignant cells invade surrounding tissue, emitting clawlike protrusions that disturb the RNA and DNA within normal cells. Disrupting these substances, which control cellular metabolism and reproduction, produces **mutant cells** that differ in form, quality, and function from normal cells.

Cancer staging is a classification system that describes how much a cancer has spread at the time it is diagnosed; it helps doctors and patients decide on appropriate treatments and

neoplasm A new growth of tissue that results from uncontrolled, abnormal cellular development and serves no physiological function.

tumor A neoplasmic mass that grows more rapidly than surrounding tissue.

malignant Very dangerous or harmful; refers to a cancerous tumor.

benign Harmless; refers to a noncancerous tumor.

biopsy Removal and examination of a tissue sample to determine if a cancer is present.

mutant cells Cells that differ in form, quality, or function from normal cells.

cancer staging A classification system that describes how far a person's disease has advanced.

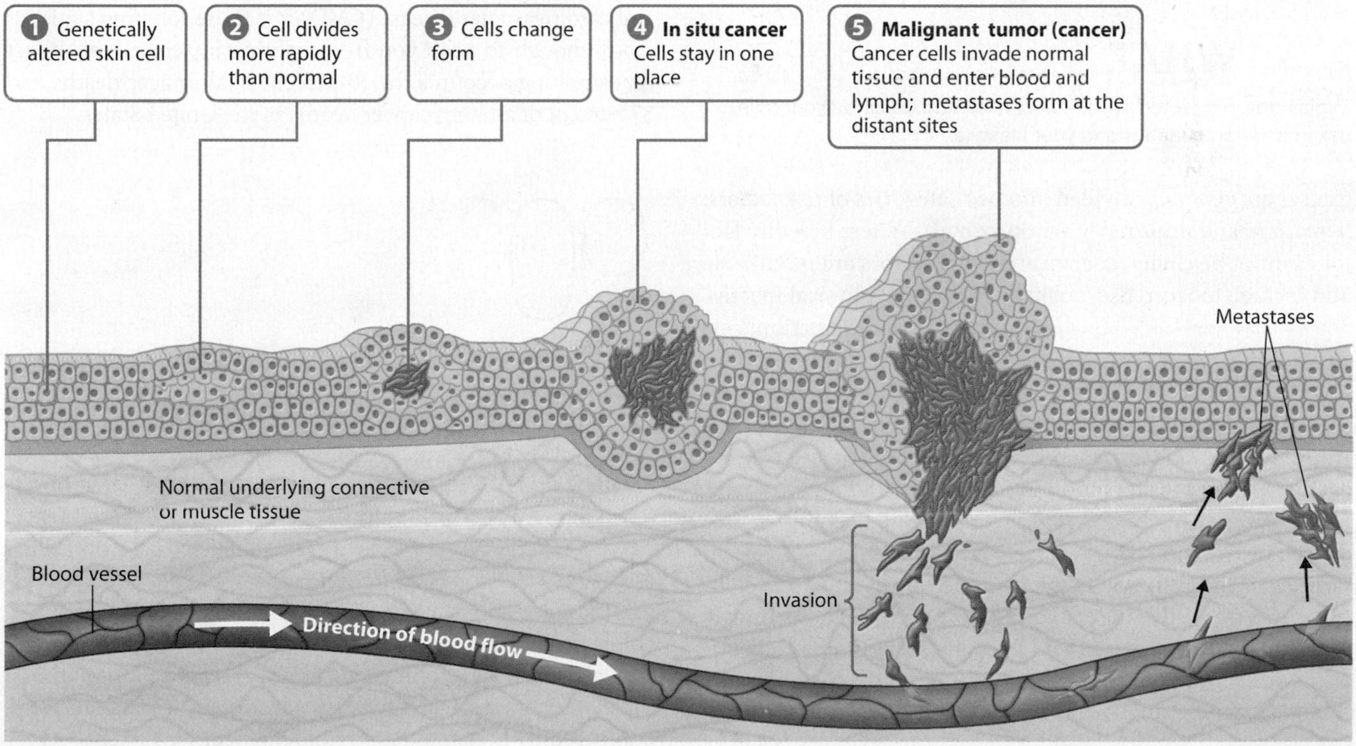

1 Genetically altered skin cell
2 Cell divides more rapidly than normal
3 Cells change form
4 In situ cancer Cells stay in one place
5 Malignant tumor (cancer) Cancer cells invade normal tissue and enter blood and lymph; metastases form at the distant sites
Metastases
Normal underlying connective or muscle tissue
Blood vessel
Invasion
Direction of blood flow

FIGURE 16.2 **Metastasis** A mutation to the genetic material of a skin cell triggers abnormal cell division and changes cell formation, resulting in a cancerous tumor. If the tumor remains localized, it is considered *in situ* cancer. If the tumor spreads, it is considered a malignant cancer.

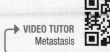

VIDEO TUTOR Metastasis

TABLE 16.1 | Cancer Stages

Stage	Definition
0	Early cancer, when abnormal cells remain only in the place they originated.
I II III	Higher numbers indicate more extensive disease: Larger tumor size and/or spread of the cancer beyond the organ in which it first developed to nearby lymph nodes and/or organs adjacent to the location of the primary tumor.
IV	Cancer has spread to other organs

Source: National Cancer Institute, National Institutes of Health, "Fact Sheet, Cancer Staging," 2013, www.cancer.gov/cancertopics/factsheet/detection/staging.

estimate a person's life expectancy. Cancers are typically staged based on the size of a tumor, how deeply it has penetrated, the number of lymph nodes that are affected, and the degree of metastasis or spread, known as the *TNM* (for ***t**umor,* ***n**ode,* and ***m**etastasis*) system. The most commonly known staging system assigns the numbers 0 to IV to the disease, with IV being most advanced. (see **TABLE 16.1**). In addition to staging, many tumors are assigned a grade based on the degree of cell abnormality. Typically, the lower the stage and grade, the better the prognosis.[6]

WHY SHOULD I CARE?

Lifestyle, tobacco use, nutrition, and activity are things you control and areas in which you can start good habits now to reduce your chances of developing cancer.

LO 3 | WHAT CAUSES CANCER?

Explain the suspected causes of cancer, and describe your own risks based on genetics and your lifestyle.

Causes are generally divided into two categories of risk factors: *hereditary* and *acquired* (environmental). Where heredity factors cannot be changed, environmental factors are modifiable and include tobacco use; quality of nutrition; physical inactivity; obesity; inflammation; certain infectious agents; certain medical treatments; drug and alcohol consumption; excessive sun exposure; and exposure to **carcinogens** (cancer-causing agents) in food, water, and air. Hereditary and environmental factors may interact to make cancer more likely, accelerate cancer progression, or increase susceptibility during certain periods of life. The mechanisms underlying cancer development are not fully understood. Two people with seemingly identical risk factors may end up with very different experiences when it comes to developing cancer, and at present the reasons for these differences remain a mystery.

carcinogens Cancer-causing agents.

Lifestyle Risks for Cancer

Cancer occurs in all age groups, but the older you are, the greater your risk. Nearly 77 percent of all cancers are diagnosed in adults over age 55.[7] Cancer researchers refer to one's cancer risk when they assess risk factors. *Lifetime risk* refers to the probability that an individual, over the course of a lifetime, will develop cancer. In the United States, men have a lifetime risk of about 1 in 2; women have a lower risk, at 1 in 3.[8] Risks also vary by race, socioeconomic status, education, occupation, geographic location, and several other factors.

Relative risk is a measure of the strength of the relationship between risk factors and a particular cancer. Basically, it compares your risk of cancer if you engage in certain known risk behaviors with that of someone who does not engage in such behaviors. For example, if you are a man and smoker, your relative risk of getting lung cancer is about twice that of a male nonsmoker.[9]

Over the years, researchers have found that diet, a sedentary lifestyle, overconsumption of alcohol, tobacco use, stress, and other factors play a key role in the incidence (number of new cases) of cancer. Keep in mind that a high relative risk does not guarantee cause and effect. It merely indicates the likelihood of a particular risk factor being related to a particular outcome.

Tobacco Use In the United States, smoking has the dubious distinction of being *the leading cause of preventable death* and is responsible for nearly 1 in 5 deaths, or about 443,000 premature deaths each year. In addition, nearly 9 million more people suffer from smoking-related diseases, such as chronic bronchitis, emphysema, and cardiovascular disease (CVD).[10] If those sobering statistics aren't enough to keep you from lighting up, consider the fact that smoking accounts for 30 percent of all cancer deaths and 87 percent of all lung cancer deaths in the United States.[11]

90%

OF ALL LUNG CANCERS COULD BE **AVOIDED** IF PEOPLE SIMPLY DID NOT SMOKE.

Smoking is associated with increased risk of at least 15 different cancers. According to the 2014 *Surgeon General Report on the Health Consequences of Smoking*, several compelling associations between smoking and cancer were reported, including causal relationships between smoking and liver cancer, colorectal polyps, and colorectal cancer.[12]

Chances of developing cancer are 23 times higher among male smokers and 13 times higher among female smokers, compared to nonsmokers.[13] Coincidence? Not likely.[14] Over the years, cigarette smoking has declined in many regions of the world, largely due to major efforts aimed at prevention and control through education, policy development, and taxation. Still, developing countries continue to be disproportionately affected by increasing numbers of cancer cases and high smoking rates. In fact, over 60 percent of the world's total cancer cases and 70 percent of cancer deaths occur in Africa, Asia, and Central and South America.[15] Lung cancer continues to be the leading cause of cancer deaths globally, in spite of massive efforts to prevent or control smoking.[16] Smoking in the home increases cancer risks for family members and pets.

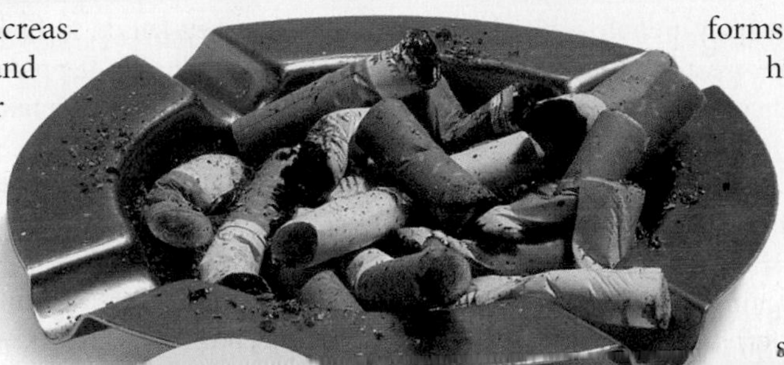

Of the several lifestyle risk factors for cancer, tobacco use is the most significant—and the most preventable.

Alcohol and Cancer Risk

Over the past decade, countless studies have implicated alcohol as a risk factor for cancer. Light to moderate alcohol intake (more than one drink per day) appears to increase risk of breast cancer among women.[17] Moderate alcohol intake (above one drink per day) in women also appears to increase the risk of cancers of the oral cavity and pharynx, esophagus, and larynx, and binge drinking may increase gastric and pancreatic cancer risk as well.[18]

Men who drink also increase their cancer risk. In a study of over 3,500 men aged 35 to 70, regular heavy consumption of alcohol increased the risk of esophageal and liver cancers more than sevenfold. The risk of colon, stomach, and prostate cancers was about 80 percent higher among heavy drinkers, while lung cancer risk rose by almost 60 percent compared to nondrinkers.[19]

Poor Nutrition, Physical Inactivity, and Obesity Mounting evidence suggests nearly one-third of annual cancer deaths in the United States may be due to lifestyle factors such as overweight or obesity, physical inactivity, and poor nutrition.[20] Aside from choosing not to use tobacco, dietary choices and physical activity are the most important modifiable determinants of cancer risk. Several studies indicate a relationship between a high body mass index (BMI) and death rates from cancers of the esophagus, colon, rectum, liver, stomach, kidney, and pancreas, and others.[21]

Just how great is the risk for someone with a high BMI? Women who gain 55 pounds or more after age 18 have almost a 50 percent greater risk of breast cancer compared to those who maintain their weight.[22] Overall, risk appears to increase with age. The good news is that, particularly for postmenopausal women, losing 10 pounds or more and keeping it off may actually reduce breast cancer risk.[23]

The relative risk of colon cancer in men is 40 percent higher for obese men than it is for nonobese men. The relative risk of gallbladder cancer is five times higher in obese individuals than in individuals of healthy weight. Numerous other studies support the link between various forms of cancer and obesity.[24] The higher the BMI, the greater the cancer risk.[25]

Stress and Psychosocial Risks Although stress has been implicated in increased susceptibility to several types of cancers, most reports of cancer being caused by stress are observational in nature, and many of these studies lack scientific rigor or are simply too small to show definitive results. A recent large meta-analytic study found no relationship between job strain and risk for colorectal, lung, breast, or prostate cancer.[26] That said, people who are under chronic, severe stress or who suffer from depression or other persistent emotional problems show higher rates of cancer than their healthy counterparts. Sleep disturbances, unhealthy diet, and emotional or physical trauma may weaken the body's immune system, increasing susceptibility to cancer. Other possible contributors to cancer are poverty and the health disparities associated with low socioeconomic status.

Genetic and Physiological Risks

If one of your close family members develops cancer, does it mean that you have a genetic predisposition for it? Scientists believe that about 5 percent of all cancers are strongly hereditary. It seems that some people may be more predisposed to the malfunctioning of genes that ultimately cause cancer.[27]

Suspected cancer-causing genes are called **oncogenes**. Although these genes are typically dormant, certain conditions such as age; stress; and exposure to carcinogens, viruses, and radiation may activate them. Once activated, oncogenes cause cells to grow and reproduce uncontrollably.

oncogenes Suspected cancer-causing genes present on chromosomes.

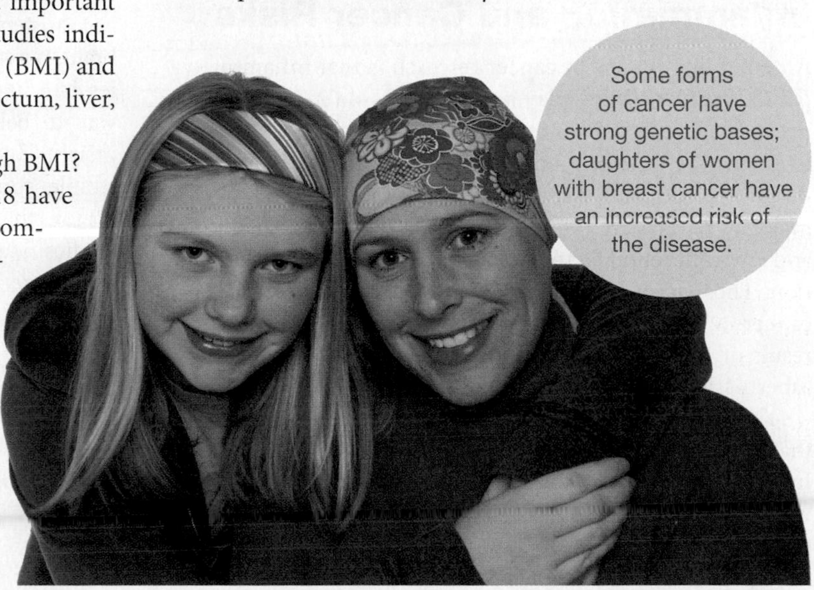

Some forms of cancer have strong genetic bases; daughters of women with breast cancer have an increased risk of the disease.

Scientists are uncertain whether only people who develop cancer have oncogenes or whether we all have genes that can become oncogenes under certain conditions.

Certain cancers, particularly those of the breast, stomach, colon, prostate, uterus, ovaries, and lungs, appear to run in families. For example, a woman runs a much higher risk of breast cancer if her mother or sisters have had the disease, particularly at a young age. Hodgkin disease and certain leukemias show similar familial patterns. Can we attribute these familial patterns to genetic susceptibility or to the fact that people in the same families experience similar environmental risks? Research in this area is inconclusive. It is possible that we can inherit a tendency toward a cancer-prone, weak immune system, or conversely, that we can inherit a cancer-fighting potential. But the complex interaction of heredity, lifestyle, and environment on the development of cancer makes it a challenge to determine a single cause. Even among those predisposed to mutations, avoiding risks may decrease chances of cancer development.

Reproductive and Hormonal Factors The effects of reproductive factors on breast and cervical cancers have been well documented. Increased numbers of fertile or menstrual cycle years (early menarche, late menopause), not having children or having them later in life, recent use of birth control pills or hormone replacement therapy, and opting not to breast-feed all appear to increase risks of breast cancer.[28] While the above factors appear to play a significant role in increased risk for non-Hispanic white women, they do not appear to have as strong an influence on Hispanic women, who may have more protective reproductive patterns (an overall lower age at first birth and greater number of births). They also use less hormone replacement therapy and have a lower utilization rate for mammograms, making comparisons difficult.[29] Although some earlier studies suggested that hormone therapy may slightly increase the risk of lung cancer, newer research has shown no significant increases in lung cancer risk owing to hormone therapy.[30]

Inflammation and Cancer Risks

An emerging theory in cancer research is that inflammatory processes in the body play a significant role in the development of cancer—from initiation and promoting cancer cells to paving the way for them to invade, spread, and weaken the immune response.[31] According to some researchers, the vast majority of cancers (90%) are caused by cellular mutations and environmental factors that occur as a result of inflammation. These same researchers believe that up to 20 percent of cancers are the result of chronic infections, 30 percent are the result of tobacco smoking and inhaled particulates such as asbestos, and 35 percent are due to dietary factors.[32]

The common denominator in these threats is inflammation that primes the system for cancer to gain a foothold and spread. Inflammation appears to be a key factor in colorectal cancer, with inflammatory bowel disease, Crohn's disease, colitis, and other gastrointestinal (GI) tract inflammatory problems having a higher risk of cancer development.[33] If inflammation is indeed a key factor, reducing inflammation via stress reduction, sleep, dietary supplements, low-dose aspirin, and other behaviors may prove beneficial in reducing cancer risks.

Occupational and Environmental Risks

Workplace hazards account for only a small percentage of all cancers, but various substances are known to cause cancer when exposure levels are high or prolonged. Asbestos—a fibrous material once widely used in the construction, insulation, and automobile industries—nickel, chromate, and chemicals such as benzene, arsenic, and vinyl chloride have been shown to be carcinogens. Also, people who routinely work with certain dyes and radioactive substances may have increased risks for cancer. Working with coal tars, as in the mining profession, or with inhalants, as in the auto-painting business, is hazardous. So is working with herbicides and pesticides, although evidence is inconclusive for low-dose exposures. Several federal and state agencies are responsible for monitoring such exposures and ensuring that businesses comply with standards designed to protect workers.

Radiation Ionizing radiation (IR)—radiation from X-rays, radon, cosmic rays, and ultraviolet radiation (primarily UVB radiation)—is the only form of radiation proven to cause human cancer. Evidence that high-dose IR causes cancer comes from studies of atomic bomb survivors, patients receiving radiotherapy, and certain occupational groups, such as uranium miners. Virtually any part of the body can be affected by IR, but bone marrow and the thyroid are particularly susceptible. Radon exposure in homes can increase lung cancer risk, especially in cigarette smokers. To reduce the risk of harmful effects, diagnostic medical and dental X-rays are set at the lowest dose levels possible.

Nonionizing radiation produced by radio waves, cell phones, microwaves, computer screens, televisions, electric blankets, and other products has been a topic of great concern in recent years, but research has not proven excess risk to date. Although a wide range of studies have been conducted, none have shown a consistent link between cell phone use and cancers of the brain, nerves, or other tissues of the head or neck. Major studies of adults from several countries and children are underway to help provide more insight. In the meantime, simple strategies can help ensure that even if future studies identify prolonged cell usage as a risk factor for cancer, you will have reduced your risk. First and foremost, use a hands-free device, and try to keep as much space as possible between your head and your phone. When hands free isn't available, limit your talk time, keep the

WHAT DO YOU THINK?

How should we determine whether a behavior or substance is a risk factor for a disease and whether programs should be enacted to reduce the risk or stop a behavior?

- Do you think that there should be federal legislation banning the use of tanning booths/beds in all 50 states? Why or why not? Would you favor such bans for minors only? Adults?

phone away from your bed, and use the speaker function on your phone to get it as far from your head/body as possible.[34] (See **Chapter 20** for more on the potential hazards of both ionizing and nonionizing radiation.)

Chemicals in Foods Much of the concern about chemicals in food centers on the possible harm caused by pesticide and herbicide residues. Whereas some of these chemicals cause cancer at high doses in experimental animals, the government considers the very low concentrations found in some foods to be safe. Continued research regarding pesticide and herbicide use is essential, and scientists and consumer groups stress the importance of a balance between chemical use and the production of high-quality food products.

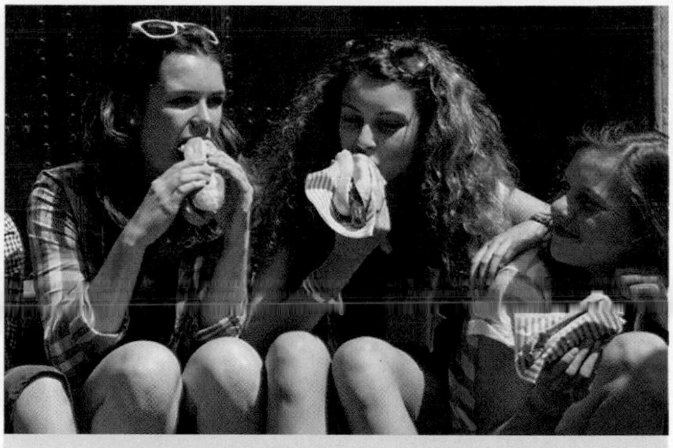

Concern about the carcinogenic properties of nitrates, which are often used to preserve hot dogs, hams, and luncheon meats, has led to the introduction of meats that are nitrate-free or contain reduced levels of the substance.

Infectious Diseases and Cancer Risks

Over 10 percent of all cancers in the United States are caused by infectious agents such as viruses, bacteria, or parasites.[35] Worldwide, approximately 15 to 20 percent of human cancers have been traced to infectious agents.[36] Infections are thought to influence cancer development in several ways, most commonly through chronic inflammation, suppression of the immune system, or chronic stimulation.

Hepatitis B, Hepatitis C, and Liver Cancer

Viruses that cause chronic forms of hepatitis B (HBV) and C (HCV) are believed to stimulate growth of cancer cells in the liver because they chronically inflame liver tissue. This may prime the liver for cancer or make it more hospitable for cancer development. Global increases in hepatitis B and C rates and concurrent rises in liver cancer rates seem to provide evidence of such an association. Vaccines that prevent hepatitis B may reduce the risk of liver damage as well as cancer.

Human Papillomavirus and Cervical Cancer

Between 70 and 100 percent of women with cervical cancer have evidence of human papillomavirus (HPV) infection, which is believed to be a major cause of cervical cancer, as well as vaginal and vulvar cancers in women and penile cancers in men. Genital warts and anal and oropharyngeal cancers in both men and women are also associated with HPV infections. Today, vaccines are available to help protect men and women from being infected with HPV and increased cancer susceptibility. While vaccines don't completely prevent all of these cancers, they seem to be effective in reducing risks of cervical and penile cancer.[37] Unfortunately, nearly one-fourth of parents in a recent survey indicated they did not intend to vaccinate their daughters.[38] Although attitudes toward vaccination and overall knowledge about risks are higher among college-educated populations, only 33 percent of females aged 9 to 26 receive the recommended three HPV shots.[39] (For more information on the HPV vaccine, see the discussion in **Chapter 14**.)

***Helicobacter pylori* and Stomach Cancer** *Helicobacter pylori* is a potent bacterium found in the stomach lining of approximately 30 to 40 percent of Americans. It causes inflammation, scarring, and ulcers, damaging the lining of the stomach and leading to cellular changes that may lead to cancer. More than half of all cases of stomach cancer are thought to be linked to *H. pylori* infection, even though most infected people don't develop cancer.[40] Treatment with antibiotics often cures the ulcers, which appears to reduce risk of new stomach cancer.[41]

Medical Factors

Some medical treatments can increase a person's risk for cancer. For example, estrogen use for relieving menopausal symptoms is now recognized to contribute to multiple cancer risks and provides fewer benefits than originally believed. Prescriptions for estrogen therapy have declined dramatically, and many women are trying to reduce or eliminate use of the hormone.

Ironically, medicines used to treat cancers, such as selected chemotherapy drugs, have been shown to increase risks for other cancers. Weighing the benefits versus harms of these treatments is always necessary.

LO 4 | TYPES OF CANCERS

Describe the different types of cancer and the risks they pose to people at different ages and stages of life, as well as key actions to prevent cancer development.

Cancers are grouped into four broad categories based on the type of tissue from which each arises:

- **Carcinomas.** Epithelial tissues (tissues covering body surfaces and lining most body cavities) are the most common sites for cancers; cancers occurring in epithelial tissue are called *carcinomas*. These cancers affect the outer layer of the skin and mouth as well as mucous membranes. They metastasize through the circulatory or lymphatic system initially and form solid tumors.

Estimated New Cases of Cancer*		Estimated Deaths from Cancer*	
Female	Male	Female	Male
Breast 232,670 (29%)	Prostate 232,670 (29%)	Lung & bronchus 72,330 (26%)	Lung & bronchus 86,930 (28%)
Lung & bronchus 108,210 (13%)	Lung & bronchus 108,210 (13%)	Breast 40,000 (15%)	Prostate 29,480 (10%)
Colon & rectum 65,000 (8%)	Colon & rectum 71,830 (9%)	Colon & rectum 24,040 (9%)	Colon & rectum 26,270 (8%)
Uterine corpus 52,630 (6%)	Urinary bladder 56,390 (7%)	Pancreas 19,420 (7%)	Pancreas 20,170 (7%)
Thyroid 47,790 (6%)	Melanoma of the skin 43,890 (5%)	Ovary 14,270 (5%)	Liver & intrahepatic bile duct 15,870 (5%)
Non-Hodgkin lymphoma 32,530 (4%)	Kidney & renal pelvis 39,140 (5%)	Leukemia 10,050 (4%)	Leukemia 14,040 (5%)
Melanoma of the skin 32,210 (4%)	Non-Hodgkin lymphoma 38,270 (4%)	Uterine corpus 8,590 (3%)	Esophagus 12,450 (4%)
Kidney & renal pelvis 24,780 (3%)	Oral cavity & pharynx 30,220 (4%)	Non-Hodgkin lymphoma 8,520 (3%)	Urinary bladder 11,170 (4%)
Pancreas 22,890 (3%)	Leukemia 30,100 (4%)	Liver & intrahepatic bile duct 7,130 (3%)	Non-Hodgkin lymphoma 10,470 (3%)
Leukemia 22,280 (3%)	Pancreas 22,289 (3%)	Brain & other nervous system 6,230 (2%)	Kidney & renal pelvis 8,900 (3%)
All Sites 810,320 (100%)	All Sites 855,220 (100%)	All Sites 275,370 (100%)	All Sites 310,010 (100%)

*Excludes basal and squamous cell skin cancers and in situ carcinoma except urinary bladder. Percentages may not total 100% due to rounding.

FIGURE 16.3 Leading Sites of New Cancer Cases and Deaths, 2014 Estimates

Source: Data from American Cancer Society, *Cancer Facts & Figures 2014*, Table (Atlanta: American Cancer Society; 2014), 10. Note that percentages do not add up to 100 due to omissions of certain rare cancers as well as rounding of statistics.

- **Sarcomas.** Sarcomas occur in the mesodermal, or middle, layers of tissue—for example, in bones, muscles, and general connective tissue. In early stages, they metastasize primarily via the blood. Sarcomas are less common but generally more virulent than carcinomas. They also form solid tumors.
- **Lymphomas.** Lymphomas develop in the lymphatic system—the infection-fighting regions of the body—and metastasize through the lymphatic system. Hodgkin disease is an example. Lymphomas also form solid tumors.
- **Leukemias.** Cancer of the blood-forming parts of the body, particularly the bone marrow and spleen, is called leukemia. A nonsolid tumor, leukemia is characterized by an abnormal increase in the number of white blood cells that the body produces.

FIGURE 16.3 shows the most common sites of cancer and the number of new cases and deaths from each type that were estimated to have occurred in 2014. A comprehensive discussion of the many different forms of cancer is beyond the scope of this book, but we will discuss the most common types in the next sections.

Lung Cancer

Lung cancer is the leading cause of cancer deaths for both men and women in the United States. It killed an estimated 160,000 Americans in 2014, accounting for nearly 27 percent of all cancer deaths.[42] The lifetime risks for males and females getting lung cancer is 1 in 13 and 1 in 16, respectively. Risks begin to rise around age 40 and continue to climb through all age groups thereafter.[43]

Since 1987, more women have died each year from lung cancer than breast cancer, which had been the leading cause of cancer deaths in women for 40 years prior. Although past reductions in smoking rates bode well for cancer statistics,

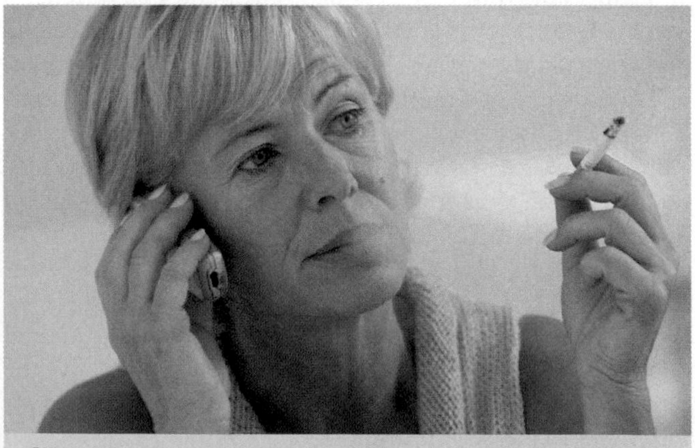

Stopping smoking at any time will reduce your risk of lung cancer. Studies show that within 5 years of quitting, women's risk of death from lung cancer decreases by 21 percent, compared to people who continue smoking.

there is growing concern about the number of young people, particularly young women and persons of low income and low educational levels, who continue to pick up the habit.

There is also growing concern about the increase in lung cancers among lifelong *never smokers*—a group of people who, as the name suggests, have never smoked, but still have as much as 15 percent of all lung cancers. Never smokers' lung cancer is believed to be related to genetic mutations that increase risk, exposure to secondhand smoke, radon gas, asbestos, indoor wood burning stoves, exposure to environmental agents that increase risk, and aerosolized oils caused by cooking with oil and deep fat frying.[44] Unfortunately, because doctors often don't think of lung cancer when a never smoker presents with a cough, patients are often put on antibiotics or cough suppressants as therapy. By the time they recognize that it's really lung cancer, their cancer is likely to be more advanced and treatment is more challenging.

Detection, Symptoms, and Treatment Symptoms of lung cancer include a persistent cough, blood streaked sputum, voice change, chest pain or back pain, and recurrent attacks of pneumonia or bronchitis. Newer computerized tomography (CAT) scans, molecular markers in saliva, and newer biopsy techniques have improved screening accuracy for lung cancer, but they have a long way to go. Treatment depends on the type (large or small scale) and stage of the cancer. Surgery, radiation therapy, chemotherapy, and targeted biological therapies are all options. If the cancer is localized, surgery is usually the treatment of choice. If it has spread, surgery is combined with radiation, chemotherapy, and other targeted drug treatments. Fewer than 15 percent of lung cancer cases are diagnosed at the early, localized stages. Early stage cancers have a 54 percent 1-year survival rate, falling to 6 to 18 percent at 5 years after diagnosis.[45]

Risk Factors and Prevention Risks for cancer increase dramatically based on the quantity of cigarettes smoked and the number of years smoked, often referred to as *pack years*. The greater the number of pack years smoked, the greater the risk of developing cancer. Quitting smoking does reduce the risk of developing lung cancer.[46] Exposure to industrial substances or radiation also highly increases the risk for lung cancer.

Breast Cancer

Breast cancer is a group of diseases that cause uncontrolled cell growth in breast tissue, particularly in the glands that produce milk and the ducts that connect those glands to the nipple. Cancers can also form in the connective and lymphatic tissues of the breast. In 2014, approximately 232,679 women and 2,360 men in the United States were diagnosed with invasive breast cancer for the first time. In addition, 63,570 new cases of *in situ* breast cancer, a more localized cancer, were diagnosed. About 40,430 women (and 430 men) died, making breast cancer the second leading cause of cancer death for women.[47] Women have a 1 in 8 lifetime risk of being diagnosed with breast cancer. From birth to age 49, the risk is 1 in 53, but between the ages of 50 and 59, the chance for breast cancer becomes 1 in 43.[48] This is why most health groups have advocated screening for breast cancer more thoroughly after age 40.

SEE IT! VIDEOS

Could you have inherited breast cancer from a female relative? Watch **Breast Cancer Patients Getting Younger** available on MasteringHealth.™

Detection The earliest signs of breast cancer are usually observable on mammograms, often before lumps can be felt. However, mammograms are not foolproof, and there is debate regarding the optimal age at which women should start regularly receiving them. Although not recommended as a screening tool, per se, a newer form of magnetic resonance imaging (MRI) appears to be even more accurate, particularly in women with genetic risks for tumors or those who have suspicious areas of the breast or surrounding tissue that warrant a clearer image. If you are referred for a breast MRI, be sure to go to a facility where they can perform a breast biopsy if there are any areas that need further investigation.[49]

Breast Awareness and Self-Exam Breast self-exam (BSE) has been recommended by major health organizations as a form of early breast cancer screening for the last two

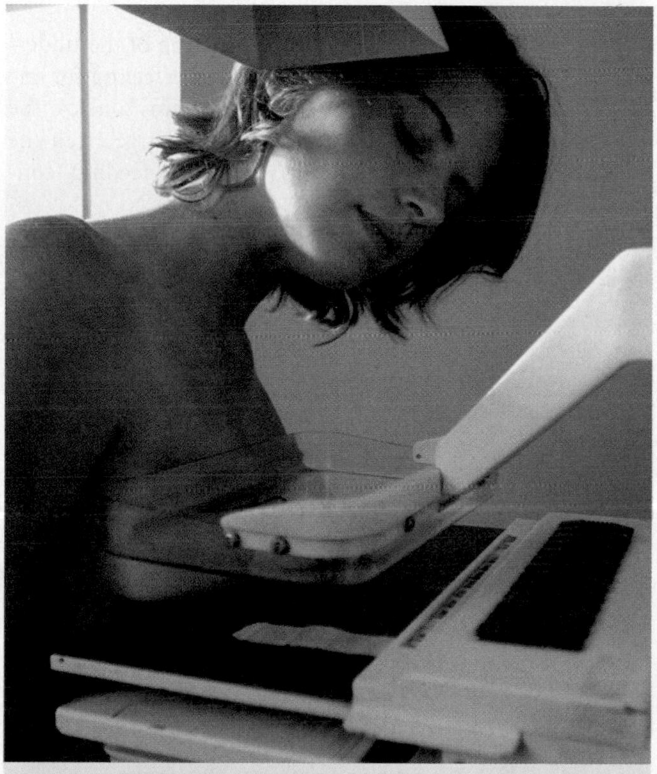

Early detection through mammography and other techniques greatly increases a woman's chance of surviving breast cancer.

decades (see **FIGURE 16.4**). However, a 2009 "study of studies" done by the U.S. Preventive Services Task Force determined that breast self-exams did not decrease suffering and death and, in fact, often lead to unnecessary worry, unnecessary tests, and increased health care costs. As a result of this research, several groups have downgraded the recommendation about BSE from "do them and do them regularly" to "learn how to do them, and if you desire, do them to know your body and be able to recognize changes."

To do a breast self-exam, begin by standing in front of a mirror to inspect the breasts, looking for their usual symmetry. Some breasts are not symmetrical, and if this is not a change, it is okay. Raise and lower both arms while checking that the breasts move evenly and freely. Next, inspect the skin, looking for areas of redness, thickening, or dimpling, which might have the appearance of an orange peel. Look for any scaling on the nipple.

To feel for lumps, raise one arm above your head while either standing or lying. This will flatten out the breast, making it easier to feel the tissue. Using the index, middle, and fourth fingers of your opposite hand, gently push down on the breast tissue and move the fingers in small circular motions, varying pressure from light to more firm. Start at one edge of the breast and move upward and then downward, working your way across the breast until all of the breast tissue has been covered. Often breast tissue will feel dense and irregular, and this is usually normal. It helps to do regular self-exams to become familiar with what your breast tissue feels like; then, if there is a change, you will notice. Cancers usually feel like a dense or firm little rock and are very different from the normal breast tissue.

Next, lower the arm and reach into the top of the underarm and pull downward with gentle pressure feeling for any enlarged lymph nodes. To complete the exam, squeeze the tissue around the nipple. If you notice discharge from the nipple and you have not recently been breast-feeding, consult your doctor. Likewise, if you notice any asymmetry, skin changes, scaling on the nipple, or new lumps in the breast, you should see your doctor for evaluation.

Symptoms and Treatment If breast cancer grows large enough, it can produce the following symptoms: a lump in the breast or surrounding lymph nodes, thickening, dimpling, skin irritation, distortion, retraction or scaliness of the nipple, nipple discharge, or tenderness.

Treatments range from a lumpectomy to radical mastectomy to various combinations of radiation or chemotherapy. Among nonsurgical options, promising results have been noted among women using *selective estrogen-receptor modulators (SERMs)* such as tamoxifen and raloxifene, particularly among women whose cancers appear to grow in response to estrogen. These drugs, as well as new *aromatase inhibitors*, work by blocking estrogen. The 5-year survival rate for people with localized breast cancer has risen from 80 percent in the 1950s to 99 percent today.[50] However, these statistics vary dramatically, based on the stage of the cancer when it is first detected and whether it has spread. If the cancer has spread to the lymph nodes or other organs, the 5-year survival rate drops to as low as 24 percent.[51] Having access to early diagnosis and treatment is key to survival.

Risk Factors and Prevention The incidence of breast cancer increases with age. Although there are many possible risk factors, those that are well supported by research include family history of breast cancer, menstrual periods that started early and ended late in life, weight gain after the age of 18, obesity after menopause, recent use of oral contraceptives or postmenopausal hormone therapy, never bearing children or bearing a first child after age 30, consuming two or more drinks of alcohol per day, and physical inactivity. In addition, there is new evidence that heavy smoking, particularly among women who started smoking before their first pregnancy, increases risk. Other factors that increase risk include having dense breasts, type 2 diabetes, high bone mineral density, and exposure to high-dose radiation.[52] Although the *BRCA1* and *BRCA2* gene mutations are rare and occur in less than 1 percent of the population, they account for approximately 5 to 10 percent of all cases of breast cancer.[53] Women who possess these genes have up to an 80 percent risk of developing breast cancer in their lives and tend to develop breast cancer at earlier ages. Cancers are also more likely to occur in both breasts in

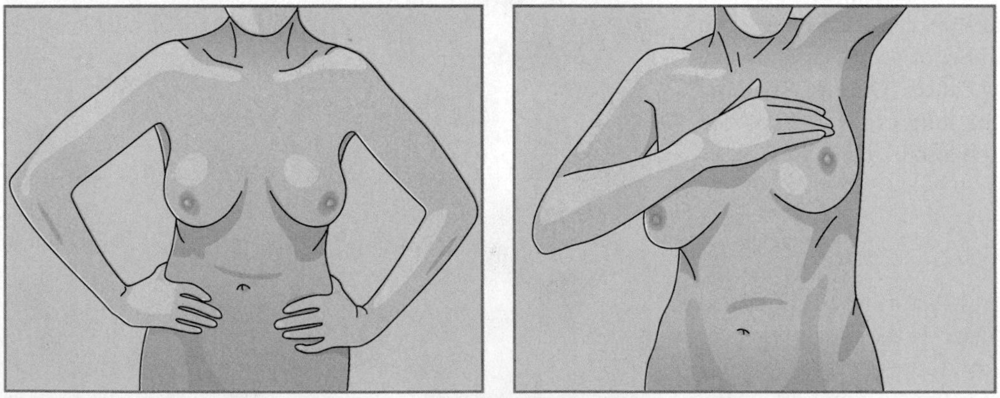

1 Face a mirror and check for changes in symmetry.

2 Either standing or lying down, use the pads of the three middle fingers to check for lumps. Follow an up-and-down pattern on the breast to ensure all tissue gets inspected.

FIGURE 16.4 Breast Awareness and Self-Exam

Source: Adapted from Breast Self-Exam Illustration Series, National Cancer Institute Visuals Online Collection, U.S. National Institutes of Health, https://visualsonline.cancer.gov.

women with the genes as compared to women without these genes. Because these genes are rare, routine screening for them is not recommended unless there is a strong family history (particularly among younger primary relatives) of breast cancer.[54]

International differences in breast cancer incidence correlate with variations in diet, especially fat intake, although a causal role for these dietary factors has not been firmly established. Sudden weight gain has also been implicated. Research also shows that regular exercise can reduce risk.[55] In particular, two large meta-analyses of studies focused on the role of dietary fiber indicate strong inverse relationships between dietary fiber and breast cancer. In short, if you eat more fiber, breast cancer rates seem to go down, and if you eat less, rates seem to increase.[56]

WHY SHOULD I CARE?

Breast cancer accounts for 1 in every 3 cancer diagnoses in women in the United States. You can take action to reduce your risk by keeping your weight within a healthy range, drinking less than one alcoholic drink a day, and exercising regularly. Starting now is your best means of prevention.

Colon and Rectal Cancers

Colorectal cancers (cancers of the colon and rectum) continue to be the third most commonly diagnosed cancer in both men and women and the third leading cause of cancer deaths, even though death rates are declining. Most cases occur in people age 50 and over, but new cases can occur at any age.[57] In 2014, there were 96,830 cases of colon cancer and 40,000 cases of rectal cancer diagnosed in the United States, as well as 50,310 deaths.[58] Ninety percent of colorectal cancers occur in individuals who are over the age of 50. From birth to age 49, men have a 1 in 305 risk of developing it, while women have a 1 in 334 chance.[59]

Detection, Symptoms, and Treatment Because colorectal cancer tends to spread slowly over a period of 10 to 20 years, the prognosis is quite good for those who receive recommended screenings and are diagnosed in early stages; in fact, when caught at an early, localized stage, 5-year survival rates are over 90 percent.[60] Through education, screening tests, and timely treatment, we've made remarkable progress in reducing the incidence and death rates of this cancer. However, the bad news is that in its early stages, colorectal cancer typically has no clear symptoms and only 39 percent of cases are caught in the earliest stage.[61] Because symptoms may not be obvious, large numbers of people lack access and/or insurance, and some individuals are fearful/embarrassed about screening tests, only 59 percent of those over age 50 who should be screened actually get screened.[62] Hispanics and non-English-speaking individuals have even lower rates of screening.[63] As such, far too many colorectal cancer diagnoses occur at later stages when 5-year survival rates are much lower. Men, who as a group are more reluctant to seek medical care early, tend to have a 30 to 40 percent higher rate of colorectal cancer incidence and mortality.[64] As the disease progresses, stool changes, bleeding, cramping or pain in the lower abdomen, unusual urges to have a bowel movement, unusual weight loss, decreased appetite, and unusual fatigue are the major warning signals.

Colonoscopies and other screening tests should begin at age 50 for most people. Virtual colonoscopies and fecal DNA testing are newer diagnostic techniques that have shown promise. However, only 10 percent of all Americans over age 50 have had the most basic screening test—the at-home *fecal occult blood* test (FBOT)—in the past year, and slightly over 50 percent have had an endoscopy test.[65] Rates are even lower in those who are non-white, have fewer years of education, lack health insurance, and are recent immigrants.[66]

Treatment often consists of radiation or surgery. Chemotherapy, although not used extensively in the past, is today a possibility.

Risk Factors and Prevention The older you are, the greater your chances of colorectal cancer. Although anyone can develop it, people who are over age 50, who are obese, who have a family history of colon and rectal cancer, who have a personal or family history of polyps (benign growths) in the colon or rectum, or who have inflammatory bowel problems such as colitis run an increased risk. A history of diabetes also seems to increase risk. Other possible risk factors include diets high in fat or low in fiber, high consumption of red and processed meats, smoking, sedentary lifestyle, high alcohol consumption, and low intake of fruits and vegetables.

59%

IS THE PERCENTAGE OF PEOPLE OVER THE AGE OF 50 WHO SHOULD HAVE RECOMMENDED **SCREENING TESTS** FOR COLORECTAL CANCER AND ACTUALLY GET THEM!

Following recommended screenings and paying attention to your own bowel activity are key factors in early diagnosis. If you have a history of inflammatory bowel problems such as irritable bowel syndrome (IBS), colitis, or Crohn's disease, and/or a history of type 2 diabetes, talk with your doctor about whether or not you should begin colorectal screening before age 50. Regular exercise, a diet with lots of fruits and other plant foods, maintaining a healthy weight, avoiding tobacco products, and moderation in alcohol consumption appear to be among the most promising prevention strategies. Consumption of milk and calcium and having higher blood levels of vitamin D decrease risks. New research suggests that nonsteroidal anti-inflammatory drugs (NSAIDs) such as aspirin, postmenopausal hormones, folic

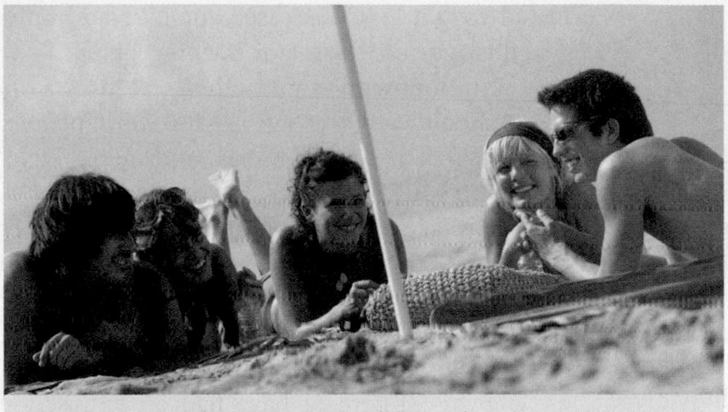

There is no such thing as a "safe" tan, because a tan is visible evidence of UV-induced skin damage. According to the American Cancer Society, tanned skin provides only the equivalent of sun protection factor (SPF) 4 sunscreen—much too weak to be protective.

acid, calcium supplements, selenium, and vitamin E may also help.[67] However, drugs are not recommended as a preventive measure as these each have other risks that might outweigh any benefit.

Skin Cancer

The exact number of basal and squamous cell skin cancers is unknown because these cases are not required to be reported to cancer registries. It is widely accepted, however, that skin cancer is the most common form of cancer in the United States today, with over 3.5 million diagnosed cases in 2014.[68] Millions more remain undiagnosed and untreated, and 1 in 5 people in the United States will be diagnosed in their lifetime! In 2014, an estimated 12,980 deaths from skin cancer will occur, 9,710 from melanoma and 3,370 from other skin cancers.[69] The two most common types of skin cancer—*basal cell* and *squamous cell carcinomas*—are highly curable. **Malignant melanoma**, the third most common form of skin cancer, is the most deadly. The majority of these deaths are in white men over the age of 50, with only rare cases among African Americans. With improved knowledge about risks, as well as greater awareness of symptoms and improved treatments, death rates are declining in whites under the age of 50. Death rates have increased slightly among those over 50, reflecting past work and recreational behaviors that put people at risk. Between 65 percent and 90 percent of melanomas are caused by exposure to ultraviolet (UV) light or sunlight. Even though death rates have declined, it is important to note that the incidence of melanoma continues to rise.[70]

malignant melanoma A virulent cancer of the melanocytes (pigment-producing cells) of the skin.

Detection, Symptoms, and Treatment Basal and squamous cell carcinomas show up most commonly on the face, ears, neck, arms, hands, and legs as warty bumps, colored spots, or scaly patches. Bleeding, itching, pain, or oozing are other symptoms that warrant attention. Surgery may be necessary to remove them, but they are seldom life threatening.

Although malignant melanoma may appear to be a harmless form of cancer initially, it's size, shape, and color often undergo distinctive changes over time. Unless one takes note of these changes, it can invade body organs and tissues with devastating consequences. Malignant melanomas account for over 75 percent of all skin cancer deaths. Like other cancers, survival is largely dependent on how advanced the cancer is when diagnosed. If melanoma has not yet penetrated the underlying layers of skin, chances of survival are over 90 percent. However, if it is diagnosed after deeper layers of skin are penetrated and it has spread to other organs, the survival rate falls to 15 percent.[71] **FIGURE 16.5** compares melanoma with basal cell and squamous cell carcinomas. The *ABCD* rule can help you remember the warning signs of melanoma:

- **Asymmetry.** One half of the mole or lesion does not match the other half.
- **Border irregularity.** The edges are uneven, notched, or scalloped.
- **Color.** Pigmentation is not uniform. Melanomas may vary in color from tan to deeper brown, reddish black, black, or deep bluish black.
- **Diameter.** Diameter is greater than 6 millimeters (about the size of a pea).

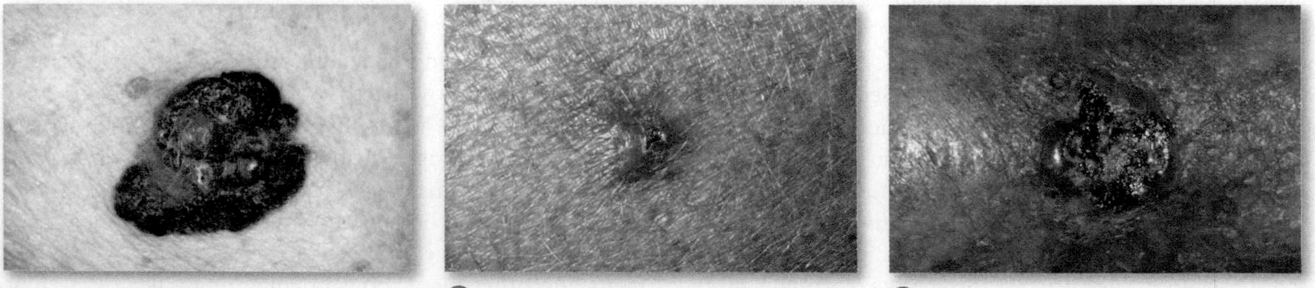

(a) Malignant melanoma (b) Basal cell carcinoma (c) Squamous cell carcinoma

FIGURE 16.5 Types of Skin Cancers Preventing skin cancer includes keeping a careful watch for any new pigmented growths and for changes to any moles. The ABCD warning signs of melanoma (a) include *a*symmetrical shapes, irregular *b*orders, *c*olor variation, and an increase in *d*iameter. Basal cell carcinoma (b) and squamous cell carcinoma (c) should be brought to your physician's attention, but they are not as deadly as melanoma.

SEE IT! VIDEOS

Is there such a thing as a "safe" tan? Watch **Extreme Tanning** available on MasteringHealth.™

Treatment of skin cancer depends on the type of cancer, its stage, and its location. Surgery, laser treatments, topical chemical agents, *electrodesiccation* (tissue destruction by heat), and *cryosurgery* (tissue destruction by freezing) are all common forms of treatment. For melanoma, treatment may involve surgical removal of the regional lymph nodes, radiation, or chemotherapy.

Risk Factors and Prevention Anyone who overexposes himself or herself to ultraviolet (UV) radiation without adequate protection is at risk for skin cancer. The risk is greatest for people who:

- Have fair skin; blonde, red, or light brown hair; blue, green, or gray eyes
- Always burn before tanning or burn easily and peel readily
- Don't tan easily but spend lots of time outdoors
- Use no or low sun protection factor (SPF) sunscreens or expired suntan lotions
- Have had skin cancer or a family history of skin cancer
- Experienced severe sunburns during childhood. Contrary to popular thinking, there is no such thing as getting a base tan that protects against damage. The greater the exposure dose and the longer the time periods of exposure, the greater the risk.

Preventing skin cancer is a matter of limiting exposure to harmful UV rays and applying broad spectrum suntan lotions liberally and often when exposed. What happens when you expose yourself to sunlight? The skin responds to photodamage by increasing its thickness and the number of pigment cells (melanocytes), which produce the "tan" look. (A tan is actually the body's way of trying to protect itself or defend against UV attack. It can fight the onslaught only for a short time before damage begins to accrue.) Ultraviolet light damages the skin's immune cells, lowering the normal immune protection of the skin and priming it for cancer. Photodamage also causes wrinkling by impairing the elastic substances (collagens) that keep skin soft and pliable. See the **Skills for Behavior Change** box for tips on staying safe in the sun.

In spite of the risks, many Americans are still "working on a tan," either outdoors or in tanning salons, prompting some psychologists to speculate that there might be a form of compulsion to tan termed "tanorexia." Tanning is thought to be addictive due to some form of brain response to UVR light, prompting physiological or psychological responses. Recent studies of young adults exposed to indoor tanning suggest a possible link to tanning dependence and activation of the reward system.[72] However, critics argue that this research is preliminary and that significant, large-scale clinical trials are necessary to confirm an association. For information on the risks of tanning salons, see the **Student Health Today** box on the next page.

SKILLS FOR BEHAVIOR CHANGE

TIPS FOR PROTECTING YOUR SKIN IN THE SUN

- Seek shade from 10 A.M. to 4 P.M., when the sun's rays are strongest. Even on a cloudy day, up to 80 percent of the sun's rays can get through.
- Apply a sunscreen with SPF 15 or higher evenly to all uncovered skin before going outside. Look for a broad-spectrum sunscreen that protects against both UVA and UVB radiation. If the sunscreen label does not specify otherwise, assume you need to apply it 15 minutes before going outside.
- Know your SPFs. You may think that a 15 SPF is only half as good as a 30 SPF and that a 100 SPF is going to block 100 percent of the damaging sun rays. Not so! An SPF 15 product typically blocks about 94 percent of UVB rays while an SPF 30 may block 97 percent. If you pay for a 70 to 100 SPF product you are probably just wasting your money. New regulations are in play designed to simply say 50+ SPF so that consumers are not led on a merry chase, paying more for no more benefit.
- Check the expiration date on your sunscreen. Sunscreens lose effectiveness over time. Ditch that suntan lotion in your medicine cabinet from 3 to 5 years ago when you went to Lake Shasta or Florida for spring break. If it doesn't *have* an expiration date, it is probably so old that they weren't required. Don't waste your time with expired products!
- Put sunscreen on your lips, nose, ears, neck, hands, and feet. If you don't have much hair, apply sunscreen to the top of your head, too. Most people do not apply sunscreen liberally enough! Did you know that you should probably apply half a typical tube of lotion at each sun outing? One to 2 ounces are suggested, applied liberally and often.
- Reapply sunscreen at least every 2 hours. It is recommended that you apply at least 15 minutes before getting into water or before lying out on the beach so that it is absorbed and likely to protect you. The label will tell you how often you need to do this. If it isn't waterproof, reapply after swimming or if you are sweating.
- Wear loose-fitting, light-colored clothing. For extra protection, in most sporting goods stores you can now purchase clothing that has SPF protection. A wide-brimmed hat will protect your head and face.
- Buy good quality sunglasses from reputable companies rather than the $5 to $10 versions available at beachside stands. Make sure they cover your entire eye and don't allow lots of sunlight in the corners and edges of your eye. Use sunglasses with 99 to 100 percent UV protection to protect your eyes. Look for polarized lenses.
- Check your skin for cancer, keeping an eye out for changes in birthmarks, moles, or sunspots.

Source: U.S. Food and Drug Administration, "FDA Sheds Light on Sunscreens," 2013, www.fda.gov/ForConsumers/ConsumerUpdates/ucm258416.htm.

STUDENT HEALTH TODAY

INDOOR TANNING

Sacrificing Health for Beauty

In our culture, being tan is equated with being healthy, chic, and attractive. In a study of nearly 3,000 adults, over 18 percent of women and nearly 6.5 percent of men report tanning in the last 12 months. Teens and 20-somethings are the most likely to be users of indoor tanning overall. Indoor tanning is a multi-billion-dollar industry. But users should know that their "glow" comes with a greatly increased cancer risk.

Many people believe—incorrectly—that tanning booths are safer than sitting in the sun. But all tanning lamps emit UVA rays, and most emit UVB rays as well. Both types of light rays cause long-term skin damage and can contribute to cancer. Consider the following:

- Studies have found that there is a 59 percent increased risk of melanoma in those exposed to regular UV radiation from tanning beds. The evidence from these studies has been so compelling that tanning devices have been listed as carcinogenic for humans.
- People who use tanning beds are 2.5 times more likely to develop squamous cell carcinoma and 1.5 times more likely to develop basal cell carcinoma.
- New high-pressure sunlamps used in some salons emit doses of UV radiation that can be as much as 12 times that of the sun.
- People who tan regularly end up with older-looking skin. Up to 90 percent of visible skin changes commonly blamed on aging are caused by the sun.
- More than 30 states have restricted access to tanning booths to minors or require parental consent for minor use. Others are considering more stringent regulations, with professional groups calling for banning sales of tanning equipment for nonmedical use.

Because of the many salons that are springing up across the country, the artificial tanning industry is difficult to monitor and proposals for federal legislation to ban minor use of tanning facilities are being considered. Some tanning facilities do not calibrate the UV output of their tanning bulbs or ensure sufficient rotation of newer and older bulbs, which can lead to more or less exposure than you paid for. And unlike most beachgoers, tanning facility patrons often try for a total body tan. This is a problem because the buttocks and genitalia are particularly sensitive to UV radiation and are prone to developing skin cancer.

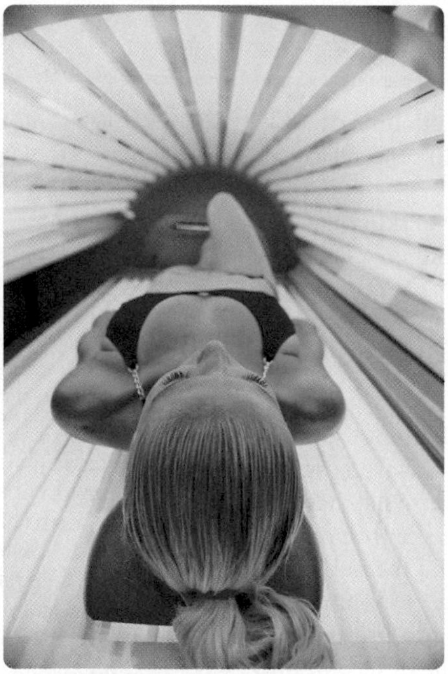

Indoor tanning—greatly increased risk of melanoma comes along with the "golden glow."

Finally, shared tanning booths and beds pose significant hygiene risks. Anytime you come in contact with body secretions from others, you run the risk of an infectious disease. Don't assume that those little colored water sprayers used to "clean" the inside of the beds are sufficient to kill organisms. The busier the facility, the more likely you are to come into contact with germs that could make you ill.

Sources: NCSL, "Indoor Tanning Restrictions for Minors—A State-by-State Comparison," May 2014, www.ncsl.org/research/health/indoor-tanning-restrictions.aspx; American College of Dermatology, "The Dangers of Indoor Tanning Beds," 2014, www.aad.org/spot-skin-cancer/understanding-skin-cancer/dangers-of-indoor-tanning; D. Lazovich et al., "Indoor Tanning and Risk of Melanoma: A Case-Control Study in a Highly Exposed Population," *Cancer Epidemiology Biomarkers and Prevention* 19, no. 6 (2010): 1557–68, DOI:10.1158/1055-9965.EPI-09-1249; National Cancer Institute, "Tanning Bed Study Shows Strongest Evidence Yet of Increased Melanoma Risk," *NCI Cancer Bulletin*, 2010, www.cancer.gov/ncicancerbulletin/060110/page2; Skin Cancer Foundation, "Skin Cancer Facts," 2012, www.skincancer.org/skin-cancer-information/skin-cancer-facts.

Prostate Cancer

After skin cancer, prostate cancer is the most frequently diagnosed cancer in American males today. It is the second leading cause of cancer deaths in men after lung cancer. In 2014, about 233,000 new cases of prostate cancer were diagnosed in the United States. Although the reasons are unclear, African American rates of prostate cancer are about 60 percent higher than in non-Hispanic whites. About 1 in 6 men will be diagnosed with prostate cancer during his lifetime. However, with improved screening and early diagnosis, 5-year survival rates are nearly 100 percent for all but the most advanced cases. Men who are obese and smoke have an increased risk of dying from prostate cancer.[73]

prostate-specific antigen (PSA) An antigen found in prostate cancer patients.

Detection, Symptoms, and Treatment The prostate is a muscular, walnut-sized gland that surrounds part of a man's urethra, the tube that transports urine and sperm out of the body. A part of the reproductive system, its primary function is to produce seminal fluid. Often, early stages of prostate cancer have no symptoms. As the disease progresses, symptoms may include weak or interrupted urine flow; difficulty starting or stopping urination; feeling the urge to urinate frequently, particularly at night; pain on urination; and blood in the urine. Prostate cancer often spreads to the bones if not treated early; unexplained pain in the hips, low back, ribs, or other areas may indicate the cancer has spread.

Men over age 40 should have an annual digital rectal prostate examination. Another screening method for prostate cancer is the **prostate-specific antigen (PSA)** test, a blood test

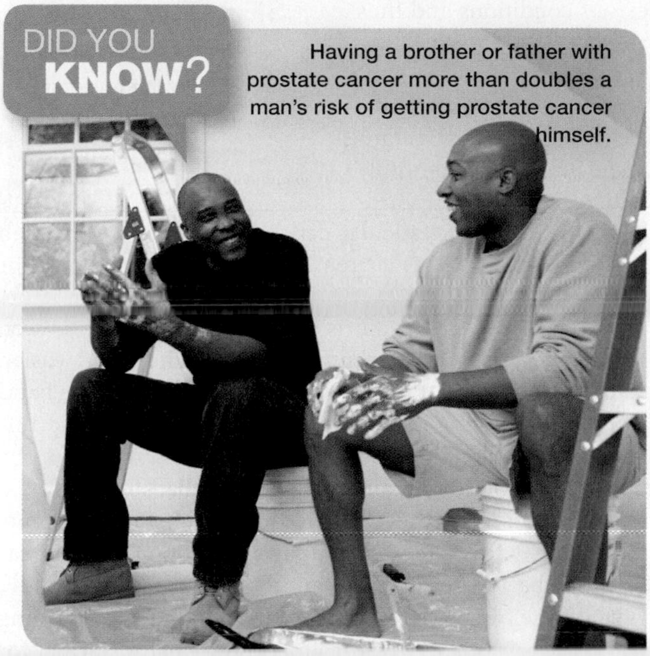

that screens for an indicator of prostate cancer. However, the United States Preventive Services Task Force recommends that otherwise asymptomatic men no longer receive the routine PSA test because, overall, it does not save lives and may in fact lead to painful, unnecessary cancer treatments. If you have a family history or other symptoms, consult with your physician.

Risk Factors and Prevention Increasing age is one of the biggest risks for prostate cancer, as is African ancestry or a family history of prostate cancer. In fact, over 97 percent of all cases occur in men over the age of 50.[74]

African American men and Jamaican men of African descent have the highest documented prostate cancer incidence rates in the world and are more likely to be diagnosed at more advanced stages than other racial groups.[75]

Having a father or brother with prostate cancer more than doubles a man's risk of getting prostate cancer. Men who have had several relatives with prostate cancer, especially those with relatives who developed prostate cancer at younger ages, are also at higher risk.[76]

Eating more fruits and vegetables, particularly those containing *lycopene*, a pigment found in tomatoes and other red fruits, may lower the risk of prostate cancer death; however, more research is necessary to determine why.[77] Diets high in processed meats or dairy and obesity also appear to increase risks.[78] The best advice is to follow the dietary recommendations of the U.S. Department of Agriculture discussed in **Chapter 7** and maintain a healthy weight.

There is some evidence that risk for prostate cancer is elevated in firefighters. Although there have been some indicators that certain infectious diseases may increase the risk of prostate cancer, research is inconclusive.[79]

Ovarian Cancer

Ovarian cancer is the fifth leading cause of cancer deaths for women, with about 22,000 diagnosed in 2012 and 14,270 dying from it.[80] Ovarian cancer causes more deaths than any other cancer of the reproductive system because women tend not to discover it until the cancer is at an advanced stage. If detected when localized, 5-year survival rates are 92 percent. If diagnosed at the regional level, rates drop to 72 percent, and if metastasis is diffuse and distant, survival rates drop to 27 percent.[81]

Detection, Symptoms, and Treatment Ovarian cancer symptoms are often not obvious, and it is common for women to have no early symptoms at all. A woman may complain of feeling bloated, having pain in the pelvic area, feeling full quickly, or feeling the need to urinate more frequently. Some may experience persistent digestive disturbances, while other symptoms include fatigue, pain during intercourse, unexplained weight loss, unexplained changes in bowel or bladder habits, and incontinence. If these vague symptoms persist for more than a week or two, prompt medical evaluation is a must.

Treatment for early-stage ovarian cancer typically includes surgery, chemotherapy, and occasionally radiation therapy. Depending on the patient's age and her desire to bear children in the future, one or both ovaries, fallopian tubes, and the uterus may be removed.

Risk Factors and Prevention Primary relatives (mother, daughter, sister) of a woman who has had breast or ovarian cancer are at increased risk, as are those with a family or personal history of breast or colon cancer (particularly those with positive *BRCA1* or *BRCA2* tests). Women who have never been pregnant are more likely to develop ovarian cancer than those who have given birth, and the more children a woman has had, the less risk she faces. The use of estrogen alone as postmenopausal therapy may increase a woman's risk, as will smoking and obesity.[82]

Research shows that long-term use of oral contraceptives, adhering to a low-fat diet, having multiple children, breastfeeding, and tubal ligation may reduce your risk of ovarian cancer.[83] So, should you get pregnant or start taking birth control pills to reduce risk? No. General prevention strategies such as focusing on diet, exercise, sleep, stress management, and weight control are good ideas for combating cancer risk.

To protect yourself, get a complete annual pelvic examination. Women over 40 should have a cancer-related checkup every year. Uterine ultrasound or a blood test is recommended for those with risk factors or unexplained symptoms.

Cervical and Endometrial (Uterine) Cancer

Most uterine cancers develop in the body of the uterus, usually in the endometrium. The rest develop in the cervix, located at the base of the uterus. In 2014, an estimated 12,360 new cases of cervical cancer and 52,630 cases of endometrial cancer were diagnosed in the United States.[84] As more women have regular **Pap test** screenings—a procedure in which cells taken from the

Pap test A procedure in which cells taken from the cervical region are examined for abnormal cellular activity.

cervical region are examined for abnormal activity—rates should decline even further in the future. As of 2013, it is recommended women get a Pap test every 2 years beginning at age 21. Between ages 30 and 65, women should have an HPV and Pap test every 5 years and a Pap test alone every 3 years. Those with parents and/or siblings with breast cancer should talk with their doctor about having tests more frequently.

Although Pap tests are very effective for detecting early-stage cervical cancer, they are less effective for detecting cancers of the uterine lining. Women have a lifetime risk of 1 in 151 for being diagnosed with cervical cancer and a 1 in 37 risk of being diagnosed with uterine corpus cancer.[85] Early warning signs of uterine cancer include bleeding outside the normal menstrual period or after menopause, or persistent unusual vaginal discharge.

Risk factors for cervical cancer include early age at first intercourse, multiple sex partners, cigarette smoking, and certain sexually transmitted infections, including HPV (the cause of genital warts) and herpes. Today, both young men and women have the option of getting vaccinated against HPV. For endometrial cancer, age is a risk factor; however, estrogen and obesity are also strong risk factors. In addition, risks are increased by treatment with tamoxifen for breast cancer, metabolic syndrome, late menopause, never bearing children, a history of polyps in the uterus or ovaries, a history of other cancers, and race (white women are at higher risk).[86]

Testicular Cancer

Testicular cancer is one of the most common types of solid tumors found in young adult men, affecting nearly 8,820 men in 2014.[87] Over one half of all cases occur between the ages of 20 and 34, with steady increases in this group over the last few years.[88] However, with a 95 percent 5-year survival rate, it is one of the most curable forms of cancer, particularly if caught in localized stages. Although the cause of testicular cancer is unknown, several risk factors have been identified. Men with undescended testicles appear to be at greatest risk, and some studies indicate a genetic influence. Risk is also higher if you are white, have HIV or AIDS, or if a primary relative (father or brother, in particular) has had testicular cancer.[89]

Testicular Self-Exam In general, testicular tumors first appear as an enlargement of the testis or thickening in testicular tissue. Some men report a heavy feeling, dull ache, or pain that extends to the lower abdomen or groin area. Testicular self-exams have long been recommended for teen boys and young men to perform monthly as a means of detecting testicular cancer (see **FIGURE 16.6**). However, recent studies discovered that findings from monthly self-exams result in testing for noncancerous conditions and thus are not cost-effective. For this reason, the U.S. Preventive Services Task Force has dropped their recommendation for monthly testicular exams. Regardless, most cases of testicular cancer are discovered through self-exam, and there is currently no other screening test for the disease.

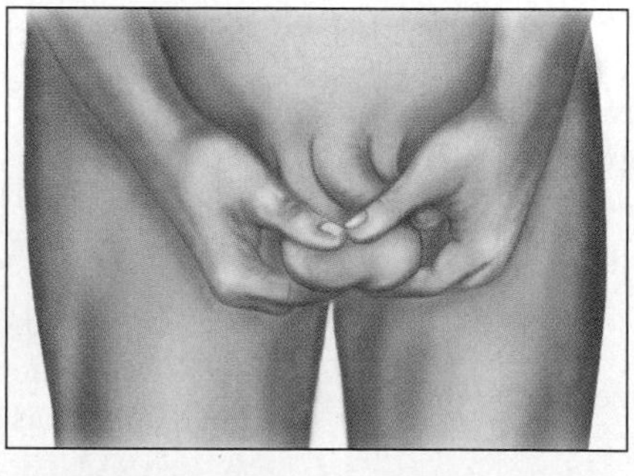

FIGURE 16.6 Testicular Self-Exam

Source: From Michael Johnson, *Human Biology: Concepts and Current Issues*, 3rd ed. Copyright © 2006. Reprinted with permission of Pearson Education, Inc.

SEE IT! VIDEOS

How can you prevent cervical cancer? Watch **Preventing Cervical Cancer** available on MasteringHealth.™

The testicular self-exam is best done after a hot shower, which will relax the scrotum and make the exam easier. Standing in front of a mirror, hold the testicle with one hand while gently rolling its surface between the thumb and fingers of your other hand. Feel underneath the scrotum for the tubes of the epididymis and blood vessels that sit close to the body. Repeat with the other testicle. Look for any lump, thickening, or pealike nodules, paying attention to any areas that may be painful over the entire surface of the scrotum. When done, wash your hands with soap and water. Doing regular self-exams will help you to know what is normal for you and to note any irregularity. Consult a doctor if you note anything that is unusual.

Leukemia

Leukemia is a cancer of the blood-forming tissues that leads to proliferation of millions of immature white blood cells. These abnormal cells crowd out normal white blood cells (which fight infection), platelets (which control hemorrhaging), and red blood cells (which carry oxygen to body cells). Resulting symptoms include fatigue, paleness, weight loss, easy bruising, repeated infections, nosebleeds, and other forms of hemorrhaging.

Leukemia can be acute or chronic and can strike both sexes and all age groups. An estimated 52,380 new cases were diagnosed in the United States in 2014.[90] Chronic leukemia can develop over several months and have few symptoms. It is usually treated with radiation and chemotherapy. Other treatments include bone marrow and stem cell transplants.

Lymphoma

Just a few short years ago, not many people had heard much about lymphomas, a group of cancers of the lymphatic system that include Hodgkin disease and non-Hodgkin lymphoma. Today, however, lymphomas are among the fastest growing cancers, with an estimated 79,990 new cases in 2014.[91] Much of this increase has occurred in women and, like many cancers, risk increases with age. The cause is unknown; however, a weakened immune system is suspected—particularly one that has been exposed to viruses such as HIV, hepatitis C, Epstein-Barr virus (EBV), and others. Treatment and prognosis for lymphoma varies by type and stage; however, chemotherapy and radiotherapy are commonly used. If detected early, survival rates are high.

Pancreatic Cancer

In 2014, nearly 46,500 people will get the dreaded diagnosis of cancer of the pancreas, one of the deadliest forms of cancer. In spite of advances in diagnosis and treatment, only 27 percent survive 1 year after diagnosis, and only 6 percent survive 5 years.[92] Although most cases occur after age 50, there are increasing numbers of cases at earlier ages. Overall, rates are higher in African Americans and in populations with lower socioeconomic status and education levels. They are also about 30 percent higher in men than women.[93]

Key risk factors appear to be tobacco use, obesity, consuming high levels of red meat, and high-fat diet. Family history, genetic links, and a history of chronic inflammation of the pancreas (*pancreatitis*) also seem to increase risk. There appears to be a greater risk among diabetics and those who have had infections with hepatitis B and C and the *Helicobacter* bacteria. Because pancreatic cancer has few early symptoms, there is no reliable test to detect it in its early stages. When symptoms begin, weight loss, stomach discomfort, and pain that may radiate to the back may occur. Often, by the time it is diagnosed via CAT or MRI examinations, it is too advanced to treat effectively.

LO 5 | FACING CANCER

Discuss cancer diagnosis and treatment, including radiotherapy and chemotherapy and other common methods of detection and treatment, indicating where we've made progress in recent decades.

There is much you can do to reduce your own risk of cancer. Make a realistic assessment of your own risk factors, avoid behaviors that put you at risk, and increase healthy behaviors. Even if you have significant risks, those are factors you can control. Avoid known carcinogens and other environmental hazards, and follow the recommendations for self-exams and medical checkups in TABLE 16.2. The earlier cancer is diagnosed, the better the prognosis will be.

magnetic resonance imaging (MRI) A device that uses magnetic fields, radio waves, and computers to generate an image of internal tissues of the body for diagnostic purposes without the use of radiation.

computerized axial tomography (CAT) scan A scan by a machine that uses radiation to view internal organs not normally visible in X-rays.

Detecting Cancer

If you are at high risk for developing cancer, or if you notice potential cancer symptoms, your health care provider might use one or more tests to diagnose or rule out cancer. **Magnetic resonance imaging (MRI)** uses a huge electromagnet to detect tumors by mapping the vibrations of the atoms in the body on a computer screen. The **computerized axial tomography (CAT) scan** uses X-rays to examine parts of the

TABLE 16.2 | Screening Guidelines for Early Cancer Detection in Average Risk and Asymptomatic People

Cancer Site	Screening Procedure	Age and Frequency of Test
Breast	Mammograms	The NCI recommends that women in their forties and older have mammograms every 1 to 2 years. Women who are at higher-than-average risk of breast cancer should talk with their health care provider about whether to have mammograms before age 40 and how often to have them.
Cervix	Pap test (Pap smear)	Women should begin having Pap tests 3 years after they begin having sexual intercourse or when they reach age 21 (whichever comes first). Most women should have a Pap test at least once every 3 years.
Colon and rectum	***Fecal occult blood test:*** Sometimes cancer or polyps bleed. This test can detect tiny amounts of blood in the stool. ***Sigmoidoscopy:*** Checks the rectum and lower part of the colon for polyps. ***Colonoscopy:*** Checks the rectum and entire colon for polyps and cancer.	People aged 50 and older should be screened. People who have a higher-than-average risk of cancer of the colon or rectum should talk with their doctor about whether to have screening tests before age 50 and how often to have them.
Prostate	Prostate-specific antigen (PSA) test	Some groups encourage yearly screening for men over age 50, and some advise men who are at a higher risk for prostate cancer to begin screening at age 40 or 45. Others caution against routine screening. Currently, Medicare provides coverage for an annual PSA test for all men age 50 and older.

Sources: National Cancer Institute, National Institutes of Health, "What You Need to Know About Cancer Screening," 2012, www.cancer.gov/cancertopics/wyntk/cancer/page4; National Cancer Institute, "Fact Sheet, Prostate-Specific Antigen (PSA) Test," 2012, www.cancer.gov/cancertopics/factsheet/detection/PSA.

stereotactic radiosurgery A type of radiation therapy that can be used to zap tumors; also known as gamma knife surgery.

gamma knife surgery *See* stereotactic radiosurgery.

radiotherapy The use of radiation to kill cancerous cells.

chemotherapy The use of drugs to kill cancerous cells.

body. In both of these painless, noninvasive procedures, cross-sectioned pictures can reveal a tumor's shape and location more accurately than can conventional X-rays. *Prostatic ultrasound* (a rectal probe using ultrasonic waves to produce an image of the prostate) is being investigated as a means to increase the early detection of prostate cancer. In 2011, the FDA approved the first 3D mammogram machines, which offer significant improvements in imaging and breast cancer detection but deliver nearly double the radiation risk of conventional mammograms.

Cancer Treatments

Cancer treatments vary according to the type and stage of cancer. Surgery, in which the tumor and surrounding tissue are removed, is one common strategy. It may be performed alone or in combination with other treatments. The surgeon may operate using traditional surgical instruments such as a scalpel, or by using a laser, laparoscope, or other tools for less invasive results. Pain and infection are the most common problems after surgery.

Stereotactic radiosurgery, also known as **gamma knife surgery**, uses a targeted dose of gamma radiation to zap tumors with pinpoint accuracy without any blood loss or ever using a scalpel. **Radiotherapy** (the use of radiation) or **chemotherapy** (the use of drugs) to kill cancerous cells are also used. Radiation destroys malignant cells or stops cell growth. It is most effective in treating localized cancer masses because it can be targeted to a particular area of the body. Over the course of several weeks, patients are treated by a machine that exposes the designated part of the body to high-energy rays. Radiotherapy usually takes place on an outpatient basis. Side effects include fatigue, changes to the skin in the affected area, and a small increase in the chance of developing another type of cancer.

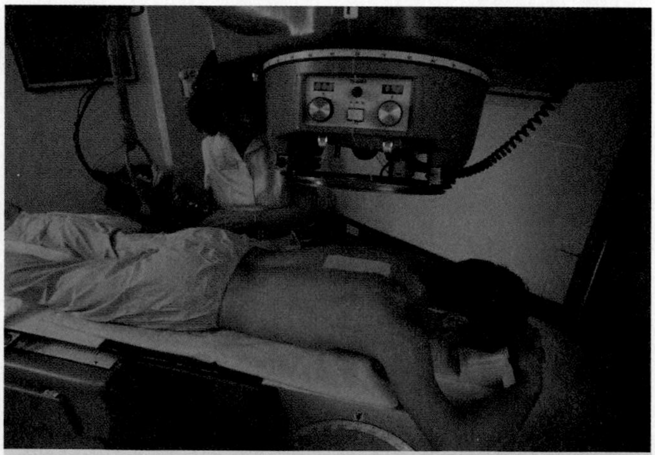

Radiation therapy is often used to target and destroy cancerous tumors. The machine in this photograph emits gamma rays, which are typically used to treat localized secondary cancers and also provide pain relief for otherwise untreatable cancers. Gamma rays are less powerful than the X-rays emitted from linear accelerators, another machine frequently used in radiation therapy.

Chemotherapy may be used to shrink a tumor before surgery or radiation therapy, after surgery or radiation therapy to kill remaining cancer cells, or on its own. Powerful drugs, often targeted for specific tumors, are given, usually in on-and-off cycles so the body can recover from their effects. Side effects may include nausea, hair loss, fatigue, increased chance of bleeding, bruising, infection, and anemia, among others. These usually diminish as the drugs leave the body after treatment. Other possible effects include loss of fertility, damage to blood vessels, and memory loss. In the process of killing malignant cells, some healthy cells are also destroyed, and long-term damage to the cardiovascular system and other body systems can be significant.

Participation in clinical trials (people-based studies of new drugs or procedures) has provided a new source of hope for many patients undergoing cancer treatment. Because of the many unknown variables, deciding whether to participate in a clinical trial can be a difficult decision. Despite the risks, thousands of clinical trial participants have benefited from treatments that would otherwise be unavailable to them.

Several newer treatments described in the **Health Headlines** box are either being used in clinical trials or have become available in selected cancer centers throughout the country. In addition, psychosocial and behavioral research has become increasingly important as health professionals learn more about lifestyle factors that influence risk and survivability. Health practitioners have begun to tailor treatment programs to meet the diverse psychological needs of patients and families.

Before beginning any form of cancer therapy, it is imperative to be a vigilant and vocal consumer. Read and seek information from cancer support groups. Check the skills of your surgeon, your radiation therapist, and your doctor in terms of clinical experience and interpersonal interactions. Look at *Oncolink* and other websites supported by the *National Cancer Institute* and the *American Cancer Society (ACS)*, and check out clinical trials, reports on effectiveness of various treatments, new experimental therapies, and other options. Although you may like and trust your family doctor, it is always a good idea to seek advice or consultation from large cancer facilities that see many patients and are well equipped to deal with all situations. Do not be afraid to question health care providers about options and their reasons for selecting one course of treatment over another. Check the credentials and specialty areas of your oncologist and try to find the best match for your type of cancer. See the **Student Health Today** box on page 474 for more on being your own advocate or an advocate for someone you love.

@ HEALTH HEADLINES

NEW TREATMENTS FOR CANCER

Surgery, chemotherapy, and radiation therapy remain the most common treatments for all types of cancer. However, newer techniques are constantly being investigated that may be more effective for certain cancers or certain patients:

- **Immunotherapy.** The goal of immunotherapy is to enhance the body's own disease-fighting systems. Biological response modifiers such as interferon and interleukin-2 are under study. Immunotherapies have been particularly effective against melanomas and certain kidney cancers.
- **Biological therapies.** One of the most exciting new approaches for spurring the immune system to ward off cancer is the use of *cancer-fighting vaccines*. These alert the body's immune defenses to good cells that have gone bad. Rather than preventing disease as other vaccines do, they help people who are already ill.
- **Gene therapies.** Research on the effectiveness of *gene therapy* has moved into early clinical trials. Scientists have found signs of a virus carrying genetic information that makes the cells it infects (such as cancer cells) susceptible to an antiviral drug. Scientists are also looking at ways to transfer genes that increase the patient's immune response to the cancerous tumor or that confer drug resistance to the bone marrow to allow higher doses of chemotherapeutic drugs.
- **Angiogenesis inhibitors.** Researchers are testing compounds that may stop tumors from forming new blood vessels, a process called *angiogenesis*. Without adequate blood supply, tumors either die or grow very slowly, giving other chemotherapeutic agents a better chance to fight them.
- **Disrupting cancer pathways.** In recent years, scientists have identified various steps in what is termed the *cancer pathway*. These include oncogene actions, hormone receptors, growth factors, metastasis, and angiogenesis. Preliminary studies are under way to design compounds that inhibit actions at these various steps.
- **Smart "bullet" drugs.** Drugs such as T-DM1 (which combines chemotherapy and targeted antibodies), Herceptin, Gleevec, and Avastin are new forms of *targeted smart-drug therapies* that deliver chemotherapy to attack only the cancer cells and avoid healthy cells, which helps patients avoid severe sickness during aggressive treatments.
- **Enzyme inhibitors.** A powerful enzyme inhibitor, TIMP2, shows promise for slowing the metastasis of tumor cells. A metastasis suppressor gene, *NM23*, has also been identified. Both of these therapies are aimed at disrupting cancer pathways.
- **Neoadjuvant chemotherapy.** This method (which uses chemotherapy to shrink the tumor and then surgically removing it) has been tried against various types of cancers.
- **Stem cell research.** When a patient's bone marrow has been destroyed by disease, chemotherapy, or radiation, transplants of stem cells from donor bone marrow may successfully restore blood stem cells (the cells that divide to produce blood cells).

LO 6 | CANCER SURVIVORS

Discuss what it really means to be a "cancer survivor" and how it means more than living cancer free for 5 years after diagnosis.

Today, an increasing number of people in the United States and globally survive cancer with less disease burden and disability, better outcomes in terms of healthy years, and fewer problems than any previous generation. Although a diagnosis of cancer is never easy, living with cancer is less traumatic than ever before, largely due to heightened public awareness, less stigma, and a much greater level of support for cancer patients. Cancer patients are much less likely to face cancer alone or make decisions about treatment in isolation. Cancer support groups, cancer information workshops, and low-cost medical consultation are widely available via a wide range of information networks. Groups such as the Susan G. Komen for the Cure Foundation have provided support for survivors and their families and have helped people realize that cancer is not a death sentence or something to be hidden. Coping with cancer can be difficult, but there are ways to ease the burden and make surviving less challenging for all concerned.[94]

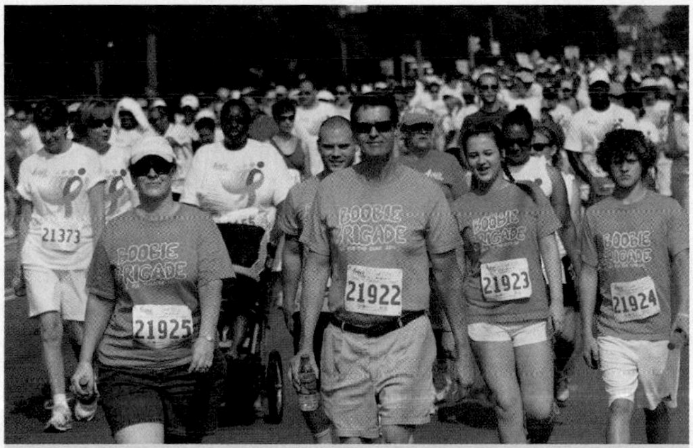

There may be physical and emotional issues as well as financial issues related to health insurance and cost of care to cope with for years after cancer diagnosis and treatment. Survivors also have to live with the possibility of a recurrence. However, cancer survivors can and do live active, productive lives despite these challenges. Many survivors and their relatives find it emotionally satisfying to participate in cancer research fund-raiser walks and other events.

STUDENT HEALTH TODAY

BEING A HEALTH ADVOCATE FOR YOURSELF OR SOMEONE YOU LOVE

When cancer is diagnosed, people often react with anxiety, fear, and anger. Emotional distress is sometimes so intense that patients and their loved ones are unable to make critical health care decisions. Sometimes, they are unable to understand how a treatment will really work or what the risks vs. benefits are. If you or a loved one is diagnosed with cancer, the following actions can help you remain calm as you check out available treatment options:

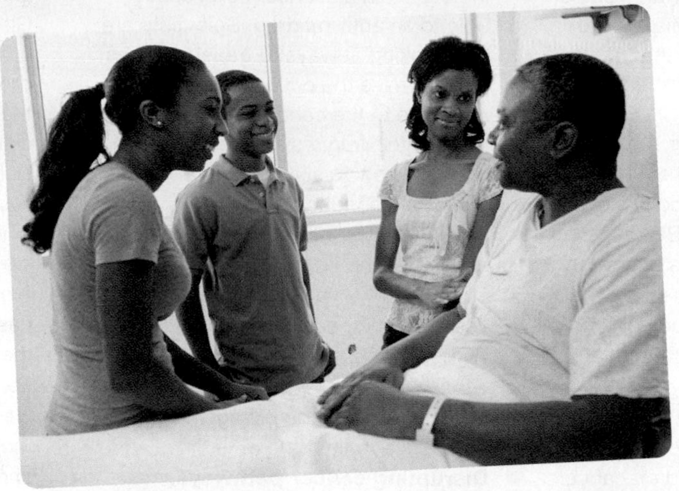

If you or someone you love is diagnosed with cancer, it is important to seek out all the help and information that you can find.

- **Pair up for doctor appointments.** Even suspecting cancer can cause fear and shock, and that can prevent a patient from asking important questions or from hearing key details. Bring a trusted friend or relative with you to the doctor, and talk together about what you heard later.
- **Find out as much as possible about the cancer.** Before you go to your appointment, *read widely* about your suspected cancer. There are numerous sources that can help you understand your treatment options, long-term prognosis, and overall options. Don't be afraid to ask questions. If your doctor acts too busy to answer or acts annoyed, find another doctor. Questions you might ask include an explanation of the type and stage of cancer, the recommended treatment plan, and the potential risks and benefits. Read about your cancer on reliable websites such as the American Cancer Society or the National Cancer Institute. If your doctor recommends that you participate in a clinical drug trial, request a copy of the documents outlining potential risks and benefits. Remember that not everyone in a clinical trial gets the experimental treatment right away. If you are in the control group (placebo) group, when will you get the treatment? Can you afford to wait?
- **Get a second opinion.** Request a copy of the diagnostic test results and get an "out of group" physician (someone unaffiliated with your original doctor) to review them. Find an oncologist (cancer specialist) at a big teaching hospital where they see a large number of patients with your type of cancer. Don't worry about hurting the original doctor's feelings. This is a common practice. Remember, it's your life!
- **Check out the credentials of the hospital, surgeon, and treatment specialist.** If surgery is recommended, find out about the patient-to-caregiver ratio in the hospital and the plan for aftercare. Ask for recommendations from patients who've had the procedures that are planned for you. When you go in for scans, ask if they have the newest generation of CT scanners and other radiation emitting equipment. Older generation scanners can expose you to more radiation than newer scanners.
- **Find local resources and support groups.** It can be helpful to talk with someone who isn't emotionally involved in your personal situation. Survivor support groups can provide information you can get only from people who have lived through cancer. Talking with a counselor is another good way to keep the focus on getting well.
- **Get your personal ducks in a row.** Write down financial information, where to find important papers, passwords for computer files, and key bits of information. It's always a good idea to have a file box with detailed documentation of the above, as well as your advanced directives and other medical wishes, even when you don't have an actual cancer diagnosis. Find someone to take care of your home and pets if you will be hospitalized and someone who can bring you home when you are released.
- **Know what insurance does and doesn't cover.** Call your insurer ahead of time and know what procedures require permission. Find out what percentage of the bill is the patient's responsibility and how this may change if you need to see specialists. If you do not have insurance, talk with social service agencies, your student health center financial director, or others who can help you come up with a plan for payment.
- **Mobilize family and friends to help.** If you or your loved one will be bedridden, ask friends to make and deliver dinners, do errands, take you for follow-up appointments, or help around the house. Don't be afraid to ask for the help you need. Friends and family usually want to have some concrete way to help in times of crisis. Let others "in." Encourage your loved ones to share thoughts and fears.

Although survival used to be measured almost exclusively by whether a person had gone 5 years without cancer symptoms, **survivorship** is now viewed much more broadly in terms of both years and the quality of life that a person experiences after diagnosis. Today, survivorship comprises the unique ways in which people survive and thrive after cancer has been diagnosed. The National Cancer Institute defines this term as the "physical, psychological, emotional, and economic issues of cancer from diagnosis until the end of life."[95]

Accumulating evidence makes clear that breast cancer survivorship, for example, is influenced by a constellation of important factors, including age, socioeconomic status, availability of support services, education level, relationship status, social support, sexual identity, race, stress level, coping style, spirituality, and depression.

survivorship Physical, psychological, emotional, and economic issues of cancer from diagnosis until the end of life.

Rather than looking only at the number of years people survive, quality of the survival experience is becoming increasingly important. In fact, quality-of-life measures may influence whether a person actually reaches the 5-year survivor milestone.

STUDY PLAN

Customize your study plan—and master your health!—in the Study Area of **MasteringHealth.**

ASSESS **YOURSELF**

Could you be at risk for cancer? Want to find out? Take the **What's Your Personal Risk for Cancer?** assessment available on MasteringHealth.™

Need help creating a plan? Follow the strategies in the **Your Plan for Change** box for short- and long-term improvements to your health.

YOUR PLAN FOR **CHANGE**

If the **ASSESS YOURSELF** activity identified particular risky behaviors you want to change, follow these steps:

TODAY, YOU CAN:

- ☐ Assess your personal risks for specific cancers, looking at lifestyle as well as your genetic risks. For which cancers might you be most at risk?
- ☐ Take advantage of the salad bar in your dining hall for lunch or dinner and load up on greens, or request veggies such as steamed broccoli or sautéed spinach.

WITHIN THE NEXT 2 WEEKS, YOU CAN:

- ☐ Buy a bottle of broad-spectrum sunscreen (with SPF 15 or higher) and begin applying it liberally as part of your daily routine. (Be sure to check the expiration date, particularly on sale items!) Also, stay in the shade from 10 A.M. to 4 P.M., as this is when the sun is strongest.
- ☐ Find out your family health history. Talk to your parents, grandparents, or an aunt or uncle to find out if family members have developed cancer. This will help you assess your own genetic risk.

BY THE END OF THE SEMESTER, YOU CAN:

- ☐ Work toward achieving a healthy weight. If you aren't already engaged in a regular exercise program, begin one now. Maintaining a healthy body weight and exercising regularly will lower your risk for cancer.
- ☐ Stop smoking, avoid secondhand smoke, and limit your alcohol intake.

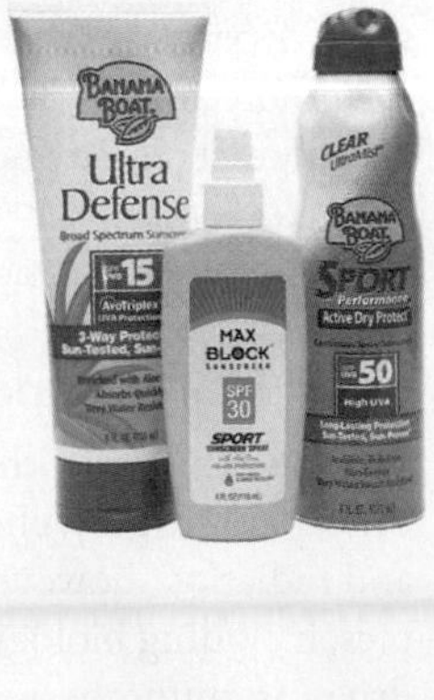

CHAPTER **REVIEW**

To hear an MP3 Tutor Session, scan here or visit the Study Area in **MasteringHealth**.

LO 1 | An Overview of Cancer

- Cancer is the second most common cause of death in the United States. The current 5-year survival rates for cancer have greatly increased from those of previous generations.

LO 2 | What Is Cancer?

- Cancer is a group of diseases characterized by uncontrolled growth and spread of abnormal cells. These cells may create tumors. Benign (noncancerous) tumors grow in size but do not spread; malignant (cancerous) tumors spread to other parts of the body.

LO 3 | What Causes Cancer?

- Lifestyle factors for cancer include smoking and obesity as well as poor diet, lack of exercise, stress, and other factors. Biological factors include inherited genes, age, and gender. Potential environmental carcinogens include asbestos, radiation, preservatives, and pesticides. Infectious agents may increase your risks for cancer; those that appear most likely to cause cancer are chronic hepatitis B and C, human papillomavirus, and genital herpes. Medical factors may elevate the chance of cancer.

LO 4 | Types of Cancers

- There are many different types of cancer, each of which poses different risks, depending on several factors. Common cancers include that of the lung, breast, colon and rectum, skin, prostate, testis, ovary, and uterus; leukemia; and lymphomas.

LO 5 | Facing Cancer

- The most common treatments for cancer are surgery, chemotherapy, and radiation; however, newer therapies, including biologicals, smart drugs, immunotherapy, and others, show promising results and should always be considered.
- Early diagnosis improves survival rate. Self-exams for breast, testicular, and skin cancer aid early diagnosis.

LO 6 | Cancer Survivors

- The number of cancer survivors is at an all-time high. Surviving cancer is viewed in terms of both the years of life and the quality of life a person experiences after diagnosis.

POP **QUIZ**

Visit **MasteringHealth** to personalize your study plan with Chapter Review Quizzes and Dynamic Study Modules.

LO 1 | An Overview of Cancer

1. Overall, which cancer has the worst 5-year survival rate today?
   a. Prostate
   b. Pancreas
   c. Melanoma
   d. Breast

LO 2 | What Is Cancer?

2. When cancer cells have *metastasized,*
   a. they have grown into a malignant tumor.
   b. they have spread to other parts of the body.
   c. the cancer is retreating and cancer cells are dying off.
   d. the tumor is localized and considered *in situ*.
3. A cancerous *neoplasm* is
   a. a type of biopsy.
   b. a form of benign tumor.
   c. a type of treatment for a tumor.
   d. a malignant group of cells or tumor.

LO 3 | What Causes Cancer?

4. "If you are male and smoke, your chances of getting lung cancer are 23 times greater than those of a nonsmoker." This statement refers to a type of risk assessed statistically, known as
   a. relative risk.
   b. comparable risk.
   c. cancer risk.
   d. genetic predisposition.
5. One of the biggest factors in increased risk for cancer is
   a. increasing age.
   b. not having children.
   c. being of long-lived parents.
   d. increased consumption of fruits and vegetables.

LO 4 | Types of Cancers

6. Who is at the highest risk for developing skin cancer?
   a. People who sunburned badly during childhood
   b. People who have dark skin
   c. People without a base tan
   d. People who wear sunscreen daily but tan easily
7. The cancer that causes the most deaths for men and women in the United States is:
   a. colorectal cancer.
   b. pancreatic cancer.
   c. lung cancer.
   d. stomach cancer.
8. The most common type of cancer in men and women in the United States is
   a. lung.
   b. bladder.
   c. oral.
   d. skin.

LO 5 | Facing Cancer

9. Which of the following treatment methods uses drugs to kill cancerous cells?
   a. radiotherapy
   b. chemotherapy
   c. stem cell therapy
   d. stereotactic radiosurgery

LO 6 | Cancer Survivors

10. What does the term cancer *survivorship* mean?
    a. the likeliness of surviving cancer during the treatment process and for 1 year following

b. the emotional and physical states of relatives who have lost loved ones to cancer
c. the likeliness of living with cancer past the 5-year survival rates
d. the physical, psychological, emotional, and economic issues of surviving cancer

Answers to the Pop Quiz can be found on page A-1. If you answered a question incorrectly, review the section identified by the Learning Outcome. For even more study tools, visit MasteringHealth.

THINK ABOUT IT!

LO 1 | An Overview of Cancer

1. What are some of the factors that account for the great increase in 5-year survival rates for people with cancer in recent years?

LO 2 | What Is Cancer?

2. What is cancer? How does it spread? What is the difference between a benign tumor and a malignant tumor?

LO 3 | What Causes Cancer?

3. List the likely causes of cancer. Which of these causes would be a risk for you, in particular? What can you do to reduce these risks? What risk factors do you share with family members? Friends?

LO 4 | Types of Cancers

4. What are the symptoms of lung, breast, prostate, and testicular cancers? How can you reduce your risk of developing these cancers or increase your chances of surviving them?
5. What are the differences between carcinomas, sarcomas, lymphomas, and leukemia? Which is the most common? Least common? Why is it important that you know the stage of your cancer?

LO 5 | Facing Cancer

6. Why are breast and testicular self-exams especially important for college students? What factors keep you from doing your own self-exams? What could you do to make sure you do regular self-exams?

LO 6 | Cancer Survivors

7. How has the idea of survivorship changed the way people think about the years after diagnosis? What are some ways people cope with and fight through a cancer diagnosis?

ACCESS YOUR HEALTH ON THE INTERNET

Visit **MasteringHealth** for links to the websites and RSS feeds.

The following websites explore further topics and issues related to personal health.

American Cancer Society. This private organization is dedicated to cancer prevention. Here you'll find information, statistics, and resources regarding cancer. **www.cancer.org**

National Cancer Institute. On this site you will find valuable information on cancer facts, results of research, new and ongoing clinical trials, and the Physician Data Query (PDQ), a comprehensive database of cancer treatment information. **www.cancer.gov**

National Women's Health Information Center (NWHIC). A wealth of information about cancer in women is presented on this site, which is cosponsored by the National Cancer Institute. **http://womenshealth.gov**

Oncolink. Sponsored by the University of Pennsylvania Cancer Center, this site educates cancer patients and their families by offering information on support services, cancer causes, screening, prevention, and common questions. **www.oncolink.com**

Susan G. Komen for the Cure. Up-to-date information about breast cancer, issues in treatment, and support groups are presented here; there is also a wealth of videos and information. This site is especially useful for diagnosed patients looking for additional support and advice. **www.komen.org**

National Coalition for Cancer Survivorship. Cancer survivors share their experiences advocating for themselves during and after cancer treatment. **www.canceradvocacy.org**

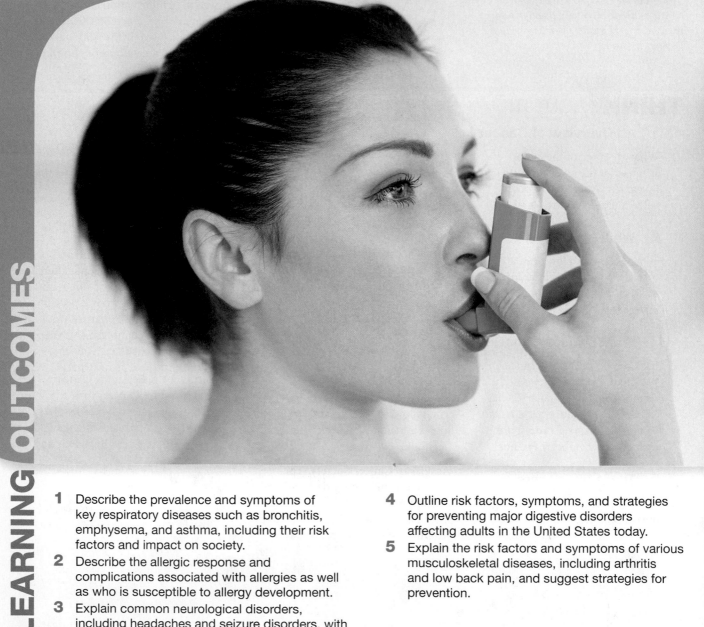

17 Reducing Risks and Coping with Chronic Conditions

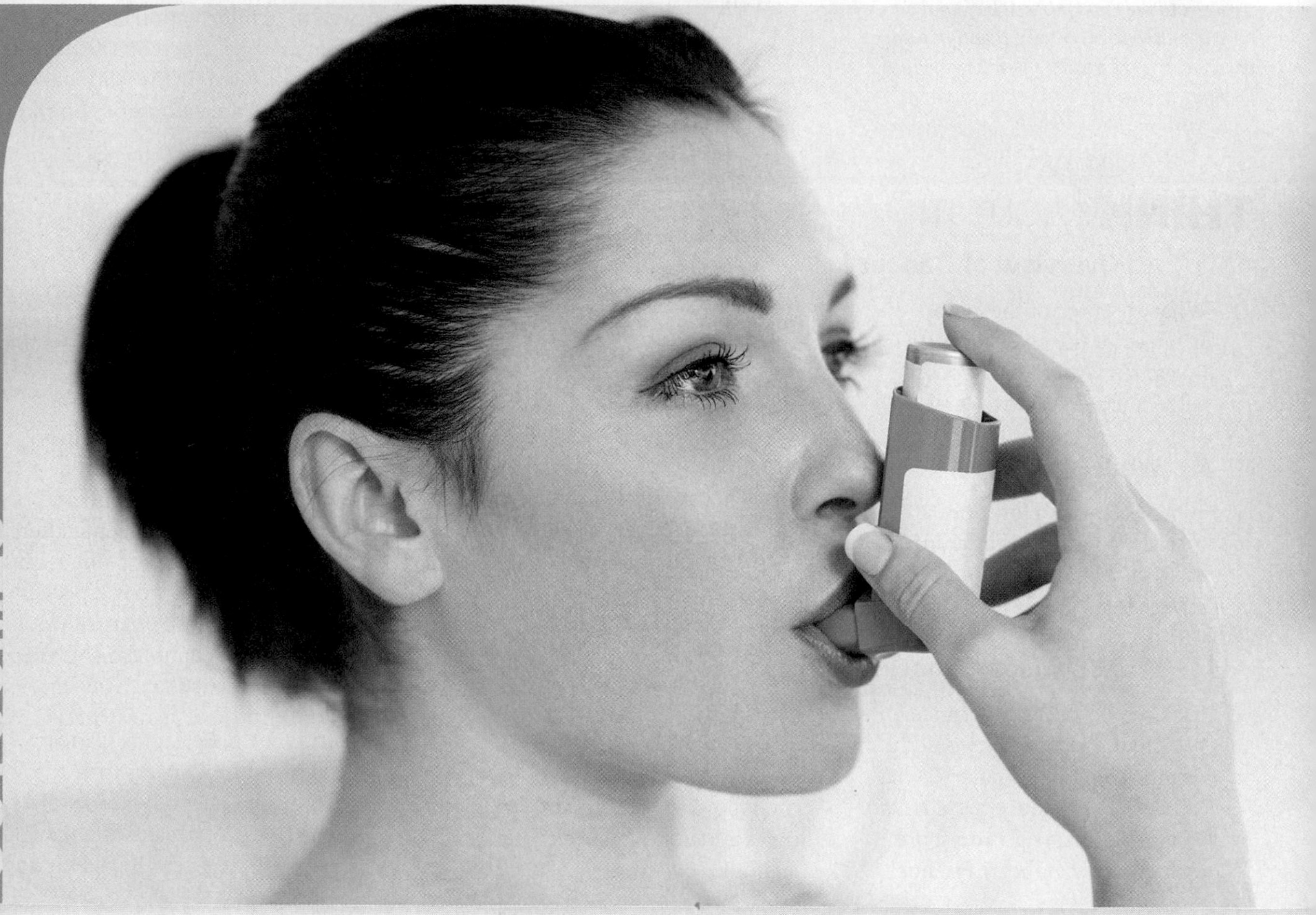

LEARNING OUTCOMES

1 Describe the prevalence and symptoms of key respiratory diseases such as bronchitis, emphysema, and asthma, including their risk factors and impact on society.

2 Describe the allergic response and complications associated with allergies as well as who is susceptible to allergy development.

3 Explain common neurological disorders, including headaches and seizure disorders, with emphasis on risk factors, possible causes, and what is being done to control them.

4 Outline risk factors, symptoms, and strategies for preventing major digestive disorders affecting adults in the United States today.

5 Explain the risk factors and symptoms of various musculoskeletal diseases, including arthritis and low back pain, and suggest strategies for prevention.

Typically, when we think of major noninfectious ailments, we think of "killer" diseases such as cancer and heart disease. Although they do make up the majority of life-threatening diseases, other chronic conditions also cause pain, suffering, and disability. Fortunately, many of them can be prevented, and their symptoms delayed or relieved.

Chronic diseases and conditions often develop over a long period of time, cause progressive damage to the body, and are not easily cured. Genetics, the environment, lifestyle, and personal health habits are often implicated as underlying causes; however, the causes of many chronic diseases and conditions remain a mystery. An increasing number of diseases are **idiopathic** (of unknown cause). In these cases, health professionals often use **palliative treatments**, those treatments designed to treat or ease symptoms but not cure the disease. In general, prevention or intervention for chronic diseases requires investment in education about risks where they are known, lifestyle changes, environmental risk reduction, and assistance via pharmaceuticals and other medical interventions. Public support in the form of targeted research is also key to reducing illness and deaths.

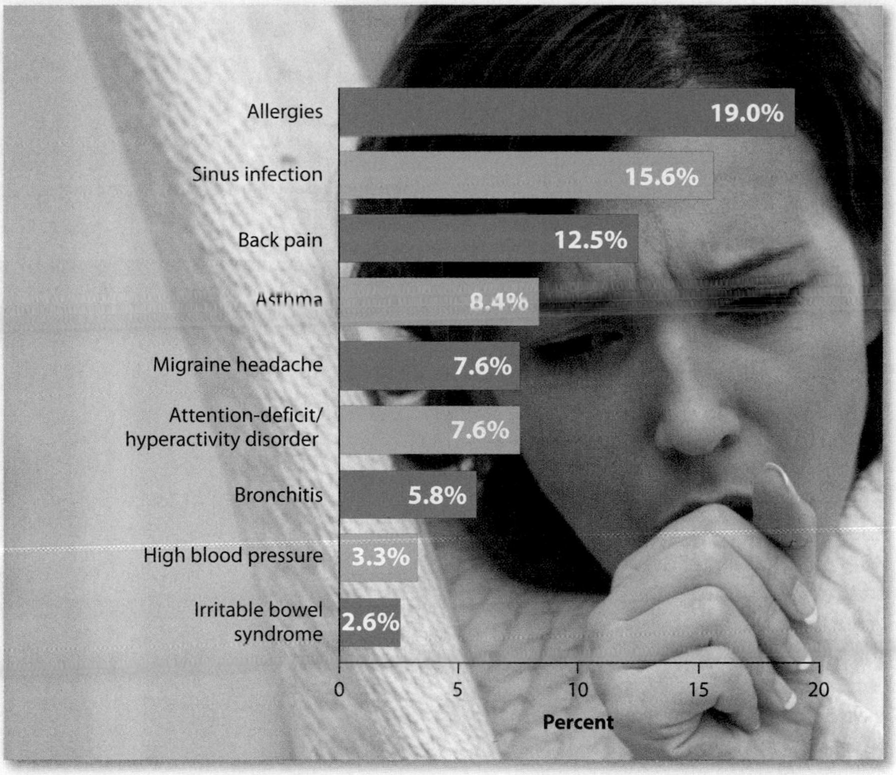

FIGURE 17.1 Proportion of College Students Diagnosed with or Treated for Chronic Conditions in the Past 12 Months Do you think chronic diseases and health problems are a concern only for older Americans? Think again. College students are affected by chronic health issues, too.

Source: Data are from American College Health Association, *American College Health Association—National College Health Assessment II (ACHA-NCHA II): Reference Group Data Report, Spring 2013* (Baltimore, MD: American College Health Association, 2014).

In this chapter, we discuss some of the leading chronic diseases, other than cardiovascular disease (CVD) and cancer, that affect millions of Americans at all ages and stages of life. (The **Health in a Diverse World** box on the next page discusses maladies specific to women.) Knowledge is a key weapon in reducing risks, preventing disease, and controlling threats to health now and in the future (see **FIGURE 17.1**).

LO 1 | COPING WITH RESPIRATORY PROBLEMS

Describe the prevalence and symptoms of key respiratory diseases such as bronchitis, emphysema, and asthma, including their risk factors and impact on society.

The normal adult takes 12 to 15 breaths per minute at rest—varying by age and overall cardiorespiratory health and fitness level.[1] Our respiratory systems move fresh air into the body and waste gases out. Breath really is *life*, but the respiratory system does much more than push air in and out. When healthy, the respiratory system is a finely tuned machine: It filters the air you breathe, and it protects you from invaders by trapping and expelling harmful particles that you inhale with a cough or a sneeze.

Unfortunately, several respiratory diseases are on the rise. **Chronic lower respiratory disease (CLRD)** (including bronchitis, emphysema, and asthma) is the third leading cause of death in the United States (right after heart disease and cancer) and is responsible for over 138,000 deaths each year.[2]

Virtually any disease or disorder that impairs lung function is considered a lung disease. The lungs can be damaged by a single exposure to a toxic chemical or severe heat or be impaired from years of inhaling the tar and chemicals in tobacco smoke. Occupational or home exposure to toxic environmental substances such as asbestos, silica dust, paint fumes and lacquers, or pesticides can cause lung deterioration. Cancers, infections, and degenerative changes can also wreak havoc with lung function. When the lungs are impaired, a condition known as **dyspnea**, a choking type of breathlessness, can occur, even with mild exertion. As the body is deprived of oxygen, the heart is forced to work harder, and over time, cardiovascular problems, suffocation, and death

idiopathic Of unknown cause.

palliative treatment Those treatments designed to treat or ease symptoms but not cure the disease.

chronic lower respiratory disease (CLRD) Lung diseases such as emphysema, asthma, and some forms of bronchitis that are long-term in nature.

dyspnea Shortness of breath, usually associated with disease of the heart or lungs.

HEALTH IN A DIVERSE WORLD

MALADIES SPECIFIC TO WOMEN

Men and women frequently experience different rates of chronic conditions. In addition, there are some conditions that are specific to one gender or the other because they affect body structures and organs associated with reproductive functions.

Fibrocystic Breast Condition

About 90 percent of all women in the United States, particularly those over the age of 30, have a noncancerous condition called *fibrocystic breast condition*. Indeed, it is so common that many experts have taken it out of the disease category and refer to it as *benign breast changes*.

Symptoms range from one small, palpable lump to large masses of irregular tissue found in both breasts. Although most cysts consist of fibrous tissue, some are filled with fluid. The underlying causes of the condition are unknown; it may relate to an imbalance between estrogen and progesterone or to hormonal changes that occur during the normal menstrual cycle. Some experts believe that caffeine raises hormone levels, which can increase susceptibility to fibrous tissue buildup. Women with certain types of fibrocystic tissue may have a slightly higher risk of breast cancer, but this may be because fibrous tissue makes it more difficult to notice an abnormal lump. Treatment, if needed, often involves removing fluid from the affected area or surgically removing the cyst.

This image, created by computerized analysis of the light absorption of tissues, shows a fibrocystic breast.

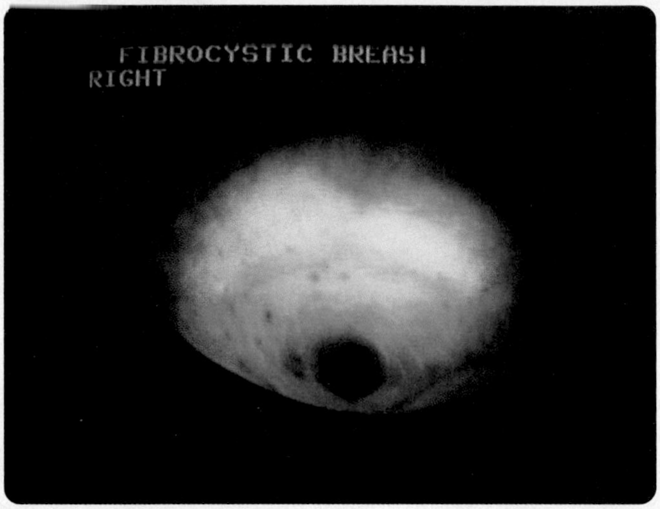

Endometriosis

Endometriosis is a hormonal and immune system disease affecting at least 8.5 million women and girls in the United States and more than 176 million worldwide. Endometriosis is characterized by abnormal growth and development of endometrial tissue (the tissue lining the uterus) in regions of the body other than the uterus. One of the top three causes of female infertility, it is readily treatable if diagnosed; however, it is often misdiagnosed. The most widely used diagnostic strategy is a laparoscopic biopsy of uterine tissue, and the average age for first diagnosis is 27 years.

Symptoms of endometriosis include severe cramping during and between menstrual cycles, irregular periods, unusually heavy or light menstrual flow, abdominal bloating, fatigue, painful bowel movements with periods, painful intercourse, constipation, blood in the urine, pelvic pain, diarrhea, infertility, and low back pain. Among the most widely accepted theories concerning the causes of endometriosis are the transmission of endometrial tissue to other regions of the body during surgery or through the birthing process, the movement of menstrual fluid backward through the fallopian tubes during menstruation, and abnormal cell migration through body-fluid movement. Women with cycles shorter than 27 days or flows longer than a week are at increased risk. The more aerobic exercise a woman engages in and the earlier she starts it, the less likely she is to develop endometriosis.

Treatment for endometriosis ranges from bed rest and stress reduction to *hysterectomy* (surgical removal of the uterus) or surgical removal of one or both ovaries and the fallopian tubes. More conservative treatments involve dilation and curettage, surgically scraping endometrial tissue off the fallopian tubes and other reproductive organs. Combinations of hormone therapy have also become more acceptable.

Sources: M. Conrad-Stoppler, "Fibrocystic Breast Condition," 2012, www.medicinenet.com/fibrocystic_breast_condition/page3.htm; Endometriosis Association, "What Is Endometriosis?," May 2012, www.endometriosisassn.org/endo.html; The Endometriosis Foundation of America. "Endometriosis," 2014, www.endofound.org/endometriosis; National Institutes of Health, Medline Plus, "Endometriosis," Updated 2014, www.nlm.nih.gov/medlineplus/endometriosis.html.

chronic obstructive pulmonary disease (COPD) A collection of chronic lung diseases, including emphysema and chronic bronchitis, where some form of obstruction interferes with a person's ability to breathe.

can occur. Compromised lungs show symptoms of distress, including prolonged coughing, shortness of breath, excess mucus production, wheezing, pain, and coughing up phlegm or blood. Fatigue, increased heart rate, and a host of other problems may occur. Keeping your lungs healthy is an important part of an overall healthy lifestyle.

Chronic Obstructive Pulmonary Disease (COPD)

Chronic obstructive pulmonary disease (COPD) is a progressive lung disease that slowly makes it more and more difficult for a person to breathe. COPD may begin with shortness of breath after little exertion, but may eventually leave patients gasping for air and needing onboard oxygen to perform even the simplest tasks. In the United States, the term COPD refers to two specific diseases, *chronic bronchitis* and *emphysema,* which

HEALTH HEADLINES

BE ECO-CLEAN AND ALLERGEN FREE

Exposure to household chemicals, dust, and pet dander may exacerbate asthma, allergies, and other respiratory problems. Reduce exposure to noxious household chemicals and create a clean, comfortable home by using cleaning supplies and household products that are less toxic to the home environment. Read labels carefully, and look for independent certifications such as the Green Seal and the Environmental Protection Agency's (EPA's) Design for the Environment program.

- For a handy glass and surface cleaner, mix 1/2 cup of white vinegar with 4 cups of water. Pour the solution into a spray bottle, and keep the remainder for a quick and cheap refill. You can make another surface cleaner by combining 2 tablespoons of lemon juice with 4 cups of water.
- Baking soda is a great deodorizer and cleaner. Use it to remove carpet odors and to scour sinks, toilets, and bathtubs.
- Because chlorine can damage lungs, skin, and eyes, and chlorine production adds toxic chemicals such as carcinogenic dioxins to our environment, use a chlorine bleach alternative. For example, use 1/2 cup of hydrogen peroxide in your laundry or try oxygen-based bleaches.
- An all-purpose cleaner can be made of 1/2 cup of borax (found in the laundry aisle) and 1 gallon of hot water.
- For green air fresheners, use essential oils, such as lemon or lavender. Many store-bought air fresheners contain phthalates, often called "fragrance," that are related to respiratory problems and other noninfectious conditions. Place a few drops of essential oils on a piece of tissue paper, in a bowl of warm water, or in a store-bought diffuser.

As you transition to green cleaning, do not just throw old products in the trash, as these can wind up polluting landfills and leaching into water supplies. Instead, take them to a hazardous chemical recycling facility.

Making your own cleansers ensures that they are not harmful to your health.

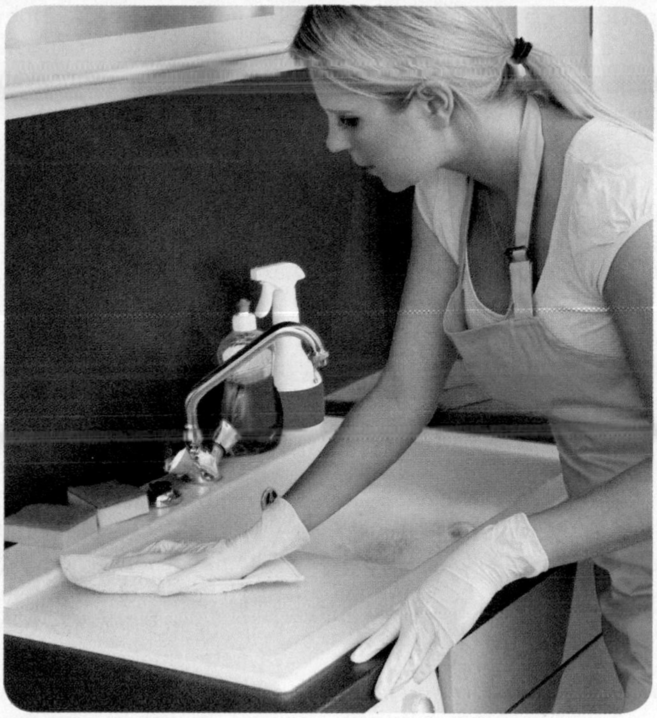

often occur together and can lead to problems with inhalation and exhalation. Currently, nearly 13 million people aged 18 and over have impaired lung function caused by COPD; however, these numbers are believed to grossly underestimate the over 24 million people believed to have undiagnosed lung impairment.[3]

Women are nearly twice as likely to be diagnosed with chronic bronchitis as their male counterparts. While men have historically been more likely to be diagnosed with emphysema, in 2011, for the first time, women surpassed men in emphysema diagnoses. In addition to having a greater chance of COPD diagnosis, women are more likely to die of these diseases.[4] The vast majority of people with COPD are either former or current smokers. Other risk factors include a history of asthma, heredity, exposure to air pollution, secondhand smoke, occupational and industrial dusts and chemicals, and other lung irritants, including childhood respiratory infections. Usually, COPD develops over time; however, one big dose of superheated air or another lung-damaging event can cause it.

There is no cure for COPD; however, there is much that can be done to prevent it, including quitting smoking, avoiding secondhand smoke, and maximizing lung function through exercise. While lifestyle changes are important, vaccines for the flu and pneumonia are also important preventive options to help reduce risk of lung damage. Some occupations continue to pose risks, but major improvements in reducing worker exposure have occurred in recent years. Reading labels, wearing protective devices, and making sure areas where toxins accumulate are ventilated when spraying chemicals and cleaning products are important. If you have symptoms, such as a chronic cough, shortness of breath, rapid heart rate, or note your lips or nail beds are gray or blue, don't wait to see a doctor. Early treatment and regular follow-up are important. There are many options for relieving symptoms, preventing further damage, and improving lung function. The **Health Headlines** box describes ways to minimize exposure to household chemicals.

Bronchitis **Bronchitis** involves inflammation and eventual scarring of the lining of the bronchial tubes (*bronchi*) that connect the windpipe to the lungs. When the bronchi become inflamed or infected with bacteria, less air is able to flow from the lungs and heavy mucus begins to form. Although some mucus is normal and necessary, bronchitis sufferers typically have numerous coughing spasms in a day as they try to rid their bodies of phlegm. Frequent clearing of the throat, a sensation of tightness in the chest, back pain, and shortness of breath are other bronchitis symptoms.

Inhaling certain chemicals such as tobacco, marijuana, or e-cigarette smoke can trigger bronchitis. Cosmetic sprays, perfumes hair sprays, household cleaners, and air fresheners can also be triggers. The more common *acute bronchitis* is often caused by other infectious diseases. Symptoms often begin to go away in a week or two once the sources are removed and any inflammation and infections are treated.

bronchitis An inflammation and eventual scarring of the lining of the bronchial tubes.

emphysema A respiratory disease in which the alveoli become distended or ruptured and are no longer functional.

alveoli Tiny air sacs of the lungs where gas exchange occurs (oxygen enters the body and carbon dioxide is removed).

asthma A chronic respiratory disease that blocks airflow into and out of the lungs, characterized by attacks of wheezing, shortness of breath, and coughing spasms.

When the symptoms of bronchitis last for at least 3 months of the year for 2 consecutive years, the condition is considered *chronic bronchitis*. In some cases, this chronic inflammation and irritation goes undiagnosed for years, particularly in smokers who feel it's a normal part of their lives. By the time these individuals receive medical care, the damage to their lungs is severe and may lead to heart and respiratory failure or to a chronic need to carry oxygen to aid in breathing. Coal miners, grain handlers, metalworkers, painters, hairdressers, and others exposed to fumes, dusts, and hazards are particularly susceptible. Nearly 10 million Americans, the majority of whom are women, suffer from chronic bronchitis; 33 percent are under age 45. In 2011, for the first time, non-Hispanic black Americans experienced more chronic bronchitis than other ethnic groups.[5]

To help prevent the problems associated with bronchitis, stop smoking and avoid particulates that trigger bronchitis attacks. Avoid smoke-filled bars or other settings that make your situation worse. If the pollution index is high, stay indoors, make sure windows and doors are closed, and use air filtration systems. See a doctor promptly if you have recurrent symptoms. Prescription drugs can reduce inflammation, prevent mucus buildup, and stop secondary bacterial infections from setting in.

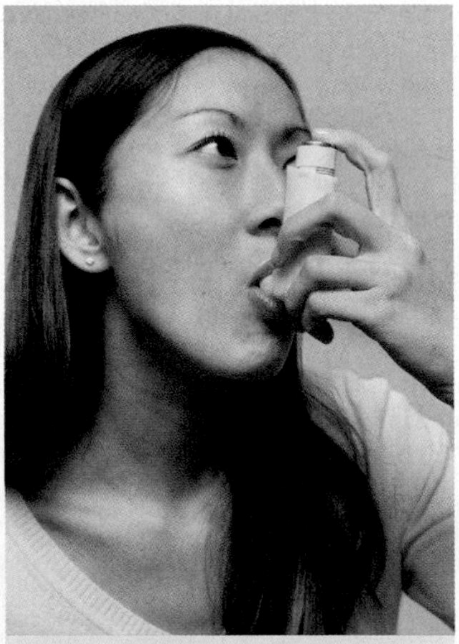

People with asthma can generally control their symptoms through the use of inhaled medications, and most asthmatics keep a "rescue" inhaler of bronchodilating medication on hand to use in case of a flare-up.

Emphysema Over 4.7 million Americans suffer from **emphysema**. Emphysema was historically a "man's disease," but today more women than men are diagnosed with emphysema. In the last 5 years, emphysema rates have risen over 63 percent for women and declined 6 percent among men.[6] Emphysema involves the gradual, irreversible destruction of the **alveoli** (tiny air sacs through which gas exchange occurs) of the lungs. Destruction of the alveoli walls impairs the transfer of oxygen and carbon dioxide into and out of the blood and makes the lungs less elastic, which makes it harder to breathe. As the alveoli are destroyed, the affected person finds it more and more difficult to exhale. People with emphysema liken this experience to engaging in heavy exercise while breathing through a straw. What most of us take for granted—the easy, rhythmic flow of air in and out of the lungs—becomes a continuous, anxious, and life-threatening struggle.

WHAT DO YOU THINK?

Have you or any of your friends or family experienced any of the conditions discussed in this section?

- Why do you think the incidence of COPD is increasing?
- What actions can you or the people in your community take to reduce risks and problems from these diseases on campus? In your homes? In your communities?

The cause of emphysema is uncertain. There is, however, a strong relationship between emphysema and long-term cigarette smoking and exposure to air pollution. (See **Chapter 11** for more on the connection between smoking and emphysema.) To avoid emphysema, don't smoke. If you smoke, quit. Avoid occupational exposure that involves inhaling chemicals and fumes. If you must take a job that involves inhaling toxins, use appropriate protection.

A key to coping with emphysema is to make sure the patient complies with doctor's orders. Prescribed medications must be taken. Healthy meals, exercise, stress management, and adequate rest are imperative to keep the body functioning at maximum capacity and keep depression at bay. Many persons on oxygen supplementation become depressed and irritable. You may need to suggest counseling or help from social services. Support groups can be very helpful, as well as respite care for the caregiver.

Asthma

Asthma is a long-term, chronic inflammatory disorder that blocks airflow into and out of the lungs. Asthma causes tiny airways in the lung to overreact with spasms in response to certain triggers (**FIGURE 17.2**). Symptoms include wheezing, difficulty breathing, shortness of

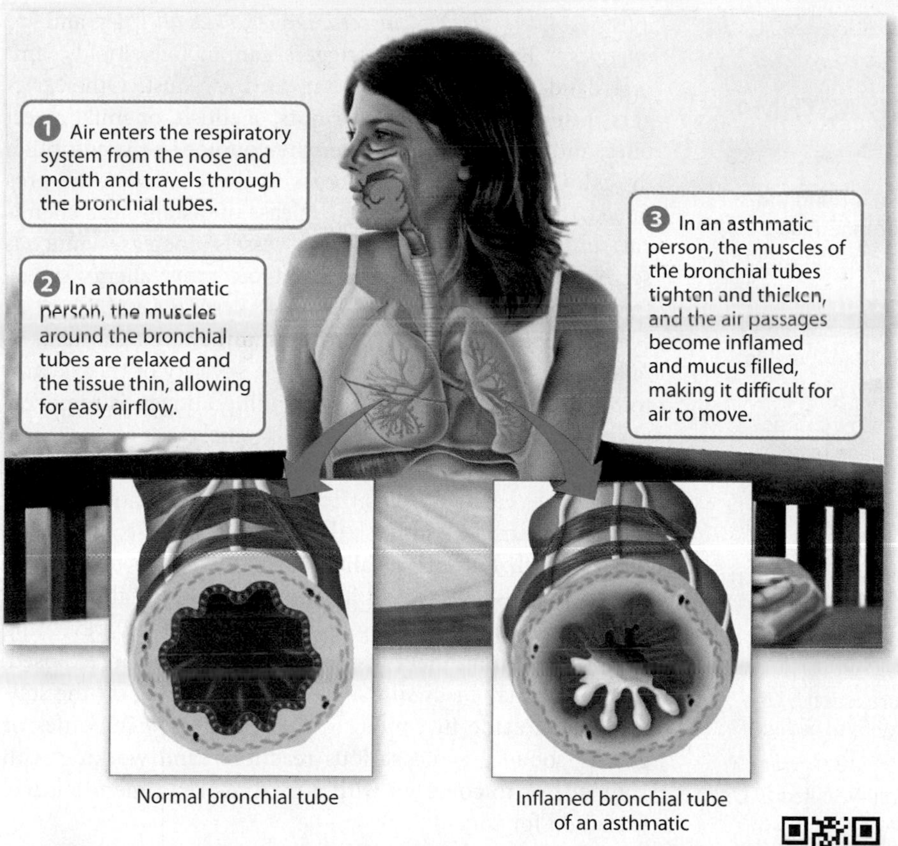

1 Air enters the respiratory system from the nose and mouth and travels through the bronchial tubes.
2 In a nonasthmatic person, the muscles around the bronchial tubes are relaxed and the tissue thin, allowing for easy airflow.
3 In an asthmatic person, the muscles of the bronchial tubes tighten and thicken, and the air passages become inflamed and mucus filled, making it difficult for air to move.
Normal bronchial tube
Inflamed bronchial tube of an asthmatic

FIGURE 17.2 **Asthma Is an Inflammation of the Airways within the Lungs**

VIDEO TUTOR
Lungs during an Asthma Attack

breath, and coughing spasms. Although most asthma attacks are mild, severe attacks can trigger bronchospasms (contractions of the bronchial tubes in the lungs) that are so severe that, without rapid treatment, death may occur. Between attacks, most people have few symptoms. Approximately 21million adults and 9 million children in the United States have asthma.[7] It is the most common chronic disease of childhood, affecting nearly 10 percent of all children in the United States today.[8]

Asthma falls into two distinctly different types. The more common form, *extrinsic* or *allergic asthma*, is typically associated with allergic triggers; it tends to run in families and develop in childhood. Often by adulthood, a person has few episodes, or the disorder completely goes away. The less common form of asthma, *intrinsic* or *nonallergic asthma,* may be triggered by anything except an allergy.

Several factors, including medical conditions, animal dander and saliva, mold, cockroach allergens, dust mites, perfumes, exercise, smoke, food allergies, weather changes, pollen, and air pollution, can trigger asthma flare-ups. In fact, even emotions such as anger, fear, or stress can trigger an asthma attack.[9] Genetics may play a role in asthma development. If your mom or dad has asthma, or if family members have a history of allergies, asthma is more likely. If you had respiratory infections when you were younger, such as colds, the flu, or sinus infections, or if you are exposed to environmental allergens and irritants, you are more likely to develop asthma.[10] Certain medications, particularly fever reducers or anti-inflammatory drugs such as NSAIDS, may also be triggers. Between 10 and 20 percent of all people with asthma are sensitive to aspirin, while others are sensitive to beta-blockers and ACE inhibitors used to treat cardiovascular problems.[11]

Asthma rates have increased over 30 percent in the last 20 years.[12] Asthma can occur at any age but is most likely to appear in children between infancy and age 5 and in adults before age 40. In childhood, asthma strikes more boys than girls; in adulthood, it strikes more women than men. Poverty, low education, and risky home and work environments as well as limited access to health care lead to clear disparities in asthma treatment and control. Puerto Ricans have the highest rates of asthma in the United States—nearly double non-Hispanic white rates (15.7% vs. 7.5%).[13] Non-Hispanic blacks have a 9.8 percent rate of diagnosed asthma, and Mexican Americans have a 6.5 percent rate.[14] Many believe that today's homes contain more triggers (such as dust mites in mattresses, chemicals in carpets and furniture, and airtight buildings for efficient cooling and heating).

The **Skills for Behavior Change** box on the next page suggests ways to reduce asthma attacks. In addition to avoiding triggers, finding the most effective medications can help asthmatics cope with their condition and avoid severe attacks.

LO 2 | COPING WITH ALLERGIES

Describe the allergic response and complications associated with allergies as well as who is susceptible to allergy development.

Allergies are diseases characterized by an overreaction of the immune system to a foreign protein substance (*allergen* or *antigen*) that is swallowed, breathed into the lungs, injected, or touched.[15] When foreign pathogens such as bacteria or viruses enter the body, the body responds by producing *antibodies* to destroy these invaders. Normally, antibody production is a positive element in the body's defense system. However, for unknown reasons, sometimes the body develops an overly elaborate protective

allergies Hypersensitivity reactions in which the body produces antibodies to a normally harmless substance in the environment.

SKILLS FOR BEHAVIOR CHANGE

PREVENTING ASTHMA ATTACKS

Although asthma rates continue to increase around the world, there is much that individuals and communities can do to reduce risk:

- Purchase a good air filter for your home, and clean furnace filters regularly. If you have a fireplace or wood-burning stove, check it regularly to make sure that it is not spewing smoke and particulate matter.
- Wash pillows and sheets regularly. Use pillow protectors and mattress protectors. Don't purchase used mattresses, which may be teeming with mites.
- If you're a pet lover but animal dander bothers you, try a nonshedding breed of dog or cat. Keep pets off your bed, and wash them and their bedding weekly. Vacuum regularly.
- Keep your home clean and pest free; cockroaches and other vermin have enzymes in their saliva or particles on their bodies that may trigger allergic reactions. Use a high-suction vacuum rather than a broom to reduce dust particles suspended in the air.
- Use antimold cleaners or run a dehumidifier to keep moisture levels down and reduce the growth of mold.
- Avoid mowing the lawn or other activities leading to excessive outdoor exposure to pollen during high-pollen times. If you must be outdoors, wear a pollen mask.
- Exercise regularly to keep your lungs functioning well.
- Avoid cigarette, cigar, and pipe smoke.
- Keep asthma medications handy. Let people close to you know that you are asthmatic, and educate them about what to do if you have an asthma attack.
- Investigate local regulations on the burning of household and yard trash, field burning, wood-burning stoves, and secondhand smoke from cigarettes—all known triggers for asthma attacks—and work to revise them as necessary.

mechanism against relatively harmless substances. The resulting *hypersensitivity reaction* to specific allergens or antigens in the environment is fairly common, as anyone who has awakened with a runny nose or itchy eyes can attest. People with severe allergies can suffer much more extreme responses, including hives, vomiting, and anaphylaxis.

histamine Chemical substance that dilates blood vessels, increases mucus secretions, and triggers other allergy symptoms.

immunotherapy Treatment strategies based on the concept of regulating the immune system, as by administering antibodies or desensitization shots of allergens.

hay fever A chronic allergy-related respiratory disorder that is most prevalent when ragweed and flowers bloom, also known as *pollen allergy*.

Allergies are grouped by the kind of trigger, time of year, or where symptoms appear on the body into *outdoor* or *indoor allergies, food and drug allergies, latex allergies, insect allergies, skin allergies,* and *eye allergies*.[16] Environmental triggers can include molds, animal dander, pollen, grasses, ragweed, or dust. Other triggers include foods such as peanuts, shellfish, or milk; insect bites; and medicines (both over-the-counter and prescription drugs). Once excessive antibodies to these antigens are produced, they, in turn, trigger the release of **histamine**, a chemical substance that dilates blood vessels, increases mucous secretions, swells tissues, and produces other allergy symptoms, particularly in the respiratory system (**FIGURE 17.3**). Many people have found that **immunotherapy** treatment, or "allergy shots," somewhat reduces the severity of their symptoms. In most cases, once the offending antigen is removed, allergy-prone people suffer few symptoms.

Globally, between 40 and 50 percent of all school-aged children are currently sensitized to one or more of the common allergens.[17] Asthma (discussed above) is a unique disease in that it is typically considered to be both a key respiratory disease as well as one of the major allergic diseases.[18] Prevention of allergies usually focuses on preventing exposure to things that cause you to react. If you are exposed, treatments may be as simple as quickly washing off the substance you came in contact with, taking antihistamines or getting shots to avoid serious reactions, and working with your doctor to come up with a treatment regimen that will work best for you.

Hay Fever

Hay fever, or *pollen allergy,* occurs throughout the world and is one of the most common chronic diseases in the United States, affecting nearly 18 million adults and 7 million children

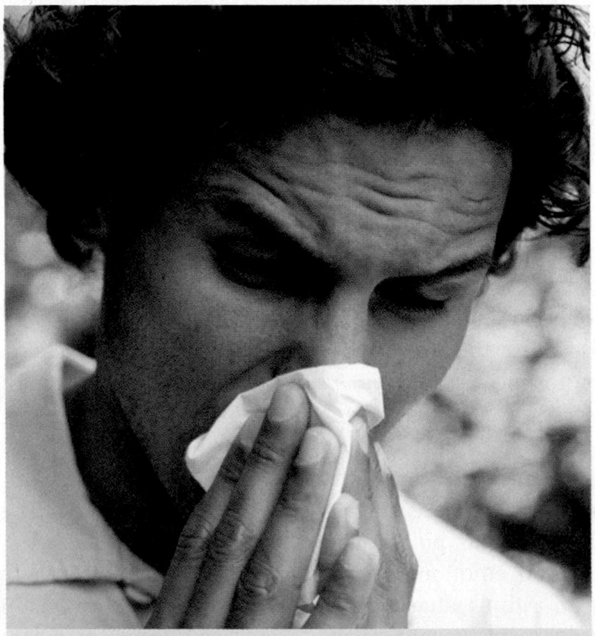

To minimize your exposure to hay fever, keep windows closed, stay indoors when pollen counts are highest (typically 10 A.M. to 4 P.M.), and change clothes after spending time outdoors.

B cell

1 Exposure to an allergen causes B cells to produce specific IgE antibodies.

— Allergen

IgE antibodies

Binding sites for IgE

Mast cell

Vesicles containing histamine

2 The IgE antibodies bind to mast cells, sensitizing them to future exposures to the same allergen.

Allergens specific for IgE

3 The next exposure to the allergen causes mast cells to release histamine.

4 Histamine causes a localized or systemic inflammatory response.

Histamine

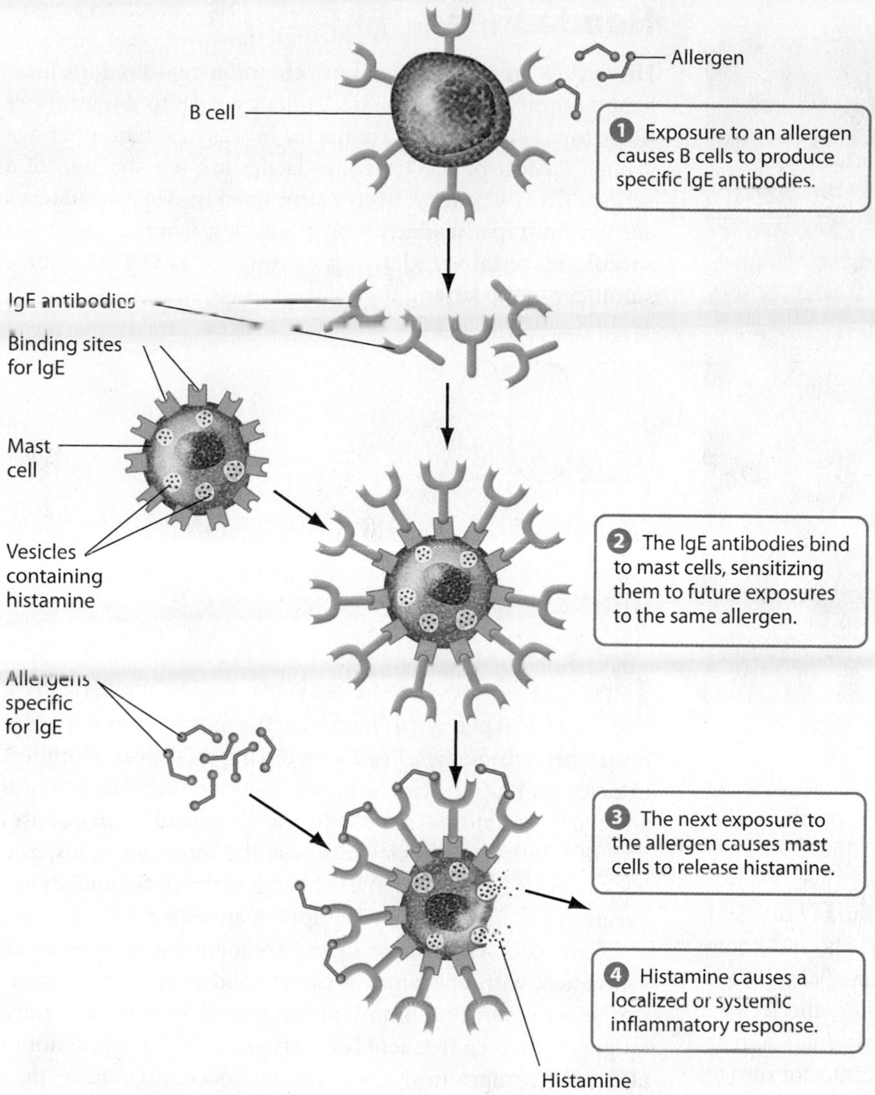

FIGURE 17.3 Steps of an Allergic Response

Source: Adapted from Johnson, Michael D., *Human Biology: Concepts and Current Issues*, 7th Ed., © 2014, p. 211. Printed and electronically reproduced by permission of Pearson Education, Inc., Upper Saddle River, New Jersey.

each year.[19] It is usually considered a seasonal disease because it is most prevalent when ragweed and flowers are blooming. Hay fever attacks are characterized by sneezing and itchy, watery eyes and nose. As with other allergies, hay fever results from an overzealous immune system that is hypersensitive to certain substances. You are more likely to

have hay fever if you have a family history of allergies, are male, were born during pollen season, are a firstborn child, were exposed to cigarette smoke during your first year of life, or are exposed to dust mites.

Typical over-the-counter treatment consists of antihistamines. These work well for mild cases, but may become less effective over time. Air conditioning, whole house air filters, and air purifiers can also help relieve symptoms. To determine if you have pollen allergy, the best bet is to get tested by an **allergist**— a doctor specializing in allergies. Typical treatments include prescription medications and/or allergy shots. While allergy shots are one of the most effective ways of treatment, side effects are possible and doctors recommend them for limited time periods.[20]

Food Allergies

A **food allergy** is an exaggerated immune response to certain foods, such as milk, eggs, peanuts, tree nuts, shellfish, fish, wheat, and soy. Symptoms of a food allergy typically include hives or rash; hoarse voice; wheezing and trouble breathing; swelling of the tongue, lips, or face; abdominal pain; diarrhea or vomiting; difficulty swallowing; and itching.[21] The reaction can be so severe that the victim goes into *anaphylactic shock,* with a rapid heart rate, changes in blood pressure, swelling of the tongue or throat, breathing difficulties, and possible death. Over 200 Americans die each year from food allergies, and another 30,000 or

more end up in the emergency room.[22] Food allergies should not be confused with **food intolerance**, which is the inability to properly digest a particular food due to problems with physical, hormonal, enzyme, or biochemical systems in your gastrointestinal (GI) tract. *Food intolerance* typically causes stomach or GI pain, gas, cramps, and/or diarrhea, but not true allergic reactions. Some estimate that 8 percent of children and 4 percent of adults may have food allergies.[23] There are increasing numbers of media reports and marketing around food allergies, even though actual diagnoses are not widely available. Sometimes, people may think

allergist Medical doctor focusing on the diagnosis and treatment of allergies.

food allergy An immune response against a specific food that the majority of people can eat without problem.

food intolerance Difficulty or inability to digest certain foods due to problems with the physical, hormonal, or biochemical systems in your digestive tract.

18 MILLION

ADULTS AND 7 MILLION CHILDREN SUFFER FROM **HAY FEVER**.

DID YOU **KNOW?**

At least 40 people per year die from insect stings. Many more have life-threatening reactions to the bites or stings from spiders, horseflies, bees, and other insects.

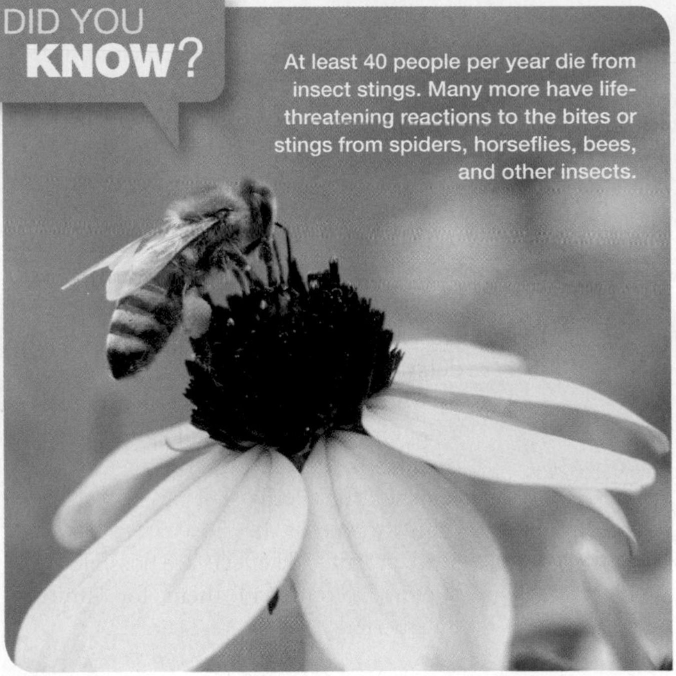

they have an allergy when they are reacting to specific pathogens in the food and really have a foodborne illness.

Although some food allergies can be outgrown, there is no cure. If you have an allergy, you can avoid many reactions by reading labels, asking questions in restaurants, and knowing exactly what you are eating. Wear a medical alert bracelet or necklace that says you have food allergies, and let your friends, family members, and instructors know that you react to certain foods. Carry antihistamines or autoinjector devices con-taining epinephrine (adrenaline) so that you can quickly respond in the event of accidental exposure.

LO 3 | COPING WITH NEUROLOGICAL DISORDERS

Explain common neurological disorders, including headaches and seizure disorders, with emphasis on risk factors, possible causes, and what is being done to control them.

While stroke is the fourth leading cause of death (see **Chapter 15**) and *Alzheimer's disease* (AD) (see **Chapter 21**) is the sixth leading cause of death, with a rapid rise in prevalence in the last decade, there are hundreds of neurological diseases and disorders responsible for a tremendous burden on family members, health care providers, social service workers, workplaces, and patients themselves.[24] More than 600 disorders can affect the nervous system, causing problems for an estimated 50 million Americans each year.[25] Some of these disorders, such as migraine headaches and epilepsy, are well known, but there are many lesser-known disorders and some that that elude diagnosis. (See the **Health Headlines** box on page 488 for pain treatment options.)

Headaches

Headaches are one of the most common reasons for emergency room visits each year. Adults aged 18 to 44 are more likely to visit emergency rooms for headaches than other age groups.[26] Most of the time, headaches are not the sign of a serious disease and go away fairly quickly. Most headaches are tension-type headaches or migraines, whereas some are specific to certain underlying causes; see **TABLE 17.1** for a summary of the latter.

20%

OF ADULTS IN THE U.S., THE MAJORITY OF WHOM ARE WOMEN, SUFFER FROM **IRRITABLE BOWEL SYNDROME.**

Tension-Type Headaches Nearly 90 percent of women and 70 percent of men have the most common type of headache, *tension-type headache,* during their lives. Numbers of cases peak up to the age of 40; however, they can occur at any age.[27] Symptoms include dull, aching head pain; a sensation of tightness or pressure across the forehead, sides, and back of your head; tenderness on the scalp, neck, and shoulder muscles; and, occasionally, loss of appetite.[28]

There is a wide range in the frequency and severity of symptoms, with occurrences categorized as episodic (occurring less than once a month and triggered by stress, anxiety, fatigue, or anger); frequent (occurring 1 to 15 days per month along with migraines); and chronic (occurring more than 15 days per month, with varying pain). While the cause(s) of tension headaches remain unknown, possible triggers include stress, depression and anxiety, jaw clenching, poor posture, or working in an awkward position. Red wine, lack of sleep, extreme fasting, hormonal changes, and certain food additives or preservatives have also been implicated.[29]

Tension-type headaches are most often prevented by reducing triggers. If stress is a trigger, try to relax with a hot bath, relaxing music, hot compresses, massage, or other relaxation techniques. Exercise can relieve some types of tension headaches, while aspirin, ibuprofen, acetaminophen, and naproxen sodium remain standby pain relievers. If headaches occur more frequently and are difficult to treat with OTC medications, they are probably *chronic tension headaches*—the result of physical or psychological problems or depression. These more difficult forms of tension headaches warrant a visit to the doctor to assess the underlying cause.

SEE IT! VIDEOS

Plagued by serious headaches? Watch **Migraine Breakthrough** available on MasteringHealth.™

Migraine Headaches Over 37 million Americans—three times more women than men—suffer from

TABLE 17.1 | Types of Headaches

Type	Symptoms	Precipitating Factors	Treatment	Prevention
Allergy	Generalized headache. Nasal congestion, watery eyes.	Seasonal allergens such as pollen, molds. Allergies to food are not usually a factor.	Antihistamine medication; topical, nasal cortisone-related sprays, or desensitization injections.	None.
Caffeine-withdrawal	Throbbing headache caused by rebound dilation of the blood vessels, occurring multiple days after consumption of large quantities of caffeine.	Caffeine.	In extreme cases, treat by terminating caffeine consumption.	Avoid excess caffeine.
Cluster	Excruciating pain in vicinity of eye. Tearing of eye, nose congestion, flushing of face. Pain frequently develops during sleep and may last for several hours. Attacks occur every day for weeks/months, then disappear for up to a year. 80% of cluster patients are male, most ages 20–50.	Alcoholic beverages, excessive smoking.	Oxygen, ergotamine, sumatriptan, or intranasal application of local anesthetic agent.	Use of steroids, ergotamine, calcium channel blockers, and lithium.
Exertion	Generalized head pain of short duration (minutes to 1 hour) during or following physical exertion (running, jumping, or sexual intercourse) or passive exertion (sneezing, coughing, moving one's bowels, etc.).	For these headaches, 10% caused by organic diseases (aneurysms, tumors, or blood vessel malformation); 90% are related to migraine or cluster headaches.	Cause must be accurately determined. Most commonly treated with aspirin, indomethacin, or propranolol. Extensive testing is necessary to determine the headache cause. Surgery to correct organic disease is occasionally indicated.	Alternative forms of exercise. Avoid jarring exercises.
Eyestrain	Usually frontal, bilateral pain, directly related to eyestrain. Rare cause of headache.	Muscle imbalance. Uncorrected vision, astigmatism.	Correction of vision.	Same as treatment.
Hangover	Migraine-like symptoms of throbbing pain and nausea not localized to one side.	Alcohol, which causes dilation and irritation of the blood vessels of the brain and surrounding tissue.	Liquids (including broth). Consumption of fructose (honey, tomato juice are good sources) to help burn alcohol.	Drink alcohol only in moderation.
Hunger	Pain strikes just before mealtime. Caused by muscle tension, low blood sugar, and rebound dilation of the blood vessels, oversleeping, or missing a meal.	Strenuous dieting or skipping meals.	Regular, nourishing meals containing adequate protein and complex carbohydrates.	Same as treatment.
New daily persistent headache (NDPH)	This headache can best be described as the rapid development (less than 3 days) of unrelenting headache, and typically presents in a person with no past history of a headache.	Typically NDPH does not evolve from migraine or episodic tension-type headache. NDPH begins as a new headache. It may be the result of a viral infection.	In some cases, NPDH can resolve on its own within several months. Other cases persist and are more refractory.	Does not respond to traditional options. However, antiseizure medications, topiramate, or gabapentin can be used.
Sinus	Gnawing pain over nasal area, often increasing in severity throughout the day. Caused by acute infection, usually with fever, producing blockage of sinus ducts and preventing normal drainage. Sinus headaches are rare. Migraine and cluster headaches are often misdiagnosed as sinus in origin.	Infection, nasal polyps, anatomical deformities, such as a deviated septum, that block the sinus ducts.	Treat with antibiotics, decongestants, surgical drainage if necessary.	None.

Source: Adapted from "The Complete Headache Chart," 2010, www.headaches.org. Reprinted by permission of the National Headache Foundation.

@ HEALTH HEADLINES

TREATING CHRONIC PAIN

Chronic pain is pain that persists and keeps neurons firing for days, weeks, or even months. For those who have it, it is a nagging, often agonizing, threat to their mental and physical health and overall well-being. Millions of people suffer from chronic pain every day, exacting a heavy toll on individuals, families, businesses, and society. The collective direct and indirect costs of unresolved pain are estimated to be over $635 billion. Chronic pain affects more Americans than diabetes, heart disease, and cancer combined. Pain disrupts activities of daily living while contributing to mental health problems such as depression and anxiety. Even with pain medications, 50 to 75 percent of patients die in moderate to severe pain.

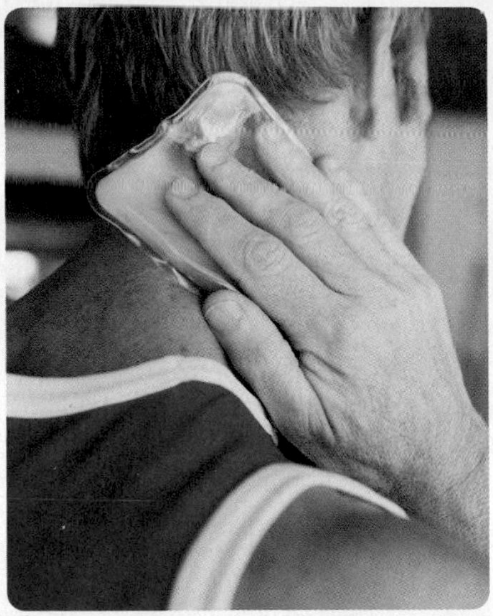

Cold packs are one of many options for pain treatment.

Who Suffers Most from Pain?

- Women are more likely to suffer from pain.
- Adults aged 18 to 44 are more likely to experience migraines or severe headaches.
- Poor or near poor families are more likely to experience pain from all causes.

Newer research suggests that two groups of people may be more likely to experience pain in their lifetimes: people with abnormalities in the structure of their brain and people who experienced chronic pain during childhood. Based on magnetic resonance imaging (MRI) scans, scientists have been able to predict with 85 percent accuracy who would experience chronic pain based on irregular markers on the axons, pathways for nerve transmission in white matter of the brain. Overall, pain from most conditions increases with age, particularly among those 65 and over.

Chronic pain sufferers have a variety of treatment options:

- **Over-the-counter (OTC) medications.** Available without prescription are medications such as acetaminophen (Tylenol) and nonsteroidal anti-inflammatory drugs (NSAIDs), including ibuprofen (Advil, Motrin), aspirin, and naproxen (Aleve).
- **Prescription medications.** A variety of these are available. They may give faster results than OTC drugs, but they also present increased risks for patients in terms of addiction and drug interactions. Prescription pain killers are the second most abused category of drugs in the United States, contributing to over 12,000 unintentional deaths each year.
- **Cold and heat treatments.** Cold packs are used to numb areas, reduce swelling, and ease joint aches. Hot packs relax muscles, bring blood to an area, and aid healing.
- **Acupuncture, acupressure, and massage.** All are designed to reduce pain, relax the patient, and speed healing. (See **Chapter 18** for more on these options and their rates of effectiveness.)
- **Physical therapy.** Physical therapists use a variety of modalities—heat and cold, electrical stimulation, stretching, and others—to work with patients experiencing a wide range of pain-related conditions, increasing core strength and range of motion, while retraining muscles to function effectively and reduce pain.
- **Local electrical stimulation.** Transcutaneous electrical nerve stimulation (TENS) blocks pain messages to the brain and modifies perceptions of pain. Brief electrical pulses to nerve endings provide pain relief.
- **Psychological treatment.** Among a small percentage of pain sufferers, pain appears to be precipitated by emotional or psychological trauma or suffering. In these cases, counseling, relaxation training, water therapy, meditation, biofeedback, aromatherapy, light therapy, dietary changes, yoga, and other mind-body techniques can reduce the severity of pain or eventually make it go away.
- **Surgery.** If someone has tried everything else and nothing seems to work, surgery may be a last option.

Sources: Institute of Medicine Committee on Advancing Pain Research, Care, and Education, *Relieving Pain in America: A Blueprint for Transforming Prevention, Care, Education and Research* (Washington, DC: The National Academies Press; 2011), Available from: http://books.nap.edu/openbook.php?record_id=13172&page=1; NINDS, "Chronic Pain Information D. Page," April 2014, www.ninds.nih.gov/disorders/chronic_pain/chronic_pain.htm; J. Gaskin and P Richard, "The Economic Costs of Pain in the United States," *The Journal of Pain* 13, no. 8 (2012): 715, DOI: 10.1016/j.jpain.2012.03.009; The American Academy of Pain Medicine, "AAPM Facts and Figures on Pain," Accessed June 2014, www.painmed.org/patientcenter/facts_on_pain.aspx; A. Mansour et al., "Brain White Matter Structural Properties Predict Transition to Chronic Pain," *PAIN* 154, no. 10 (2013): 2160, DOI: 10.1016/j.pain.2013.06.044; American Pain Society, "Links of Childhood Pain to Adult Chronic Pain, Fibromyalgia," *ScienceDaily*, December 19, 2013, www.sciencedaily.com/releases/2013/12/131219162532.htm.

migraine A type of headache characterized by debilitating symptoms that possibly results from alternating dilation and constriction of blood vessels.

migraines, vascular headaches that often have debilitating symptoms.[30] Symptoms include moderate to severe pain on one or both sides of the head, head pain with a pulsating or throbbing quality, pain that worsens with physical activity or interferes with regular activity, nausea with or without vomiting, and sensitivity to light and sound. In fact, 1 out of 4 households has a migraine sufferer. Usually, migraine incidence peaks in young adulthood (between ages 20 and 45).

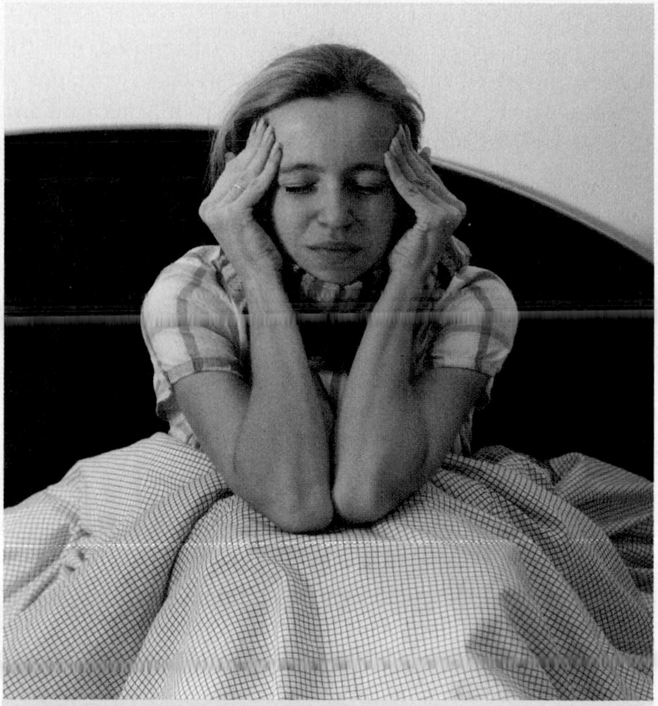

Patients report that migraines can be triggered by emotional stress, fatigue, too much or not enough sleep, fasting, caffeine, chocolate, alcohol, menses, hormone changes, altitude, weather, and certain foods. What triggers a migraine in one person may relieve it in another.

Migraine appears to run in families: If both your parents experience migraines, you have a 75 percent chance of experiencing them, too; if only one parent has them, you have a 50 percent chance.[31] If any of your relatives have them, you have a 20 percent risk.[32]

Whereas all headaches can be painful, migraines can be disabling. Symptoms vary greatly by individual, and attacks can last anywhere from 4 to 72 hours, with distinct phases of symptoms. In about 25 percent of cases, migraines are preceded by a sensory warning sign called an *aura,* which includes flashes of light, flickering vision, blind spots, tingling in arms or legs, or a sensation of odor or taste.[33] The triggers of a migraine vary widely from one person to the next and include stress, fatigue, too much or too little sleep, fasting or missing meals, food or drugs that change blood vessel diameter, caffeine, chocolate, alcohol (particularly red wine), menses, hormonal changes, changes in humidity, and altitude changes, as well as certain food additives such as MSG, nitrates, and nitrites.[34] Although vascular abnormalities in the brain have long been thought to be underlying causes, experts are beginning to believe that migraines may be triggered within the brain itself as a result of a complex biochemical and inflammatory process.[35]

WHAT DO YOU THINK?

Have you ever experienced a migraine or tension-type headache? How did you alleviate the pain?

- What actions can you take to reduce your risks of severe headaches in the future?

Because triggers for migraine vary by individual, treatment also varies. Keeping a careful diary and noting when migraine occurs is important in identifying your triggers and making appropriate changes in behavior where possible. Healthy lifestyle in the form of diet and exercise is important. When true migraines occur, relaxation is only minimally effective as a treatment. Often, prescription pain relievers are necessary. See your doctor for more information or go to the National Headache Foundation website (www.headaches.org) for the latest information on treatments.

Cluster Headaches The severe pain of a cluster headache has been described as "killer" or "suicidal." Usually, these headaches cause excruciating, stabbing pain on one side of the head, behind the eye, or in one defined spot. Fortunately, cluster headaches are relatively rare, affecting less than 1 percent of people, usually men. Young adults in their twenties tend to be particularly susceptible.[36]

Cluster headaches can last for weeks and disappear quickly. More commonly, they last for 40 to 90 minutes and often occur in the middle of the night, usually during rapid eye movement (REM) sleep. Oxygen therapy, drugs, and even surgery have been used to treat severe cases.

Seizure Disorders

Approximately 3 million people in the United States suffer from **epilepsy** or some other seizure-related disorder (the word *epilepsy* derives from the Greek *epilepsia,* meaning "seizure"). Approximately 1 percent of the population will develop epilepsy by age 20, and 3 percent by age 75.[37] An estimated 10 percent of the population will experience at least one seizure in their lives.[38] Each year, there are between 150,000 and 200,000 new cases of epilepsy diagnosed.[39] Males have a slightly greater risk than females do.[40]

epilepsy A neurological disorder caused by abnormal electrical brain activity; can be accompanied by altered consciousness or convulsions.

Seizure disorders are generally caused by abnormal electrical activity in the brain and are characterized by loss of control of muscular activity and unconsciousness. Risk factors include taking certain drugs, withdrawing from drugs, having a high fever and abnormal blood levels of sodium or glucose, or experiencing physical, chemical, or temperature trauma. Symptoms vary widely and can range from temporary confusion to major seizure activity.

Although causes of nearly half of seizure disorders are unknown, likely contributors include stroke, congenital abnormalities, injury or illness resulting in inflammation of the brain or spinal column, high fever, drug reactions, tumors, nutritional deficiency, and heredity. (See the appendix at the end of this book for information on providing first aid to someone experiencing a seizure.)

Public ignorance and stigma associated with seizure disorders can have a significant impact on sufferers and their families as they cope with the challenges of treatment and daily living. In most cases, people with these disorders can lead normal, seizure-free lives as a result of advancements in diagnosis and treatment.

LO 4 | COPING WITH DIGESTION-RELATED DISORDERS AND DISEASES

Outline risk factors, symptoms, and strategies for preventing major digestive disorders affecting adults in the United States today.

The *gastrointestinal tract* (GI tract), otherwise known as the *digestive system,* is a remarkable and fine-tuned machine, responsible for the breakdown of food into smaller molecules for absorption, fueling the body, and eliminating waste products. Although you may already know that the digestive system is about 9 feet long, what you may not know is that the inner surface of your GI tract is about as large as a small studio apartment, or between 100 and 130 square feet.[41] Every inch of that system has a job to do in keeping you healthy and maintaining bodily function. When any of several key indicators of digestive problems shows up—severe abdominal pain and cramping, bloody stool, diarrhea/constipation, weight loss, and changes in bowel habits—it should tell you something has run amuck and a visit to the doctor might be in your cards.

inflammatory bowel disease (IBD) A group of disorders in which the intestines become inflamed.

ulcerative colitis An inflammatory bowel disease that affects the mucous membranes of the large intestine and can lead to ulcers, erosion of the outer lining of the colon, and serious bleeding.

Crohn's disease An autoimmune inflammatory bowel disease that can affect several parts of the gastrointestinal tract as well as other body organs and systems.

irritable bowel syndrome (IBS) A functional bowel disorder caused by certain foods or stress that is characterized by nausea, pain, gas, or diarrhea.

Today, digestive disorders are among the fastest growing and most costly problems that Americans of all ages and stages of life face. Last year, over 70 million people suffered from one or more digestive problems, with nearly 49 million visiting a doctor.[42] Unfortunately, the causes of digestive disorders are often complex, symptoms are often subtle, and there is great variability in type of treatment and effectiveness. Two of the most common reported disorders are *lactose intolerance* and *celiac disease* (gluten intolerance) (discussed in **Chapter 7**); disorders that are not related to a specific nutrient are described below. See **TABLE 17.2** for discussion of gallbladder disease, another common digestive disorder, as well as several other modern maladies.

Inflammatory Bowel Disease

Inflammatory bowel disease (IBD) is an umbrella term for a group of disorders in which the intestines become inflamed. Causes are not known, but symptoms tend to come and go. Typically, they are severe, with stomach cramping, bloating, pain, and bloody bouts of diarrhea (as many as 20 bouts a day). The most common types of IBD are *ulcerative colitis* and *Crohn's disease.* About 25 percent of those with IBD develop it before age 20, with the majority of additional cases in the 15- to 35-year-old age range, especially among those who have a family history of the disease.[43] More than 1 million people in the United States have been diagnosed, with the majority of cases being among whites, particularly persons of Jewish descent.[44] Numbers of cases in African Americans and Latinos are increasing without clear patterns by geographical region. Asian Americans tend to have lower rates than do whites and African Americans.[45]

Ulcerative Colitis

Ulcerative colitis affects the colon and large intestine. It often first flares in the teens and can continue for life.[46] Although some experts believe that colitis occurs more frequently in people with high stress levels, this theory is controversial. Smokers have a higher risk of ulcerative colitis, as do those who have had measles and certain bacterial infections. Ulcerative colitis appears to have a genetic component and is slightly more common in males than females. Other risks appear to be exposure to a foodborne illness or allergy or infection in the gastrointestinal tract.[47] Determining the cause of colitis is difficult because the disease can go into remission and then recur without apparent reason. This pattern often continues over periods of years and may be related to later development of colorectal cancer.

Because the cause is unknown, it is important to treat symptoms and avoid substances that may trigger attacks. Keeping a food diary and recording potential flare-ups of colitis is an important part of prevention. Treatment focuses on relieving the symptoms by decreasing foods that are hard to digest (raw vegetables, seeds, nuts, and high-fiber foods); taking probiotics; and taking anti-inflammatory drugs, steroids, and other medications to reduce inflammation and soothe irritated intestinal walls.

Crohn's Disease

Crohn's disease primarily affects the small intestine, resulting in major inflammation and swelling. It is usually diagnosed in men and women in their twenties and thirties. It is characterized by intense stomach pain, often in the lower right area, fever, weight loss, joint pain, mouth ulcers, and watery diarrhea. Intestinal bleeding may also occur and can be serious enough to cause anemia, fatigue, and immune system dysfunction. The most common complication is actually bowel obstruction due to swelling and scar tissue and ulcers that erode and form little infection-prone out-pouches known as fistula. Those diagnosed with this disease must carefully monitor their diet to ensure adequate nutrition, be "tuned in" to their body and changes that may occur, see their doctors if symptoms develop, and take medications to reduce inflammation and prevent infection.[48] Surgery to remove damaged or obstructed portions of the bowel may be necessary.

Irritable Bowel Syndrome (IBS)

Inflammatory bowel disease (IBD) and **irritable bowel syndrome (IBS)** are not the same condition, although they may sound as if they were. Irritable bowel syndrome is a *functional bowel disorder* (affecting how the bowel, including the colon and rectum, works). The exact cause is unknown, but

TABLE 17.2 | Other Modern Maladies

Disease	Who Is Affected?	Causes and Risk Factors	Symptoms	Treatment	Prevention
Fibromyalgia Extreme fatigue; painful, aching joints and muscles.	Affects 2% of the population. Rates increase with age.	Unknown. Affects primarily women in their thirties and forties.	Numbness, tingling, pain, headache, dizziness.	Pain medications, anti-inflammatories, rest, stress management.	Rest, dietary adjustments. Avoid extreme temperatures.
Gallbladder diseases Most common are cholecystitis (inflammation) and cholelithiasis (gallstones).	Affects 10%–15% of the population, twice as many women as men. Highest in Mexican Americans and Native Americans.	Chemical exposure, infections, traumatic injury, obesity, cirrhosis of liver, rapid weight loss, diabetes, cholesterol-lowering drugs.	Acute pain in the upper right quadrant of abdomen, particularly after eating fatty food; nausea, vomiting. Often asymptomatic.	Medications to relieve inflammation or cause of inflammation; removal of gallstones through lithotripsy or surgery.	Reduce dietary fat; avoid alcohol, fried foods, whole grains.
Multiple sclerosis Degenerative, autoimmune neurological disease caused by breakdown of protective sheath around nerves.	Over 400,000 cases, most between ages of 20 and 40. Over 10,000 new cases per year.	Suspected causes include genetics, viruses, allergies, and environmental toxins. Caucasians are at greatest risk.	From minor numbness, blurred vision, fatigue, balance issues to severe disability. Intermittent course for some.	No cure, but drug therapy, climate change, and lifestyle choices can reduce symptoms and increase healthy years.	Flare-up prevention possible with healthy lifestyle, adequate sleep, healthy diet, stress management, and avoidance of temperature extremes.
Parkinson's disease Chronic, progressive, neurological disease that affects motor function.	There are 50,000–60,000 new cases per year. Nearly 2 million total, mostly over age 50.	Cause currently unknown.	Tremors of limbs and head; rigidity, postural instability, slowness, balance issues, shuffling gait; speech difficulties.	No cure, but medications can relieve symptoms. Deep brain stimulation and gamma knife surgery may help.	None obvious. Healthy lifestyle may help slow progression.
Raynaud's syndrome Exaggerated constriction of small arteries in the extremities.	Affected are 5%–10% of adults, primarily women.	Unknown.	Fingers and toes become numb, turn white or purple; throbbing pain.	Topical medications to reduce symptoms.	More common in those exposed to extreme cold repeatedly, so avoid frostbite or medications that affect blood flow.
Rosacea Inflammatory skin condition causing redness and small red bumps or pustules on the face.	Affects over 16 million Americans; more common in menopausal women and people with fair skin/sensitive skin.	Still unknown, but many suspects, ranging from genetic predisposition to blushing, skin mites, bacteria. None conclusive.	Can progress from flushing and spider veins on face to lumps and bumps. Skin thickening, red itchy eyes, bulbous nose in later stages.	No cure, but controls include prescription medications and lotions, less irritating soaps, surgery, laser treatments, freezing.	Unknown.
Systemic lupus erythematosus Autoimmune disease in which antibodies destroy or injure organs such as kidneys, brain, and heart.	Affected are 1 in 700 Caucasians, 1 in 250 African Americans; 90% of patients are women between ages 18 and 45. Ratio of females to males is 10:1.	Cause unknown. Possible genetic predisposition combined with environment and hormones.	Sensitivity to light, arthritis, swelling, tendency toward increased infections, butterfly-shaped rash across nose and cheeks.	Medications such as steroids to reduce symptoms and complications.	Healthy lifestyle; other possible preventive measures unknown.

Sources: NIH, Medline Plus, "Fibromyalgia," 2014, www.nlm.nih.gov/medlineplus/fibromyalgia.html; L. Stinton and E. Shaffer, "Epidemiology of Gall Bladder Diseases," *Gut and Liver* 6, no. 2 (2012): 172–87; National Multiple Sclerosis Society, "Who Gets MS?," 2013, www.nationalmssociety.org/What-is-MS/Who-Gets-MS; National Multiple Sclerosis Society, "What Causes MS?," www.nationalmssociety.org/about-multiple-sclerosis/what-we-know-about-ms/who-gets-ms/index.aspx; P. Sweeney, Cleveland Clinic, Center for Continuing Education, "Parkinson's Disease," www.clevelandclinicmeded.com/medicalpubs/diseasemanagement/neurology/parkinsons-disease; The National Rosacea Society, "The Many Faces of Rosacea," www.rosacea.org/rr/2013/winter/article_1.php; What Health?, "Rosacea Statistics," www.whathealth.com/rosacea/incidence.html; American College of Rheumatology, "Systemic Lupus Erythematosus (Lupus)," 2013, www.rheumatology.org/practice/clinical/patients/diseases_and_conditions/lupus.asp.

in individuals with IBS, the normal muscular contractions in the intestines don't work properly and food isn't processed or eliminated as it should be.[49] Irritable bowel syndrome affects up to 20 percent of adults in the United States—particularly women—and usually begins in adolescence or early adulthood, with those under 35 being most susceptible.[50] It is also the second leading cause of work absenteeism after the common cold.[51]

Irritable bowel syndrome may begin after an infection, a stressful life event, or onset of maturity, without any other medical indicators. Characterized by nausea, pain, gas, diarrhea, bloating, or cramps after eating certain foods or during unusual stress, IBS can be uncomfortable, but usually does not permanently harm the intestines unless symptoms are severe. Symptoms may vary from week to week and can fade for long periods of time. Researchers suspect that people with IBS have digestive systems that are overly sensitive to what they eat and drink, to stress, and to certain hormonal changes. Often, because symptoms are so similar to other gastrointestinal tract diseases, IBS is only diagnosed after all the other gastrointestinal diseases have been ruled out.

Although there is no cure for IBS, treatments attempt to relieve symptoms; stress management, relaxation techniques, regular activity, and diet changes can control it in the vast majority of cases. Problems with diarrhea can be reduced by cutting down on fat and avoiding caffeine and *sorbitol,* a sweetener found in diet foods and chewing gum. Constipation can be relieved by a gradual increase in fiber and increased fluid consumption. Some sufferers benefit from drugs that relax the intestinal muscle or from antidepressant drugs and counseling to reduce stress.

Gastroesophageal Reflux Disease

Gastroesophageal reflux disease (GERD), commonly referred to as *heartburn* or *acid reflux,* affects millions of people throughout the world. Risk factors include age, diet, alcohol use, obesity, pregnancy, and smoking. At any given time, people of all ages and stages of life suffer from a sensation of heartburn, or backflow of stomach acid into the esophagus, characterized by discomfort or a burning sensation behind the breastbone. Symptoms usually occur after a meal and can include coughing, choking, or vomiting. When these symptoms are severe and occur more than two to three times per week, GERD is often the diagnosis.

Prevention of GERD focuses on determining which foods or beverages trigger symptoms (coffee, sodas, high-acid food and juices, and alcohol are the big culprits) and avoiding spicy or fried foods. Dietary control is often a key in reducing heartburn symptoms. Also, it is important to find out whether there are mechanical causes of reflux, such as sleeping or sitting in positions that exacerbate symptoms. It may be helpful to elevate your upper body if acid rushes into the esophagus when you lie down. If repositioning doesn't work, taking medications to reduce stomach acids can help. If heartburn persists, see your doctor.

gastroesophageal reflux disease (GERD) Chronic condition in which stomach acid backflows into the esophagus, causing heartburn and potential damage to the esophagus.

arthritis Painful inflammatory disease of the joints.

LO 5 | COPING WITH MUSCULOSKELETAL DISEASES

Explain the risk factors and symptoms of various musculoskeletal diseases, including arthritis and low back pain, and suggest strategies for prevention.

Musculoskeletal diseases—including back pain, arthritis, bodily injuries, and osteoporosis—are more common than any other health condition in the United States and exact a tremendous toll in disability, pain, and suffering. Every year, more than half of all days of work missed due to a major medical condition result from musculoskeletal problems such as joint pain, arthritis, and back/neck pain (**FIGURE 17.4**). As the population ages and becomes increasingly overweight and sedentary, the musculoskeletal system has seen epidemic increases in problems.

Arthritis and Related Conditions

Nearly 23 percent of Americans, or 53 million people, have one of the doctor-diagnosed forms of **arthritis**.[52] With the aging of the baby boomers, these numbers are projected to soar to 67 million or 25 percent of the population by 2030.[53] Arthritis consists of more than 100 conditions that wreak havoc on joints, bones, muscles, cartilage, and connective tissues, leading to disability and pain. Osteoarthritis and rheumatoid arthritis are the most common types, with symptoms

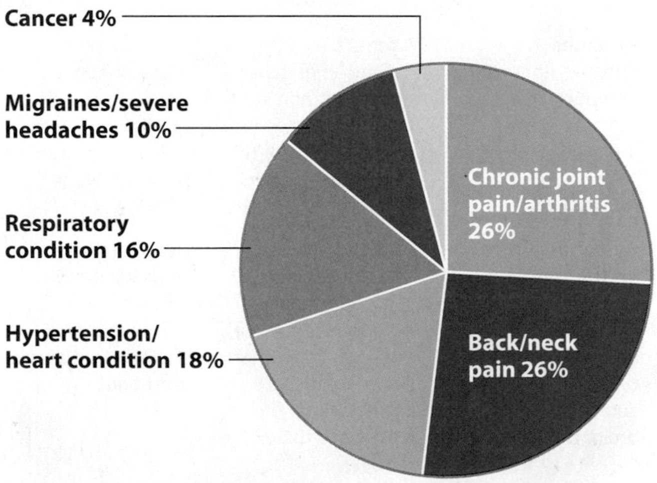

FIGURE 17.4 Proportion of Lost Work Days for Persons Age 18 and Older by Major Medical Condition

Sources: © 2008, American Academy of Orthopaedic Surgeons, Modified with permission from *The Burden of Musculoskeletal Diseases in the United States.* Source of data: National Center for Health Statistics, National Health Interview Survey, Adult Sample, 2005.

that range from minor aches and pains to crippling disability. Arthritis is not just a disease of old age; in fact, two-thirds of those with arthritis are under the age of 65, with over 300,000 children affected.[54] Each year, arthritis costs over $128 billion in direct and indirect costs.[55]

Osteoarthritis Also called *degenerative joint disease,* **osteoarthritis (OA)** is the most common form of arthritis, affecting over 27 million adults in the United States.[56] If you notice that your parents or grandparents are slow to get up or walk stiffly after getting out of bed, they may be showing early signs of OA. Before age 45, more men than women have osteoarthritis; after age 45, more women have it.[57] This progressive deterioration of cartilage, bones, and joints has been associated with the "wear-and-tear" theory of aging.

Although age and injury are undoubtedly factors in osteoarthritis, heredity, abnormal joint use, diet and excess weight, abnormalities in joint structure, and impaired blood supply to the joint may also contribute. For most people, anti-inflammatory drugs and pain relievers such as aspirin and cortisone-related agents ease discomfort. In some sufferers, applications of heat, mild exercise, and massage also relieve the pain. When joints become so distorted that they impair activity, surgical intervention is often necessary. Joint replacement and bone fusion are increasingly common.

WHAT DO YOU THINK?

Do you know anyone who currently has problems with arthritis?

- Which joints seem to be most affected?
- What factors do you think might have contributed to their problems?
- What could they have done to reduce their risks?

Rheumatoid Arthritis The most crippling form of arthritis, **rheumatoid arthritis (RA)** is an autoimmune disease involving chronic inflammation. Over 1.3 million people have RA, with nearly three times as many women as men.[58] It typically affects women at younger ages than men. Increasing numbers of cases are occurring in people in their twenties.[59] Symptoms include stiffness, pain, redness, and swelling of multiple joints, particularly those of the hands and wrists, and can be gradually progressive or sporadic, with occasional unexplained remissions. Although the cause of rheumatoid arthritis is unknown, some believe that invading microorganisms take over the joint and cause the immune system to begin attacking the body's own tissues. Exposure to toxic chemicals and stress are also possible triggers, as are hormonal influences.[60] Genetic markers that seem to increase risk have also been identified.

Treatment of rheumatoid arthritis emphasizes pain relief and improved functional mobility. In some instances, immunosuppressant drugs can reduce the inflammatory response, and in advanced cases, surgery may be necessary. Advanced rheumatoid arthritis often involves destruction of the bony ends of joints. The remedy for this condition is typically bone fusion, which leaves the joint immobile. In some instances, joint replacement may be a viable alternative.

osteoarthritis (OA) Progressive deterioration of bones and joints that has been associated with the wear-and-tear theory of aging; also called *degenerative joint disease.*

rheumatoid arthritis An autoimmune inflammatory joint disease.

osteoporosis A disease in which bones become brittle and break easily.

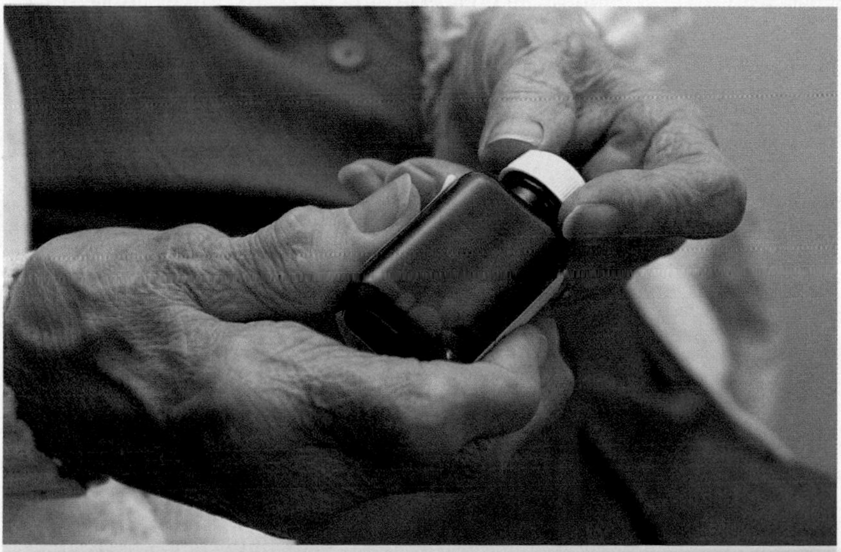

Arthritis can make even a simple task painful and difficult.

Osteoporosis

Osteoporosis is a disease in which bones become brittle and weak and break easily. Most commonly, bones in the spine fracture, which results in back pain, loss of height over time, and a stooped posture. Ultimately, bones in other parts of the body fracture easily, too, including the hands, wrists, and hip.

Osteoporosis affects men and women of all races. But white and Asian women—especially those who are past menopause—are at highest risk.

The good news is that recent research has shown significant decreases in osteoporosis in persons 50 and over in recent years, due to improved early diagnosis, medications, and lifestyle changes. Nevertheless, an estimated 200 million people globally have osteoporosis.[61] Nearly 40 percent of women with osteoporosis and 15 to 30 percent of men will have one or more fragility fractures in their lifetimes.[62] Prevention strategies, including regular exams, adequate amounts of calcium and vitamin D, and regular weight-bearing exercise and strength training, are among key recommendations to reduce risks of developing osteoporosis.

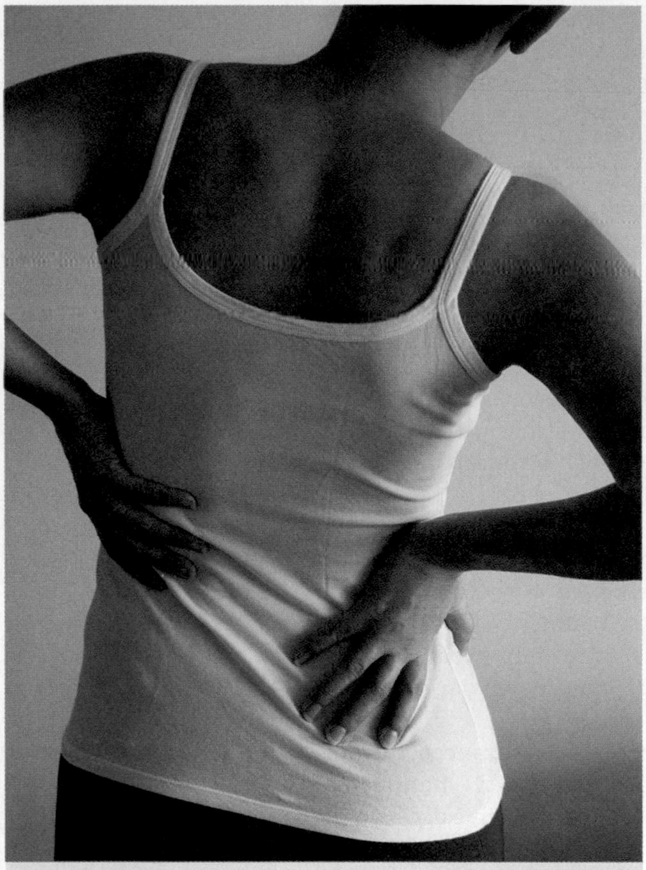

In the United States, low back pain is the major cause of disability for people age 20 to 45, who suffer more frequently and severely from this problem than older people do. It is one of the most common chronic ailments among college students.

Low Back Pain

If you're like 85 percent of the population, at some point you will experience **low back pain (LBP)**, the number one cause of activity limitation and work absence worldwide.[63] The resulting pain may be mild, involving short-lived muscle spasms, or it may be more severe, involving damage to discs, dislocation, a fracture, or another form of spinal trauma. In about 23 percent of LBP cases, pain is chronic and comes and goes with activities as varied as sneezing, bending over, and lifting heavy objects.[64] About 12 percent of those with LBP become permanently disabled.[65] Treatment may involve medication, rehabilitation, injections, and surgery.

Low back pain is increasingly common, especially among young adults (see the **Student Health Today** box for one possible cause).[66] These injuries tend to be shorter lived initially, but over time they progress toward more recurrent and long-term disability and costs.[67] Overall costs of diagnosing and treatment, as well as costs to employers and other indirect costs, may be up to $200 billion a year.[68] LBP causes more disability in Americans under 45 years old than any other condition, with over 26 million Americans aged 20 to 64 years reporting frequent episodes.[69] As a result, employers throughout the country have become increasingly interested in preventing these injuries.

low back pain (LBP) Pain or discomfort in the lumbosacral region (lowest vertebrae) of the back.

The following factors contribute to LBP:

- **Age.** People between the ages of 20 and 45 run the greatest risk of LBP. At age 50, the condition becomes less common. After age 65, the incidence again rises, apparently because of bone and joint deterioration. For college students, heavy purses or backpacks can be major precipitators of back problems, particularly among those who are primarily sedentary or who have weak core muscles.
- **Body type.** Many studies indicate that people who are very tall, have a high body mass index (BMI), or have a lanky body type run an increased risk of LBP. Other sources say that being slightly overweight helps reduce the risk of LBP, as the weight helps strengthen core muscles. However, much of this research is controversial.
- **Posture.** Poor posture may be one of the greatest contributors to LBP. If you routinely slouch, particularly over a computer or workstation, you run an increased risk of LBP.
- **Strength and fitness.** People with LBP tend to have less overall core strength than other people. The total level of fitness and conditioning is also a factor—the fitter you are, the better. Sedentary people who suddenly decide to "get fit" often are among those most at risk for LBP, as they engage in strenuous activity without first strengthening supporting muscles.
- **Psychological factors.** Numerous psychological factors appear to increase risk for LBP. Depression, apathy, inattentiveness, boredom, emotional upsets, drug abuse, and family and financial problems all heighten risk.
- **Occupational risk.** The type of work you do and the conditions you do it in greatly affect risk. For example, truck drivers, who must endure the bumps and jolts of the road while in a sitting position, frequently suffer from back pain.

Repetitive Motion Disorders

It's the end of the term, and you have finished the last of several papers. After hours of nonstop typing, your hands are numb and you feel an intense, burning pain that makes the thought of typing one more word almost unbearable. If this happens, you may be suffering from a *repetitive motion disorder* (RMD). Repetitive motion disorders include carpal tunnel syndrome, bursitis, tendonitis, ganglion cysts, and others.[70] Twisting of the arm or wrist, overexertion, and incorrect posture or position are usually contributors. The areas most likely to be affected are the hands, wrists, elbows, and shoulders, but the neck, back, hips, knees, feet, ankles, and legs can be affected, too. Over time, repetitive motion can cause permanent damage to nerves, soft tissue, and joints.

STUDENT HEALTH TODAY

COLLEGE STUDENTS AND LOW BACK PAIN *Oh, My Aching Backpack?*

Did you know that more than half of your college peers suffer from back problems? Why are there so many issues with the back? Although athletics, exercise regimens, sitting for hours while studying, and other normal activities can cause problems, modern conveniences may also be a huge factor. Look no further than the backpacks, messenger bags, and supersized purses in vogue today. Laptops, tablets, books, water bottles, wallets, smartphones, headphones, snacks, and a change of shoes or a T-shirt are but a few of the items that can be found in the typical "portable locker" students tote on their backs or sling over their shoulder. Not surprisingly, lugging such an assortment around each day can inflame muscles and other soft tissues. According to one study, 85 percent of college students report neck or back pain attributable to carrying heavy backpacks or laptops.

Whereas hikers have long recognized the importance of internal frames and heavy-duty hip straps to displace the weight of heavy packs, most college students carry less supportive (and cheaper) daypacks that contain as much as 30 to 40 pounds of stuff, supported with only one shoulder strap. Over time, this weight can wreak havoc on even the most fit and healthy backs and shoulders. Increasing numbers of students are experiencing knee and foot problems related to backpack overload. Neuromas, flat feet, plantar foot pressure injuries, and other problems are on the increase among those who add unnecessary weight to their packs.

College students are not alone; even elementary schoolchildren are toting heavy backpacks—sometimes carrying amounts that are 10 to 15 percent of their total body weight. Because such repetitive strain on the back can result in a lifetime of pain and disability, prevention is imperative. If you must carry a pack all day, protect your back by following this advice:

- Opt for the lightest pack available and make sure that it has a heavy-duty hip strap so that you are not carrying the bulk of the weight around your back and shoulders. Adjust the strap so the weight is primarily on your hips.
- If you can afford a small internal-frame pack, buy one. There are many excellent packs available from outdoor recreation supply companies, or consider a rolling computer case.
- If your pack has two straps, use them both, rather than putting additional strain on one side of your body.
- Use and carry the lightest computer possible. If you have to carry larger devices, don't let your ego get in the way. Let a roller bag take the weight rather than your back! Don't bring your books to class unless your instructor asks you to. Plan ahead and bring only those study materials to campus that you can complete while you're there; carry a smaller notepad; store files on a jump drive and upload to a campus computer to do work.
- Limit the amount of personal items you carry each day. Wallets, makeup, hair products, and so on should be kept to a minimum.

Overstuffed backpacks can lead to a lifetime of back pain.

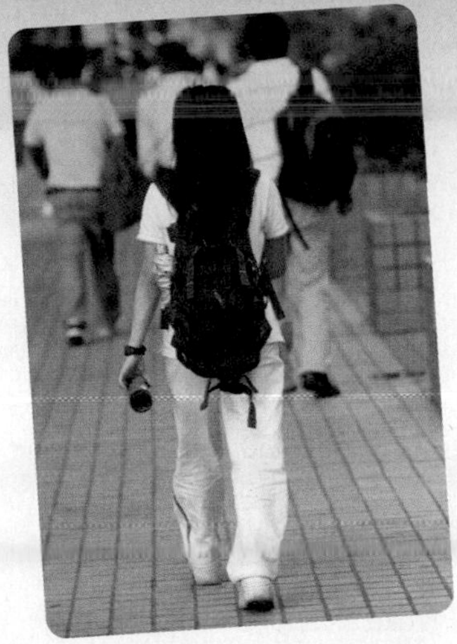

- When lifting your pack to put it on your back, stand with both feet on the ground, knees slightly flexed, and your back straight. Twisting the back while swinging up the load can cause back injuries.
- Pack heavy items on the bottom and as close to your back as possible.
- Once you're ready to go, weigh the pack. If it's over 15 pounds, reassess what is necessary and ditch the rest.

Sources: H. Son, "The Effect of Backpack Load on Muscle Activities of the Trunk and Lower Extremities and Plantar Foot Pressure in Flatfoot," *Journal of Physical Therapy Science* 25, no. 11 (2013): 1383–1386; D. Gilkey et al., "Risk Factors Associated with Back Pain: A Cross-Sectional Study of College Students," *Journal of Manipulative and Physiological Therapeutics* 33, no. 2 (2010): 88–95.

One of the most common RMDs is **carpal tunnel syndrome**, a product of spending hours typing, texting, gaming, or using the latest media device repetitively. RMDs are not limited to leisure or office job activities. Motions such as flipping groceries through computerized scanners or other tasks requiring repeated hand and wrist movements can irritate the median nerve in the wrist, causing numbness, tingling, and pain in the fingers and hands. Although carpal tunnel syndrome risk can be reduced by proper placement of the keyboard, mouse, wrist pads, and other techniques, it is often overlooked until significant damage has been done. Better education and ergonomic workplace designs can eliminate many injuries of this nature. Newer endoscopic surgical techniques have been effective in reducing or eliminating pain and discomfort. Physical and occupational therapy is an important part of treatment and eventual recovery.

carpal tunnel syndrome An occupational injury in which the median nerve in the wrist becomes irritated, causing numbness, tingling, and pain in the fingers and hands.

STUDY PLAN

Customize your study plan—and master your health!—in the Study Area of **MasteringHealth.**

ASSESS **YOURSELF**

Could you be at risk for chronic illness? Want to find out? Take the **Are You at Risk for Chronic Illness?** assessment available on MasteringHealth.™

Need help creating a plan? Follow the strategies in the **Your Plan for Change** box for short- and long-term improvements to your health.

YOUR PLAN FOR **CHANGE**

Now that you have completed the **ASSESS YOURSELF** activity and considered your results, you may need to take further steps to understand and address your risks.

TODAY, YOU CAN:

- ☐ Make an appointment with your doctor to find out more about any symptoms you've been having or discuss your potential risk factors.
- ☐ Call your parents and find out if they have ever had similar problems or if they know of anyone in your family who has had these problems.
- ☐ Weigh your full backpack or purse; if it's more than 10 percent of your body weight, decide what you can leave at home.

WITHIN THE NEXT 2 WEEKS, YOU CAN:

- ☐ Find out more about your family history of chronic illness and what you can do to cut down your risk. Ask your parents what sorts of illnesses your family members have had and use that information for planning your own prevention strategies. If your parent has low back pain, find out what they have done to reduce their risks.
- ☐ If you suffer from migraines, keep a diary, pay attention to what triggers them for you, and then work on creating a routine that keeps you out of harm's way.
- ☐ If you suffer from heartburn, identify the foods or situations (such as sleeping postures) that bring it on. Make an effort to eliminate problematic foods or positions.

BY THE END OF THE SEMESTER, YOU CAN:

- ☐ Adjust your routine to avoid environmental toxins. Avoid going to parties where people smoke, for example.
- ☐ Keep track of allergy-related symptoms to see if you can identify any likely triggers.
- ☐ Replace all of your cleaning products for your house, apartment, or dorm room with less toxic ones made from vinegar, lemon juice, and other natural ingredients (see the **Health Headlines** box on page 481 for tips on how to make these yourself). Find out how to safely dispose of the chemical-intensive products that you previously used.

CHAPTER **REVIEW**

LO 1 Coping with Respiratory Problems

- Chronic lower respiratory disease (CLRD) (including bronchitis, emphysema, and asthma) is the third leading cause of death in the United States (right after heart disease and cancer).

LO 2 Coping with Allergies

- Allergies occur as the immune system responds to allergens. They can be triggered by pollens, foods, or other substances.

LO 3 Coping with Neurological Disorders

- Neurological conditions include headaches and seizure disorders such as epilepsy. The most common types of headache are tension and migraine.

LO 4 Coping with Digestion-Related Disorders

- Inflammatory bowel disease includes ulcerative colitis and Crohn's disease. Irritable bowel syndrome (IBS) and other digestive problems affect increasing numbers of adults.

LO 5 Coping with Musculoskeletal Disorders

- Musculoskeletal problems such as arthritis, repetitive motion disorders, low back pain, and osteoporosis cause significant pain and disability in millions of people. Many of these problems are preventable.

POP **QUIZ**

Visit **MasteringHealth** to personalize your study plan with Chapter Review Quizzes and Dynamic Study Modules.

LO 1 Coping with Respiratory Problems

1. The gradual destruction of the alveoli in a smoker's lung usually causes which COPD characterized by difficulty in exhaling?
   a. Dyspnea
   b. Bronchitis
   c. Emphysema
   d. Asthma
2. Margaret experiences occasional wheezing, shortness of breath, and coughing spasms. What chronic respiratory disorder is she likely suffering from?
   a. Sleep apnea
   b. Bronchitis
   c. Asthma
   d. COPD
3. The leading chronic disease in school-aged children today is
   a. bronchitis.
   b. common cold.
   c. attention-deficit disorder.
   d. asthma.

LO 2 Coping with Allergies

4. Julie has found that she cannot eat nuts without suffering from itching and nausea. What condition is she likely to be suffering from?
   a. Irritable bowel syndrome
   b. Ulcerative colitis
   c. Food allergy
   d. Diabetes mellitus
5. Which of the following statements is correct?
   a. Lactose intolerance is an example of a food allergy.
   b. Children are more likely than adults to outgrow allergies to foods.
   c. Food allergies and food intolerance are the same thing.
   d. Food allergies appear to be decreasing in the United States.

LO 3 Coping with Neurological Disorders

6. If you experience an aura, a sensory warning sign that may include flickering vision or blind spots, you are likely to
   a. have an asthma attack.
   b. have a migraine headache.
   c. have a tension-type headache.
   d. be showing symptoms of glaucoma.
7. Which of the following is correct?
   a. Migraine incidence usually peaks in older adulthood (between ages 60 and 80).
   b. Women have more migraine headaches; men have more cluster headaches.
   c. Tension-type headaches are often preceded by an aura.
   d. If untreated, migraines can progress into epilepsy or another seizure-related disorder.

LO 4 Coping with Digestion-Related Disorders

8. Which of the following is correct?
   a. Inflammatory bowel syndrome often occurs before age 35.
   b. Inflammatory bowel disease and inflammatory bowel syndrome are the same.
   c. Consuming fruit juices lessens heartburn associated with gastroesophageal reflux disease.
   d. Smokers have a lower risk of ulcerative colitis.

LO 5 Coping with Musculoskeletal Disorders

9. Which of the following conditions is the leading cause of employee sick time and lost productivity in the United States?
   a. Low back pain
   b. Upper respiratory infections
   c. Asthma
   d. On-the-job injuries
10. After Dylan spent 5 hours typing his term paper, he noticed numbness, tingling, and pain in his left wrist. Dylan is most likely experiencing
    a. rheumatoid arthritis.
    b. osteoporosis.
    c. osteoarthritis.
    d. carpal tunnel syndrome.

Answers to the Pop Quiz can be found on page A-1. If you answered a question incorrectly, review the section identified by the Learning Outcome. For even more study tools, visit MasteringHealth.

THINK ABOUT IT!

LO 1 Coping with Respiratory Problems

1. List common respiratory diseases affecting Americans. Which of these has a genetic basis? An environmental basis? An individual basis?

LO 2 Coping with Allergies

2. What is the difference between a food allergy and food intolerance?

LO 3 Coping with Neurological Disorders

3. Compare and contrast the different types of headaches.

LO 4 Coping with Digestion-Related Disorders

4. Compare the symptoms of ulcerative colitis, gastroesophageal reflux disease, and Crohn's disease. How can you tell whether your stomach is reacting to final exams or telling you that you have a serious medical condition?

LO 5 Coping with Musculoskeletal Disorders

5. What are the major disorders of the musculoskeletal system? Describe the difference between osteoarthritis and rheumatoid arthritis.

ACCESS YOUR HEALTH ON THE INTERNET

Visit **MasteringHealth** for links to the websites and RSS feeds.

The following websites explore further topics and issues related to personal health.

American Academy of Allergy, Asthma, and Immunology. This site presents an overview of asthma and allergy information, particularly as it applies to children with allergies. It also offers interactive quizzes to test your knowledge and an ask-the-expert section. **www.aaaai.org**

American Lung Association. The latest news on asthma and lung disease is available here. **www.lungusa.org**

National Center for Chronic Disease Prevention and Health Promotion. A wide range of information is available from this organization, which is dedicated to chronic diseases and health promotion. The organization is linked to the Centers for Disease Control and Prevention. **www.cdc.gov/chronicdisease**

National Institute of Neurological Disorders and Stroke. This site contains up-to-date information to help individuals cope with pain-related difficulties. **www.ninds.nih.gov**

National Institute for Diabetes and Digestive and Kidney Diseases (NIDDK). This valuable resource provides key information about diabetes and the major digestive and kidney diseases, as well as resources for prevention and treatment options. **www2.niddk.nih.gov**

18 Becoming a Responsible Health Care Consumer

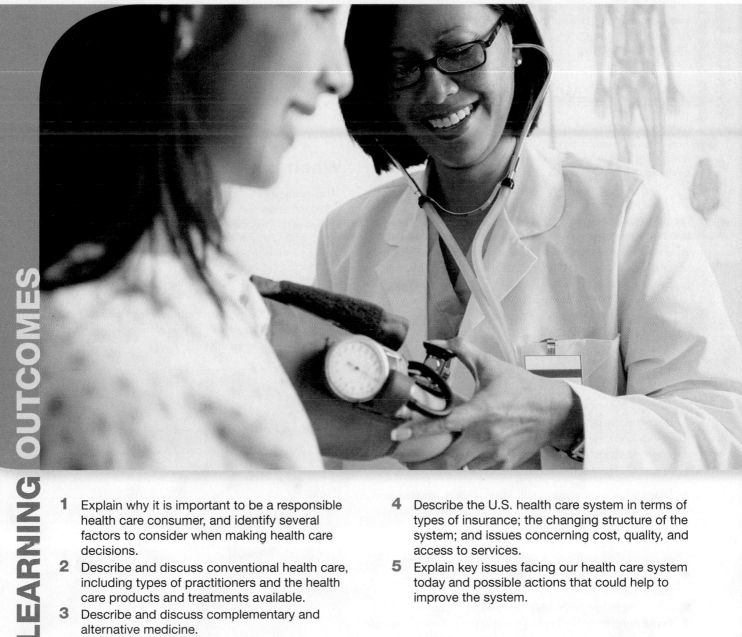

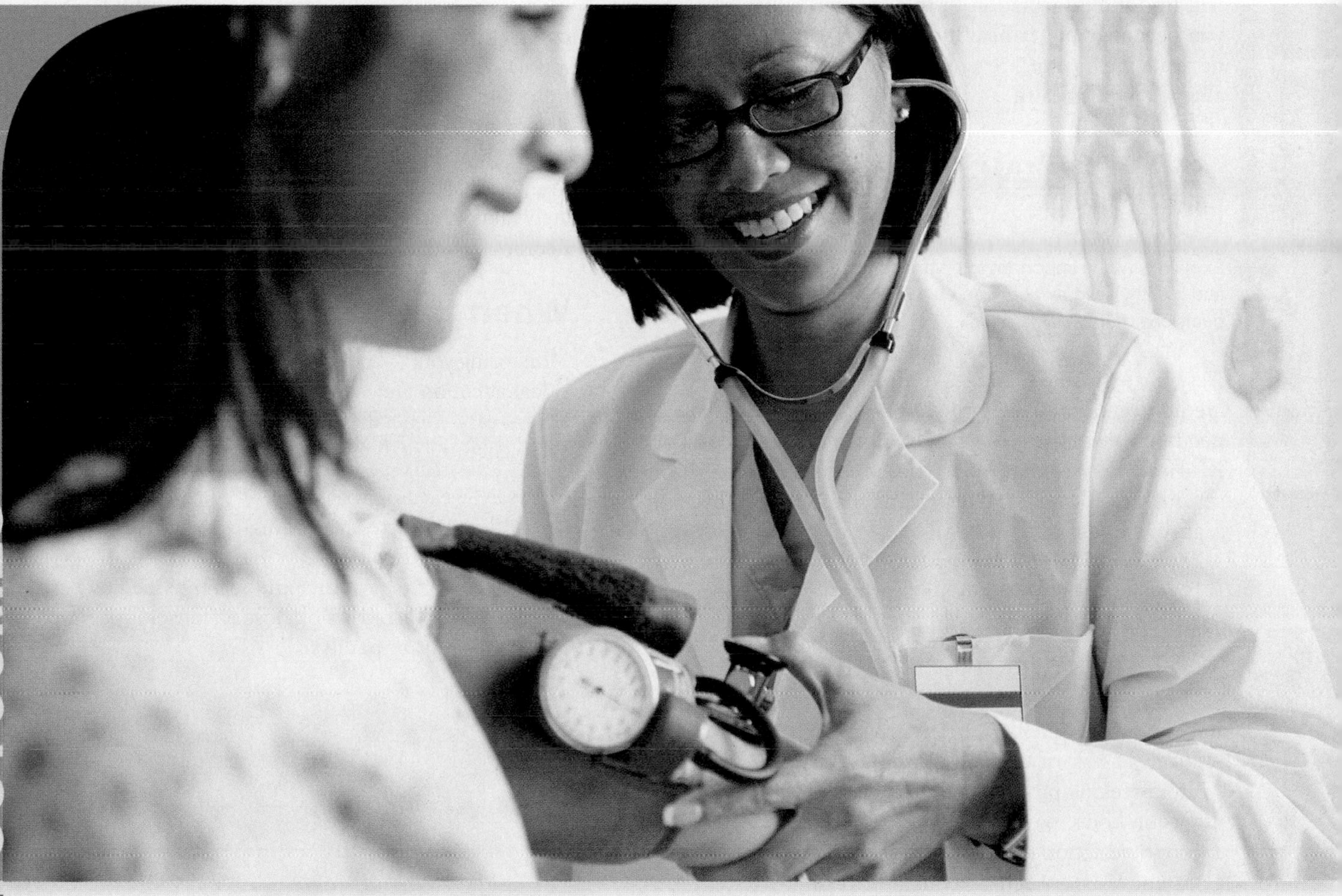

LEARNING OUTCOMES

1 Explain why it is important to be a responsible health care consumer, and identify several factors to consider when making health care decisions.

2 Describe and discuss conventional health care, including types of practitioners and the health care products and treatments available.

3 Describe and discuss complementary and alternative medicine.

4 Describe the U.S. health care system in terms of types of insurance; the changing structure of the system; and issues concerning cost, quality, and access to services.

5 Explain key issues facing our health care system today and possible actions that could help to improve the system.

Have there been times when you wondered whether you were sick enough to go to your campus health clinic? Have you left visits with your health care provider feeling that the doctor didn't give you a thorough exam or that you had more questions than you did when you arrived? Do you engage in risky behaviors, such as riding your bike without a helmet, and don't know where or how you would be treated if you were injured? Have you ever had to help a family member or loved one make health care decisions? Are you one of the 7.5 percent of college students without health insurance?[1]

If the answer to any of these questions is yes, then you will find the information in this chapter valuable in helping you become a better health care consumer. Learning how to navigate the health care system is an important part of taking charge of your health.

LO 1 | TAKING RESPONSIBILITY FOR YOUR HEALTH CARE

Explain why it is important to be a responsible health care consumer, and identify several factors to consider when making health care decisions.

Acting responsibly in times of illness can be difficult. If you are not feeling well, you must first decide whether you really need to seek medical advice. For ailments like colds or minor injuries, self-care may be the best course of action. In more serious cases, not seeking treatment, whether because of high costs or limited coverage, or trying to medicate yourself when a professional diagnosis and treatment are needed, is potentially dangerous. It's important to know the benefits and limits of self-care.

Self-Care

Individuals can practice behaviors that promote health and reduce the risk of disease as well as treat minor afflictions without seeking professional help. Self-care consists of knowing your body, paying attention to its signals, and taking appropriate action to stop the progression of illness or injury. Common forms of self-care include the following:

- Diagnosing symptoms or conditions that occur frequently but may not require physician visits (e.g., the common cold, minor abrasions)
- Using over-the-counter remedies to treat mild, infrequent, and unambiguous pain and other symptoms
- Performing first aid for common, uncomplicated injuries and conditions
- Checking blood pressure, pulse, and temperature
- Performing monthly breast or testicular self-examinations
- Doing periodic checks for blood glucose, cholesterol, or other levels as prescribed by a physician
- Learning from reliable self-help books, websites, and DVDs
- Performing meditation and other relaxation techniques
- Maintaining a healthful diet, getting adequate rest, and exercising

In addition, a vast array of at-home diagnostic kits are now available to test for pregnancy, allergies, HIV, genetic disorders, and many other conditions. Caution is in order here: diagnoses from these devices and kits may not always be accurate—or you may not have the ability to understand the ramifications of what you learn without professional interpretation. Moreover, home health tests are not substitutes for regular, complete examinations by a trained practitioner.

HEAR IT! PODCASTS
Want study podcasts for this chapter? Download **Consumerism: Selecting Health Care Products and Services** and **Complementary** and **Alternative Medicine** available on MasteringHealth.™

Many people also use self-care treatment methods inappropriately. Taking prescription drugs used for a previous illness to treat your current illness, using unproven self-treatment, or using other people's medications are examples of inappropriate self-care. Using self-care methods appropriately takes effort, education, and the ability to make informed decisions that are based on scientific evidence.

When to Seek Help

Monitoring your symptoms and deciding which warrant professional attention and which you can take care of yourself is not always easy. Generally, you should consult a physician if you experience *any* of the following:

- A serious accident or injury
- Sudden or severe chest pains, especially if they cause breathing difficulties
- Trauma to the head or spine accompanied by persistent headache, blurred vision, loss of consciousness, vomiting, convulsions, or paralysis

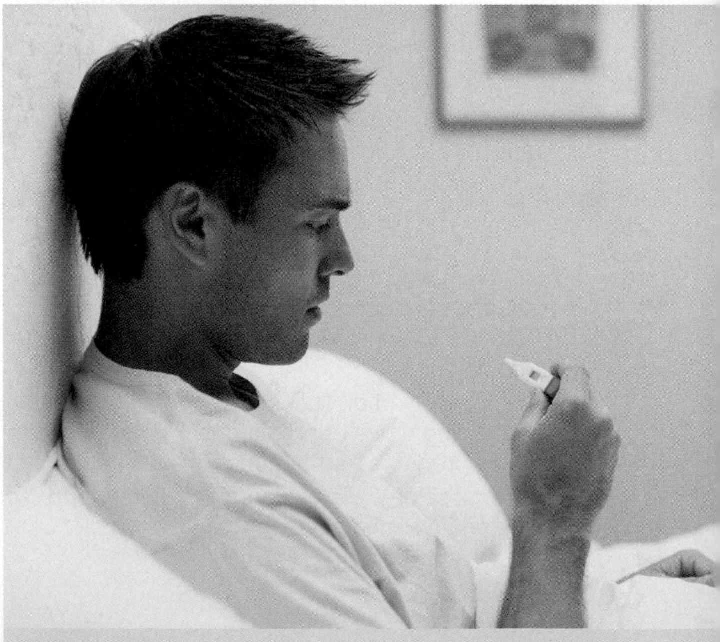

Deciding when to contact a physician can be difficult. Most people first try to diagnose and treat a condition themselves.

35 MILLION

AMERICANS ARE ADMITTED TO THE **HOSPITAL** EACH YEAR.

- Sudden high fever or recurring high temperature (over 102°F for children and 103°F for adults) and/or sweats
- Tingling sensation in the arm accompanied by slurred speech or impaired thought processes
- Adverse reactions to a drug or insect bite (shortness of breath, severe swelling, dizziness)
- Unexplained sudden weight loss
- Persistent or recurrent diarrhea or vomiting
- Blue-colored lips, eyelids, or nail beds
- Any lump, swelling, thickness, or sore that does not subside or that grows for over a month
- Any blood in the stool or urine, or significant pain, or marked, persistent change in bowel or bladder habits
- Yellowing of the skin or the whites of the eyes
- Sudden severe pain that has no apparent cause
- Any symptom that is unusual and recurs over time
- Pregnancy

See the **Skills for Behavior Change** box for information on taking an active role in your own health care.

Assessing Health Professionals

Suppose you decide that you do need medical help. How should you go about assessing the qualifications of a health care provider? Numerous studies document the importance of good communication skills: The most satisfied patients are those who feel their health care provider explains diagnosis and treatment options thoroughly and demonstrates competency as well as a genuine concern for you.[2]

When evaluating health care providers, consider the following questions:

- Do they listen to you, respect you as an individual, and give you time to ask questions? Do they return your calls, and are they available to answer questions between visits? How long would it take you to get in to see them if you really needed an appointment?
- What professional education and training have they had? What license or board certification(s) do they hold? Note that there is a difference between "board certified" and "board eligible" physicians. *Board certified* indicates that the physician has passed the national board examination for his or her specialty (e.g., pediatrics) and has been certified as competent in that specialty. In contrast, *board eligible* merely means that the physician is eligible to take the specialty board's exam, but not necessarily that he or she has passed it.
- Are they affiliated with an accredited medical facility or institution? The Joint Commission is an independent nonprofit organization that evaluates and accredits more than 15,000 health care organizations and programs in the United States. Accreditation requires that these institutions verify all education, licensing, and training claims of their affiliated practitioners.
- Are they open to complementary or alternative strategies? Would they refer you for different treatments if

SEE IT! VIDEOS

How do you avoid misdiagnosed medical advice online? Watch **Misdiagnosis on the Web** available on MasteringHealth.

SKILLS FOR BEHAVIOR CHANGE

BE PROACTIVE IN YOUR HEALTH CARE

The more you know about your body and the factors that can affect your health, the better you will be at communicating with health care providers. The following points can help:

- Know your own and your family's medical history.
- Research your condition—causes, physiological effects, possible treatments, and prognosis. Don't rely solely on the health care provider for this information.
- Write out your questions in advance. Don't feel awkward asking them, and don't accept a defensive response: Asking questions is your right as a patient.
- Bring someone with you to appointments to listen, take notes, and ask for clarification if necessary. If you go alone, take notes.
- Ask the practitioner to explain the problem and possible tests, treatments, and medications in a clear and understandable way. If you don't understand something, ask for clarification.
- If the health care provider prescribes any medications, ask whether you can take generic equivalents that cost less.
- Ask for a written summary of the results of your visit and any lab tests.
- Seek a second opinion about important tests or treatment recommendations.
- After your health care visit, you will likely receive an e-mail with a link to the provider's record of your visit. Read the record carefully, and contact the provider if you have any questions or concerns. Otherwise, store it with your other health care files. If your doctor doesn't provide this sort of service, write down an accurate account of what happened and what was said. Be sure to include the names of the provider and all other people involved in your care, the date, and the place.
- When filling prescriptions, the pharmacist will provide you with a drug information sheet that lists medical considerations and details about potential drug and food interactions. Read it.

appropriate? Are they willing to refer you to a larger facility or specialist if you want to go out of their group, or do they try to keep their business "in house"?

- Do they indicate clearly what your treatment options might be, the pros and cons of each, and the effectiveness of a given treatment in the short and long terms? What might be the side effects of a treatment, and what possible symptoms might you expect?
- Who will be responsible for your care when your physician is on vacation or off call?
- Are there professional reviews and information on any lawsuits against them available online?

Questions to ask yourself about the quality of care you are receiving include the following:

- Did your health care provider take a thorough health history, give you more than a "managed care moment" when examining you, and ask for any recent updates to your health history? Was your examination thorough?
- Did your health care provider seem comfortable talking with you and engaged in the relationship or was he or she cool or detached?
- Did you feel comfortable asking questions? Did your health care provider answer thoroughly, in a way that was easy to understand? Did his or her knowledge of your conditions and treatment options seem up to date? Did he or she admit to not knowing an answer to your question when appropriate?
- Would you feel comfortable seeing the health care provider again, or did you leave feeling that the visit was too fast and too impersonal—that you'd rather have seen someone else?

Bottom line: If you don't feel that the physician was a good fit for you, do your homework and look for another. Unfortunately, most people spend more time searching for a car than they do taking the time to find a good physician. Ask people you trust whom they might recommend. Being proactive and finding the best doctor for your situation is key.

Another critical factor in your decision-making process is whether or not a physician is covered by your insurance plan and whether the facility where they work is included in your "in network" approved facility list. Today, many clinics, hospitals, and their emergency departments use contracted services from independent providers who may or may not belong to their "in network" insurance-eligible provider group. So don't assume that because a facility is in your network, all providers at that facility are as well. Confirm in advance that the provider you're seeing is covered by your plan. Health care insurance is discussed in more detail later in this chapter.

Active participation in your treatment is the only sensible course in a health care environment that encourages **defensive medicine**, an approach to health care in which practitioners order tests or treatments, or avoid high-risk patients or procedures, largely to reduce their liability to malpractice suits. In a recent survey of physicians, 58 percent indicated that they have ordered a test or procedure for primarily defensive medicine reasons.[3] Unwarranted tests and treatments to protect against malpractice exposure are two significant factors driving up the cost of medicine. It is estimated that at least $500 billion per year is spent on medical tests and procedures that do not improve health outcomes.[4]

defensive medicine The use of medical practices designed to avert the possibility of malpractice suits in the future.

informed consent Acknowledgment that you have been told of the potential risks and benefits of a recommended test or treatment, understand what you have been told, and agree to the care.

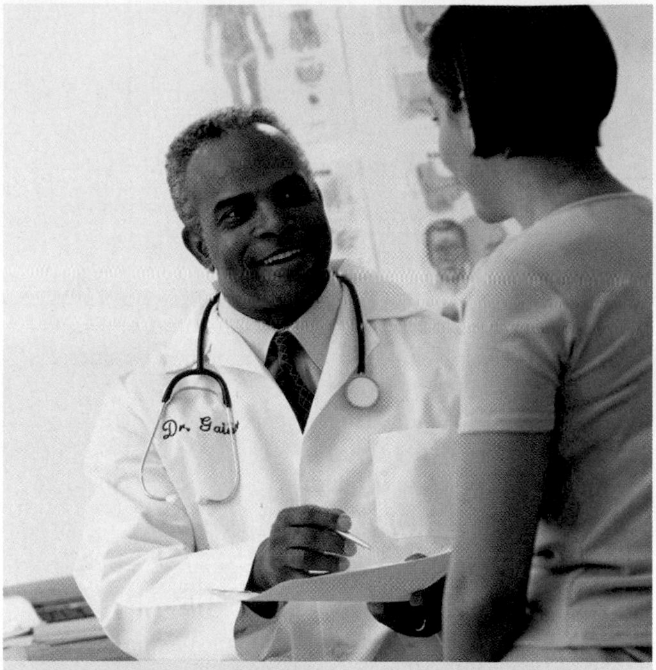

It's important to understand recommendations that your health care provider makes. Questions to ask include how often the practitioner has performed a procedure, the proportion of successful outcomes for the treatment or procedure, and why a test has been ordered.

72%

OF U.S. PHYSICIANS SAY THE AVERAGE MD ORDERS AN **UNNECESSARY** TEST OR PROCEDURE AT LEAST ONCE A WEEK.

Your Rights as a Patient

In addition to asking the suggested questions above, being proactive in your health care also means that you should be aware of your rights as a patient, as follows:[5]

1. The right of **informed consent** means that before receiving any care, you should be fully informed of what is being planned; the risks and potential benefits; and

STUDENT HEALTH TODAY

THE PLACEBO EFFECT

Mind Over Matter?

The *placebo effect* is an apparent cure or improved state of health brought about by a substance, product, or procedure that has no generally recognized therapeutic value. Patients often report improvements in a condition based on what they expect, desire, or were told would happen after receiving a treatment, even though the treatment was, for example, simple sugar pills instead of powerful drugs. Placebo-controlled studies are often used to determine the effectiveness of medications. Patients with a particular condition are given either the drug that is being tested or a placebo. If a significantly greater number of patients receiving the drug have a significantly better outcome than the patients receiving the placebo, then the treatment can be considered effective. Most such studies are double-blind; that is, neither the patients nor the doctors involved in the study are told until the study ends who had the real treatment and who had the placebo.

There is also a *nocebo* effect, in which a practitioner's negative assessment of a patient's symptoms leads to a worsening of the condition, such as increased anxiety and pain. Similarly, a negative assessment of a treatment's potential efficacy induces a failure to respond to that treatment.

Researchers are investigating how and why expectation appears to change physiology. Evidence from pain studies suggests that use of a placebo for pain control causes

Is it a real medicine or a placebo? In some cases, it may not make a difference.

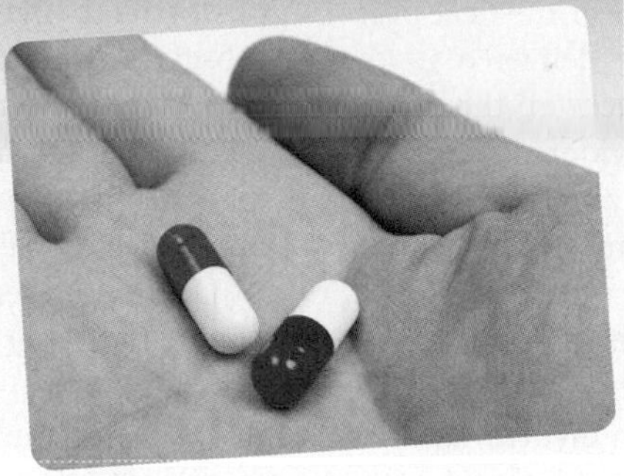

the brain to release the same endogenous (natural) opioids it releases when the study participant uses a pain medication with an active ingredient. But pain is not the only factor to respond to expectation. Let's look at a few more examples:

- A study of resting tremor (such as involuntary finger tapping) in patients with Parkinson's disease found that positive or negative expectations of a treatment's effectiveness reduced or increased patient tremor when they were given the same valid medication or the same placebo.
- A study of patients with clinical depression found no significant difference in effectiveness of a commonly prescribed antidepressant, an herbal remedy often used for depression, and a placebo after 26 weeks of therapy.
- Several studies have found a significant placebo effect in trials of medications to treat alcohol dependency; that is, alcohol-dependent patients who believe they have been taking medication consume fewer alcoholic drinks and report less alcohol dependence and cravings, regardless of whether they are receiving the drug or a placebo.

If you're curious to learn more about the scientific evidence behind a drug prescribed for you, get online. A quick search using the exact name of the medication and the words "drug studies" should provide links to the information you're looking for.

Sources: L. Colloca and C. Grillon, "Understanding Placebo and Nocebo Responses for Pain Management," *Current Pain and Headache Reports* 18, no. 6 (2014): 419, DOI: 10.1007/s11916-014-0419-2; A. Keitel et al., "Expectation Modulates the Effect of Deep Brain Stimulation on Motor and Cognitive Function in Tremor-Dominant Parkinson's Disease," *PLoS One* 8, no. 12 (2013): e81878, DOI: 10.1371/journal.pone.0081878; J. Sarris, M. Fava, I. Schweitzer, and D. Mischoulon, "St. John's Wort (*Hypericum perforatum*) versus Sertraline and Placebo in Major Depressive Disorder: Continuation Data from a 26-Week RCT," *Pharmacopsychiatry* 45, no. 7 (2012): 275–8, DOI: 10.1055/s-0032-1306348; R. A. Litten et al., "The Placebo Effect in Clinical Trials for Alcohol Dependence: An Exploratory Analysis of 51 Naltrexone and Acamprosate Studies," *Alcoholism, Clinical and Experimental Research* 37, no. 12 (2013): 2128–37, DOI: 10.1111/acer.12197; G. L. Petersen et al., "The Magnitude of Nocebo Effects in Pain: A Meta-Analysis," *Pain*, (April 26, 2014), pii: S0304-3959(14)00195-X, DOI: 10.1016/j.pain.2014.04.016.

possible alternative forms of treatment, including the option to refuse treatment. Your consent must be voluntary and without any form of coercion. It is critical that you read any consent forms carefully and amend them as necessary before signing.

2. You are entitled to know whether the treatment you are receiving is standard or experimental. In experimental conditions, you have the legal and ethical right to know if any drug is being used in the research project for a purpose not approved by the Food and Drug Administration (FDA) and whether the study is one in which some people receive treatment whereas others receive a placebo. (See the **Student Health Today** box for more on placebos and the placebo effect.)
3. You have the right to make decisions regarding the health care that is recommended by the physician.
4. You have the right to confidentiality. This means that you do not have an obligation to reveal the source of payment for your treatment. It also means you have the right to make personal decisions concerning all reproductive matters.
5. You have the right to receive adequate health care, as well as to refuse treatment and to cease treatment at any time.
6. You are entitled to have access to all of your medical records and to have those records remain confidential.
7. You have the right to continuity of health care.
8. You have the right to seek the opinions of other health care professionals regarding your condition.
9. You have the right to courtesy, respect, dignity, responsiveness, and timely attention to health needs.

LO 2 | CONVENTIONAL HEALTH CARE

Describe and discuss conventional health care, including types of practitioners and the health care products and treatments available.

Conventional health care, also called **allopathic medicine**, mainstream medicine, or traditional Western medical practice, is the dominant type of health care delivered in the United States, Canada, Europe, and much of the developed world. Among U.S. health care providers, the majority receive conventional medical training and treat patients using conventional medicine. Allopathic medicine is based on the premise that illness is a result of exposure to harmful environmental agents, such as infectious microorganisms and pollutants, or organic changes in the body. The prevention of disease and the restoration of health involve vaccines, drugs, surgery, and other treatments.

Be aware, however, that not all allopathic treatments have had the benefit of the extensive clinical trials and long-term studies of outcomes necessary to conclusively prove effectiveness in different populations. Even when studies appear to support the health benefits of a particular treatment or product, other studies with equal or better scientific validity often refute these claims. Also, today's recommended treatment may change dramatically in the future as new technologies and medical advances replace older practices. Like other professionals, health care providers must stay informed of advances in their field.

allopathic medicine Conventional, Western medical practice; in theory, based on scientifically validated methods and procedures.

evidence-based medicine Decisions regarding patient care based on clinical expertise, patient values, and current best scientific evidence.

primary care practitioner (PCP) A medical practitioner who treats routine ailments, advises on preventive care, gives general medical advice, and makes appropriate referrals when necessary.

osteopath General practitioner who receives training similar to a medical doctor's but with an emphasis on the skeletal and muscular systems; often uses spinal manipulation as part of treatment.

ophthalmologist Physician who specializes in the medical and surgical care of the eyes, including prescriptions for glasses.

optometrist Eye specialist whose practice is limited to prescribing and fitting lenses.

dentist Specialist who diagnoses and treats diseases of the teeth, gums, and oral cavity.

nurse Health professional who provides many services for patients and who may work in a variety of settings.

Health care providers strive to ensure the quality of care they provide to their patients, and one of the ways they do this is by practicing **evidence-based medicine.** Decisions regarding patient care are based on clinical expertise, patient values, and current best scientific evidence. Clinical expertise refers to the clinician's cumulative experience, education, and clinical skills. The patient brings his or her own personal and unique concerns, expectations, and values. The best evidence is usually found in clinically relevant research that has been conducted using sound methodology.

Conventional Health Care Practitioners

Selecting a **primary care practitioner (PCP)**—a medical practitioner whom you can visit for routine ailments, preventive care, general medical advice, and appropriate referrals—is not an easy task. The PCP for most people is a family practitioner, an internist, or for women, an obstetrician-gynecologist (ob-gyn). Many people routinely see nurse practitioners or physician assistants who work for an individual doctor or a medical group, and others use nontraditional providers as their primary source of care. As a college student, you may opt to visit a PCP at your campus health center.

SEE IT! VIDEOS
Knowing your medical history can keep you informed of health risks. Watch **Your Medical History** available on MasteringHealth.™

Doctors undergo rigorous training before they can begin practicing. After 4 years of undergraduate work, students typically spend 4 years studying for their medical degree (MD). After this general training, some students choose a specialty, such as pediatrics, cardiology, cancer, radiology, or surgery, and spend 1 year in an internship and several years doing a residency. Some doctors receive additional training in order to specialize in certain elective surgeries (see the **Student Health Today** box). Some specialties also require a fellowship; in all, the time spent in additional training after receiving a medical degree can be up to 8 years.

Osteopaths are general practitioners who receive training similar to that of a medical doctor but place special emphasis on the skeletal and muscular systems. Their treatments may involve manipulation of the muscles and joints. Osteopaths receive the degree of doctor of osteopathy (DO) rather than MD.

Eye care specialists can be either ophthalmologists or optometrists. An **ophthalmologist** holds a medical degree and can perform surgery and prescribe medications. An **optometrist** typically evaluates visual problems and fits glasses but is not a trained physician. If you have an eye infection, glaucoma, or other eye condition needing diagnosis and treatment, you need to see an ophthalmologist.

Dentists are specialists who diagnose and treat diseases of the teeth, gums, and oral cavity. They attend dental school for 4 years and receive the title of doctor of dental surgery (DDS) or doctor of medical dentistry (DMD). They must also pass both state and national board examinations before receiving a license to practice. The field of dentistry includes many specialties. For example, *orthodontists* specialize in the alignment of teeth. *Oral surgeons* perform surgical procedures to correct problems of the mouth, face, and jaw.

Nurses are trained health care professionals who provide a wide range of services for patients and their families, including patient education, counseling, community health and disease prevention information, and administration of medications. They may choose from several training options. Registered nurses (RNs) in the United States complete either a 4-year program leading to a bachelor of science in nursing (BSN) degree or a 2-year program leading to an associate degree in nursing (ADN). They must then pass a national certification exam. Lower-level licensed practical or vocational nurses (LPN or LVN) complete a 1-year training program, which may be based in either a community college or a hospital, and take a licensing exam.

STUDENT HEALTH TODAY

CHOOSING SURGERY

Elective Procedures

The National Center for Health Statistics states that over 40 million elective medical procedures—surgeries and treatments that are planned, nonemergency procedures—are performed every year, and that number seems to be growing. Although not considered medically necessary, many types of elective procedures, from musculoskeletal to weight loss surgeries, greatly improve people's health and functioning, and some can reduce the patient's risk for chronic disease. Even purely cosmetic surgeries can enhance the patient's self-esteem.

If a procedure is considered not medically necessary, it may not be covered by insurance. In some cases, insurance companies may require a second opinion before approving payment on elective surgical procedures. If you are considering elective surgery, review your coverage requirements with your health insurance carrier before scheduling the procedure.

An elective surgical procedure is typically performed by a surgeon or qualified physician in either a hospital or an ambulatory center. Some simple, minimally invasive procedures may even be performed in a doctor's office. The type of surgery will mandate the qualifications and background of the surgeon or physician who performs it. The following are some of the more common elective surgeries.

Lasik

Millions of Americans have had surgery to reduce their dependence on contact lenses or glasses. The most common technique is called Lasik (*laser-assisted in situ keratomileusis*), in which a surgeon uses a razor-like instrument or laser to cut a flap in the cornea, the clear covering on the front of the eye, and then reshapes the exposed area using a laser. The surgery alters the way the eye focuses light, correcting nearsightedness, farsightedness, and some astigmatism. However, Lasik is not effective at treating close-up vision problems in middle-aged and older adults.

The procedure usually takes less than 5 minutes, is painless, and the patient is awake the entire time. Postoperative complications can include infection or night glare—starbursts or halos that appear when you are viewing lights at night.

Cosmetic Surgery

Cosmetic surgery is performed to enhance appearance. Over the past 15 years, the number of cosmetic surgeries performed in the United States has nearly doubled. In 2013, approximately 1.8 million were performed. The five most common, in order, are as follows:

- Liposuction, the removal of pockets of fatty tissue with a vacuum-like device, to slim the hips, thighs, abdomen, or other areas
- Breast augmentation, the surgical placement of an implant behind each breast to increase breast volume and enhance shape
- Blepharoplasty, to improve the appearance of the eyelids
- Abdominoplasty, commonly called a "tummy tuck," to remove excess abdominal skin and fat and restore weakened or separated muscles
- Rhinoplasty, correction and reconstruction of the nose

Among adults age 65 and older, rhytidectomy, commonly called a facelift, is the procedure most frequently performed. It improves signs of aging such as sagging skin in the face and neck. Risks and complications of cosmetic surgery include infection, bruising, numbness, bleeding, and poor healing.

Nonsurgical cosmetic procedures are even more common than cosmetic surgeries, and their rate has increased more than fivefold over the past 15 years. These include procedures such as dermabrasion, a surgical scraping of the top layers of the skin to remove fine wrinkles, acne scars, and skin growths, and botulinum toxin injections to reduce facial wrinkles.

If you have imperfect vision and want to ditch your glasses or contact lenses for good, you may want to consider Lasik laser eye surgery.

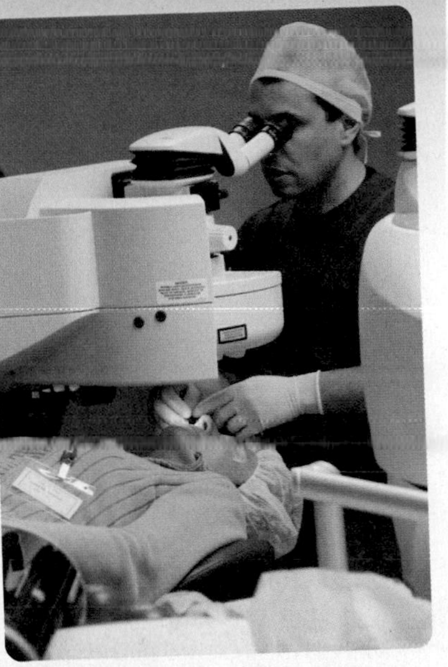

Sources: U.S. Food and Drug Administration, "LASIK," December 9, 2011, www.fda.gov/MedicalDevices/ProductsandMedicalProcedures/SurgeryandLifeSupport/LASIK/default.htm; American Society for Aesthetic Plastic Surgery, "Quick Facts," 2013, www.surgery.org/sites/default/files/2013-quick-facts_0.pdf.

Nurse practitioners (NPs) are nurses with advanced training obtained through either a master's degree program or a specialized nurse practitioner program. Nurse practitioners have the training and authority to conduct diagnostic tests and prescribe medications (in some states). They work in a variety of settings, particularly in HMOs (health maintenance organizations), clinics, and student health centers. Nurses and nurse practitioners may also earn the clinical doctor of nursing degree (ND), doctor of nursing science (DNS and DNSc degrees), or a research-based PhD in nursing.

Physician assistants (PAs) are licensed to examine and diagnose patients, offer treatment, and write prescriptions under a physician's supervision. An important difference between a PA and a NP is that the PA must practice under a physician's supervision. Like other health care providers, PAs are licensed by state boards of medicine.

nurse practitioner (NP) Professional nurse with advanced training obtained through either a master's degree program or a specialized nurse practitioner program.

physician assistant (PA) A midlevel practitioner trained to handle most standard cases of care under the supervision of a physician.

TABLE 18.1 | Common Over-the-Counter Drugs, Their Uses, and Potential Side Effects

Type/Name of Drug	Use	Examples	Potential Hazards/Common Side Effects
Acetaminophen	Pain reliever, fever reducer.	Tylenol	Bloody urine, painful urination; skin rash; bleeding and bruising; yellowing of the eyes or skin; difficulty in diagnosing overdose because reaction may be delayed up to a week; liver damage from chronic low-level use.
Antacids	Relieve "heartburn."	Tums, Maalox	Reduced mineral absorption from food; possible concealment of ulcer; reduced effectiveness of anticlotting medications; interference with the function of certain antibiotics (for antacids that contain aluminum); worsened high blood pressure (for antacids that contain sodium); aggravated kidney problems.
Anticholinergics	Often added to cold preparations to reduce nasal secretions and tears.	atropine, scopolamine	None of the preparations tested by the FDA has been found to be Generally Recognized as Effective (GRAE) or Generally Recognized as Safe (GRAS). Some cold compounds contain alcohol in concentrations greater than 40%.
Antihistamines	Central nervous system depressants that dry runny noses, clear postnasal drip and sinus congestion, and reduce tears.	Claritin, Benadryl, Xyzal	Drowsiness, sedation, dizziness, disturbed coordination.
Aspirin	Pain reliever; reduces fever and inflammation.	Bayer, Bufferin	Stomach upset and vomiting; stomach bleeding; worsening of ulcers; enhancement of the action of anticlotting medications; hearing damage from loud noise; severe allergic reaction; association with Reye's syndrome in children and teenagers; prolonged bleeding when combined with alcohol.
Decongestants	Reduce nasal stuffiness due to colds.	Sudafed, DayQuil, Allermed	Nervousness, restlessness, excitability, dizziness, drowsiness, headache, nausea, weakness, sleep problems.
Diet pills, caffeine	Aid to weight loss.	Dexatrim	Organ damage or death from cerebral hemorrhage; nervousness; irritability; dehydration.
Expectorants	Loosen phlegm, which allows the user to cough it up and clear congested respiratory passages.	Mucinex	Safety issues may arise when combined with other medications, particularly in frail or very ill individuals. Effectiveness is sometimes in question.
Ibuprofen	Pain reliever; reduces fever and inflammation.	Advil, Motrin	Allergic reaction in some people with aspirin allergy; fluid retention or swelling (edema); liver damage similar to that from acetaminophen; enhancement of anticlotting medications; digestive disturbances.
Laxatives	Relieve constipation.	ex-lax, Citrucel	Reduced absorption of minerals from food; dehydration; dependency.
Naproxen sodium	Pain reliever; reduces fever and inflammation.	Aleve, Naprosyn	Potential bleeding in the digestive tract; possible stomach cramps or ulcers.
Sleep aids and relaxants	Help relieve occasional sleeplessness.	Nytol, Sleep-Eze, Sominex	Drowsiness the next day; dizziness; lack of coordination; reduced mental alertness; constipation; dry mouth and throat; dependency.

Conventional Health Products

Prescription drugs can be obtained only with a written prescription from a physician, whereas over-the-counter drugs can be purchased without a prescription. Just as making wise decisions about providers is an important aspect of responsible health care, so is making wise decisions about medications.

Prescription Drugs In about three-fourths of doctor visits, the physician administers or prescribes at least one medication.[6] In fact, prescription drug use has increased steadily over the past decade, and over 68 percent of Americans now use one or more prescription drugs.[7] Even though these drugs are administered under medical supervision, the wise consumer still takes precautions. Adverse effects and complications arising from the use of prescription drugs are common, as is failure to respond to a medication.

Consumers have a variety of resources available to help them determine the risks of various prescription medicines and to make educated decisions about whether to take a certain drug. One of the best resources is the FDA's Center for Drug Evaluation and Research website (www.fda.gov/drugs). This consumer-specific section of the FDA website provides current information on risks and benefits of prescription drugs. Being knowledgeable about what you are taking or thinking about taking is a sound strategy to ensure safety.

Common types of prescription drugs discussed in this text include antidepressants and antianxiety drugs (**Chapter 2**), hormonal contraceptives (**Chapter 6**), weight-loss aids (**Chapter 8**), smoking-cessation aids (**Chapter 11**), stimulants and sedatives (**Chapter 12**), antibiotics (**Chapter 13**), and statins and other cholesterol-lowering drugs (**Chapter 15**).

Generic drugs, medications sold under a chemical name rather than a brand name, contain the same active ingredients as brand-name drugs but are usually much less expensive. Not all drugs are available as generics. If your doctor prescribes a medication, always ask if a generic equivalent exists and if it would be safe and effective for you to try.

Although generic medications behave very similarly to brand-name versions and show a similar efficacy, there is some concern that substitutions made in minor ingredients might reduce a patient's response to the drug or cause side effects such as an allergic reaction in some patients.[8] Always note any reactions you have to medications and tell your doctor about them.

Many consumers choose to have prescriptions filled online. Although many websites are operating legally and observe the safeguards of traditional procedures for dispensing drugs, some sell counterfeit drugs of inconsistent quality or sidestep required consumer protections. The FDA advises that if you buy medications online, buy only from state-licensed pharmacy sites based in the United States. Purchase only from sites that require a valid, current prescription from your doctor and have a licensed pharmacist available to answer your questions. Don't provide any personal health or financial information, including a Social Security number, unless you are sure the website will keep your information safe and private.[9]

generic drugs Medications sold under chemical names rather than brand names.

Over-the-Counter (OTC) Drugs

Medications available without a prescription are referred to as *over-the-counter (OTC)* drugs. Although physicians often recommend OTC remedies to patients for common conditions such as muscle pain or constipation, OTC drugs are also used in the course of self-diagnosis and self-treatment. American consumers spend billions of dollars yearly on OTC preparations for relief of everything from runny noses to ingrown toenails. Those most commonly used are pain relievers; cold, cough, and allergy medications; stimulants; sleeping aids and relaxants; and dieting aids (**TABLE 18.1**).

Despite a common belief that OTC products are safe and effective, indiscriminate use and abuse can occur with these drugs as with all others. For example, people who frequently drop medication into their eyes to "get the red out" or pop antacids after every meal are likely to become dependent. Many people also experience adverse side effects because they ignore the warnings on labels or simply do not read them.

The FDA has developed a standard label that appears on most OTC products (**FIGURE 18.1**). It includes directions for use, active and inactive ingredients, warnings, and other useful information.

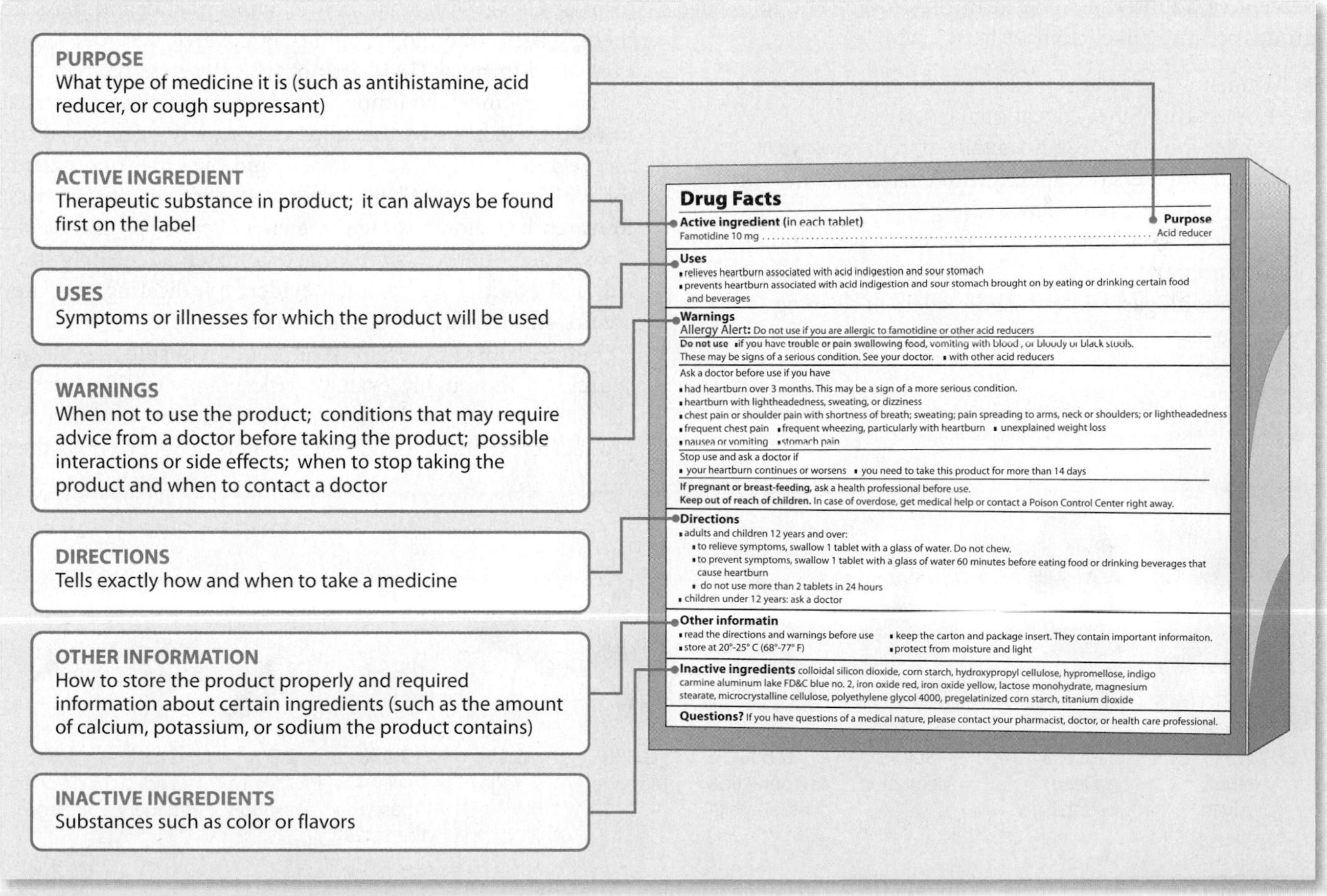

FIGURE 18.1 The Over-the-Counter Medicine Label

Source: Consumer Healthcare Products Association, OTC Label, www.otcsafety.org. Used with permission.

VIDEO TUTOR
Being a Good Health Care Consumer

LO 3 | COMPLEMENTARY AND ALTERNATIVE MEDICINE (CAM)

Describe and discuss complementary and alternative medicine.

Although the terms *complementary* and *alternative* are often used interchangeably when referring to therapies, there is a distinction between them. **Complementary medicine** is used *together with* conventional medicine as part of the modern integrative-medicine approach.[10] An example of complementary medicine is to use massage therapy along with prescription medicine to treat anxiety. **Alternative medicine** has traditionally been used *in place of* conventional medicine, such as following a special diet or herbal remedy to treat cancer instead of using radiation, surgery, or other conventional treatments.

complementary medicine Treatment used in conjunction with conventional medicine.

alternative medicine Treatment used in place of conventional medicine.

holistic Relating to or concerned with the whole body and the interactions of systems, rather than treatment of individual parts.

The National Center for Complementary and Alternative Medicine (NCCAM), part of the National Institutes of Health (NIH), funds research into CAM practices and provides reliable information about CAM safety and effectiveness to health care providers and consumers. Nearly 40 percent of adults use some form of CAM.[11] The following groups are more likely to have used CAM:

- Women
- People with higher educational levels
- People who have been hospitalized in the past year
- Former smokers (compared with current smokers or those who have never smoked)
- People with back, neck, head, or joint aches or other painful conditions
- People with gastrointestinal disorders or sleeping problems

Many people seek CAM therapies as alternatives to the conventional Western system of medicine, which some people regard as too invasive, too high-tech, and too toxic in terms of laboratory-produced medications. In contrast, most CAM therapies incorporate a **holistic** approach that focuses on treating the whole person, rather than just an isolated part of the body. Some CAM patients believe that alternative practices will give them greater control over their health care.

Types and Domains of Complementary and Alternative Medicine

Practitioners of most complementary and alternative therapies spend years learning their practice. In addition, various forms of CAM are increasingly being taught in U.S. medical schools. Similar to conventional medicine, there is no national training, certification, or licensure standard for CAM practitioners, and state regulations differ. Whereas practitioners of conventional medicine have graduated from U.S.-sanctioned schools of medicine or are licensed medical practitioners recognized by the American Medical Association (AMA)—the governing body for all physicians—each CAM domain has a different set of training standards, guidelines for practice, and licensure procedures.

Nearly all health insurance providers cover at least one form of CAM, with acupuncture, chiropractic, and massage therapy being the most commonly covered services. However, other forms of CAM are not typically covered.

The ten most common CAM therapies are identified in **FIGURE 18.2**. CAM therapies vary widely in terms of the nature and extent of the treatment and the types of problems for which they offer help. They also vary in effectiveness. Research has shown some to be effective for specific conditions, whereas others simply have not been adequately studied, and others have research evidence indicating that they are not effective for any specific condition.[12]

Before considering any treatments, consult reliable resources to thoroughly evaluate risks, the scientific basis of claimed benefits, and any contraindications to using the product or service. Avoid practitioners who promote their

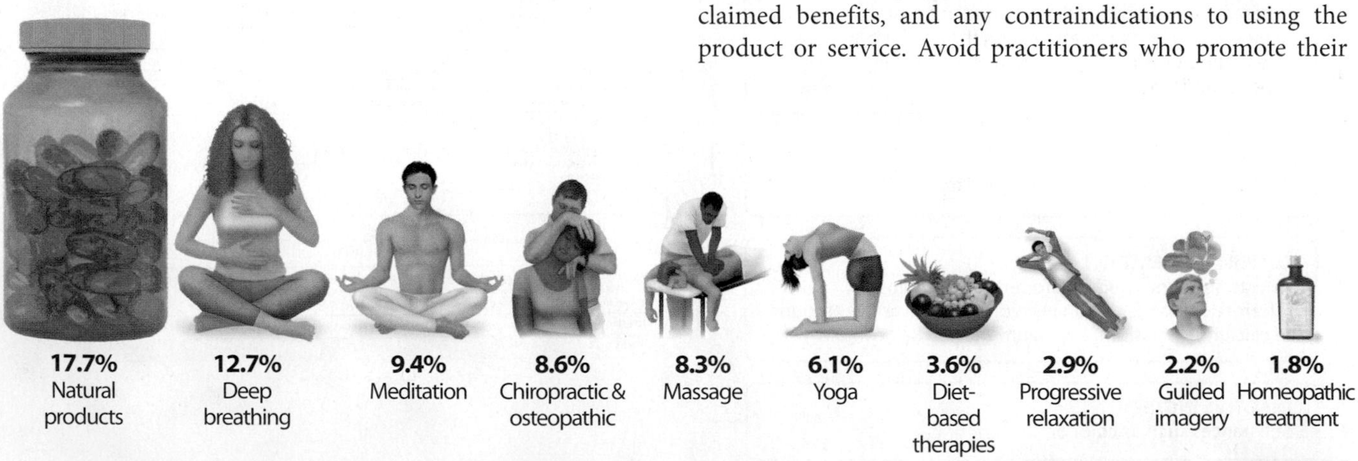

FIGURE 18.2 The Ten Most Common CAM Therapies among U.S. Adults

Source: Data are from P. M. Barnes, B. Bloom, and R. Nahin, "Complementary and Alternative Medicine Use among Adults and Children: United States, 2007," *CDC National Health Statistics Report,* no. 12 (December 2008).

VIDEO TUTOR
CAM: Risks vs. Benefits

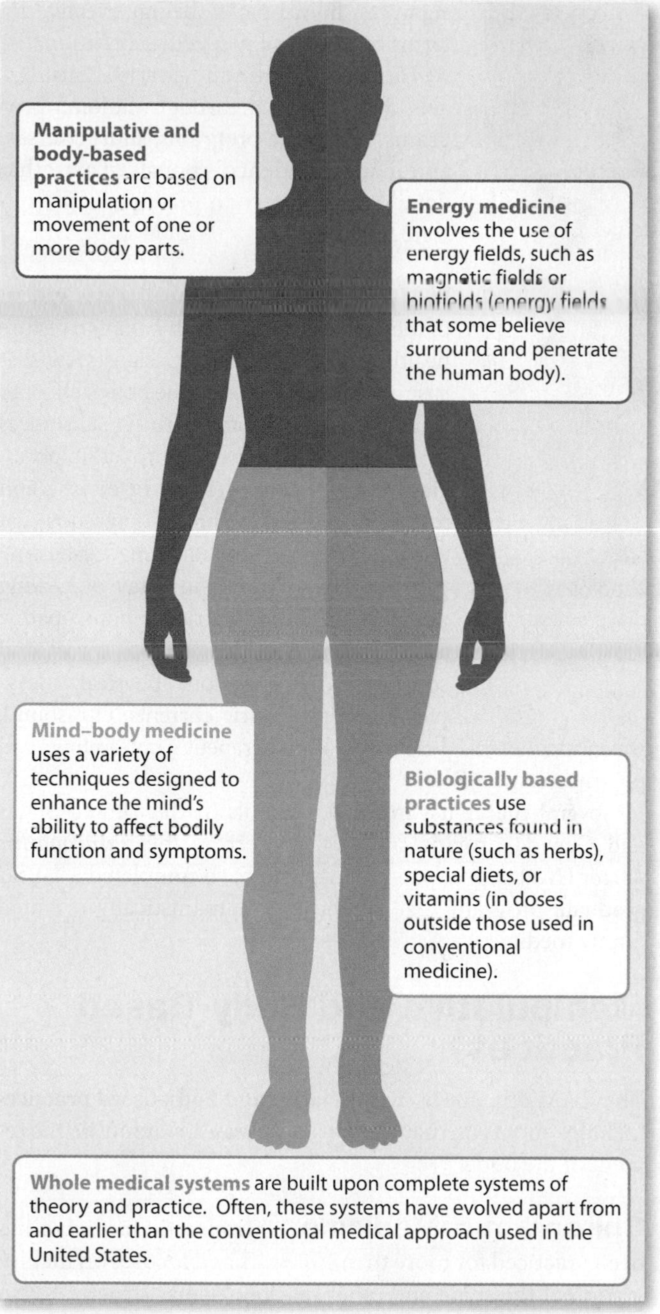

Manipulative and body-based practices are based on manipulation or movement of one or more body parts.
Energy medicine involves the use of energy fields, such as magnetic fields or biofields (energy fields that some believe surround and penetrate the human body).
Mind–body medicine uses a variety of techniques designed to enhance the mind's ability to affect bodily function and symptoms.
Biologically based practices use substances found in nature (such as herbs), special diets, or vitamins (in doses outside those used in conventional medicine).
Whole medical systems are built upon complete systems of theory and practice. Often, these systems have evolved apart from and earlier than the conventional medical approach used in the United States.

FIGURE 18.3 The Domains of Complementary and Alternative Medicine (CAM) NCCAM groups CAM practices into five domains, recognizing that there can be some overlap. In particular, CAM whole medical systems cut across all domains.

Source: National Center for Complementary and Alternative Medicine, "The Use of Complementary and Alternative Medicine in the United States," NCCAM Publication no. D347, Updated May 2012, http://nccam.nih.gov.

treatments as a cure-all for every health problem or who seem to promise remedies for ailments that have thus far defied the best scientific efforts of mainstream medicine. In short, apply the same strategies to researching CAM as you would to choosing allopathic care.

The NCCAM has grouped the many varieties of CAM into five general domains of practice, recognizing that domains may overlap (**FIGURE 18.3**).

36%

OF 18- TO 29-YEAR-OLDS REPORT HAVING USED SOME FORM OF **CAM**.

Alternative Medical Systems

Alternative (whole) medical systems reflect specific theories of health and balance that have developed outside the influence of conventional medicine. Many have been practiced by various cultures throughout the world for centuries. For example, Native American, Aboriginal, African, Middle Eastern, South American, and Asian cultures have their own unique healing systems. Here, we discuss only a few of the most commonly available options.

Traditional Chinese Medicine The concept of *qi* (pronounced "chee"), or vital energy, is foundational to **traditional Chinese medicine (TCM)**. When *qi* is in balance, the person is in a state of health; imbalance of *qi* results in disease. Diagnosis is based on personal history, observation of the body (especially the tongue), palpation, and pulse diagnosis, a detailed procedure requiring considerable skill and experience by the practitioner. Techniques such as acupuncture, herbal medicine, massage, and *qigong* (a form of energy therapy) are among the TCM approaches to health and healing. TCM is complex, and research into its effectiveness is limited.[13]

Traditional Chinese medicine practitioners within the United States must have completed a graduate program at a college or university approved by the Accreditation Commission for Acupuncture and Oriental Medicine (ACAOM). Graduate programs vary based on the specific area of concentration within TCM but usually involve an extensive 3- or 4-year clinical internship. In addition, an examination by the National Commission for the Certification of Acupuncture and Oriental Medicine, a standard for licensing in the United States, must be completed. Specific practices incorporated in TCM are discussed later in the chapter under the different CAM domains.

alternative (whole) medical systems Specific theories of health and balance that have developed outside the influence of conventional medicine.

traditional Chinese medicine (TCM) Ancient comprehensive system of healing that uses herbs, acupuncture, and massage to bring vital energy, *qi*, into balance and to remove blockages of *qi* that lead to disease.

ayurveda (ayurvedic medicine) A comprehensive system of medicine, derived largely from ancient India, that places equal emphasis on the body, mind, and spirit, and strives to restore the body's innate harmony through diet, exercise, meditation, herbs, massage, exposure to sunlight, and controlled breathing.

Ayurveda The "science of life," **ayurveda (ayurvedic medicine)** is an alternative medical system that has evolved over thousands of years in India. Ayurveda seeks to integrate and balance the body, mind, and spirit and to restore harmony

Shirodhara—a traditional ayurvedic treatment in which warm herbalized oil is poured over the forehead in guided rhythmic patterns—is said to relieve stress and anxiety, treat insomnia and chronic headaches, and improve memory.

in the individual.[14] Ayurvedic practitioners use various techniques, including questioning, observation, and pulse palpation, to determine which of three vital energies, or *doshas,* is dominant in the particular patient. They then establish a treatment plan to bring the doshas into balance, thereby reducing the patient's symptoms. Dietary modification and herbal remedies drawn from the botanical wealth of the Indian subcontinent are common. Research into ayurveda is limited, but studies have shown some of the herbal remedies to be effective.[15] Treatments may also include certain yoga postures, meditation, massage, steam baths, changes in sleep patterns and sun exposure, and controlled breathing.

Training of ayurvedic practitioners varies. There is no national standard for certification, although professional groups are working toward creating licensing guidelines.

Homeopathy

Homeopathic medicine is an unconventional Western system of medicine developed in Germany in the late 1700s. It is based on the principle that "like cures like." In other words, the same substance that in a large dose produces the symptoms of an illness—and may even be fatal—will in a small dose prompt the body's own defenses to cure the illness. Many homeopathic remedies are derived from toxic substances such as arsenic and belladonna; however, the preparation of the remedy may be so diluted that no actual molecules of the original substance remain.[16] The NCCAM reports that little evidence supports homeopathy being effective in terms of treating any specific condition.[17]

Homeopathic training varies considerably and is offered through diploma programs, certificate programs, short courses, and correspondence courses. Laws that detail requirements to practice vary from state to state.

homeopathic medicine Unconventional Western system of medicine based on the principle that "like cures like."

naturopathy (naturopathic medicine) System of medicine in which practitioners work with nature to restore people's health.

manipulative and body-based practices Treatments involving manipulation or movement of one or more body parts.

chiropractic medicine Manipulation of the spine and neuromuscular structure to promote proper energy flow.

Naturopathy

Naturopathy is a system of medicine that works with nature to restore health.[18] Naturopathic physicians view disease as a manifestation of the body's effort to ward off impurities and harmful substances from the environment. Naturopathic physicians emphasize prevention of disease and restoration of health through methods that encourage the person's inherent self-healing process. They employ an array of healing practices, including nutrition; homeopathy; acupuncture; herbal medicine; spinal and soft-tissue manipulation; physical therapies involving electric currents, ultrasound, water, magnets, and light therapy; therapeutic counseling; and pharmacology.

Several major naturopathic schools in the United States and Canada provide training, conferring the *naturopathic doctor* (*ND*) degree on students who have completed a 4-year graduate program that emphasizes humanistically oriented family medicine.

Manipulative and Body-Based Practices

The CAM domain of **manipulative and body-based practices** includes methods that are based on manipulation or movement of the body.

Chiropractic Medicine

Chiropractic medicine has been practiced for more than 100 years and focuses on manipulation of the spine and other neuromuscular structures.[19] A century ago, allopathic medicine and chiropractic medicine were in direct competition. Today, however, many health care organizations work closely with chiropractors, and many insurance companies will pay for chiropractic treatment, particularly if it is recommended by a medical doctor.

Chiropractic medicine is based on the idea that a life-giving energy flows through the nervous system, including the spinal cord. If the spine is partly misaligned or dislocated, that force is disrupted. Chiropractors use a variety of techniques to manipulate the spine back into proper alignment so the energy can flow unimpeded. It has been established that their treatment can be effective for back pain, neck pain, and headaches.

SEE IT! VIDEOS

Is acupuncture right for you? Watch **Health Benefits of Acupuncture** available on MasteringHealth.™

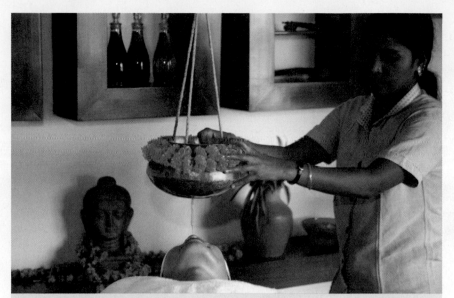

The average chiropractic training program includes intensive courses in biochemistry, anatomy, physiology, diagnostics, pathology, nutrition, and related topics, combined with hands-on clinical training. Many chiropractors continue their training to obtain specialized certification, for instance, in neurology, geriatrics, or pediatrics. Although states vary, increasing numbers require a 4-year undergraduate degree prior to entrance into a 4-year chiropractic program. After completion of these requirements, applicants must pass an extensive licensing examination given by the National Board of Chiropractic Examiners. The practice of chiropractic medicine is licensed and regulated in all 50 states.[20]

WHY SHOULD I CARE?

The ultimate choice about health care remains with you. In order to make sound decisions about what is best for your health, you need to understand as much as you can about your options.

Massage Therapy References to massage exist in numerous ancient texts, including those of Greece, Rome, Japan, China, Egypt, and India.[21] **Massage therapy** is soft tissue manipulation by trained therapists for relaxation and healing. Therapists manipulate the patient's muscles and connective tissues to loosen the fibers and break up adhesions, improve the body's circulation, and remove waste products. The NCCAM reports that research evidence supports the effectiveness of massage therapy to treat painful conditions, promote relaxation, reduce stress and anxiety, and relieve depression. Some of the more popular types of massage therapy are as follows:

- *Swedish massage* uses long strokes, kneading, and friction on the muscles and moves the joints to aid flexibility.
- *Deep tissue massage* uses patterns of strokes and deep finger pressure on parts of the body where muscles are tight or knotted, focusing on layers of muscle deep under the skin.
- *Sports massage* is performed to prevent athletic injury and keep the body flexible. It is also used to help athletes recover from injuries.
- *Trigger point massage* (also called *pressure point massage*) uses a variety of strokes but applies deeper, more focused pressure on myofascial trigger points—"knots" that can form in the muscles, are painful when pressed, and cause symptoms elsewhere in the body as well.
- *Shiatsu massage* is a traditional healing art from Japan that applies firm finger pressure to specified points on the body that are believed to be important for the flow of vital energy.

The course of study in massage schools typically covers sciences such as anatomy and physiology as well as massage techniques and business, ethical, and legal considerations.[22] The programs vary in length, quality, and whether they are accredited. For licensing, many states require a minimum of 500 hours of training and a passing grade on a national certification exam. Massage therapists work in private studios and health spas, as well as in medical and chiropractic offices, studios, hospitals, nursing homes, and fitness centers.[23]

WHAT DO YOU THINK?

Why do you think more and more people are opting for complementary and alternative treatments?

- What are the potential benefits of these treatments?
- What are the potential risks?

Bodywork CAM encompasses a broad range of movement-based approaches from East and West, and is used to promote well-being—physical, emotional, mental, and spiritual. Examples include movement re-education techniques, exercise modalities, and techniques in which the therapist induces movement of the patient's body. Some commonly available approaches are as follows:

- The *Alexander technique* is a movement education method designed to release harmful tension in the body to improve ease of movement, balance, and coordination.
- The *Feldenkrais Method* is a system of gentle movements and exercises. It is designed to improve movement, flexibility, coordination, and overall functioning through techniques that enhance awareness and retrain the nervous system.
- *Pilates* is a popular exercise method focused on improving flexibility, strength, and body awareness. It involves a series of controlled movements, some of which are performed using special equipment.

massage therapy Soft tissue manipulation by trained therapists for relaxation and healing.

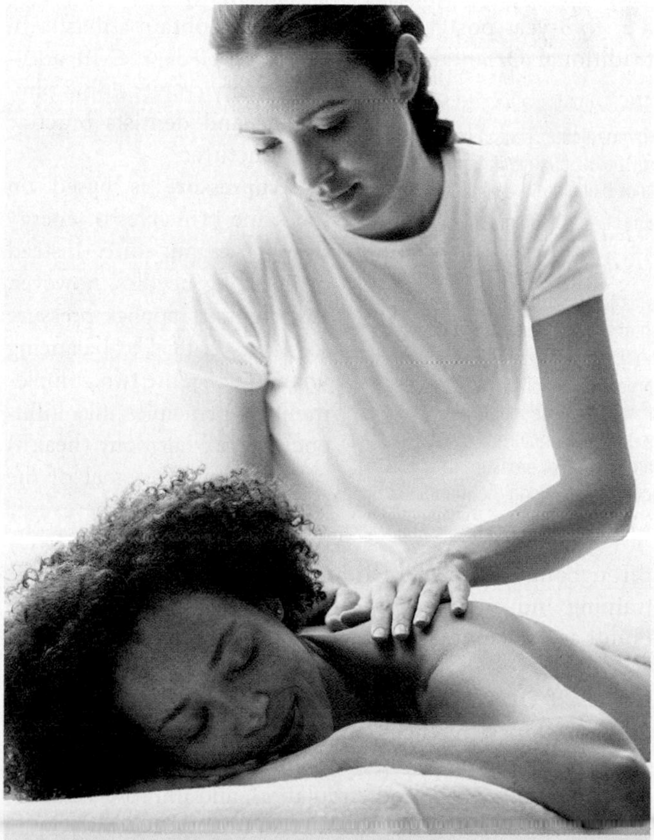

Oh, my aching back? Try massage!

Energy Medicine

Energy medicine therapies focus either on energy fields thought to originate within the body (biofields) or on fields from other sources (electromagnetic fields). The existence of these fields has not been experimentally proven. Most forms of energy therapy manipulate biofields by applying pressure and/or manipulating the body by placing the hands in, or through, these fields.[24] Popular examples of biofield therapy include acupuncture, acupressure, qigong, Reiki, and therapeutic touch.

Acupuncture and Acupressure

Acupuncture, one of the oldest and most popular TCM therapies, is used to relieve a wide variety of health conditions, from musculoskeletal dysfunction to depression. The therapist stimulates various points on the body with a series of precisely placed and extremely fine needles. The stimulation of these acupuncture points is thought to increase the flow of *qi* through the *meridians,* or energy pathways, in the body (**FIGURE 18.4**).

Following acupuncture, most participants in clinical studies report high levels of satisfaction with the treatment and improvement in their condition; however, extensive research has been inconclusive, and there is significant controversy over whether or not such results are simply a placebo response.[25] A 2012 study provided further evidence of a modest but significant reduction in chronic pain among people receiving acupuncture, particularly when they believe it will work and when needles are used in a specific way.[26]

Most U.S. acupuncturists are state licensed; however, licensing requirements vary by state. Many have completed a 2- to 3-year postgraduate program to obtain a master of traditional Oriental medicine (MTOM) degree. In addition, many conventional physicians and dentists practice acupuncture.[27]

energy medicine Therapies using energy fields, such as magnetic fields or biofields.

acupuncture Technique of traditional Chinese medicine that involves the placement of long, thin needles to affect flow of energy (*qi*) along energy pathways (meridians) within the body.

acupressure Technique of traditional Chinese medicine related to acupuncture that uses the application of pressure to selected points along the meridians to balance energy.

Acupressure is based on the same principles of energy flow as acupuncture. Instead of inserting needles, however, the therapist applies pressure to points critical to balancing *yin* and *yang,* the two complementary principles that influence overall harmony (health) of the body. The goal of the therapy is for *qi* to be evenly distributed and flow freely throughout the body. Practitioners must have the same basic training and understanding of meridians and acupuncture points as do acupuncturists.

Other Forms of Energy Therapy

Qigong, a traditional Chinese medicine technique, brings together movement, meditation, and regulation of breathing to increase the flow of *qi,* enhance blood circulation, and improve immune function. Recent research shows that qigong, and the related practice *tai chi,* are effective for promoting bone health, cardiopulmonary fitness, and balance.[28]

Reiki is a hands-on energy therapy that originated in Japan. The name is derived from the Japanese words representing "universal" and "vital energy," or *ki.* Reiki is based on the belief that by channeling *ki* to the patient, the practitioner facilitates healing. In two related therapies, *therapeutic touch* and *healing touch,* the therapist attempts to perceive, through his or her hands held just above the patient's body, imbalances in the patient's energy. The therapist promotes healing by increasing the flow of the body's energies and bringing them into balance. Research supporting the effectiveness of these therapies is limited.[29]

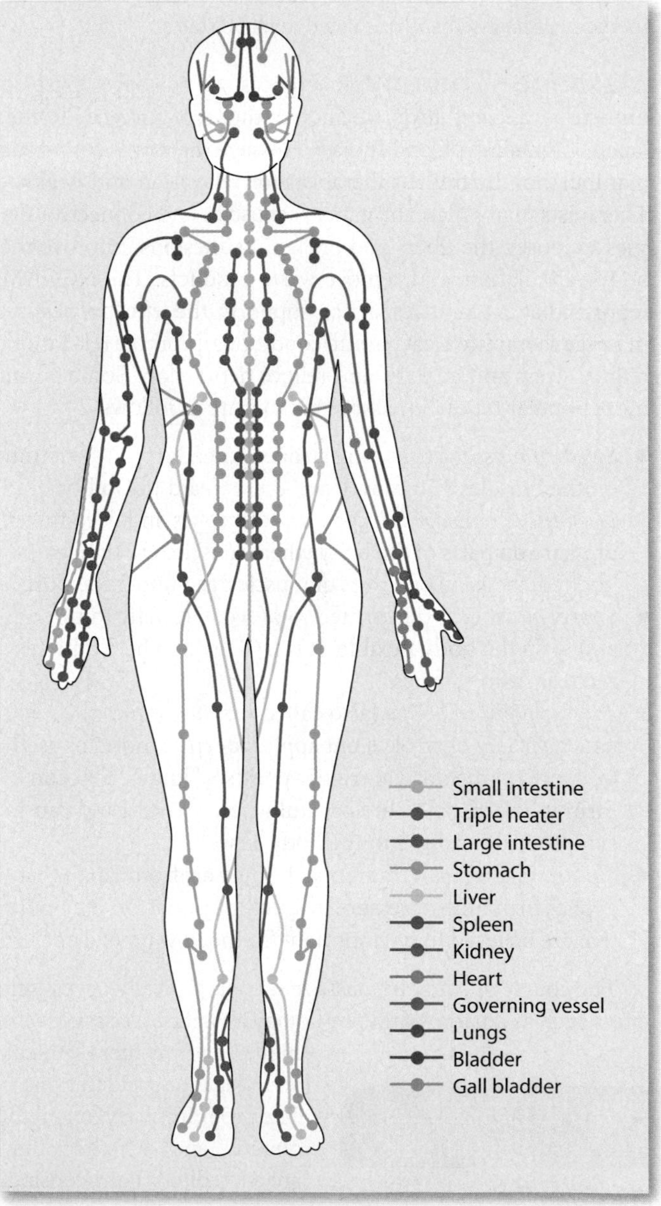

FIGURE 18.4 The Main Meridian Channels Acupuncture and acupressure are two therapies within traditional Chinese medicine based on the belief that vital energy flows through meridian channels in the body.

Source: Courtesy of the Association for Energy and Meridian Therapies (The AMT), East Sussex, UK, http://theamt.com.

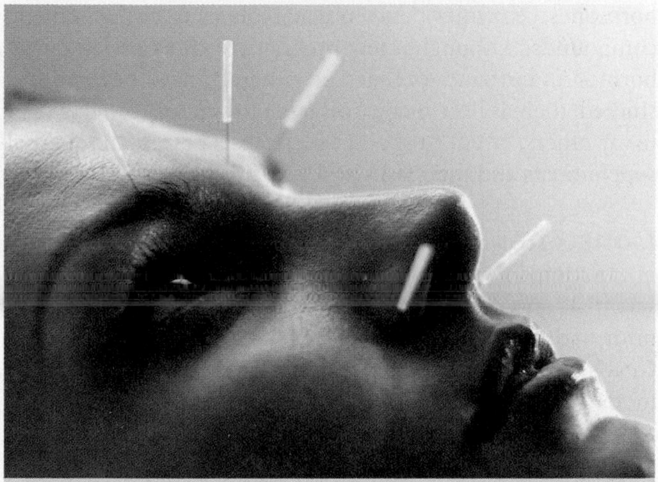

In acupuncture, long, thin needles are inserted into specific points along the body. This is thought to increase the flow of life-force energy, providing many physical and mental benefits.

Mind-Body Medicine

Mind-body medicine employs a variety of techniques to enhance the mind's capacity to affect bodily functions and symptoms and promote health. At present, mind-body techniques include deep breathing, meditation, yoga, progressive relaxation, and guided imagery—all commonly used CAM therapies in the United States. (See **Chapter 9** for more on yoga and tai chi, and **Chapters 2** and **3** and **Focus On: Cultivating Your Spiritual Health** for more on the mind-body connection.)

Research on *psychoneuroimmunology (PNI)* supports the effectiveness of mind-body therapies. PNI studies the interrelationships among behavioral, neural, endocrine, and immune processes.[30] (PNI is covered in greater detail in **Chapter 3**.) Many researchers have postulated that excessive stress and maladaptive coping can lead to immune system dysfunction and increase the risk of disease. Scientists are exploring ways in which relaxation, biofeedback, meditation, yoga, tai chi, and activities that involve either conscious or unconscious mind "quieting" may counteract negative stressors. For example, a recent review study of PNI found that psychological support—including relaxation therapies—can improve wound healing,[31] whereas inflammatory molecules such as C-reactive protein, which is a risk factor for heart disease, were found to be reduced in older adults after 16 weeks of *tai chi*.[32] Studies have also shown promising positive effects of mind-body techniques that encourage relaxation and other stress-reduction strategies for people with cancer.[33]

Dietary Products

Dietary products, including specially formulated foods and dietary supplements, are perhaps the most controversial domain of CAM therapies because of the sheer number of options available and the many claims that are made about their effects. Many of these claims have not been thoroughly investigated, and many of the products are not currently regulated.

Functional Foods Dietary changes are often part of CAM therapies, and such changes commonly involve increased intake of certain *functional foods*—foods said to improve some aspect of physical or mental functioning beyond the contribution of their specific nutrients. Both whole foods, such as broccoli and nuts, and modified foods, such as an energy bar said to enhance memory, are classified as functional foods.[34] Food producers sometimes refer to their functional foods as **nutraceuticals** to emphasize their combined nutritional and pharmaceutical benefits. For example, the label on a package of cocoa may state that the product provides antioxidants. The claim is backed up by research: Cocoa contains antioxidant phytochemicals called flavonoids, which have been shown to modestly reduce blood pressure.[35] The FDA regulates claims made on food labels; however, the FDA does not test functional foods prior to their coming to market and can only remove a product from the market if it is found to be unsafe.

Other common functional foods and their benefits include the following:

- **Plant stanols/sterols.** Reduces "bad" low-density lipoprotein (LDL) cholesterol.
- **Oat fiber.** Can lower LDL cholesterol; serves as a natural soother of nerves; stabilizes blood sugar levels.
- **Soy protein.** May lower heart disease risk by reducing LDL cholesterol and triglycerides.
- **Garlic.** Lowers cholesterol and reduces clotting tendency of blood; lowers blood pressure; may serve as a form of antibiotic.
- **Ginger.** May prevent motion sickness, stomach pain, and stomach upset; discourages blood clots; may relieve rheumatism.
- **Probiotics.** Yogurt and other fermented dairy foods that are labeled "live and active cultures" contain active, friendly bacteria called *probiotics*. Normal residents of the large intestine, probiotics in foods are thought to reduce inflammation and lower risk for certain types of infections, including opportunistic yeast infections and those associated with acute diarrhea. The National Institutes of Health (NIH) is currently funding extensive research into the therapeutic effects of probiotics on human health.[36]

Herbal Remedies and Other Dietary Supplements The Office of Dietary Supplements, part of the NIH, defines a dietary supplement as a "product (other than tobacco) that is intended to supplement or add to the diet; contains one or more dietary ingredients (including vitamins, minerals, herbs or other botanicals, amino acids, and other substances) or their constituents; is intended to be taken by mouth as a pill, capsule, tablet, or liquid; and is labeled on the front panel as being a dietary supplement."[37] Typically, people take dietary supplements—often without guidance from

mind-body medicine Techniques designed to enhance the mind's ability to affect bodily functions and symptoms.

nutraceuticals Food or food-based supplements that have combined nutritional and pharmaceutical benefits; used interchangeably with the term *functional foods*.

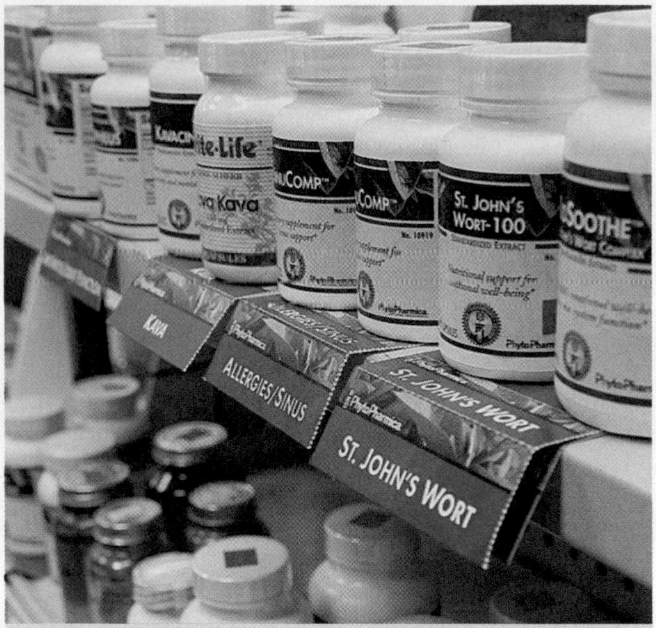

Herbs do have the potential to cause negative side effects. St. John's wort, for example, has potentially dangerous interactions with some prescription antidepressants and should never be taken with them.

any CAM practitioner—to improve health, prevent disease, or enhance mood.

Herbal remedies, often referred to as botanicals, are among the most common dietary supplements sold. People have been using herbal remedies for thousands of years. Herbs were the original sources for compounds found in approximately 25 percent of the pharmaceutical drugs we use today, including aspirin (white willow bark), the heart medication digitalis (foxglove), and the cancer treatment Taxol (Pacific yew tree). In addition, scientists continue to make pharmacological advances by studying the herbal remedies used in cultures throughout the world.

It's tempting to assume herbal remedies are safe because they are natural, but natural does not mean safe. For example, in recent years, the NCCAM has warned that certain herbal products containing kava may be associated with severe liver damage.[38] Even rigorously tested products can be risky. Many plants are poisonous, and some can be toxic if ingested in high doses. Others may be dangerous when combined with prescription or over-the-counter drugs, could disrupt the normal action of the drugs, or could cause unusual side effects.[39]

In general, herbal medicines tend to be milder than synthetic medications and produce their effects more slowly. But too much of any herb, particularly from nonstandardized extracts, can cause problems. **TABLE 18.2** provides an overview of some of the most common herbal supplements on the market.

Not all the supplements on the market today are directly derived from plant sources. In recent years, there have been increasing media claims on the health benefits of various hormones, enzymes, and other biological and synthetic compounds. Although a few products, such as melatonin (a hormone) and zinc lozenges (a mineral), have been widely studied, there is little quality research to support the claims of many others. **TABLE 18.3** on page 516 lists popular nonherbal supplements and their risks and benefits.

Consumer Protection The burgeoning popularity of functional foods and dietary supplements concerns many scientists and consumers. It is important to gather whatever information you can on both the safety and efficacy of any CAM treatment you are considering. In the case of functional foods and dietary supplements, start your own research with NCCAM (www.nccam.nih.gov) and the Cochrane Collaboration's review on complementary and alternative medicine (www.cochrane.org).

Dietary supplements can currently be sold without FDA approval. This raises issues of consumer safety. Even when products are dispensed by CAM practitioners, the situation can be risky. Products sold in "health food" stores and over the Internet may have varying levels of the active ingredient or may contain additives to which the consumer may have an adverse reaction.

As a result of such concerns, pressure has mounted to establish an approval process for dietary supplements similar to the process the FDA uses for drugs. In the meantime, if you're considering purchasing a dietary supplement, look for the USP Verified Mark on the label (**FIGURE 18.5**). The USP (United States Pharmacopeia) is a nonprofit, scientific organization. It does not regulate or determine the safety of medications, foods, or dietary supplements, but it does offer verification services to manufacturers of dietary supplement products. Dietary supplement products must meet stringent quality and manufacturing criteria to earn the USP Verified Mark.[40]

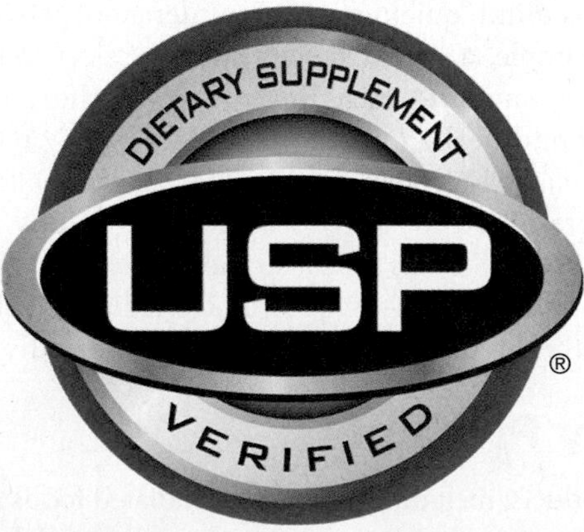

FIGURE 18.5 The U.S. Pharmacopoeia Verified Mark

Source: Used with permission of The United States Pharmacopeial Convention, www.uspverified.org.

TABLE 18.2 | Common Herbs and Herbal Supplements: Benefits, Research, and Risks

	Herb	Claims of Benefits	Research Findings	Potential Risks
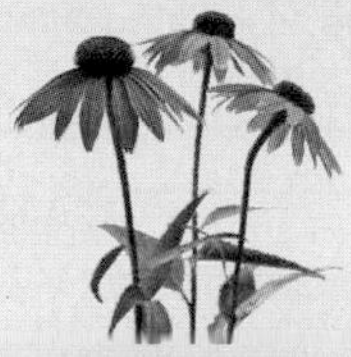	Echinacea (purple coneflower, *Echinacea purpurea, E. angustifolia, E. pallida*)	Stimulates the immune system and helps fight infection. Used to both prevent and treat colds and flu.	Some studies have provided preliminary evidence of its effectiveness in treating respiratory infections, but two recent studies found no benefit either for prevention or treatment.	Allergic reactions, including rashes, increased asthma, gastrointestinal problems, and anaphylaxis (a life-threatening allergic reaction).
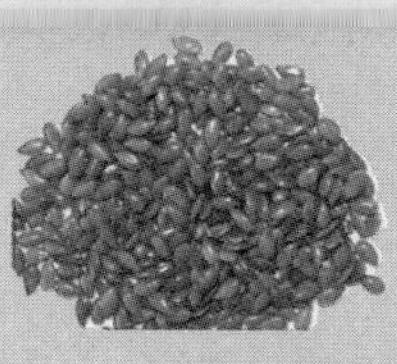	Flaxseed (*Linum usitatissimum*) and flaxseed oil	Used as a laxative and for hot flashes and breast pain, as well as to reduce cholesterol levels and risk of heart disease and cancer.	Flaxseed contains soluble fiber and may have a laxative effect. Study results are mixed on whether flaxseed decreases hot flashes. Insufficient data are available on the effect of flaxseed on cholesterol levels, heart disease, or cancer risks.	Delays absorption of medicines, but otherwise has few side effects. Oil taken in excess could cause diarrhea. Should be taken with plenty of water.
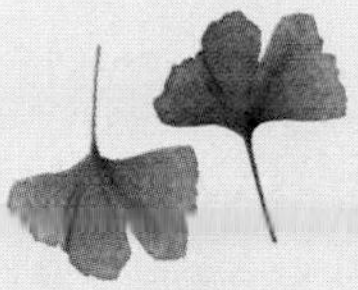	Ginkgo (*Ginkgo biloba*)	Popularly used to prevent cognitive decline, dementia, and Alzheimer's disease, and general vascular disease.	Although some small studies have had promising results, the large Ginkgo Evaluation of Memory study found ginkgo did not reduce Alzheimer's disease or dementia, slow cognitive decline, or reduce blood pressure.	Gastric irritation, headache, nausea, dizziness, difficulty thinking, memory loss, and allergic reactions. Ginkgo seeds are highly toxic; only products made from leaf extracts should be used.
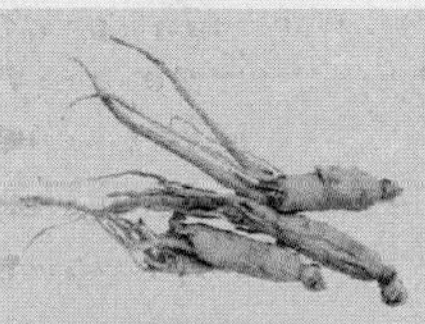	Ginseng (*Panax ginseng*)	Claimed to increase resistance to stress, boost the immune system, lower blood glucose and blood pressure, and improve stamina and sex drive.	Some studies suggest that ginseng may improve immune function and lower blood glucose; however, research overall is inconclusive.	Headaches, insomnia, and gastrointestinal problems are the most commonly reported adverse effects.
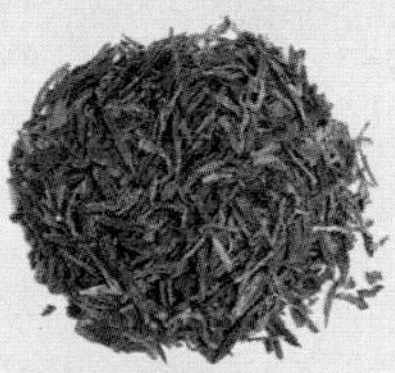	Green tea (*Camellia sinensis*)	Useful for lowering cholesterol and risk of some cancers, protecting the skin from sun damage, bolstering mental alertness, and boosting heart health.	Although some studies have shown promising links between green and white tea consumption and cancer prevention, recent research questions the ability of tea to significantly reduce the risk of breast, lung, or prostate cancer.	Insomnia, liver problems, anxiety, irritability, upset stomach, nausea, diarrhea, or frequent urination.

Sources: National Center for Complementary and Alternative Medicine, "Herbs at a Glance," January 2014, http://nccam.nih.gov/health/herbsataglance.htm; American Cancer Society, "Green Tea," May 2012, www.cancer.org.

LO 4 | HEALTH INSURANCE

Describe the U.S. health care system in terms of types of insurance; the changing structure of the system; and issues concerning cost, quality, and access to services.

Whether you're visiting your regular doctor, consulting a specialist, or preparing for a hospital stay, chances are you'll be using some form of health insurance to pay for your care. Insurance typically allows you, the consumer, to pay into a pool of funds and then bill the insurance carrier for health care charges you incur. The fundamental principle of insurance underwriting is that the cost of health care can be predicted for large populations. This is how health care **premiums**, payments made by the policyholders and/or their employer to the insurance company, are calculated. Policyholders pay premiums into a pool of funds, from which insurance companies pay claims. When you are sick or injured, the insurance company pays your care provider out of the pool regardless of your total contribution. Depending on circumstances, you may never pay for what your medical care costs, or you may pay much more for insurance than your medical bills ever total. The idea is that you pay affordable premiums so that you never have to face catastrophic bills. In profit-oriented systems, insurers prefer to have healthy people in their plans who pour money into risk pools without taking money out.

premium Payment made to an insurance carrier, usually in monthly installments, that covers the cost of an insurance policy.

Private Health Insurance

Originally, health insurance consisted solely of coverage for hospital costs (it was called *major medical*), but gradually it was extended to cover routine physicians' treatment and other

TABLE 18.3 | Common Nonherbal Supplements: Benefits, Research, and Risks

Supplement	Claims	Research Findings	Potential Risks
Coenzyme Q10 (antioxidant enzyme found in the heart, liver, kidneys, and pancreas)	Used to improve heart function and reduce blood pressure; also used to increase male fertility and to prevent cancer.	Appears to improve heart function in patients with heart failure. Research on blood-pressure reduction is mixed. May improve sperm quality and count. No proven cancer-prevention benefits.	Does not appear to be associated with serious side effects. Some common side effects include nausea, headaches, insomnia, and heartburn. May reduce effectiveness of anticoagulant medications.
Vitamin E	Claimed to reduce risk of heart disease and age-related vision impairment and slow cognitive decline.	Research into the role of vitamin E in heart disease and vision loss is mixed. There is no evidence supporting its use for improving brain function.	High doses cause bleeding when taken with blood thinners.
Glucosamine (biological substance that helps the body grow cartilage)	Used to relieve pain and inflammation in arthritis and related degenerative joint diseases.	Research shows no significant difference in effectiveness between glucosamine and a placebo. For moderate-to-severe joint pain, glucosamine may be effective when taken with chondroitin sulfate.	Few side effects noted.
Carnitine (amino acid derivative)	Used to improve athletic performance and slow cognitive decline.	Extensive research finds no evidence it improves performance in healthy athletes. Limited evidence suggests that it may enhance mental function in older adults with mild cognitive impairment.	Interacts with some drugs. Common side effects include nausea, vomiting, abdominal cramps, diarrhea, "fishy" body odor. Some evidence of increased risk for cardiovascular disease.
Melatonin (hormone)	Used to regulate circadian rhythms (to prevent jet lag) and treat insomnia; claims of antiaging benefits.	Some evidence supports its usefulness in regulating sleep patterns. No scientific support for antiaging claims.	Nausea, headaches, dizziness, blood vessel constriction; possibly a danger for people with high blood pressure or other cardiovascular problems.
SAMe (pronounced "sammy") (biological compound that aids over 40 functions in the body)	Used in treatment of mild to moderate depression and in treatment of arthritis pain.	Studies have supported its usefulness in treating depression and arthritis pain.	Fewer side effects than prescription antidepressants, but questions remain over correct dosage, form, and long-term side effects.
Zinc (mineral)	Supports immune system; lozenges used to lessen duration and severity of cold symptoms.	Some research suggests that zinc lozenges can reduce the severity and duration of a cold if taken within 24 hours of onset of symptoms.	Use of zinc lozenges can cause nausea. Excessive use can reduce immune function.

Source: Office of Dietary Supplements, National Institutes of Health, "Dietary Supplement Fact Sheets," April 2014, http://ods.od.nih.gov/Health_Information/Information_About_Individual_Dietary_Supplements.aspx.

services, such as dental, vision care, and pharmaceuticals. These payment mechanisms laid the groundwork for today's steadily rising health care costs. Hospitals were reimbursed for the costs of providing care plus an amount for profit. This system provided no incentive to contain costs, limit the number of procedures, or curtail capital investment in redundant equipment and facilities. Physicians were reimbursed on a fee-for-service (indemnity) basis determined by "usual, customary, and reasonable" fees. This system encouraged physicians to charge high fees, raise them often, and perform as many procedures as possible. Until the middle to late twentieth century, most insurance did not cover routine or preventive services, and consumers generally waited until illness developed to see a doctor instead of seeking preventive care. Consumers were also free to choose any provider or service they wished, including even inappropriate—and often very expensive—levels of care.

WHAT DO YOU THINK?

Why is it important that private insurance cover preventive or lower-level care as well as hospitalization and high-technology interventions?

- What kinds of incentives would cause you to seek care early rather than delay care?

To limit potential losses, private insurance companies began increasingly employing several mechanisms: cost sharing (in the form of deductibles, co-payments, and coinsurance), waiting periods, exclusions, "preexisting condition" clauses, and upper limits on payments:

- *Deductibles* are payments (which can range from about $500 to $5000 annually) you make for health care before insurance coverage kicks in to pay for eligible services.
- *Co-payments* are set amounts that you pay per service or product received, regardless of the total cost (e.g., $20 per doctor visit or per prescription filled).

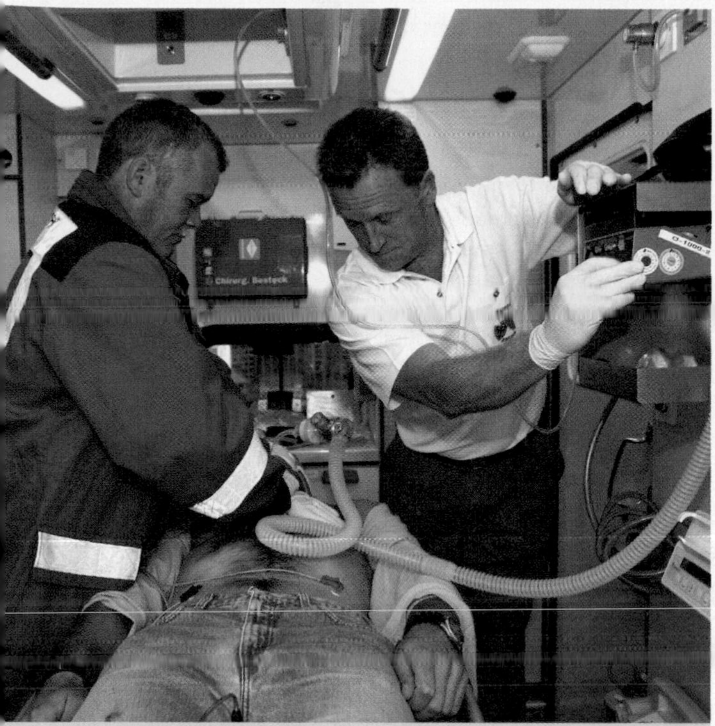

People without insurance can't gain access to preventive care, so they seek care only in an emergency or crisis. Because emergency care is extraordinarily expensive, they often are unable to pay, and the cost is absorbed by those who can pay—the insured or taxpayers.

- *Coinsurance* is the percentage of costs that you must pay based on the terms of the policy (e.g., 20% of the total bill).
- Some group plans specify a *waiting period* that cannot exceed 90 days before they will provide coverage. Waiting periods do not apply to plans purchased by individuals.
- All insurers set some limits on the types of *covered services* (e.g., most exclude cosmetic surgery, private rooms, and experimental procedures).
- *Preexisting condition clauses* once limited the insurance company's liability for medical conditions that a consumer had before obtaining coverage. For example, if a person applying for insurance had cancer, the insurer could deny the application entirely, or agree to cover the applicant, but only for conditions unrelated to the cancer. Under the 2010 Patient Protection and Affordable Care Act (ACA), no one can be discriminated against due to a preexisting condition.
- Some insurance plans also imposed an *annual upper limit* or *lifetime limit,* after which coverage would end. The ACA makes this practice illegal.

Managed Care

Managed care describes a health care delivery system consisting of the following elements:

- A network of physicians, hospitals, and other providers and facilities linked contractually to deliver comprehensive health benefits within a predetermined budget, sharing economic risk for any budget deficit or surplus
- A budget based on an estimate of the annual cost of delivering health care for a given population
- An established set of administrative rules requiring patients to follow the advice of participating health care providers in order to have their health care paid for under the terms of the health plan

Types of managed care plans include health maintenance organizations (HMOs), preferred provider organizations (PPOs), and point of service (POS). More than 73 million Americans are enrolled in HMOs, the most common type.[41]

Many managed care plans pay their contracted health care providers through **capitation**, that is, prepayment of a fixed monthly amount for each patient without regard for the type or number of health services provided. Some plans pay health care providers a salary, and some are still fee-for-service plans. As with other insurance plans, enrollees are members of a risk pool, and it is expected that some persons will use no services, some will use a modest amount, and others will have high-cost usage over a given year. Doctors have the incentive to keep their patient pool healthy and avoid catastrophic ailments that are preventable; usually such incentives come back in terms of increased salaries, bonuses, and other benefits. As such, prevention and health education to reduce risk and

managed care Cost-control procedures used by health insurers to coordinate treatment.

capitation Prepayment of a fixed monthly amount for each patient without regard to the type or number of services provided.

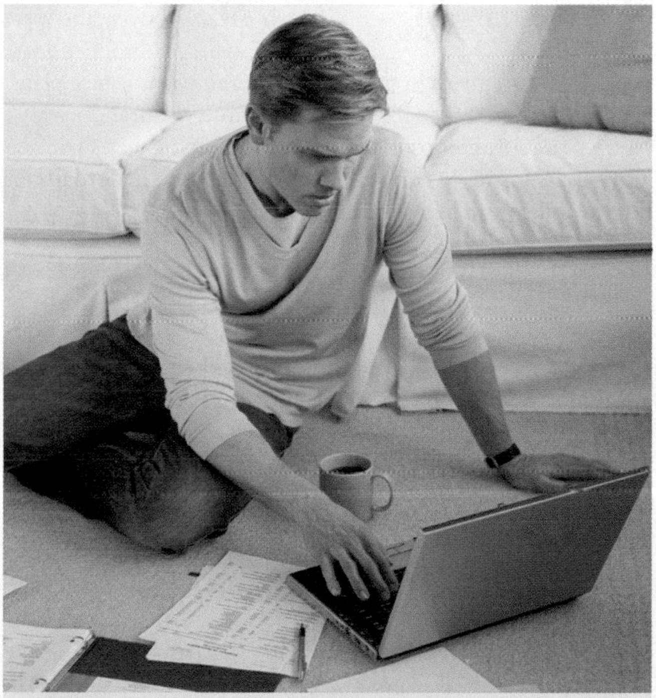

Choosing a health insurance plan can be confusing. Some things to think about include how comprehensive your coverage needs to be, how much you are willing to spend on premiums and co-payments, and whether the services of the plan meet your needs.

MONEY & HEALTH | HEALTH CARE SPENDING ACCOUNTS

A Flexible Spending Account (FSA) for health care and a Health Savings Account (HSA) are savings plans that give you the opportunity to save money tax free to be used toward qualified health care expenses. As long as you're not claimed as a dependent on someone else's tax return, you can open one, either an FSA through your employer or an HSA through your bank.

What expenses can you pay for with the money in your FSA or HAS account? Deductibles, co-payments, eyeglasses, contact lenses, and prescription drugs are all allowed. Visits to approved health care providers, including dentists and optometrists, also are payable from your account if you have no health insurance coverage for them. You can even use the funds to pay for OTC drugs such as pain relievers or allergy medications, as long as you have a written statement from your care provider that the OTC item is being purchased for a specific medical condition.

If you work in a job with an FSA benefit, upon enrollment you identify the amount you want diverted from your paycheck into your FSA before taxes are withheld. The maximum you can contribute varies with different employers and health plans. One drawback to the FSA is that any funds still in the account at the end of the plan year are forfeited. This is known as the "use it or lose it" rule. Therefore, you need to estimate carefully what your out-of-pocket health expenses will be during the plan year.

With an HSA, there is no time limit on when the funds have to be used. Contributions to the account can be made from your paycheck by your employer as pre-tax deductions, or you can make them yourself, in which case you can claim them as an "above-the-line" deduction (a deduction from your gross income) when you file your tax return.

Does a health care spending account make sense for you? If you currently pay out-of-pocket for more than one or two health care visits a year, a few prescriptions, contact lenses, etc., and the money you use for these expenses comes from taxable income, then a health care savings plan might be worth a closer look. Contact your employee benefits specialist, your tax preparer, or a customer service provider at your bank.

Medicare A federal health insurance program that covers people age 65 and older, the permanently disabled, and people with end-stage kidney disease.

intervene early to avoid major problems are often capstone components of such plans.

Managed care plans have grown steadily over the past decade with a proportionate decline of enrollment in traditional indemnity insurance plans. The reason for this shift is that indemnity insurance, which pays providers and hospitals on a fee-for-service basis with no built-in incentives to control costs, has become unaffordable or unavailable for many Americans.

Health Maintenance Organizations Health maintenance organizations (HMOs) provide a wide range of covered health benefits (e.g., physician visits, laboratory tests, surgery, and usually a prescription drug benefit) for a fixed amount prepaid by the patient, the employer, Medicaid, or Medicare (discussed later). Usually, HMO premiums are the least expensive form of managed care (saving between 10% and 40% more than other plans), but they are also the most restrictive (offering little or no choice in doctors and certain services). These premiums are 8 to 10 percent lower than for traditional plans, there are low or no deductibles or coinsurance payments, and co-payments are modest.

The downside of HMOs is that patients are typically required to use the plan's doctors and hospitals. Within an HMO, the PCP serves as a "gatekeeper," coordinating the patient's care and providing referrals to specialists and other services. As more and more people enroll in HMOs, concerns have arisen about care allocation and access to services, profit-motivated medical decision making, and the degree of focus on prevention and intervention.

Preferred Provider Organizations Preferred provider organizations (PPOs) are networks of independent doctors and hospitals that contract to provide care at discounted rates. Although they offer greater choices in doctors than HMOs do, they are less likely to coordinate a patient's care. Members may choose to see doctors who are not on the preferred list, but this choice may involve having to pay a higher percentage of the cost of care.

Point of Service Point of service (POS) plans—a hybrid of HMO and PPO plans—provide a more familiar form of managed care for people used to traditional indemnity insurance, which may explain why it is among the fastest growing of managed care plans. Under POS plans, members select an in-network PCP, but they can go to nonnetwork providers for care without a referral and pay the extra cost.

No matter what type of plan you're in, a special savings account for health-related expenses could save you money. How do such accounts work, and are they right for you? See the **Money & Health** box and find out.

Government-Funded Programs

The federal government, through programs such as Medicare and Medicaid, currently funds 45 percent of total U.S. health care spending.[42]

Medicare **Medicare** is a federal insurance program that employees and employers pay into over the course of a person's working life at a rate of approximately 3 percent of salary per year. The more a person makes, the more they pay. The funds are used to cover a broad range of services but not long-term care. Medicare covers 99 percent of Americans over age 65, all totally and permanently disabled people (after a waiting period), and all people with end-stage kidney failure; together, these groups comprise over 60 million people, or 1 in 6 Americans.[43]

Since its inception in 1965, Medicare has faced increasing funding challenges. Many factors have contributed, including rising health care costs; an aging population, which means more enrollees removing money from the system at the same time that fewer young workers are paying into the system, and diversion of funds to other government programs. As the costs of medical care have continued to increase, Medicare has placed limits on the amount of reimbursement to providers. As a result, some providers no longer accept Medicare patients, creating a potential two-tiered system where Medicare patients may not be able to access the best health care providers.

To control hospital costs, the federal government set up a prospective payment system based on *diagnosis-related groups (DRGs)* for Medicare. Nearly 500 groupings were created to establish how much a hospital would be reimbursed for caring for a patient diagnosed with a particular condition or combination of conditions. DRGs are based on the assumption that patients with similar health status and conditions will require a similar amount of hospital resources. If the costs of treating a patient are less than the predetermined amount, the hospital can keep the difference. However, if a patient's care costs more than the set amount, the hospital must absorb the difference (with a few exceptions that must be reviewed by a panel). This system motivates hospitals to discharge patients quickly, to provide more ambulatory care, and to admit patients classified into the most favorable (profitable) DRGs. Many private health insurance companies have also adopted reimbursement rates based on DRGs.

The Centers for Medicare and Medicaid Services (CMS) has encouraged the growth of HMO plans for Medicare-eligible persons. Under this system, commercial managed care insurance plans receive a fixed per capita premium from CMS and then offer more preventive services with lower out-of pocket co-payments. These managed care plans encourage providers and patients to utilize health care resources under administrative rules similar to commercial HMO plans.

Medicaid In contrast to Medicare, **Medicaid**, covering approximately 62 million people, is a federal-state matching funds program that provides health insurance for people defined as low-income, including many who are blind, disabled, elderly, pregnant, or eligible for Temporary Assistance for Needy Families (TANF). Medicaid relies on funds provided by both federal and state sources. Because each state determines income eligibility, covered services, and payments to providers, there are vast differences in the way Medicaid operates from state to state. The ACA provides generous federal subsidies to states that expand Medicaid coverage to all Americans living below 133 percent of the federal poverty level (in 2014, the poverty level was $19,790 for a three-person household).[44] Although states are responsible for only a small percentage of the funding to expand Medicaid, some have refused; however, those states complying with Medicaid expansion are expected to have increased enrollment in Medicaid by over 17 million Americans by 2016.[45]

The Children's Health Insurance Program (CHIP) was created in 1997 and reauthorized through new legislation in 2009. It provides health insurance coverage to nearly 8 million uninsured children whose family income is too high to qualify for Medicaid.[46] Like Medicaid, it is jointly funded by federal and state funds and is administered by state governments.

Insurance Coverage by the Numbers

In 2014, the average family's annual health insurance premium was more than $16,000.[47] For workers employed in organizations that offer health care insurance, most of this cost is hidden: The worker pays 15 percent to 25 percent of the full premium, usually as a deduction from his or her paycheck, and earns lower wages in return for the remaining cost of the coverage. However, people who are self-employed or work in companies that do not provide group health insurance must pay their premiums independently, often at extremely high rates. Millions of employed but uninsured Americans do not find them affordable. In total, about 31 million Americans—15.8 percent—are uninsured; that is, they have no private health insurance and are not eligible for Medicare, Medicaid, or other subsidized government health programs.[48] The vast majority of the uninsured work or are dependents of employed people.

Not having health insurance has been associated with individuals delaying health care, as well as increased mortality. *Underinsurance*—the inability to pay for expenses despite being covered—can also cause poor health outcomes. In a 2013 national survey of college students, 7.5 percent of respondents said they did not have health insurance.[49] However, those who are covered only under their school's health care plan—17 percent according to the same survey—may not realize that such plans are usually short term and have a low upper limit of benefits, which would be problematic if the student were to have a severe illness or injury. However, few students buy higher-level catastrophic plans.

Racial and ethnic minorities are overly represented in the number of uninsured Americans. Almost a third of all Hispanic Americans are uninsured compared to 15.1 percent of African Americans and 11.5 percent of whites.[50] Issues such as citizenship and language barriers contribute to some of the disparities in access to health insurance for many in our country.

Why should all Americans be concerned about those who are uninsured and underinsured? People without adequate health care coverage are less likely than other Americans to have their children immunized, seek early prenatal care, obtain annual blood pressure checks and other screenings, and seek attention for symptoms of health problems. Experts believe that this ultimately leads to higher system costs because their conditions go undetected

Medicaid A federal-state matching funds program that provides health insurance to low-income people.

at their earliest, most treatable stage, deteriorating to a more debilitating and costly stage before they are forced to seek help, often in an emergency room. Because emergency care is far more expensive than clinic care, uninsured and underinsured patients are often unable to pay, and the cost is absorbed by "the system" in the form of higher hospital costs, insurance premiums, and taxes.

LO 5 | ISSUES FACING TODAY'S HEALTH CARE SYSTEM

Explain key issues facing our health care system today and possible actions that could help to improve the system.

In recent decades, the number of Americans without health insurance increased dramatically as costs and restrictions on eligibility for coverage rose. In 2010, Congress passed the Patient Protection and Affordable Care Act (ACA) to provide a means for these and all Americans to obtain affordable health care. In addition to increasing access to care, the ACA is expected to address America's high cost of care and to improve the overall quality of care. Here, we examine these three key issues, as well as the potential impact of the ACA.

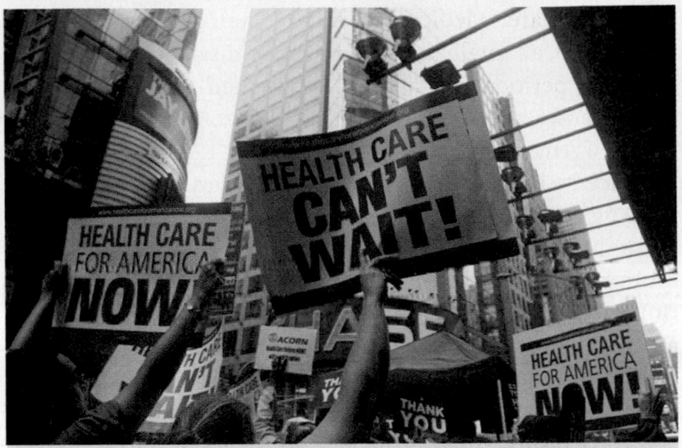

The debate over healthcare for all rages as millions remain uninsured or underinsured.

Access

Access to health care is determined by numerous factors, the most significant of which are the supply and proximity of providers and facilities and insurance coverage.

Access to Providers, Facilities, and Treatments In 2012, there were almost 700,000 physicians in the United States.[51] However, there is an oversupply of higher-paid specialists and a shortage of lower-paid primary care physicians (family practitioners, internists, pediatricians, etc.). Inner cities and some rural areas face constant shortages of physicians. Similarly, of the nearly 5,000 non-federal hospitals in the United States, over 60 percent serve urban areas, leaving many rural communities without readily accessible care.[52]

Managed care health plans determine access on the basis of participating providers, health plan benefits, and administrative rules. Often this means that consumers do not have the freedom to choose specialists, facilities, or treatment options beyond those contracted with the health plan and recommended by their primary care provider.

WHAT DO YOU THINK?

Do you believe prospective patients should have access to information about practitioners' and facilities' malpractice records?

- How about their success and failure rates or outcomes of various procedures?

Access to Quality Health Insurance Even if care providers and facilities are only a few miles away, not all Americans have equal access to them. A key disparity is the quality of the patient's health insurance plan. Otis W. Brawley, Chief Medical Officer for the American Cancer Society, uses the term "wallet biopsy" to describe the assessment a physician makes of a patient's—or his or her insurance company's—ability to pay for prescribed tests and procedures. Patients with excellent insurance coverage may then be encouraged to undergo expensive tests and treatments (a practice that can lead to useless or even harmful overtreatment, which we address shortly), whereas patients with poor insurance may not be informed of the full variety of diagnostic and treatment options.[53]

Key provisions in the ACA aim to increase access to quality health insurance among Americans. These include the following:

- Insurers are now required to cover several preventive services, such as health screenings for cancer, diabetes and cardiovascular disease screenings for patients at increased risk, and counseling on topics such as losing weight, quitting smoking, treating depression, and reducing alcohol use.
- Insurers are required to cover young adults on a parent's plan through age 26. Coverage is in place for prescription medications, including psychotropic medications.
- Americans with preexisting conditions cannot be denied coverage.
- No annual and lifetime limits on benefits are allowed.
- Affordable Insurance Exchanges (AIEs) facilitate consumer shopping and enrollment in plans with the same kinds of choices that members of Congress have.
- Small businesses, which typically paid as much as 18 percent more than large businesses for health insurance coverage for their employees, now qualify for special tax credits to help fund insurance plans.

Even before passage of the ACA, Congress provided assistance with insurance coverage for employees who change jobs. Under the Consolidated Omnibus Budget Reconciliation Act (COBRA), former employees, retirees, spouses, and dependents have the option to continue their insurance for up to 18 months at group rates. People who enroll in COBRA pay a higher amount than they did when they were employed, as they're covering both the personal premium and the amount previously covered by the employer.

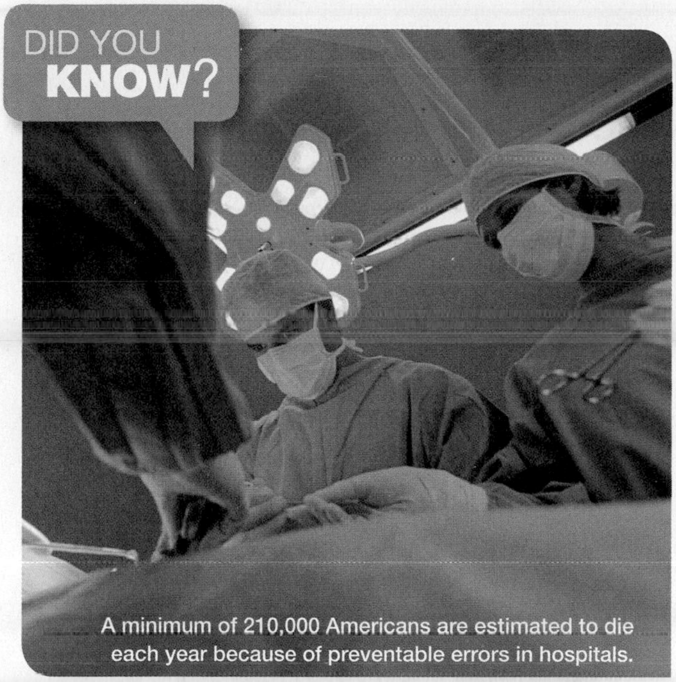

DID YOU KNOW?
A minimum of 210,000 Americans are estimated to die each year because of preventable errors in hospitals.

Source: J. T. James, "A New, Evidence-Based Estimate of Patient Harms Associated with Hospital Care," *Journal of Patient Safety* 9, no. 3 (2013): 122–8, DOI: 10.1097/PTS.0b013e3182948a69.

Cost

Both per capita and as a percentage of gross domestic product (GDP), the United States spends more on health care than any other nation. In 2014, our national health expenditures were projected to reach $3.1 trillion, nearly $9,700 for every man, woman, and child.[54] Does this sound like a lot? Consider that health care expenditures are projected to grow by 5.8 percent each year, reaching over $5 trillion annually by 2022—nearly 20 percent of our projected GDP.[55]

Why are America's health care costs so high? Many factors are involved: duplication of services; an aging population; growing rates of obesity, inactivity, and related health problems; demand for new diagnostic and treatment technologies; an emphasis on crisis-oriented care instead of prevention; stock-owned pharmaceutical companies that are accountable to stock holders for increasing profits, leading to increases in prescription drug costs; physician overtreatment, whether to avoid malpractice suits or to increase income; and inappropriate use of services by consumers, including use of emergency services for routine care and family demands for futile and expensive procedures for patients who are dying.

Our insurance system is also to blame. Currently, more than 2,000 companies provide health insurance in the United States, each with different coverage structures and administrative requirements. This lack of uniformity prevents our system from achieving the *economies of scale* (bulk purchasing at a reduced cost) and administrative efficiency realized in countries where there is a single-payer delivery system. According to the trade association for America's Health Insurance Plans (AHIP), commercial insurance companies commonly experience administrative costs greater than 12 percent of the total health care insurance premium.[56] These administrative expenses contribute to the high cost of health care and force companies to require employees to share more of the costs, cut back on benefits, and drop some benefits altogether. These costs are largely passed on to consumers in the form of higher prices for goods and services. See **FIGURE 18.6** for a breakdown of how health care dollars are spent.

The ACA's provision for Affordable Insurance Exchanges would increase bulk purchasing and reduce administrative costs, thus achieving some savings. Moreover, the ACA mandates the following cost-control measures:

- Insurance companies that spend less than 80 percent of premium dollars on medical care in a given year have to send enrollees a rebate.
- All insurance companies have to publicly justify their actions if they plan to raise rates by 10 percent or more.
- Tougher screening procedures and penalties are helping to reduce health care fraud.

See the **Money & Health** box on the following page for ways you can maximize your care while minimizing the costs.

Quality

The United States has several mechanisms for ensuring quality services: Providers are assessed according to education, licensure, certification/registration, accreditation, peer review, and the legal system of malpractice litigation. Over-the-counter

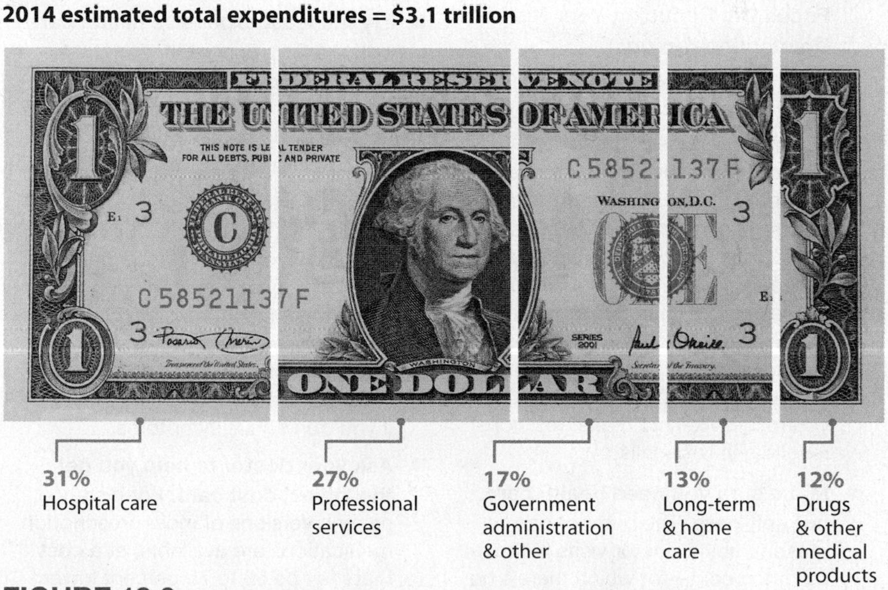

FIGURE 18.6 Where Do We Spend Our Health Care Dollars?

Source: Data are from Centers for Medicare & Medicaid Services, "National Health Expenditure Projections 2012–2022: Forecast Summary," November 2013, www.cms.gov/Research-Statistics-Data-and-Systems/Statistics-Trends-and-Reports/NationalHealthExpendData/Downloads/proj2012.pdf.

MONEY & HEALTH | MAXIMIZING CARE WHILE MINIMIZING COSTS

Maybe you're like the 7.5 percent of college students who reported in a 2013 survey that they had no health insurance. Or maybe you're on your parents' plan or one sponsored by your college or university, but there's a hefty deductible or co-payment. Or the test or medication you need isn't covered. Whatever your situation, following a few strategies will help you get the best care for the lowest cost.

- **Preserve your health.** Remember that four behaviors—poor nutrition, failing to exercise, smoking, and abusing alcohol—account for the majority of preventable disease. Your most important cost-sparing strategy is to take care of your health in the first place.
- **Avoid unnecessary risks.** Unintentional injuries aren't just the top cause of death in young adults, they're also a primary reason young adults seek emergency care. (For additional information, see **Focus On: Reducing Your Risk of Unintentional Injury**.)
- **Do your research.** If you have health care insurance, read the summary plan description (SPD). This explains what types of care providers, tests, and treatments are covered and also specifies if vision, dental, or prescription benefits are included. The SPD also outlines any co-payments, annual deductibles, and in- and out-of-network rules for seeing specialists. When you know the answers to these questions, you're less likely to make decisions resulting in large bills.
- **Make sure you need health care, not self-care.** The number one reason behind doctor visits is the common cold—for which there's no treatment. For many conditions, rest, nutritious fluids, and the passage of time are the only healers. So think before you spend money on health care you don't need.
- **Try the least expensive health care options first.** For instance, your student health center may be able to provide exactly the level of care you need for little or no cost. Or call the nurse hotline available on your insurance plan.
- **Go prepared.** When you do visit your doctor, come with a list of symptoms, concerns, and questions. If you think you need a diagnostic test, request it and explain why. If you're sexually active, ask your doctor what tests you should have for sexually transmitted infections, even if you don't have symptoms.
- **Ask your doctor to help you get the lowest cost care.** For instance, generic versions of most prescription medications are available, at a cost that may be 50 to 75 percent lower than that of the brand-name drug. Ask the doctor for the generic version of the drug, when possible.

If you are uninsured or underinsured, ask your doctor for generic prescriptions to save on your costs.

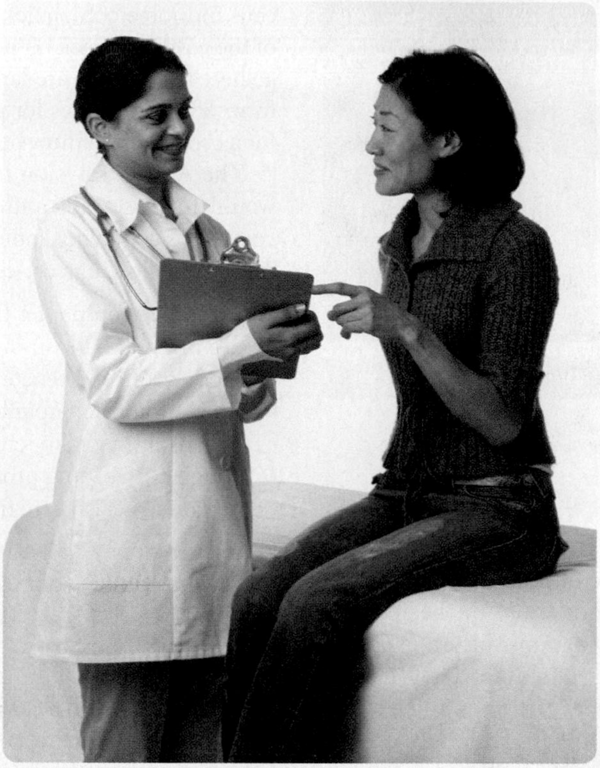

- **Find out what assistance is available to pay for medications.** If you can't afford a medication you need, and you are thinking about not taking it, find out if you qualify for assistance by visiting the website of the Partnership for Prescription Assistance at www.pparx.org. Also talk to your pharmacist. Most large drugstore chains sponsor prescription discount programs, or your pharmacist may be able to direct you to online coupons for commonly prescribed drugs.
- **Use the emergency room (ER) only for emergencies.** Studies show that almost 70 percent of ER visits are not really emergencies at all—and care in an ER can cost ten times as much as the same care in a walk-in clinic.
- **When you get a bill from your provider, check it for accuracy.** Medical bill errors are common, especially duplicated charges and simple typos. Also review the statements you get from your plan to make sure that you received the care described and the right reimbursements.
- **Be aware that if your plan denies coverage for a test or treatment that your physician says is necessary, you have the right to appeal the decision.** Check your SPD for your plan's appeals process, which typically involves writing a letter explaining your grievance. Copy both your physician and your state insurance commissioner, and keep a copy for your own records.

Sources: American College Health Association, *American College Health Association-National College Health Assessment II: Reference Group Executive Summary, Spring 2013* (Baltimore, MD: American College Health Association, 2013); U.S. Department of Labor; *Top 10 Ways to Make Your Health Benefits Work for You*, www.dol.gov/ebsa/publications/10working4you.html; Aetna, *Six Ways to Save Money with Your Aetna Student Health Benefits*, Aetnastudenthealth.com, www.aetnastudenthealth.com/schools/SavingMoneyFlyer.pdf.

and prescription medications, as well as medical devices, must be approved by the FDA. Insurance companies and government payers may also require a higher level of quality by linking payment to whether a practitioner is board certified, a facility is accredited, or a treatment is an approved therapy. In addition, most insurance plans now require prior authorization and/or second opinions, not only to reduce costs, but also to improve quality of care.

Although our health care spending far exceeds that of any other nation, we rank far below many other nations in key indicators of quality. For example, in 2014, the Central Intelligence Agency ranked the United States 42nd in life expectancy. At a projected 79.5 years, U.S. life expectancy was a full decade below that of the top-ranked country, Monaco.[57] And our infant mortality rate, at 6.2 deaths per every 1,000 live births, is higher than that of 55 other nations.[58] The ACA is intended to improve the quality of health care in the United States. As a first step, in 2011 the Department of Health and Human Services released to Congress a National Strategy for Quality Improvement in Health Care. Its priorities include a new emphasis on promoting the safest, most preventive, and most effective care; increasing communication and coordination among providers; and ensuring that patients and families are engaged as partners in their care.[59]

Although many health experts feel that the ACA does not go far enough in addressing the unequal access, high cost, and poor quality of our health care system, others believe that it is a step in the right direction. They contend that gradual improvements in technology and implementation and increased state acceptance of federal funding will help the ACA achieve its overall goals of improved cost, quality, and access to care for all Americans.

As consumers, the best strategy is to read the accumulated evidence on what is and is not working in the health care system and base your decisions on a rational unbiased approach that considers others, as well as yourself, as we work to improve health care delivery in the United States.

STUDY PLAN

Customize your study plan—and master your health!—in the Study Area of **MasteringHealth.**

ASSESS **YOURSELF**

What could you do to become a better health care consumer? Want to find out? Take the **Are You a Smart Health Care Consumer?** assessment available on MasteringHealth.™

Need help creating a plan? Follow the strategies in the **Your Plan for Change** box for short- and long-term improvements to your health.

YOUR PLAN FOR **CHANGE**

Once you have considered your responses to the **ASSESS YOURSELF** questions, you may want to change or improve certain behaviors in order to get the best treatment from your health care provider and the health care system.

TODAY, YOU CAN:

- ☐ Research your insurance plan. Find out which health care providers and hospitals you can visit in your area, your options for medical care when traveling outside your area, the amounts of co-payments and premiums you are responsible for, and the drug coverage of your plan.
- ☐ Update your medicine cabinet. Dispose properly of any expired prescriptions or OTC medications. Keep on hand a supply of basic items, such as pain relievers, antiseptic cream, bandages, cough suppressants, and throat lozenges.

WITHIN THE NEXT 2 WEEKS, YOU CAN:

- ☐ Find a regular health care provider if you do not already have one and make an appointment for a general checkup.
- ☐ Check with your insurance provider and see what CAM practitioners and therapies are covered.
- ☐ Find out what alternative therapies your college's health clinic offers.

BY THE END OF THE SEMESTER, YOU CAN:

- ☐ Become an advocate for others' health. Write to your congressperson or state legislature to express your interest in health care reform.
- ☐ Make relaxation and mind-body stress-reducing techniques a part of your everyday life. This can simply mean practicing meditation, deep breathing, or even taking long walks in nature. You don't need to visit a CAM practitioner or follow a specific therapeutic practice to benefit from methods of relaxation, meditation, and spiritual awakening.

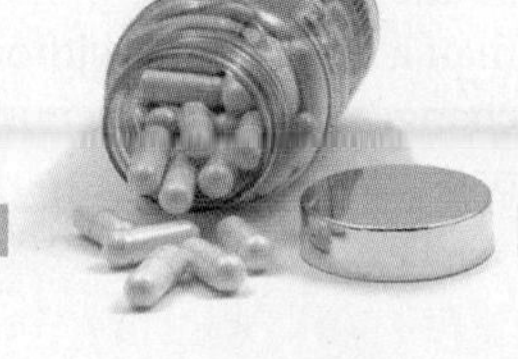

CHAPTER REVIEW

To hear an MP3 Tutor Session, scan here or visit the Study Area in **MasteringHealth.**

LO 1 Taking Responsibility for Your Health Care

- Knowing when and how to take care of yourself and when to seek professional health care will save you money and improve your health status. Advance planning can help you navigate health care treatment in unfamiliar situations or emergencies. Assess health professionals by considering their qualifications, their record of treating similar problems, and their ability to work with you.

LO 2 Conventional Health Care

- In theory, conventional Western (allopathic) medicine is based on scientifically validated methods and procedures. Medical doctors, specialists of various kinds, nurses, physician assistants, and other health care professionals practice allopathic medicine.
- Prescription drugs are obtained through a written prescription from a physician, whereas over the-counter-drugs can be purchased without a prescription.

LO 3 Complementary and Alternative Medicine (CAM)

- Throughout the world, people are using complementary and alternative medicine (CAM) in increasing numbers. Alternative medical systems include traditional Chinese medicine (TCM), ayurveda, homeopathy, and naturopathy. CAM also includes manipulative and body-based practices, energy medicine, mind-body medicine, and natural products.
- Consumers need to understand that the FDA does not study and approve dietary supplements before they are brought to market. Thus, there is no guarantee of their safety or effectiveness. However, the USP Verified Mark does indicate that a supplement has met certain criteria for product purity and manufacturing standards.

LO 4 Health Insurance

- Health insurance is based on the concept of spreading risk. Insurance is provided by private insurance companies (which charge premiums) and the government Medicare and Medicaid programs (which are funded by taxes). Managed care (in the form of HMOs, PPOs, and POS plans) attempts to control costs by streamlining administrative procedures and promoting preventive care, among other initiatives.

LO 5 Issues Facing Today's Health Care System

- Concerns about the U.S. health care system include access, cost, and quality. The Patient Protection and Affordable Care Act was passed by Congress in 2010 to address these issues. Many public health experts feel that it does not go far enough in addressing the fundamental flaws in the system.

POP QUIZ

Visit **MasteringHealth** to personalize your study plan with Chapter Review Quizzes and Dynamic Study Modules.

LO 1 Taking Responsibility for Your Health Care

1. Of the following conditions, which would be appropriately managed by self-care?
   a. A persistent temperature of 104°F or higher
   b. Sudden weight loss of more than a few pounds without changes in diet or exercise patterns
   c. A sore throat, runny nose, and cough that persist for several days
   d. Yellowing of the skin or the whites of the eyes

LO 2 Conventional Health Care

2. What medical practice is based on procedures whose objective is to heal by countering the patient's symptoms?
   a. Allopathic medicine
   b. Homeopathic medicine
   c. Ayurvedic medicine
   d. Chiropractic medicine
3. Which of the following health care providers holds a medical degree?
   a. Doctor of science in nursing
   b. Ophthalmologist
   c. Osteopath
   d. Naturopathic physician
4. Diego's doctor suggests he take Tums, an antacid, to reduce heartburn. Tums is an example of a(n)
   a. over-the-counter medication.
   b. prescription drug.
   c. homeopathic medication.
   d. nutraceutical.

LO 3 Complementary and Alternative Medicine (CAM)

5. CAM therapies focus on treating the mind and the whole body, which makes them part of a
   a. natural approach.
   b. psychological approach.
   c. holistic approach.
   d. gentle approach.
6. What type of medicine addresses imbalances of *qi*?
   a. Chiropractic medicine
   b. Ayurvedic medicine
   c. Traditional Chinese medicine
   d. Homeopathic medicine
7. Which of the following is a form of energy medicine?
   a. Alexander technique
   b. Psychoneuroimmunology
   c. Reiki
   d. Shiatsu

LO 4 Health Insurance

8. What mechanism used by private insurance companies requires that the subscriber pay a certain amount for health care before the insurance company will begin paying for services?
   a. Coinsurance
   b. Cost sharing
   c. Co-payments
   d. Deductibles
9. Deborah, 28, is a single parent who is unemployed. Her medical bills are paid by a federal health insurance program for the poor. This agency is
   a. an HMO.
   b. Social Security.
   c. Medicaid.
   d. Medicare.

LO 5 Issues Facing Today's Health Care System

10. Which of the following is a key provision of the ACA?
    a. Insurers are only required to cover major medical emergencies.
    b. Lifetime limits on benefits are allowed if costs exceed a set amount.
    c. Insurers are required to cover young adults on a parent's plan through age 21.
    d. Americans with preexisting conditions can't be denied coverage.

Answers to the Pop Quiz can be found on page A-1. If you answered a question incorrectly, review the section identified by the Learning Outcome. For even more study tools, visit MasteringHealth.

THINK ABOUT IT!

LO 1 Taking Responsibility for Your Health Care

1. List several conditions (resulting from illness or accident) for which you wouldn't need to seek medical help. When would you consider each condition to be bad enough to require medical attention? How would you decide where to go for treatment?

LO 2 Conventional Health Care

2. Describe your rights as a patient. Have you ever received treatment that violated these rights? If so, what action, if any, did you take?

LO 3 Complementary and Alternative Medicine (CAM)

3. What are some of the potential benefits and risks of CAM? Why do you think these practices and products are so popular?
4. What can you do to ensure that you are receiving accurate information regarding CAM treatments or medicines? Which U.S. government agency sponsors research into CAM?

ACCESS YOUR HEALTH ON THE INTERNET

Visit **MasteringHealth** for links to the websites and RSS feeds.

The following websites explore further topics and issues related to personal health.

Agency for Healthcare Research and Quality (AHRQ). AHRQ's website is a gateway to consumer health information. It provides links to sites that can address health care concerns and provide information on what questions to ask, what to look for, and what you should know when making critical decisions about personal care. **www.ahrq.gov**

Food and Drug Administration (FDA). The FDA provides news on the latest government-approved home health tests and other health-related products. **www.fda.gov**

PubMed. Find research abstracts—and increasingly entire studies—on health care topics of interest to you. This site is a service of the National Library of Medicine at the National Institutes of Health. **www.ncbi.nlm.nih.gov/pubmed**

National Committee for Quality Assurance (NCQA). The NCQA assesses and reports on the quality of managed care plans, including HMOs. **www.ncqa.org**

HealthCare.Gov. This site provides up-to-date information regarding the 2010 Patient Protection and Affordable Care Act, which mandates health insurance for previously uninsured Americans. **www.healthcare.gov**

National Center for Complementary and Alternative Medicine (NCCAM). A division of the National Institutes of Health, NCCAM is dedicated to providing the latest information and research on complementary and alternative practices. **http://nccam.nih.gov**

National Institutes of Health, Office of Dietary Supplements. This excellent resource includes access to a database of federally funded research projects pertaining to dietary supplements. **http://ods.od.nih.gov**

19 Preventing Violence and Abuse

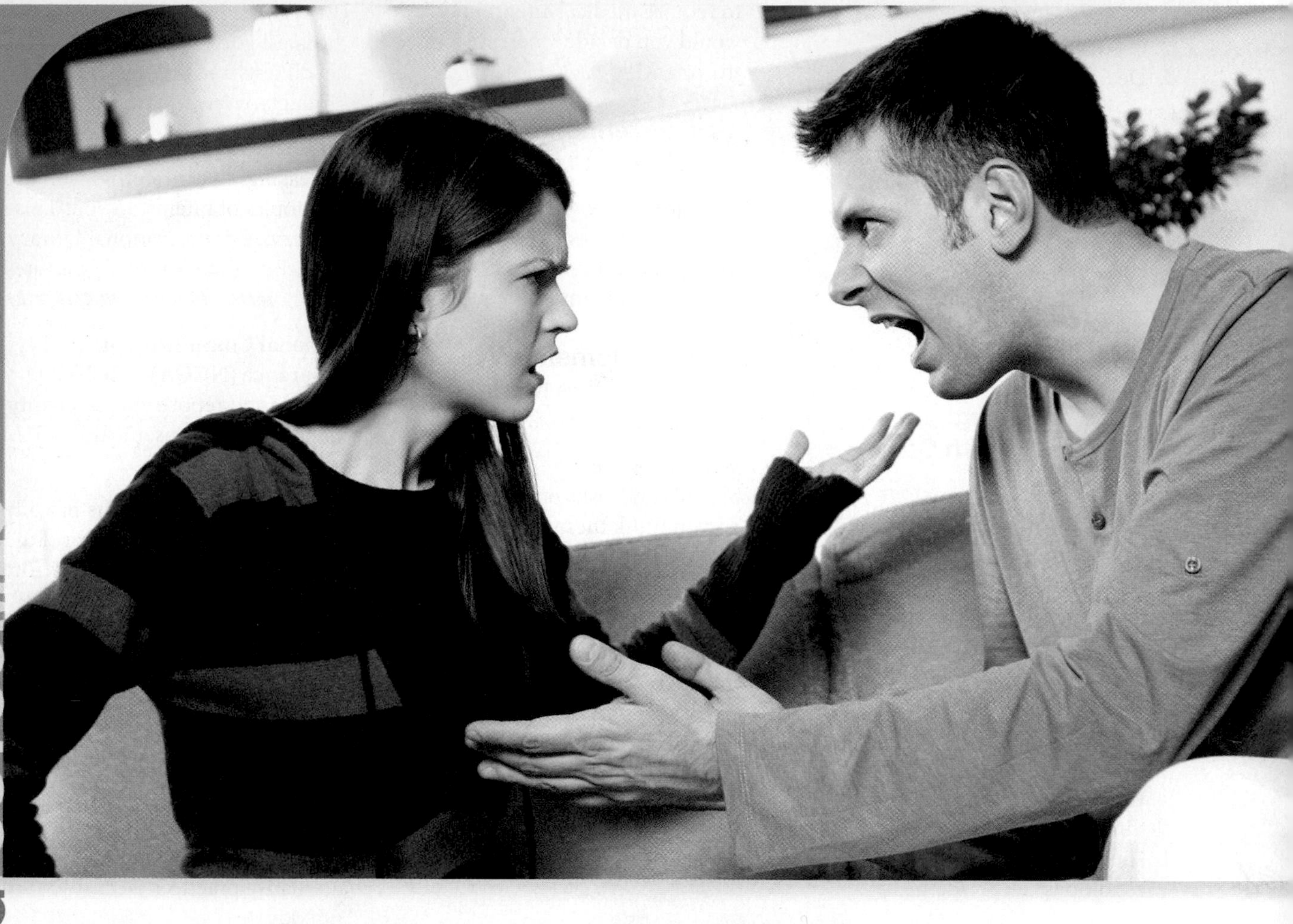

LEARNING OUTCOMES

1. Differentiate between intentional and unintentional injuries and discuss societal and personal factors that contribute to violence in American society and on college campuses.
2. List and explain factors that contribute to homicide, domestic violence, intimate partner violence, sexual victimization, and other intentional acts of violence.
3. Explain the prevalence and common causes of homicide, hate crimes, domestic violence, child abuse, sexual victimization, and other forms of interpersonal violence.
4. Describe factors that contribute to gang violence and to terrorist activities.
5. Articulate personal strategies for minimizing the risk of violence.
6. Explain potential strategies that campus leaders, law enforcement officials, and individuals can develop to prevent students from becoming victims.
7. Describe community-wide strategies for preventing violence.

Fear follows crime, and is its punishment.
—Voltaire, 1694–1778[1]

Violence is not a new phenomenon. In fact, throughout history violence has played a major role in human lives as they sought to dominate others or react to real or perceived threats. Today, national and international violence permeates the media. News coverage of war, terrorist acts, school shootings, interpersonal violence, and other crimes invade our homes and thoughts. In this environment, many people live in fear and feel increasingly frustrated by what seems to be an increasingly violent world. Some worry that they might become victims while walking down the street, going to concerts or athletic events, traveling internationally, or even sitting in classrooms. Are these fears justified? Is violence in the United States worse than ever? And to which kinds of violence are college students particularly vulnerable? What can we do to reduce our risk?

Before we can discuss the extent and nature of violence, it's important to understand what the word *violence* means. The World Health Organization (WHO) defines **violence** as "the intentional use of physical force or power, threatened or actual, against oneself, another person, or a group or community that results in or has a high likelihood of resulting in injury, death, psychological harm, maldevelopment or deprivation."[2] Today, most experts realize that emotional and psychological forms of violence can be as devastating as physical blows to the body.

The U.S. Public Health Service historically categorized violence resulting in injuries as either intentional or unintentional, based on the intent to cause harm. Today, experts recognize that intent is not always completely clear and that distinguishing cause and intent can be difficult. Typically, **intentional injuries**—those committed with intent to harm—include assaults, homicides, self-inflicted injuries, and suicides. **Unintentional injuries** are those committed without apparent intent to harm, such as motor vehicle crashes and other types of accidents. (See **Focus On: Reducing Your Risk of Unintentional Injury**.)

Intentional injury can be categorized into three major types: *interpersonal violence, collective violence,* and *self-directed violence,* although there is some degree of overlap among these groups.[3] Interpersonal violence and collective violence are discussed later in the chapter. (Self-directed violence is discussed in **Chapter 2**.)

Why do we focus attention on violence in an introductory health text? The answer is simple: Young adults are disproportionately affected by violence and injury. In fact, homicide and suicide are the second and third leading causes of death of young adults in the United States.[4] Globally, violence is a leading cause of death for young adults aged 15 to 44.[5] When intimate partner violence, assaults, harassment, and psychological abuse occur on campuses, there can be major threats to emotional, mental, and physical health.

LO 1 | VIOLENCE IN THE UNITED STATES

Differentiate between intentional and unintentional injuries and discuss societal and personal factors that contribute to violence in American society and on college campuses.

Violence has been a part of the American landscape since colonial times. However, it wasn't until the 1980s that the U.S. Public Health Service identified violence as a leading cause of death and disability and gave it *chronic disease status*, indicating that it was a pervasive threat to society. Violent crimes involve force or threat of force, and include four offenses: *murder and nonnegligent manslaughter, forcible rape, robbery,* and *aggravated assault.* Statistics from the Federal Bureau of Investigation (FBI) have shown that, after steadily increasing from 1973 to 2006, the rates of overall crime and certain types of violent crime have been slowly decreasing in recent years.[6] However, in October 2012, the news media caused confusion by running conflicting headlines about violence. Some outlets reported a 4 percent decline in violent crime, while others claimed there had been a huge jump in violent crime—*up 18 to 22 percent in 1 year.*[7]

violence Aggressive behaviors that produce injuries and can result in death.

intentional injuries Injury, death, or psychological harm inflicted with the intent to harm.

unintentional injuries Injury, death, or psychological harm caused unintentionally or without premeditation.

Which report was right? Actually, both! Historically, we use two measures for violence in the United States: the FBI's *Uniform Crime Reporting (UCR) Program* and the Bureau of Justice Statistics *National Crime Victimization Survey (NCVS).* While the FBI's UCR collects data on violent crimes involving force or threat *reported* to law enforcement agencies, the Bureau of Justice statistics collects detailed information on the frequency and nature of certain crimes twice a year through *surveys* of over 100,000 people.[8] In addition to using different methods, the Bureau of Justice Statistics does not track homicides or crimes against businesses. See **FIGURE 19.1** for the percent change of violent crimes reported in 2013 and **FIGURE 19.2** for the frequency of different types of crimes.

Violence trends are difficult to assess, but whether total rates of crime are up or down, there are huge disparities in crime rates based on race, sex, age, socioeconomic status, location, crime type, and other factors. Additionally, over 50 percent of violent victimizations are not reported to the police.[9] Rates of nonreporting are even higher for some offenses such as rape. If those nonreports suddenly become reported crimes, we might have a

HEAR IT! PODCASTS
Want a study podcast for this chapter? Download the podcast **Violence and Abuse: Creating Healthy Environments** available on MasteringHealth.™

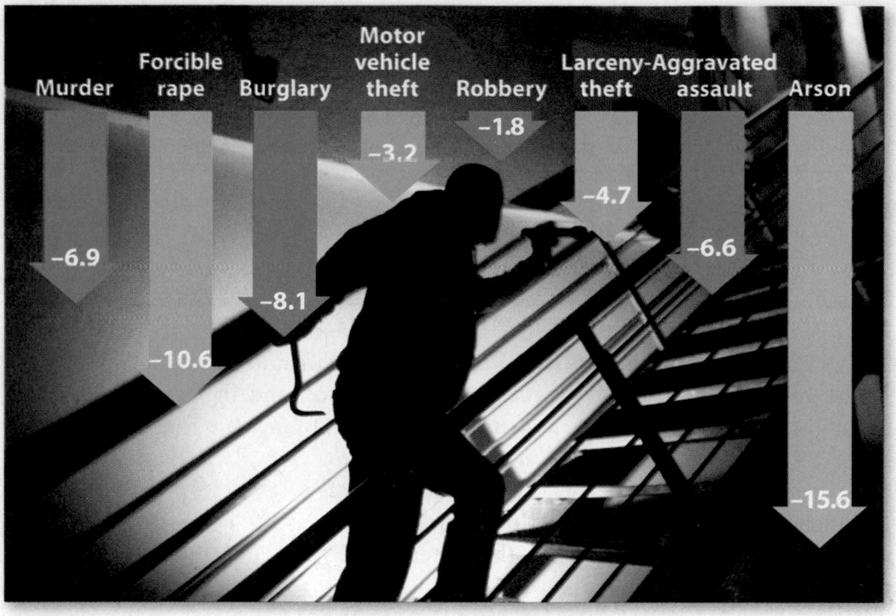
Murder
-6.9
Forcible rape
-10.6
Burglary
-8.1
Motor vehicle theft
-3.2
Robbery
-1.8
Larceny-theft
-4.7
Aggravated assault
-6.6
Arson
-15.6

FIGURE 19.1 **Changing Crime Rates** FBI statistics show reported violent crimes decreasing in early 2013. Although numbers of violent crimes reported to police have decreased in recent years, surveys of Americans indicate that overall crime rates have increased in the last 2 years, particularly as identity theft, burglaries, theft, simple assaults, and other crimes have increased.

Source: FBI Crime in the United States, 2013, "Preliminary Semiannual Uniform Crime Report, January–June 2013," May 2014, www.fbi.gov.

very different profile. What is clear is that after two decades of declines, overall rates of crime increased in 2011 and 2012, even though rates of FBI reported violent crimes appear to have declined. Also, overall crime rates are considerably lower (nearly one-third less) than they were in the early 1990s.[10]

Even if we have never been victims ourselves, we all are victimized by violent acts that cause us to be fearful; impinge on our liberty; and damage the reputation of our campus, city, or nation. If you don't go out for a walk or run at night, have to keep your doors and windows locked at all times, or avoid an international vacation because you are worried about being attacked, you are a victim of societal violence.

Violence on U.S. Campuses

Campus gun violence has made headline news far too many times in recent years. Whether at Virginia Tech University, where 32 people died in the deadliest mass shooting in U.S. history; at University of California–Santa Barbara, where 7 people were gunned down and many more injured in 2014; or at Sandy Hook Elementary, where 26 elementary school students and teachers were gunned down by a 20-year-old, campus shootings are on the rise, and no age group is immune. Tragedies like these have sparked dialogue and action across the nation, prompting increases in campus security and safety measures. Today, it would be hard to find a campus without some form of safety plan in place to prevent and respond to violent attacks. Campuses have stepped up to protect their students and their images, but many forms of campus violence continue to be hidden behind a veil of secrecy, with many victims reluctant to report assaults.

Relationship violence is one of the most prevalent problems on campus. In the most recent American College Health Association survey, 10.7 percent of women and 7.1 percent of men reported being emotionally abused in the past 12 months by a significant other. Almost 7 percent of women and 3.6 percent of men reported being stalked, and 2.3 percent of women and 2.2 percent of men reported being involved in a physically abusive relationship. Nearly 1 percent of men and over 2 percent of women reported being in a sexually abusive relationship.[11]

The statistics on reported campus violence represent only a glimpse of the big picture. It is believed that fewer than 25 percent of campus crimes in general are reported to *any* authority.[12] Even though over 20 percent of college women will be raped or sexually assaulted before they graduate, 95 percent of them never report these crimes.[13]

Why do so many never report these assaults? Typical reasons include concerns over privacy, fear of retaliation, embarrassment or shame, lack of support, perception that the crime was too minor or they were somehow at fault, or uncertainty that it was a crime. This is particularly true in situations where a victim knew her rapist or where drinking was involved and crime details were fuzzy, as well as instances of stalking and hazing. See the **Student Health Today** box for more on hazing.

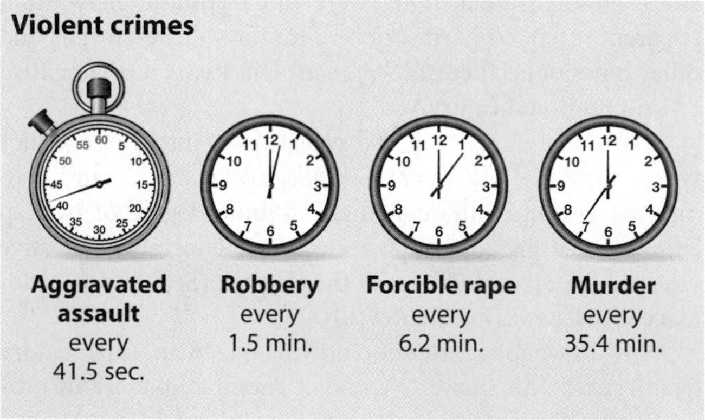
Violent crimes
Aggravated assault every 41.5 sec.
Robbery every 1.5 min.
Forcible rape every 6.2 min.
Murder every 35.4 min.

FIGURE 19.2 **Crime Clock** The crime clock represents the annual ratio of crime to fixed time intervals. The crime clock should not be taken to imply a regularity in the commission of crime.

Source: Adapted from Federal Bureau of Investigation, "Crime in the United States, 2012," Accessed June 2014, www.fbi.gov/about-us/cjis/ucr/crime-in-the-u.s/2012/crime-in-the-u.s.-2012/offenses-known-to-law-enforcement/crime-clock.

STUDENT HEALTH TODAY

HAZING

Over the Top and Dangerous for Many

We've all seen instances of hazing—those silly, humiliating things sorority or fraternity initiates, rookie team members, or new club recruits are asked to do. However, with the death of Robert Cameron, a 26-year-old drum major at Florida A&M in 2011, and a death of a fraternity member at Arizona State in 2012, the issue of hazing became headline news. Currently, hazing is considered a crime in 39 states. Most institutions have policies against hazing, but few students ever report it, and only when high-profile cases make it into the media do most of us pay attention.

Just what is hazing? Essentially it is "any activity expected of someone joining or participating in a group that humiliates, degrades, abuses, or endangers them regardless of a person's willingness to participate." Typically, it involves forcing students to consume excessive alcohol; dress in humiliating garb; undergo forced sleep deprivation; endure verbal abuse from group members; or physical abuse in the form of beatings, heat or cold exposure, or forced sexual acts. For those who are victimized and don't find their forced hazing humorous, psychological and physical damage can be serious.

According to a recent national study, 55 percent of college students involved in clubs, teams, and organizations experience hazing, and 47 percent of students come to college already having experienced hazing. Yet many students are unaware of its dangers or legal implications, and 9 out of 10 students who experience hazing in college do not realize they've been hazed.

In 95 percent of cases in which students identified their experience as hazing, they did not report the events to campus officials. There may be several reasons for this underreporting, but one reason seems to be that more students perceive positive rather than negative outcomes of hazing, for example, feeling a sense of accomplishment or belonging. Students also report that school administrators do little to prevent hazing beyond maintaining a "hazing is not tolerated" stance. If schools are to have an impact on the prevalence of hazing on their campuses, they need to implement broader prevention and intervention efforts and work to educate their campus community on the physical and legal perils of hazing.

Source: Adapted from E. Allan and M. Madden, *Hazing in View: College Students at Risk* (Orono, ME: National Collaborative for Hazing Research and Prevention, 2008), www.hazingstudy.org. Reprinted by permission of Elizabeth Allan. *Emory Law Journal*, "Am I My Brother's Keeper? Reforming Criminal Hazing Laws Based on Assumption of Care," 2014, www.law.emory.edu/fileadmin/journals/elj/63/63.4/Chamberlin.pdf.

LO 2 | FACTORS CONTRIBUTING TO VIOLENCE

List and explain factors that contribute to homicide, domestic violence, intimate partner violence, sexual victimization, and other intentional acts of violence.

No single criterion can explain what causes people to become violent offenders. Multiple negative factors appear to collide when violence erupts. Key risk factors include the following:[14]

- **Community contexts.** Environments where interactions with unsafe neighborhoods, schools, and workplaces predominate increase risks of exposure to drugs, guns, and gangs. Inadequately staffed police and social services add to risks.[15]
- **Societal factors.** Policies and programs that seek to remove inequality/disparity and discourage discrimination decrease risks; social and cultural norms that support male dominance over women and violence as a means of settling problems increase risks.[16]
- **Religious beliefs and differences.** Extreme religious beliefs can lead people to think that violence against others is justified.
- **Political differences.** Civil unrest and differences in political party affiliations and beliefs have historically been triggers for violent acts.
- **Breakdowns in the criminal justice system.** Overcrowded prisons, lenient sentences, early releases, and inadequate availability of mental health services can encourage repeat offenses and future violence.
- **Stress.** People who are in crisis or under stress are more apt to be highly reactive, striking out at others, displaying anger, or acting irrationally.[17]

What Makes Some Individuals Prone to Violence?

In addition to the broad, societal-based factors that contribute to crime, personal factors also can increase risks for violence. Emerging evidence suggests that the family and home environment in general may be the greatest contributor to eventual violent behavior among family members.[18] The following are among key predictors of aggressive behavior, including anger and irrational beliefs, genetic predispositions toward anger, and influences of coercive and contagious peers.[19]

Anger Anger is a well-known catalyst for violence. Anger typically occurs when there is a *triggering event* or a person has learned that acting out in angry ways can get him or her what he or she wants. Anger tends to be an active, attack-oriented emotion in which people feel powerful and in control for

SEE IT! VIDEOS

What would you do if you saw someone being bullied for being gay? Watch **Teen Bullied for Being Gay** available on MasteringHealth.™

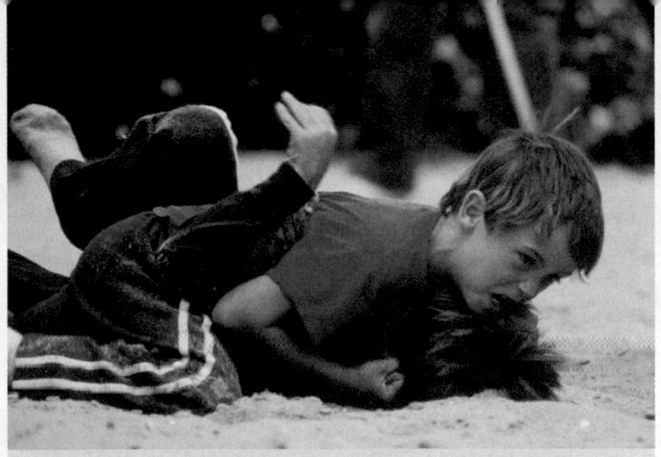

Most adults learn to control outbursts of anger in a rational manner. However, some people act out their aggressive tendencies in much the same way they did as children—with anger and violence that are a form of self-assertion or a response to frustration.

primary aggression Goal-directed, hostile self-assertion that is destructive in nature.

reactive aggression Hostile emotional reaction brought about by frustrating life experiences.

a short period.[20] Learning to assess the underlying "self-talk" or the beliefs that lead to anger is an important part of prevention. (For more suggestions on anger management, see **Chapter 3**, on stress.)

People who anger quickly often have a low tolerance for frustration and jump before thinking of the consequences. The cause may be genetic or physiological; there is evidence that some people are born with strong tendencies toward anger.[21] Typically, anger-prone people come from families that are disruptive, chaotic, and unskilled in emotional expression and where anger, domestic violence and abuse occur regularly.[22] Those who have been bullied in school may also be prone to react with violence in future situations.[23]

Aggressive behavior is often a key aspect of violent interactions. **Primary aggression** is goal-directed, hostile self-assertion that is destructive in nature. **Reactive aggression** is more often part of an emotional reaction brought about by frustrating life experiences. Whether aggression is reactive or primary, it is most likely to flare up in times of acute stress.

Substance Abuse Alcohol and drug abuse are often catalysts for violence at all levels of society, both nationally and internationally.[24]

- Consumption of alcohol precedes over half of all violent crimes and is a major factor in domestic violence at all levels.[25]
- Men who are heavier drinkers and more frequently drink to intoxication are the most likely to be perpetrators of sexual violence.[26]
- Research indicates higher rates of alcohol use and violence in some athlete populations when compared to nonathlete populations. Masculinity, antisocial norms, and violent social identity connected to certain sports may contribute to violence among athletes.[27]
- Alcohol abuse, particularly binge drinking, is associated with physical victimization among males and sexual victimization among females on campuses.[28]
- Numbers of suicide attempts and completions are highly correlated to drug and alcohol intake.[29]

WHY SHOULD I CARE?

The amount you drink tonight can directly affect your chances of becoming a victim of injury or assault. College students are particularly at risk for crimes committed under the influence of alcohol, including assault, rape, and intimate partner violence, but understanding the impact of alcohol in escalating potentially violent situations can help you stay out of harm's way.

How Much Impact Do the Media Have?

After massacres at Sandy Hook elementary, UC–Santa Barbara, and countless other incidents, people invariably ask *why* such things happen to innocent people. The media focus their attention squarely on what are widely perceived to be causes of violence: (1) too many high-capacity assault rifles and handguns, as well as a faulty system of monitoring who has access to guns; (2) inadequate mental health resources; and (3) a daily dose of media violence. Does a regular diet of heinous crimes and bloody massacres from video games, TV, and movies make people more likely to engage in murder and mayhem? Is there such a thing as becoming so desensitized to violence that life and death scenarios feel commonplace?

WHAT DO YOU THINK?

Do you think the media influence your behavior? If so, in what ways?

- Could that influence lead to your becoming violent? Why or why not?
- Are there instances in which curtailing violent viewing or restricting the nature and extent of violence and sex in the media is warranted? If so, under what circumstances?

Although the media are blamed for having a major role in the escalation of violence, this association has been challenged continuously. While early studies seemed to support a link between excessive exposure to violent media and subsequent violent behavior, much of this research has now been called into question for methodological problems such as poor measures of violence, biased subject selection, and sample size issues.[30] More recent studies of a possible relationship between media violence and violent acts seem to point a weak finger toward a connection between media violence and short-term aggression; however, the link to homicides and assaults is much less clear.[31] Other researchers continue to point out that exposure to violent videos has neither long- nor short-term effects of either positive or negative behaviors.[32] Although there appears to be an association between celebrity suicide depicted in the media and subsequent increases in fan suicides, it is no stronger than the increase in suicides that occur when a peer suicide occurs.[33]

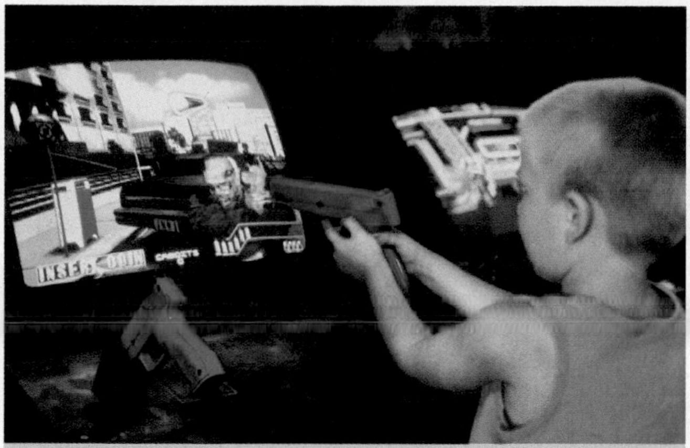

Arguably, Americans today—especially children—are exposed to more depictions of violence than ever before, but research has not shown a clear link between a person's exposure to violent media and his or her propensity to engage in violent acts.

Despite evidence to the contrary, some continue to believe that viewing violent media somehow numbs people to humanity, allows people to commit violence without empathy or regret, or even triggers violent events.[34] Several potential restrictions have been proposed to ban violent media for youth. The Supreme Court has steadfastly rejected them, echoing the claims that a relationship between violent acts and the consumption of violent media has not been proven through consistent, rigorous research. President Obama and several professional groups have called for more research to better understand the complex factors that prompt violence and what might be done to reduce risks.

Critics of previous studies point out that today's young people are exposed to more media violence—on the Internet and TV, and in movies and video games—than any previous generation, yet rates of violent crime among youth have fallen to 40-year lows.[35] Still, concerns have been raised about those who spend a disproportionate amount of time online instead of interacting in real-time, face-to-face communication. Will they miss the important lessons that come from talking with people in person and learning to get along with others? What will be the result of a generation that opts out of significant "live" interactions with their peers? When problems arise in face-to-face interactions and we can't click delete, will we know how to respond?

LO 3 | INTERPERSONAL VIOLENCE

Explain the prevalence and common causes of homicide, hate crimes, domestic violence, child abuse, sexual victimization, and other forms of interpersonal violence.

Interpersonal violence includes intentionally using "physical force or power, threatened or actual," to inflict violence against an individual that results in injury, death, or psychological harm.[36] Homicide, hate crimes, domestic violence, child abuse, elder abuse, and sexual victimization all fit into this category.

Homicide

Homicide, defined as murder or nonnegligent manslaughter (killing another human), is the fifteenth leading cause of death in the United States, the second leading cause of death for persons aged 15 to 24, and the fourth leading cause of death for those 25 to 44. Overall, it is among the top five leading causes of death for ages 1 to 44.[37] It accounts for over 16,000 premature deaths in the United States annually, the majority of which are caused by firearms.[38] Over half of all homicides occur among people who know one another. In two-thirds of these cases, the perpetrator and the victim are friends or acquaintances; in one-third, they are family members.[39]

Homicide rates reveal clear disparities across races and ages. Whereas overall homicide rates in the United States have fluctuated minimally and have even decreased in some populations, those involving young victims and perpetrators, particularly young black males, have surged. Based on the most recent data, homicide rates were nearly 52 per 100,000 for African American males aged 10 to 24, compared with almost 14 per 100,000 for Hispanic males and only 3 per 100,000 for white males.[40] The rates of homicide in the United States are higher than in many other developed nations, as shown in **TABLE 19.1**. See the **Health Headlines** box on the next page for a discussion of guns and violence.

interpersonal violence Violence inflicted against one individual by another or by a small group of others.

homicide Death that results from intent to injure or kill.

TABLE 19.1 | Per Capita Homicide Rates in Selected Nations

Rank	Country	Homicide Rate
1	Colombia	0.617847 per 1,000 people
2	South Africa	0.496008 per 1,000 people
5	Russia	0.201534 per 1,000 people
6	Mexico	0.130213 per 1,000 people
16	Zimbabwe	0.0749938 per 1,000 people
24	United States	0.042802 per 1,000 people
26	India	0.0344083 per 1,000 people
40	France	0.0173272 per 1,000 people
43	Australia	0.0150324 per 1,000 people
44	Canada	0.0149063 per 1,000 people
55	Ireland	0.00946215 per 1,000 people
00	Japan	0.00499933 per 1,000 people
61	Saudi Arabia	0.00397456 per 1,000 people

@ HEALTH HEADLINES

BRINGING THE GUN DEBATE TO CAMPUS

On average, each year in the United States 100,000 people are shot. Over 31,000 of them die, and of those who survive, many experience significant physical and emotional repercussions. Some facts about guns and gun violence include the following:

- Handguns are consistently responsible for more murders than any other type of weapon.
- Today, 35 percent of American homes have a gun on the premises, with nearly 300 million privately owned guns registered—and millions more that are unregistered and/or illegal.
- Firearms are the weapons most often used in attacks on American campuses. The most common reason for an incident is "related to an intimate relationship," followed by "retaliation for a specific action."
- The presence of a gun in the home triples the risk of a homicide in that location and increases suicide risk more than five times.

What factors contribute to gun deaths in the United States? Gun critics argue that large numbers of guns in the United States as well as relatively lax gun-control laws are the culprits. However, gun-rights advocates say that the problem lies not with guns, but with the people who own them, and point to countries such as Canada, with similar numbers of guns as in the United States, but with much lower gun-related crime rates.

High-profile shootings at schools and other public places have brought the gun debate to campuses. The National Conference on State Legislatures reported that 22 states ban carrying a concealed weapon on a college campus. But in 25 other states, the decision to ban or allow concealed carry weapons on campuses is made by each institution. Mississippi and Wisconsin passed some form of concealed weapon bills in 2011, and in 2012, so did 16 other states. Proponents argue that there is no evidence that legally allowing guns on campus would increase the risk of campus violence. What do you think?

- How would you feel about students in your classes having guns? Would it make you feel more or less safe? What about bringing a gun to a sporting event, party on campus, or other venue?
- Do you think making guns illegal on campus would prevent students from bringing guns to school? Why or why not?
- What factors should be taken into consideration as states vote on guns on campus?

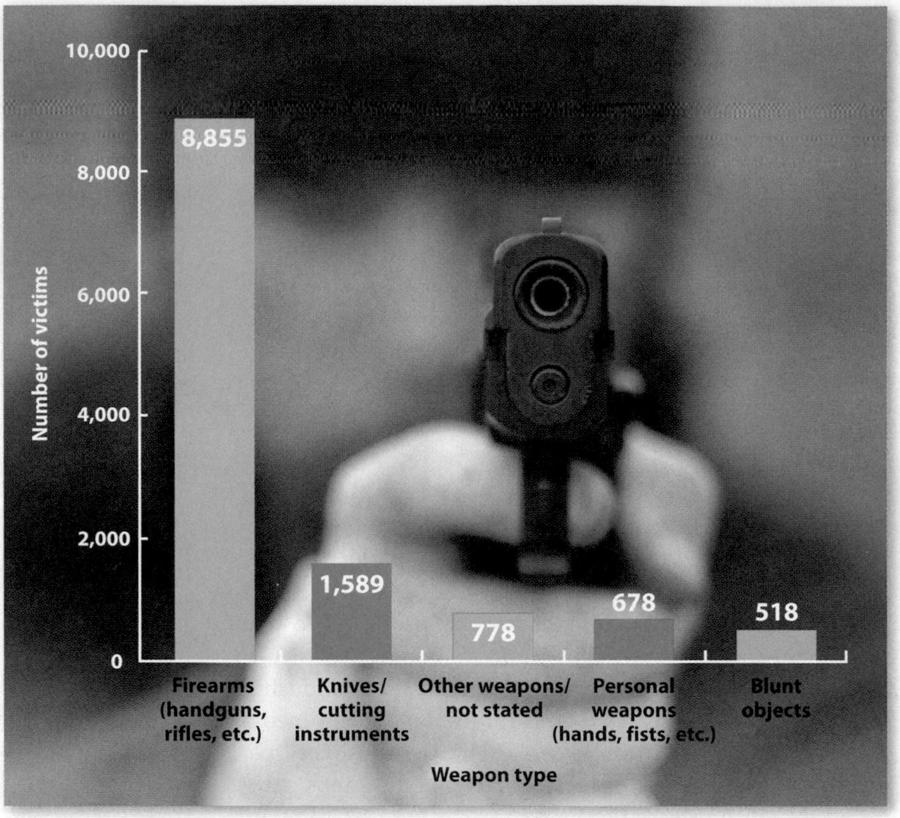

Homicide in the United States by Weapon Type, 2012

Sixty-seven percent of murders in the United States are committed using firearms, far outweighing all other weapons combined.

Source: Data from U.S. Department of Justice, Federal Bureau of Investigation, *Crime in the United States, 2012*, "Expanded Homicide Data," Table 8, www.fbi.gov.

Sources: D. Drysdale, W. Modzeleski, and A. Simons, *Campus Attacks: Targeted Violence Affecting Institutions of Higher Learning* (Washington DC: United States Secret Service, United States Department of Education, and the Federal Bureau of Investigation, 2010); National Conference of State Legislatures, "Guns on Campus: Overview," 2013, http://www.ncsl.org/research/education/guns-on-campus-overview.aspx; Brady Campaign to Prevent Gun Violence, "Facts: Gun Violence," Revised 2010, www.bradycampaign.org; S. Lewis, "Concealed Carry on Campus—Guns on Campus—College Campus Carry," CNN Report, 2011, www.campuscarry.com.

Hate and Bias-Motivated Crimes

A **hate crime** is a crime committed against a person, property, or group of people that is motivated by the offender's bias against a race, religion, disability, sexual orientation, or ethnicity. As a result of national efforts to promote understanding and appreciation of diversity, reports of hate crimes have declined to an all-time low of 5,790 reported incidents in 2012, according to the FBI[41] (**FIGURE 19.3**). Of these hate crimes, over 48 percent were a result of bias toward a particular race, nearly 20 percent were motivated by bias based on sexual orientation, 19 percent toward religion, 11.5 percent by ethnicity/national origin bias, and nearly 1.6 percent reflected bias toward disabilities. In 2012, *gender* and *gender identity* were added to hate crime statistics.[42]

In sharp contrast, when a representative sample of Americans completed the anonymous National Crime Victimization Survey, an estimated 294,000 violent and property hate crimes occurred in 2012![43] Fear of retaliation keeps many hate crimes hidden. While 60 percent of hate crimes may never be reported, only about one-fourth of those reported are reported by victims themselves.[44]

Bias-related crime, sometimes referred to as **ethnoviolence**, describes violence based on prejudice and discrimination among ethnic groups in the larger society. **Prejudice** is an irrational attitude of hostility directed against an individual, group, or race or the supposed characteristics of an individual, group, or race. **Discrimination** constitutes actions that deny equal treatment or opportunities to a group of people, often based on prejudice. Often prejudice and discrimination stem from a fear of change and a desire to blame others when forces such as the economy and crime seem out of control. Teaching tolerance, understanding, and respect for people from different backgrounds can reduce bias-related crimes.

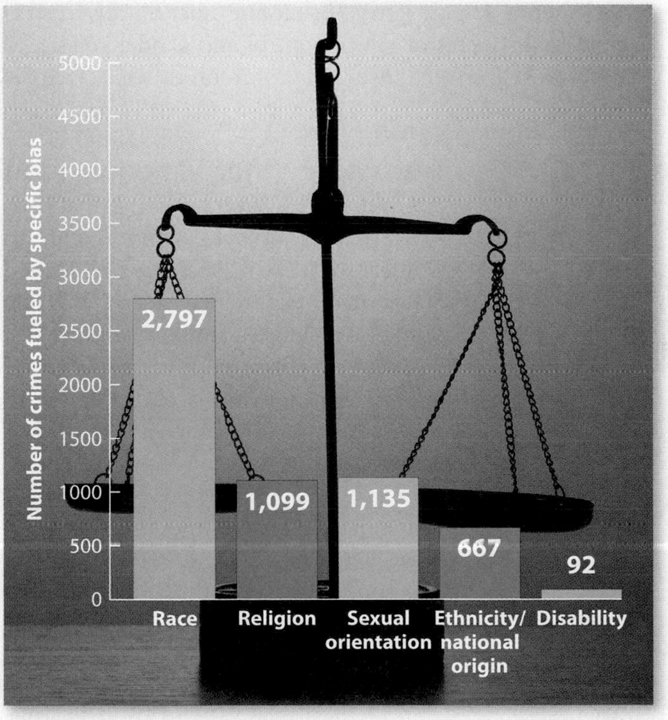

FIGURE 19.3 Bias-Motivated Crimes, Single-Bias Incidence, 2012

Source: Data from Federal Bureau of Investigation, "Hate Crime Statistics, 2012" Table 1, www.fbi.gov.

Common reasons given to explain bias-related and hate crimes include (1) *thrill seeking* by multiple offenders through a group attack; (2) *feeling threatened* that others will take their jobs or property or beset them in some way; (3) *retaliating* for some real or perceived insult or slight; and (4) *fearing the unknown or differences.* For other people, hate crimes are a part of their mission in life, either due to religious zeal, lack of understanding, or distorted moral beliefs.

Statistics on bias and hate crimes on campus are difficult to find, but increasing media attention has put these issues in the national spotlight. Campuses have responded to reports of hate crimes by offering courses that emphasize diversity, having zero tolerance for violations, training faculty appropriately, and developing policies that enforce punishment for hate crimes.

Domestic Violence

Domestic violence refers to the use of force to control and maintain power over another person in the home environment. It can occur between parent and child, between spouses or intimate partners, or between siblings or other family members. The violence may involve emotional abuse, verbal abuse, threats of physical harm, and physical violence ranging from slapping and shoving to beatings, rape, and homicide.

Intimate Partner Violence and Women

Intimate partner violence (IPV) describes physical, sexual, or psychological harm done by a current or former partner or spouse. This type of violence can occur among heterosexual or same-sex couples and does not require sexual intimacy. Over the course of a year, millions of women and men are victims of rape, physical and psychological abuse, stalking, and other offenses by an intimate partner. Homicide committed by a current or former intimate partner is the leading cause of death of pregnant women in the United States.[45] In addition, 74 percent of all murder-suicides in the United States involve an intimate partner.[46]

hate crime Crime targeted against a particular societal group and motivated by bias against that group.

ethnoviolence Violence directed at persons affiliated with a particular ethnic group.

prejudice A negative evaluation of an entire group of people that is typically based on unfavorable and often wrong ideas about the group.

discrimination Actions that deny equal treatment or opportunities to a group, often based on prejudice.

domestic violence The use of force to control and maintain power over another person in the home environment, including both actual harm and the threat of harm.

intimate partner violence (IPV) Describes physical, sexual, or psychological harm by a current or former partner or spouse.

Nearly half of all women and men in the United States have experienced psychological aggression by an intimate partner in their lifetime. This abuse can take the form of constant criticism, verbal attacks, displays of explosive anger meant to intimidate, and controlling behavior. Psychological abusers seek to intimidate and debase their partners, thereby gaining control over the partner and the relationship. Those who have experienced this violence are more likely to report depression, difficulty in intimate relationships, frequent headaches, chronic pain, difficulty with sleeping, activity limitations, poor physical health, irritable bowel syndrome, and other health problems.[47]

1 IN 3 WOMEN AND 1 IN 10 MEN

HAVE BEEN **VICTIMS** OF INTIMATE PARTNER VIOLENCE IN THE FORM OF RAPE, STALKING, OR PHYSICAL VIOLENCE IN THEIR LIFETIMES.

The Cycle of IPV and Battered Woman Syndrome Have you ever heard of a woman who is repeatedly beaten by her partner and wondered, "Why doesn't she just leave him?" There are many reasons some women find it difficult to break their ties with abusers. Some women, particularly those with small children, are financially dependent on their partners. Others fear retaliation against themselves or their children. Some hope the situation will change with time, and others stay because cultural or religious beliefs forbid divorce. Finally, some women still love the abusive partner and are concerned about what will happen to him if they leave.

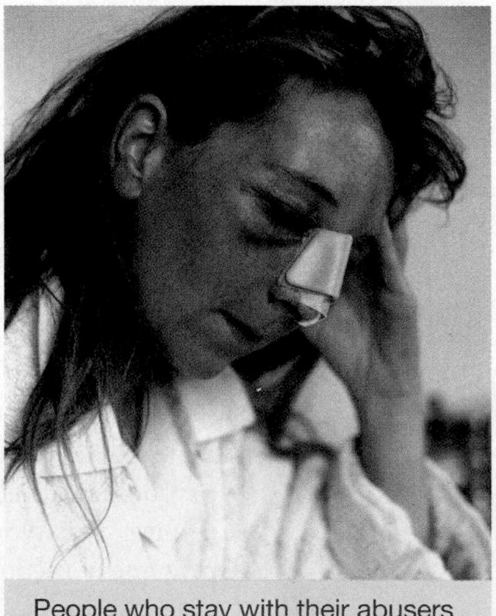
People who stay with their abusers may do so because they are dependent on the abuser, because they fear the abuser, or even because they love the abuser. In some cultures, women may not be free to leave an abusive relationship because of restrictive laws, religious beliefs, or social mores.

In the 1970s, psychologist Lenore Walker developed a theory called the *cycle of violence* that explained predictable, repetitive patterns of psychological and/or physical abuse that seemed to occur in abusive relationships. The cycle consisted of three major phases:[48]

1. **Tension building.** Prior to the overtly abusive act, tension building includes breakdowns in communication, anger, psychological aggression, growing tension, and fear.
2. **Incident of acute battering.** When the acute attack is over, he may respond with shock and denial about his own behavior or blame her for making him do it.
3. **Remorse/reconciliation.** During a "honeymoon" period, the batterer may be kind, loving, and apologetic, swearing that he will work to change his behavior.

Walker's initial work was criticized by some for its lack of scientific rigor and for what appeared to be a simplified approach to a complex problem. In her most recent book, *The Battered Woman Syndrome,* Walker's conclusions were based on improved quantitative analysis, reviews of recent research, and an extensive list of experts in the field of violence.[49] Today, *battered woman syndrome* is considered to be a subgrouping of post-traumatic stress disorder (PTSD). For a woman who gets caught in this cycle, it is often very hard to summon the resolution to extricate herself. Most need effective outside intervention.[50] Many experts believe that some of the same issues occur for battered men.

Causes of Domestic Violence and IPV There is no single reason that will explain abuse in relationships. Alcohol abuse is often associated with such violence, as are having a history of family violence and marital dissatisfaction. Numerous studies also point to differences in communication patterns between abusive and nonabusive relationships. Stress, mental health issues, economic uncertainty/frustration, jealousy, issues of power/control and gender roles, and issues with self-esteem are among common reasons given for IPV.[51]

Intimate Partner Violence: Men as Victims We may think that intimate partner violence happens only to women, but every year in the United States men experience nearly 830,000 domestic violence assaults by an intimate partner or spouse, male or female. In fact, gay men appear to be just as susceptible to male-perpetrated violence as are women in heterosexual relationships, and abuse of heterosexual men by their female partners is likely more common than statistics show. Between 1994 and 2010, about 1 in 5 victims of overall intimate partner violence were men. However, men's assaults tended to be less severe and less likely to end in fatality.[52]

Why don't men report abuse? Reasons include the following:

- A sense of humiliation and/or fear that no one will believe them
- Abuse that has reached the point that they believe they deserve bad treatment

- Belief that not hitting back is a sign of honor, strength, or masculinity
- Lack of awareness and support services for men in abusive relationships

Recognizing that a problem exists, communities across the nation are responding with education and awareness programs and resources such as support groups and counseling to help male victims protect themselves and make positive changes in their lives.

Child Abuse and Neglect

Children living in families in which domestic violence or sexual abuse occurs are at great risk for damage to personal health and well-being. **Child maltreatment** is defined as any act or series of acts of commission or omission by a parent or caregiver that results in harm, potential for harm, or threat of harm to a child.[53] **Child abuse** refers to *acts of commission,* which are deliberate or intentional words or actions that cause harm, potential harm, or threat of harm to a child. The abuse may be sexual, psychological, physical, or any combination of these. **Neglect** is an *act of omission,* meaning a failure to provide for a child's basic physical, emotional, or education needs or to protect a child from harm or potential harm. Failure to provide food, shelter, clothing, medical care, or supervision, or exposing a child to unnecessary environmental violence or threat are examples of neglect. Last year, over 75 percent of reported cases of maltreatment or abuse were for neglect, more than 15 percent for physical abuse, and nearly 10 percent for sexual abuse. Although exact figures for child abuse are difficult to obtain, in 2013 an estimated 3.8 million cases of child abuse were reported, involving the alleged maltreatment of approximately 6 million children.[54] **FIGURE 19.4** shows the rates of abuse among children in different age groups.

There is no single profile of a child abuser. Frequently, the perpetrator is a young adult in his or her mid-twenties without a high school diploma, living at or below the poverty level, depressed, socially isolated, with a poor self-image, and having difficulty coping with stressful situations. In many instances, the perpetrator has experienced violence and is frustrated by life.

It is important to remember that child abuse occurs at every socioeconomic level, across ethnic and cultural lines, within all religions, and at all levels of education. Not all violence against children is physical. Health can be severely affected by psychological violence—assaults on personality, character, competence, independence, or general dignity as a human being. Negative consequences of this kind of victimization can include depression, low self-esteem, and a pervasive fear of offending the abuser.

WHAT DO YOU THINK?

Why do you think rates of violence in the United States are so much higher than those of other developed nations, such as Great Britain and Japan?

- What do you think is the single greatest cause of violence?
- What could be done to reduce risk from this factor?

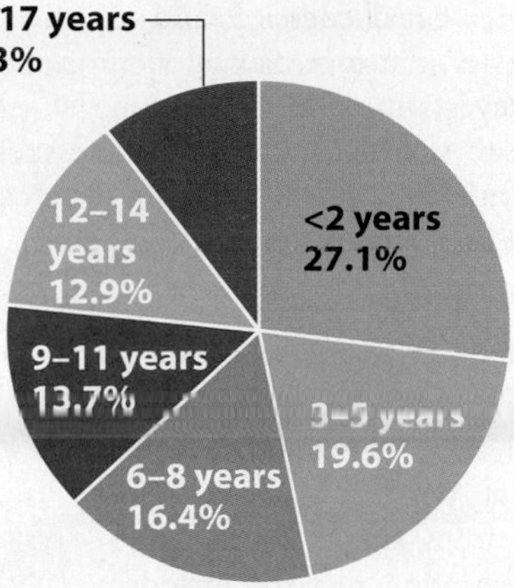

FIGURE 19.4
Child Abuse and Neglect Victims by Age, 2011

Source: U.S. Department of Health and Human Services, Administration on Children, Youth and Families, *Child Maltreatment 2011* (Washington, DC: U.S. Government Printing Office, 2012).

child maltreatment Any act or series of acts of commission or omission by a parent or caregiver that results in harm, potential for harm, or threat of harm to a child.

child abuse Deliberate, intentional words or actions that cause harm, potential for harm, or threat of harm to a child.

neglect Failure to provide a child's basic needs such as food, clothing, shelter, and medical care.

Elder Abuse

By 2030, the number of people in the United States over the age of 65 will exceed 71 million—nearly double their number in 2000. Each year, hundreds of thousands of adults over the age of 60 are abused, neglected, or financially exploited as they enter the later years of life, and these statistics are likely an underestimate.[55] Many victims fail to report abuse because they are embarrassed or because they don't want the abuser to get in trouble or retaliate by putting them in a nursing home or escalating the abuse. Some do not report due to feeling guilty because someone has to take care of them. Others suffer from dementia and may not be aware of the abuse. A variety of social services focus on protecting our seniors, just as we endeavor to protect other vulnerable populations.

Sexual Victimization

The term *sexual victimization* refers to any situation in which an individual is coerced or forced to comply with or endure another's sexual acts or overtures. It can run the gamut from harassment to stalking to assault and rape by perpetrators known or unknown to the victim. It can

SEE IT! VIDEOS

Should strangers step into prevent partner abuse? Watch **Will Anyone Confront Abusive Boyfriend?** available on MasteringHealth.™

even include sexual coercion and rape by spouses within the confines of marriage. Sexual victimization and violence can have devastating and far-reaching effects on people of any age. Fear, sexual avoidance, sleeplessness, anxiety, and depression are just a few of the long-term consequences for victims of sexual victimization.[56]

Sexual Assault and Rape **Sexual assault** is any act in which one person is sexually intimate with another person without that person's consent. This may range from simple touching to forceful penetration and may include, for example, ignoring indications that intimacy is not wanted, threatening force or other negative consequences, and actually using force. Although the exact prevalence of sexual violence is not known, a new survey sheds some light:[57]

- Bisexual women have the highest lifetime prevalence of rape by any perpetrator (46.1%).
- Heterosexual women have the second highest lifetime prevalence of rape (17.4 percent).
- Lesbians have the next highest lifetime prevalence of rape (13.1%).
- For a lifetime prevalence of sexual violence *other than rape*, the reported rates are 74 percent for bisexual women, 46.4 percent for lesbians, and 43.4 percent for heterosexual women,
- Rape percentages were too small to estimate for gay and bisexual men, and heterosexual men reported a lifetime prevalence of rape of less than 1 percent.
- For a lifetime prevalence of sexual violence other than rape, the reported rates are 47.4 percent for bisexual men, 40.2 percent for gay men and 20.8 percent for heterosexual men.
- Males were the perpetrators in rape 98.3 percent of the time for bisexual women and 99.1 percent of the time for heterosexual women.

WHY SHOULD I CARE?

You may be too young to be at risk for elder abuse, but your parents and grandparents could become victims—of domestic violence; abusive caregivers; financial fraud; or sexual, physical, or emotional abuse. If you're aware of this possibility, you may be able to help identify a problem and take steps to fix it.

Considered the most extreme form of sexual assault, **rape** is defined as penetration without the victim's consent. Incidents of rape generally fall into one of two types—aggravated or simple. An **aggravated rape** is any rape involving one or multiple attackers, strangers, weapons, or physical beatings. A **simple rape** is a rape perpetrated by one person, whom the victim knows, and does not involve a physical beating or use of a weapon. Most rapes are classified as simple rape, but that terminology should not be taken to mean that a simple rape is any less violent or criminal.

sexual assault Any act in which one person is sexually intimate with another without that person's consent.

rape Sexual penetration without the victim's consent.

aggravated rape Rape that involves one or multiple attackers, strangers, weapons, or physical beating.

simple rape Rape by one person, usually known to the victim, that does not involve physical beating or use of a weapon.

acquaintance rape Any rape in which the rapist is known to the victim (replaces the formerly used term *date rape*).

By most indicators, reported cases of rape appear to have declined in the United States since the early 1990s, even as reports of other forms of sexual assault have increased. This decline is thought to be due to shifts in public awareness and attitudes about rape, combined with tougher crime policies, major educational campaigns, and media attention. These changes enforce the idea that rape is a violent crime and should be treated as such. However, numerous sources indicate that rape is among one of the most underreported crimes, particularly on college campuses.[58]

Acquaintance Rape The terms *date rape* and *acquaintance rape* have been used interchangeably in the past. However, most experts now believe that the term *date rape* is inappropriate because it implies a consensual interaction in an arranged setting and may, in fact, minimize the crime of rape when it occurs. Today, **acquaintance rape** refers to any rape in which the rapist is known to the victim. Acquaintance rape is more common when drugs or alcohol have been consumed by the offender or victim, making the campus party environment a high-risk venue. Alcohol is frequently involved in rape, as are a growing number of rape-facilitating drugs such as Rohypnol and gamma-hydroxybutyrate (GHB).

OVER 20%

OF UNDERGRADUATE WOMEN HAVE BEEN **SEXUALLY ASSAULTED** ONE OR MORE TIMES DURING THEIR UNDERGRADUATE YEARS.

Rape on U.S. Campuses In 1992, Congress passed the Campus Sexual Assault Victim's Bill of Rights, known as the *Ramstad Act.* The act gave victims the right to call in off-campus authorities to investigate serious campus crimes and required universities to develop educational programs and notify students of available counseling. More recent provisions of the act specify notification procedures and options for victims, rights of victims and accused perpetrators, and consequences, including possible loss of federal support, if schools do not comply. It also asks campuses to conduct climate surveys, report rapes, and provide assessments of prevention activities to the U.S. Department of Education.[59]

With a flurry of national media exposure, President Obama has raised the issue of rape on campus to the level of a

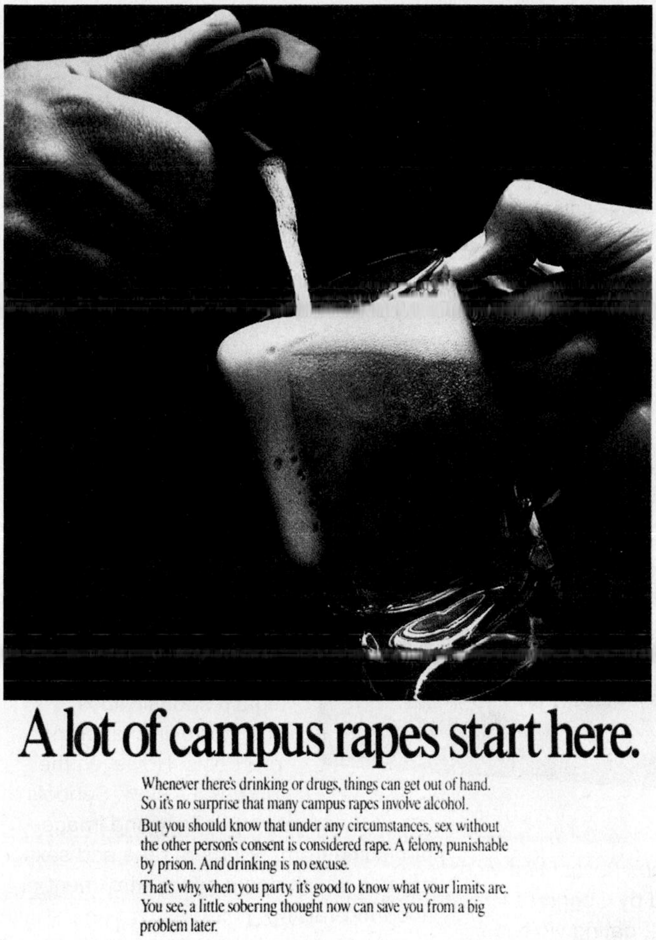

A lot of campus rapes start here.
Whenever there's drinking or drugs, things can get out of hand. So it's no surprise that many campus rapes involve alcohol.
But you should know that under any circumstances, sex without the other person's consent is considered rape. A felony, punishable by prison. And drinking is no excuse.
That's why, when you party, it's good to know what your limits are. You see, a little sobering thought now can save you from a big problem later.

Acquaintance rape is particularly common on college campuses, where alcohol and drug use can impair young people's judgment and self-control.

VIDEO TUTOR Acquaintance Rape on Campus

national crisis.[60] For more information, see the **Health Headlines** box on the next page on sexual assault on campus.

Marital Rape Although its legal definition varies within the United States, *marital rape* can be any unwanted intercourse or penetration (vaginal, anal, or oral) obtained by force, threat of force, or when the spouse is unable to consent. This problem has undoubtedly existed since the origin of marriage as a social institution, and it is noteworthy that marital rape did not become a crime in all 50 states until 1993.

78%

OF **SEXUAL VIOLENCE** INVOLVES AN OFFENDER WHO IS A FAMILY MEMBER, INTIMATE PARTNER, FRIEND, OR ACQUAINTANCE OF THE VICTIM.

Even more noteworthy is the fact that 30 states still allow exemptions from marital rape prosecution, meaning that the judicial system may treat it as a lesser crime.[61]

Although research in this area is scarce, it has been estimated that 10–14 percent of married women are raped by their husbands in the United States. About one-third of women report having had "unwanted sex" with their partner.[62] In general, women under the age of 25 and those from lower socioeconomic groups are at highest risk of marital rape. Internationally, women raised in cultures where male dominance is the norm and women are treated as property tend to have higher rates of forced sex within the confines of marriage. Women who are pregnant, ill, separated, or divorced have higher rates, as do women from homes where other forms of domestic violence are common and where there is a high rate of alcoholism or substance abuse.

Child Sexual Abuse Sexual abuse of children by adults or older children includes sexually suggestive conversations; inappropriate kissing; touching; petting; oral, anal, or vaginal intercourse; and other kinds of sexual interaction. Recent studies indicate that the rates of sexual abuse in children range from 3 to 32 percent of all children, with girls being at greater risk than young boys, even though young boys are abused in significant numbers.[63] Internationally, the prevalence of child sexual abuse ranges from 8 to 31 percent for girls and 3 to 17 percent for boys.[64]

The shroud of secrecy surrounding this problem makes it likely that the number of actual cases is grossly underestimated both in the United States and globally. Unfortunately, the programs taught in schools today, often with an emphasis on "stranger danger," may give children the false impression that they are more likely to be assaulted by a stranger. In reality, 90 percent of child sexual abuse victims know their perpetrator, with nearly 70 percent of children abused by family members, usually an adult male.[65]

People who were abused as children bear spiritual, psychological, and/or physical scars. Studies have shown that child sexual abuse has an impact on later life: Children who experience sexual abuse are at increased risk for anxiety disorders, depression, eating disorders, PTSD, and suicide attempts.[66] Youth who have been sexually abused are 25 percent more likely to experience teen pregnancy, 30 percent more likely to abuse their own children, and are much more likely to have problems with alcohol abuse or drug addiction.[67]

sexual harassment Any form of unwanted sexual attention related to any condition of employment, education, or performance evaluation.

Sexual Harassment **Sexual harassment** is defined as unwelcome sexual conduct that is related to any condition of employment or evaluation of student performance. Unwelcome sexual advances, requests for sexual favors, and other

HEALTH HEADLINES

SEXUAL ASSAULT *Changing the Culture of Silence?*

The reluctance to report sexual assault on campus and the difficulty of pursuing criminal proceedings in the campus environment can create turmoil in victims' lives while too rarely leading to punishment of offenders.

Responding to increased evidence of major issues and increased pressure to take action, President Obama formed a National Task Force to study sexual assault and make recommendations for change. Its report notes that over 20 percent of college students are sexually assaulted as undergraduates. As part of its recommendations, colleges are being asked to do the following:

- Identify the problem. Consider using mandatory anonymous surveys where experiences with unwanted sexual contact, sexual assault, rape, and sexual harassment are reported.
- Teach the definition of consent and the legal ramifications of any actions that are undertaken without clear consent.
- Effectively respond when there is a report.
- Increase transparency and improve enforcement.
- Teach "bystander education" to show students how to intervene in potentially harmful situations.

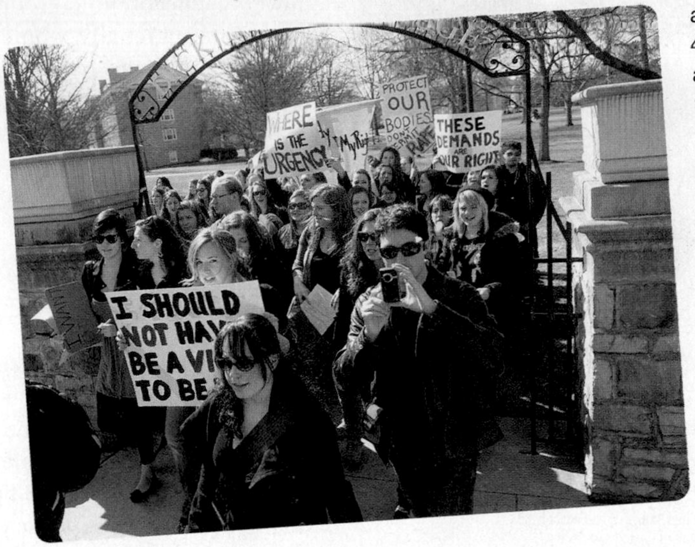

As part of the *Campus Sexual Violence Elimination Act*, passed by Congress last year, domestic violence, dating violence, sexual assault and stalking cases must be reported on annual campus crime reports. The White House is asking for measures that would levy harsh penalties for not taking strong action to prevent assaults.

Ironically, as campuses improve education/awareness, increase reporting, and call for zero tolerance, the number of reported forcible rapes and assaults has increased 49 percent between 2008 and 2012! It is likely that these increases are not real increases in events per se, but rather, an increased willingness of victims to come forward. Efforts are underway to change campus culture by educating students about their options, informing counselors and support staff of their legal responsibilities, and improving reporting protocols. However, the process is slow. Schools fear negative publicity and image tarnishing from reports of rape and sexual assault, which could affect enrollment and fund-raising.

Source: White House Task Force to Protect Students from Sexual Assault, *Not Alone: First Report of White House Task Force to Protect Students from Sexual Assault*, April 2014, www.whitehouse.gov/sites/default/files/docs/report_0.pdf.

verbal or physical conduct of a sexual nature constitute sexual harassment when:

- Submission to such conduct is made either explicitly or implicitly a term or condition of an individual's employment or education;
- Submission to or rejection of such conduct by an individual is used as the basis for employment or education-related decisions affecting such an individual; or
- Such conduct is sufficiently severe or pervasive that it has the effect, intended or unintended, of unreasonably interfering with an individual's work or academic performance because it has created an intimidating, hostile, or offensive environment and would have such an effect on a reasonable person of that individual's status.[68]

SEE IT! VIDEOS

Is there a hidden culture of sexual harassment on campuses across the country? Watch **Sexual Harassment on Campus** available on MasteringHealth.™

Commonly, people think of harassment as involving only faculty members or persons in power, where sex is used to exhibit control of a situation. However, peers can harass one another too. Sexual harassment may include unwanted touching; unwarranted sex-related comments or subtle pressure for sexual favors; deliberate or repeated humiliation or intimidation based on sex; and gratuitous comments, jokes, questions, or remarks about clothing or bodies, sexuality, or past sexual relationships.

Most schools and companies have sexual harassment policies in place, as well as procedures for dealing with harassment problems. If you feel you are being harassed, the most important thing you can do is be assertive:

- **Tell the harasser to stop.** Be clear and direct. Tell the person if it continues that you will report it. If the harassing is via phone or Internet, block the person.
- **Document the harassment.** Make a record of each incident. If the harassment becomes intolerable, a record of exactly what occurred (and when and where) will help

DID YOU **KNOW?**

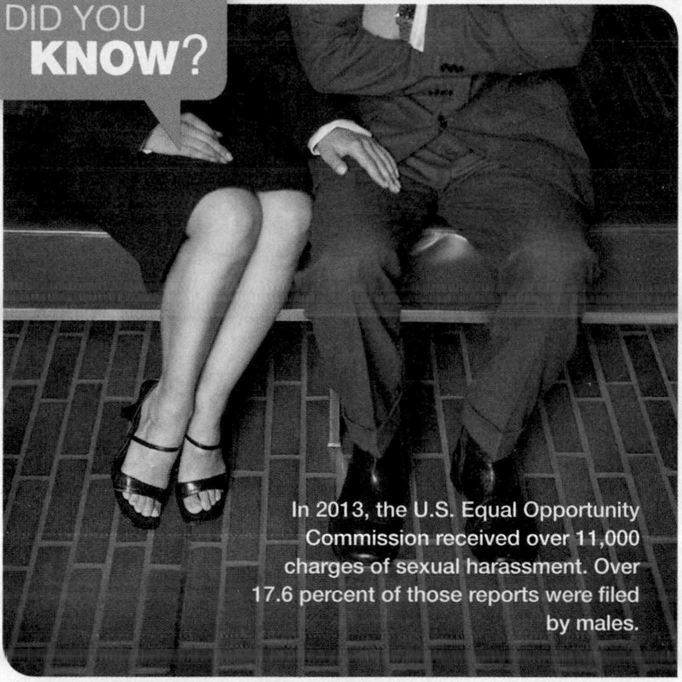

Source: Data are from U.S. Equal Employment Opportunity Commission, "Sexual Harassment," 2013, www.eeoc.gov.

make your case. Save copies of all communication from the harasser.

- **Try to make sure you aren't alone in the harasser's presence.** Witnesses to harassment can ensure appropriate validation of the event.
- **Complain to a higher authority.** Talk to legal authorities or your instructor, adviser, or counseling center psychologist about what happened.
- **Remember that you have not done anything wrong.** You will likely feel awful after being harassed (especially if you have to complain to superiors). However, feel proud that you are not keeping silent.

Stalking **Stalking** can be defined as a course of conduct directed at a specific person that would cause a reasonable person to feel fear. This may include repeated visual or physical proximity, nonconsensual written or verbal communication, and implied or explicit threats.[69] Stalking can even occur online (see the **Tech & Health** box on the next page for information on staying safe when using social networking sites).

More than 1 in 4 victims report being stalked through the use of some form of technology. The most common stalking behaviors included unwanted phone calls and messages, spreading rumors, spying on the victim, and showing up at the same places as the victim without having a reason to be there.[70] Millions of women and men are stalked annually in the United States, and the vast majority of stalkers are persons involved in relationship breakups or are other dating acquaintances; fewer than 10 percent of stalkers are strangers to their victims.[71] Adults between the ages of 18 and 24 experience the highest rates of stalking. Like sexual harassment, stalking is an underreported crime. Often students do not think a stalking incident is serious enough to report, or they worry that the police will not take it seriously.

WHAT DO **YOU** THINK?

What policies does your school have regarding consensual relationships between faculty members and students?

- Should consenting adults have the right to become intimate or interact socially, regardless of their positions within a school system or workplace?
- What are the potential dangers of such interactions? Are such interactions ever okay?

Social Contributors to Sexual Violence Sexual violence and intimate partner violence share common factors that increase the likelihood of their occurrence. Certain societal assumptions and traditions can promote sexual violence, including the following:

- **Trivialization.** Many people think that rape committed by a husband or intimate partner doesn't count as rape.
- **Blaming the victim.** In spite of efforts to combat this type of thinking, there is still the belief that a scantily clad woman "asks" for sexual advances.
- **Pressure to be macho.** Males are taught from a young age that showing emotions is a sign of weakness. This portrayal often depicts men as aggressive and predatory and females as passive targets.
- **Male socialization.** Many still believe ideas like "sowing wild oats" and "boys will be boys" are merely a normal part of male development. Women are often *objectified* (treated as sexual objects) in the media, which contributes to the idea that it's natural for men to be predatory.
- **Male misperceptions.** With media implying that sex is the focus of life, it's not surprising that some men believe that when a woman says no, she is really asking to be seduced. Later, these same men may be surprised when the woman says she was raped.
- **Situational factors.** Dates in which the male makes all the decisions, pays for everything, and generally controls the entire situation are more likely to end in an aggressive sexual scenario. Alcohol and other drugs increase the risk and severity of assaults.

LO 4 | COLLECTIVE VIOLENCE

Describe factors that contribute to gang violence and to terrorist activities.

Collective violence is violence perpetrated by groups against other groups and includes violent acts related to political, governmental, religious, cultural, or social clashes. Gang violence and terrorism are two forms of collective violence that have become major threats in recent years.

stalking Willful, repeated, and malicious following, harassing, or threatening of another person

collective violence Violence perpetrated by groups against other groups.

TECH & HEALTH | SOCIAL NETWORKING SAFETY

More than 15 million Americans became victims of identity fraud in 2012, the majority of which involved the fraudulent use of existing account information or the unauthorized use or attempted use of personal information to open a new account under a different identity. The largest groups of identity theft victims were aged 20 to 29, followed by those 30 to 39.

Very real threats to health, reputation, financial security, and future employment lie in wait for those who post indiscriminately and unwisely to the Web or who fail to do regular checks of their accounts and credit ratings. The following tips will help you remain safe and protect your identity when you express yourself online:

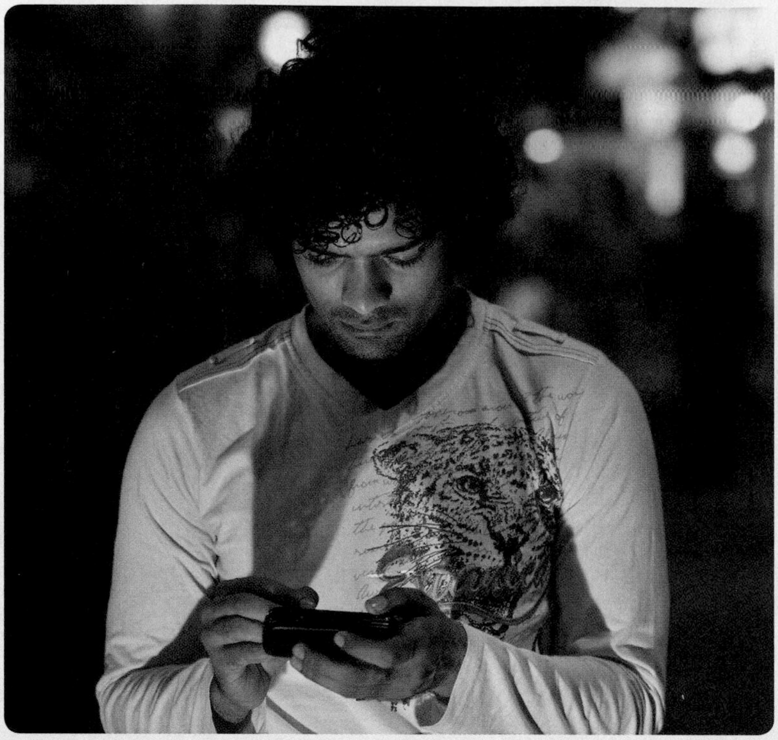

To stay safe online, think before you tweet.

- Don't post compromising pictures, videos, or other things that you wouldn't want your mother or coworkers to see.
- Never agree to meet a stranger in person whom you've met only online without bringing a trusted friend, or at the very least, notifying a close friend or family member of where you will be and when you will return. Choose a well-established, public place and only meet during daylight hours. Don't give your address or traceable phone numbers to the person you are meeting.
- Change your passwords and security questions often, and don't write them all down where someone can find them.
- Avoid banking or accessing sensitive personal financial documents when using public WiFi servers. Make sure your cell phone is not posting your location publically.
- Check for software updates for your devices and run full scans often.
- When you get rid of phones or other devices, make sure you wipe them of your data and close all accounts in your name.
- Never give credit card information or personal information over the phone.
- Invest in a shredder.
- Invest in high-quality locking mailboxes.
- Only leave small amounts of money in an overdraft fund. If you have a larger savings account, don't let it be a source of overdraft funds.

Source: NCVRW, *2012 NCVRW Resource Guide*, "Internet Victimization," February 2013, Available at www.ncjrs.gov.

Gang Violence

Gang violence is increasing in many regions of the world; U.S. communities face escalating threats from gang networks engaged in drug trafficking, sex trafficking, shootings, beatings, thefts, carjackings, and the killing of innocent victims caught in the crossfire. Currently, there are between 30,000 and 33,000 gangs in the United States, with membership in excess of 1.4 million.[72] Gangs are believed to be responsible for 48 percent of U.S. violent crime overall, and in some locations, as much as 90 percent.[73]

Why do young people join gangs? Often, gangs give members a sense of self-worth, companionship, security, and excitement. In other cases, gangs provide economic security through drug sales, prostitution, and other types of criminal activity. Friendships with delinquent peers, lack of parental monitoring, negative life events, and alcohol and drug use appear to increase risks for gang affiliation. Other risk factors include low self-esteem, academic problems, low socioeconomic status, alienation from family and society, a history of family violence, and living in gang-controlled neighborhoods.[74] It becomes difficult to leave gangs once youth become involved, but prevention strategies appear to offer promise.

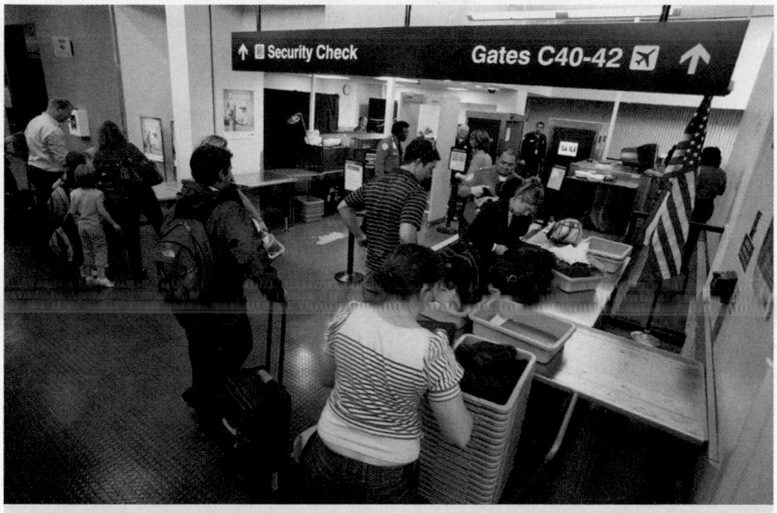

The threat of terrorism has affected many aspects of our daily lives.

Terrorism

Numerous terrorist attacks around the world reveal the vulnerability of all nations to domestic and international threats. Effects on our economy, travel restrictions, additional security measures, and military buildups are but a few of the examples of how terrorist threats have affected our lives. As defined in the U.S. Code of Federal Regulations, **terrorism** is the "unlawful use of force or violence against persons or property to intimidate or coerce a government, the civilian population, or any segment thereof in furtherance of political or social objectives."[75]

Over the past decade, the Centers for Disease Control and Prevention (CDC) established the *Emergency Preparedness and Response Division*. This group monitors potential public health problems, such as bioterrorism, chemical emergencies, radiation emergencies, mass casualties, national disaster, and severe weather; develops plans for mobilizing communities in case of emergency; and provides information about terrorist threats. In addition, the Department of Homeland Security works to prevent future attacks, and the FBI and other government agencies work to ensure citizens' health and safety.

LO 5 | MINIMIZE YOUR RISK OF BECOMING A VICTIM OF VIOLENCE

Articulate personal strategies for minimizing the risk of violence.

It is far better to prevent a violent act than to recover from it. Both individuals and communities can play important roles in preventing violence and intentional injuries.

Self-Defense against Personal Assault and Rape

Assault can occur no matter what preventive actions you take, but commonsense self-defense tactics can lower the risk. Self-defense is a process that includes increasing your awareness, developing self-protective skills, taking reasonable precautions, and having the judgment necessary to respond quickly to changing situations. It is important to know ways to avoid and extract yourself from potentially dangerous situations.

Most attacks by unknown assailants are planned in advance. Many rapists use certain ploys to initiate their attacks. Examples include asking for help, offering help, staging a deliberate "accident" such as bumping into you, or posing as a police officer or other authority figure. Sexual assault frequently begins with a casual, friendly conversation.

Trust your intuition. Be assertive and direct to someone who is getting out of line or becoming threatening—this may convince a would-be attacker to back off. Don't try to be nice, and don't fear making a scene. Use the following tips to let a potential assailant know that you are prepared to defend yourself:

terrorism Unlawful use of force or violence against persons or property to intimidate or coerce a government, civilian population, or any segment thereof in furtherance of political or social objectives.

- **Speak in a strong voice.** State, "Leave me alone!" rather than, "Will you please leave me alone?" Sound like you mean it.
- **Maintain eye contact.** This keeps you aware of the person's movements and conveys an aura of strength and confidence.
- **Stand up straight, act confident, and remain alert.** Walk as though you own the sidewalk.

If you are attacked, act immediately. Draw attention to yourself and your assailant. Scream "Fire!" as loudly as you can. Research has shown that passersby are much more likely to help if they hear the word *fire* rather than just a scream.

What to Do if Rape Occurs

If you are a rape victim, report the attack. This gives you a sense of control. Follow these steps:

- Call 9-1-1.
- Do not bathe, shower, douche, clean up, or touch anything the attacker may have touched.
- Save the clothes you were wearing, and do not launder them. They will be needed as evidence. Bring a clean change of clothes to the clinic or hospital.
- Contact the rape assistance hotline in your area, and ask for advice on counseling if you need additional help.

If a friend is raped, here's how you can help:

- Believe the rape victim Don't ask questions that may appear to imply that she/he is at fault in any way for the assault.
- Recognize that rape is a violent act and that the victim was not looking for this to happen.

- Encourage your friend to see a doctor immediately, because she may have medical needs but feel too embarrassed to seek help on her own. Offer to go with her.
- Encourage her to report the crime.
- Be understanding, and let her know you will be there for her.
- Recognize that this is an emotional recovery, and it may take time for her to bounce back.
- Encourage your friend to seek counseling.

LO 6 | CAMPUS-WIDE RESPONSES TO VIOLENCE

Explain potential strategies that campus leaders, law enforcement officials, and individuals can develop to prevent students from becoming victims.

Increasingly, campuses have become microcosms of the greater society, complete with the risks, hazards, and dangers that people face in the world. Many college administrators have been proactive in establishing violence-prevention policies, programs, and services. Campuses have begun to take a careful look at the aspects of campus culture that promote and tolerate violent acts.

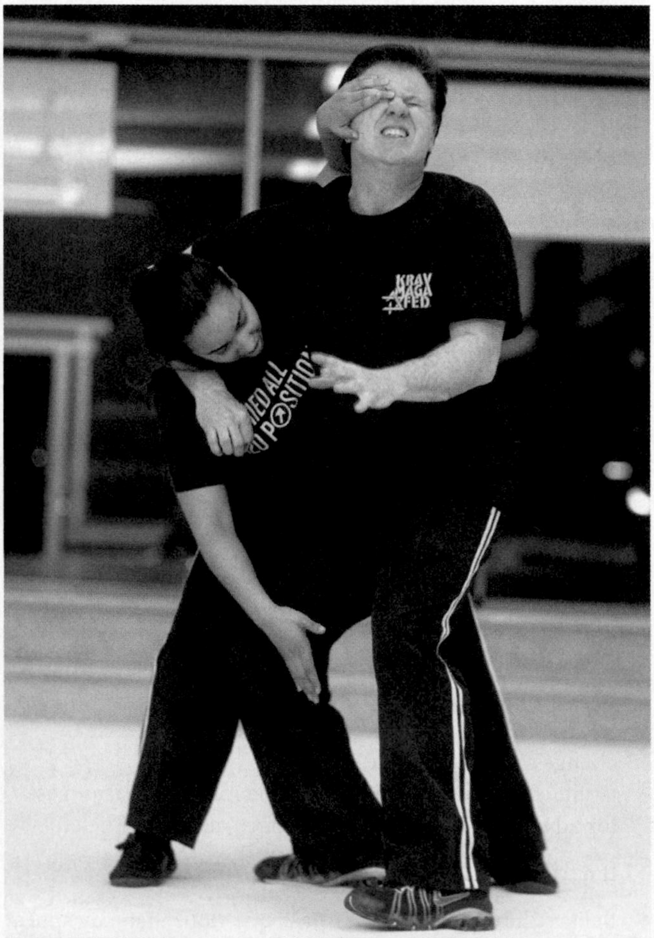

College campuses often offer safety workshops and self-defense classes to arm students with the physical and mental skills that may help them repel or deter an assailant.

Prevention and Early Response Efforts

Campuses are conducting emergency response drills and reviewing the effectiveness of emergency messaging systems, including mobile phone alert systems. The REVERSE 9-1-1 system uses database and geographic information system (GIS) mapping technologies to notify campus police and community members in the event of problems, and other systems allow administrators to send out alerts in text, voice, e-mail, or instant message format. Some schools program the phone numbers, photographs, and basic student information for all incoming first-year students into a university security system so that in the event of a threat, students need only hit a button on their phones, whereupon campus police will be notified and tracking devices will pinpoint their location.

Changes in the Campus Environment

There are many changes that can be made to the campus environment to improve safety. Campus lighting, parking lot security, emergency call boxes, removal of overgrown shrubbery, and stepped-up security are increasingly on the radar of campus safety personnel. Buildings can be designed with better lighting and enhanced security features, and security cameras can be installed in hallways, classrooms, and public places. Safe rides can be provided for students who have consumed too much alcohol, and health promotion programs can step up their violence prevention efforts through seminars on acquaintance rape, sexual assault, harassment, and other topics.

Campus Law Enforcement

Campus law enforcement has changed over the years by increasing both its numbers and its authority to prosecute student offenders. In fact, many campuses now hire state troopers or local law enforcement officers to deal with campus issues rather than maintain a separate police staff.

Coping in the Event of Campus Violence

Although schools have worked tirelessly to prevent violence, it can and does still occur. In its aftermath, some may find it difficult to remain on campus, as it represents a place of violation and lack of safety; others may experience problems with concentration, studying, and other daily activities. Although there is no "fix" for these traumatic events, several strategies can be helpful. First, members of the campus community should be allowed to mourn. Memorial services and acknowledgment of grief, fear, anger, and other emotions are critical to healing. Second, students, faculty, and staff should

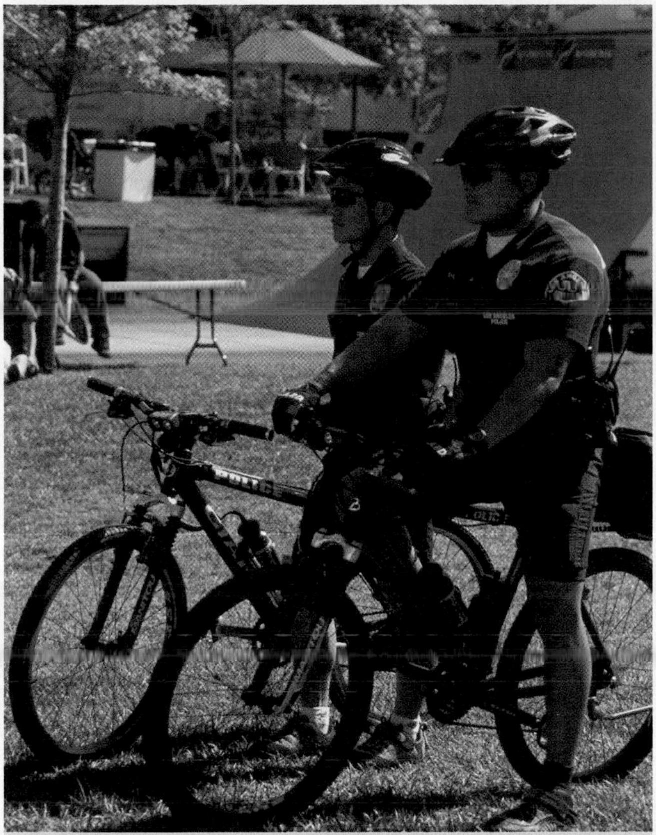

Presence and visibility of campus law enforcement have increased recently.

be involved in planning to prevent future problems—it can help to impart a feeling of control. Third, students should seek out support groups, therapists who specialize in treating PTSD, and trusted family members or friends if they need to talk and work through their feelings. Journaling or writing about feelings can also help.

LO 7 | COMMUNITY STRATEGIES FOR PREVENTING VIOLENCE

Describe community-wide strategies for preventing violence.

There are many steps you can take to ensure your personal safety (see the **Skills for Behavior Change** box); however, it is also necessary to address the issues of violence and safety at a community level. Strategies recommended by the CDC's injury response initiatives include the following:

- Inoculate children against violence in the home. Teaching youth principles of respect and responsibility are fundamental to the health and well-being of future generations.
- Develop policies and laws that prevent violence. Enforce laws so offenders know you mean business in your settings.
- Develop skills-based educational programs that teach the basics of interpersonal communication, elements of healthy relationships, anger management, conflict resolution,

SKILLS FOR BEHAVIOR CHANGE

STAY SAFE ON ALL FRONTS

Follow these tips to protect yourself from assault.

OUTSIDE ALONE

- Carry a cell phone and keep it turned on, but stay off it. Be aware of what is happening around you. Don't walk to your car in a dark parking lot while chatting to others. Stay alert.
- If you are being followed, don't go home. Head for a location where there are other people. If you decide to run, run fast and scream loudly to attract attention.
- Vary your routes. Stay close to other people.
- Park in lighted areas; avoid dark areas where someone could hide.
- Carry pepper spray or other deterrents. Consider using your campus escort service.
- Tell others where you are going and when you expect to be back.

IN YOUR CAR

- Lock your doors. Do not open your doors or windows to strangers.
- If someone hits your car, drive to the nearest gas station or other public place if you are able. Call the police or road service for help, and stay in your car until help arrives.
- If a car appears to be following you, do not drive home. Drive to the nearest police station.

IN YOUR HOME

- Install dead bolts on all doors and locks on all windows. Make sure the locks work, and don't leave a spare key outside.
- Lock doors when at home, even during the day. Close blinds and drapes whenever you are away and in the evening when you are home.
- Rent apartments that require a security code or clearance to gain entry, and avoid easily accessible apartments, such as first-floor units. When you move into a new residence, pay a locksmith to change the keys and locks.
- Don't let repair people in without asking for identification, and have someone else with you when repairs are being made.
- Keep a cell phone near your bed and call 9-1-1 in emergencies. Buy phones that have E911 locators so that emergency personnel can find you even when you can't respond or don't know where you are.
- If you return home to find your residence has been broken into, don't enter. Call the police. If you encounter an intruder, it is better to give up money or valuables than to resist.

appropriate assertiveness, stress management, and other health-based behaviors.

- Involve families, schools, community programs, athletics, music, faith-based organizations, and other community groups in providing experiences that help young people to develop self-esteem and self-efficacy.
- Promote tolerance and acceptance and establish and enforce policies that forbid discrimination. Offer diversity training and mandate involvement.
- Improve community services focused on family planning, mental health services, day care and respite care, and alcohol and substance abuse prevention.
- Make sure walking trails, parking lots, and other public areas are well lit, unobstructed, and patrolled regularly to reduce threats.
- Improve community-based support and treatment for victims and ensure that individuals have choices available when trying to stop violence in their lives.

STUDY PLAN

Customize your study plan—and master your health!—in the Study Area of **MasteringHealth.**

ASSESS **YOURSELF**

How often are you at risk of being a victim of violence? Want to find out? Take the **Are You at Risk for Violence?** assessment available on MasteringHealth.™

Need help creating a plan? Follow the strategies in the **Your Plan for Change** box for short- and long-term improvements to your health.

YOUR PLAN FOR **CHANGE**

The **ASSESS YOURSELF** activity gave you the chance to consider symptoms of abuse in your relationships and signs of unsafe behavior in other realms of your life. Now that you are aware of these signs and symptoms, you can work on changing behaviors to reduce your risk.

TODAY, YOU CAN:

- ☐ Pay attention as you walk your normal route around campus: Is it well lit? Do you walk in areas that receive little foot traffic? Are there emergency phone boxes along the way? Does campus security patrol the area? If part of your route seems unsafe, look around for alternate routes. Vary your route when possible.
- ☐ Look at your residence's safety features. If you notice any potential safety hazards, report them to your landlord or campus residential life administrator right away.

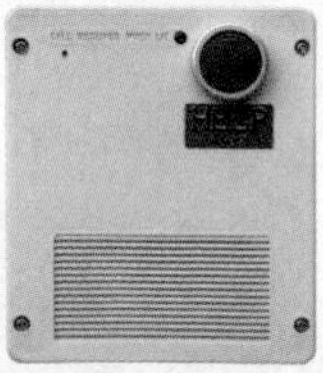

WITHIN THE NEXT 2 WEEKS, YOU CAN:

- ☐ Speak up when you hear comments that belittle or demean others. Let people know you don't like that kind of talk and why it bothers you.
- ☐ If you are worried about potentially abusive behavior in a partner or a friend's partner, visit the campus counseling center and ask about resources on campus or in your community that can be of help. Consider talking to a counselor about your concerns or sitting in on a support group.
- ☐ The next time you go out to a party or bar, decide ahead of time on the number of drinks you will have, arrange with a friend to monitor each other's behavior, and be sure you have a reliable, safe way of getting home. If you see your friend drinking too much, ask him/her to leave with you.

BY THE END OF THE SEMESTER, YOU CAN:

- ☐ Sign up for a self-defense or violence prevention class or workshop.
- ☐ Get involved in an on-campus or community group dedicated to promoting safety. You might want to attend a meeting of an antiviolence group, join in a Take Back the Night rally, or volunteer at a local rape crisis center or battered women's shelter.

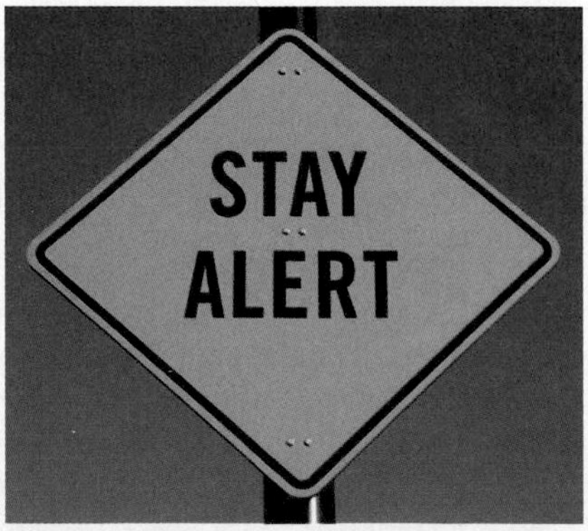

CHAPTER REVIEW

To hear an MP3 Tutor Session, scan here or visit the Study Area in **MasteringHealth**.

LO 1 Violence in the United States

- Violence affects everyone in society—from the direct victims, to children and families who witness it, to those who modify their behaviors because they are fearful.

LO 2 Factors Contributing to Violence

- Factors that lead to violence include poverty or economic difficulties, unemployment, parental and family influences, cultural beliefs, discrimination or oppression, religious or political differences, breakdowns in the criminal justice system, and stress. Mental health problems, anger, and substance abuse can contribute to violence and aggression.

LO 3 Interpersonal Violence

- Interpersonal violence includes homicide, domestic violence, child abuse, elder abuse, and sexual victimization. Each of these causes significant emotional, social, and physical risks to health.

LO 4 Collective Violence

- Forms of collective violence, including gang violence and terrorism, result in fear, anxiety, and issues of discrimination.

LO 5 Minimize Your Risk of Becoming a Victim of Violence

- Individual strategies to reduce the risk of becoming a victim of violence include the following: Recognize how to protect yourself and your friends; know where to turn for help; and have honest, straightforward dialogue about sexual matters in dating situations. Alcohol moderation is another key factor in reducing your risks.

LO 6 Campus-wide Responses to Violence

- With increasing reports of violence on campus, national attention has sharply focused what we can do to change a culture of violence. New recommendations by the White House are designed to encourage campuses to report, respond, engage, and support victims of violence and prevent violent assaults.

LO 7 Community Strategies to Prevent Violence

- Preventing violence is a public health priority that involves community activism, prioritizing mental and emotional health, and providing skills training in anger management, stress management, conflict resolution, and other key coping skills. Policies and procedures designed to increase security and enforce penalties are key to success.

POP QUIZ

Visit **MasteringHealth** to personalize your study plan with Chapter Review Quizzes and Dynamic Study Modules.

LO 1 Violence in the United States

1. ________ is an example of an *intentional injury*.
   a. A car accident
   b. Murder
   c. Accidental drowning
   d. Road rage

LO 2 Factors Contributing to Violence

2. An emotional reaction brought about by frustrating life experience is called
   a. reactive aggression.
   b. primary aggression.
   c. secondary aggression.
   d. tertiary aggression.

LO 3 Interpersonal Violence

3. When Jane began a new job with all male coworkers, her supervisor told her that he enjoyed having an attractive woman in the workplace, and he winked at her. His comment constitutes
   a. poor judgment, but not a problem if Jane likes compliments.
   b. sexual assault.
   c. sexual harassment.
   d. sexual battering.
4. In a sociology class, some students were discussing sexual assault. One student commented that some women dress too provocatively. The assumption this student made is
   a. minimization.
   b. trivialization.
   c. blaming the victim.
   d. "boys will be boys."
5. Which of the following statements is *correct*?
   a. In 8 out of 10 homicides, the victim is male.
   b. The majority of all sexual assaults against women are by men who the women barely know or don't know at all.
   c. "Date rape" is the appropriate ("politically correct") label for a rape by a person the woman knows well.
   d. A new White House report and recommendations on campus violence make sexual assault a federal offense.
6. Jack beats his wife Melissa "to teach her a lesson." Afterward, he denies attacking her. This illustrates which phase of the cycle of violence?
   a. Acute battering
   b. Fear/depression
   c. Remorse/reconciliation
   d. Tension building

LO 4 Collective Violence

7. Which of the following is an example of collective violence?
   a. Sexual assault
   b. Homicide
   c. Domestic violence
   d. Terrorism

LO 5 Minimize Your Risk of Becoming a Victim of Violence

8. Which of the following is recommended in the case of rape?
   a. Wait 24 hours before seeing a doctor.
   b. Call 9-1-1 immediately.
   c. Wash clothes the attacker touched.
   d. Shower immediately.

LO 6 Campus-wide Responses to Violence

9. Which of the following is *true* regarding responses to violence on campus?
   a. "Bystander" education is one of the new strategies for helping prevent a sexual assault.
   b. Most sexual assault programs should focus their money/effort on women only because they are the ones most likely to be victims.
   c. E-mail alerts and campus lockdowns are not effective ways of preventing a possible violent attack on campus.
   d. In the aftermath of media attention and White House reports designed to curb sexual violence, campus reports of violence have dropped dramatically.

LO 7 Community Strategies to Preventing Violence

10. Which of the following is a tip to protect yourself from assault?
    a. If a car is following you, drive home, go in, and lock your doors.
    b. If you get home and find your residence has been broken into, go inside, assess damages, and call the police.
    c. Talk or text on your phone when you're outside alone to look busy.
    d. If you're going somewhere alone, tell others where you are going and when you expect to be back.

Answers to the Pop Quiz can be found on page A-1. If you answered a question incorrectly, review the section identified by the Learning Outcome. For even more study tools, visit MasteringHealth.

THINK ABOUT IT!

LO 1 Violence in the United States

1. What forms of violence do you think are most significant or prevalent in the United States today? Why? What programs/policies are in effect on your campus to prevent violent attacks? Would you know what to do if a campus lockdown occurred?

LO 2 Factors Contributing to Violence

2. Why do some people develop into violent or abusive adults and others become pacifists or peaceful adults? What key factors influence violent offenders to be violent?

LO 3 Interpersonal Violence

3. Have you known anyone personally who has been sexually assaulted on campus? What actions were taken to help him or her cope with the assault? What campus services, if any, were used?

LO 4 Collective Violence

4. Have you been affected by acts of terrorism or gang violence? What strategies can you take to discourage collective violence, as an individual and as a community?

LO 5 Minimize Your Risk of Becoming a Victim of Violence

5. What are some everyday decisions you can make to minimize your risk of becoming a victim of violence? How can you be a good friend to someone who has become a victim of violence?

LO 6 Campus-wide Responses to Violence

6. Is your campus safe? What steps has your campus administration and community taken to reduce levels of campus-wide violence?

LO 7 Community Strategies to Preventing Violence

7. What actions need to be taken to stem the tide of violence in the United States at the individual level? At the community level? In schools? On college campuses? Nationally?

ACCESS YOUR HEALTH ON THE INTERNET

Visit **MasteringHealth** for links to the websites and RSS feeds.

The following websites explore further topics and issues related to personal health.

Not Alone. This site houses the report of the White House Task Force to Protect Students from Sexual Assault and recommendations for reporting, responding, and preventing future assaults. Detailed recommendations and action plans. **www.whitehouse.gov/sites/default/files/docs/report_0.pdf**

Communities against Violence Network. This site provides an extensive, searchable database for information about violence against women, with articles about everything from domestic violence to legal information and statistics. **www.cavnet.com**

Men Can Stop Rape. Practical suggestions for men interested in helping to protect women from sexual predators and assault are provided on this site. **www.mencanstoprape.org**

National Center for Injury Prevention and Control. The Web-based Injury Statistics Query and Reporting System (WISQARS) database of this CDC section provides statistics and information on fatal and nonfatal injuries, both intentional and unintentional. **www.cdc.gov/injury**

National Sexual Violence Resource Center. This is an excellent resource for victims of sexual violence. **www.nsvrc.org**

FOCUS ON

Reducing Your Risk of Unintentional Injury

Taking simple precautions, such as wearing a safety belt when you are in a car and using appropriate caution and common sense in all your activities, can go a long way in keeping you safe and injury free.

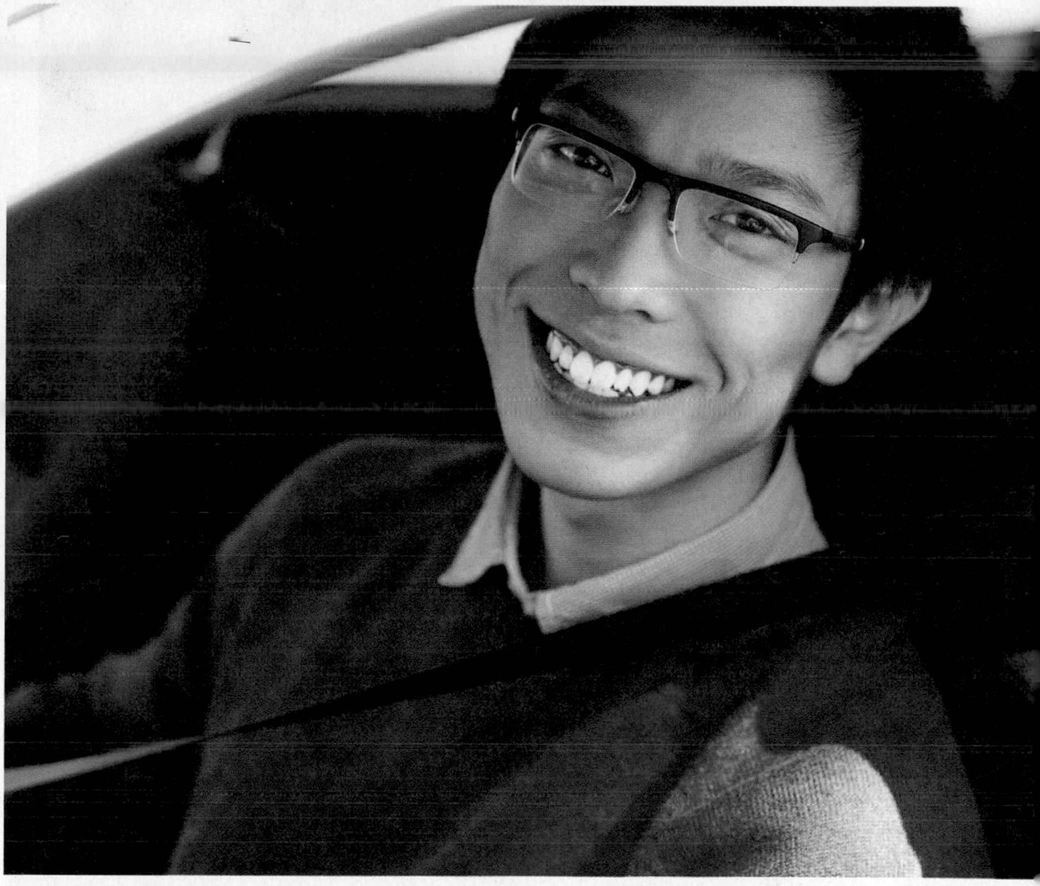

LEARNING OUTCOMES

1 Discuss factors that contribute to motor vehicle accidents and how to reduce their occurrence.

2 Explain safety guidelines for recreational activities that are particularly prone to cause injury.

3 Discuss injuries that occur in the home and what you can do to prevent them.

4 Describe work-related injuries and what you can do to prevent them.

5 Identify which natural disasters affect different regions of the U.S., and explain ways to prepare for and respond to natural disasters.

When Matt planned his birthday trip for spring break, he never thought he'd be spending part of the day in a hospital room. After drinking for several hours at the cantina on the beach, he and his friends started back to their hotel to continue the party by the swimming pool. They had all been drinking heavily, and they were in a celebratory mood when two of Matt's friends picked him up and threw him into the water, shouting, "Happy Birthday!" When he hit the water, Matt started thrashing, but he was too drunk to understand what was happening or figure out what to do. All he knew was an all-consuming panic as he inhaled the water. Then he passed out. Fortunately, another hotel patron sitting by the pool recognized what his friends were too intoxicated to realize: Matt was drowning. She jumped into the water and pulled Matt's limp body to the edge, screaming to his friends, "Dial 9-1-1!" Then she started cardiopulmonary resuscitation (CPR). As the ambulance arrived, Matt regained consciousness, but even hours later, in his hospital room, he had no memory of what had really happened to him.

Drowning is just one of many unintentional injuries in which alcohol commonly plays a role. Alcohol reduces your ability to stay alert, to maintain an awareness of your surroundings, and to make good decisions. Other factors—such as drowsiness, distraction, and failing to take sensible precautions—increase your risk of injury for similar reasons. In fact, although the term **unintentional injury** might sound academic, most health professionals shy away from the more familiar term *accidental injury* because it implies that these injuries occur without individuals having any control over their situation. As we saw with Matt's near-drowning, "accidents" often occur as a consequence of people's poor choices. Car "accidents," for example, often occur because the driver was speeding; distracted by cell phone use or another activity; or impaired by substance abuse, sleep deprivation, or other circumstances.

How big a problem is unintentional injury? Among Americans age 1 through 44, unintentional injuries are the leading cause of death, killing nearly 45,000 people in the prime of life.[1] In fact, unintentional injuries are responsible for almost 30 percent of all deaths in this age group.[2] Until recently, motor vehicle accidents (MVAs) were responsible for the greatest number of unintentional injury deaths each year. However, unintentional drug overdose has recently overtaken MVAs as the number one cause.[3] Other mechanisms responsible for significant mortality each year include falls, chokings, drownings, and fires.

16,451

AMERICANS DIED IN 2010 AFTER TAKING AN UNINTENTIONAL OVERDOSE OF A **PRESCRIPTION DRUG**.

In this chapter, we'll discuss the most common unintentional injuries, beginning with motor vehicle crashes, which are the leading cause of death among teens and adults through age 27.[4] For each injury type, we'll identify steps you can take to reduce your risk as well as strategies for managing an injury situation should one occur.

unintentional injury Any injury committed or sustained without intent of harm.

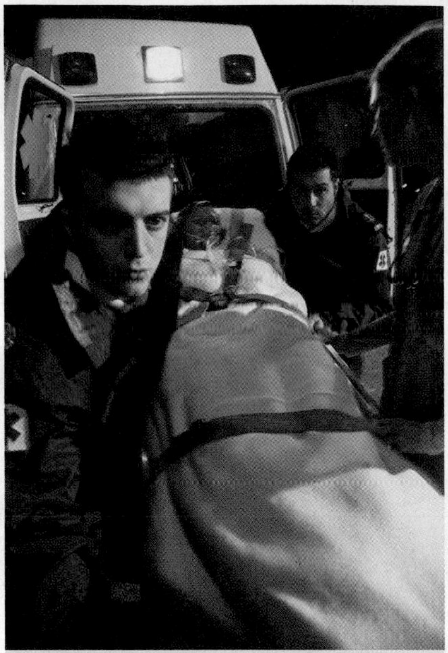

Unintentional injuries killed over 127,792 Americans in 2012. That's 350 people a day. Most strategies for preventing unintentional injuries focus on changing something about the person, the environment, or the circumstances that put people in harm's way.

Source: Centers for Disease Control and Prevention, "Fatal Injury Reports, National and Regional, 1999–2012," 2013, http://webappa.cdc.gov/sasweb/ncipc/mortrate10_us.html.

LO 1 | ARE YOU AT RISK ON THE ROAD?

Discuss factors that contribute to motor vehicle accidents and how to reduce their occurrence.

In 2012, over 33,500 Americans of all ages died in the over 5.6 million motor vehicle accidents reported by police.[5] That's an average of 92 people every day. What factors contribute to MVAs? And how can you reduce your risk?

Your Choices Affect Motor Vehicle Safety

In the blink of an eye, your actions could transform your vehicle from a pleasant mode of transportation into a deadly weapon. Factors within your control—distracted driving, impaired driving, speeding, and vehicle safety issues such as failure to wear your seat belt—contribute to the great majority of MVAs.[6]

Distracted Driving

Four types of activities constitute distracted driving: looking at something other than the road, hearing something not related to driving, manipulating something other than the steering wheel, and thinking about something other than driving.[7] In 2012, over 3,300 Americans died and over 420,000 were injured in distraction-affected crashes.[8]

Although there's no conclusive evidence identifying the forms of distraction most likely to contribute to MVAs, the behaviors of greatest concern are texting and talking on a cell phone. Overall, 31 percent of U.S. drivers age 18 to 64 report texting while driving, and 69 percent report that they talk on their cell phone while driving.[9] How do these behaviors contribute to MVAs? In 2012, 3,328 Americans died in MVAs involving distracted drivers, representing nearly 10 percent of all MVA fatalities.[10] Texting is particularly deadly: Highway safety experts estimate that the average time a person's eyes are off the road while texting is about 5 seconds. At 55 mph, that's the equivalent of driving the length of a football field blindfolded.[11] Given these statistics, it's no wonder that laws regulating cell phone use while driving have been passed in several states: At this time, 43 states ban text-messaging for all drivers, and 12 states ban all handheld cell phone use of any kind.[12]

Other common distractions for drivers include manipulating handheld music and Internet devices; adjusting CD players, the radio, or the mirror; and eating. Engaging in manual tasks like these triples your risk of getting into a crash.[13] The next time you're tempted to text, make a call, or even swat an insect while driving, don't do it. Pull over. Handle the distraction. Then rejoin the traffic when you're ready to give it your full attention.

Impaired Driving

In 2012, over 10,300 people in the United States died in MVAs that involved an alcohol-impaired driver. This represents an average of one such death every 51 minutes. Viewed another way, 31

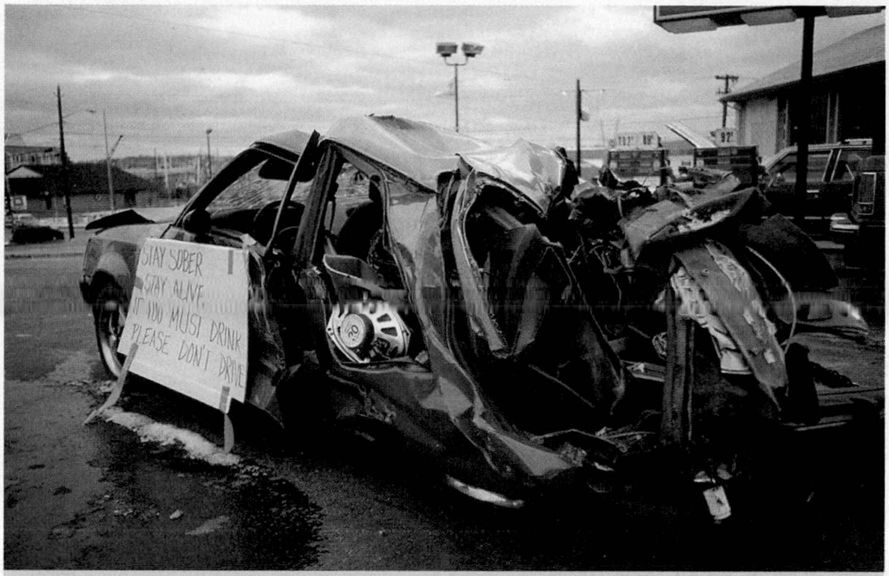

Driving under the influence of alcohol greatly increases the risk of being involved in a motor vehicle crash. Of all drivers between the ages of 21 and 24 involved in fatal crashes, nearly 1 out of 3 was legally drunk.

Source: NHTSA, "Traffic Safety Facts 2012 Data: Alcohol-Impaired Driving," DOT HS 811 870, December 2013, www-nrd.nhtsa.dot.gov/Pubs/811870.pdf.

percent of all MVA fatalities are due to alcohol impairment.[14] If you think these deaths occur mainly among teens, think again: The age group with the highest percentage of alcohol-impaired drivers involved in fatal crashes is that of people age 21 through 24.[15]

95%

OF COLLEGE STUDENTS SURVEYED REPORTED THAT THEY MOSTLY OR ALWAYS WEAR A **SEAT BELT** WHEN DRIVING OR RIDING IN A CAR.

Although alcohol is the primary cause of impairment while driving, other substances and situations are also responsible. For example, use of drugs other than alcohol, including marijuana, cocaine, and prescription medications, is an increasing problem among young adult drivers and is a significant cause of MVA injury and death.[16] In one study, 18 percent of fatally injured drivers tested positive for at least one illicit, prescription or over-the-counter drug.[17] Drowsiness can impair driving, too; many researchers contend that driving while sleep deprived is as dangerous as driving drunk. Drowsy driving causes an estimated 5,000–6,000 fatal MVAs each year.[18]

Both public health and law enforcement agencies are cooperating on several measures to keep impaired drivers off the road. These include the following:

- Promotion of community-based designated driver programs, including measures such as public funding of "safe rides" for people who have been drinking and training restaurant and bar staff to enforce drink limits and recognize and deny alcohol to impaired customers
- Strict enforcement of existing laws defining impaired driving and the legal drinking age
- Implementation of measures to prevent repeat offenses by anyone previously convicted of driving while impaired, whether due to alcohol or other drugs or to drowsiness: mandatory alcohol or other drug abuse treatment; installation of ignition interlock systems that prevent vehicle operation by anyone with a blood alcohol concentration above a specified safe level; revoking the driver's license.

SEE IT! VIDEOS

Are you at risk of falling asleep at the wheel? Watch **Dozing and Driving: 1 in 24 Asleep at Wheel** available on MasteringHealth.™

Speeding

Driver surveys suggest that many people speed because they don't perceive it as dangerous; they believe that traffic laws are overly restrictive and don't apply to them. But every day, 25–30 Americans die in speed-related car crashes; in 2012, speeding was a factor in 30 percent of all MVA fatalities, resulting in over 10,200 deaths.[19]

Vehicle Safety Issues

Wearing a safety belt cuts your risk of death or serious injury in a crash by almost half.[20] In 2012, 52 percent of the passenger vehicle occupants killed in traffic crashes were unrestrained.[21]

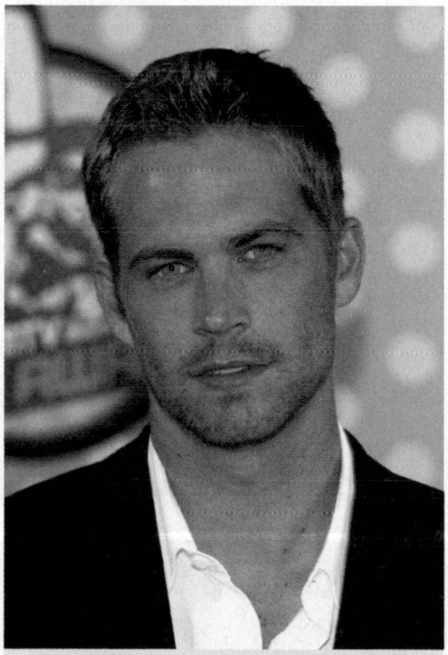

In November 2013 actor Paul Walker was killed when the Porsche driven by his friend Roger Rodas hit an electricity pole and a tree. Both men died within seconds of impact. Official police reports estimated that Rodas had been driving at a speed of more than 90 mph in a 45 mph zone.

Buckle up, and insist any passengers do the same. If you're transporting an infant or child in your vehicle, follow state laws governing use and location of age-appropriate safety seats.

Vehicles can include many safety features, from air bags to stability control. Unfortunately, people who don't have the financial resources to drive vehicles with all of the state-of-the-art features—and that group often includes college students—are at increased risk during MVAs. Still, the next time you're planning to purchase a car, new or used, look for the following features recommended by the Insurance Institute for Highway Safety:

1. Does the car have front air bags? Side air bags? Remember, air bags do not eliminate the need for everyone to wear safety belts.
2. Does the car have antilock brakes? Traction and electronic stability control? Each of these features can mean the difference between life, injury, or death.
3. Does the car have impact-absorbing crumple zones?
4. Are there strengthened passenger compartment side walls?
5. Is there a strong roof support? (The center doorpost on four-door models gives you an extra roof pillar.)

Another factor in MVA safety is the size of the vehicles involved. All cars sold in the United States must meet U.S. Department of Transportation standards for crashworthiness, no matter their size. However, in 2012 there were nearly four times as many deaths per vehicle among minicars as compared to very large cars, and 23 of the top 26 cars with the lowest rates of driver deaths were midsize or larger.[22] Many college students drive minicars because they are more affordable and use less gas, but the laws of physics make such cars more dangerous.

Motorcyclists Face Unique Risks

Per vehicle mile traveled, motorcyclists are about 26 times more likely than passenger car occupants to die in an MVA, and 5 times more likely to be injured. In 2012, this translated into over 4,900 motorcyclist deaths and 93,000 injuries.[23]

The National Highway Traffic Safety Administration (NHTSA) estimates that helmets saved the lives of 1,699 motorcyclists in 2012. If all motorcyclists had worn helmets, an additional 781 lives would have been saved.[24] Although the benefits of helmets and protective clothing are well established, only 19 states have full helmet requirements for anyone riding a motorcycle.[25] To find out what your state requirements are, go to www.iihs.org/iihs/topics/laws/helmetuse.

Practice Risk-Management Driving Techniques

Although you can't control what other drivers are doing, you can reduce your risk of injury in an MVA by practicing risk-management driving techniques. These include the following:

- Don't use electronic devices while driving. Avoid talking on a cell phone while driving, even if the phone is hands free.
- Don't drink and drive—take a taxi or arrange for someone to be the designated driver.
- Don't drive when tired, highly emotional, or highly stressed.
- Never tailgate. The rear bumper of the car ahead of you should be at least 3 seconds worth of distance away, making stopping safely possible. Increase the distance when visibility is reduced, speed is increased, or roads are slick.
- Scan the road ahead of you and to both sides.
- Drive with your low-beam headlights on, *day and night,* to make your car more visible to other drivers.
- Drive defensively. Be on the alert for unsignaled lane changes, sudden braking, or other unexpected maneuvers.
- Obey all traffic laws.
- Always wear a seat belt, whether you're the driver or the passenger.

Even the most careful drivers may find themselves having to avoid an accident at some time in their lives. See the **Skills for Behavior Change** box for tips on how to manage your risk.

SKILLS FOR BEHAVIOR CHANGE

MINIMIZING THE CHANCE OF INJURY DURING A CAR ACCIDENT

If a car accident is unavoidable, you can still behave in a way that lessens the chance of serious injury. Some tips include the following:

- Generally, it's safer to veer right rather than left.
- Steer, don't skid, off the road to avoid rolling your vehicle.
- If you have to hit a vehicle, better to sideswipe one moving in your direction than to hit one in the oncoming lane.
- Avoid hitting pedestrians, motorcyclists, and bicyclists at all costs.

LO 2 | CAN YOU PLAY IT SAFE AND STILL HAVE FUN?

Explain safety guidelines for recreational activities that are particularly prone to cause injury.

Recreational activities among young people that commonly involve injury include biking, skateboarding, snow sports, swimming and boating, and using fireworks. By following some basic guidelines while doing these activities, you can have fun and be safe.

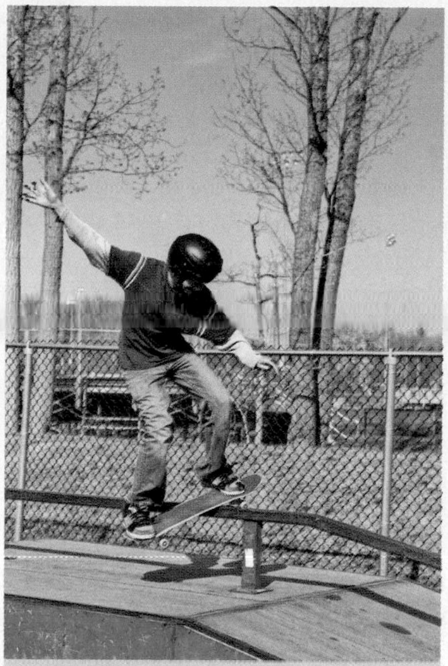

Many skateboarding injuries occur among people who have been practicing the sport for more than a year, often when they attempt a stunt beyond their level of skill. Wearing a helmet will help protect you in case of a fall.

Follow Bike Safety Rules

The NHTSA reports that, in 2011, 677 people died in cycling accidents, and 48,000 were injured. The fatality rate is six times higher for males than females, and males age 45 to 54 had the highest number of cycling-related deaths.[26] Most fatal collisions are due to cyclists' errors, usually failure to yield at intersections. However, alcohol also plays a significant role in bicycle deaths and injuries: In 2011, nearly one-fourth (23%) of cyclists killed were legally drunk, and in 37 percent of all fatal accidents between motor vehicles and bicycles, either the driver or the cyclist was drunk.[27]

All cyclists should wear a properly fitted bicycle helmet every time they ride (**FIGURE 1**). In spite of this, only 34 percent of all college students report "mostly or always" wearing a helmet while biking.[28] The NHTSA reports that a helmet is the single most effective way to prevent head injury resulting from a bicycle crash. Moreover, cyclists are considered vehicle operators; they are required to obey the same rules of the road as drivers.

Cyclists should consider the following suggestions:

- Wear a helmet approved by the American National Standards Institute (ANSI) or the Snell Memorial Foundation.
- Watch the road and listen for traffic sounds! Never listen to an MP3 player or talk on a cell phone, even hands free, while cycling.
- Don't drink and ride.
- Follow all traffic laws, signs, and signals.
- Ride with the flow of traffic.
- Wear light or brightly colored reflective clothing that is easily seen at dawn, dusk, and during full daylight.
- Avoid riding after dark. If you must ride at night, use a front light and a red reflector or flashing rear light, as well as reflective tape or other markings on your bike and clothing.
- Know and use proper hand signals.
- Keep your bicycle in good condition.
- Use bike paths whenever possible.
- Stop at stop signs and traffic lights.

Stay Safe on Your Board

According to the U.S. Consumer Product Safety Commission (CPSC), skateboard-related injuries are commonly due to riding in traffic, trick riding, excessive speed, and consumption of alcohol. Lack of protective equipment, poor board maintenance, riding on irregular road surfaces, inexperience, and overconfidence also play a role.[29] Skateboard safety tips from the CPSC include the following:[30]

- Wear an approved helmet designed for skateboarding, as well as gloves, wrist guards, knee and elbow pads, and flat-soled shoes.
- Maintain your board. Between uses, check it for loose, broken, sharp, or cracked parts.
- Examine the surface where you'll be riding for holes, bumps, and debris.
- Never skateboard in the street, and never hitch a ride from another vehicle.
- Don't speed.
- Don't ride alone.
- Don't drink and ride.

Stay Safe in the Snow

The National Ski Areas Association (NSAA) reports that, on average during the past 10 years, there have been about 40 fatalities per year in U.S. ski areas.[31] Severe nonfatal injuries, such as head trauma and spinal cord injury, also occur at a similarly low rate. This makes snow sports much safer, overall, than bicycling, swimming, and many others. More good news is that the rate of fatal and nonfatal injuries has been declining for decades, largely because

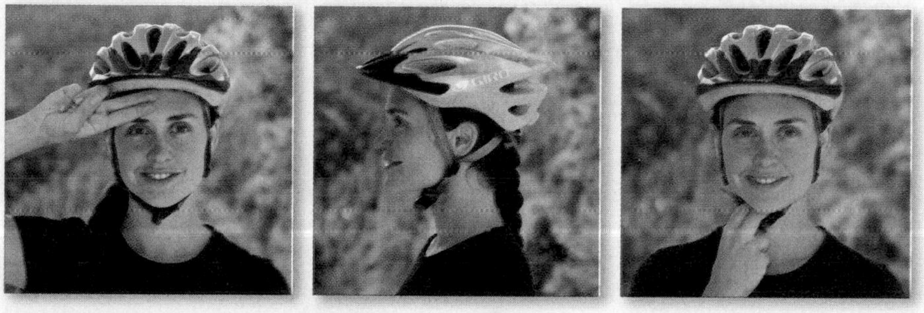

1 The helmet should sit level on your head and low on your forehead—one or two finger-widths above your eyebrows.

2 The sliders on the side straps should be adjusted to form a "V" shape under, and slightly in front of, your ears. Lock the sliders if possible.

3 The chin strap buckle should be centered under your chin. Tighten the strap until it is snug, so that no more than two fingers fit under the strap.

FIGURE 1 Fitting a Bicycle Helmet When your helmet is fitted correctly, opening your mouth wide in a yawn should cause the helmet to pull down on your head. Also, you should not be able to rock the helmet back more than the width of two fingers above the eyebrows or forward into your eyes.

VIDEO TUTOR Biking Safety

personal flotation device A device worn to provide buoyancy and keep the wearer, conscious or unconscious, afloat with the nose and mouth out of the water; also known as a life jacket.

of the use of shorter skis, improved safety features on equipment, and increased safety efforts at resorts, such as having more monitors on the slopes, setting aside special family skiing areas, and encouraging helmet use.

One of the most important ways to protect yourself while skiing or snowboarding is to wear an approved helmet. The NSAA reports that helmet use reduces the risk of any head injury by 30 to 50 percent.[32] However, the use of a helmet does not appear to protect against severe head injuries and fatalities; therefore, skiers are warned against assuming that it's safe to take risks on the slopes because they're wearing a helmet. It's also important to keep skis and snowboards in good condition and to ski according to your ability. Pay attention to the locations of other skiers, and if you stop, move to the side of the trail. Finally, observe all posted signs and warnings.

The sun's ultraviolet (UV) rays can be up to eight times stronger on ski slopes than elsewhere.[33] When skiing in bright sunlight, wear sunscreen on exposed skin, as well as glasses or goggles designed for winter sports.

Stay Safe in the Water

About ten Americans die every day from drowning, making this the fifth leading cause of unintentional injury death among Americans of all ages. Males are four times more likely than females to die from drowning, and as we saw with Matt at the beginning of this chapter, alcohol plays a significant role in many drownings: Up to 70 percent of all deaths associated with water recreation among adolescents and adults involve alcohol.[34]

Swimming

The American Red Cross reports that almost half of adults surveyed say they've had an experience in which they nearly drowned.[35] Most drownings occur during water recreation—swimming, diving, or just simply having fun—in unorganized or unsupervised areas, such as ponds or pools without lifeguards present. Many drowning victims were strong swimmers, so all swimmers should take the following precautions:

- Don't drink alcohol before or while swimming.
- Don't enter the water without a lifejacket unless you can swim at least 50 feet unassisted.
- Know your limitations; get out of the water when you start to feel even slightly fatigued.
- Never swim alone, even if you are a skilled swimmer. You never know what might happen.
- Never leave a child unattended, even in extremely shallow water.
- Before entering the water, check the depth. Most neck and back injuries result from diving into water that is too shallow.
- Never swim in a river with currents too swift for easy, relaxed swimming.
- Never swim in muddy or dirty water that obstructs your view of the bottom. Water that is discolored and choppy or foamy may indicate a rip current.
- If you are caught in a rip current, swim parallel to the shore. Once you are free of the current, swim toward the shore.
- Learn cardiopulmonary resuscitation (CPR). In the event of an emergency, your CPR skills could make a difference in someone's life. CPR performed by bystanders while waiting for paramedics to arrive has been shown to improve outcomes in drowning victims.[36]

Boating

In 2013, the U.S. Coast Guard received reports of 2,620 injured boaters and 560 deaths.[37] About 77 percent of these boating fatalities were drownings, and among those who drowned, 84 percent were not wearing a **personal flotation device**—that is, a lifejacket.[38] Although operator inattention, inexperience, excessive speed, and mechanical failure also contributed to these deaths, alcohol consumption was the leading factor.[39]

In any given year, about one-third of all boating fatalities involve alcohol.[40] In fact, the effects of alcohol can be more pronounced during boating than they are during driving. This is due to boat and engine noise, vibration, wind, sun, glare, temperature, and wave action. When boat operators are drinking, both collisions with other boats and falls overboard are much more likely. If someone who has been drinking does fall overboard, he or she is more likely to drown or to die of hypothermia. Unfortunately, the "designated driver" concept does not apply to boating because intoxicated passengers often cause or directly contribute to boating accidents. The U.S. Coast Guard and every state have "Boating under the Influence" (BUI) laws that carry stringent

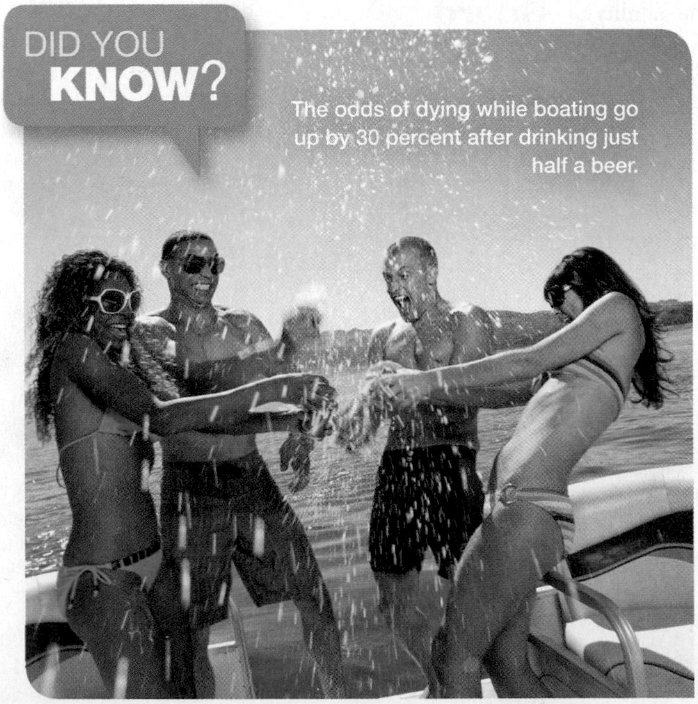

DID YOU KNOW?
The odds of dying while boating go up by 30 percent after drinking just half a beer.

Source: Data are from American Boating Association, "Alcohol Sharply Raises Death Risk for Boaters," 2013, www.americanboating.org/alcohol_in_deadly_accidents.asp.

penalties for violation, including fines, license revocation, and even jail time.[41]

The following boating safety tips are from the American Boating Association:[42]

- Share your plans for your outing. Before leaving home, let others know where you are going, who will be with you, and when you expect to return.
- Check the weather. Listen to boating advisories regarding high winds, storms, and other environmental factors.
- Make sure your boat is seaworthy. Even if you are just going for a short trip, make sure the vessel doesn't leak, has enough fuel (if powered), and has the proper safety equipment.
- Make sure you have enough life jackets for all who are on board and that they are easily accessible.
- Carry an emergency radio and cell phone.
- Don't drink alcohol before you leave, and don't bring any aboard.

In addition, the U.S. Coast Guard recommends that before setting out, you put on your life jacket. Most modern life jackets are thin and flexible and can be worn comfortably all day. Children must wear a life jacket once the vessel is under way, unless they are below deck. Even if you and your companions decide not to put on life jackets initially, a life jacket must be immediately available for every person aboard. Bear in mind that you need to wear a life jacket not only when sailing or motorboating, but also when canoeing, kayaking, and rafting.

Like the snow, water reflects UV rays. Wear sun-protective clothing, sunscreen on exposed skin, a hat, and sunglasses with UV protection. For more on sun safety, see **Chapter 16**.

Have Fun with Fireworks—Safely

It's the Fourth of July, and you plan to celebrate with friends. Should you bring along some fireworks? If you do, play it safe: Each year, fireworks cause between 7,000 and 12,000 injuries in the United States, often the loss of fingers or hands. In 2011, four people died after suffering traumatic injuries from exploded fireworks.[43] Here are some safety tips from the National Council on Fireworks Safety:[44]

- Only use fireworks outdoors in an open area, at least 50 feet from spectators, buildings, dry grasses, and the like.
- Have plenty of water handy—either a hose or a bucket.
- When lighting fireworks, crouch down and reach out. Never bend over them. Don't hold onto them or throw them: Light the fuse and step away.
- Use only commercial fireworks, never homemade ones: They can kill you.
- Never tamper with fireworks, for example, trying to combine the powders. Use them only as intended.
- Never try to relight a "dud" firework. It could explode in your hand. Set it aside for 20 minutes, then soak it in a bucket of water.
- Alcohol and fireworks don't mix. Anyone who has been drinking should keep away from fireworks.

Before using any type of fireworks, check your state laws. You can find a state-by-state directory of fireworks-related laws at www.fireworksafety.com.

LO 3 | HOW CAN YOU AVOID INJURIES AT HOME?

Discuss injuries that occur in the home and what you can do to prevent them.

Injuries within the home typically occur in the form of poisonings, falls, or burns. Some populations, such as the elderly, are particularly vulnerable. However, older adults are not the only victims; each year, thousands of young adults, teens, and children are brought to hospital emergency rooms for treatment of such injuries.

Prevent Poisoning

A **poison** is any substance that is harmful to your body when ingested, inhaled, injected, or absorbed through the skin. Any substance can be poisonous if too much is taken; however, nine out of ten poisoning deaths now result from drug overdose. After rising steadily over the past two decades, these deaths have recently become the leading cause of unintentional injury death in the United States. Every day, 105 Americans die as a result of an accidental drug overdose, and more than 6,700 are treated in hospital emergency departments. The drugs most commonly involved in these deaths and injuries are prescription medications—whether or not they were prescribed for the victim.[45]

> **poison** Any substance harmful to the body when ingested, inhaled, injected, or absorbed through the skin.

Over-the-counter (OTC) drugs are also commonly implicated in overdose incidents. These include cough syrups, sleep medications, and aspirin and other pain relievers. In fact, use of the pain reliever acetaminophen—sold under the brand name Tylenol and a component of several other drugs—is associated with an increased risk of severe liver injury. In 2014, the U.S. Food and Drug Administration issued a safety warning recommending that health care providers discontinue prescribing or dispensing doses over 325 mg.[46]

Tips to Prevent Poisonings

In 2012, the 57 poison control centers in the United States logged more than 2.2 million calls for assistance with a poisoning.[47] The safety tips below were adapted from the American Association of Poison Control Centers:[48]

- Read and follow all usage and warning labels before taking medications or working with chemicals, including household products.
- Never share or sell your prescription drugs. Don't take prescriptions meant for others.
- Never take more than one medication at the same time without the approval of your health care provider. Mixing medications, such as a prescription drug and an OTC

remedy, can result in poisoning. Also follow medication guidelines for alcohol consumption. Acetaminophen, for example, is much more dangerous when taken with even a modest amount of alcohol.

- Never mix household products together, as combinations of products can give off toxic fumes.
- When working with chemicals, wear a protective mask and make sure the area in which you are working is well ventilated. Wear gloves and other protective clothing if there is any possibility of skin contact and eyeglasses or an eye guard if splashing could occur.
- Be especially careful with medications, dietary supplements, and alcohol around children. Keep such items out of sight, preferably in a locked cabinet, and never refer to medication as "candy."
- If you use e-cigarettes, make sure to keep all nicotine vials out of reach of children or pets because drinking these can result in poisoning and death.
- If you live where poisonous reptiles or arachnids are present, keep clothing off of the floors and check inside shoes before putting them on.
- Program the national poison control number, 1-800-222-1222, into your cell phone. The line is open 24 hours a day, 7 days a week.

What to Do in Case of Poisoning

If you suspect you have ingested or inhaled a poison, are stung/bitten by a venomous animal, or are with someone who has collapsed, dial 9-1-1. If you are with someone who is not breathing and you are trained in CPR, provide CPR until paramedics arrive. If the victim is awake and alert, dial the poison control hot line (1-800-222-1222). Follow the instructions you are given: If you are told to take the person to a hospital emergency room, bring along the suspected drug or other agent, if possible.

Avoid Falls

Falls are the third most common cause of death from unintentional injury, and a very common source of injury in the home. About 20 to 30 percent of people who fall suffer moderate to severe injury such as bruises, a fracture, a dislocation, or a head injury. In fact, falls are the most common cause of traumatic brain injury.[49] Although falls are most common among older adults, people of all ages experience them, and many are preventable.

Observe the following measures to reduce your risk of falls:

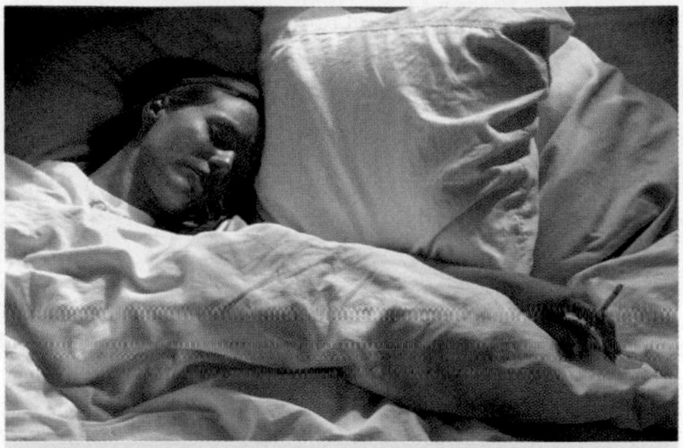

Smoking is the number one cause of fire-related deaths. If you fall asleep with a lit cigarette, bedding and clothing can quickly ignite. If you can't quit, take it outside.

Source: CDC, "Fire Deaths and Injuries: Fact Sheet," October 2011, www.cdc.gov/HomeandRecreationalSafety/Fire-Prevention/fires-factsheet.html.

- Keep the floor and the stairs clear from all objects; don't leave anything lying around.
- Avoid using small scatter rugs and mats, which can slide out from under your feet. Use rubberized liners or strips to secure large rugs to the floor.
- Train your pets to stay away from your feet.
- Install slip-proof mats, treads, or decals in showers and tubs and on the stairs.
- If you need to reach something in a high cupboard or closet, or to change a ceiling light, use an appropriate step stool or short ladder. Don't try to balance on a ledge or on any piece of furniture not designed to bear and balance body weight.
- When using a ladder, make sure it's stable and rated for your body weight before climbing.
- Wear supportive shoes. Flip-flops and shoes without laces can trip you up.

Reduce Your Risk of Fire

In 2010, more than 2,600 Americans—not including firefighters—died in a fire.[50] Although fire-related deaths are less common on college campuses in the United States, a total of 85 fatal fires have occurred on campuses over the past 15 years, claiming the lives of 122 students and staff.[51] The primary causes of fires in campus housing are cooking, use of candles, careless disposal of smoking materials, faulty wiring, and arson.[52] However, impaired judgment from alcohol consumption is also considered a major contributor to campus fires and fire deaths, in part because of delays in responding, calling 9-1-1, and evacuating.[53] Disabled or broken smoke alarms and lack of automatic sprinklers in buildings is also a common factor.

Fire Prevention

Tips to prevent fires include the following:

- Extinguish all cigarettes in ashtrays before bed, and never smoke in bed!
- Set lamps and candles away from curtains, linens, paper, and other combustibles. Never leave candles unattended or burning while you sleep.
- In the kitchen, keep hot pads and kitchen cloths away from stove burners; avoid reaching over hot pans. Use caution when lighting barbecue grills.
- Avoid overloading electrical circuits with appliances and cords. Older buildings are at particular risk for fire from such overloads.
- Have the proper fire extinguishers ready in case of fire, and replace batteries in smoke alarms and test them periodically.

What to Do in a Fire

If a fire breaks out in your dorm or apartment, your priority is to get out. Don't take time to phone before leaving. Don't gather up your stuff. First, feel the door handle: If it's hot, don't open the door! Go to a window, open it as fully as possible, and call for help. Hang a sheet from the window to let rescuers know where you are. If no one is outside, call 9-1-1. If smoke is entering your room, seal the cracks in the door with blankets or towels. Then stay low until you're rescued—there is less smoke close to the floor.

If the door handle is not hot, open the door cautiously. If the hallway is clear to the exit, get out, yelling, "Fire!" and knocking on doors as you leave. If you encounter smoke, stay low to the floor—crawl if necessary—to make your way out. If you pass a fire alarm on your way out, pull it. Always use the stairs, never an elevator. Once you're outside, dial 9-1-1.

The same tips apply when you're staying in a hotel or motel. Always bring a flashlight with you when traveling, and study the evacuation plan posted in your room. Before going to bed, locate the two exits nearest your room and the fire alarms on your floor.

Learn First Aid and CPR

If you were to encounter someone who is injured, would you offer assistance? Many bystanders don't because they lack training and are afraid their efforts will do more harm than good. However, one simple action can help any injury victim: Dial 9-1-1. As soon as your call is answered, describe the situation, then follow the advice you're given. (First aid measures are provided in **Appendix B**, "Providing Emergency Care.")

If you witness someone who has collapsed and you cannot detect a pulse, the American Heart Association advises that you call 9-1-1 and then begin chest compressions.[54] This technique simply requires you to push down in the middle of the victim's chest hard and fast (about 100 compressions per minute). Traditional **cardiopulmonary resuscitation (CPR)**, which includes mouth-to-mouth resuscitation as well as chest compression, is preferable for victims of near-drowning and other forms of respiratory collapse. Everyone is encouraged to get training in CPR, and the course is offered on most college campuses.

Limit Your Exposure to Loud Noise

Our modern society is too often filled with excessive noise. Take a look at **FIGURE 2**, which shows the decibel (dB) levels of various common sounds.

cardiopulmonary resuscitation (CPR) Emergency technique to provide lifesaving chest compression and mouth-to-mouth resuscitation when an individual has stopped breathing and has no pulse.

In general, chronic exposure to noise levels above 85 dB (about as loud as a diesel truck) can result in hearing loss. When you consider the many such noises people are exposed to every day, it should be no surprise that hearing

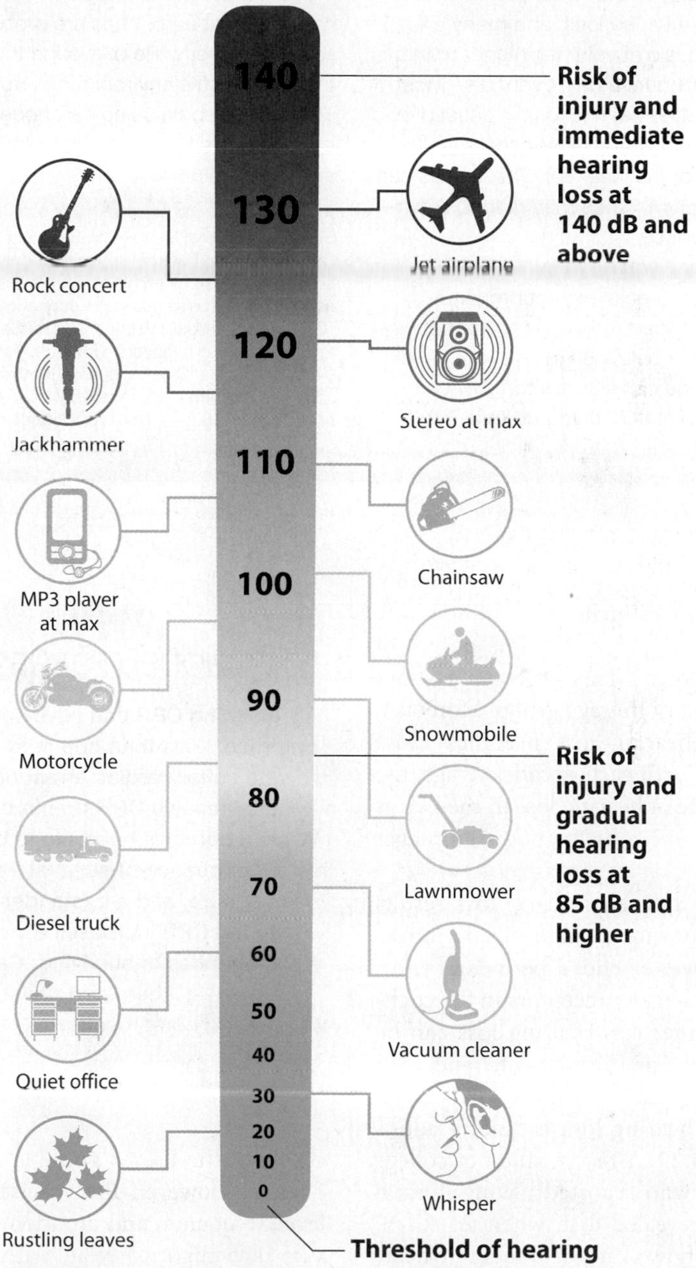

FIGURE 2 Noise Levels of Various Sounds (dB) Decibels increase logarithmically, so each increase of 10 dB represents a tenfold increase in loudness.

Source: Adapted from National Institute on Deafness and Other Communication Disorders, "How Loud Is Too Loud? Bookmark," Updated July 2011, www.nidcd.nih.gov/health/hearing/ruler.asp.

STUDENT HEALTH TODAY

TURNING DOWN THE TUNES

Increasingly, children and young adults experience hearing loss due to use of portable music devices such as MP3 players. High frequency, duration of use, and high volume all make hearing loss a high-risk side effect when using earphones. Long or repeated exposure to any sound at or above 85 decibels (dB) can cause hearing loss, and many people listen to music at volumes higher than this for several hours a day, every day. Most noise-induced hearing loss is caused by damage to delicate sensory cells (called hair cells) of the inner ear. These cells cannot regenerate: Once they're lost, they're gone for good.

What can you do to avoid hearing loss while still enjoying your music? The most important step is to keep the volume at or below 80 dB—or at a level at which you can still comfortably carry on a conversation. If you do that, you won't need to limit the amount of time you spend listening to music. Another way to tell if your volume is set too loud is to ask people nearby if they can hear your music. If they can, it's definitely too loud. Finally, debate continues over the relative safety of over-the-ear earphones versus in-the-ear ear buds. Research indicates, however, that earphones are probably safer because, while delivering the music, they also muffle environmental noise. Therefore, people using earphones in noisy environments tend to set their MP3 players at a lower volume.

Sources: National Institute on Deafness and Other Communication Disorders, "Noise-Induced Hearing Loss," April 2014, www.nidcd.nih.gov/health/hearing/pages/noise.aspx; P. Henry and A. Foots, "Comparison of User Volume Control Settings for Portable Music Players with Three Earphone Configurations in Quiet and Noisy Environments," *Journal of the American Academy of Audiology* 23, no. 3 (2012): 182–91, DOI: 10.3766/jaaa.23.3.5.

Hearing loss is becoming more frequent as music lovers increase the frequency, duration, and volume of their listening time.

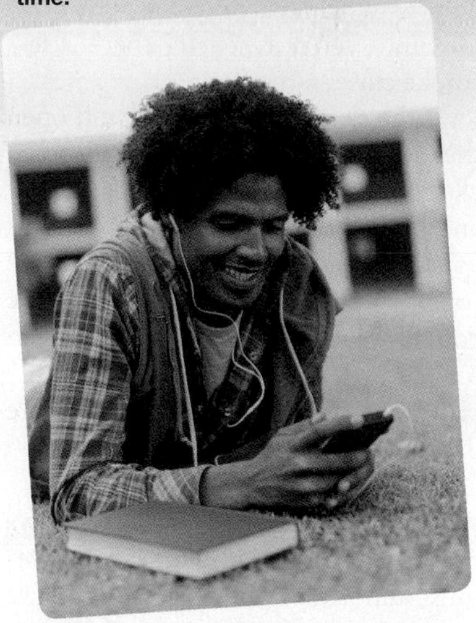

loss is becoming increasingly common. In fact, an estimated 48 million U.S. teens and adults have some degree of hearing loss.[55] This represents about 20 percent of this age group. Moreover, because hearing loss becomes more common with each decade we age, the prevalence of hearing loss in the U.S. is expected to rise as the population ages overall.

Noise-induced hearing loss results when exposure to high-decibel noise, usually over extended periods of time, damages sensory receptors in the cochlea, or inner ear. Hearing loss can be temporary or permanent, and one of the highest rates of sudden noise-induced hearing loss is among adults age 20 to 29. A recent study of college students who reported having normal hearing revealed that, when tested, 12 percent showed at least moderate hearing loss.[56] The study authors identified a correlation between use of a personal music player and increased risk for hearing loss. Several other studies have also linked hearing loss in young adults to the use of portable listening devices. However, the precise decibel level, frequency, and duration of exposure that might correlate with hearing loss is currently under investigation.[57] Check out the **Student Health Today** box for more details and tips for protecting your hearing while enjoying your tunes.

WHY SHOULD I CARE?

Knowing CPR can save someone's life. Less than one third of people who suffer cardiac arrest outside of a hospital receive CPR from a bystander. When a person's heart stops beating, his or her chance of survival decreases each minute, and a bystander administering CPR increases a victim's chances of surviving. Call 9-1-1, then start chest compressions.

Another source of hearing impairment is frequent concert attendance. Most rock musicians use earplugs when performing or rehearsing, and their audiences would be wise to do the same. Hearing loss may result from one evening in front of huge speakers at a rock concert. If you can't hear the person standing next to you at a concert, then you should put in earplugs or look for a quieter spot. In addition, you should rest your ears between nights out partying or attending concerts or loud sporting events.

LO 4 | HOW CAN YOU AVOID INJURY WHILE WORKING?

Describe work-related injuries and what you can do to prevent them.

American adults spend most of their waking hours on the job. Although most job situations are pleasant and productive, others pose hazards. Over

4,300 fatal work injuries occurred in the United States in 2012. Transportation incidents made up the largest number of fatal work injuries (more than 40%). In addition, workers in material moving, construction, and extraction (mining) and those in the service industry are at high risk of fatal injuries. Farmers, fishing workers, and loggers are also at high risk.[58]

Although on-the-job deaths capture media attention, workers may also be seriously injured or disabled at their jobs. Common work injuries include cuts and lacerations, chemical burns, fractures, sprains and strains (often of the back), and repetitive motion disorders. Because so many work injuries are due to overexertion, poor body mechanics, or repetitive motion, they are largely preventable. We discuss these problems and share some prevention strategies here.

Protect Your Back

Low back pain (LBP), usually as a result of injury, is epidemic throughout the world and is the major cause of disability for people age 30 to 50 in the United States; this age group suffer more frequently and severely from this problem than older people do.[59] It is one of the most commonly experienced chronic ailments among college students. In a recent survey, 12.5 percent of college students reported having seen their doctor in the previous year because of back pain.[60]

Because most injuries to the back are in the lumbar spine area (lower back), strengthening core muscle groups and stretching muscles to avoid cramping and spasms are key strategies to reduce risks. Frequently, sports injuries, stress on spinal bones and tissues, or the sudden jolt of a car accident are the culprits. Other times, sitting too long in the same position or hunching over your computer while you're pulling an all-nighter can leave you with pain so severe that you can't stand up or walk comfortably. Carrying heavy backpacks between classes is another frequent source of LBP.

You can avoid typical risks by using common sense and thinking "safety" when engaging in activities that could injure your back. Getting up and stretching after a few hours in a static position is another great strategy to avoid problems. Maintaining good posture can also reduce back problems.

Other measures you can take to reduce the risk of back pain include the following:

- Invest in a high-quality, supportive mattress.
- Avoid high-heeled shoes, which tilt the pelvis forward.
- Control your weight. Extra weight puts increased strain on your knees, hips, and back.
- Warm up and stretch before exercising or lifting heavy objects.
- When lifting something heavy, use your leg muscles and use proper form (**FIGURE 3**). Do not bend from the waist or take the weight load on your back.
- Buy a desk chair with good lumbar support.
- Move your car seat forward so your knees are elevated slightly.
- Engage in exercise regularly, particularly in core exercises that strengthen the abdominal muscles and stretch the back muscles.
- Downsize your backpack.

Maintain Alignment while Sitting

How many hours have you spent today glued to a laptop, tablet, smartphone, or book? Were you slouching, hunched over, or sitting up straight? Your answers are probably reflected in the degree of aching and stiffness you may be feeling right now. Try these strategies to maintain a healthy alignment while you sit and work:

1. Sit comfortably with your feet flat on the floor or on a footrest, and your knees level with your hips. Raise or lower your chair, or move to a different chair, to achieve this position.
2. Your middle back should be firmly against the back of the chair. The small of your back should be supported, too. If you can't feel the chair back supporting your lumbar region, try placing a small cushion or even a rolled towel behind the curve of your lower back.
3. Keep your shoulders relaxed and straight, not rolled or hunched forward.
4. The angle of your elbows should be 90 degrees to your upper arms. Change your position or the position of your device to achieve this angle.
5. Ideally, you should be looking straight ahead, not peering down at a screen or book.

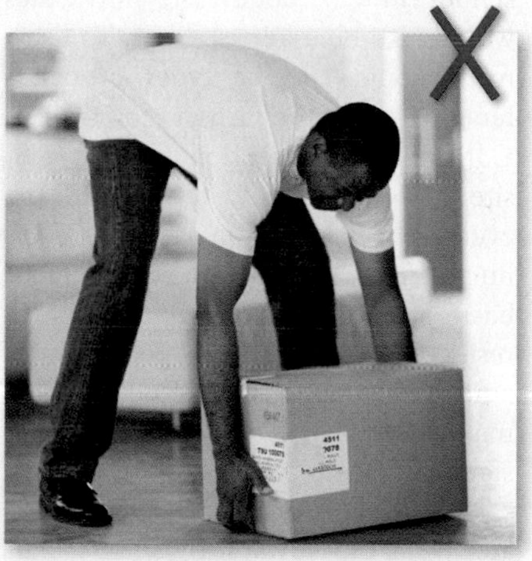

(a) Attempting to lift a heavy object by bending at your waist is a common cause of back injury.

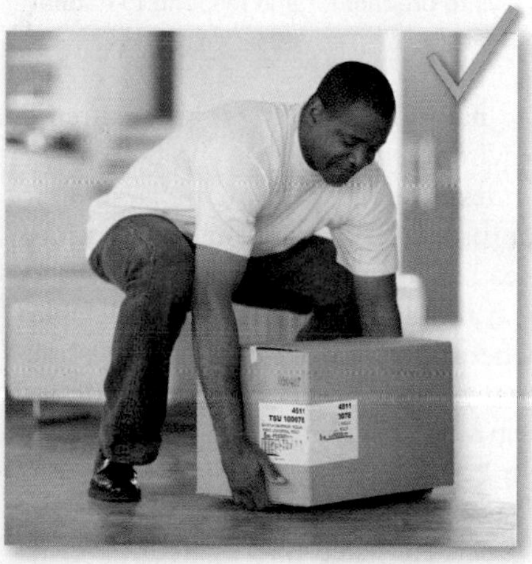

(b) Start as close to the object as possible, with it positioned between your knees as you squat down. Keep your feet parallel, or stagger one foot in front of the other. Keep the object close to your body as you stand, using your legs, not your back, to lift.

FIGURE 3 Lifting a Heavy Object

repetitive motion disorder (RMD) An injury to soft tissue, tendons, muscles, nerves, or joints due to the physical stress of repeated motions.

carpal tunnel syndrome A common occupational injury in which the median nerve in the wrist becomes irritated, causing numbness, tingling, and pain in the fingers and hands.

natural disaster Any extreme environmental event that causes widespread destruction of land and/or property, injuries, and sometimes deaths.

Avoid Repetitive Motion Disorders

It's the end of the term, and you have finished the last of several papers. After hours of nonstop typing, your hands are numb and you feel an intense pain that makes the thought of typing one more word almost unbearable. If this happens, you may be suffering from one of several **repetitive motion disorders (RMDs)**, sometimes called *overuse syndrome, cumulative trauma disorders*, or *repetitive stress injuries*. These refer to a family of painful soft tissue injuries that begin with inflammation and gradually become disabling.

Repetitive motion disorders include carpal tunnel syndrome, bursitis, tendonitis, and ganglion cysts, among others. Twisting of the arm or wrist, overexertion, and incorrect posture or position are usually contributors. The areas most likely to be affected are the hands, wrists, elbows, and shoulders, but the neck, back, hips, knees, feet, ankles, and legs can be affected, too. Over time, RMDs can cause permanent damage to nerves, soft tissue, and joints. Usually, RMDs are associated with repeating the same task in an occupational setting and gradually irritating the area in question. However, certain sports (tennis, golf, and others), gripping the wheel while driving, keyboarding or texting, and a number of newer technology-driven activities can also result in RMDs.

Because many of these injuries occur in everyday work, play, and athletics, they are often not reported to national agencies that keep track of injury statistics. Many people just pop over-the-counter pain remedies and continue working until the pain becomes unbearable. Nevertheless, reports of increasing numbers of cases of disorders like "BlackBerry thumb," carpal tunnel syndrome, and other maladies are widespread.

One of the most common RMDs is **carpal tunnel syndrome (CTS)**, an inflammation of the soft tissues within the "tunnel" through the carpal bones of the wrist (**FIGURE 4**). This puts pressure on the median nerve, which runs down the forearm through the tunnel to innervate the hand. Symptoms include numbness, tingling, and pain in the fingers and hands. Carpal tunnel syndrome typically results from spending hours typing at the computer keyboard, flipping groceries through computerized scanners, or manipulating other objects in jobs "made simpler" by technology. The risk for CTS can be reduced by proper design of workstations, protective wrist pads, and worker training. Physical and occupational therapy is an important part of treatment and recovery.

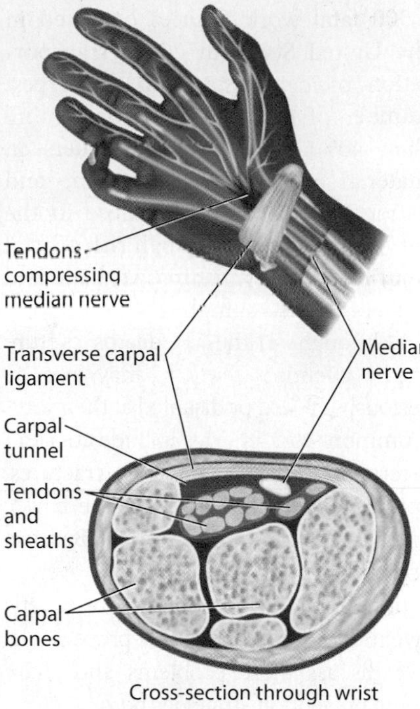

FIGURE 4 Carpal Tunnel Syndrome
The carpal tunnel is a space beneath the transverse carpal ligament and above the carpal bones of the wrist. The median nerve and the tendons that allow you to flex your fingers run through this tunnel. Carpal tunnel syndrome occurs when repetitive use prompts inflammation of the tissues and fluids of the tunnel. This in turn compresses the median nerve.

LO 5 | ARE YOU PREPARED FOR ENVIRONMENTAL EVENTS?

Identify which natural disasters affect different regions of the U.S., and explain ways to prepare for and respond to natural disasters.

A **natural disaster** is any extreme environmental event that causes widespread destruction of land and/or property, injuries, and sometimes deaths. Some, such as hurricanes and volcanic eruptions, may be predictable, whereas others, like earthquakes and many tornadoes, can occur without warning. If a natural disaster were to strike without warning in your region, would you be prepared?

The first step in preparedness is to learn what types of natural disasters typically affect the area where you live. If you've relocated from New England to the Midwest to attend school, for example, you may want to learn about tornado preparedness. If you attend school in the Southeast, hurricanes would also be a key concern. To learn more about specific types of disasters, log on to the Centers for Disease Control and Prevention (CDC) website at www.cdc.gov and search the event name. For instance, the CDC's hurricane page provides key facts; basic steps to prepare yourself, your residence, and even your pets; a list of emergency supplies you'd need; information on how to evacuate safely; and steps to take to get through the storm safely if you're ordered *not* to evacuate. You can always find advisories and other information about weather-related events in your area—from blizzards to gales to flash floods—by visiting the National Weather Service website at www.weather.gov.

ASSESS **YOURSELF**

What could you do to be safer on the road? Want to find out? Take the **Are You at Risk for a Motor Vehicle Accident?** assessment available on MasteringHealth.™

Need help creating a plan? Follow the strategies in the **Your Plan for Change** box for short- and long-term improvements to your health.

YOUR PLAN FOR **CHANGE**

The **ASSESS YOURSELF** activity helped you identify the ways you take risks on the road. Depending on your responses, you might choose to make some of the following changes.

TODAY, YOU CAN:

- ☐ Fasten your seat belt before you turn the ignition key, and ask everyone in your vehicle to do the same.
- ☐ Commit to turning off your cell phone and other handheld devices before you drive.
- ☐ Drive within the posted speed limit.

WITHIN THE NEXT 2 WEEKS, YOU CAN:

- ☐ Offer to be the designated driver the next time you go out with friends.
- ☐ Get 7 to 8 hours of sleep before setting out on a long drive.

BY THE END OF THE SEMESTER, YOU CAN:

- ☐ Bring your car in for a tune-up, and have the mechanic check that the seat belts and air bags are functioning properly.

20 Preserving and Protecting Your Environment

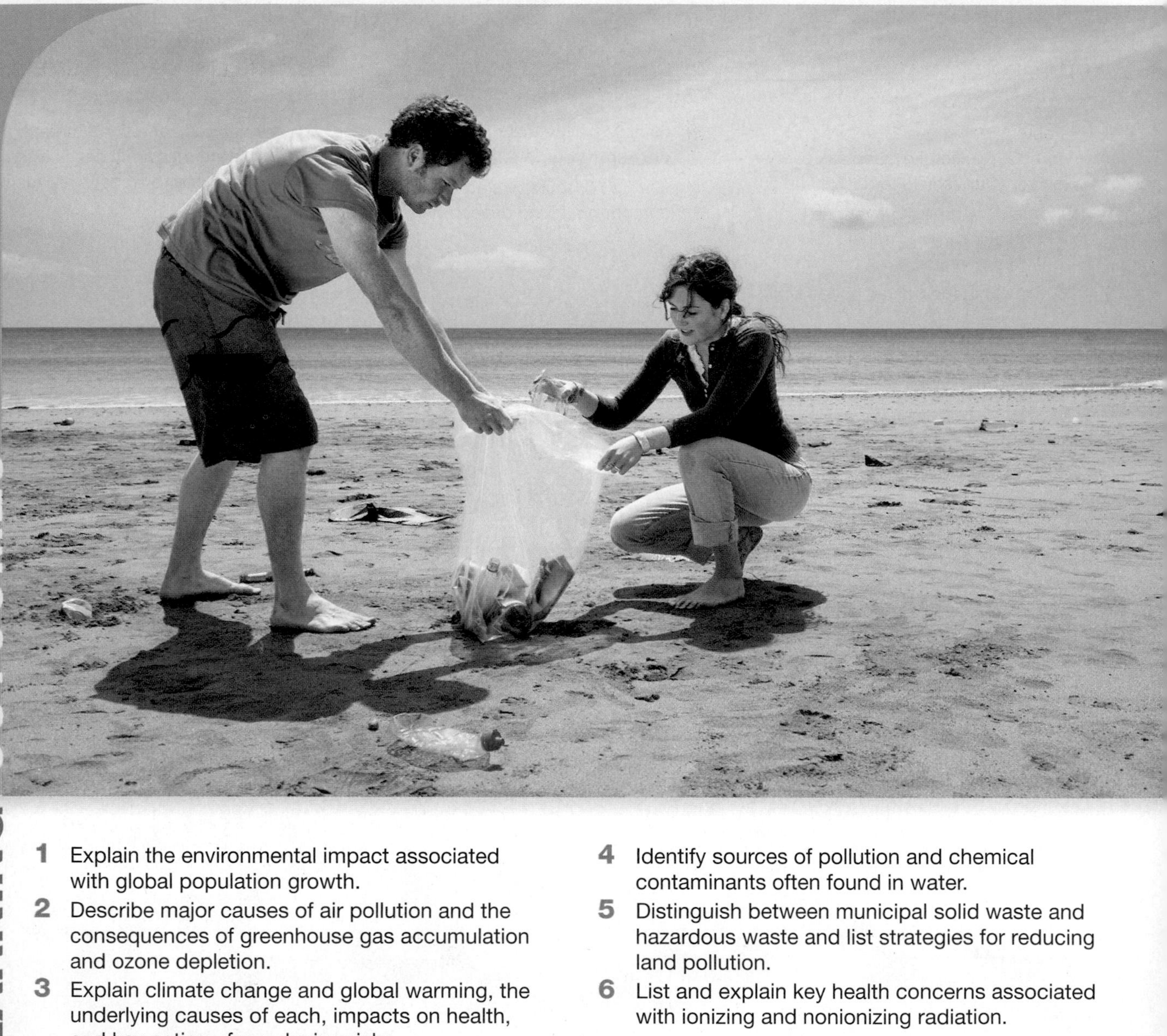

LEARNING OUTCOMES

1 Explain the environmental impact associated with global population growth.

2 Describe major causes of air pollution and the consequences of greenhouse gas accumulation and ozone depletion.

3 Explain climate change and global warming, the underlying causes of each, impacts on health, and key actions for reducing risks.

4 Identify sources of pollution and chemical contaminants often found in water.

5 Distinguish between municipal solid waste and hazardous waste and list strategies for reducing land pollution.

6 List and explain key health concerns associated with ionizing and nonionizing radiation.

"*... [T]he fact is, the 12 hottest years on record have all come in the last 15. Heat waves, droughts, wildfires, and floods—all are now more frequent and intense. We can choose to believe that Superstorm Sandy, and the most severe drought in decades, and the worst wildfires some states have ever seen were all just a freak coincidence. Or we can choose to believe in the overwhelming judgment of science—and act before it's too late.*"

—President Barack Obama, 2013 State of the Union Address, February 12, 2013.

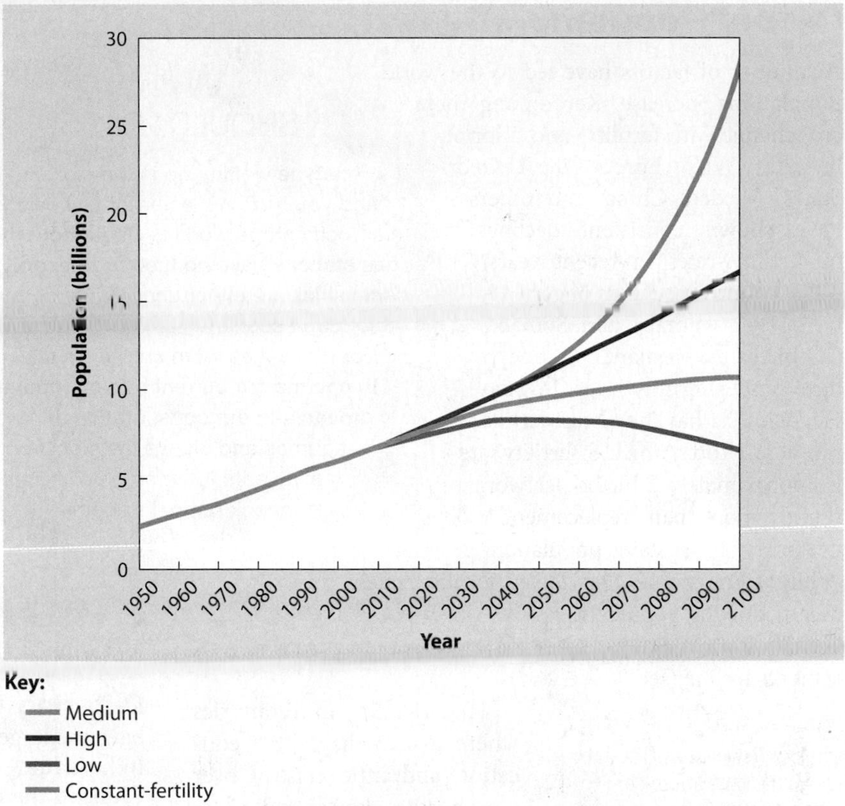

FIGURE 20.1 Projected World Population Growth, 1950–2100, According to Different Projections

Source: Population Division of the Department of Economic and Social Affairs of the United Nations Secretariat, *World Population Prospects: The 2012 Revision* (New York, NY: United Nations, 2013).

We live in an especially dangerous time. The global population has grown more in the past 50 years than at any other time in human history. More people pose a potentially devastating threat to the water we drink, the air we breathe, the food we eat, and our capacity to survive. Polar ice caps and glaciers are melting at rates that surpass even the most dire predictions of a decade ago, and threats of rising sea levels loom large. One in four species of mammals in the world is now threatened with extinction as humans destroy habitat, exacerbate drought and flooding through climate change, and pollute the environment. Clean water is becoming scarce, fossil fuels are being depleted, and the amount of solid and hazardous waste is growing. In short, our collective disregard for the planet's life-sustaining resources may ultimately put all living things in peril unless we take action now.

This chapter provides an overview of the factors contributing to the global environmental crisis. It also provides a blueprint for action—by individuals, communities, policymakers, and governments. Staying informed and becoming an advocate for a healthy environment are key things you can do to help.

LO 1 | OVERPOPULATION: THE PLANET'S GREATEST THREAT

Explain the environmental impact associated with global population growth.

As anthropologist Margaret Mead put it, "*Every human society is faced not with one population problem but two: how to beget and rear enough children and how not to beget and rear too many.*"[1]

The United Nations projects that the world population will grow from its current 7.2 billion to 9.6 billion in 2050 and 10.9 billion in 2100, assuming a fairly *constant* **fertility rate**—the average number of births per woman in a specific country or region.[2] Current population projections have assumed a low, declining, or constant fertility rate. However, recent data indicate that these rates have increased significantly, particularly in developing regions of the world, leading many to believe that our population projections may grossly underestimate the reality of our global population in the next decades. Add increasing fertility rates to increases in overall survival and increases in life expectancy at birth and other variables, and you have created a perfect storm whereby future populations may skyrocket to nearly 28 billion by 2100 (see **FIGURE 20.1**).[3] Tomorrow's population will be significantly larger, younger, more industrialized, consume more resources, and produce even more waste than previous generations unless actions are taken to control population growth.[4]

fertility rate Average number of births a female in a certain population has during her reproductive years.

97%

OF **GLOBAL GROWTH** IN THE NEXT FOUR DECADES WILL HAPPEN IN ASIA, AFRICA, LATIN AMERICA, AND THE CARIBBEAN.

Global Population Growth

A number of factors have led to the world population's increase. Key among them are changes in fertility and mortality rates. While Europe, the United States, Mexico, China, and others have shown consistent declines in fertility rates in recent years, other countries such as Niger (7.8 births per woman) and Somalia (7.1 births per woman) continue to have higher fertility rates. Bosnia-Herzegovina has the lowest fertility rate at 1.2. Today, the U.S. fertility rate is approximately 2 births per woman, slightly more than "replacement" values necessary to sustain population growth. While some argue that lower fertility rates means slowing population growth, sheer population size can cause major increases, even if fertility rates remain constant or decline (see **TABLE 20.1**).[5]

WHY SHOULD I CARE?

Imagine waking up in the morning to find you have no water for a shower, the electricity stops working throughout the day, gas stations have no fuel for sale, and basic necessities are either unavailable or unaffordable. Such scenarios are not science fiction. Major difficulties loom unless we take action to change our current rate of population growth and our consumption of natural resources and unless the global community acts to enforce policies to check rampant population growth.

carrying capacity of the earth The largest population that can be supported indefinitely given the resources available in the environment.

Historically, in countries where women have little education and little control over reproductive choices and where birth control is either not available or frowned upon, pregnancy rates continue to rise. As women become more educated, obtain higher socioeconomic status, work more outside of the home, and have more control over reproduction—as birth control becomes more accessible—fertility rates decline. Recognizing that population control will be essential in the decades ahead, many countries have enacted strict population control measures or have encouraged their citizens to limit the size of their families. Proponents of *zero population growth* believe that each couple should produce only two offspring, allowing the population to stabilize.

Mortality rates from chronic and infectious diseases have declined as a result of improved public health infrastructure, increased availability of drugs and vaccines, better disaster preparedness, and other factors. As people live longer, they add more years of resource consumption and add to the overall human footprint on the environment.

TABLE **20.1** | Selected Total Fertility Rates Worldwide, 2013

Country	Number of Children Born per Woman*
Niger	7.6
Chad	7.0
Somalia	6.8
Congo, Dem Republic	6.3
India	2.4
Mexico	2.2
United States	1.9
Australia	1.9
Canada	1.6
China	1.6
Russia	1.7
Germany	1.4
Japan	1.4

*Indicates average number of children that would be born per woman if all women lived to the end of their childbearing years and bore children according to a given fertility rate at each age.

Source: Data from Population Reference Bureau, "World Population Data Sheet," 2014, www.prb.org/Publications/Datasheets/2013/2013-world-population-data-sheet.aspx.

Differing Growth Rates The country projected to have the largest increase in population in coming decades is India, adding another 600 million people by 2050, surpassing China as the most populous nation on earth.[6]

With a current population of over 318 million and a net gain of one person every 13 seconds, the United States leads most other industrialized nations in growth, even though fertility rates are down.[7] It also has one of the largest "ecological footprints," exerting a greater impact on many of the planet's resources than do most other nations.[8]

WHAT DO YOU THINK?

Should individuals get tax breaks for having fewer children?

- How would such policies compare to our current policies?
- Can you think of other policies that might be effective in encouraging population control and resource conservation in the United States?

Measuring the Impact of People

Today, experts are analyzing the **carrying capacity of the earth**—the largest population that can be supported indefinitely, given the resources available in the environment. At what point will we be unable to restore the balance between humans and nature? Since 1996, the global demand for natural resources has doubled. It now takes 1.5 years to regenerate the renewable resources used in 1 year by humans. A significant report indicates that by 2030 it will take the equivalent of two planets to meet the demand for resources, and by 2100, we may need more than four planets to support human needs. Simply put, we are running out of the natural resources necessary to sustain us, and the problem is growing at an unprecedented rate.[9] Vast

HEAR IT! PODCASTS

Want a study podcast for this chapter? Download the podcast **Environmental Health** available on MasteringHealth.™

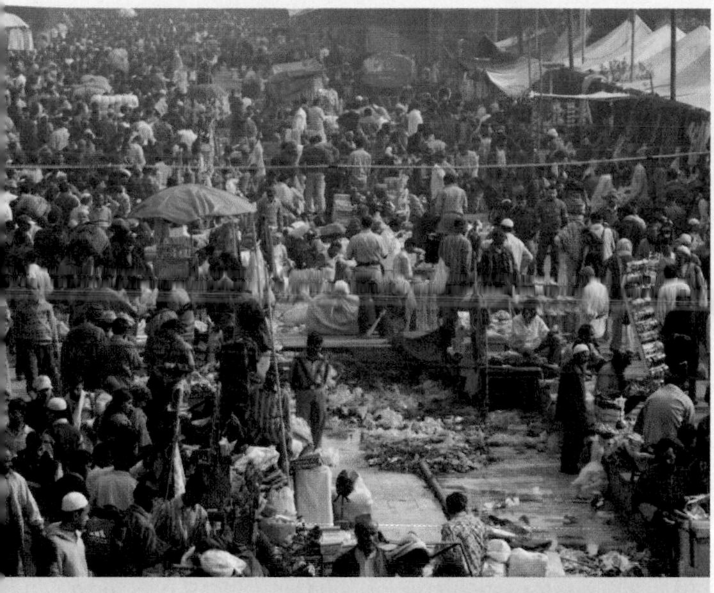

Every year the global population grows by 90 million, but Earth's resources are not expanding. Population increases are believed to be a key factor in our escalating pressure on increasingly scarce natural resources and climate change.

differences exist between countries that have the *biocapacity* to sustain their growth and those that are draining the global capacity to sustain life. Evidence of the effects of unchecked population growth is everywhere:

- **Impact on other species.** Changes in the **ecosystem** are resulting in mass destruction of many species and their habitats.[10] Twelve percent of all birds are threatened, with seabirds taking the greatest hit (over 38% are threatened). More than 75 species of mammals are already extinct, with others, such as tigers, already having populations decline by 95 percent in the last century.[11] In spite of major efforts to stop organized crime's international killing of elephants for ivory, nearly 20,000 African elephants were slaughtered in Africa in 2013, causing many to question their ultimate survival.[12] About a third of amphibians (frogs, toads, and salamanders) are threatened or extinct, and many of those that survive have chemically induced ailments or genetic mutations that will hasten their demise.[13] Along with mammals, rapid declines in plant species are reasons for concern.[14]
- **Impact on the food supply.** We are currently fishing the oceans at rates that are 250 percent more than they can regenerate, and scientists project a global collapse of all fish species by 2050.[15]

Aquatic ecosystems continue to be heavily contaminated by chemical and human waste. Recent reports indicate that our oceans are 30 percent more acidic now than they were just 200 years ago, largely due to human-caused pollutants. Living coral reefs that support aquatic life have declined by over 50 percent in the last 27 years, with virtual dead zones stretching for miles on ocean floors.[16] Massive storms, earthquakes, radiation, invasive species, and other threats hasten the demise of natural sea life and lead to increased aquaculture and fish farms rather than wild fish catches.

Today, our global quest for food means that increasing amounts of the earth's surface are used for agriculture. Because agriculture accounts for over 90 percent of our global water footprint, groundwater withdrawals have tripled in the last 50 years, which puts increased pressure on dwindling water reserves.[17] Drought and erosion and natural disasters make growing food increasingly difficult, and food shortages and famine are occurring in many regions of the world with increasing frequency.

ecosystem Collection of physical (nonliving) and biological (living) components of an environment and the relationships between them.

fossil fuels Carbon-based material used for energy; includes oil, coal, and natural gas.

- **Land degradation and contamination of drinking water.** The per capita availability of freshwater is declining rapidly, and contaminated water remains the greatest single environmental cause of human illness. Unsustainable land use and climate change are increasing land degradation, including erosion, toxic chemical infiltration, nutrient depletion, deforestation, and other problems that will inevitably affect human life.
- **Energy consumption.** "Use it *and* lose it" is an apt saying for our use of nonrenewable energy sources in the form of **fossil fuels** (oil, coal, natural gas). Although we are seeing a shift toward renewable energy sources, such as hydropower, solar and wind power, and biomass power, the predominant energy sources are still fossil fuels. The United States is the largest consumer of liquid fossil fuels and natural gas and among the top four consumers of nuclear power, coal, and hydroelectric power.[18] In many developing regions of the world, greater industrialization and more citizen affluence has resulted in skyrocketing demand for limited fossil fuels (see **FIGURE 20.2**).

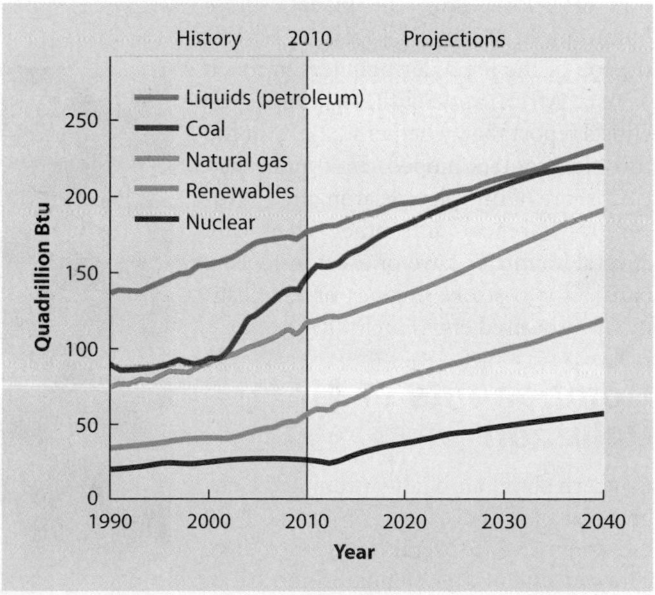

FIGURE 20.2 World Energy Consumption by Fuel Type, 1990–2040 (Quadrillion Btu) Liquid fuels include petroleum. The last year with real data is 2010; years thereafter are projected estimates.

Source: U.S. Energy Information Administration, *International Energy Outlook 2013*, Figure 2, Page 2, www.eia.gov/forecasts/ieo/pdf/0484%282013%29.pdf.

LO 2 | AIR POLLUTION

Describe major causes of air pollution and the consequences of greenhouse gas accumulation and ozone depletion.

The term *air pollution* refers to the presence, in varying degrees, of substances (suspended particles and vapors) not found in clean air. From the beginning of time, natural events, living creatures, and toxic by-products have polluted the environment. Air pollution is not new, but the vast array of **pollutants** that exist today and their potential interactive effects are.

Air pollutants are either *naturally occurring* or *anthropogenic* (caused by humans). Naturally occurring air pollutants include *particulate matter*, such as ash from volcanic eruptions, soil, and dust. Anthropogenic sources include those caused by *stationary sources* (e.g., power plants, factories, and refineries) and *mobile sources*, such as vehicles. Mobile sources are *on-road* vehicles (cars, trucks, and buses) or *off-road* sources (such as construction equipment). Planes, trains, and watercraft are considered *nonroad* sources.[19] According to Environmental Protection Agency estimates, mobile sources are the major contributors of key air pollutants, such as carbon monoxide (CO), sulfur oxides (SO_X), and nitrogen oxides (NO_X). Motor vehicles alone contribute nearly 30 percent of all CO emissions.[20]

pollutant Substance that contaminates some aspect of the environment and causes potential harm to living organisms.

smog Brownish haze that is a form of pollution produced by the photochemical reaction of sunlight with hydrocarbons, nitrogen compounds, and other gases in vehicle exhaust.

temperature inversion Weather condition that occurs when a layer of cool air is trapped under a layer of warmer air, preventing the air from circulating.

A new study focused on commuting polluters may surprise urbanites who think that gas-sipping mopeds are their way of helping save the planet. Those humming little two-stroke engines are at the top of the list of air polluters in much of Asia, Africa, and Southern Europe. Scientists report that, whether idling or at full throttle, scooters/mopeds emit more than their share of fine particle aromatic hydrocarbons (arenes) and other chemicals. Several countries have or are considering bans on two-stroke engines or establishment of lowered emission limits.[21]

Components of Air Pollution

Concern about air quality prompted Congress to pass the *Clean Air Act* in 1970 and to amend it several times since then. The act established standards for six of the most widespread air pollutants that seriously affect health: sulfur dioxide, particulates, carbon monoxide, nitrogen dioxide, ground-level ozone, and lead. There have been major decreases in these six criteria pollutants, even as populations have increased in the United States. However, ozone and particulate matter continue to be present at significant levels.[22] See TABLE 20.2 for an overview of the sources and effects of these pollutants.

Photochemical Smog

Smog is a brownish haze produced by the photochemical reaction of sunlight with hydrocarbons, nitrogen compounds, and other gases in vehicle exhaust. It is sometimes called *ozone pollution* because ozone is a main component of smog. Smog tends to form in areas that experience a **temperature inversion**, in which a cool layer of air is trapped under a layer of warmer air, preventing the air from circulating. Smog is more likely to occur in valley areas surrounded by hills or mountains, such as Los Angeles or Mexico City. The most noticeable adverse effects of smog are difficulty breathing, burning eyes, headaches, and nausea. Long-term exposure poses serious health risks, particularly for children, older adults, pregnant women, and people with chronic respiratory disorders.

Air Quality Index

The Air Quality Index (AQI) is a measure of how clean or polluted the air is on a given day and if there are any health concerns related to air quality. The AQI focuses on health effects that can happen within a few hours or days after breathing polluted air.

The AQI scale is from 0 to 500: The higher the AQI value, the greater the level of air pollution and associated health risks. An AQI value of 100 generally corresponds to the national air quality standard for the pollutant, which is the level the EPA has set to protect public health. AQI values below 100 are generally considered satisfactory. When AQI values rise above 100, air quality is considered unhealthy

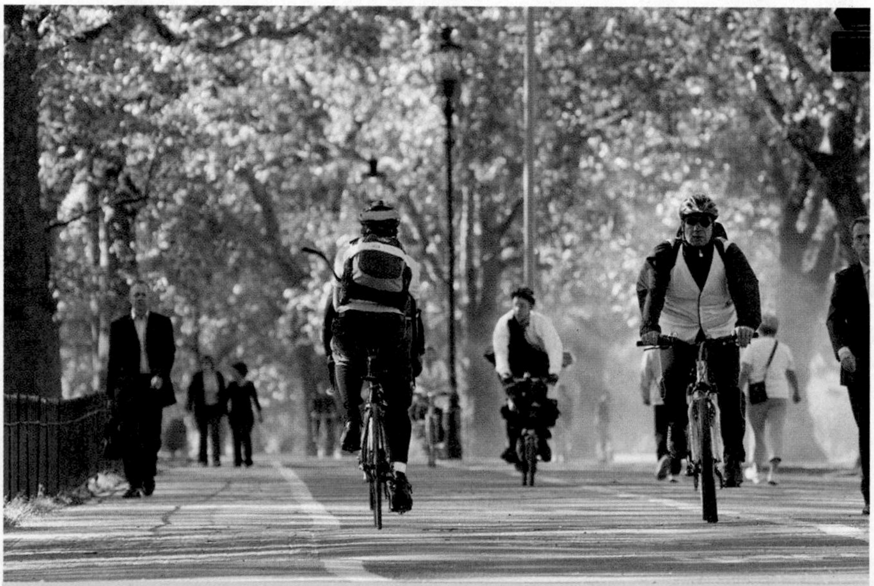

Making small changes such as driving less, riding your bike more, taking public transportation or carpooling, turning off lights, recycling, and composting can all help to reduce your carbon footprint.

TABLE 20.2 | Sources, Health Effects, and Environmental Impacts of Six Major Air Pollutants

Pollutant	Description	Sources	Health Effects	Welfare Effects
Carbon monoxide (CO)	Colorless, odorless gas	Motor vehicle exhaust; indoor sources include kerosene and wood-burning stoves	Headaches, reduced mental alertness, heart attack, cardiovascular diseases, impaired fetal development, death	Contributes to the formation of smog
Sulfur dioxide (SO_2)	Colorless gas that dissolves in water vapor to form acid and interacts with other gases and particles in the air	Coal-fired power plants, petroleum refineries, manufacture of sulfuric acid, and smelting of ores containing sulfur	Eye irritation, wheezing, chest tightness, shortness of breath, lung damage	Contributes to the formation of acid rain, visibility impairment, plant and water damage, aesthetic damage
Nitrogen dioxide (NO_2)	Reddish brown, highly reactive gas	Motor vehicles, electric utilities, and other industrial, commercial, and residential sources that burn fuels	Susceptibility to respiratory infections, irritation of the lungs and respiratory symptoms (e.g., cough, chest pain, difficulty breathing)	Contributes to the formation of smog, acid rain, water quality deterioration, global warming, and visibility impairment
Ozone (O_3)	Gaseous pollutant when formed near the ground	Vehicle exhaust and certain other fumes; formed from other air pollutants in the presence of sunlight	Eye and throat irritation, coughing, respiratory tract problems, asthma, lung damage	Plant and ecosystem damage, global warming
Lead (Pb)	Metallic element	Metal refineries, lead smelters, battery manufacturers, iron and steel producers	Anemia, high blood pressure, brain and kidney damage, neurological disorders, cancer, lowered IQ	Affects animals, plants, and the aquatic ecosystem
Particulate matter (PM)	Very small particles of soot, dust, or other matter, including tiny droplets of liquids	Diesel engines, power plants, industries, windblown dust, wood stoves	Eye irritation, asthma, bronchitis, lung damage, cancer, heavy metal poisoning, cardiovascular effects	Visibility impairment, atmospheric deposition, aesthetic damage

Source: U.S. Environmental Protection Agency, "Air and Radiation: Air Pollutants," 2012, www.epa.gov/air/urbanair/ and www.epa.gov/air/airpollutants.html.

at certain levels for specific groups of people and at higher levels for everyone. As shown in **FIGURE 20.3**, the EPA has divided the AQI scale into six categories with corresponding color codes. National and local weather reports generally include information on the day's AQI.

When the AQI is in this range:	... air quality conditions are	... as symbolized by this color:
0 to 50	Good	Green
51 to 100	Moderate	Yellow
101 to 150	Unhealthy for sensitive groups	Orange
151 to 200	Unhealthy	Red
201 to 300	Very unhealthy	Purple
301 to 500	Hazardous	Maroon

FIGURE 20.3 Air Quality Index The EPA provides individual air quality indexes (AQIs) for ground-level ozone, particle pollution, carbon monoxide, sulfur dioxide, and nitrogen dioxide. All of the AQIs are presented using the general values, categories, and colors of this figure.

Source: U.S. Environmental Protection Agency, "Air Quality Index: A Guide to Air Quality and Your Health," Updated May 2014, www.airnow.gov/index.cfm?action=aqibasics.aqi.

Acid Deposition and Acid Rain

Acid deposition is replacing the term *acid rain* in scientific circles; it refers to the deposition of *wet* (rain, snow, sleet, fog, cloud water, and dew) and *dry* (acidifying particles and gases) acidic components that fall to the earth in dust or smoke.[23] Sulfur dioxide (SO_2) and nitrogen oxide (NO_x) cause damage to plants, aquatic animals, forests, and humans over time. In the United States, roughly two-thirds of all sulfur dioxides and one-fourth of all nitrogen oxides come from electric power generation that relies on burning fossil fuels such as coal.[24] When coal-powered plants, oil refineries, and other facilities burn these fuels, sulfur and nitrogen in the emissions combine with oxygen and sunlight to become sulfur dioxide and nitrogen oxide. Small acid particles are carried by the wind and combine with moisture to produce acidic rain or snow.[25]

acid deposition Acidification process that occurs when pollutants are deposited by precipitation, clouds, or directly on the land.

Acid deposition gradually acidifies ponds, lakes, and other bodies of water. Once the acid content of the water reaches a certain level, plant and animal life cannot survive.[26] Ironically, acidified lakes and ponds become a crystal-clear deep blue, giving the illusion of beauty and health even as they wreak destruction. Every year, acid deposition destroys millions of trees in Europe and North America. Sugar maples and other trees in the northeastern United States appear to be the newest victims of acid deposition, as they are having difficulty regenerating seedlings destroyed by these deposits. Scientists have concluded that much of the world's forestlands are now experiencing damaging levels of acid deposition.[27]

Acid deposition aggravates and may even cause bronchitis, asthma, and other respiratory problems, and people with emphysema or heart disease may suffer from exposure.[28] It may also be hazardous to fetuses. Acid deposition can cause metals such as aluminum, cadmium, lead, and mercury to **leach** out of the soil. If these metals make their way into water or food supplies, they can cause cancer in humans.

leach To dissolve and filter through soil.

Although there have been substantial reductions in SO_2 and NO_x emissions from power plants that use the fossil fuels coal, gas, and oil in the last decade, full recovery is still years away. Global pressure to reduce use and invest in technology to dramatically reduce emissions from coal production and burning is a key aspect of 2012 global environmental meetings in Rio de Janeiro and in other parts of the world. Although coal is "cleaner" than it was a decade ago from a production standpoint, the idea of "clean coal" is far from reality.[29]

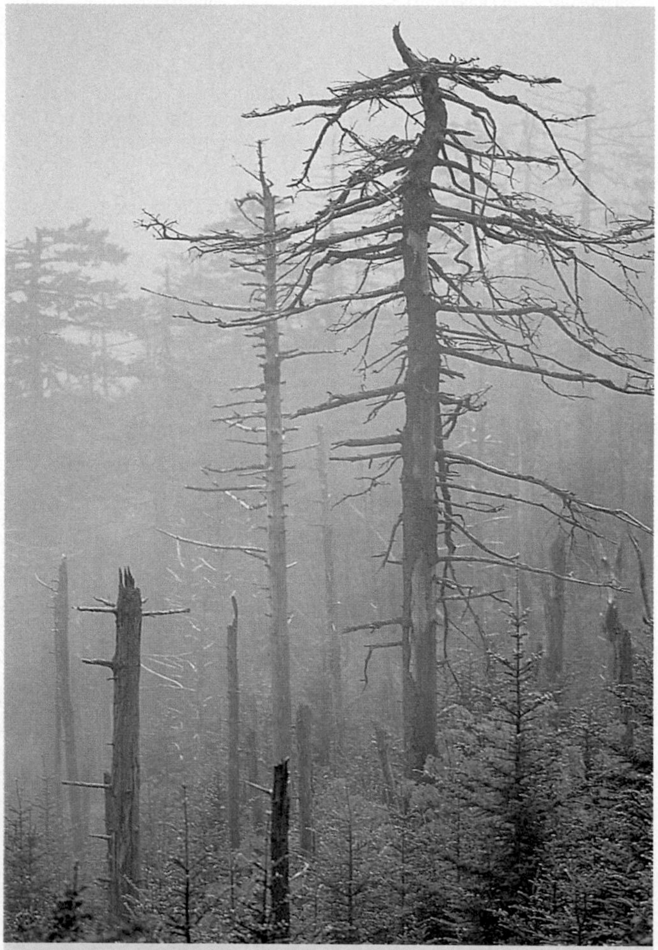

Acid deposition has many harmful effects on the environment. Because its toxins seep into groundwater and enter the food chain, it also poses health hazards to humans.

SKILLS FOR BEHAVIOR CHANGE

SHOPPING TO SAVE THE PLANET

- Look for products with less packaging or with refillable, reusable, or recyclable containers.
- Bring your own reusable cloth grocery bags to the store. Be sure to wash them after transporting uncooked meat, fish, or poultry.
- Buy foods that are produced sustainably.
- Purchase organic foods or foods produced with fewer chemicals and pesticides.
- Do not buy plastic bottles of water. Use a refillable water bottle.
- Do not use caustic cleaning products. Simple vinegar is usually just as effective and less harsh on your home and the environment. Also, many natural products are available.
- Buy laundry products that are free of dyes, fragrances, and sulfates.
- Purchase appliances with the Energy Star logo.
- Use reusable cups, mugs, plates, and utensils rather than disposable products.
- Buy recycled paper products.
- Purchase bed linens and bath towels that are made from bamboo, hemp, or organic cotton.

Indoor Air Pollution

A growing body of scientific evidence indicates that the air within homes and other buildings can be 10 to 40 times more hazardous than outdoor air, even in the most industrialized cities. Potentially dangerous chemical compounds can increase risks of cancer, contribute to respiratory problems, reduce the immune system's ability to fight disease, and increase problems with allergies and allergic reactions. According to a spokesperson for the EPA, "Indoor air pollution causes 50 percent of illnesses globally. That's more than all cancers and heart diseases combined."[30]

Indoor air pollution comes primarily from cooking stoves and furnaces, woodstoves and space heaters, household cleaners and solvents, mold, pesticides, asbestos, formaldehyde, radon, and lead. Today, more and more manufacturers are offering green building products and furnishings, such as natural fiber fabrics, untreated wood for furniture and floors, low-VOC (low-volatile organic compound) paints, and many other products, in an attempt to reduce potential pollutants. See the **Skills for Behavior Change** box for ideas on how to become a more environmentally conscious consumer.

Multiple factors, including age, individual sensitivity, preexisting medical conditions, liver function, and the condition of the immune and respiratory systems contribute to a person's risk for being affected by indoor air pollution.[31] Those with allergies may be particularly vulnerable, as may those living in newer, airtight, energy-efficient homes. Health effects may develop over years of exposure or may occur in response to toxic levels of pollutants. Room temperature and humidity also play a role. **TABLE 20.3** lists major sources of indoor air pollution and possible health effects.

Preventing indoor air pollution should focus on three main areas: *source control* (eliminating or reducing individual contaminants), *ventilation improvements* (increasing the amount of outdoor air coming indoors), and *air cleaners* (removing particulates from the air).[32]

TABLE 20.3 | Health Effects of Indoor Air Pollution

Pollutant	Sources	Health Effects
Asbestos	Deteriorating or damaged insulation; fireproofing, acoustical materials, and floor tiles	Long-term risk of chest and abdominal cancers and lung diseases. Smokers are at higher risk of developing asbestos-induced lung cancer.
Lead	Lead-based paint, contaminated soil, dust, and drinking water	At or above 80 μg/dL of blood (high levels) it can cause convulsions, coma, and death. Lower levels can cause central nervous system, kidney, and blood disorders. Blood lead levels as low as 10 μg/dL can impair mental and physical development.
Radon	Uranium in the soil or rock on which homes are built can lead to air exposure inside. Well water also can be a source.	A major nontobacco cause of lung cancer from air and drinking water exposure; it also has a synergistic effect with smoking exposure.
Environmental tobacco smoke	Smoke from the burning end of cigarettes, pipes, or cigars or smoke exhaled by a smoker; consists of a complex mixture of 4,000+ compounds	Over 40 compounds linked to increased risk of lung cancer; asthma, lower respiratory infections; sudden infant death syndrome (SIDS), and heart disease
Biological contaminants (molds, mildew, viruses, animal dander, cat saliva, dust mites, cockroaches, and pollen)	Improper ventilation and moisture buildup, lack of cleanliness/sanitation, contaminated heating systems, faulty construction, household pets, rodents, insects, damp carpets	Allergic reactions, including hypersensitivity, rhinitis, asthma, infectious illnesses, sneezing, watering eyes, coughing, shortness of breath, dizziness, lethargy, fever, digestive problems
Combustion products	Unvented kerosene heaters, woodstoves, fireplaces, gas stoves	Carbon monoxide causes headaches, dizziness, weakness, nausea, confusion and disorientation, chest pain, death. Nitrogen dioxide causes irritation of nose and eyes, respiratory distress. Particles cause lung damage and irritation.
Benzene	Paint, new carpet, new drapes, upholstery, fast-drying glues, caulks	Headaches, eye/skin irritation, fatigue, cancer
Formaldehyde	Tobacco smoke, plywood, cabinets, furniture, particleboard, new carpet and drapes, wallpaper, ceiling tile, paneling	Headaches, eye/skin irritation, drowsiness, fatigue, respiratory problems, memory loss, depression, gynecological problems, cancer
Chloroform	Paint, new drapes, new carpet, upholstery	Headaches, asthma attacks, dizziness, eye/skin irritations
Toluene	All paper products, most finished wood products	Headaches, eye/skin irritation, sinus problems, dizziness, cancer
Hydrocarbons	Tobacco smoke, gas burners and furnaces	Headaches, fatigue, nausea, dizziness, breathing difficulty
Ammonia	Tobacco smoke, cleaning supplies, animal urine	Eye/skin irritation, headaches, nosebleeds, sinus problems
Trichloroethylene	Paints, glues, caulking, vinyl coatings, wallpaper	Headaches, eye/skin irritation, upper respiratory irritation

Source: U.S. Environmental Protection Agency, "The Inside Story: A Guide to Indoor Air Quality," Updated November 18, 2013, www.epa.gov/iaq/pubs/insidest.html.

Environmental Tobacco Smoke Perhaps the greatest source of indoor air pollution is *environmental tobacco smoke* (*ETS*), also known as secondhand smoke, which contains carbon monoxide and cancer-causing particulates. The level of carbon monoxide in cigarette smoke in enclosed spaces has been found to be 4,000 times higher than that allowed in the clean air standard established by the EPA. Secondhand smoke is made up of more than 7,000 chemicals, hundreds of which are toxic and around 70 of which are carcinogenic.[33] Itchy eyes, breathing difficulties, headaches, nausea, and dizziness often occur in those with sensitivities. Children, the elderly, and those who are ill are especially vulnerable to secondhand smoke. The only truly effective way to eliminate ETS in public places is to enact strict no-smoking policies. Thirty-eight states currently have 100 percent smoking bans in restaurants, and 32 states have total bans in bars.[34] In addition, many major cities and municipalities have banned indoor smoking. To date, as many as 82 percent of U.S. workers have some form of smoking ban in their workplace, and many cities have banned outdoor smoking in public places, including parks and beaches.[35] To protect vulnerable children from smoking parents, bans on smoking in automobiles while children are present are on the increase.

asbestos Mineral compound that separates into stringy fibers and lodges in the lungs, where it can cause disease.

formaldehyde Colorless, strong-smelling gas released through outgassing; causes respiratory and other health problems.

radon Naturally occurring radioactive gas resulting from the decay of certain radioactive elements.

lead Highly toxic metal found in emissions from lead smelters and processing plants; also sometimes found in pipes or paint in older buildings.

Home Heating Woodstoves emit significant levels of particulates and carbon monoxide in addition to other pollutants, such as sulfur dioxide. If you rely on wood for heating, make sure that your stove is properly installed, vented, and maintained. Burning properly seasoned wood reduces particulates. People who rely on oil- or gas-fired furnaces also need to make sure that these appliances are properly installed, ventilated, and maintained. Inexpensive monitors are available to detect high carbon monoxide levels in the home.

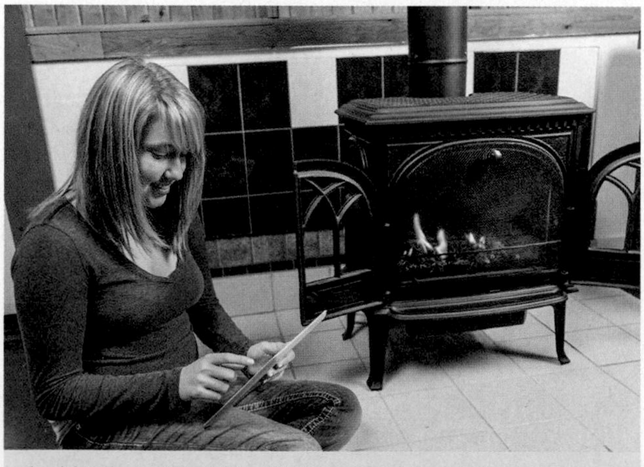

Inside air can be 10 to 40 times more hazardous than outside air. Indoor air pollution comes from woodstoves, furnaces, tobacco smoke, asbestos, formaldehyde, radon, lead, mold, and household chemicals.

WHAT DO YOU THINK?

Think of the products you use each day. How many of these could you do without?

- What options do you have for cleaning products or personal care products that won't pollute the water supply or contaminate the air in your home?

Asbestos The mineral compound **asbestos** was once commonly used in insulating materials and also found its way into vinyl flooring, shingles/roofing materials, heating pipe coverings, and many other products in buildings constructed before 1970. When bonded to other materials, asbestos is relatively harmless, but if its tiny fibers become loosened and airborne, they can embed themselves in the lungs. Their presence leads to cancer of the lungs, stomach, and chest lining and other life-threatening lung diseases called *mesothelioma* and *asbestosis*. If asbestos is detected in the home, it must be removed or sealed off by a professional.

Formaldehyde **Formaldehyde** is a colorless, strong-smelling gas present in some carpets, draperies, furniture, particleboard, plywood, wood paneling, countertops, and many adhesives. It is released into the air in a process called *outgassing*. Outgassing is highest in new products, but the process can continue for many years. Exposure to formaldehyde can cause respiratory problems, dizziness, fatigue, nausea, and rashes. Long-term exposure can lead to central nervous system disorders and cancer. Ask about the formaldehyde content of products you are considering for your home, and avoid those that contain it.

Radon **Radon** is an odorless, colorless gas that penetrates homes through cracks, pipes, or sump pits, and other openings in the basement or foundation. The U.S. Surgeon General warns that radon is the second leading cause of lung cancer, after smoking, each year.[36] The EPA estimates that as many 20,000 lung cancer deaths per year are attributable to excess radon in the home. As many as 1 in 3 homes may have elevated radon levels.[37] Since 1988, the EPA and the Office of the Surgeon General have recommended that homes be tested for radon below the third floor and that Americans test their homes every 2 years or when they move into a new home. Low-cost radon test kits are available online, in hardware stores, and through other retail outlets.

Lead **Lead** is a highly toxic metal common in paints used in many American homes before its banning in 1978. By some estimates, as many as 25 percent of U.S. homes still have lead-based paint hazards, and nearly 535,000 children aged 1 to 5 years old in the United States have blood lead levels that are high.[38] It is also found in batteries, soils, drinking water, older

SKILLS FOR BEHAVIOR CHANGE

AVOIDING MOLD

- Keep the humidity level between 40 and 60 percent.
- Be sure your living space has adequate ventilation, including exhaust fans in the kitchen and bathrooms. If there are no fans, open windows for air circulation when the weather permits.
- Add mold inhibitors to paints or buy paints with mold-resistant properties. If you notice a musty smell, call your landlord. If you see mold, call your landlord!
- Do not carpet bathrooms and basements.
- Use a dehumidifier in damp rooms or basements.
- Many antimold products commonly used on lawns, roofs, and other outdoor areas are extremely toxic and require wearing masks and gloves when applying them. Use them sparingly or not at all.
- Get rid of mattresses and other furniture that may have been exposed to moisture or other situations where slow drying may occur.
- Dry clothing thoroughly before folding and placing in drawers or hanging in closets.
- When buying or renting a house, have a mold inspection performed and check regularly thereafter.

pipes, dishes, and other items. In recent years, toys produced in China and other regions of the world have been recalled owing to unsafe levels of lead. Low-income individuals living in older homes that may not be in compliance with newer recommended levels of lead exposure are at higher risk. Risk in general appears to be greatest during home remodeling and for persons with occupations in fields such as construction, e-waste/recycling, and demolition.[39]

Lead affects the circulatory, reproductive, urinary, kidneys, and nervous systems, and it can accumulate in bone and other tissues. It is particularly detrimental to children and fetuses, and can cause birth defects, learning problems, behavioral abnormalities, and other health problems. To reduce unsafe exposure at home, use water filters, keep areas where children play clean and dust free, regularly wash children's hands and toys, leave lead-based paint undisturbed if it is in good condition, or hire a professional contractor to remove it.

Mold Molds are fungi that live both indoors and outdoors in most regions of the country. They produce tiny reproductive spores, which waft through the indoor and outdoor air. When they land on a damp spot indoors, they may begin growing and digesting whatever they are on, including wood, paper, carpet, and food. In general, molds are harmless; however, some people are sensitive or allergic to them. In such people, exposure to molds may lead to nasal stuffiness, eye irritation, wheezing, or skin irritation. For those who are very sensitive, molds may cause fever or shortness of breath.[40] Before purchasing a home, having a mold inspection is a wise decision. A history of mold can wreak havoc on home values as well as your health. For ways to reduce your exposure to mold, see the **Skills for Behavior Change** box.

Sick Building Syndrome **Sick building syndrome (SBS)** occurs when people occupying a building experience severe health effects correlated to spending time in the building, but no specific source of the effects can be identified.[41] Poor ventilation is a primary cause, along with faulty furnaces, pet dander, mold, and dust. Volatile compounds from products such as hair spray, cleaners, and adhesives can cause problems, as can heavy metals such as lead, particularly in older buildings. Symptoms include eye irritation, sore throat, queasiness, and worsening of asthma.

Indoor air pollution and SBS are increasing concerns in the classroom and workplace. Studies show that significant numbers of U.S. schools have unsatisfactory indoor air quality, often due to poor ventilation, construction techniques that block outside air, and the use of synthetic materials.[42] Long-term exposure to poor air quality can affect student learning as well as trigger allergies, asthma, and other health problems among students.[43]

Ozone Layer Depletion

The ozone layer forms a protective stratum in the stratosphere—the highest level of Earth's atmosphere, located 12 to 30 miles above the surface. The ozone layer protects our planet and its inhabitants from ultraviolet B (UVB) radiation, a primary cause of skin cancer. Such radiation damages DNA and weakens immune systems.

In the 1970s, scientists began to warn of a breakdown in the ozone layer. Instruments developed to test atmospheric contents indicated that certain chemicals, especially **chlorofluorocarbons (CFCs)**, were contributing to the ozone layer's rapid depletion. The U.S. government banned the use of aerosol sprays containing CFCs in the 1970s. The discovery of an ozone "hole" over Antarctica led to treaties whereby the United States and other nations agreed to further reduce the use of CFCs and other ozone-depleting chemicals. Today, more than 197 United Nations countries have agreed to basic protocols designed to preserve and protect the ozone layer.[44] Although the ban on CFCs is believed to be responsible for slowing the depletion of the ozone layer, some CFC replacements may also be damaging because they contribute to the **enhanced greenhouse effect.**

sick building syndrome (SBS) Describes a situation in which occupants of a building experience acute health effects linked to time spent in a building, but no specific illness or cause can be identified

chlorofluorocarbons (CFCs) Chemicals that contribute to the depletion of the atmospheric ozone layer.

enhanced greenhouse effect Warming of the earth's surface due to increases in greenhouse gas concentration in the atmosphere, which traps more of the sun's radiation than is normal.

LO 3 | CLIMATE CHANGE

Explain climate change and global warming, the underlying causes of each, impacts on health, and key actions for reducing risks.

Climate change refers to a shift in typical weather patterns across the world. These changes can include fluctuations in seasonal temperatures, rain or snowfall amounts, and the occurrence of catastrophic storms. **Global warming** is a type of climate change in which average temperatures increase. Over 97 percent of scientists now agree the planet is warming, and over the last 50 years, this warming has been driven largely by the burning of fossil fuels.[45] Over the last 100 years, the average temperature of the earth has increased by 1.5°F, with projections of another 2° to 11.5°F rise in the next 100 years.[46] According to the National Aeronautics and Space Administration (NASA), the National Oceanic and Atmospheric Administration (NOAA), and the National Research Council, climate change poses major risks to lives, and excess **greenhouse gases** are a key culprit.[47] The *greenhouse effect* is a natural phenomenon in which greenhouse gases such as carbon dioxide, nitrous oxide, methane, CFCs, and hydrocarbons form a layer in the atmosphere, allowing solar heat to pass through and trapping some of the heat close to the surface, where it warms the planet (**FIGURE 20.4**). Excess carbon dioxide accounts for 82 percent of greenhouse gases emitted through human activity in the United States.[48]

climate change A shift in typical weather patterns that includes fluctuations in seasonal temperatures, rain or snowfall amounts, and the occurrence of catastrophic storms.

global warming A type of climate change in which average temperatures increase.

greenhouse gases Gases that accumulate in the atmosphere, where they contribute to global warming by trapping heat near the earth's surface.

Scientific Evidence of Climate Change and Human-Caused Global Warming

According to data from U.S. and international sources, climate responds to changes in naturally occurring greenhouse gases as well as solar output and the earth's orbit; however, recent

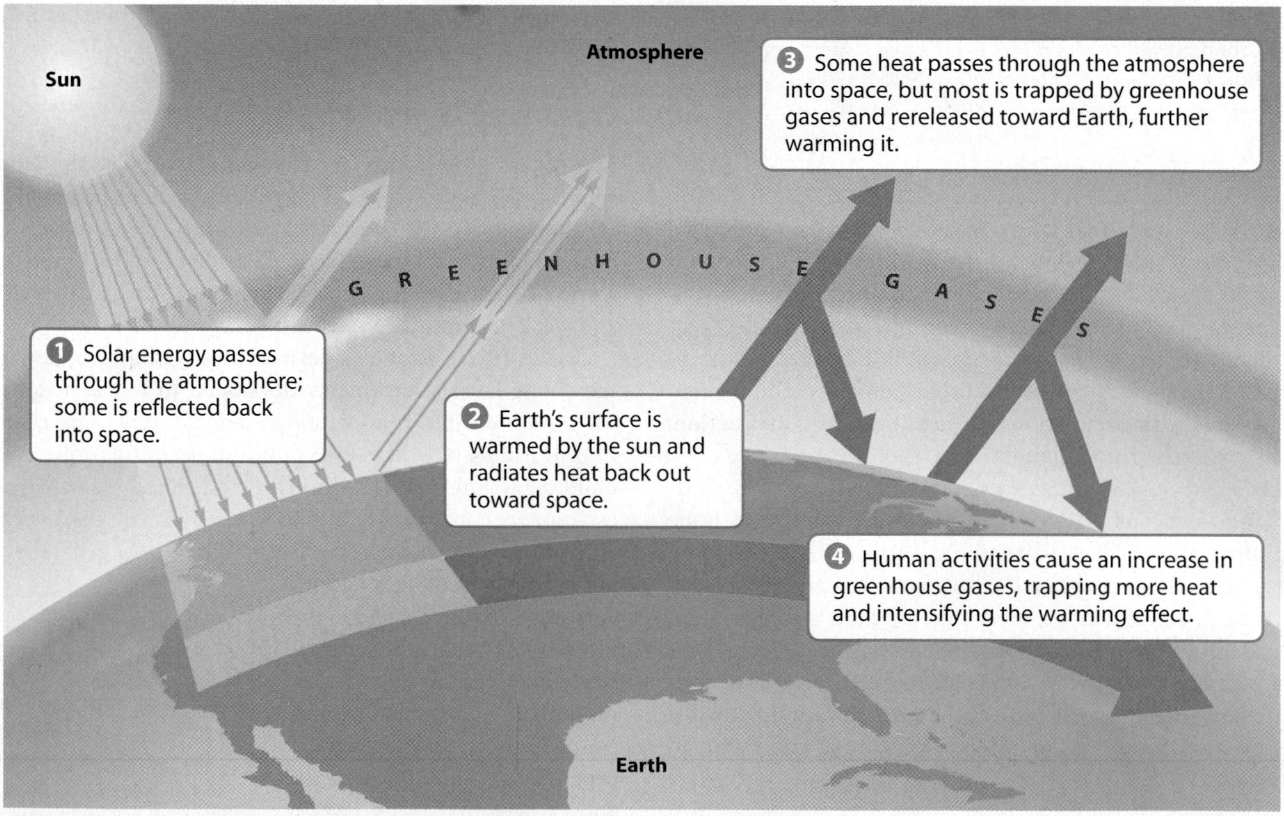

FIGURE 20.4 The Enhanced Greenhouse Effect The natural greenhouse effect is responsible for making Earth habitable; it keeps the planet 33°C (60°F) warmer than it would otherwise be. An increase in greenhouse gases resulting from human activity is creating the *enhanced greenhouse effect*, trapping more heat and causing dangerous global climate change.

Source: OzCoasts (Geoscience Australia), "The enhanced greenhouse effect (Global warming)," 2013, http://www.ozcoasts.gov.au/indicators/greenhouse_effect.jsp.

VIDEO TUTOR
Enhanced Greenhouse Effect

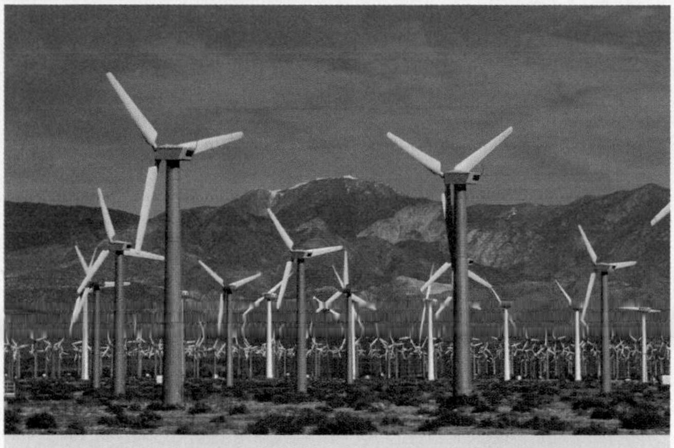

By reducing your use of fossil fuels, using high-efficiency vehicles, and supporting increased use of renewable resources such as solar, wind, and water power, you can help combat global warming.

evidence points to unusual changes in climate that go beyond predictable natural causes. So, what evidence do we have that climate change and global warming are real and human activity is a major contributor? Consider the following:[49]

- Global sea levels rose 6.7 inches in the last 100 years, mostly in the last decade. With accelerated glacial and ice sheet melts, this rise is likely to increase dramatically.
- Since 1981, 20 of the warmest years ever have occurred, and all of the 10 warmest years have been during the last 12 years.
- Greenland is losing 36 to 60 cubic miles of ice per year; Antarctica is losing 36 cubic miles of ice per year.
- Glaciers are receding at unprecedented and rapid rates.

Multiple reconstructions of the earth's climate history show that the amounts of greenhouse gases in the atmosphere went up dramatically around the time of the industrial revolution—when humans began burning fossil fuels on a large scale—and correlates very closely with temperature increases.[50] Studies also indicate that large changes in climate can occur in decades rather than centuries or thousands of years.[51]

Reducing the Threat of Global Warming

Climate change problems are largely rooted in our energy, transportation, and industrial practices.[52] However, the problem isn't just one of increased CO_2 production. Rapid deforestation contributes to the rise in greenhouse gases. Trees take in carbon dioxide, transform it, store the carbon for food, and release oxygen into the air. As we lose forests at the rate of hundreds of acres per hour, we lose the capacity to store and dissipate carbon dioxide.[53] Population increases and human destruction of natural resources pose additional threats.

SEE IT! VIDEOS

How is climate change affecting the weather during winter? Watch **Snowstorms in the Forecast** available on MasteringHealth.™

Toward Sustainable Development

To slow climate change, most experts agree that reducing consumption of fossil fuels, shifting to alternative energy sources, and using mass transportation are all crucial, but clean energy, green factories, improved energy efficiency, and governmental regulation are also key. The United Nations Conference on Sustainable Development (known as RIO+20) took place in 2012 in Rio de Janeiro and outlined a plan for protecting the environment (called "The World We Want") through **sustainable development**—development that meets the needs of the present without compromising the needs of future generations.[54] However, leaders of many nations, including the United States, France, Germany, and the United Kingdom, opted not to attend, and the resulting plan includes a list of general goals to work toward, but without the "teeth" necessary to motivate nations to comply with sustainable development needs.

Promising Trends?

Although getting the nations of the world to come up with a plan that all can work toward may seem a bit like "herding cats," some glimmers of progress by individual nations may be occurring. In 2012, some of the major CO_2-emitting countries contributed to what appears to be a "slowing" of this trend. In fact, after years of double-digit carbon emission increases, overall emissions increased only about 1.1 percent. The United States had a 12 percent reduction in coal and a shift to cleaner burning natural gas in 2013.[55] More wind, solar, and bioenergy use, reductions in natural gas prices, more strict emission standards, and public concerns about smog and pollution are likely reasons for these improvements in many regions.[56] Although stricter laws on vehicular carbon emissions and the development of cars that operate on electricity, hydrogen, biodiesel, ethanol, or other alternative energy sources are promising, we have a long way to go to reduce fossil fuel consumption. While hybrid cars often use much less gasoline, in areas where coal is the major source of electricity, issues arise as to whether using coal for electricity rather than gas really makes a car "green."

Many communities and campuses have established plans to reduce their carbon footprint. Creating user-friendly bicycle lanes and monitored bike garages to prevent theft/vandalism, and holding "bike to work" days, motivate students to leave cars at home. Some campuses have raised fees for parking permits in the hopes of discouraging students from bringing cars to campus. You can participate in this effort by finding ways to reduce your own **carbon footprint**, or the amount of CO_2 emissions you contribute to the atmosphere in your daily life.

sustainable development Development that meets the needs of the present without compromising the ability of future generations to meet their own needs.

carbon footprint Amount of greenhouse gases produced, usually expressed in equivalent tons of carbon dioxide emissions.

LO 4 | WATER POLLUTION AND SHORTAGES

Identify sources of pollution and chemical contaminants often found in water.

Seventy-five percent of Earth is covered with water, but only 2.5 percent of all Earth's water is drinkable freshwater.[57] Approximately 1.2 percent of freshwater is surface water that comes from lakes, ground ice, swamps, marshes, rivers, and soil moisture.[58] Another 30.1 percent is groundwater from underwater wells and aquifers, and the rest of the freshwater (68.7 percent) is locked in glaciers and ice caps.[59] We draw our drinking water from groundwater and surface water; however, much of this water is too polluted or too difficult to reach.[60]

We cannot take the safety of our water supply for granted. Over half the global population faces a shortage of clean water. More than 2.6 billion people, about 40 percent of the planet's population, have no access to basic sanitation or adequate toilet facilities. More than 1 billion have no access to clean water, and more than 4,500 children die every day from illnesses caused by lack of safe water and sanitation.[61] Water issues will only get worse, as demand for freshwater is projected to exceed current supply by over 40 percent by 2030, increasing competition for scarce reserves and posing a major risk to global food supplies, energy supplies, and human survival.[62] Some areas of the world will be at high risk due to extended drought, population increases, and dwindling supply. Poor sanitation, consumer waste, agricultural enterprises and development in areas that are historically arid, and public apathy all add to the burden.[63] The **Skills for Behavior Change** box presents simple conservation measures that you can adopt to save water where you live.

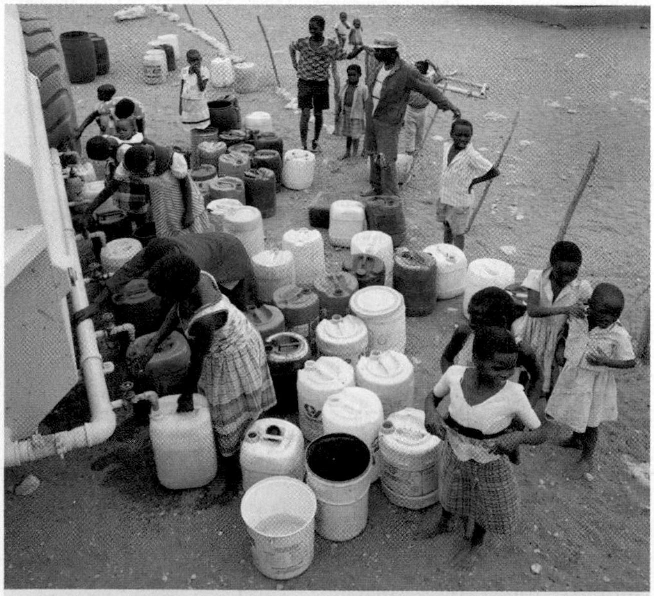

The lack of clean water and sanitation is a major global problem. *Closed basins* are regions where existing water cannot meet the agricultural, industrial, municipal, and environmental needs. The Stockholm International Water Institute estimates that 1.4 billion people live in a closed basin, and the problem is worsening.

SKILLS FOR BEHAVIOR CHANGE

WASTE LESS WATER!

IN THE KITCHEN

- Turn off the tap while washing dishes. Use only half a sink full, and don't run rinse water until you need it.
- Repair leaky pipes and faucets. More than 3,000 gallons of water each year are lost to leaks.
- Equip faucets with aerators to reduce water use by 4 percent.
- Run dishwashers only when they are full, and use the energy-saving mode.

IN THE LAUNDRY ROOM

- Ask yourself, "can I wear this again before washing?" If you didn't sweat in it, soil it, or get it smelly, hang it in "the not quite clean" section of your closet and wear it again.
- Wash only full loads or use a washing machine that adjusts to allow a reduced water level for smaller loads. Use cold water whenever possible to save energy. Upgrade to a high-efficiency washer to use 30 percent less water per load and run the shortest cycle.
- Limit the use of the dryer and line dry clothing when possible. Buy a drying rack for your room.
- Buy soaps that are dye free, fragrance free, and biodegradable whenever possible.

IN THE BATHROOM

- Detect and fix leaks. A leaky toilet can waste about 200 gallons of water per day.
- Replace old toilets with a high-efficiency models that use 60 to 80 percent less water per flush.
- Take showers instead of baths, and limit showers to the time it takes to lather up and rinse off. Ideally, get wet, shut off water, lather up, and turn on water to rinse.
- Replace old showerheads with efficient models that use 60 percent less water per minute.
- Turn off the tap while brushing your teeth to save up to 8 gallons of water per day.

Water Contamination

Any substance that gets into the soil can potentially enter the water supply. Industrial pollutants and pesticides eventually work their way into the soil, then into groundwater. Underground storage tanks for gasoline may leak. U.S. Geological Survey researchers discovered the presence of low levels of many chemical compounds in a network of 139 targeted

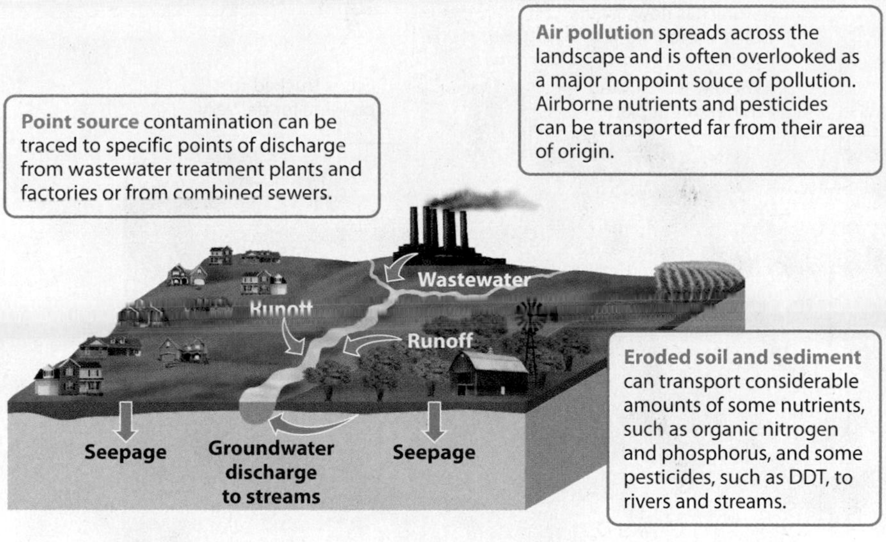

Point source contamination can be traced to specific points of discharge from wastewater treatment plants and factories or from combined sewers.
Air pollution spreads across the landscape and is often overlooked as a major nonpoint souce of pollution. Airborne nutrients and pesticides can be transported far from their area of origin.
Wastewater
Runoff
Runoff
Eroded soil and sediment can transport considerable amounts of some nutrients, such as organic nitrogen and phosphorus, and some pesticides, such as DDT, to rivers and streams.
Seepage
Groundwater discharge to streams
Seepage

FIGURE 20.5 Potential Sources of Groundwater Contamination

Source: Adapted from U.S. Geological Survey, Wisconsin Water Science Center, "Learn More about Groundwater," 2008, http://wi.water.usgs.gov/gwcomp/learn.

streams across the United States. Steroids, pharmaceuticals, personal care products, hormones, insect repellent, and wastewater compounds were all detected.[64]

Tap water in the United States is among the safest in the world. The Safe Drinking Water Act (SDWA) is the main federal law that ensures the quality of Americans' drinking water. Under the SDWA, the EPA sets standards for drinking water quality and oversees the states, localities, and water suppliers who implement those standards. Cities and municipalities have strict policies and procedures governing water treatment, filtration, and disinfection to screen out pathogens and microorganisms. However, their ability to filter out increasing amounts of chemical by-products and other substances is in question. According to a recent study of over 50 large wastewater sites in the United States, over half of the samples tested positive for at least 25 of the 56 prescription and over-the-counter drugs monitored![65] These levels of drugs have been shown to have significant effects on aquatic life; however, more research needs to be done to examine human risks, particularly for more vulnerable populations.[66]

Congress has coined two terms that describe general sources of water pollution. **Point source pollutants** enter a waterway at a specific location through a pipe, ditch, culvert, or other conduit. The major sources of point source pollution are sewage treatment plants and industrial facilities. **Nonpoint source pollutants**—commonly known as *runoff* and *sedimentation*—drain or seep into waterways from broad areas of land. Nonpoint source pollution results from a variety of land use practices, including soil erosion and sedimentation, construction and engineering project wastes, pesticide and fertilizer runoff, urban street runoff, acid mine drainage, septic tank leakage, and sewage sludge (**FIGURE 20.5**).

SEE IT! VIDEOS

Is bottled water better for you? Watch **Americans' Obsession with Bottled Water** available on MasteringHealth.™

Pollutants causing the greatest potential harm are the following:

- **Gasoline and petroleum products.** There are more than 2 million underground storage tanks for gasoline and petroleum products in the United States, most located at gasoline filling stations.[67] Tank leaks allow petroleum to contaminate the ground and water. Fortunately, cleanup procedures have reduced this contamination dramatically in the last decade, with over 70 percent compliance among violators.[68]
- **Chemical contaminants.** *Organic solvents* are chemicals designed to dissolve grease and oil. These extremely toxic substances are used to clean clothing, painting equipment, plastics, and metal parts. Consumers often dump leftover products into the toilet or into street drains. Industries pour leftovers into barrels, which are then buried. Eventually, the chemicals eat through the barrels and leach into groundwater. Hydraulic fracturing, more commonly known as *fracking*, is a method of extracting natural gas from the ground by forcing pressurized liquids into underground rock, allowing oil and gas to flow to the surface for extraction.[69] Chemicals used in fracking pose the risk of contaminating underground wells, surface waters, and aquifers.[70] (See **FIGURE 20.6**.)
- **Polychlorinated biphenyls.** Fire resistant and stable at high temperatures, **polychlorinated biphenyls (PCBs)** were used for many years as insulating materials in high-voltage electrical equipment, such as transformers and older fluorescent lights. The human body does not excrete ingested PCBs but rather stores them in the liver and fatty tissues. PCB exposure is associated with birth defects, cancer, and skin problems. As of 1977, PCBs are no longer manufactured in the United States, but approximately 500 million pounds have been dumped into landfills and waterways, where they continue to pose an environmental threat.[71]
- **Dioxins.** **Dioxins** are found in herbicides (chemicals used to kill vegetation) and are produced during certain industrial processes. Dioxins have the ability to accumulate in

point source pollutant Pollutant that enters waterways at a specific location.

nonpoint source pollutant Pollutant that runs off or seeps into waterways from broad areas of land.

polychlorinated biphenyls (PCBs) Toxic chemicals that were once used as insulating materials in high-voltage electrical equipment.

dioxins Highly toxic chlorinated hydrocarbons contained in herbicides and produced during certain industrial processes.

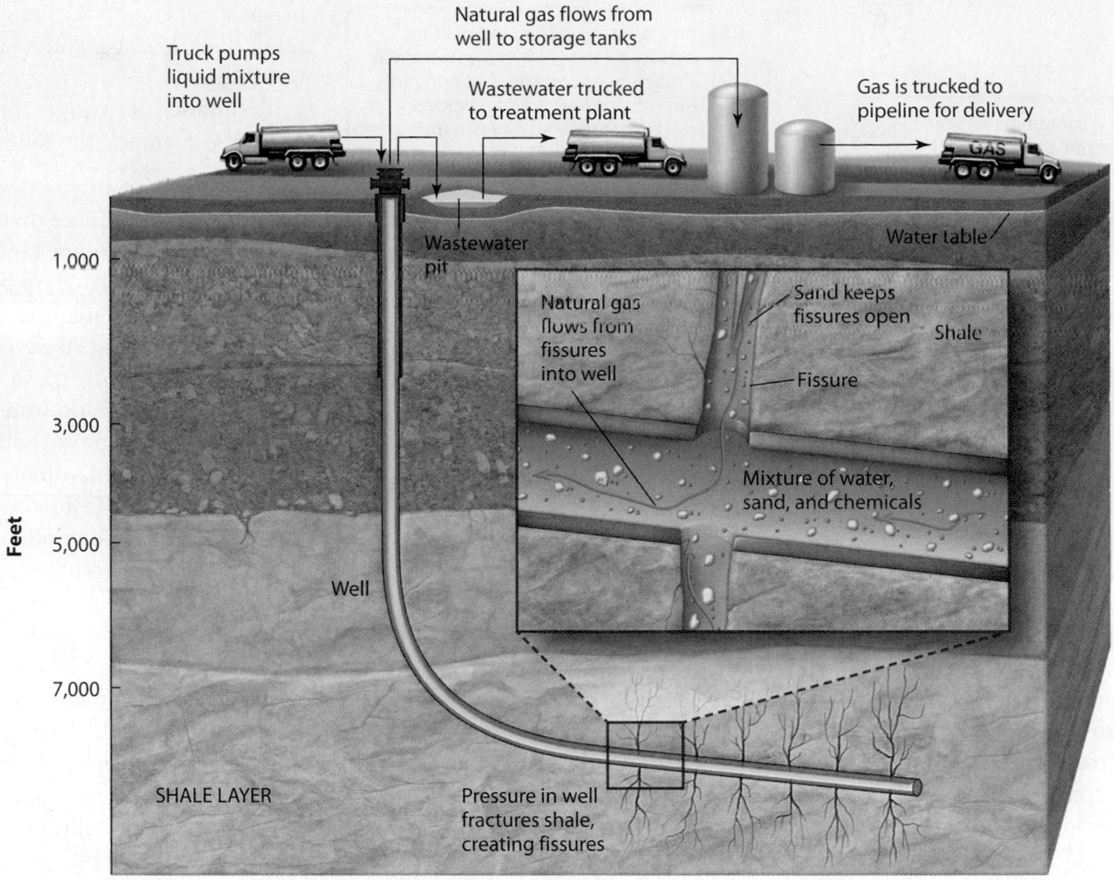
Natural gas flows from well to storage tanks
Truck pumps liquid mixture into well
Wastewater trucked to treatment plant
Gas is trucked to pipeline for delivery
GAS
Water table
Wastewater pit
1,000
3,000
5,000
7,000
Feet
Natural gas flows from fissures into well
Sand keeps fissures open
Shale
Fissure
Mixture of water, sand, and chemicals
Well
SHALE LAYER
Pressure in well fractures shale, creating fissures

FIGURE 20.6 Hydraulic Fracturing (Fracking)

Source: Adapted from schematic found in "Potential Relationships Between Hydraulic Fracturing and Drinking Water Resources," U.S. Environmental Protection Agency, 2010, http://www.epa.gov/ogwdw/uic/pdfs/presentations_hf_public_meetings_presentation.pdf.

the body and are much more toxic than PCBs. Long-term effects include possible immune system damage and increased risk of infections and cancer. Exposure to high concentrations of PCBs or dioxins for a short period of time can also have severe consequences, including nausea, vomiting, diarrhea, painful rashes and sores, and chloracne, an ailment in which the skin develops hard, black, painful pimples that may never heal.

- **Pesticides.** **Pesticides** are chemicals designed to kill insects, rodents, plants, and fungi. Americans use more than a billion pounds of pesticides each year, the majority of which settle on the land and in our air and water.[72] Pesticides evaporate readily and are often dispersed by winds over a large area or carried out to sea. In tropical regions, many farmers use pesticides heavily, and the climate promotes their rapid release into the atmosphere. Pesticide residues cling to fruits and vegetables and can accumulate in the body. Potential hazards associated with exposure to pesticides include birth defects, liver and kidney damage, and nervous system disorders.

pesticides Chemicals that kill pests such as insects or rodents.

municipal solid waste (MSW) Solid waste such as durable and nondurable goods, containers and packaging, food waste, yard waste, and miscellaneous waste from residential, commercial, institutional, and industrial sources.

LO 5 | LAND POLLUTION

Distinguish between municipal solid waste and hazardous waste and list strategies for reducing land pollution.

Much of the waste that ends up polluting water starts out polluting the land. Growing population creates more pressure on the land to accommodate increasing amounts of refuse, much of which is nonbiodegradable and some of which is directly harmful to living organisms.

Solid Waste

Each day, every person in the United States generates nearly 4.4 pounds of **municipal solid waste (MSW)**, more commonly known as trash or garbage, totaling about 251 million tons of

251 MILLION

TONS OF MUNICIPAL SOLID **WASTE** WAS GENERATED IN THE U.S. IN 2012.

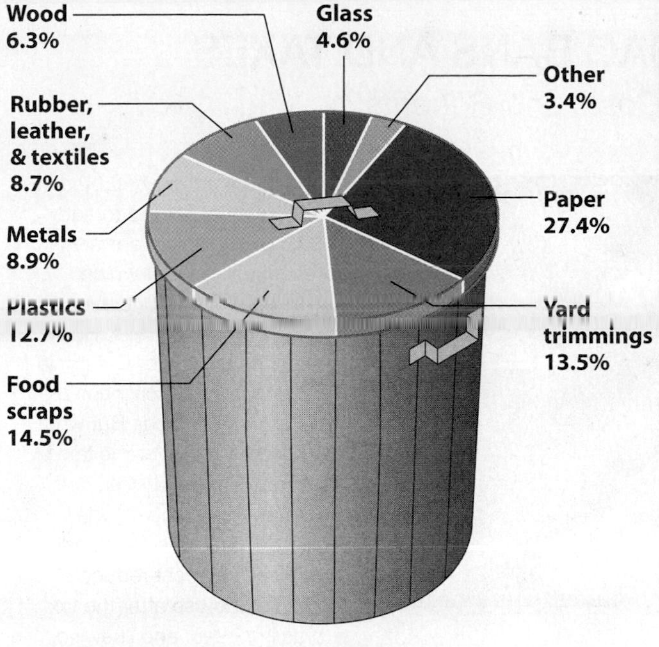

Wood 6.3%
Glass 4.6%
Other 3.4%
Rubber, leather, & textiles 8.7%
Paper 27.4%
Metals 8.9%
Plastics 12.7%
Yard trimmings 13.5%
Food scraps 14.5%

FIGURE 20.7 What's in Our Trash?

Source: Data are from U.S. Environmental Protection Agency, *Municipal Solid Waste Generation, Recycling, and Disposal in the United States: Facts and Figures for 2012*, EPA-530-F-14-001, February 2014, www.epa.gov/wastes/nonhaz/municipal/pubs/msw_2012_rev_factsheet.pdf.

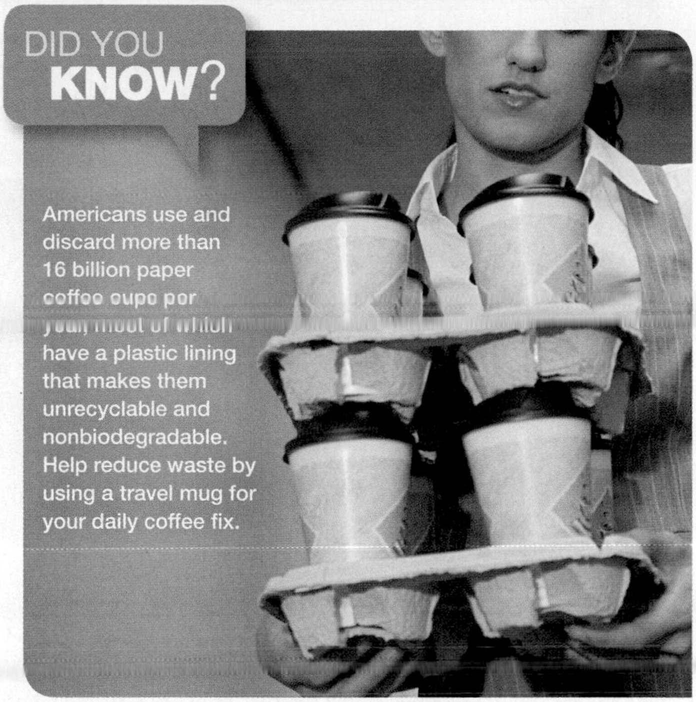

trash each year, with organic materials making up the largest share. Paperboard accounts for just over 27 percent, and yard trimmings and food scraps account for another 28 percent (**FIGURE 20.7**).[73]

Although we recycle only slightly over one-third of the waste we generate, experts believe we could recycle up to 90 percent of trash (**FIGURE 20.8**).[74] Currently, 34.8 percent of all MSW in the United States is recycled or composted, over 14 percent is burned at combustion facilities, and the remaining 54 percent is disposed of in landfills.[75]

The number of U.S. landfills has actually decreased in the past decade, but their sheer mass has increased. Many people worry that we are rapidly losing our ability to dispose of all of the waste we create. As communities run out of landfill space, it is becoming common to haul garbage to other states or to dump it illegally in woods, waterways, or oceans, where it contaminates ecosystems, or to ship it to landfills in developing countries, where it becomes someone else's problem. In today's throwaway society, we need to become aware of the amount of waste we generate and to look for ways to recycle, reuse, and—most desirable of all—reduce what we consume.

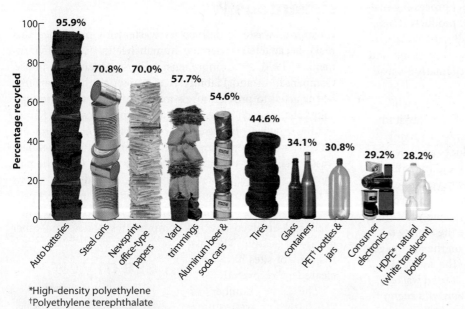

Percentage recycled
100
80
60
40
20
0
95.9%
70.8%
70.0%
57.7%
54.6%
44.6%
34.1%
30.8%
29.2%
28.2%
Auto batteries
Steel cans
Newsprint, office-type papers
Yard trimmings
Aluminum beer & soda cans
Tires
Glass containers
PET† bottles & jars
Consumer electronics
HDPE* natural (white translucent) bottles
*High-density polyethylene
†Polyethylene terephthalate

FIGURE 20.8 How Much Do We Recycle?

Source: Data are from U.S. Environmental Protection Agency, *Municipal Solid Waste Generation, Recycling, and Disposal in the United States: Facts and Figures for 2012*, EPA-530-F-14-001, February 2014, www.epa.gov/wastes/nonhaz/municipal/pubs/msw_2012_rev_factsheet.pdf.

Communities, businesses, and individuals can adopt several strategies to reduce MSW:

- *Source reduction (waste prevention)* involves altering the design, manufacture, or use of products and materials to reduce the amount and toxicity of waste. The most effective waste-reducing strategy is preventing waste from being generated in the first place. Do we really need to buy products that have three outer shells of plastic? Consumers can help by boycotting such packaging strategies. See the **Money & Health** box on plastic bag bans and use taxes.

MONEY & HEALTH | PLASTIC BAG BANS AND TAXES

What Are the Costs and Benefits?

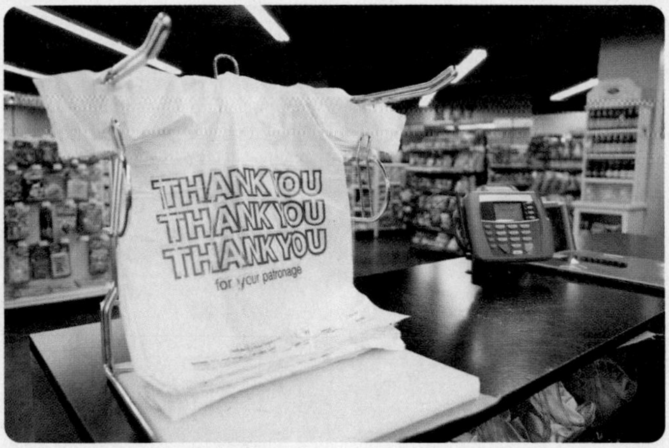

There is a growing list of places across the United States that have enacted taxes or bans on plastic bags at the checkout counter or fees for paper bags when you fail to bring in your own bags. In September 2014, California became the first state to totally ban plastic bags. Complete or partial bans are increasing in cities and states throughout the U.S. Proponents of the bans and taxes say plastic bags are bad for the environment because they are made from nonbiodegradable petroleum, are infrequently recycled, and are commonly littered, ending up in waterways where they become a wildlife hazard. When thrown away as trash, they sit in landfills for decades. But how do bag bans and taxes impact our wallets?

Many locations with bag taxes require stores to charge customers a nominal fee, often a nickel per single-use plastic bag. By contrast, reusable cloth bags are usually sold for several dollars apiece. Of course, the upfront costs of the reusable bags are recouped over time.

How much tax revenue is collected by communities with bag taxes varies widely. In Washington, DC, a 5-cent disposable bag tax at grocery, convenience, and liquor stores instituted in 2010 was expected to add $3.6 million to government revenues, most of which was earmarked for cleanup efforts on a local river. However, the District of Columbia reported the tax only netted $2 million that year. But what wasn't so good for the tax coffers appeared to pay off for the environment: One survey of DC residents indicated 75 percent reduced plastic bag use after the tax was imposed, and likewise, local businesses reported that bag use was down about 50 percent.

Sources: "D.C. Bag Tax Nets $2 Million," Associated Press, January 5, 2011, http://voices.washingtonpost.com/local-breaking-news/dc/dc-bag-tax-nets-2m.html; Alice Ferguson Foundation, "Public Perceptions and Willingness to Address Litter in the District of Columbia," funded by Washington's District Department of Environment (DDOE), 2011, www.fergusonfoundation.org/trash_initiative/AFF_DC_%20ResearchMemo021511.pdf.

- *Recycling* involves sorting, collecting, and processing materials to be reused in manufacturing new products. This process diverts items such as paper, cardboard, glass, plastic, and metals from the waste stream. Be responsible and recycle everything that is recyclable, particularly e-waste and paper.
- *Composting* involves collecting organic waste, such as food scraps and yard trimmings, and allowing it to decompose with the help of microorganisms (mainly bacteria and fungi). This process produces a nutrient-rich substance used to fertilize gardens and for soil enhancement. Many communities now have yard carts that allow you to mix your food scraps in with yard trimmings. Find out what options are available in your area. Not all organic waste is composted; see the **Money & Health** box on the next page for more on the cost and prevalence of food waste.
- *Combustion with energy recovery* typically involves the use of boilers and industrial furnaces to incinerate waste and use the burning process to generate energy.

hazardous waste Toxic waste that poses a hazard to humans or to the environment.

Superfund Fund established under the Comprehensive Environmental Response, Compensation, and Liability Act to be used for cleaning up toxic waste dumps.

Hazardous Waste

Hazardous waste is defined as waste with properties that make it capable of harming human health or the environment. In 1980, the Comprehensive Environmental Response, Compensation and Liability Act, known as the **Superfund**, was enacted to provide funds for cleaning up what are typically "abandoned" hazardous waste dump sites. This Superfund is financed by taxes on the chemical and petroleum industries, payments by those responsible for dumping waste, federal tax revenues, and other sources. Over the past three decades, the Superfund has located and assessed tens of thousands of hazardous waste sites, worked to protect people and the environment from contamination at the worst sites, and involved affected communities, states, and other groups in cleanup. The vast majority of sites have been cleared or "recovered."[76]

The large number of U.S. hazardous waste dump sites indicates the severity of our toxic chemical problem. American manufacturers and individuals

SEE IT! VIDEOS

What do those numbers on the bottoms of plastic bottles mean? Watch **Crack Those Recycling Codes** available on MasteringHealth.™

MONEY & HEALTH | ARE YOU A FOOD WASTER?

At a time when starvation, hunger, and food insecurity plague people throughout the world, a new study by Britain's Institute of Mechanical Engineers indicates that *up to half of the food produced worldwide never makes it into consumer's mouths*. Over 2 billion tons of food could feed millions, but never reaches them.

Global consumer behaviors in more affluent nations are responsible for much of the waste. Big box stores that promote "bigger size is cheaper" entice people to buy more than they can eat before it spoils. Freezers in homes encourage waste as food dries up before it is eaten, while other food sits on shelves until past its expiration date.

It isn't just our behaviors that contribute to the waste, however. When fresh produce is in surplus and demand is low, crops languish in fields. If weather or insects cause produce to be blemished, we reject it in stores and it is tossed in the trash. Americans are among the worst of the food wasters, wasting over 40 percent of all edible food. The average person in the United States dumps about 20 pounds of food each month, equivalent to between $28 and $43 per month. If we cut our food waste by just 15 percent, some estimate 26 million food-insecure people in the United States could be fed.

From an environmental perspective, when we waste food, we waste all of the time, effort, and resources that went into production and put unnecessary stress on the environment. By wasting less, we put less pressure on our vulnerable habitat.

What can you do?

- Be a better food planner. Make a list when shopping, and only buy what you will use.
- Buy locally.
- Don't be picky. Buy fruit and vegetables even if they don't have a perfect shape, and eat them before they rot.
- Eat leftovers. Make a rule that you can't buy fast food or eat out when there is good food in your fridge.
- Eat lower on the food chain. By eating more vegetables, nuts, legumes, and other food crops, and reducing consumption of meat, dairy, and other animal products, you have a smaller footprint stomping on the planet.

Sources: Institute of Mechanical Engineers, "Global Food: Waste Not, Want Not," 2013, Available at www.imeche.org; J. Bloom, *American Wasteland* (Cambridge: DeCapo Press, 2010); National Resource Defense Council, "Food Facts: Your Scraps Add Up," March 2013, www.nrdc.org.

WHAT DO YOU THINK?

Do you know people who throw away recyclable items rather than recycling them?

- What do you think motivates their behavior?
- How might you encourage them to recycle more than they do now?

generate around 40 million tons of hazardous waste each year, including commercial chemical refuse, solvents and oils, petroleum refining by-products, and household wastes such as batteries, cleaning products, and paints.[77] Many wastes are now banned from land disposal or are being treated to reduce their toxicity before they become part of land disposal sites. The EPA has developed protective requirements for land disposal facilities, such as double liners, detection systems for substances that may leach into groundwater, and groundwater-monitoring systems.

LO 6 | RADIATION

List and explain key health concerns associated with ionizing and nonionizing radiation.

Radiation is energy that travels in waves or particles. There are many different types of radiation, ranging from radio waves to gamma rays, all making up the electromagnetic spectrum. Exposure to radiation is an inescapable part of life on this planet, but only some of it poses a threat to human health.

Nonionizing Radiation

Nonionizing radiation is radiation at the lower end of the electromagnetic spectrum. This radiation moves in relatively long wavelengths and has enough energy to move atoms around or cause them to vibrate, but not enough to alter molecular structure. Examples of nonionizing radiation are radio waves, TV signals, microwaves, infrared waves, and visible light. Concerns have been raised about the safety of radio frequency waves generated by cell phones (see the **Health Headlines** box on the next page).

Ionizing Radiation

Ionizing radiation is caused by the release of particles and electromagnetic rays from atomic nuclei during the normal process of disintegration. This type of radiation has enough energy to remove electrons from the atoms it passes through. Some naturally occurring elements, such as uranium, emit ionizing radiation. The sun is another source of ionizing radiation, in the form of high-frequency ultraviolet rays—those against which the ozone layer protects us.

nonionizing radiation Electromagnetic waves having relatively long wavelengths and enough energy to move atoms around or cause them to vibrate.

ionizing radiation Electromagnetic waves and particles having short wavelengths and energy high enough to ionize atoms.

HEALTH HEADLINES

E-CONCERNS

Given that cell phone use has skyrocketed and billions of people are hanging out with their phones 24/7, only the most apathetic wouldn't be concerned about *radio (RF) frequency*. But what is the real risk? In theory, RF energy has the potential to penetrate the skull, neck, and upper torso. For the very young, whose skulls have not yet sufficiently hardened, the risk might be even greater. However, after over a decade of research trying to prove a solid link between cell phone use and some type of disease, very little conclusive evidence exists. More research looking at superusers may provide the missing link. In the interim, it makes good sense to use caution. Go hands free. Check out the specific absorption rate (SAR) charts online or from your phone company before buying.

Cable or satellite TV box guzzling your electricity? While you are in class, out to dinner, or in bed sound asleep, your cable box is using more electricity than almost any appliance in your house! Surprised by that? A recent report indicates that a set-top cable or satellite box can consume as much as 35 watts of power and cost about $8.00 a month in certain regions of the country. It is estimated that the nearly quarter of a million boxes currently in U.S. homes use as much electricity together as four nuclear power plants generate. Even when turned off, hard drives keep running, downloading, and updating. Unplugging can help, but depending on location, it can require a long reboot when you want to use the system. The answer might be to use fewer boxes in your home or do more streaming on lower-energy-use devices such as laptops.

The global burden of e-waste (trashed computers, televisions, and other electronic devices) has also skyrocketed in recent years. Although there are many avenues for disposing of items like cell phones, hang on to your TV, phone, or other device for as long as possible. "Use it and *don't* lose it," so to speak. When you are thinking about *e-recycling*, check out www.ecyclingcentral.com for a state-by-state listing of e-recyclers in your area.

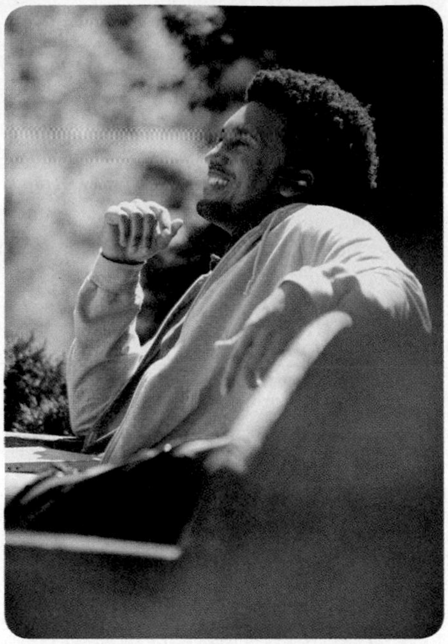

A hands-free device lets you keep your phone—and any radio-frequency energy it may emit—away from your head.

Sources: National Cancer Institute, Factsheet, "Cell Phones and Cancer Risk," 2013, www.cancer.gov/cancertopics/factsheet/Risk/cellphones; R. Vartabedian, "Cable TV Boxes Become 2nd Biggest Energy Users in Many Homes," *LA Times*, June 19, 2014, www.latimes.com/nation/la-na-power-hog-20140617-story.html#page=1.

Radiation exposure is measured in **radiation absorbed doses** or **rads** (also called *roentgens*). Radiation can cause damage at dosages as low as 100 to 200 rads. At this level, signs of radiation sickness include nausea, diarrhea, fatigue, anemia, sore throat, and hair loss. At 350 to 500 rads, these symptoms become more severe, and death may result because the radiation hinders bone marrow production of the white blood cells we need to protect us from disease. Dosages above 600 to 700 rads are fatal.

radiation absorbed dose (rad) Unit of measure of radiation exposure.

Recommended maximum "safe" exposure ranges from 0.5 to 5 rads per year.[78] Approximately 50 percent of the radiation to which we are exposed comes from background sources, including natural and human-made sources. Natural sources include radon gas in the air and cosmic radiation. Human-made sources include certain building materials. Another 45 percent comes from medical and dental X-rays. The remaining 5 percent is nonionizing radiation that comes from such sources as computer monitors, microwave ovens, televisions, and radar screens.[79] Most of us are exposed to far less radiation than the safe maximum dosage per year. The effects of long-term exposure to relatively low levels of radiation are unknown. Some scientists believe that such exposure can cause lung cancer, leukemia, skin cancer, bone cancer, and skeletal deformities.

Nuclear Power Plants

Currently, nuclear power plants account for less than 1 percent of the total radiation to which we are exposed; however, the number of U.S. plants may increase in the next decade, so that percentage of exposure may increase. Proponents of nuclear energy believe that it is a safe and efficient way to generate electricity. Initial costs of building nuclear power plants are high, but actual power generation is relatively inexpensive. A 1,000-megawatt reactor produces enough energy for 650,000 homes and saves 420 million gallons of fossil fuels each year. In some areas where nuclear power plants were decommissioned, electricity bills tripled when power companies turned to hydroelectric or fossil fuel sources to generate electricity. Nuclear reactors discharge fewer carbon oxides into the air than do fossil fuel–powered generators. Advocates believe that converting to nuclear power could help slow global warming.

HEALTH HEADLINES

THE NUCLEAR EMERGENCY AFTER THE JAPANESE TSUNAMI

On March 11, 2011, an earthquake registering 9.0 on the Richter scale occurred off the coast of Japan. The earthquake, the largest to strike Japan in recorded history, initiated a devastating tsunami that leveled cities and washed over farmlands in northern Japan. The combined damaging effects of the earthquake and tsunami also triggered the worst nuclear emergency since Chernobyl. The Fukushima Daiichi Nuclear Power Station, positioned in the region hardest hit by the tsunami, suffered several explosions, multiple fires, radioactive gas leaks, and a partial meltdown in three of its reactors. Despite continued exposure to toxic radioactive material and risk to their lives, nuclear plant workers labored for weeks to stave off a full-scale meltdown and to minimize the destruction to the public and surrounding region by attempting to cool and repair the damaged reactors.

There continues to be significant concern for public safety due to exposure to radioactive materials through the air, food, and water supplies. Of all the hundreds of dangerous radioactive chemicals released during the Fukushima Daiichi nuclear emergency, scientists expressed the most concern about the levels of iodine, plutonium, cesium, and strontium in the atmosphere, water, and food supplies. According to reports of tests on food and drinking water samples made in late March 2011, iodine and cesium were detected, but the majority of measurements remained below regulation values. Additionally, small amounts of plutonium were found in the soil outside the plant, though not enough to pose a significant health risk. Now research indicates that radiation levels in seafood, particularly tuna, in the Pacific Northwest are elevated as a result of Fukushima; however, levels thus far appear to be low enough that they do not pose a significant risk to humans. The long-term effects on oceans and sea life remain unknown.

This emergency has spurred Japan and other nations to reconsider the safety of nuclear power plants and the policies necessary to protect the environment and public health.

Testing a resident for radiation in Fukushima, Japan.

Sources: "Japan's Nuclear Emergency," *Washington Post*, 2011, www.washingtonpost.com/wp-srv/special/world/japan-nuclear-reactors-and-seismic-activity/; "Earthquake, Tsunami, and Nuclear Crisis," *New York Times*, 2011, http://topics.nytimes.com/top/news/international/countriesandterritories/japan/index.html; P. Knight, Oregon State University, "Ongoing study finds more albacore with traces of Fukushima radiation," *Breaking Waves*, April 2014, http://blogs.oregonstate.edu/breakingwaves/?cat=2296.

The advantages of nuclear energy must be weighed against the disadvantages. Disposal of nuclear waste is extremely problematic. In addition, a reactor core meltdown could pose serious threats to the immediate environment and to the world in general. A **nuclear meltdown** occurs when the temperature in the core of a nuclear reactor increases enough to melt the nuclear fuel and breach the containment vessel. Most modern facilities seal the reactors and containment vessels in concrete buildings with pools of cold water on the bottom. If a meltdown occurs, the building and the pool are supposed to prevent radiation from escaping.

The International Atomic Energy Agency ranks nuclear and radiological accidents and incidents by severity on a scale of 1 to 7. To date, we have had two major nuclear disasters that resulted in a 7, the highest severity rating, meaning that there was a major release of radioactive material with widespread health and environmental consequences. The first was the 1986 reactor core fire and explosion at the Chernobyl nuclear power plant in Russia, which has led to conservative estimates of from 2,000 to as many as 724,000 deaths. Many regions surrounding the area may be uninhabitable for decades.[80] The damage to the Fukushima Daiichi Nuclear Power Station in northern Japan caused by the March 2011 earthquake and tsunami was also listed as a level 7 nuclear disaster and has awakened worldwide fears about nuclear power. Even so, the use of nuclear power worldwide is expected to double in the next 20 to 25 years.[81] Some research suggests that there may be as many as 400,000 additional cancer patients and over 40,000 deaths from thyroid cancer alone among those within 200 kilometers of the Fukushima Daiichi plant; however, exact information is difficult to obtain.[82] See the **Health Headlines** box for a look at recent events surrounding nuclear energy.

nuclear meltdown Accident that results when the temperature in the core of a nuclear reactor increases enough to melt the nuclear fuel and breach the containment vessel.

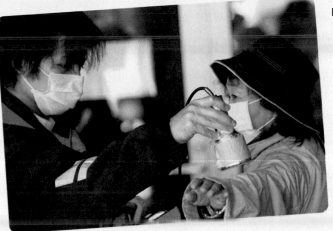

STUDY PLAN

Customize your study plan—and master your health!—in the Study Area of **MasteringHealth.**

ASSESS **YOURSELF**

What measures can you take to preserve your environment? Want to find out? Take the **Are You Doing All You Can Do to Protect the Environment?** assessment available on MasteringHealth.™

Need help creating a plan? Follow the strategies in the **Your Plan for Change** box for short- and long-term improvements to your health.

YOUR PLAN FOR **CHANGE**

Now that you have considered your results from the **ASSESS YOURSELF** activity, you can take steps to become more environmentally responsible.

TODAY, YOU CAN:

- [ ] Find out how much energy you are using. Visit http://footprint.wwf.org.uk/ to find out what your carbon footprint is and how your behaviors would affect the planet if others lived like you. Learn about things you can do to change your carbon footprint.
- [ ] Reduce paper waste in your mailbox. The Direct Marketing Association's Mail Preference Service site (www.dmachoice.org), 1-888-5-OPT-OUT, and www.catalogchoice.org are all free services that help cut down on unsolicited catalogs, credit card offers, and advertisements.

WITHIN THE NEXT 2 WEEKS, YOU CAN:

- [ ] Take part in a local cleanup day or recycling drive or sign up for an environmental science–focused course.

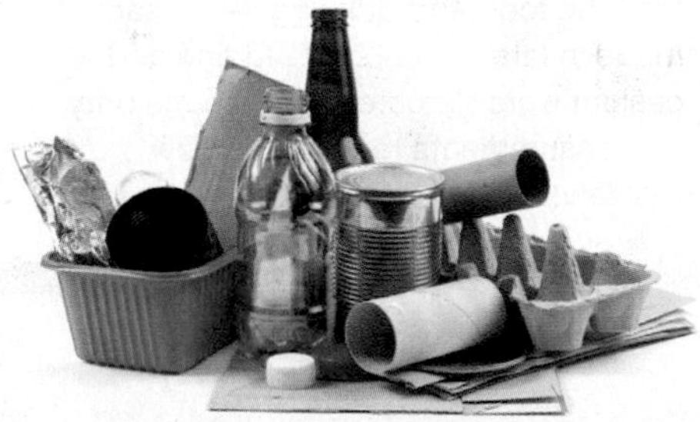

BY THE END OF THE SEMESTER, YOU CAN:

- [ ] Check if your campus dining hall composts. If it doesn't, ask the managers to start.
- [ ] Make a habit of recycling everything you can, from bottles to batteries.
- [ ] Take part in an environmental activism group on campus or in your community. Let your legislators know how you feel about environmental issues and vote for candidates with pro-environment records.

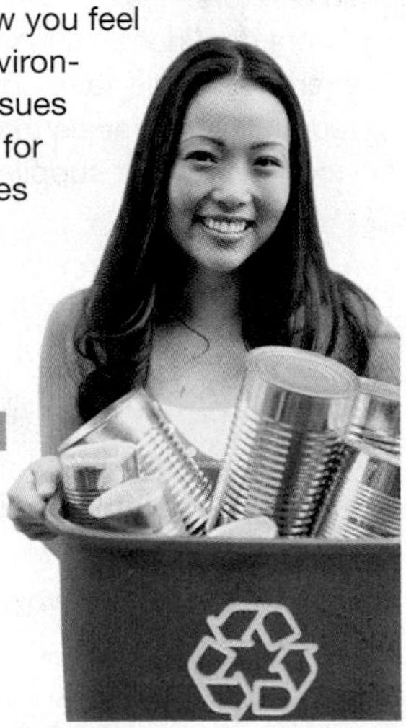

CHAPTER **REVIEW**

To hear an MP3 Tutor Session, scan here or visit the Study Area in **MasteringHealth.**

LO 1 The Threat of Overpopulation

- Population growth is the single largest factor affecting the environment. Demand for more food, water, and energy—as well as places to dispose of waste—puts unsustainable strain on Earth's resources.

LO 2 Air Pollution

- The primary constituents of air pollution are sulfur dioxide, particulate matter, carbon monoxide, nitrogen dioxide, ozone, lead, carbon dioxide, and hydrocarbons. Indoor air pollution is caused primarily by tobacco smoke, woodstove smoke, furnace emissions, asbestos, formaldehyde, radon, lead, and mold.

LO 3 Climate Change

- Air pollution is depleting Earth's protective ozone layer and contributing to global warming, a type of climate change, by enhancing the greenhouse effect.

LO 4 Water Pollution and Shortages

- Water pollution can be caused by either point sources (direct entry) or nonpoint sources (runoff or seepage). Major contributors to water pollution include petroleum products, organic solvents, polychlorinated biphenyls (PCBs), dioxins, pesticides, and lead.

LO 5 Land Pollution

- Municipal solid waste (MSW) includes household trash, plastics, glass, metals, and paper. Many of these items can be recycled. Limited landfill space creates problems in dealing with growing volumes of MSW. Hazardous waste is toxic; improper disposal creates health hazards for people in surrounding communities.

LO 6 Radiation

- Nonionizing radiation comes from electromagnetic fields, such as those around power lines. Ionizing radiation results from the erosion of atomic nuclei. The disposal and storage of radioactive waste from nuclear power plants pose potential public health problems.

POP **QUIZ**

Visit **MasteringHealth** to personalize your study plan with Chapter Review Quizzes and Dynamic Study Modules

LO 1 The Threat of Overpopulation

1. The largest population that can be supported indefinitely given the resources available is known as Earth's
   a. maximum fertility rate.
   b. fertility capacity.
   c. maximum population growth.
   d. carrying capacity.

LO 2 Air Pollution

2. One source of indoor air pollution is a gas present in some carpets and home furnishings known as
   a. lead.
   b. asbestos.
   c. radon.
   d. formaldehyde.
3. Which substance separates into stringy fibers that can become embedded in the lungs and cause disease?
   a. Asbestos
   b. Particulate matter
   c. Radon
   d. Formaldehyde
4. The air pollutant that originates primarily from motor vehicle emissions is
   a. particulates.
   b. nitrogen dioxide.
   c. sulfur dioxide.
   d. carbon monoxide.
5. Which gas can potentially become cancer causing when it seeps into a home?
   a. Carbon monoxide
   b. Radon
   c. Hydrogen sulfide
   d. Ozone

LO 3 Climate Change

6. When gases such as carbon dioxide, nitrous oxide, methane, CFCs, and hydrocarbons form a layer in the atmosphere, allowing solar heat to pass through and trapping some of the heat close to the surface to warm the planet, what is it called?
   a. Photochemical smog
   b. The ozone layer
   c. Gray air smog
   d. The greenhouse effect

LO 4 Water Pollution and Shortages

7. The terms *point source* and *nonpoint source* are used to describe the two general sources of
   a. water pollution.
   b. air pollution.
   c. noise pollution.
   d. ozone depletion.
8. Some herbicides contain toxic substances known as
   a. THMs.
   b. PCPs.
   c. dioxins.
   d. PCBs.

LO 5 Land Pollution

9. A DVD you recently purchased had less packaging than those you had bought previously. This change in packaging design is an example of reducing municipal solid waste by
   a. source reduction.
   b. recycling.
   c. composting.
   d. incineration.

LO 6 | Radiation

10. What is the recommended safe level of rads exposure per year?
    a. 0.5 to 5 rads
    b. 5 to 100 rads
    c. 100 to 200 rads
    d. 200 to 350 rads

Answers to the Pop Quiz can be found on page A-1. If you answered a question incorrectly, review the section identified by the Learning Outcome. For even more study tools, visit MasteringHealth.

THINK ABOUT IT!

LO 1 | The Threat of Overpopulation

1. How are the rapid increases in global population and consumption of resources related? What are options for controlling population and less consumption of resources? Is population control the best solution? Why or why not?

LO 2 | Air Pollution

2. What are the primary sources of air pollution? What can be done to reduce air pollution?

LO 3 | Climate Change

3. What are the causes and consequences of global warming? What can individuals do to reduce the threat of global warming?

LO 4 | Water Pollution and Shortages

4. What are point and nonpoint sources of water pollution? What can be done to reduce or prevent water pollution?

LO 5 | Land Pollution

5. How do you think communities and governments could encourage recycling efforts? Or should industry be forced to reduce packaging and waste? Which do you think would have the biggest impact? Why?

LO 6 | Radiation

6. What can be done, personally, to reduce your amount of radiation exposure? On the community level? On the national level?

ACCESS YOUR HEALTH ON THE INTERNET

Visit **MasteringHealth** for links to the websites and RSS feeds.

The following websites explore further topics and issues related to personal health.

Environmental Literacy Council. This website is an excellent source of information about environmental issues in general. Topics range from how the ozone layer works to why the rain forests are important ecosystems. **www.enviroliteracy.org**

Environmental Protection Agency (EPA). The EPA is the U.S. government agency responsible for overseeing environmental regulation and protection issues. **www.epa.gov**

National Center for Environmental Health (NCEH). This site provides information on a wide variety of environmental health issues and includes a series of helpful fact sheets. **www.cdc.gov/nceh**

National Environmental Health Association (NEHA). This organization provides educational resources and opportunities for environmental health professionals. **www.neha.org**

Environmental Working Group (EWG). This organization provides resources for consumers, such as a guide to fruits and vegetables that ranks the best to worst in terms of pesticide contaminants. It also works for national policy change. **www.ewg.org**

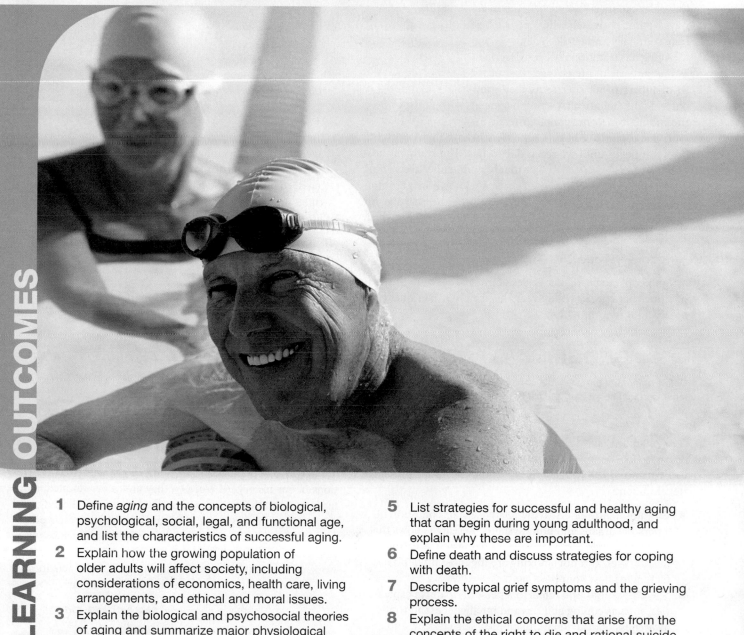

21 Preparing for Aging, Death, and Dying

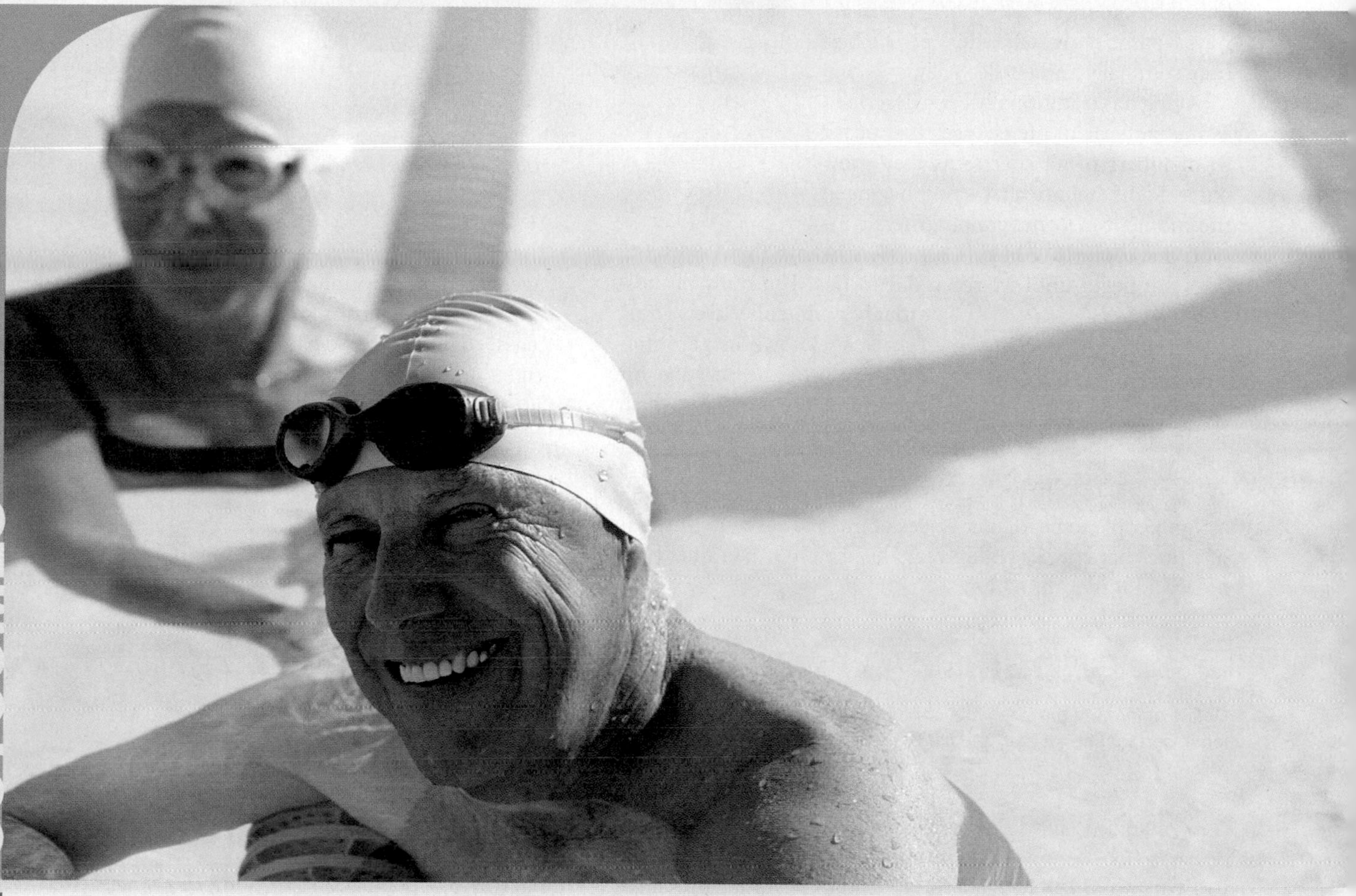

LEARNING OUTCOMES

1. Define *aging* and the concepts of biological, psychological, social, legal, and functional age, and list the characteristics of successful aging.
2. Explain how the growing population of older adults will affect society, including considerations of economics, health care, living arrangements, and ethical and moral issues.
3. Explain the biological and psychosocial theories of aging and summarize major physiological changes that occur as a result of the normal aging process.
4. Describe unique health challenges faced by older adults.
5. List strategies for successful and healthy aging that can begin during young adulthood, and explain why these are important.
6. Define death and discuss strategies for coping with death.
7. Describe typical grief symptoms and the grieving process.
8. Explain the ethical concerns that arise from the concepts of the right to die and rational suicide.
9. Review the decisions that need to be made when someone is dying or has died, including hospice care, funeral arrangements, wills, and organ donation.

In a society that seems to worship youth, researchers have begun to offer good—even revolutionary—news about the aging process. Health promotion, disease prevention, and wellness-oriented activities can prolong vigor and productivity in older people, even among those who haven't always led model lifestyles or made healthful habits a priority. Numerous research studies show that people who make even modest lifestyle changes can reap significant health benefits. In fact, getting older can mean getting better in many ways—particularly socially, psychologically, spiritually, and intellectually.

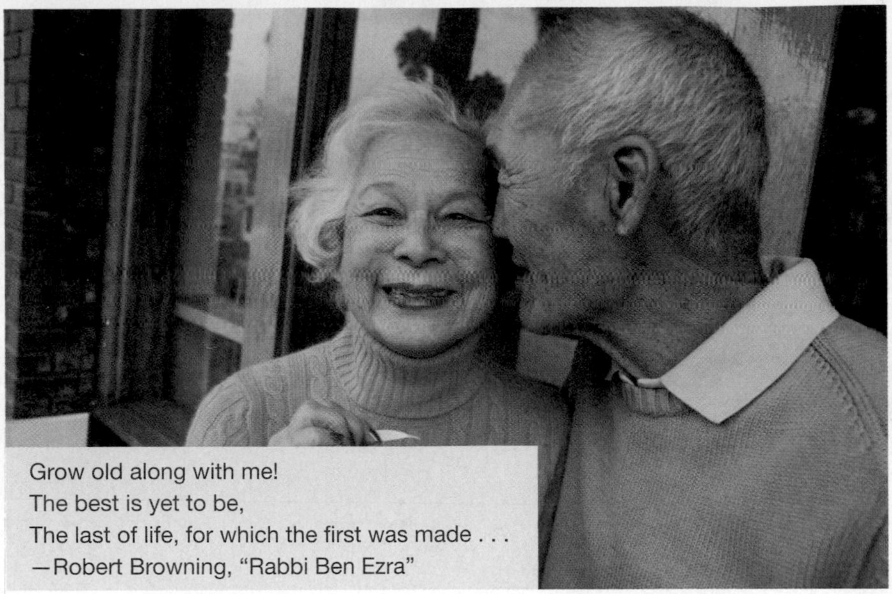

Grow old along with me!
The best is yet to be,
The last of life, for which the first was made . . .
—Robert Browning, "Rabbi Ben Ezra"

Aging has traditionally been described as the patterns of life changes that occur in members of all species as they grow older. Some believe that aging begins at the moment of conception. Others contend that it starts at birth. Still others believe that true aging does not begin until we reach our forties. The study of individual and collective aging processes, known as **gerontology,** explores the reasons for aging and the ways in which people cope with and adapt to this process. Chronological age has traditionally been used to assign people to particular stages of life. However, definitions of aging that consider only years lived rather than quality of life warrant reexamination.

aging Patterns of life changes that occur in members of all species as they grow older.
gerontology The study of individual and collective aging processes.

LO 1 | REDEFINING AGING

Define *aging* and the concepts of biological, psychological, social, legal, and functional age, and list the characteristics of successful aging.

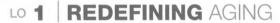

Gerontologists have identified several age-related characteristics that define where a person is in terms of biological, psychological, social, legal, and functional life-stage development:[1]

- **Biological age** refers to the relative age or condition of a person's organs and body systems. Research shows that healthy lifestyle behaviors such as being active, eating a healthy diet, and not smoking are the most influential factors for how your body ages.[2]
- **Psychological age** refers to a person's adaptive capacities, such as coping abilities and intelligence, and to the awareness of individual capabilities, self-efficacy, and general ability to adapt to new situations. Research demonstrates that many older adults maintain a positive attitude and successfully cope with the physical and cognitive changes associated with aging.[3]
- **Social age** refers to a person's habits and roles relative to society's expectations.
- **Legal age** is probably the most common definition of age. Based on chronological years lived, legal age is used as a factor in determining voting rights, driving privileges, eligibility for Social Security payments, and other rights and obligations.
- **Functional age** refers to a person's status in terms of physical and mental performance.

3.5%

OF **SENIOR CITIZENS** AGED 65 AND ABOVE LIVE IN INSTITUTIONAL SETTINGS SUCH AS NURSING HOMES.

What Is Successful Aging?

Today's elderly population is among the longest lived generations in our history. As a group, they are more educated, more likely to report that they are in excellent or very good health, and more engaged in leisure or physical activities than their predecessors. They also drink less alcohol and smoke much less than previous generations. The majority of those over 65 continue to work, care for and help others, and engage in social activities, in spite of chronic conditions that may limit them in various ways.[4]

While there are major disparities by race and socioeconomic status, people who "age successfully" have the following characteristics:

- They stay active, through leisure activities and regular exercise.

HEAR IT! PODCASTS
Want a study podcast for this chapter? Download **Life's Transitions: The Aging Process** available on MasteringHealth.™

SKILLS FOR BEHAVIOR CHANGE
AGING WELL

Many older Americans lead active, productive lives. The majority of adults over 65 continue to work, care for and help others, engage in social activities, and remain otherwise active.

The following characteristics, as indicated by older adults, can help with successful aging:

- Stay active through leisure activities and regular exercise.
- Maintain a normal weight range.
- Eat a healthy diet containing low levels of saturated fats, with plenty of fruits, vegetables, and whole grains.
- Participate in meaningful activities, like volunteering and other social activities.
- Don't smoke, and consume alcohol in moderation.

Sources: Federal Interagency Forum on Aging Related Statistics, "Older Americans 2012: Key Indicators of Well-Being," 2012, www.agingstats.gov; National Institute on Aging, "Healthy Aging: Lessons from the Baltimore Longitudinal Study of Aging," July 2010, www.nia.nih.gov.

- They maintain a normal weight range.
- They eat a healthy diet containing low levels of saturated fats, with plenty of fruits, vegetables, and whole grains.
- They participate in meaningful activities, such as volunteering and other social activities.
- They don't smoke, and they consume alcohol in moderation.[5]

The question is not how many years someone has lived, but how much life the person has packed into those years. This quality-of-life index, combined with the chronological process, appears to be the best indicator of "aging gracefully." Most experts agree that the best way to experience a productive, full, and satisfying old age is to lead a productive, full, and satisfying life prior to old age. See the **Skills for Behavior Change** box for some characteristics shared among those who have aged well.

LO 2 | OLDER ADULTS: A GROWING POPULATION

Explain how the growing population of older adults will affect society, including considerations of economics, health care, living arrangements, and ethical and moral issues.

The United States and much of the developed world are on the brink of a *longevity revolution,* one that will affect society in many ways. Medical care breakthroughs and improved understanding of fitness and nutrition have steadily increased lifespan. According to the latest statistics, life expectancy for

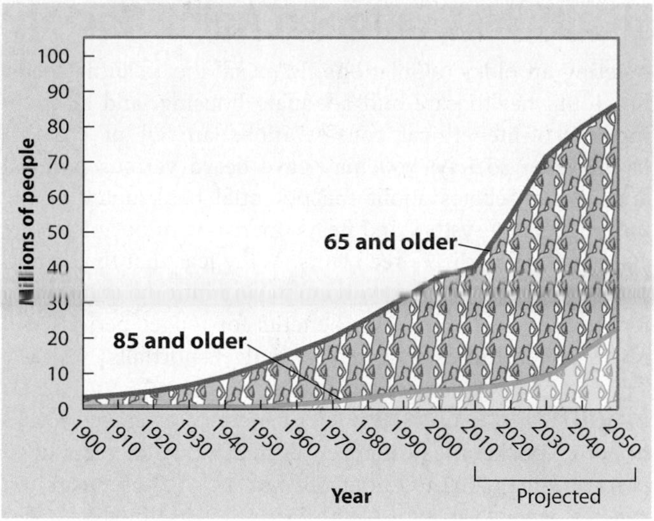

FIGURE 21.1 Number of Americans 65 and Older (in millions), Years 1900–2008 and Projected 2010–2050

Source: Data from U.S. Census Bureau, Decennial Census, Population Estimates and Projections. Available at www.census.gov

Note: Data for 2010–2050 are projections of the population.

a child born in 2013 is 78.9 years—more than 30 years longer than for a child born in 1900.[6] Today there are 43.1 million people age 65 or older in the United States, making up over 13 percent of the total population.[7] In comparison, a mere 3 million people were age 65 and older in 1900 (**FIGURE 21.1**).[8] Similar trends are true throughout the world, with the number of people over age 60 expected to increase to 22 percent by 2050.[9]

Within the United States, the population of those over 65 will increase substantially over the next two decades due to the aging "baby boomer" generation, an especially large segment of the population born during the period of economic prosperity that began after World War II in the late 1940s and continued through the early 1960s. The oldest of the Baby Boomers are just beginning to retire, and their impact on the economy, housing market, health care system, and Social Security will be profound in coming decades.

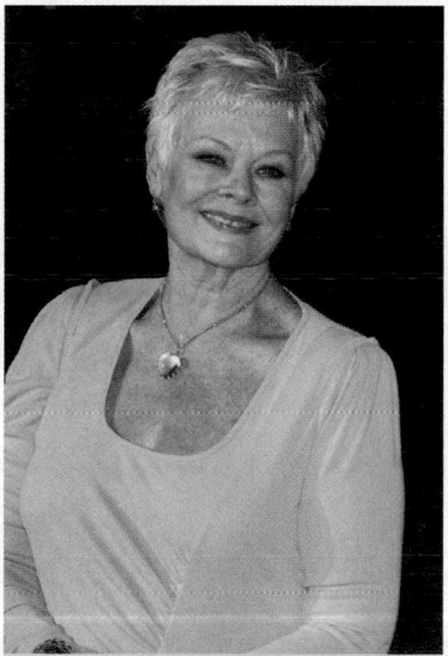

The people we often think of as aging gracefully—such as actress Dame Judi Dench—are those who continue to be active and productive; who are not frightened or ashamed of growing older; who adapt to the changing circumstances of their lives; and who strive to be healthy, vibrant, and alive at any age.

Health Issues for an Aging Society

Meeting an older population's financial and medical needs, providing health care and adequate housing, and addressing end-of-life ethical considerations are all of concern in an aging society. You may have heard various political and media debates about the potential bankruptcy of the Social Security system and heavy increases in out-of-pocket expenses for Medicare recipients. Many fear that the combination of fewer younger workers paying into the system and more older people drawing benefits for longer periods will result in tremendous government budget shortfalls.

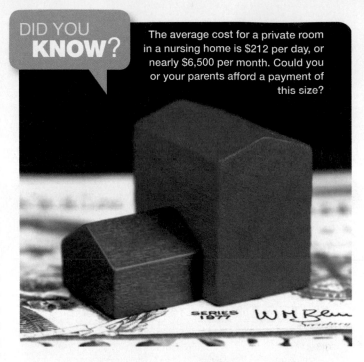

DID YOU KNOW?

The average cost for a private room in a nursing home is $212 per day, or nearly $6,500 per month. Could you or your parents afford a payment of this size?

Health Care Costs Older Americans averaged $5,118 in out-of-pocket medical expenses in 2012, an increase of 43 percent since 2002.[10] About 65 percent of those costs, on average, went to pay for health insurance itself, while drugs or medical services not covered by insurance premiums accounted for roughly one-third of the costs.[11] As people live longer, the chances of developing a costly chronic disease increase, and as technology improves, chronic illnesses that once were quickly fatal may now be treated successfully for years. Most older adults have at least one chronic condition, and many have multiple conditions. It is estimated that 34 percent of older adults have hypertension, 50 percent have been diagnosed with arthritis, 32 percent with heart disease, 23 percent with cancer, and 19 percent with diabetes.[12]

Housing and Living Arrangements Most older adults never live in a nursing home. Many live with a spouse, partner, or friend; others live with family or friends or pay for home health services. An increasing number opt for assisted living in apartments, foster homes, or individual homes with supportive services like meals, help with housekeeping and medication, or other options that help seniors live independently (**FIGURE 21.2**). Other communities and facilities include 24/7 monitoring of unique needs, such as Alzheimer's or other disabilities. Newer, technologically advanced housing includes physiological monitoring that records heart rate and other life indicators to ensure prompt emergency services in case of problems. With increasing age comes an increased likelihood of some form of institutional setting, with just over 1 percent of those aged 65 to 74, 3.5 percent of those aged 75 to 85, and 13.2 percent of those over 85 living in nursing homes.[13]

If you have the money, the sky's the limit in terms of superb care during your later years. Savings plans, long-term care insurance, supportive family members, and progressive communities provide many options for those who know how to maneuver in an increasingly complex, costly system. The average cost for institutional care varies tremendously by state and level of care, ranging from $80,000 to $125,000 or more per year for a private room in a nursing home to $40,000 to $50,000 for an assisted living facility room.[14] Tremendous income-based disparities exist in caring for the elderly, and even with significant savings, many elderly budgets will be stretched to the limit. Many American seniors live on small fixed incomes, and in 2012 the *supplemental poverty measure* calculated by the government estimated that about 9.1 percent of seniors lived in poverty in the United States.[15] Those without means are more likely to be shut out of all but the most meager care situations.

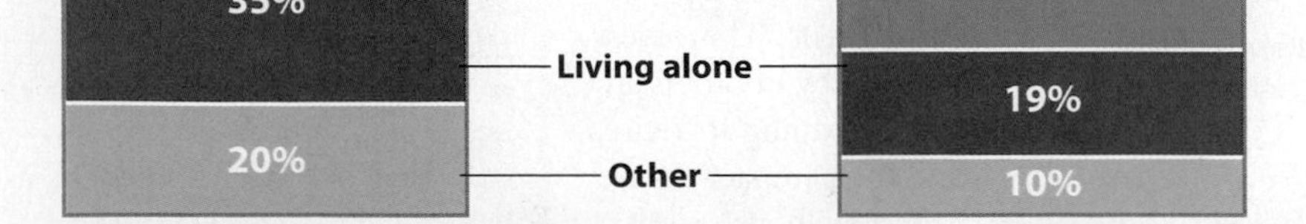

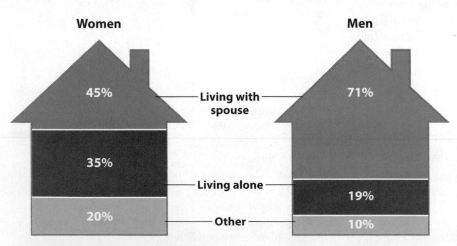

FIGURE 21.2 Living Arrangements of Americans Age 65 and Older Percentages may not total 100% due to rounding.

Source: Administration on Aging, U.S. Dept. of Health and Human Services, "A Profile of Older Americans: 2013," 2014, www.aoa.gov/Aging_Statistics/Profile/2013/docs/2013_Profile.pdf.

Ethical and Moral Considerations Difficult ethical questions arise when we consider the implications of an already overburdened health care system. The cost of care versus the quality and length of life it buys, particularly for terminally ill older people, is something each society must weigh. Is prolonging life at all costs a moral imperative, or will future generations devise a set of criteria for deciding who will be helped and who will not? Such debates leave much room for careful thought and discussion.

LO 3 | THEORIES OF AGING

Explain the biological and psychosocial theories of aging and summarize major physiological changes that occur as a result of the normal aging process.

Social gerontologists, behaviorists, biologists, geneticists, and physiologists continue to explore various potential explanations for why the body breaks down over time. One explanation for the biological cause of aging is the *wear-and-tear theory,* which states that, like everything else in the world, the human body wears out. Inherent in this theory is the idea that the more you abuse your body, the faster it will wear out.

Another theory, the *cellular theory,* proposes that at birth we have only a certain number of usable cells, which are genetically programmed to reproduce a limited number of times. Once cells reach the end of their reproductive cycle, they die, and the organs they build begin to deteriorate, ultimately leading to body system failures and death.

According to the *genetic mutation theory,* the number of body cells exhibiting unusual or different characteristics increases with age. Proponents of this theory believe that aging is related to the amount of mutational damage within the genes. The more mutation there is, the greater the chance that cells will not function properly.

SEE IT! VIDEOS
Why do some people live longer than others? Watch **Myth-Busting Longevity** available on MasteringHealth.™

Finally, the *autoimmune theory* attributes aging to the decline of the body's immunological system. Studies indicate that as we age, the ability to produce necessary antibodies declines, and our immune systems become less effective in fighting disease. At the same time, the white blood cells active in the immune response become less able to recognize foreign invaders and more likely to mistakenly attack the body's own proteins.

LO 4 | PHYSICAL AND MENTAL CHANGES OF AGING

Describe unique health challenges faced by older adults.

Although the physiological consequences of aging can differ in severity and timing, certain standard changes occur as a result of the aging process. Many of these changes are physical (see **FIGURE 21.3**), whereas others are mental or psychosocial.

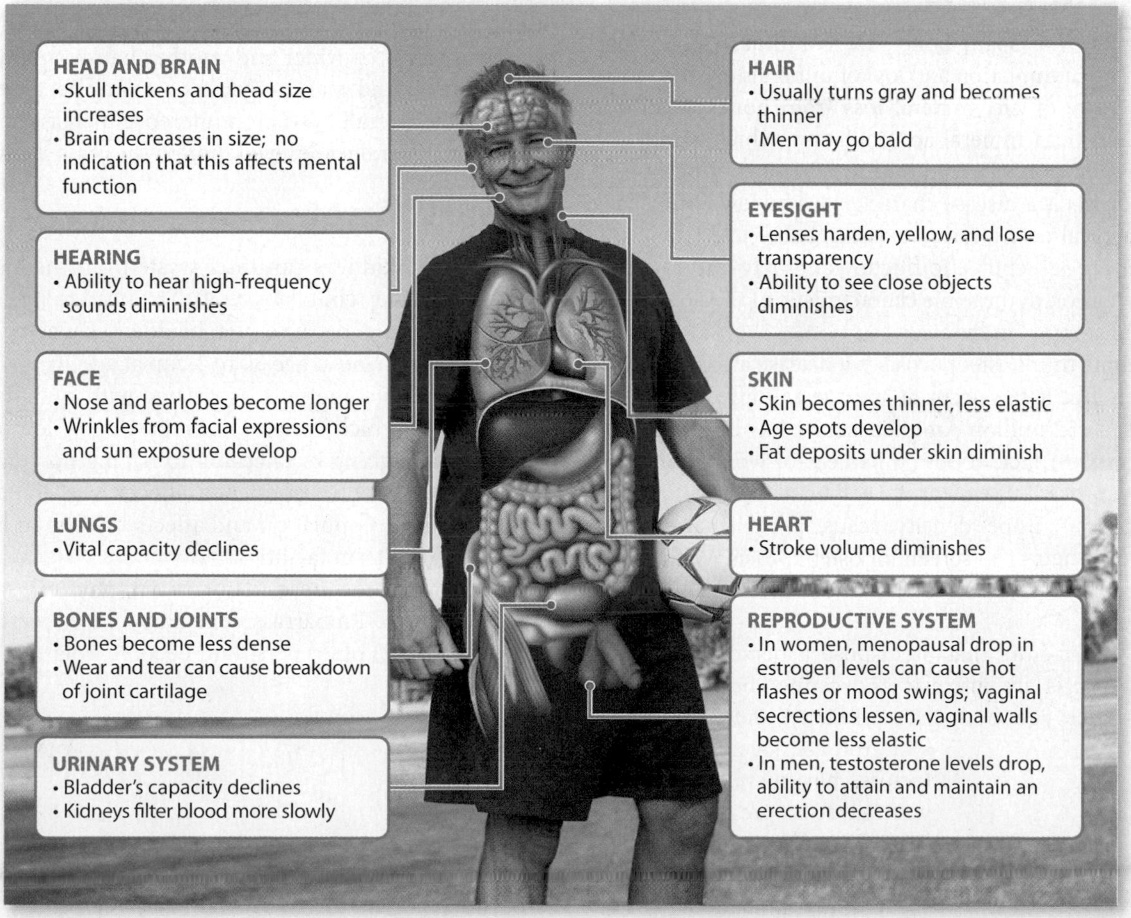

HEAD AND BRAIN
• Skull thickens and head size increases
• Brain decreases in size; no indication that this affects mental function
HEARING
• Ability to hear high-frequency sounds diminishes
FACE
• Nose and earlobes become longer
• Wrinkles from facial expressions and sun exposure develop
LUNGS
• Vital capacity declines
BONES AND JOINTS
• Bones become less dense
• Wear and tear can cause breakdown of joint cartilage
URINARY SYSTEM
• Bladder's capacity declines
• Kidneys filter blood more slowly
HAIR
• Usually turns gray and becomes thinner
• Men may go bald
EYESIGHT
• Lenses harden, yellow, and lose transparency
• Ability to see close objects diminishes
SKIN
• Skin becomes thinner, less elastic
• Age spots develop
• Fat deposits under skin diminish
HEART
• Stroke volume diminishes
REPRODUCTIVE SYSTEM
• In women, menopausal drop in estrogen levels can cause hot flashes or mood swings; vaginal secretions lessen, vaginal walls become less elastic
• In men, testosterone levels drop, ability to attain and maintain an erection decreases

FIGURE 21.3 Normal Effects of Aging on the Body

VIDEO TUTOR
Effects of Aging on Body

The Skin

As a normal part of aging, the skin becomes thinner and loses elasticity, particularly in the outer surfaces. Fat deposits, which add to the soft lines and shape of the skin, diminish. Because of the loss of body fat, thinning of the epithelium, and diminished glandular activity, older adults experience greater difficulty regulating body temperature. This limits their ability to withstand extreme cold or heat, which increases the risks of hypothermia, heatstroke, and heat exhaustion.

Starting at about age 30, lines develop on the forehead as a result of smiling, squinting, and other facial expressions. During the forties, these lines become more pronounced, with added "crow's feet" around the eyes. In a person's fifties and sixties, the skin begins to sag and lose color, which leads to pallor in the seventies. Body fat in underlying layers of skin continues to be redistributed away from the limbs and extremities into the body's trunk region. Age spots become more numerous because of excessive pigment accumulation under the skin, particularly in areas of the skin exposed to heavy sun.

WHY SHOULD I CARE?

Aging isn't a distant process somewhere in the future—it's something that is happening to every one of us every day of our lives. The way you live your life now has a direct impact on how you will live it in the future. Learning to cope with challenges and changes early in life develops attitudes and skills that contribute to a full and satisfying old age.

Bones and Joints

Throughout the life span, bones are continually changing because of the accumulation and loss of minerals. By the third or fourth decade of life, mineral loss from bones becomes more prevalent than mineral accumulation, which results in a weakening and porosity (diminishing density) of bony tissue. **Osteoporosis** is a disease characterized by low bone density and structural deterioration of bone tissue. These porous, fragile bones are susceptible to fracture and may lead to crippling malformation of the spine characteristic of the dowager's hump seen in stooped individuals.

Many people think osteoporosis is a disease affecting only older women, but it can occur at any age and affects men as well. More than 52 million Americans have low bone density or osteoporosis. In fact, about 50 percent of women and 25 percent of men over 50 years of age will break a bone because of osteoporosis.[16] Bone density scans using dual-energy X-ray absorptiometry can screen for osteoporosis. With early detection, steps can be taken to reverse bone loss and prevent fractures.

Some of the factors that predispose a person to developing osteoporosis are intrinsic and cannot be controlled, including gender, age, body size, ethnicity, and family history. You cannot modify these factors, but there *are* things you can do to prevent the disease. During your lifetime, bone is constantly being added (formation) and being broken down and removed (reabsorption). At around age 30, a person reaches *peak bone mass*. After this point, a slow and steady decline occurs. Individuals who develop strong, dense, healthy bones through proper diet and exercise can minimize this decline and reduce their risk for osteoporosis.

osteoporosis Degenerative bone disorder characterized by increasingly porous bones.

urinary incontinence Inability to control urination.

Adequate calcium intake is important, as is vitamin D, which helps the body absorb and use calcium more efficiently. Bone is a living tissue that grows stronger with exercise and weight bearing activity; therefore, bone loss can be slowed or prevented with regular weight-bearing exercise, such as walking, jogging, and dancing, as well as through strength training. Unhealthy behaviors that contribute to bone loss include smoking, excessive alcohol consumption, and anorexia nervosa.

Another bone condition that afflicts almost 27 million Americans is *osteoarthritis*, a progressive breakdown of joint cartilage that becomes more common with age and is a major cause of disability in the United States.[17]

Head and Face

With age, features of the head enlarge and become more prominent. Increased cartilage and fatty tissue cause the nose to grow a half inch wider and another half inch longer. Earlobes get fatter and grow longer. As the skull becomes thicker with age, the overall head circumference increases one quarter of an inch per decade, even though the brain itself shrinks.

Urinary Tract

At age 70, the kidneys can filter waste from the blood only half as fast as they could at age 30. The need to urinate more frequently occurs because the bladder's capacity declines from 2 cups of urine at age 30 to 1 cup at age 70.

One problem sometimes associated with aging is **urinary incontinence,** which ranges from passing a few drops of urine while laughing or sneezing to having no control over urination. Urinary incontinence affects 30 percent of the general geriatric population and affects more than half of all persons in long-term facilities.[18]

Incontinence can pose major social, physical, and emotional problems. Embarrassment and fear of wetting oneself may cause an older person to become isolated and avoid

6.7 MILLION

SENIOR CITIZENS ARE IN THE **LABOR FORCE.**

social functions. Caregivers may become frustrated with incontinent patients. Prolonged wetness and the inability to properly care for oneself can lead to tissue irritation, infections, and other problems.

However, incontinence is not an inevitable part of aging. Most cases are caused by persistent infections, medications, treatable neurological problems that affect the central nervous system, weakness in the pelvic wall, and so on. When the problem is treated, the incontinence is usually resolved.[19]

Heart and Lungs

Resting heart rate stays about the same over the course of a person's life, but the stroke volume (the amount of blood the heart pushes out per beat) diminishes as heart muscle deteriorates. Vital capacity, or the amount of air that moves when you inhale and exhale at maximum effort, also declines with age. Exercise can do a great deal to preserve heart and lung function. Not smoking and avoiding smoke-filled environments are important ways of reducing risks.

The Senses

With aging, the senses (vision, hearing, touch, taste, and smell) become less acute. By age 30, the lens of the eye begins to harden, which can cause problems by the early forties. The lens begins to yellow and lose transparency, and the pupil shrinks, allowing less light to penetrate. By age 60, depth perception declines, and farsightedness often develops. **Cataracts** (clouding of the lens) and **glaucoma** (elevated pressure within the eyeball) become more likely. Eventually, a tendency toward color blindness may develop, especially for shades of blue and green. **Macular degeneration** is the breakdown of the light-sensitive area of the retina responsible for the sharp, direct vision needed to read or drive. Its effects can be devastating to independent older adults and causes are still being investigated.

Presbycusis, or age-related hearing loss, is one of the most common chronic conditions of the elderly—affecting an estimated 28 million Americans by 2030.[20] It appears that hearing loss may play a much greater role in maintaining health in the elderly than was thought. A new study has found that hearing loss and mental decline may be related—showing that older people with hearing deficits were more likely than those with normal hearing to develop problems with memory and thinking.[21]

For some people, the need for reading glasses is one of the earliest signs of aging.

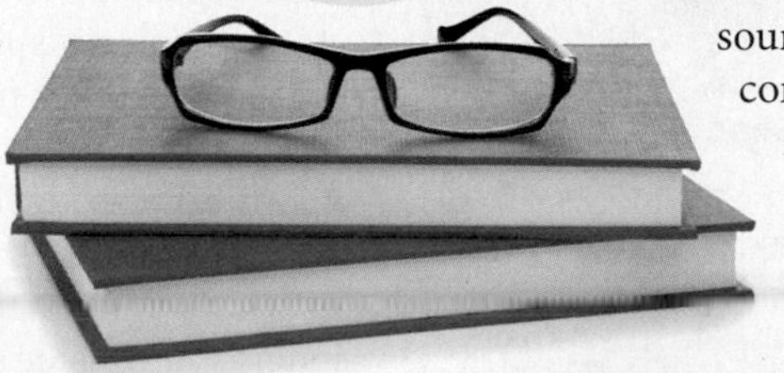

With age, the ear structure also experiences changes and often deteriorates. The eardrum thickens, and the inner ear bones are affected. The inner ear is the portion that controls balance (equilibrium). As a result, it often becomes difficult for a person to maintain balance. Studies have shown that exercises including resistance/strength training, yoga, and tai chi can improve balance in older adults.[22] The ability to hear high-frequency consonants (e.g., *s, t,* and *z*) also diminishes with age. Much of the actual hearing loss lies in the inability to distinguish extreme ranges of sound rather than an inability to distinguish normal conversational tones.

Many studies have indicated that with age, there is a reduced or changed sensation of pain, vibration, cold, heat, pressure, and touch. Some of these changes may be caused by decreased blood flow to touch receptors or to the brain and spinal cord.[23] It may become difficult, for example, to tell the difference between cool and cold. Decreased temperature sensitivity increases the risk of injuries such as hypothermia and frostbite.

The senses of taste and smell are closely connected. The number of taste buds decreases starting at about age 40 in women and age 50 in men. Each remaining taste bud also begins to atrophy (lose mass). The sense of smell may diminish, especially after age 70. This may be related to loss of nerve endings in the nose. Studies on the cause of decreased sense of taste and smell have conflicting results. Some studies have indicated that normal aging produces very little change in taste and smell.[24] Therefore, changes may be related to chronic diseases, smoking, and environmental exposures over a lifetime.

cataracts Clouding of the lens that interrupts the focusing of light on the retina, resulting in blurred vision or eventual blindness.

glaucoma Elevation of pressure within the eyeball, leading to hardening of the eyeball, impaired vision, and possible blindness.

macular degeneration Breakdown of the macula, the light-sensitive part of the retina responsible for sharp, direct vision.

Sexual Function

As men age, they experience noticeable alterations in sexual function. Although the degree and rate of change vary greatly from man to man, several changes generally occur, including a slowed ability to obtain an erection, diminished ability to maintain an erection, and a decline in angle of the erection. Men may also experience a longer refractory period between orgasms and shortened duration of orgasm.[25]

Women also experience several changes in sexual function as they age. Menopause usually occurs between the ages of 45 and 55. Women may experience hot flashes, mood swings, weight gain, development of facial hair, or other hormone-related symptoms. The walls of the vagina become less elastic, and the epithelium thins, possibly making intercourse painful. Vaginal secretions, particularly during sexual activity, diminish. The breasts become less firm, and loss of fat in various areas leads to fewer curves, with a decrease in the soft lines of body contours.

Although these physiological changes may sound discouraging, sex is still an essential component in the lives of those in their mid-fifties and older, and many people remain sexually active throughout their entire adult lives. According to a recent study, more than 80 percent of 50–90 year olds are sexually active.[26]

With that, cases of sexually transmitted diseases have more than doubled in the past 10 years.[27] With the advent of drugs such as Viagra and medical interventions designed to treat sexual dysfunction, many older adults are able to be sexually active. However, older adults also report low percentages of condom use, signifying a need for education regarding the spread of STIs.

Mental Function and Memory

Given an appropriate length of time, older people learn and develop skills in a manner similar to younger people. Researchers have also determined that what many older adults lack in speed of learning they make up for in practical knowledge—that is, the "wisdom of age." Memory loss is not necessarily a normal part of aging; however, as a person ages, drug interactions, vascular deficiencies, hormonal or biochemical imbalances, and other physiological changes can make memory lapses occur more frequently. Although short-term memory may fluctuate on a daily basis, in the absence of disease, the ability to remember events from past decades seems to remain largely unchanged.

dementias Progressive brain impairments that interfere with memory and normal intellectual functioning.

Alzheimer's disease (AD) Chronic condition involving changes in nerve fibers of the brain that results in mental deterioration.

What can you do to help improve memory and overall mental functioning as you age? Generally, those who maintain their memory in old age have exercised and kept their cardiovascular system and other body systems healthy over the years. Another key to maintaining memory is keeping your mind active as well. People who foster their creative side and engage their minds by reading books, solving mental puzzles, playing musical instruments, volunteering, and doing other brain-sharpening activities seem to fare much better in the memory department. As with the physical aspects of the body, "use it or lose it" applies to your brain acuity.

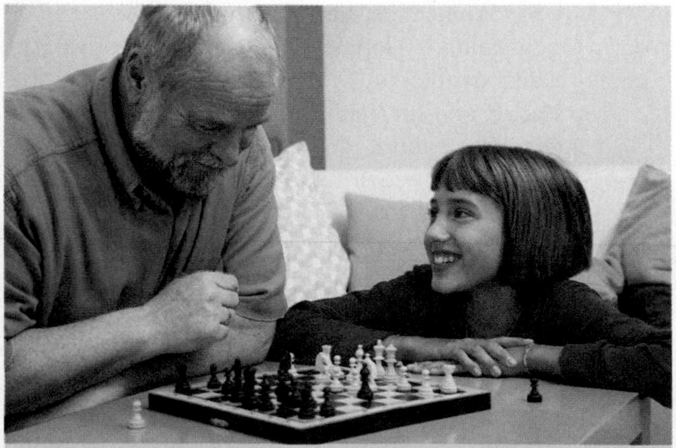

Certain physiological conditions or diseases may cause older people to experience memory loss, but in general the knowledge and memories gained through a lifetime remain intact.

Depression

Most older adults lead healthy, fulfilling lives. However, while research indicates that depression is the most common psychological problem affecting this population, the rate of major depression is actually lower among older people than it is among younger adults. Regardless of age, people who have a poor perception of their health, have multiple chronic illnesses, take a lot of medications, abuse alcohol or other drugs, lack social support, and do not exercise face more challenges to their emotional resilience.

Dementias and Alzheimer's Disease

Memory failure, errors in judgment, disorientation, or erratic behavior can occur at any age and for various reasons, including nutrient deficiency (such as vitamin B deficiency), alcohol abuse, medication interactions, vascular problems, tumors, hormonal or metabolic imbalances, or any number of problems. Often, when the underlying issues are corrected, the memory loss and disorientation also improve. The terms *dementing diseases,* or **dementias,** are used to describe either reversible symptoms or progressive forms of brain malfunctioning.

Although there are many types of dementia, one of the most common forms is **Alzheimer's disease (AD).** Affecting an estimated 5.4 million Americans, this disease is one of the most painful and devastating conditions that families can endure.[28] It kills its victims twice: first through a slow loss of personhood (memory loss, disorientation, personality changes, and eventual loss of independent functioning), and then through the deterioration of body systems as they gradually succumb to the powerful impact of neurological problems. Patients with AD live for an average of 4 to 6 years after diagnosis, although the disease can last for up to 20 years.[29] The number of individuals with AD has significantly increased in the United States. Because of the growing number of people over 65 in the United States, the annual total number of new cases of Alzheimer's and other dementias is projected to almost triple by 2050.[30] An estimated 15 million family members and friends cared for a person with Alzheimer's disease or another dementia in 2011.[31] Caring for a person with AD can be a heavy financial burden; the average cost of full-time nursing care is about $80,000 a year.[32] Most people associate the disease with the aged, but AD has been diagnosed in people in their late forties.

Alzheimer's disease is a degenerative illness that involves areas of the brain developing "tangles" that impair the way nerve cells communicate, eventually causing them to die. This degeneration occurs in the sections of the brain that affect memory, speech, and personality, leaving the parts that control other functions, such as heartbeat and breathing, functioning at near-normal levels. Thus, the mind begins to go while the body lives on.

This disease characteristically progresses in stages, each of which is marked by increasingly impaired memory and judgment. In later stages of the disease, these symptoms can be accompanied by agitation and restlessness (especially at night), loss of sensory perceptions, muscle twitching, and repetitive actions. Many patients become depressed, combative, and aggressive. In the final stage, disorientation is often complete. The person becomes dependent on others for eating, dressing, and other activities. Identity loss and speech problems are common. Eventually, control of bodily functions may be lost.

Researchers are investigating several possible causes of AD, including genetic predisposition, immune system malfunction, a slow acting virus, chromosomal or genetic defects, chronic inflammation, uncontrolled hypertension, and neurotransmitter imbalance. There is no treatment that can stop the progression of AD, but there are medications that can prevent some symptoms from progressing for a short period of time or relieve symptoms such as sleeplessness, anxiety, and depression. Some researchers are looking at anti-inflammatory drugs, theorizing that AD may develop in response to an inflammatory ailment. Others are focusing on studying deposits of protein called plaques and their role in damaging and killing nerve cells.[33]

Alcohol and Drug Use and Abuse

Those who are prone to alcoholism in their younger years are likely to continue drinking later in life. Alcohol abuse is more common among older men than it is among older women. Yet those age 65 and older have the lowest rates of drinking among any age group. Typically, those who do drink do so less than younger persons.[34]

However, older adults who binge drink reported engaging in this behavior more frequently than their younger counterparts—on average 5–6 times per month. They also reported drinking six drinks when they binge drank.[35]

If recent studies are accurate, the reason there aren't many heavy drinkers among older adults may be that very heavy drinkers tend to either die of alcoholic complications before they grow old or because they are afraid of combining alcohol with their prescription drugs. Most older adults who consume alcohol are not alcoholics but rather social drinkers.

Prescription medication misuse and abuse are growing problems among older adults. Older adults are at a high risk for medication misuse because they tend to use a greater number of medications that other age groups. Because of increased medication sensitivity slower metabolism, and slower elimination, older adults are also likely to have problems with smaller quantities of medications. Pain, sleep disorders, and anxiety are just some conditions that increase the likelihood of medication misuse or abuse.[36]

People also must be aware of the possible effects of medications they take, alone or in combination. It is estimated that almost 100,000 Americans are hospitalized for adverse drug reactions each year, with most of these events linked to drugs for treatment of diabetes or to blood thinners.[37] Nearly two-thirds of the hospitalizations were due to unintentional overdoses. The risks of adverse effects are even greater for people with impaired circulation and declining kidney and liver function.

Currently, there is no one system that tracks all of a patient's prescriptions. To avoid drug interactions and other problems, older adults should use the same pharmacy consistently, ask questions about medicines, dosages, and possible drug interactions, and read directions carefully.

LO 5 | STRATEGIES FOR HEALTHY AGING

List strategies for successful and healthy aging that can begin during young adulthood, and explain why these are important.

You can do many things to prolong and improve the quality of your life. To provide for healthy older years, make each of the following part of your younger years.

Improve Fitness

Just about any moderate-intensity exercise that gets your heart beating faster and increases strength and/or flexibility will maximize your physical health and functional years. One of the physical changes that the body undergoes is *sarcopenia,* age-associated loss of muscle mass. The less muscle you have, the less energy you will burn even while resting. The lower your metabolic rate, the more likely you will gain weight. With regular strength training, you can increase your muscle mass, boost your metabolism, strengthen your bones, prevent osteoporosis, feel better, and function more efficiently.

Both aerobic and muscle-strengthening activities are critical for healthy aging. **TABLE 21.1** lists basic recommendations for aerobic and strength-training exercises for older adults. In addition to these, the Centers for Disease Control and Prevention recommends that people who are at risk of falling perform regular balance exercises.[38] It is also recommended that older adults or individuals with chronic conditions develop an activity plan with a health professional to manage risks and take therapeutic needs into account. This will maximize the benefits of physical activity and ensure your

TABLE 21.1 | Exercise Recommendations for Adults over Age 65

Option 1	Option 2	Option 3
Moderate-intensity aerobic activity (e.g., brisk walking) at least 2 hours and 30 minutes every week	Vigorous-intensity aerobic activity (e.g., jogging or running) at least 1 hour and 15 minutes every week	An equal mix of moderate- and vigorous-intensity aerobic activity
and	***and***	***and***
muscle-strengthening activity, working all major muscle groups, on 2 or more days a week	muscle-strengthening activity, working all major muscle groups, on 2 or more days a week	muscle-strengthening activity on 2 or more days a week

Source: Centers for Disease Control, "How Much Physical Activity Do Older Adults Need?," 2014, www.cdc.gov/physicalactivity/everyone/guidelines/olderadults.html.

HEALTH IN A DIVERSE WORLD

KEEPING FIT AS WE AGE

Physical activity is the key for maintaining health and independence as people age, but regular physical activity is not widespread among older adults. According to the National Institutes of Health, regular physical activity is reported by only 30 percent of Americans age 45 to 64, 25 percent of those age 65 to 74, and 11 percent of those age 85 and older.

The Centers for Disease Control and Prevention identifies regular physical activity as one of the most important things that can be done to maintain your health as you age. The benefits include the following:

- Maintenance and improvement of physical strength and fitness
- Improvement of balance
- Better management of diseases such as diabetes, heart disease, and osteoporosis
- Reduction in feelings of depression and improved mood and overall well-being

Many forms of activity can improve physical fitness.

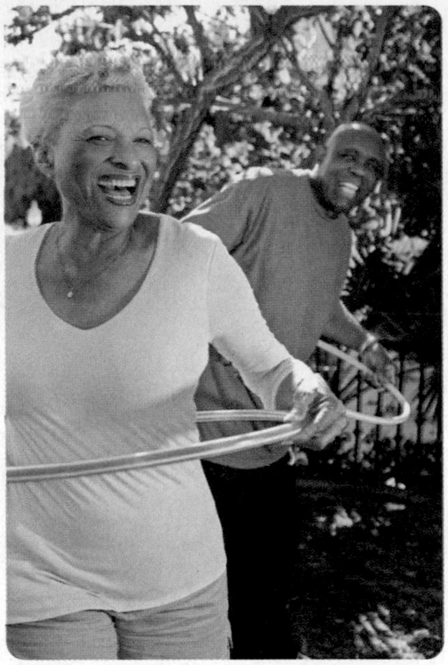

Recent studies have found that older adults who keep active may reduce their odds of losing their mental abilities. "If we want to become a healthy and fit nation, we need to increase the number of Americans who are healthy at every stage of life," former U.S. Surgeon General Dr. Regina Benjamin stated.

A new program called Go4Life (http://go4life.nia.nih.gov) is meant to encourage people 50 and older to become and stay active to improve their health. Go4Life provides to older adults resources to be physically active, such as sample exercise programs and videos. Go4Life is based on studies demonstrating the benefits of exercise and physical activity for older people, including those with chronic health conditions. This program shows them that, even with physical limitations, it is possible to exercise safely. Programs like Go4Life are also important because they are able to reach out to older adults who have traditionally not been physically active.

Source: National Institute on Aging, "Go4Life," Accessed October, 2014, http://go4life.nia.nih.gov.

safety. The **Health in a Diverse World** box describes more of the benefits of physical activity.

Eat for Longevity

Certain nutrients are especially essential for healthy aging:

- **Calcium.** Bone loss tends to increase in women, particularly in the hip region, shortly before menopause. During perimenopause and menopause, this bone loss accelerates rapidly, with an average of about 3 percent skeletal mass lost per year over a 5-year period. The result is an increased risk for fracture and disability. Adequate consumption of calcium throughout one's life can help prevent bone loss.
- **Vitamin D.** Vitamin D is necessary for adequate calcium absorption, yet as people age, particularly in their fifties and sixties, they do not absorb vitamin D from foods as readily as before. If vitamin D is unavailable, calcium levels are also likely to be lower.
- **Protein.** As some older adults become concerned about cholesterol and fatty foods and others face a limited food budget, they often cut back on protein. Meat and seafood products cost more and have the "fat" stigma associated with animal products. Yet protein is necessary for muscle mass, and protein insufficiencies can spell trouble.

Other nutrients, including vitamin E, folic acid (folate), iron, potassium, CoQ10, and vitamin B_{12} (cobalamin), are important to the aging process, and most of these are readily available in any diet that follows the U.S. Department of Agriculture's (USDA) MyPlate recommendations (www.choosemyplate.gov).

Develop and Maintain Healthy Relationships

Social bonds lend vigor and energy to life. Be willing to give to others, and seek variety in your relationships rather than befriending only people who agree with you. By interacting with diverse people and considering different points of view, we gain a new perspective on life. Positive relationships are important for well being at any age, but as people age, support systems decrease, making it particularly important to remain socially active.

Enrich the Spiritual Side of Life

Although we often take the spiritual side of life for granted, cultivating a relationship with nature, the environment, a higher being, and yourself is a key factor in personal growth and development. Take time for thought and quiet contemplation, and enjoy the sunsets, sounds, and energy of life. Setting aside

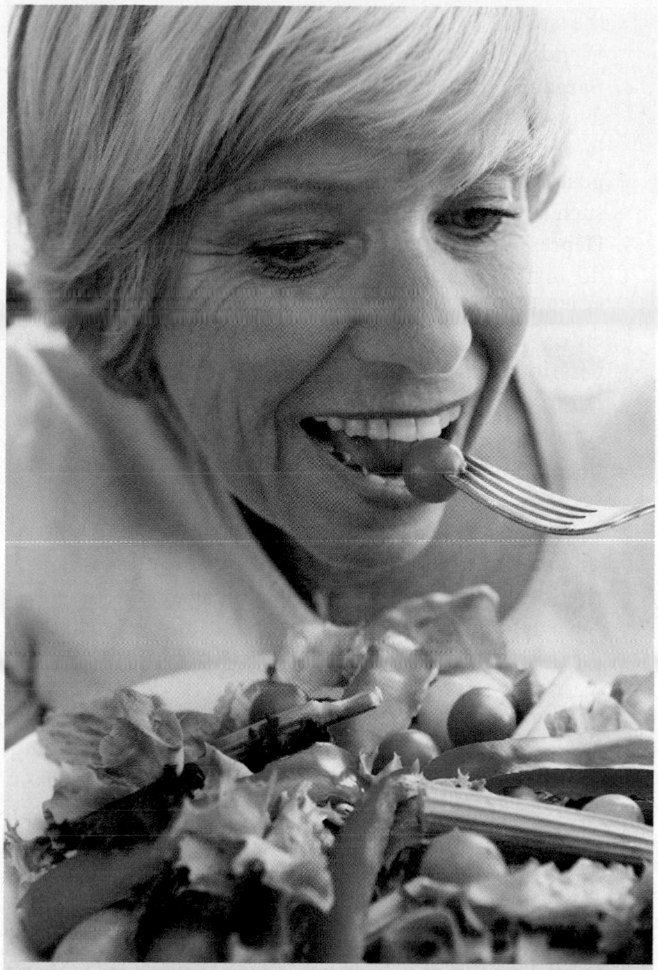

Aging is inevitable, but if you take good care of your body, mind, and spirit, you can prevent disease and delay the deterioration of abilities that can lead to disability or a poor quality of life in old age.

time for quiet, meaningful moments will leave you invigorated and refreshed—better able to cope with life's ups and downs.

Financial Planning for Retirement

Financial planning for retirement should begin early in life. Retirement generally means a change in finances. It may mean a stricter budget or even financial hardship if older adults have not been good financial planners. Starting early by putting aside small amounts of money in retirement savings accounts is one of the many ways to prepare for a comfortable retirement. Financial planning for retirement is especially important for women. Women are much less likely to be covered by pension plans. Women are also more likely to have worked at lower paying jobs, or worked part-time during childbearing years. While the gap is narrowing, women still outlive men and are more likely to develop chronic disease later in life. To be sure they will be provided for as they age, women need to take a proactive role in both the day-to-day management of their finances and their retirement planning.

LO 6 | UNDERSTANDING THE FINAL TRANSITIONS: DYING AND DEATH

Define death and discuss strategies for coping with death.

Throughout history, humans have attempted to determine the nature and meaning of death. Individuals' feelings about death vary widely, depending on many factors, including age, religious beliefs, family orientation, health, personal experience with death, and the circumstances of the death itself.

53,364

IS THE NUMBER OF PEOPLE **100** YEARS OLD OR OLDER IN THE U.S. IN 2010.

Defining Death

According to the *Merriam Webster Dictionary,* **death** can be defined as "a permanent cessation of all vital functions: the end of life."[39] This definition has become more significant as medical advances make it increasingly possible to postpone death. Legal and ethical issues led to the Uniform Determination of Death Act in 1981. This act, which several states have adopted, reads as follows: "An individual who has sustained either (1) irreversible cessation of circulatory and respiratory functions, or (2) irreversible cessation of all functions of the entire brain, including the brainstem, is dead. A determination of death must be made in accordance with accepted medical standards."[40]

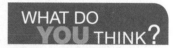

WHAT DO YOU THINK?

Why is there so much concern over the definition of death?

- How does modern technology complicate the understanding of when death occurs?

The concept of **brain death,** defined as the irreversible cessation of all functions of the entire brainstem, has gained increasing credence. As defined by the Ad Hoc Committee of the Harvard Medical School, brain death occurs when the following criteria are met:[41]

- Unreceptivity and unresponsiveness—that is, no response even to painful stimuli
- No movement for a continuous hour after observation by a physician, and no breathing after 3 minutes off a respirator
- No reflexes, including brainstem reflexes; fixed and dilated pupils
- A "flat" electroencephalogram (EEG, which monitors electrical activity of the brain) for at least 10 minutes

death The permanent ending of all vital functions.

brain death Irreversible cessation of all functions of the entire brainstem.

- All of these tests repeated at least 24 hours later with no change
- Certainty that hypothermia (extreme loss of body heat) or depression of the central nervous system caused by use of drugs such as barbiturates are not responsible for these conditions

The Harvard report provides useful guidelines; however, the exact definition of death remains somewhat controversial.

The Dying Process

Dying is the process of decline in body functions that results in the death of an organism. It is a complex process that includes physical, intellectual, social, spiritual, and emotional dimensions. Now that we have examined the physical indicators of death, we must consider the emotional aspects of dying and "social death."

dying Process of decline in body functions that results in the death of an organism.

thanatology The study of death and dying.

Coping Emotionally with Death

Science and medicine have enabled us to understand many changes throughout the life span, but they have not fully explained the nature of death. This may explain why the transition from life to death evokes so much mystery and emotion. Although emotional reactions to dying vary, many people share similar experiences during this process.

Kübler-Ross and the Stages of Dying Much of our knowledge about reactions to dying is based on the work of Elisabeth Kübler-Ross, a pioneer in **thanatology,** the study of death and dying. In 1969, Kübler-Ross published *On Death and Dying,* a sensitive analysis of the reactions of terminally ill patients. This pioneering work encouraged the development of death education as a discipline and prompted efforts to improve the care of dying patients. Kübler-Ross identified five psychological stages (**FIGURE 21.4**) that people coping with death often experience.[42]

1. **Denial.** ("Not me, there must be a mistake.") A person intellectually accepts the impending death but rejects it emotionally and feels a sense of shock and disbelief. The patient is too confused and stunned to comprehend "not being" and thus rejects the idea.
2. **Anger.** ("Why me?") The person becomes angry at having to face death when others, including loved ones, are healthy and not threatened. The dying person perceives the situation as unfair or senseless and may be hostile to friends, family, physicians, or the world in general.
3. **Bargaining.** ("If I'm allowed to live, I promise ...") The dying person may resolve to be a better person in return for an extension of life or may secretly pray for a short postponement of death to experience a special event, such as a family wedding or birth.
4. **Depression.** ("It's really going to happen, and I can't do anything about it.") Depression eventually sets in as vitality diminishes and the person begins to experience symptoms with increasing frequency. The person's deteriorating condition becomes impossible for him or her to deny. Common feelings experienced during this stage include doom, loss, worthlessness, and guilt over the emotional suffering of loved ones and arduous but seemingly futile efforts of caregivers.
5. **Acceptance.** ("I'm ready.") This is often the final stage. The patient stops battling with emotions and becomes tired and weak. With acceptance, the person does not "give up" and become sullen or resentfully resigned to death, but rather becomes passive.

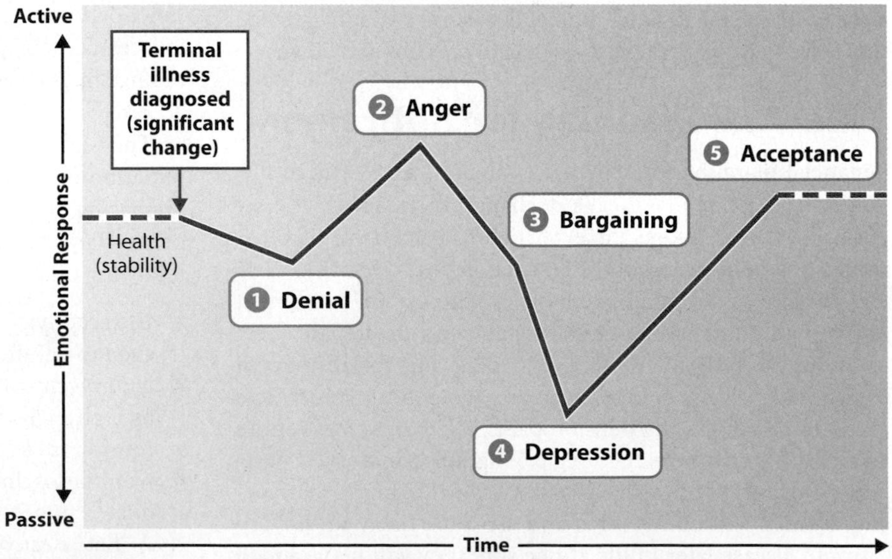

FIGURE 21.4 Kübler-Ross's Stages of Dying Kübler-Ross developed this model while working with terminally ill patients. She later expanded the model to apply to people experiencing grief or significant loss of any kind.

Some of Kübler-Ross's contemporaries consider her stage theory too neat and orderly. Subsequent research has indicated that the experiences of dying people do not fit easily into specific stages, and patterns vary from person to person. Some people never go through this process and instead remain emotionally calm; others may shift back and forth between various stages. Even if it is not accurate in all its particulars, Kübler-Ross's theory does offer valuable insights for those seeking to understand or deal with the process of dying.

Corr's Coping Approach Charles Corr developed an alternative model based on the idea that there are unique challenges and responses for the dying person and those who love him or her.[43] He suggests four dimensions of coping with loss: *physical*—doing everything possible to make oneself comfortable and minimize pain; *psychological*—living to the fullest, focusing on life accomplishments, and seeking satisfaction in daily activities; *social*—nurturing relationships, keeping loved ones involved, and sharing emotions; and *spiritual*—identifying what matters in life and reaffirming meaningful experiences.

Social Death The need for recognition and appreciation within a social group is nearly universal. Loss of being valued or appreciated by others can lead to **social death**, a situation in which a person is not treated like an active member of society. Numerous studies indicate that people are treated differently when they are dying, leading them to feel more isolated and unable to talk about their feelings: The dying person may be excluded from conversations or referred to as if he or she were already dead.[44] Dying patients are often moved to terminal wards and may be given minimal care; medical personnel may make degrading or impersonal comments about dying patients in their presence. In addition, inadequate pain control may contribute to patient suffering and anger or hostility, making caregiver assistance more difficult.

A decrease in meaningful social interaction often strips dying and bereaved people of their identity as valued members of society at a time when being able to talk, share, and make important decisions or say important things is critical.

LO 7 | COPING WITH LOSS

Describe typical grief symptoms and the grieving process.

Coping with the loss of a loved one is extremely difficult. The dying person, as well as close family and friends, frequently suffers emotionally and physically from the loss of critical relationships and roles.

Bereavement is generally defined as the loss or deprivation that a survivor experiences when a loved one dies. The death of a parent, spouse, sibling, child, friend, or pet will result in different kinds of feelings for different people. We should not make assumptions about the value a person places on his or her relationship with the deceased or the nature of his or her feelings about the loss. For example, often people fail to recognize the importance a pet can have, especially in single people's lives; for some, the loss of a pet may be as significant as the loss of a child. The loss of a loved one leaves "holes" and inevitable changes. Loneliness and despair may envelop the survivors. Understanding these normal reactions, along with time, patience, and support from loved ones, can do much to help the bereaved heal and move on, even though they will not forget.

Grief occurs in reaction to significant loss, including one's own impending death, the death of a loved one, or a *quasi-death* experience (a significant loss such as the end of a relationship or job, which involves separation, rejection, or a change in personal identity). Grief may be experienced as a mental, physical, social, or emotional reaction and often includes changes in patterns of eating, sleeping, working, and even thinking.

SKILLS FOR BEHAVIOR CHANGE: TALKING TO FRIENDS WHEN SOMEONE DIES

DO . . .

- Let your genuine concern and caring show; say you are sorry about their loss and pain.
- Be available to listen, run errands, help with children, or whatever else seems needed at the time.
- Allow them to express as much grief as they are feeling at the moment and are willing to share.
- Encourage them to be patient with themselves and not worry about things they should be doing.
- Allow them to talk about the person who has died as much and as often as they want to.
- Reassure them that they did everything they could, that the medical care given was the best, or whatever else you know to be true and positive about the care given.

DON'T . . .

- Let your own sense of helplessness keep you from reaching out to those who are bereaved.
- Avoid them because you are uncomfortable.
- Say you know how they feel (unless you've suffered a similar loss, you probably don't).
- Say, "You ought to be feeling better by now" or anything else that implies judgment about their feelings or what they should be doing.
- Change the subject when they mention the person who has died.

When a person experiences a loss that cannot be openly acknowledged, publicly mourned, or socially supported, coping may be much more difficult. This type of grief is referred to as *disenfranchised grief.* It may occur among people who experience a miscarriage, who are developmentally disabled, or who are close friends rather than blood relatives of the deceased. It may also include relationships that are not socially approved, such as extramarital affairs or homosexual relationships.

Symptoms of grief vary in severity and duration, depending on the situation and the individual. However, the bereaved person can benefit from emotional and social support from family, friends, clergy, employers, and traditional support organizations. The larger and stronger the support system, the easier readjustment is likely to be. See the **Skills for Behavior Change** box to learn how you can best help a grieving friend.

social death A seemingly irreversible situation in which a person is not treated as an active member of society.

bereavement Loss or deprivation experienced by a survivor when a loved one dies.

grief An individual's reaction to significant loss, including one's own impending death, the death of a loved one, or a quasi-death experience; grief can involve mental, physical, social, or emotional responses.

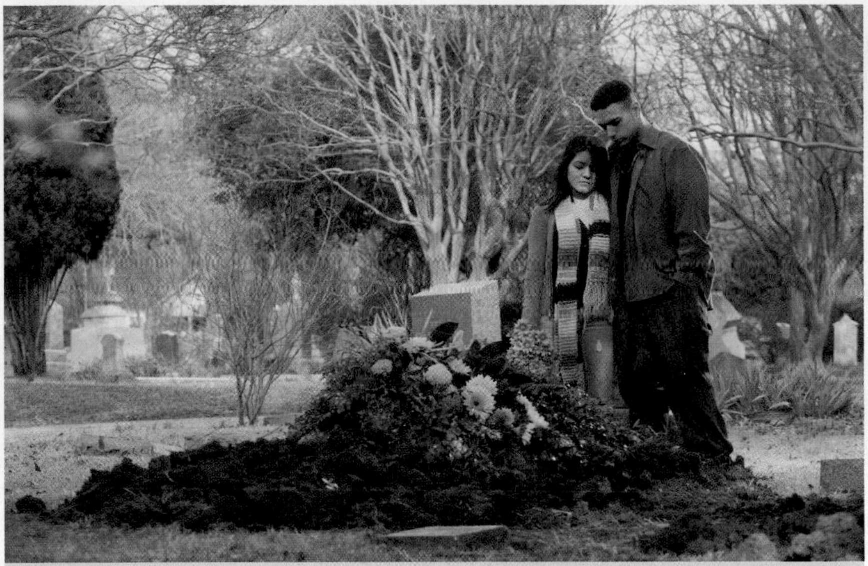

The most important thing you can do for a grieving friend is offer emotional support and a caring presence. Knowing what to say is less important than knowing how to listen.

The term *mourning* is often incorrectly equated with the term *grief*. As we have noted, *grief* refers to a wide variety of feelings and actions that occur in response to bereavement. **Mourning,** in contrast, refers to culturally prescribed and accepted time periods and behavior patterns for the expression of grief. In Judaism, for example, *sitting shivah* is a designated mourning period of 7 days that involves prescribed rituals and prayers. Depending on a person's relationship with the deceased, various other rituals may continue for up to a year.

What Is "Typical" Grief?

A bereaved person may suffer emotional pain and exhibit a variety of grief responses for many months after the death. Grief responses vary widely from person to person but frequently include such symptoms as periodic waves of prolonged physical distress, a feeling of tightness in the throat, choking or shortness of breath, sighing, feelings of emptiness, muscular weakness, or intense anxiety that is described as actually painful. Other common symptoms of grief include insomnia, memory lapses, loss of appetite, difficulty concentrating, a tendency to engage in repetitive or purposeless behavior, a feeling of being removed from reality, difficulty making decisions, lack of organization, excessive talking, social withdrawal or hostility, guilty feelings, and preoccupation with the image of the deceased. Susceptibility to disease increases with grief and may even be life threatening in severe and enduring cases.

mourning Culturally prescribed behavior patterns for the expression of grief.

grief work Process of accepting the reality of a person's death and coping with memories of the deceased.

The rate of the healing process depends on the amount and quality of grief work that a person does. **Grief work** is the process of integrating the reality of the loss into everyday life and learning to feel better. Often, a bereaved person must deliberately and systematically work at reducing denial and coping with the pain that comes from remembering the deceased.

Grief and Trauma

Disasters, war, and other events can leave many people suddenly bereaved of spouses, children, parents, close friends, and coworkers. In the immediate aftermath of the event, some bereaved survivors feel numb or unable to accept the loss. Many feel shocked, lost, anxious, and depressed. For many, the pain from their loss can be intense and unrelenting. These emotional and bodily reactions may be very strong and can themselves be traumatizing, especially if they are unfamiliar and unexpected. This secondary reaction can further amplify the pain caused by the loss.

It is important to realize that intense and unfamiliar emotionality is entirely normal and does not necessarily have implications for long-term emotional stability or health. However, if the symptoms linger and become increasingly debilitating, the condition turns into what is now being referred to as *unresolved, traumatic,* or *complicated grief,* which has features of both depression and post-traumatic stress disorder (PTSD). The most characteristic symptoms are intrusive thoughts and images of the deceased person and a painful yearning for his or her presence. Other complications are denial of the death, imagining that the dead person is alive, desperate loneliness and helplessness, anger and bitterness, and wanting to die. Treatment requires professional therapy and can include a promising new treatment called *traumatic grief therapy*, which uses cognitive behavioral methods for traumatic symptoms and stress relief, along with interpersonal techniques to encourage reengagement with the world.

Worden's Model of Grieving Tasks

William Worden, a researcher into the death process, developed an active grieving model that suggests four developmental tasks that a grieving person must complete in the grief work process:[45]

1. **Accept the reality of the loss.** This task requires acknowledging and realizing that the person is dead. Traditional rituals, such as the funeral, help many bereaved people move toward acceptance.
2. **Work through the pain of grief.** It is necessary to acknowledge and work through the pain associated with loss, or it will manifest itself through other symptoms or behaviors.
3. **Adjust to an environment in which the deceased is missing.** The bereaved may feel lonely and uncertain

about a new identity without the person who has died. This loss confronts them with the challenge of adjusting their own sense of self.

4. **Emotionally relocate the deceased and move on with life.** Individuals never lose memories of a significant relationship. They may need help in letting go of the emotional energy that used to be invested in the person who has died, and they may need help in finding an appropriate place for the deceased in their emotional lives.

Children and Death

Children are highly valued in our society, and their deaths are considered major tragedies. No matter what the cause of death—miscarriage, fatal birth defects, childhood illness, accident, suicide, homicide, natural disaster, neglect, or war injuries—the grief experienced when a child dies may be overwhelming.

Siblings of a deceased child may have a particularly hard time with grief work. Because so much attention and energy are devoted to the deceased child, the surviving children may feel emotionally abandoned by their parents. They may feel uncomfortable talking about death, and they may also receive less social support and sympathy than their parents do.

Bereaved children usually have limited experience with death and therefore have not yet learned how to deal with major loss. Often, when children suffer a loss, they will continue to behave "normally" to the adult observer. When it comes to complex emotional issues, children do not always show their feelings as openly as adults. Children tend to experience more prolonged grieving periods. They worry about whether they caused the death and whether they will die or will lose someone else they love, and they worry about what will happen to them and to the person who died. It can be helpful for family members to involve children in the dying process and to talk with them about the death while reassuring them of their safety. A professional counselor may also be of help in assisting children who are coping with loss.

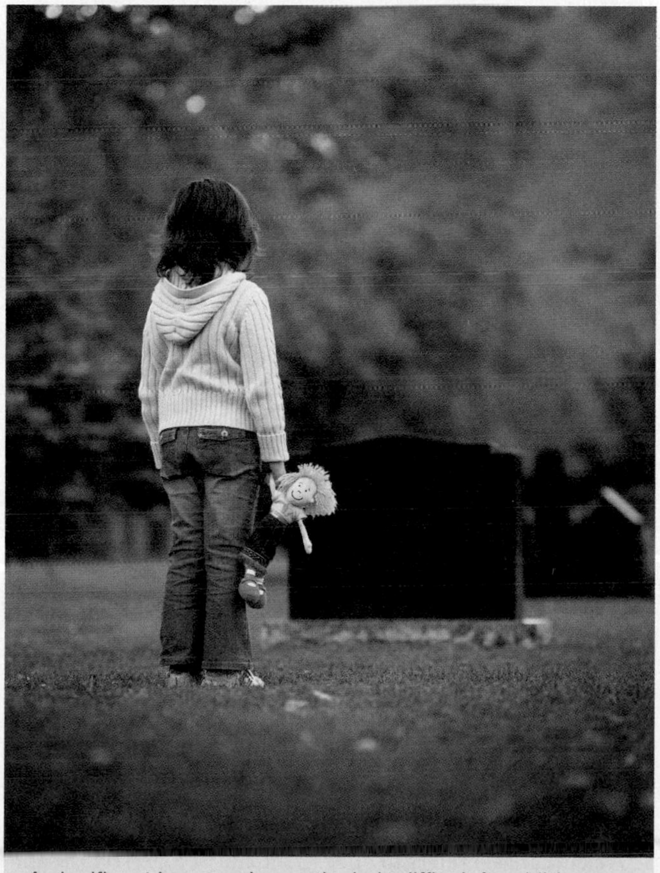

A significant loss can be particularly difficult for children.

WHAT DO YOU THINK?

If you have experienced a death among your family or friends, how did you grieve?

- Did you accomplish Worden's tasks?
- Did any of the models discussed match your experience?

LO 8 | LIFE-AND-DEATH DECISION MAKING

Explain the ethical concerns that arise from the concepts of the right to die and rational suicide.

When a loved one is dying, many complex and emotional—and often expensive—life-and death decisions must be made during a highly distressing period.

The Right to Die

Few people would object to the right to a dignified death. Going beyond that concept, however, many people today believe that they should be allowed to die if their condition is terminal and their existence depends on mechanical life-support devices or artificial feeding or hydration systems. Artificial life-support techniques that may be legally refused by competent patients include electrical or mechanical heart resuscitation, mechanical respiration by machine, nasogastric tube feedings, intravenous nutrition, gastrostomy (tube feeding directly into the stomach), and medications to treat life-threatening infections.

As long as a person is conscious and competent, he or she has the legal right to refuse treatment, even if this decision will hasten death. However, when a person is in a coma or otherwise incapable of speaking on his or her own behalf, medical personnel, family members, and administrative policy will dictate treatment. This issue has evolved into a battle involving personal freedom, legal rulings, health care administration policy, and physician responsibility. The living will and other **advance directives** were developed to assist in solving these conflicts. See **Student Health Today** on the next page for a list of documents that you can put in order while you're in good health.

advance directive Document that stipulates an individual's wishes about medical care; used to make treatment decisions when an individual becomes physically unable to voice his or her preferences.

STUDENT HEALTH TODAY

PREPARING FOR ENDINGS

While college and those years immediately following graduation are not typically times we think about needing to prepare for death, we do know that life circumstances can change quickly for anyone. Here is a list of documents you should pull together in a central location, whether on a computer or in an old fashioned file box.

Source: *The Wall Street Journal*, "25 Documents You Need before You Die," Accessed June 2014, http://online.wsj.com/news/interactive/DOC110702?ref=SB10001424052702303627104576410234039258092.

Marriage and Divorce
- Marriage license
- Divorce papers

Life Insurance/Retirement
- Life insurance policies
- Individual retirement accounts
- 401(k) accounts

Health Care
- Personal and family medical history
- Authorization to release health care information
- Durable power of attorney
- Living will
- Do-not-resuscitate order

Bank Accounts
- List of bank accounts
- List of all user names and passwords
- List of safe-deposit boxes

Proof of Ownership
- Vehicle titles
- Proof of loans and debts owed
- Stock certificates and savings bonds

The Essentials
- Will
- Trust documents

living will Type of advance directive.

rational suicide The decision to kill oneself rather than endure constant pain and slow decay.

active euthanasia "Mercy killing" in which a person or organization knowingly acts to end the life of a terminally ill person.

Even young, apparently healthy people need a **living will.** Consider Terri Schiavo, who collapsed at age 26 from heart failure that led to irreversible brain damage. Schiavo, unable to survive without life support, never left any written guidelines about her wishes should she become incapacitated. After a 15-year legal battle between her parents, who wanted her to be kept alive, and her husband, who felt she should be allowed to die, the courts sided with her husband, and she was removed from life support.

Many legal experts suggest that you take the following steps to ensure that your wishes are carried out.[46]

- **Be specific.** Complete an advance directive that permits you to make very specific choices about a variety of procedures, including cardiopulmonary resuscitation (CPR); being placed on a ventilator; being given food, water, or medication through tubes; being given pain medication; and organ donation.
- **Name a health care proxy.** You may want to appoint a family member or friend to act as your agent, or *proxy,* by completing a form known as either a *durable power of attorney for health care* or a *health care proxy.* This allows the person you designate to make medical decisions for you in the event you are incapacitated.
- **Discuss your wishes.** Discuss your preferences in detail with your proxy and your doctor.
- **Deliver the directive.** Distribute several copies, not only to your doctor and your agent, but also to your lawyer and to immediate family members or a close friend. Make sure *someone* knows to bring a copy to the hospital in the event you are hospitalized.

One alternative to the traditional advance directive or living will is a document called *Five Wishes* that is written in uncomplicated language and meets the legal requirements for advance directive statutes in most states. This document differs from most other living wills because it addresses personal, emotional, and spiritual needs, as well as medical needs.[47] It is available at low cost online at www.agingwithdignity.org.

Rational Suicide and Euthanasia

It is estimated that thousands of terminally ill people every year decide to kill themselves rather than endure constant pain and slow decay. This alternative to the extended dying process is known as **rational suicide.** To these people, the prospect of an undignified death is unacceptable. This issue has been complicated by advances in death prevention techniques that allow terminally ill patients to exist in an irreversible disease state for extended periods of time.

According to public opinion polls, most Americans believe that suicide is morally wrong but are divided on whether physician-assisted suicide is morally acceptable. Roughly 70 percent of Americans believe doctors should be allowed to help end an incurably ill patient's life painlessly at the patient's request.[48]

Physician-assisted suicide is not a new phenomenon. It has been practiced in many societies throughout history and currently is legal in some European countries, such as Belgium and the Netherlands. Legalization of assisted suicide has been debated in many U.S. states. Currently, more than 30 states have statutes explicitly prohibiting assisted suicide and only three states—Oregon, Washington, and Montana—have laws allowing for physician-assisted suicide under certain circumstances.[49]

Euthanasia is often referred to as "mercy killing." The term **active euthanasia** refers to ending the life of a person (or animal) who is suffering greatly and has no chance of recovery. An example might be a physician-prescribed lethal injection, as in physician-assisted suicide. **Passive euthanasia** refers to the intentional withholding of treatment that would prolong life. Deciding not to place a person with massive brain trauma on life support is an example of passive euthanasia. Advance directives, such as "do not resuscitate" orders, can provide legal justification for various forms of passive euthanasia.

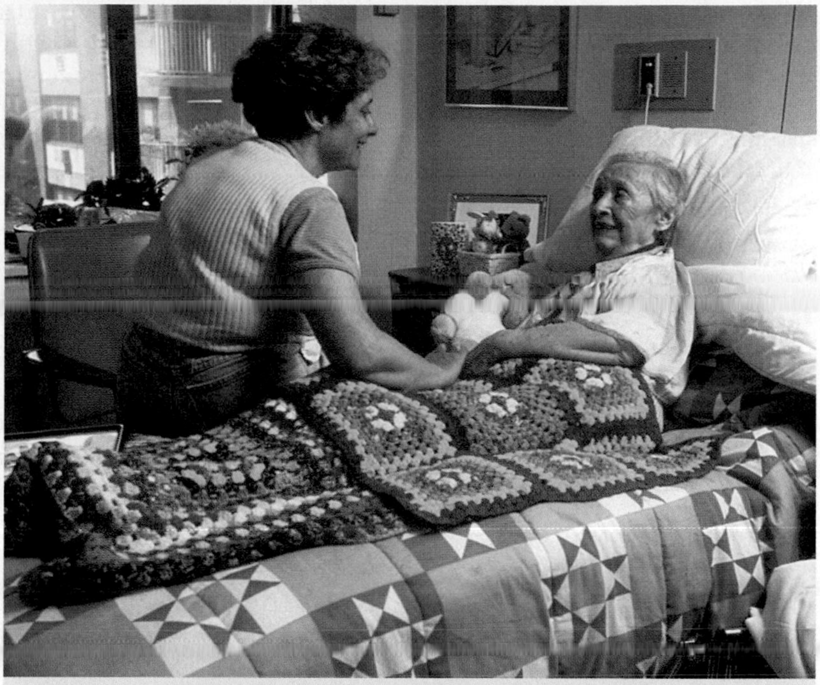

A hospice program provides support services to family members, ensures that the dying loved one is comfortable, and allows family and friends to be involved in their loved one's care.

LO 9 | MAKING FINAL ARRANGEMENTS

Review the decisions that need to be made when someone is dying or has died, including hospice care, funeral arrangements, wills, and organ donation.

Caring for a dying person and his or her loved ones involves a wide variety of psychological, legal, social, spiritual, economic, and interpersonal issues.

Hospice Care: Positive Alternatives

Since the mid-1970s, hospice programs in the United States have grown from a mere handful to more than 5,300 and are available in nearly every community.[50] These programs are a form of **palliative care** that focus on reducing pain and suffering while attending to the emotional and spiritual needs of dying individuals and their caregivers. Hospice care may help the survivors cope better with the death experience. Hospice volunteers provide much needed "respite" care for caregivers, who often face emotional and physical challenges in caring for dying loved ones.

The primary goals of **hospice** programs are to relieve the dying person's pain; offer emotional support to the dying person and loved ones; and restore a sense of control to the dying person, family, and friends. Hospice programs usually include the following characteristics:

- There is overall medical direction of the program, with all health care provided under the direction of a qualified physician. Emphasis is placed on symptom control, primarily the alleviation of pain.
- Services are provided by an interdisciplinary team.
- Coverage is provided 24 hours a day, 7 days a week, with emphasis on the availability of medical and nursing skills.
- Carefully selected and extensively trained volunteers who augment but do not replace staff service are an integral part of the health care team.
- Care of the family extends through the bereavement period.
- Patients are accepted on the basis of their health needs, not their ability to pay.

Despite the growing number of individuals and families who consider hospice facilities, some people prefer to die in a hospital, and others choose to die at home. In some communities, hospice services are available as in-home care. Individuals and families should decide as early as possible what type of terminal care is most desirable and feasible to allow time for the necessary emotional, physical, and financial preparations.

passive euthanasia Intentional withholding of treatment that would prolong life.

palliative care Any form of medical care focused on relieving the pain, symptoms, and stress of serious illness to improve the quality of life for patients and their families.

hospice Type of end-of-life care designed to maximize quality of life and help dying people have peace, comfort, and dignity.

Making Funeral Arrangements

Anthropological evidence indicates that all cultures throughout human history have developed some sort of funeral ritual. For this reason, social scientists agree that funerals assist survivors in coping with their loss. In the United States, with its diversity of religious, regional, and ethnic customs, funeral practices vary. In some faiths, the deceased may be displayed to formalize last respects and increase social support of the bereaved. This part of the funeral ritual is referred to as a *wake* or *viewing*. The funeral service may be held in a church, a funeral chapel, or at the burial site. Some people choose to replace the funeral service with a simple memorial service held within a few days of the burial. Social interaction that is part of funeral and memorial services is valuable in helping survivors cope.

SEE IT! VIDEOS

Caring for the elderly can be hard. Watch **Understanding the Difficulties of Caregivers** available on MasteringHealth.™

In addition to details related to the type of funeral or memorial service and the method of burial or body disposition, loved ones must also consider the cost of funeral and memorial options. They usually have to contact friends and relatives, plan for the arrival of guests, choose markers, submit obituary information to newspapers, and deal with many other details. Even though funeral directors are available to facilitate decision making, the bereaved may experience undue stress, especially if the death is unexpected. People who make their own funeral arrangements ahead of time can save their loved ones the difficulty of having to make these decisions during a very stressful time.

Wills

The issue of inheritance should be resolved before a person dies to reduce both conflict and needless expense. Unfortunately, many people are so intimidated by the thought of making a will that they never do so and die **intestate** (without a will). This is tragic, especially because the procedure for establishing a legal will is relatively simple and inexpensive. In addition, if you don't make a will before you die, the courts (as directed by state laws) will make a will for you. Legal issues, rather than your wishes, will preside. Furthermore, settling an estate takes longer when a person dies without a will.

Trusts

Trusts are estate-planning tools that can help you manage property during your life if you are disabled by accident or illness and ensure a smooth transition of affairs after your death. While a trust sounds appealing, there are some aspects to be aware of. A living trust is more expensive to set up than a typical will because it must be actively managed after it is created. Most importantly, however, a living trust is useless unless it is funded, and it can only control those assets that have been placed into it. If your assets have not been transferred or if you die without funding the trust, the trust will be of no benefit: Your estate will still be subject to probate, and there may be significant estate tax issues.[51]

Organ Donation

Organ donation takes healthy organs and tissues from one person for transplantation into another. Experts say that the organs from one donor can save or help as many as 50 people. You can donate internal organs (kidneys, heart, liver, pancreas, intestines, lungs); skin; bone and bone marrow; and corneas. Most organ and tissue donations occur after the donor has died, but some organs and tissues can be donated while the donor is alive.[52]

Organ donation saves lives: Approximately 79 people receive organ transplants every day. However, an average of 18 people die each day waiting for transplants because of the shortage of donated organs. The number of patients waiting for organs continues to significantly outnumber the donor organs available, and the gap is increasing (**FIGURE 21.5**).

People of all ages and backgrounds can be organ donors. It's especially important to consider becoming an organ donor if you are African American, Asian or Pacific Islander, Native American, or Hispanic. Members of these groups have a higher prevalence of certain chronic conditions that affect the kidney, heart, lung, pancreas, and liver, all of which can be treated with organ transplantation. Matching blood type is necessary for transplants, and because certain blood types are more common in particular ethnic groups, the need for minority donor organs is especially high.[53]

intestate Dying without a will.

If you want to be an organ donor, the most important thing to do is to enroll in your state's donor registry. Go to www.organdonor.gov to sign up under your state. It is also a good idea to indicate your decision on your driver's license, tell your family about your donation decision, tell your physician, and include the donation in your will and living will. Uniform donor cards are available through the U.S. Department of Health and Human Services and through many health care foundations and nonprofit organizations (**FIGURE 21.6**).

Although some people are opposed to organ transplants and tissue donation, others experience personal fulfillment from knowing that their organs may extend and improve someone else's life after their own death.

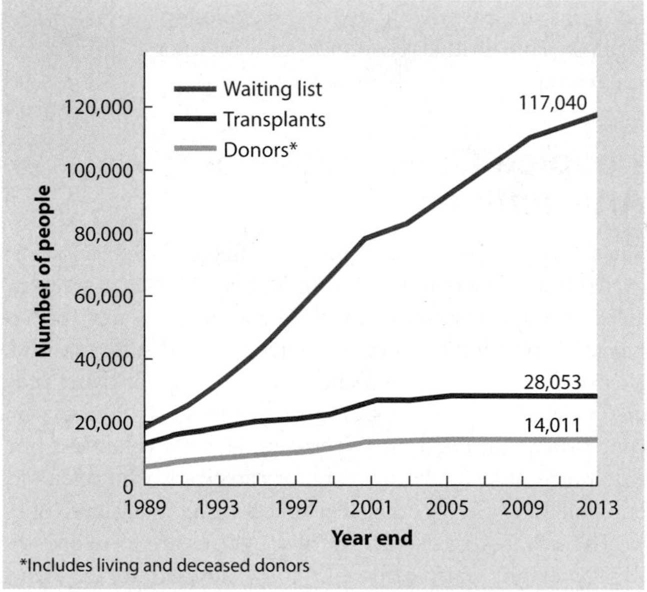

FIGURE 21.5 Organ Donors and Patients Needing and Receiving Transplants, 1989–2012

Source: U.S. Department of Health and Human Services, Organ Procurement and Transplantation Network, October, 2014, http://optn.transplant.hrsa.gov.

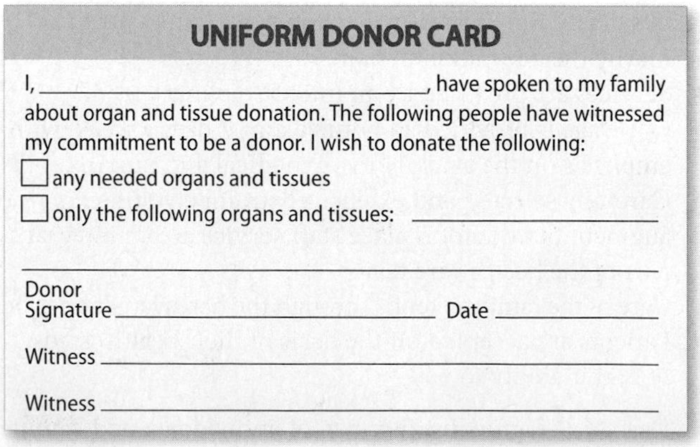
UNIFORM DONOR CARD

I, ________________, have spoken to my family about organ and tissue donation. The following people have witnessed my commitment to be a donor. I wish to donate the following:

☐ any needed organs and tissues

☐ only the following organs and tissues: __________

Donor Signature __________ Date __________

Witness __________

Witness __________

FIGURE 21.6 Organ Donor Card Each organ and tissue donor can save or improve the lives of as many as 50 people.

STUDY PLAN

Customize your study plan—and master your health!—in the Study Area of **MasteringHealth.**

ASSESS **YOURSELF**

What are your attitudes and feelings towards death? Want to find out? Take the **Are You Afraid of Death?** assessment available on MasteringHealth.

Need help creating a plan? Follow the strategies in the **Your Plan for Change** box for short- and long-term improvements to your health.

YOUR PLAN FOR **CHANGE**

After completing the "Are You Afraid of Death?" **ASSESS YOURSELF** activity, you can begin to change beliefs that may be causing you anxiety on the subject of death and dying.

TODAY, YOU CAN:

- ☐ Learn about advance directives. Visit a low-cost legal clinic for information and a sample. You can also locate samples online, including the Five Wishes document, which is available at www.agingwithdignity.org.
- ☐ Fill out an organ donation card. Knowing that you may be able to prolong another person's life after your death can help you feel more at peace with your mortality.

WITHIN THE NEXT 2 WEEKS, YOU CAN:

- ☐ Consider how you would like to be remembered. Are you living in a way that you want to be remembered? What actions can you take now to help ensure that your eulogy reflects your ideal life course?
- ☐ Talk to family members about their life goals. What have they achieved, and what do they wish they had done differently? What can you learn from their experiences?

BY THE END OF THE SEMESTER, YOU CAN:

- ☐ Consider how you feel about various medical techniques that might be used in the event you become incapacitated. Do you feel comfortable being kept alive by a machine? Make your wishes on these matters known to family members and friends, and put them in writing.
- ☐ Talk to your parents or grandparents about the arrangements they prefer in the event of their death. Do they want a burial or cremation? A full funeral or a small service? Making these decisions now will save you and your loved ones stress later.

CHAPTER **REVIEW**

To hear an MP3 Tutor Session, scan here or visit the Study Area in **MasteringHealth.**

LO 1 Redefining Aging

- Aging can be defined in terms of biological age, psychological age, social age, legal age, or functional age.

LO 2 Older Adults: A Growing Population

- The growing number of older adults (age 65 and older) has an increasing impact on society in terms of the economy, health care, housing, and ethical considerations.

LO 3 Theories of Aging

- Biological explanations of aging include the wear-and-tear theory, the cellular theory, the genetic mutation theory, and the autoimmune theory. Psychosocial theories center on adaptation and adjustments related to self-development.

LO 4 Physical and Mental Changes of Aging

- Aging changes the body and mind in many ways. Physical changes occur in the skin, bones and joints, head, urinary tract, heart and lungs, senses, sexual function, and temperature regulation. Major physical concerns are osteoporosis, urinary incontinence, and changes in eyesight and hearing. Most older people maintain a high level of mental functioning and memory. Potential mental problems include depression and Alzheimer's disease.

LO 5 Strategies for Healthy Living

- Lifestyle choices we make today will affect health status later in life. Choosing to exercise, eat a healthy diet, foster lasting relationships, engage in spiritual development, and avoid unhealthy habits such as smoking will contribute to healthy aging.

LO 6 Understanding the Final Transitions: Dying and Death

- *Death* can be defined biologically in terms of brain death or the cessation of vital functions. Dying is a multifaceted emotional process, and individuals may experience emotional stages such as denial, anger, bargaining, depression, and acceptance. Social death results when a person is no longer treated as an active member of society.

LO 7 Coping with Loss

- Grief is the state of distress felt after loss. People differ in their responses to grief. Children need to be helped through the process of grieving.

LO 8 Life-and-Death Decision Making

- The right to die by rational suicide involves ethical, moral, and legal issues.

LO 9 Making Final Arrangements

- Hospice services are available to provide care for the terminally ill and their caregivers. After death, funeral arrangements must be made quickly and customs vary by family, region, religious affiliation, and cultural background.
- Decisions made in advance of illness and death through advance directives, wills, trusts, and organ donation cards make the process easier for survivors.

POP **QUIZ**

Visit **MasteringHealth** to personalize your study plan with Chapter Review Quizzes and Dynamic Study Modules.

LO 1 Redefining Aging

1. The study of death and dying is known as
   a. thanatology.
   b. gerontology.
   c. biology.
   d. geriatrics.

LO 2 Older Adults: A Growing Population

2. Which of the following is true?
   a. The majority of men aged 65 and older live with a spouse.
   b. The number of adults aged 65 and older is decreasing the United States.
   c. The majority of women aged 65 and older live alone.
   d. The majority of men and women aged 65 and older live in nursing homes.

LO 3 Theories of Aging

3. Which biological theory of aging supports the concept that body cells are able to reproduce only so many times throughout life?
   a. Wear-and-tear theory
   b. Cellular theory
   c. Autoimmune theory
   d. Genetic mutation theory

LO 4 Physical and Mental Changes of Aging

4. Martha's ophthalmologist tells her she has a condition that involves the breakdown of the light-sensitive area of the retina that is affecting her sharp, direct vision. What is this condition?
   a. Cataracts
   b. Glaucoma
   c. Macular degeneration
   d. Nearsightedness

LO 5 Strategies for Healthy Living

5. The keys to successful aging include
   a. Drinking red wine regularly
   b. Reducing protein intake
   c. Avoiding weight-bearing activities
   d. Eating sufficient calcium and vitamin D

LO 6 Understanding the Final Transitions: Dying and Death

6. The Kübler-Ross stage of dying in which the individual rejects death

emotionally and feels a sense of shock and disbelief is known as
a. acceptance.
b. bargaining.
c. denial.
d. anger.

LO 7 | Coping with Loss

7. A culturally prescribed and accepted period of grief for someone who has died is known as
   a. bereavement.
   b. grief work.
   c. coping with loss.
   d. mourning.
8. Grief work is
   a. the process of integrating the reality of a loss with everyday life and learning to feel better.
   b. the total acceptance that a loved one has died.
   c. assigning feelings to the loss of a loved one.
   d. completing the cultural rituals required to express one's grief.

LO 8 | Life-and-Death Decision Making

9. Kerri's elderly grandmother is terminally ill and wants to die without medical intervention. Her family has agreed to withhold treatment that may prolong her life. This is called
   a. rational suicide.
   b. health care proxy.
   c. passive euthanasia.
   d. active euthanasia.

LO 9 | Making Final Arrangements

10. Destiny's grandfather dies intestate. This means he
    a. had a health care proxy.
    b. did not have a will.
    c. received hospice care.
    d. did not have a trust.

Answers to the Pop Quiz can be found on page A-1. If you answered a question incorrectly, review the section identified by the Learning Outcome. For even more study tools, visit MasteringHealth.

THINK ABOUT IT!

LO 1 | Redefining Aging

1. What are some of the different ways aging is defined? How are they different? How are they similar? How do you see it?

LO 2 | Older Adults: A Growing Population

2. As the older population grows, how will it affect your life? Would you be willing to pay higher taxes to support government programs for older adults? Why or why not?

LO 3 | Theories of Aging

3. What are the biological explanations of how and why we age? What do psychosocial theories focus on as important factors in aging?

LO 4 | Physical and Mental Changes of Aging

4. List the major physical and mental changes that occur with aging. Which of these, if any, can you change? Discuss actions you can start taking now to ensure a healthier aging process.

LO 5 | Strategies for Healthy Living

5. How do the lifestyle choices we make now affect our health status later in life? What are some of the healthy choices and changes you could make today that will contribute to healthy aging later?

LO 6 | Understanding the Final Transitions: Dying and Death

6. Explain why so many of us deny death. How could death become a more acceptable topic to discuss?

LO 7 | Coping with Loss

7. How do people differ in their responses to grief? What are some things you could do, and some things you shouldn't do, to support a friend or loved one who is grieving?

LO 8 | Life-and-Death Decision Making

8. Discuss when you think people should start deciding whether to have an advance directive. What are some important considerations when preparing an advance directive?
9. Debate whether rational suicide should be legalized for the terminally ill. What restrictions would you include in a law?

LO 9 | Making Final Arrangements

10. Are you an organ donor? What are some reasons why people decide to become organ donors? What might be some common hesitations?

ACCESS YOUR HEALTH ON THE INTERNET

Visit **MasteringHealth** for links to the websites and RSS feeds.

The following websites explore further topics and issues related to personal health.

AARP. This site includes comprehensive information on issues related to aging, including longevity and caregiving. **www.aarp.org**

Administration on Aging. This U.S. Department of Health and Human Services link is dedicated to addressing the health needs of older adults. **www.aoa.gov**

Alzheimer's Association. This site includes media releases, position statements, fact sheets, and research on Alzheimer's disease. **www.alz.org**

Grieving.com. This forum site addresses all aspects of grief and loss, including terminal illness, non-death losses, and caregiving. **http://forums.grieving.com**

APPENDIX A ANSWERS TO CHAPTER REVIEW QUESTIONS

Chapter 1

1. b; 2. d; 3. b; 4. a; 5. d; 6. a; 7. a; 8. a; 9. a; 10. c

Chapter 2

1. b; 2. a; 3. a; 4. b; 5. c; 6. c; 7. c; 8. b; 9. b; 10. b; 11. a; 12. b; 13. b

Chapter 3

1. c; 2. b; 3. c; 4. a; 5. d; 6. d; 7. c; 8. d; 9. b; 10. c

Chapter 4

1. b; 2. c; 3. a; 4. d; 5. a; 6. a; 7. b; 8. d; 9. a; 10. d

Chapter 5

1. c; 2. b; 3. c; 4. a; 5. b; 6. d; 7. a; 8. d; 9. c; 10. a

Chapter 6

1. c; 2. b; 3. b; 4. d; 5. c; 6. b; 7. a; 8. d; 9. b; 10. a; 11. b; 12. b; 13. c; 14. d; 15. a; 16. a

Chapter 7

1. d; 2. a; 3. a; 4. b; 5. b; 6. a; 7. b; 8. c; 9. b; 10. d

Chapter 8

1. a; 2. c; 3. c; 4. b; 5. b; 6. a; 7. b; 8. a; 9. d; 10. a

Chapter 9

1. d; 2. a; 3. c; 4. c; 5. a; 6. b; 7. d; 8. c; 9. b; 10. a

Chapter 10

1. c; 2. d; 3. c; 4. b; 5. d; 6. d; 7. b; 8. a; 9. a; 10. b

Chapter 11

1. c; 2. b; 3. d; 4. c; 5. c; 6. d; 7. b; 8. b; 9. a; 10. a

Chapter 12

1. b; 2. c; 3. c; 4. c; 5. b; 6. a; 7. d; 8. b; 9. d; 10. a

Chapter 13

1. b; 2. c; 3. a; 4. a; 5. c; 6. a; 7. c; 8. b; 9. c; 10. b

Chapter 14

1. d; 2. b; 3. c; 4. d; 5. c; 6. a

Chapter 15

1. c; 2. b; 3. d; 4. c; 5. d; 6. a; 7. a; 8. b; 9. c; 10. c

Chapter 16

1. b; 2. b; 3. d; 4. a; 5. a; 6. a; 7. c; 8. d; 9. b; 10. d

Chapter 17

1. c; 2. c; 3. d; 4. c; 5. b; 6. b; 7. b; 8. a; 9. a; 10. d

Chapter 18

1. c; 2. a; 3. b; 4. a; 5. c; 6. c; 7. c; 8. d; 9. c; 10. d

Chapter 19

1. b; 2. a; 3. c; 4. c; 5. a; 6. a; 7. d; 8. b; 9. a; 10. d

Chapter 20

1. d; 2. d; 3. a; 4. d; 5. b; 6. d; 7. a; 8. c; 9. a; 10. a

Chapter 21

1. a; 2. a; 3. b; 4. c; 5. d; 6. c; 7. d; 8. a; 9. c; 10. b

Ideally, first-aid procedures should be performed only by someone who has received formal training from the American Red Cross or another reputable institution. (There are numerous classes and opportunities in most communities for updating your skills in these areas. Check for such classes at your university or local community college.) If you do not have such training, contact a physician or call your local emergency medical service (EMS) by dialing 9-1-1 or your local emergency number. In life-threatening situations, however, you may need to begin first aid immediately and continue until help arrives. This section contains basic information for various emergency situations. Simply reading these directions, however, may not prepare you fully to handle these situations. For this reason, you may want to enroll in a first aid course.

CALLING FOR EMERGENCY ASSISTANCE

When calling for emergency assistance, be prepared to give exact details. Be clear and thorough, and do not panic. Never hang up until the dispatcher has informed you that he or she has all the information needed. Be ready to answer the following questions:

- Where are you and the victim located? (This is the most important information that the EMS will need.)
- What is your phone number and name?
- What has happened? Was there an accident, or is the victim ill?
- How many people need help?
- What is the nature of the emergency? What is the victim's apparent condition?
- Are there any life-threatening situations that the EMS should know about (for example, fires, explosions, or fallen electrical lines)?
- Is the victim wearing a medic-alert tag (a tag indicating a specific medical condition such as diabetes)?

ADMINISTERING FIRST AID

According to the laws in most states, you are not required to administer first aid unless you have a special obligation to the victim. For example, parents must provide first aid for their children, and a lifeguard must provide aid to a swimmer.

Before administering first aid, you should obtain the victim's consent. If the victim refuses aid, you must respect that person's rights. However, you should make every reasonable effort to persuade the victim to accept your help. In emergency situations, consent is *implied* if the victim is unconscious. Once you begin to administer first aid, you are required by law to continue. You must remain with the victim until someone of equal or greater competence takes over.

Can you be held liable if you fail to provide adequate care or if the victim is further injured? To protect people who render first aid, most states have Good Samaritan laws, which grant immunity (protection from civil liability) if you act in good faith to provide care to the best of your ability, according to your level of training. Because these laws vary, you should become familiar with the Good Samaritan laws in your state.

First-Aid Supplies

Every home, car, and boat should be supplied with a basic first-aid kit, which should be stored in a convenient place but kept out of the reach of children. Following is a list of supplies that should be included:

- Bandages, including triangular bandages (36 inches by 6 inches), butterfly bandages, a roller bandage, rolled white gauze bandages (2- and 3-inch widths), adhesive bandages
- Sterile gauze pads and absorbent pads
- Adhesive tape (2- and 3-inch widths)
- Cotton-tip applicators
- Scissors
- Thermometer
- Antibiotic ointment
- Aspirin
- Calamine lotion
- Antiseptic cream or petroleum jelly
- Safety pins
- Tweezers
- Latex gloves
- Flashlight
- Paper cups
- Blanket

You cannot be prepared for every medical emergency, but these essential tools and a knowledge of basic first aid will help you cope with many emergency situations, including the ones discussed below.

Cessation of Breathing

If someone has stopped breathing, you should perform mouth-to-mouth resuscitation. This involves the following steps:

1. Check for responsiveness by gently tapping or shaking the victim. Ask loudly, "Are you okay?"
2. Call the local EMS for help (usually 9-1-1).
3. Gently roll the victim onto his or her back.
4. Open the airway by tilting the victim's head back—place your hand nearest the victim's head on the victim's forehead, and apply backward pressure to tilt the head back and lift the chin.

5. Check for breathing (3 to 5 seconds): look, listen, and feel for breathing.
6. Give two slow breaths.
   - Keep the victim's head tilted back.
   - Pinch the victim's nose shut.
   - Seal your lips tightly around the victim's mouth.
   - Give two slow breaths, each lasting 1.5 to 2 seconds.
   - Watch for the chest to rise and fall.
7. Check for pulse at side of neck; feel for pulse for 5 to 10 seconds.
8. Begin rescue breathing.
   - Keep the victim's head tilted back.
   - Pinch the victim's nose shut.
   - Give one breath about every 5 seconds (12 breaths per minute).
   - Look, listen, and feel for breathing between breaths.
9. Recheck pulse every minute.
   - Keep the victim's head tilted back.
   - Feel for pulse for 5 to 10 seconds.
   - If the victim has a pulse but is not breathing, continue rescue breathing. If there is no pulse, begin CPR (see below).

There are some variations when performing this procedure on infants and children. For infants, at step 8, you should give one slow breath every 3 seconds. You should not pinch the nose. Instead, seal your lips tightly around the infant's nose and mouth. For children aged 1 to 8, at step 8, give one slow breath every 4 seconds.

Sudden Collapse

If an adult has a sudden cardiac arrest, his or her survival depends largely on being given immediate cardiopulmonary resuscitation (CPR). People are often afraid to offer aid for fear of doing something wrong or making matters worse. In addition, some people are squeamish about performing the artificial respiration that is part of traditional CPR. However, studies have shown that simply providing hands-only CPR to an adult who has collapsed can double that person's chance of survival. The American Heart Association now recommends that anyone, trained or untrained, who witnesses an adult's sudden collapse should call 9-1-1 and then immediately begin hands-only CPR. That means uninterrupted chest compressions—pushing hard in the center of the victim's chest—at a rate of about 100 per minute until the EMS arrives.

Conventional CPR, a technique that involves a combination of artificial respiration and chest compressions, is still recommended for infants or children, drowning victims, drug overdose, or other respiratory problems, and on adult victims who are found already unconscious and not breathing normally. The American Red Cross, the American Heart Association, and other organizations offer courses in mouth-to-mouth resuscitation and CPR as well as general first aid. If you have taken a CPR course in the past, you should be aware that certain changes have been made in the procedure. Consider taking a refresher course.

Choking

Choking occurs when an object obstructs the trachea (windpipe), thus preventing normal breathing. Failure to expel the object and restore breathing can lead to death within 6 minutes. The universal signal of distress related to choking is the clasping of the throat with one or both hands. Other signs of choking include not being able to talk and/or noisy and difficult breathing. If a victim can cough or speak, do not interfere. The most effective method for assisting choking victims is the Heimlich maneuver (**FIGURE 1**), which involves the application of pressure to the victim's abdominal area to expel the foreign object, as described below.

If the Choking Victim Is Standing or Seated

1. Recognize that the victim is choking. Without startling him or her, approach from behind.
2. Wrap your arms around the victim's waist, making a fist with one hand.
3. Place the thumb side of the fist on the middle of the victim's abdomen, just above the navel and well below the tip of the sternum.
4. Cover your fist with your other hand.
5. Press fist into victim's abdomen, with up to five quick upward thrusts.

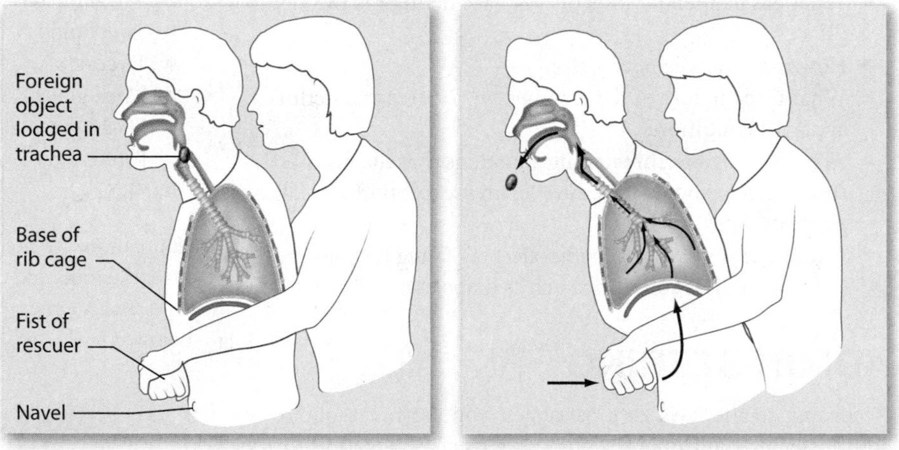

a Standing behind the victim, place a fist thumb-side in just above the victim's navel and cover it with your other hand.

b Press sharply upward and inward, using enough force to push the diaphragm and lungs up and create air pressure that will expel the object.

FIGURE 1 Heimlich Maneuver
The Heimlich maneuver can be used to dislodge an object that is blocking a person's airway, causing him or her to choke. The technique shown here is appropriate for use on a person who is either sitting or standing.

Source: Adapted from Johnson, Michael D., *Human Biology: Concepts and Current Issues*, 5th, © 2010. Printed and Electronically reproduced by permission of Pearson Education, Inc., Upper Saddle River, New Jersey.

6. After every five abdominal thrusts, check the victim and your technique.
7. If the victim becomes unconscious, gently lower him or her to the ground.
8. Try to clear the airway by using your finger to sweep the object from the victim's mouth or throat.
9. Give two rescue breaths. If the passage is still blocked and air will not go in, repeat the Heimlich maneuver.

If the Choking Victim Is Lying Down

1. Facing the person, kneel with your legs astride the victim's hips. Place the heel of one hand against the abdomen, slightly above the navel and well below the tip of the sternum. Put the other hand on top of the first hand.
2. Press inward and upward using both hands with up to five quick abdominal thrusts.
3. Repeat the following steps in this sequence until the airway becomes clear or the EMS arrives:
   - Finger sweep.
   - Give two rescue breaths.
   - Do up to five abdominal thrusts.

Alcohol Poisoning

Alcohol overdose is considered a medical emergency when an irregular heartbeat or coma occurs. The two immediate causes of death in such cases are cardiac arrhythmia and respiratory depression. If a person is seriously uncoordinated and has possibly also taken a depressant, the risk of respiratory failure is serious enough that a physician should be contacted. When dealing with someone who is drunk, remember these points:

1. Stay calm. Assess the situation.
2. Keep your distance. Before approaching or touching the person, explain what you intend to do.
3. Speak in a clear, firm, reassuring manner.
4. Keep the person still and comfortable.
5. Stay with the person if she or he is vomiting. When helping him or her to lie down, turn the head to the side to prevent it from falling back. This helps to keep the person from choking on vomit.
6. Monitor the person's breathing.

Seizures

If you are with someone experiencing a seizure, there are several steps you can take to help ensure his or her safety during and after the episode:

1. Note the length of the attack. Seizures in which a person remains unconscious for long periods of time should be monitored closely. If medical help arrives, be sure to tell them how long the person has been unconscious.
2. Remove obstacles that could harm the victim. Because seizure victims may lose motor control during a convulsion, they inadvertently thrash around. To reduce the chances of serious injury, clear away any objects that could pose a threat.
3. Loosen clothing, and turn the victim's head to the side. This will help ensure that the person can breathe freely and will allow fluids or vomit to drain from the mouth.
4. Do not force objects into the victim's mouth. Although seizure victims may bite their tongues, causing possible damage, they will not swallow them. If the victim's mouth is clamped shut, forcing objects into the mouth may break teeth or cause more harm than doing nothing.
5. Get help. After you have completed steps 1 through 4, get help or send someone for help. This is particularly important if the victim does not regain consciousness within a few minutes.
6. Reassure the victim. Too often, the seizure victim regains consciousness only to face a crowd of staring people. When administering first aid, try to dissuade curious bystanders from hanging around. Calmly reassure the victim that everything is okay.
7. Allow the person to rest. After a seizure, many people will be exhausted. Allow them to sleep if possible.

Bleeding

External Bleeding Control of external bleeding is an important part of emergency care. Survival is threatened by the loss of 1 quart of blood or more. There are three major procedures for the control of external bleeding:

- **Direct pressure.** The best method is to apply firm pressure by covering the wound with a sterile dressing, bandage, or clean cloth. Wearing disposable latex gloves or an equally protective barrier, apply pressure for 5 to 10 minutes to stop bleeding.
- **Elevation.** Elevate the wounded section of the body to slow the bleeding. For example, a wounded arm or leg should be raised above the level of the victim's heart.
- **Pressure points.** Pressure points are sites where an artery that is close to the body's surface lies directly over a bone (**FIGURE 2**). Pressing the artery against the bone can limit the flow of blood to the injury. This technique should be used only as a last resort when direct pressure and elevation have failed to stop bleeding.

For serious wounds, seek medical attention immediately.

Internal Bleeding Although internal bleeding may not be immediately obvious, you should be aware of the following signs and symptoms:

- Symptoms of shock (discussed below)
- Coughing up or vomiting blood
- Bruises or contusions of the skin
- Bruises on chest or fractured ribs
- Black, tarlike stools
- Abdominal discomfort or pain (rigidity or spasms)

In some cases, a person who has suffered an injury (such as a blow to the head, chest, or abdomen) that does not cause external bleeding may bleed internally. If you suspect internal bleeding, follow these steps:

1. Have the person lie on his or her back on a flat surface with knees bent.
2. Treat for shock. Keep the victim warm. Cover the person with a blanket, if possible.

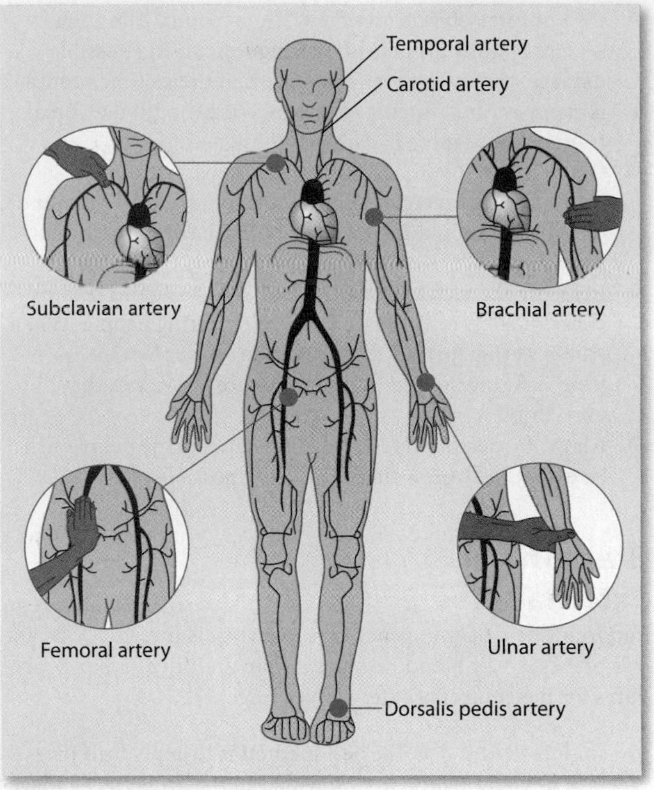

FIGURE 2 Pressure Points
Pressure can be applied to these points to stop bleeding. However, unless absolutely necessary, avoid applying pressure to the carotid arteries, which supply blood to the brain. Never apply pressure to both carotid arteries at the same time.

3. Expect vomiting. If this occurs, keep the victim on his or her side for drainage, to prevent inhalation of vomit, and to prevent expulsion of vomit from the stomach.
4. Do *not* give the victim any medications or fluids.
5. Send someone to call for emergency medical help immediately.

Nosebleeds

1. Have the victim sit down and lean slightly forward to prevent blood from running into the throat. If you do not suspect a fracture, pinch the person's nose firmly closed using the thumb and forefinger. Keep the nose pinched for at least 5 minutes.
2. While the nose is pinched, apply a cold compress to the surrounding area.
3. If pinching does not work, gently pack the nostril with gauze or a clean strip of cloth. Do not use absorbent cotton, which will stick. Be sure that the ends of the gauze or cloth hang out so that it can be easily removed later. Once the nose is packed with gauze, pinch it closed again for another 5 minutes.
4. If the bleeding persists, seek medical attention.

Shock

Shock is a condition in which the cardiovascular system fails to provide sufficient blood circulation to all parts of the body. Victims of shock display some or all of the following symptoms:

- Dilated pupils
- Cool, moist skin
- Weak, rapid pulse
- Vomiting
- Delayed or unrelated responses to questions

All injuries result in some degree of shock. Therefore, treatment for shock should be given after every major injury. The following are basic steps for treating shock:

1. Have the victim lie flat with his or her feet elevated approximately 8 to 12 inches. (In the case of chest injuries, difficulty breathing, or severe pain, the victim's head should be slightly elevated if there is no sign of spinal injury.)
2. Keep the victim warm. If possible, wrap him or her in blankets or other material. Keep the victim calm and reassured.
3. Seek medical help.

Treatment for Burns

Minor Burns For minor burns caused by fire or scalding water, apply running cold water or cold compresses for 20 to 30 minutes. Never put butter, grease, salt water, aloe vera, or topical burn ointments or sprays on burned skin. If the burned area is dirty, gently wash it with soap and water, and blot it dry with a sterile dressing.

Major Burns For major burn injuries, call for help immediately. Wrap the victim in a clean, dry sheet. Do not clean the burns or try to remove any clothing attached to burned skin. Remove jewelry near the burned skin immediately, if possible. Keep the victim lying down and calm.

Chemical Burns Remove clothing surrounding the burn. Wash skin that has been burned by chemicals by flushing with water for at least 20 minutes. Seek medical assistance as soon as possible.

Electrical Shock

Do not touch a victim of electrical shock until the power source has been turned off. Approach the scene carefully, avoiding any live wires or electrical power lines. Pay attention to the following:

1. If the victim is holding onto the live electrical wire, do not remove it unless the power has been shut off at the plug, circuit breaker, or fuse box.
2. Check the victim's breathing and pulse. Electrical current can paralyze the nerves and muscles that control breathing and heartbeat. If necessary, give mouth-to-mouth resuscitation. If there is no pulse, CPR might be necessary. (Remember that only trained people should perform CPR.)
3. Keep the victim warm and treat for shock. Once the person is breathing and stable, seek medical help or send someone else for help.

Poisoning

Among adults, almost all poisonings are caused by an overdose of a prescription drug, most commonly an opioid pain medication, or an illegal drug, such as cocaine or heroin. Among children, the majority of poisonings are caused by household products.

You should keep emergency telephone numbers for the poison control center and the local EMS close at hand. Many people keep these numbers on labels on their telephones. Check the front of your telephone book for these numbers. Be prepared to answer the following questions and to give the following information when calling for help:

- What was ingested? Have the container of the product and the remaining contents ready so you can describe it. Bring the container with you to the emergency room.
- When was the substance taken?
- How much was taken?
- Has vomiting occurred? If the person has vomited, save a sample to take to the hospital.
- Are there any other symptoms?
- How long will it take to get to the nearest emergency room?

When caring for a person who has ingested poison, keep these basic principles in mind:

1. Maintain an open airway. Make sure the person is breathing.
2. Call the local poison control center. Follow their advice for neutralizing the poison.
3. If the poison control center or another medical authority advises you to induce vomiting, then do so.
4. If a corrosive or caustic (that is, acid or alkali) substance was swallowed, immediately dilute it by having the victim drink at least one or two 8-ounce glasses of cold water or milk.
5. Place the victim on his or her left side. This position will delay advancement of the poison into the small intestine, where absorption into the victim's circulatory system is faster.

Injuries of Joints, Muscles, and Bones

Sprains Sprains result when ligaments and other tissues around a joint are stretched or torn. The following steps should be taken to treat sprains:

1. Elevate the injured joint to a comfortable position.
2. Apply an ice pack or cold compress to reduce pain and swelling.
3. Wrap the joint firmly with a roller bandage.
4. Check the fingers or toes periodically to ensure that blood circulation has not been obstructed. If the bandage is too tight, loosen it.
5. Keep the injured area elevated, and continue ice treatment for 24 hours.
6. Apply heat to the injury after 48 hours if there is no further swelling.
7. If pain and swelling continue or if a fracture is suspected, seek medical attention.

Fractures Any deformity of an injured body part usually indicates a fracture. A fracture is any break in a bone, including chips, cracks, splinters, and complete breaks. Minor fractures (e.g., hairline cracks) might be difficult to detect and might be confused with sprains. If there is doubt, treat the injury as a fracture until X-rays have been taken.

Do not move the victim if a fracture of the neck or back is suspected, because this could result in a spinal cord injury. If the victim must be moved, splints should be applied to immobilize the fracture in order to prevent further damage and to decrease pain. Following are some basic steps for treating fractures and applying splints to broken limbs:

1. If the person is bleeding, apply direct pressure above the site of the wound.
2. If a broken bone is exposed, do not try to move it back into the wound. This can cause contamination and further injury.
3. Do not try to straighten out a broken limb. Splint the limb as it lies.
4. The following materials are needed for splinting:
   - *Splint:* wooden board, pillow, or rolled up magazines and newspapers
   - *Padding:* towels, blankets, socks, or cloth
   - *Ties:* cloth, rope, or tape
5. Place splints and padding above and below the joint. Never put padding directly over the break. Padding should protect bony areas and the soft tissue of the limb.
6. Tie splints and padding into place.
7. Check the tightness of the splints periodically. Pay attention to the skin color, temperature, and pulse below the fracture to make sure the blood flow is adequate.
8. Elevate the fracture and apply ice packs to prevent swelling and reduce pain.

Head Injuries

All head injuries can potentially lead to brain damage, which may result in a cessation of breathing and pulse.

Minor Head Injuries

1. For a minor bump on the head resulting in a bruise without bleeding, apply ice to decrease the swelling.
2. If there is bleeding, apply even, moderate pressure. Do not use excessive pressure because the skull may be fractured.
3. Observe the victim for a change in consciousness.

Observe the size of pupils, including whether both pupils are dilated to the same degree, and note signs of inability to think clearly. Check for any signs of numbness or paralysis. Allow the victim to sleep, but wake him or her periodically to check for awareness.

Severe Head Injuries

1. If the victim is unconscious, check the airway for breathing. If necessary, perform mouth-to-mouth resuscitation.
2. If the victim is breathing, check the pulse. If it is less than 55 or more than 125 beats per minute, the victim may be in danger.
3. Check for bleeding. If fluid is flowing from the ears or nose, do not stop it.
4. Do not remove any objects embedded in the victim's skull.
5. Cover the victim with blankets to maintain body temperature, but guard against overheating.
6. Seek medical help as soon as possible.

Temperature-Related Emergencies

Frostbite Frostbite is damage to body tissues caused by intense cold, generally occurring at temperatures below 32°F. When skin is exposed to the cold, ice crystals form beneath the skin. Avoid rubbing frostbitten tissue, because the ice crystals can scrape and break blood vessels. The body parts most likely to suffer frostbite are the toes, ears, fingers, nose, and cheeks. To treat frostbite, follow these steps:

1. Bring the victim to a medical facility as soon as possible.
2. Cover and protect the frostbitten area. If possible, apply a steady source of external warmth, such as a warm compress. Avoid walking if the feet are frostbitten.
3. If the victim cannot be transported, warm the body part by immersing it in warm water (100°F to 105°F). Continue to warm until the frostbitten area is warm to the touch when removed from the bath. Do not allow the body part to touch the sides or bottom of the water container. After warming, dry gently and wrap the body part in bandages to protect from refreezing.

Hypothermia Hypothermia is a condition of generalized cooling of the body, resulting from exposure to cold temperatures or immersion in cold water. It can occur at any temperature below 65°F and can be made more severe by wind chill and moisture. The following are key symptoms of hypothermia:

- Shivering
- Vague, slow, slurred speech
- Poor judgment
- A cool abdomen
- Lethargy, or extreme exhaustion
- Slowed breathing and heartbeat
- Numbness and loss of feeling in extremities

After contacting the EMS, take the following steps:

1. Get the victim out of the cold.
2. Keep the victim in a flat position. Do not raise the legs.
3. Squeeze as much water as possible from wet clothing, and layer dry clothing over wet clothing. Removal of clothing may jostle the victim and lead to other problems.
4. Give the victim warm drinks only if he or she is able to swallow. Do not give the victim alcohol or caffeinated beverages, and do not allow the victim to smoke.
5. Do not allow the victim to exercise.

Heatstroke Heatstroke, the most serious heat-related disorder, results from the failure of the brain's heat-regulating mechanism (the hypothalamus) to cool the body. The following are signs and symptoms of heatstroke:

- Rapid pulse
- Hot, dry, flushed skin (absence of sweating)
- Disorientation leading to unconsciousness
- High body temperature

Body temperature should be reduced as quickly as possible. Immerse the victim in a cool bath, lake, or stream. If there is no water nearby, loosen clothing and use a fan to help lower the victim's body temperature.

Heat Exhaustion Heat exhaustion results from excessive loss of salt and water. The onset is gradual, with the following symptoms:

- Fatigue and weakness
- Anxiety
- Nausea
- Profuse sweating and clammy skin
- Normal body temperature

Move the victim to a cool place and have him or her lie down flat, with feet elevated 8 to 12 inches. Replace lost fluids slowly and steadily. Sponge or fan the victim.

Heat Cramps Heat cramps result from excessive sweating, resulting in an excessive loss of salt and water. Although heat cramps are the least serious heat-related emergency, they are the most painful. The symptoms include muscle cramps, usually starting in the arms and legs. To relieve symptoms, the victim should drink electrolyte-rich beverages or a light saltwater solution or eat salty foods.

APPENDIX C NUTRITIVE VALUE OF SELECTED FOODS AND FAST FOODS

This section presents nutritional information about a wide array of foods, including many fast foods. Values are given for calories, protein, carbohydrates, fiber, fat, saturated fat, and cholesterol for common foods and serving sizes. Use this information to assess your diet and make improvements. This is only a sampling of the most common foods. See the MyDietAnalysis database for a more extensive list of foods.

MDA Code	Food Name	Amt	Wt (g)	Ener (kcal)	Prot (g)	Carb (g)	Fiber (g)	Fat (g)	Sat (g)	Chol (g)
Beverages										
Alcoholic Beverages										
22831	Beer	12 fl. oz	360	157	1	13		0	0	0
34053	Beer, light	12 fl. oz	353	105	1	5	0	0	0	0
22606	Beer, nonalcoholic	12 fl. oz	353	73	1	14	0	0	0	0
22884	Wine, red	1 fl. oz	29	24	0	1		0	0	
22861	Wine, white	1 fl. oz	29	24	0	1		0	0	
22514	Gin, 80 proof	1 fl. oz	28	64	0	0	0	0	0	0
22593	Rum, 80 proof	1 fl. oz	28	64	0	0	0	0	0	0
22515	Tequila, 80 proof	1 fl. oz	28	64	0	0	0	0	0	0
22594	Vodka, 80 proof	1 fl. oz	28	64	0	0	0	0	0	0
22670	Whiskey, 80 proof	1 fl. oz	28	64	0	0	0	0	0	0
Coffee, Tea, and Dairy Drink Mixes										
20012	Coffee, brewed	1 cup	237	2	0	0	0	0	0	0
20686	Coffee, decaffeinated, brewed	1 cup	237	0	0	0	0	0	0	0
20439	Coffee, espresso	1 cup	237	5	0	0	0	0	0.2	0
20402	Coffee, from mix, French vanilla, sugar & fat free	1 ea	7	25	0	5	0	0	0.1	0
85	Chocolate milk, prepared w/ syrup	1 cup	282	254	9	36	1	8	4.7	25
46	Hot cocoa, w/ aspartame, sodium, vitamin A, prepared w/ water	1 cup	256	74	3	14	2	1	0.4	0
48	Hot cocoa, prep from dry mix w/ water	1 cup	275	151	3	32	1	2	0.9	0
166	Hot cocoa, w/ marshmallows, from dry packet	1 ea	28	112	1	21	1	4	4.2	0
39	Chocolate flavor, dry mix, prepared w/ milk	1 cup	266	226	9	32	1	9	4.9	24
41	Strawberry flavor, dry mix, prepared w/ milk	1 cup	266	234	8	33	0	8	5.1	32
20014	Tea, brewed	1 cup	237	2	0	1	0	0	0	0
20036	Tea, herbal (not chamomile) brewed	1 cup	237	2	0	0	0	0	0	0
Fruit and Vegetable Beverages and Juices										
71080	Apple juice, canned or bottled, unsweetened	1 ea	262	121	0	30	1	0	0.1	0
20277	Capri Sun All Natural Juice Drink, Fruit Punch	1 ea	210	99	0	26	0	0	0	0
5226	Carrot juice, canned	1 cup	236	94	2	22	2	0	0.1	0
3042	Cranberry juice cocktail	1 cup	253	137	0	34	0	0	0	0
20024	Fruit punch, canned	1 cup	248	117	0	30	0	0	0	0
20035	Fruit punch, from frozen concentrate	1 cup	247	114	0	29	0	0	0	0
20101	Grape drink, canned	1 cup	250	152	0	39	0	0	0	0
3053	Grapefruit juice, from frozen concentrate, unsweetened	1 cup	247	101	1	24	0	0	0	0
20045	Lemonade flavor drink, from dry mix	1 cup	266	72	0	18	0	0	0	0
20047	Lemonade w/ aspartame, low kcal, from dry mix	1 cup	237	7	0	2	0	0	0	0
20070	Orange drink, canned	1 cup	248	122	0	31	0	0	0	0
20004	Orange flavor drink, from dry mix	1 cup	248	122	0	31	0	0	0	0
71108	Orange juice, canned, unsweetened	1 ea	263	124	2	29	1	0	0	0
3090	Orange juice, fresh	1 cup	248	112	2	26	0	0	0.1	0
3091	Orange juice, from frozen concentrate, unsweetened	1 cup	249	112	2	27	0	0	0	0
5397	Tomato juice, canned w/o salt	1 cup	243	41	2	10	1	0	0	0
20849	Vegetable and fruit, mixed juice drink	4 oz	113	33	0	8	0	0	0	0
20080	Vegetable juice cocktail, canned	1 cup	242	46	2	11	2	0	0	0

Ener = energy (kilocalories); **Prot** = protein; **Carb** = carbohydrate; **Fiber** = dietary fiber; **Fat** = total fat; **Sat** = saturated fat; **Chol** = cholesterol.

MDA Code	Food Name	Amt	Wt (g)	Ener (kcal)	Prot (g)	Carb (g)	Fiber (g)	Fat (g)	Sat (g)	Chol (g)
Soft Drinks										
20006	Club soda	1 cup	237	0	0	0	0	0	0	0
20685	Low-calorie cola, w/ aspartame, caffeine free	12 fl. oz	355	4	0	1	0	0	0	0
20843	Cola, w/ higher caffeine	12 fl. oz	370	152	0	39	0	0	0	0
20008	Ginger ale	1 cup	244	83	0	21	0	0	0	0
20032	Lemon-lime soft drink	1 cup	246	98	0	25	0	0	0	0
20027	Pepper-type soft drink	1 cup	246	101	0	26	0	0	0.2	0
20009	Root beer	1 cup	246	101	0	26	0	0	0	0
Other										
20033	Soy milk	1 cup	245	132	8	15	1	4	0.5	0
20041	Water, tap	1 cup	237	0	0	0	0	0	0	0
Breakfast Cereals										
40095	All-Bran/Kellogg	0.5 cup	30	78	4	22	9	1	0.2	0
40032	Cap'n Crunch/Quaker	0.75 cup	27	109	1	23	1	2	1.1	0
40297	Cheerios/Gen Mills	1 cup	30	110	3	22	3	2	0.3	0
40126	Cinnamon Toast Crunch/Gen Mills	0.75 cup	30	130	2	24	1	3	0.4	0
40195	Corn Flakes/Kellogg	1 cup	28	101	2	24	1	0	0	0
40089	Corn Grits, instant, plain, prepared/Quaker	1 pkg	137	104	2	22	2	1	0.1	
40206	Corn Pops/Kellogg	1 cup	31	117	1	28	0	0	0.1	0
40179	Cream of Rice, prepared w/ salt	1 cup	244	127	2	28	0	0	0	0
40182	Cream of Wheat, instant, prepared w/ salt	1 cup	241	149	4	32	1	1	0.1	0
40104	Crispix/Kellogg	1 cup	29	109	2	25	0	0	0.1	0
40218	Froot Loops/Kellogg	1 cup	30	112	2	26	3	1	0.6	0
40217	Frosted Flakes/Kellogg	0.75 cup	31	114	1	28	1	0	0	0
11916	Frosted Mini-Wheats, bite size/Kellogg	1 cup	55	189	6	45	6	1	0.2	0
40209	Raisin Bran/Kellogg	1 cup	61	196	5	47	7	1	0.2	0
40210	Rice Krispies/Kellogg	1.25 cup	33	128	2	28	0	0	0.1	0
60887	Shredded wheat, large biscuit	2 ea	38	127	4	30	5	1	0.2	0
40211	Special K/Kellogg	1 cup	31	117	7	22	1	0	0.1	0
Dairy and Cheese										
500	Cream, half & half	2 Tbs	30	39	1	1	0	3	2.1	11
11	Milk, condensed, sweetened, canned	2 Tbs	38	123	3	21	0	3	2.1	13
19	Milk, lowfat, 1% fat, chocolate	1 cup	250	158	8	26	1	2	1.5	8
218	Milk, 2%, w/ added vitamins A & D	1 cup	245	130	8	13	0	5	3	20
6	Milk, nonfat/skim, w/ added vitamin A	1 cup	245	83	8	12	0	0	0.1	5
1	Milk, whole, 3.25%	1 cup	244	149	8	12	0	8	4.6	24
20	Milk, whole, chocolate	1 cup	250	208	8	26	2	8	5.3	30
72088	Yogurt, fruit variety, nonfat	1 cup	245	233	11	47	0	0	0.3	5
1287	American cheese, nonfat slices	1 pce	21	32	5	2	0	0	0.1	3
13349	Cheez Whiz cheese sauce/Kraft	2 Tbs	33	91	4	3	0	7	4.3	25
1014	Cottage cheese, 2% fat	0.5 cup	113	97	13	4	0	3	1.1	11
1015	Cream cheese	2 Tbs	29	99	2	1	0	10	5.6	32
1452	Cream cheese, fat free	2 Tbs	29	30	5	2	0	0	0.2	3
1016	Feta, crumbled	0.25 cup	38	99	5	2	0	8	5.6	33
47887	Mozzarella, whole milk, slice	1 ea	34	102	8	1	0	8	4.5	27
1075	Parmesan, grated	1 Tbs	5	22	2	0	0	1	0.9	4
1024	Ricotta, part skim	0.25 cup	62	86	7	3	0	5	3.1	19
1064	Ricotta, whole milk	0.25 cup	62	108	7	2	0	8	5.1	32
Eggs and Egg Substitutes										
19525	Egg substitute, liquid	0.25 cup	63	53	8	0	0	2	0.4	1
19506	Egg, white, raw	1 ea	33	16	4	0	0	0	0	0
19509	Egg, whole, fried	1 ea	46	90	6	0	0	7	2	210
19515	Egg, whole, hard boiled	1 ea	37	57	5	0	0	4	1.2	157
19521	Egg, whole, poached	1 ea	37	53	5	0	0	4	1.1	156
19516	Egg, whole, scrambled	1 ea	61	102	7	1	0	7	2.2	215
19508	Egg, yolk, raw, fresh	1 ea	17	53	3	1	0	4	1.6	205

MDA Code	Food Name	Amt	Wt (g)	Ener (kcal)	Prot (g)	Carb (g)	Fiber (g)	Fat (g)	Sat (g)	Chol (g)
Fruit										
72101	Apricots, canned, heavy syrup, drained	1 cup	182	151	1	39	5	0	0	0
3164	Fruit cocktail canned in juice	1 cup	237	109	1	28	2	0	0	0
71079	Apple w/ skin, raw	1 cup	125	65	0	17	3	0	0	0
3331	Applesauce w/ added vitamin C	0.5 cup	128	97	0	25	2	0	0	0
3657	Apricot, raw	1 cup	165	79	2	18	3	1	0	0
3210	Avocado, California, peeled, raw	1 ea	173	289	3	15	12	27	3.7	0
71002	Banana, peeled, raw	1 ea	81	72	1	19	2	0	0.1	0
71976	Grapefruit, fresh	0.5 ea	154	60	1	16	6	0	0	0
3055	Grapes, Thompson seedless, fresh	0.5 cup	80	55	1	14	1	0	0	0
3642	Melon, fresh, wedge	1 pce	69	23	1	6	1	0	0	0
3168	Mixed fruit (prune, apricot, & pear) dried	1 oz	28	69	1	18	2	0	0	0
3216	Nectarine, raw	1 cup	138	61	1	15	2	0	0	0
3726	Peach, peeled, raw	1 ea	79	31	1	8	1	0	0	0
3106	Pear, raw	1 ea	209	121	1	32	6	0	0	0
3766	Raisins, seedless	50 ea	26	78	1	21	1	0	0	0
72113	Pineapple, fresh, slice	1 pce	84	38	0	10		0		
3085	Orange, fresh	1 ea	184	86	2	22	4	0	0	0
3135	Strawberries, halves/slices, raw	1 cup	166	53	1	13	3	0	0	0
Grain Products										
Breads, Rolls, and Bread Crumbs										
71170	Bagel, cinnamon-raisin	1 ea	26	71	3	14	1	0	0.1	0
71167	Bagel, egg	1 ea	26	72	3	14	1	1	0.1	6
71152	Bagel, plain/onion/poppy/sesame, enriched	1 ea	26	67	3	13	1	0	0.1	0
42433	Biscuit, w/ butter	1 ea	82	273	5	28	1	16	3.9	1
71192	Biscuit, plain or buttermilk, refrig dough, baked, reduced fat	1 ea	21	63	2	12	0	1	0.3	0
42004	Bread crumbs, dry, plain, grated	1 Tbs	7	27	1	5	0	0	0.1	0
49144	Bread, crusty Italian w/ garlic	1 pce	50	186	4	21		10	2.4	6
70964	Bread, garlic, frozen/Campione	1 pce	28	101	2	12	1	5	0.8	
42069	Bread, oat bran	1 pce	30	71	3	12	1	1	0.2	0
42095	Bread, wheat, reduced kcal	1 pce	23	46	2	10	3	1	0.1	0
71247	Bread, white, commercially prepared, crumbs/cubes/slices	1 pce	9	24	1	5	0	0	0.1	0
42084	Bread, white, reduced kcal	1 pce	23	48	2	10	2	1	0.1	0
26561	Buns, hamburger, Wonder	1 ea	43	117	3	22	1	2	0.4	
42021	Hamburger/hot dog bun, plain	1 ea	43	120	4	21	1	2	0.5	0
42115	Cornbread, prepared from dry mix	1 pce	60	188	4	29	1	6	1.6	37
71227	Pita bread, white, enriched	1 ea	28	77	3	16	1	0	0	0
71228	Pita bread, whole wheat	1 ea	28	74	3	15	2	1	0.1	0
71368	Roll, dinner, plain, homemade w/ reduced fat (2%) milk	1 ea	43	136	4	23	1	3	0.8	15
42161	Roll, French	1 ea	38	105	3	19	1	2	0.4	0
71056	Roll, hard/kaiser	1 ea	57	167	6	30	1	2	0.3	0
42297	Tortilla, corn, w/o salt, ready to cook	1 ea	26	58	1	12	1	1	0.1	0
90645	Taco shell, baked	1 ea	5	23	0	3	0	1	0.3	0
Crackers										
71451	Cheez-its/Goldfish crackers, low sodium	55 pce	33	166	3	19	1	8	3.2	4
43507	Oyster/soda/soup crackers	1 cup	45	189	4	33	1	4	0.9	0
70963	Ritz crackers/Nabisco	5 ea	16	79	1	10	0	4	0.9	
43587	Saltine crackers, original premium/Nabisco	5 ea	14	56	1	10	0	1	0	0
43545	Sandwich crackers, cheese filled	4 ea	28	134	3	17	1	6	1.7	1
43546	Sandwich crackers, peanut butter filled	4 ea	28	138	3	16	1	7	1.4	0
44677	Snackwell Wheat Cracker/Nabisco	1 ea	15	62	1	12	1	2		
43581	Wheat Thins, baked/Nabisco	16 ea	29	140	3	20	1	6	0.9	0
43508	Whole wheat cracker	4 ea	32	137	3	22	3	5	0.7	0

MDA Code	Food Name	Amt	Wt (g)	Ener (kcal)	Prot (g)	Carb (g)	Fiber (g)	Fat (g)	Sat (g)	Chol (g)
Muffins and Baked Goods										
42723	English muffin, plain	1 ea	57	132	5	26		1	0.2	
62916	Muffin, blueberry, commercially prepared	1 ea	11	43	1	5	0	2	0.4	4
44521	Muffin, corn, commercially prepared	1 ea	57	174	3	29	2	5	0.8	15
44514	Muffin, oatbran	1 ea	57	154	4	28	3	4	0.6	0
44518	Toaster muffin, blueberry	1 ea	33	103	2	18	1	3	0.5	2
Noodles and Pasta										
38048	Chow mein noodles, dry	1 cup	45	237	4	26	2	14	2	0
38047	Egg noodles, enriched, cooked	0.5 cup	80	110	4	20	1	2	0.3	23
38060	Spaghetti, whole wheat, cooked	1 cup	140	174	7	37	6	1	0.1	0
38251	Egg noodles, enriched, cooked w/ salt	0.5 cup	80	110	4	20	1	2		23
38102	Macaroni noodles, enriched, cooked	1 cup	140	221	8	43	3	1	0.2	0
38118	Spaghetti noodles, enriched, cooked	0.5 cup	70	111	4	22	1	1	0.1	0
Grains										
38076	Couscous, cooked	0.5 cup	78	88	3	18	1	0	0	0
38080	Oats	0.25 cup	39	152	7	26	4	3	0.5	0
38010	Rice, brown, long grain, cooked	1 cup	195	216	5	45	4	2	0.4	0
38256	Rice, white, long grain, enriched, cooked w/ salt	1 cup	158	205	4	45	1	0	0.1	0
38019	Rice, white, long grain, instant, enriched, cooked	1 cup	165	193	4	41	1	1	0	0
Pancakes, French Toast, and Waffles										
42156	French toast, homemade, w/reduced fat (2%) milk	1 pce	65	149	5	16		7	1.8	75
45192	Pancake/waffle, buttermilk/Eggo/Kellogg	1 ea	42	99	3	16	0	3	0.6	5
45117	Pancakes, plain, homemade	1 ea	77	175	5	22	1	7	1.6	45
45193	Waffle, lowfat, homestyle, frozen	1 ea	35	83	2	15	0	1	0.3	9
Meat and Meat Substitutes										
Beef										
10093	Beef, average of all cuts, lean & fat (1/4" trim), cooked	3 oz	85	260	22	0	0	18	7.3	75
10705	Beef, average of all cuts, lean (1/4" trim), cooked	3 oz	85	184	25	0	0	8	3.2	73
10133	Beef, whole rib, roasted, 1/4" trim	3 oz	85	305	19	0	0	25	10	71
58129	Ground beef (hamburger), 25% fat, cooked, pan-browned	3 oz	85	236	22	0	0	15	6	76
58119	Ground beef (hamburger), 15% fat, cooked, pan-browned	3 oz	85	218	24	0	0	13	5	77
58109	Ground beef (hamburger), 5% fat, cooked, pan-browned	3 oz	85	164	25	0	0	6	2.9	76
10791	Porterhouse steak, lean & fat (1/4" trim), broiled	3 oz	85	280	19	0	0	22	8.7	61
58257	Rib eye steak, small end (ribs 10–12), 0" trim, broiled	3 oz	85	210	23	0	0	13	4.9	94
58094	Skirt steak, trimmed to 0" fat, broiled	3 oz	85	187	22	0	0	10	4	51
58328	Strip steak, top loin, 1/8" trim, broiled	3 oz	85	171	25	0	0	7	2.7	67
10805	T-Bone steak, lean & fat (1/4" trim), broiled	3 oz	85	260	20	0	0	19	7.6	55
11531	Veal, average of all cuts, cooked	3 oz	85	197	26	0	0	10	3.6	97
Chicken										
15057	Chicken breast, w/o skin, fried	3 oz	85	159	28	0	0	4	1.1	77
15080	Chicken, dark meat, w/ skin, roasted	3 oz	85	215	22	0	0	13	3.7	77
15026	Chicken, dark meat, w/o skin, fried	3 oz	85	203	25	2	0	10	2.7	82
15042	Chicken drumstick, w/o skin, fried	3 oz	85	166	24	0	0	7	1.8	80
15048	Chicken, wing, w/o skin, fried	3 oz	85	180	26	0	0	8	2.1	71
15059	Chicken, wing, w/o skin, roasted	3 oz	85	173	26	0	0	7	1.9	72
Turkey										
51151	Turkey bacon, cooked	1 oz	28	108	8	1	0	8	2.4	28
51098	Turkey patty, breaded, fried	1 ea	42	119	6	7	0	8	2	32
16110	Turkey breast w/ skin, roasted	3 oz	85	130	25	0	0	3	0.7	77
16038	Turkey breast, no skin, roasted	3 oz	85	115	26	0	0	1	0.2	71
16101	Turkey, dark meat w/ skin, roasted	3 oz	85	155	24	0	0	6	1.8	100
16003	Turkey, patty, ground, cooked	1 ea	82	193	22	0	0	11	2.8	84
Lamb										
13604	Lamb, average of all cuts (1/4" trim), cooked	3 oz	85	250	21	0	0	18	7.5	83
13616	Lamb, average of all cuts, lean (1/4" trim), cooked	3 oz	85	175	24	0	0	8	2.9	78

MDA Code	Food Name	Amt	Wt (g)	Ener (kcal)	Prot (g)	Carb (g)	Fiber (g)	Fat (g)	Sat (g)	Chol (g)
Pork										
12000	Bacon, broiled, pan-fried, or roasted	3 pcs	19	103	7	0	0	8	2.6	21
28143	Canadian bacon	1 pce	56	68	9	1		3	1	27
12211	Ham, cured, boneless, regular fat (11% fat), roasted	1 cup	140	249	32	0	0	13	4.4	83
12309	Pork, average of retail cuts, cooked	3 oz	85	203	22	0	0	12	4.2	75
12097	Pork, ribs, backribs, roasted	3 oz	85	315	21	0	0	25	9.4	100
12099	Pork, ground, cooked	3 oz	85	253	22	0	0	18	6.6	80
Lunchmeats										
13000	Beef, thin slices	1 oz	28	33	5	1	0	1	0.3	14
58275	Bologna, beef and pork, low fat	1 ea	14	32	2	0	0	3	1	5
13157	Chicken breast, oven roasted deluxe	1 oz	28	29	5	1	0	1	0.2	14
13306	Corned beef, cooked, chopped, pressed	1 ea	71	101	14	1	0	5	2	46
13264	Ham, slices, regular (11% fat)	1 cup	135	220	22	5	2	12	4	77
13101	Pastrami, beef, cured	1 oz	28	42	6	0	0	2	0.8	19
13215	Salami, beef, cotto	1 oz	28	59	4	1	0	4	1.9	24
16160	Turkey breast slice	1 pce	21	22	4	1	0	0	0.1	9
58279	Turkey ham, sliced, extra lean, prepackaged or deli-sliced	1 cup	138	171	27	4	0	5	1.5	92
Sausage										
13070	Chorizo, pork & beef	1 ea	60	273	14	1	0	23	8.6	53
57877	Frankfurter, beef	1 ea	45	148	5	2	0	13	5.3	24
13012	Frankfurter, turkey	1 ea	45	100	6	2	0	8	1.8	35
57890	Italian sausage, pork, cooked	1 ea	83	286	16	4	0	23	8	47
13021	Pepperoni sausage	1 pce	6	27	1	0	0	2	0.8	6
13185	Pork sausage links, cooked	2 ea	48	165	8	0	0	15	5.1	37
58227	Sausage, pork, precooked	3 oz	85	321	12	0	0	30	9.9	63
58007	Turkey sausage, breakfast links, mild	2 ea	56	132	9	1	0	10	2.1	90
Meat Substitutes										
7509	Bacon substitute, vegetarian, strips	3 ea	15	46	2	1	0	4	0.7	0
7722	Garden patties, frozen/Worthington, Morningstar	1 ea	67	118	12	9	3	4	0.5	1
7674	Harvest burger, original flavor, vegetable protein patty	1 ea	90	138	18	7	6	4	1	0
90626	Sausage, vegetarian, meatless	1 ea	28	72	5	3	1	5	0.8	0
7726	Spicy black bean burger/Worthington, Morningstar	1 ea	78	133	13	15	5	4	0.6	1
Nuts										
4519	Cashews, dry roasted w/ salt	0.25 cup	34	196	5	11	1	16	3.1	0
4728	Macadamia nuts, dry roasted, unsalted	1 cup	134	962	10	18	11	102	16	0
4592	Mixed nuts, w/ peanuts, dry roasted, salted	0.25 cup	34	203	6	9	3	18	2.4	0
4626	Peanut butter, chunky w/ salt	2 Tbs	32	188	8	7	3	16	2.6	0
4756	Peanuts, dry roasted w/o salt	30 ea	30	176	7	6	2	15	2.1	0
4696	Peanuts, raw	0.25 cup	36	207	9	6	3	18	2.5	0
4540	Pistachio nuts, dry roasted, salted	0.25 cup	32	182	7	9	3	15	1.8	0
Seafood										
17029	Bass, freshwater, cooked w/ dry heat	3 oz	85	124	21	0	0	4	0.9	74
17037	Cod, Atlantic, baked/broiled (dry heat)	3 oz	85	89	19	0	0	1	0.1	47
19036	Crab, Alaskan King, boiled/steamed	3 oz	85	83	16	0	0	1	0.1	45
17090	Haddock, baked or broiled (dry heat)	3 oz	85	95	21	0	0	1	0.1	63
17291	Halibut, Atlantic & Pacific, baked or broiled (dry heat)	3 oz	85	119	23	0	0	3	0.4	35
17181	Salmon, Atlantic, farmed, cooked w/ dry heat	3 oz	85	175	19	0	0	11	2.1	54
17099	Salmon, Sockeye, baked or broiled (dry heat)	3 oz	85	184	23	0	0	9	1.6	74
71707	Squid, fried	3 oz	85	149	15	7	0	6	1.6	221
17066	Swordfish, baked or broiled (dry heat)	3 oz	85	132	22	0	0	4	1.2	43
56007	Tuna salad, lunchmeat spread	2 Tbs	26	48	4	2	0	2	0.4	3
17151	White tuna, canned in water, drained	3 oz	85	109	20	0	0	3	0.7	36
17083	White tuna, canned in oil, drained	3 oz	85	158	23	0	0	7	1.1	26

MDA Code	Food Name	Amt	Wt (g)	Ener (kcal)	Prot (g)	Carb (g)	Fiber (g)	Fat (g)	Sat (g)	Chol (g)
Vegetables and Legumes										
Beans										
7038	Baked beans, plain or vegetarian, canned	1 cup	254	239	12	54	10	1	0.2	0
5197	Bean sprouts, mung, canned, drained	1 cup	125	15	2	3	1	0	0	0
7012	Black beans, boiled w/o salt	1 cup	172	227	15	41	15	1	0.2	0
5862	Beets, boiled w/ salt, drained	0.5 cup	85	37	1	8	2	0	0	0
90018	Cowpeas, cooked w/ salt	1 cup	171	198	13	35	11	1	0.2	0
7081	Hummus, garbanzo or chickpea spread, homemade	1 Tbs	15	27	1	3	1	1	0.2	0
7087	Kidney beans, canned	1 cup	256	215	13	37	14	2	0.3	0
7006	Lentils, boiled w/o salt	1 cup	198	230	18	40	16	1	0.1	0
7051	Pinto beans, canned	1 cup	240	206	12	37	11	2	0.4	0
6748	Snap green beans, raw	10 ea	55	17	1	4	1	0	0	0
5320	Snap yellow beans, raw	0.5 cup	55	17	1	4	2	0	0	0
90026	Split peas, boiled w/ salt	0.5 cup	98	114	8	20	8	0	0.1	0
7054	White beans, canned	1 cup	262	299	19	56	13	1	0.2	0
Fresh Vegetables										
9577	Artichokes (globe or French), boiled w/ salt, drained	1 ea	20	11	1	2	2	0	0	0
6033	Arugula/roquette, raw	1 cup	20	5	1	1	0	0	0	0
90406	Asparagus, raw	10 ea	35	7	1	1	1	0	0	0
5558	Broccoli stalks, raw	1 ea	114	32	3	6	3	0	0.1	0
5036	Cabbage, raw	1 cup	70	18	1	4	2	0	0	0
90605	Carrots, baby, raw	1 ea	15	5	0	1	0	0	0	0
5049	Cauliflower, raw	0.5 cup	50	12	1	2	1	0	0	0
90436	Celery, raw	1 ea	17	3	0	1	0	0	0	0
7202	Corn, white, sweet, ears, raw	1 ea	73	63	2	14	2	1	0.1	0
5900	Corn, yellow, sweet, boiled w/ salt, drained	0.5 cup	82	79	3	17	2	1	0.2	0
5908	Eggplant (brinjal), boiled w/ salt, drained	1 cup	99	33	1	8	2	0	0	0
5087	Lettuce, looseleaf, raw	2 pcs	20	3	0	1	0	0	0	0
51069	Mushrooms, brown, Italian, or crimini, raw	2 ea	28	6	1	1	0	0	0	0
90472	Onions, chopped, raw	1 ea	70	28	1	7	1	0	0	0
5116	Peas, green, raw	1 cup	145	117	8	21	7	1	0.1	0
7932	Peppers, jalapeno, raw	1 cup	90	27	1	5	2	1	0.1	0
90493	Peppers, sweet green, chopped/sliced, raw	10 pcs	27	5	0	1	0	0	0	0
6990	Pepper, sweet red, raw	1 ea	10	3	0	1	0	0	0	0
9251	Potatoes, red, flesh and skin, baked	1 ea	138	123	3	27	2	0	0	0
9245	Potatoes, russet, flesh and skin, baked	1 ea	138	134	4	30	3	0	0	0
5146	Spinach, raw	1 cup	30	7	1	1	1	0	0	0
90525	Squash, zucchini w/ skin, slices, raw	1 ea	118	20	1	4	1	0	0.1	0
6924	Sweet potato, baked in skin w/ salt	0.5 cup	100	92	2	21	3	0	0.1	0
5180	Tomato sauce, canned	0.5 cup	123	30	2	7	2	0	0	0
90532	Tomato, red, ripe, whole, raw	1 pce	15	3	0	1	0	0	0	0
5306	Yam, peeled, raw	0.5 cup	75	88	1	21	3	0	0	0
Soy and Soy Products										
7564	Tempeh	0.5 cup	83	160	15	8		9	1.8	0
7015	Soybeans, cooked	1 cup	172	298	29	17	10	15	2.2	0
7542	Tofu, firm, silken, 1" slice	3 oz	85	53	6	2	0	2	0.3	0
Meals and Dishes										
92216	Tortellini with cheese filling	1 cup	108	332	15	51	2	8	3.9	45
57658	Chili con carne w/ beans, canned entree	1 cup	222	269	16	25	9	12	3.9	29
57703	Chili, vegetarian chili w/ beans, canned entree/Hormel	1 cup	247	205	12	38	10	1	0.1	0
57068	Macaroni and cheese, unprepared/Kraft	1 ea	70	260	9	48	1	4	2	15
70958	Stir fry, rice & vegetables, w/ soy sauce/Hanover	1 cup	137	130	5	27	2	0		
70943	Beef & bean burrito/Las Campanas	1 ea	114	296	9	38	1	12	4.2	13
16195	Chicken & vegetables/Lean Cuisine	1 ea	297	232	20	26	4	5	1.9	30
70917	Hot Pockets, beef & cheddar, frozen	1 ea	142	403	16	39		20	8.8	53
70918	Hot Pockets, croissant pocket w/ chicken, broccoli, & cheddar, frozen	1 ea	128	301	11	39	1	11	3.4	37

MDA Code	Food Name	Amt	Wt (g)	Ener (kcal)	Prot (g)	Carb (g)	Fiber (g)	Fat (g)	Sat (g)	Chol (g)
56757	Lasagna w/ meat sauce/Stouffer's	1 ea	215	249	17	27	2	8	4.1	28
11029	Macaroni & beef in tomato sauce/Lean Cuisine	1 ea	283	326	21	40	3	9	3.7	32
5587	Mashed potatoes, from granules w/ milk, prep w/ water & margarine	0.5 cup	105	122	2	17	1	5	1.2	2
70898	Pizza, pepperoni, frozen	1 ea	146	432	16	42	3	22	7	22
56703	Spaghetti w/ meat sauce/Lean Cuisine	1 ea	326	284	14	49	5	4	1.1	13
Snack Foods										
10051	Beef jerky	1 pce	20	81	7	2	0	5	2.1	10
63331	Breakfast bars, oats, sugar, raisins, coconut	1 ea	43	200	4	29	1	8	5.5	0
61251	Cheese puffs and twists, corn based, low fat	1 oz	28	123	2	21	3	3	0.6	0
44032	Chex snack mix	1 cup	42	180	4	32	2	4	0.6	
23059	Granola bar, hard, plain	1 ea	24	115	2	16	1	5	0.6	0
23104	Granola bar, soft, plain	1 ea	28	126	2	19	1	5	2.1	0
44012	Popcorn, air-popped	1 cup	8	31	1	6	1	0	0	0
44076	Potato chips, plain, no salt	1 oz	28	152	2	15	1	10	3.1	0
5437	Potato chips, sour cream & onion	1 oz	28	151	2	15	1	10	2.5	2
44015	Pretzels, hard	5 pcs	30	114	3	24	1	1	0.1	0
44021	Rice cake, brown rice, plain, salted	1 ea	9	35	1	7	0	0	0.1	0
44058	Trail mix, regular	0.25 cup	38	173	5	17		11	2.1	0
Soups										
50398	Beef barley, canned/Progresso Healthy Classics	1 cup	241	142	11	20	3	2	0.7	19
50081	Chicken noodle, chunky, canned	1 cup	240	89	8	10	1	2	1	12
50085	Chicken rice, chunky, ready to eat, canned	1 cup	240	127	12	13	1	3	1	12
50088	Chicken vegetable, chunky, canned	1 cup	240	166	12	19		5	1.4	17
90238	Chicken, chunky, canned	1 cup	240	170	12	17	1	6	1.9	29
50697	Cup of Noodles, ramen, chicken flavor, dry/Nissin	1 ea	64	296	6	37		14	6.3	
50009	Minestrone, canned, made w/ water	1 cup	241	82	4	11	1	3	0.6	2
92163	Ramen noodle, any flavor, dehydrated, dry	0.5 cup	38	166	4	24	1	6	2.9	0
50043	Tomato vegetable, from dry mix, made w/ water	1 cup	253	56	2	10	1	1	0.4	0
50028	Tomato, canned, made w/ water	1 cup	244	73	2	16	1	1	0.2	0
50014	Vegetable beef, canned, made w/ water	1 cup	244	76	5	10	2	2	0.8	5
50013	Vegetarian vegetable, canned, made w/ water	1 cup	241	67	2	12	1	2	0.3	0
Desserts										
62904	Brownie, commercially prepared, square, lrg, 2-3/4" × 7/8"	1 ea	56	227	3	36	1	9	2.4	10
46062	Cake, chocolate, homemade, w/o icing	1 pce	95	352	5	51	2	14	5.2	55
46091	Cake, yellow, homemade, w/o icing	1 pce	68	245	4	36	0	10	2.7	37
71337	Doughnut, cake, w/ chocolate icing, lrg, 3 1/2"	1 ea	57	258	3	29	1	14	7.7	11
45525	Doughnut, cake, glazed/sugared, med, 3"	1 ea	45	192	2	23	1	10	2.7	14
47026	Animal crackers/Arrowroot/Tea Biscuits	10 ea	12	56	1	9	0	2	0.4	0
90636	Chocolate chip cookie, commercially prepared 3.5" to 4"	1 ea	40	190	2	26	1	9	4	0
47006	Chocolate sandwich cookie, creme filled	3 ea	30	141	2	21	1	6	1.9	0
62905	Fig bar, 2 oz	1 ea	57	197	2	40	3	4	0.6	0
90640	Oatmeal cookie, commercially prepared, 3-1/2" to 4"	1 ea	25	112	2	17	1	5	1.1	0
47010	Peanut butter cookie, homemade, 3"	1 ea	20	95	2	12		5	0.9	6
62907	Sugar cookie, refrigerated dough, baked	1 ea	23	111	1	15	0	5	1.4	7
57894	Pudding, chocolate, ready to eat	1 ea	113	160	2	26	0	5	1.4	1
2612	Pudding, vanilla, ready to eat	1 ea	113	147	2	26	0	4	1.1	1
2651	Rice pudding, ready to eat	1 ea	142	168	5	28	1	4	2.5	26
57902	Tapioca pudding, ready to eat	1 ea	113	147	2	25	0	4	1.1	1
71819	Frozen yogurts, chocolate, nonfat	1 cup	186	199	8	37	4	1	0.9	7
72124	Frozen yogurts, flavors other than chocolate	1 cup	174	221	5	38	0	6	4	23
2010	Ice cream, light, vanilla, soft serve	0.5 cup	88	111	4	19	0	2	1.4	11
90723	Ice popsicle	1 ea	59	47	0	11	0	0	0	0
42264	Cinnamon rolls w/ icing, refrigerated dough/Pillsbury	1 ea	44	145	2	23	0	5	1.5	0
71299	Croissant, butter	1 ea	67	272	5	31	2	14	7.8	45
45572	Danish, cheese	1 ea	71	266	6	26	1	16	4.8	16
45593	Toaster pastry, Pop Tart, apple-cinnamon/Kellogg	1 ea	52	205	2	37	1	5	0.9	0

MDA Code	Food Name	Amt	Wt (g)	Ener (kcal)	Prot (g)	Carb (g)	Fiber (g)	Fat (g)	Sat (g)	Chol (g)
23014	Chocolate syrup, fudge-type	2 Tbs	38	133	2	24	1	3	1.5	0
510	Whipped cream topping, pressurized	2 Tbs	8	19	0	1	0	2	1	6
54387	Whipped topping, frozen, low fat	2 Tbs	9	21	0	2	0	1	1.1	0
Fats, Oils, and Condiments										
90210	Butter, unsalted	1 Tbs	14	100	0	0	0	11	7.2	30
8084	Oil, vegetable, canola	1 Tbs	14	124	0	0	0	14	1	0
8008	Oil, olive, salad or cooking	1 Tbs	14	119	0	0	0	14	1.9	0
8111	Oil, safflower, salad or cooking, greater than 70% oleic	1 Tbs	14	120	0	0	0	14	0.8	0
44483	Shortening, household	1 Tbs	13	113	0	0	0	13	3.2	0
1708	Barbecue sauce, original	2 Tbs	36	63	0	15		0		
27001	Ketchup	1 ea	6	6	0	2	0	0	0	0
53523	Cheese sauce, ready to eat	0.25 cup	63	110	4	4	0	8	3.8	18
54388	Cream substitute, powdered, light	1 Tbs	6	25	0	4	0	1	0.2	0
50939	Gravy, brown, homestyle, canned	0.25 cup	60	25	1	3		1	0.3	2
23003	Jelly	1 Tbs	19	51	0	13	0	0	0	0
25002	Maple syrup	1 Tbs	20	52	0	13	0	0	0	0
44476	Margarine, regular, 80% fat, with salt	1 Tbs	14	101	0	0	0	11	2	0
8145	Mayonnaise, safflower/soybean oil	1 Tbs	14	99	0	0	0	11	1.2	8
8502	Miracle Whip, light/Kraft	1 Tbs	16	37	0	2	0	3	0.5	4
435	Mustard, yellow	1 tsp	5	3	0	0	0	0	0	0
23042	Pancake syrup	1 Tbs	20	47	0	12	0	0	0	0
23172	Pancake syrup, reduced kcal	1 Tbs	15	25	0	7	0	0	0	0
53524	Pasta sauce, spaghetti/marinara	0.5 cup	125	109	2	17	3	3	0.9	2
53646	Salsa picante, mild	2 Tbs	30	8	0	1	0	0		0
504	Sour cream, cultured	2 Tbs	29	56	1	1	0	6	3.3	15
53063	Soy sauce	1 Tbs	18	11	2	1	0	0	0	0
53652	Taco sauce, red, mild	1 Tbs	16	7	0	1	0	0		0
53004	Teriyaki sauce	1 Tbs	18	16	1	3	0	0	0	0
8024	Thousand Island, regular	1 Tbs	16	58	0	2	0	5	0.8	4
8013	Blue/Roquefort cheese, regular	2 Tbs	31	146	0	1	0	16	2.5	9
90232	French, regular	1 Tbs	12	56	0	2	0	6	0.7	0
44498	Italian, fat-free	1 Tbs	14	7	0	1	0	0	0	0
44696	Ranch, reduced fat	1 Tbs	15	29	0	3	0	2	0.2	2
8035	Vinegar & oil, homemade	2 Tbs	31	140	0	1	0	16	2.8	0
Fast Food										
6177	Baked potato, topped w/ cheese sauce	1 ea	296	474	15	47		29	10.6	18
56629	Burrito w/ beans & cheese	1 ea	93	189	8	27		6	3.4	14
66023	Burrito w/ beans, cheese, & beef	1 ea	102	166	7	20		7	3.6	62
66024	Burrito w/ beef	1 ea	110	262	13	29		10	5.2	32
56600	Biscuit w/ egg sandwich	1 ea	136	373	12	32	1	22	4.7	245
66029	Biscuit w/ egg, cheese, & bacon sandwich	1 ea	144	433	17	35	0	25	8.5	239
66013	Cheeseburger, double, condiments & vegetables	1 ea	166	417	21	35		21	8.7	60
56649	Cheeseburger, large, one meat patty w/ condiments & vegetables	1 ea	219	451	25	37	3	23	8.5	74
15063	Chicken, breaded, fried, dark meat (drumstick or thigh)	3 oz	85	248	17	9		15	4.1	95
15064	Chicken, breaded, fried, light meat (breast or wing)	3 oz	85	258	19	10		15	4.1	77
56000	Chicken filet, plain	1 ea	182	515	24	39		29	8.5	60
56635	Chimichanga w/ beef & cheese	1 ea	183	443	20	39		23	11.2	51
5461	Cole slaw	0.75 cup	99	151	1	15	2	10	1.6	4
56606	Croissant w/ egg & cheese sandwich	1 ea	127	368	13	24		25	14.1	216
56607	Croissant w/ egg, cheese, & bacon sandwich	1 ea	129	413	16	24		28	15.4	215
66021	Enchilada w/ cheese	1 ea	163	319	10	29		19	10.6	44
66020	Enchirito w/ cheese, beef, & beans	1 ea	193	344	18	34		16	7.9	50
66031	English muffin w/ cheese & sausage sandwich	1 ea	115	389	15	29	1	24	9.4	49
66010	Fish sandwich w/ tartar sauce	1 ea	158	431	17	41		23	5.2	55
90736	French fries fried in vegetable oil, medium	1 ea	134	427	5	50	5	23	5.3	0
56638	Frijoles (beans) w/ cheese	0.5 cup	84	113	6	14		4	2	18

MDA Code	Food Name	Amt	Wt (g)	Ener (kcal)	Prot (g)	Carb (g)	Fiber (g)	Fat (g)	Sat (g)	Chol (g)
56664	Ham & cheese sandwich	1 ea	146	352	21	33		15	6.4	58
56662	Hamburger, large, double, w/ condiments & vegetables	1 ea	226	540	34	40		27	10.5	122
56659	Hamburger, one patty w/ condiments & vegetables	1 ea	110	279	13	27		13	4.1	26
66007	Hamburger, plain	1 ea	90	266	13	30	1	10	3.2	30
5463	Hash browns	0.5 cup	72	235	2	23	2	16	3.6	0
66004	Hot dog, plain	1 ea	98	242	10	18		15	5.1	44
2032	Ice cream sundae, hot fudge	1 ea	158	284	6	48	0	9	5	21
6105	Mashed potatoes	0.5 cup	121	100	3	20		1	0.0	2
56639	Nachos w/ cheese	7 pcs	113	346	9	36		19	7.8	18
6176	Onion rings, breaded, fried	8 pcs	78	259	3	29		15	6.5	13
6173	Potato salad	0.33 cup	95	108	1	13		6	1	57
56619	Pizza w/ pepperoni 12"	1 pce	108	275	15	30		11	3.4	22
66003	Roast beef sandwich, plain	1 ea	139	346	22	33		14	3.6	51
56671	Submarine sandwich, cold cuts	1 ea	228	456	22	51		19	6.8	36
57531	Taco	1 ea	171	371	21	27		21	11.4	56
71129	Shake, chocolate, 12 fl. oz	1 ea	250	318	8	51	5	9	5.8	32
71132	Shake, vanilla, 12 fl. oz	1 ea	250	370	8	49	2	16	9.9	58

Source: This food composition table has been prepared for Pearson Education, Inc., and is copyrighted by ESHA Research in Salem, Oregon, the developer of the MyDietAnalysis software program.

GLOSSARY

5-year survival rates The percentage of people in a study or treatment group who are alive 5 years after they were diagnosed with or treated for a disease, such as cancer.

% Daily Values (%DVs) Percentages listed as "% DV" on food and supplement labels; identify how much of each listed nutrient or other substance a serving of food contributes to a 2,000 calorie/day diet.

abortion Termination of a pregnancy by expulsion or removal of an embryo or fetus from the uterus.

abstinence Refraining from a behavior.

accountability Accepting responsibility for personal decisions, choices, and actions.

acid deposition Acidification process that occurs when pollutants are deposited by precipitation or clouds, or directly on the land.

acquaintance rape Any rape in which the rapist is known to the victim (replaces the formerly used term *date rape*).

acquired immunodeficiency syndrome (AIDS) A disease caused by a retrovirus, the human immunodeficiency virus (HIV), that attacks the immune system, reducing the number of helper T cells and leaving the victim vulnerable to infections, malignancies, and neurological disorders.

active euthanasia "Mercy killing" in which a person or organization knowingly acts to end the life of a terminally ill person.

acupressure Technique of traditional Chinese medicine related to acupuncture that uses the application of pressure to selected points along the meridians to balance energy.

acupuncture Technique of traditional Chinese medicine that involves the placement of long, thin needles to affect flow of energy (*qi*) along energy pathways (meridians) within the body.

acute stress The short-term physiological response to an immediate perceived threat.

adaptive response The physiological adjustments the body makes in an attempt to restore homeostasis.

adaptive thermogenesis Theoretical mechanism by which the brain regulates metabolic activity according to caloric intake.

addiction Persistent, compulsive dependence on a behavior or substance, including mood-altering behaviors or activities, despite ongoing negative consequences.

advance directive Document that stipulates an individual's wishes about medical care; used to make treatment decisions when an individual becomes physically unable to voice his or her preferences.

aerobic capacity (or power) The functional status of the cardiorespiratory system; refers specifically to the volume of oxygen the muscles consume during exercise.

aerobic exercise Prolonged exercise that requires oxygen to make energy for activity.

aggravated rape Rape that involves one or multiple attackers, strangers, weapons, or physical beating.

aging Patterns of life changes that occur in members of all species as they grow older.

alcohol abuse Use of alcohol in a way that interferes with work, school, or personal relationships or that entails violations of the law.

alcohol poisoning (acute alcohol intoxication) Potentially lethal BAC that inhibits the brain's ability to control consciousness, respiration, and heart rate; usually occurs as a result of drinking a large amount of alcohol in a short period of time.

alcoholic hepatitis Condition resulting from prolonged use of alcohol in which the liver is inflamed; can be fatal.

Alcoholics Anonymous (AA) Organization whose goal is to help alcoholics stop drinking; includes auxiliary branches such as Al-Anon and Alateen.

alcoholism (alcohol dependence) Condition in which personal and health problems related to alcohol use are severe, and stopping alcohol use results in withdrawal symptoms.

allele One of potentially several variants of the same gene.

allergen An antigen that induces a hypersensitive immune response.

allergist Medical doctor focusing on the diagnosis and treatment of allergies.

allergy Hypersensitive reaction to a specific antigen in which the body produces antibodies to a normally harmless substance.

allopathic medicine Conventional, Western medical practice; in theory, based on scientifically validated methods and procedures.

allostatic load Wear and tear on the body caused by prolonged or excessive stress responses.

alternative (whole) medical systems Specific theories of health and balance that have developed outside the influence of conventional medicine.

alternative insemination Fertilization procedure accomplished by depositing semen from a partner or donor into a woman's vagina via a thin tube.

alternative medicine Treatment used in place of conventional medicine.

altruism Giving of oneself out of genuine concern for others.

alveoli Tiny air sacs of the lungs where gas exchange occurs (oxygen enters the body and carbon dioxide is removed).

Alzheimer's disease (AD) Chronic condition involving changes in nerve fibers of the brain that results in mental deterioration.

amino acids The nitrogen-containing building blocks of protein.

amniocentesis Medical test in which a small amount of fluid is drawn from the amniotic sac to test for Down syndrome and other genetic abnormalities.

amniotic sac Protective pouch surrounding the fetus.

amphetamines A large and varied group of synthetic agents that stimulate the central nervous system.

anabolic steroids Artificial forms of the hormone testosterone that promote muscle growth and strength.

anal intercourse Insertion of the penis into the anus.

androgyny Combination of traditional masculine and feminine traits in a single person.

anemia Condition that results from the body's inability to produce adequate hemoglobin.

aneurysm A weakened blood vessel that may bulge under pressure and, in severe cases, burst.

angina pectoris Chest pain occurring as a result of reduced oxygen flow to the heart.

angiography A technique for examining blockages in arteries or veins supplying the heart, lungs, head and neck, or limbs, utilizing a small camera on a catheter and dye passed through key vessels.

angioplasty A technique in which a catheter with a balloon at the tip is inserted into a clogged artery; the balloon is inflated to flatten fatty deposits against artery walls, and a stent is typically inserted to keep the artery open.

annual percentage rate (APR) The yearly cost of a credit card account, including interest and certain fees, expressed as a percentage.

anorexia nervosa Eating disorder characterized by deliberate food restriction, self-starvation, or extreme exercising to achieve weight loss, and an extremely distorted body image.

antagonism A drug interaction in which two drugs compete for the same available receptors, potentially blocking each other's actions.

antibiotic resistance The ability of bacteria or other microbes to withstand the effects of an antibiotic.

antibiotics Medicines used to kill microorganisms, such as bacteria.

antibodies Substances produced by the body that are individually matched to specific antigens.

antigen Substance capable of triggering an immune response.

antioxidants Substances believed to protect against oxidative stress and resultant tissue damage.

anxiety disorders Mental illness characterized by persistent feelings of threat and worry in coping with everyday problems.

appetite The learned desire to eat; normally accompanies hunger but is more psychological than physiological.

appraisal The interpretation and evaluation of information provided to the brain by the senses.

arrhythmia An irregularity in heartbeat.

arteries Vessels that carry blood away from the heart to other regions of the body.

arterioles Branches of the arteries.

arthritis Painful inflammatory disease of the joints.

asbestos Mineral compound that separates into stringy fibers and lodges in the lungs, where it can cause disease.

asthma A chronic respiratory disease that blocks airflow into and out of the lungs, characterized by attacks of wheezing, shortness of breath, and coughing spasms.

atherosclerosis Condition characterized by deposits of fatty substances (plaque) on the inner lining of an artery.

atria (singular: *atrium*) The heart's two upper chambers, which receive blood.

autoerotic behaviors Sexual self-stimulation.

autoimmune disease Disease caused by an overactive immune response against the body's own cells.

autoinoculate Transmit a pathogen from one part of your body to another part.

autonomic nervous system (ANS) The portion of the central nervous system regulating body functions that a person does not normally consciously control.

autosomal dominant disorder Single-gene disorder that occurs in individuals who have inherited at least one copy of an autosome with the affected dominant allele.

autosomal recessive disorder Single-gene disorder that occurs in individuals who have inherited two copies of an autosome with the affected recessive allele.

ayurveda (ayurvedic medicine) A comprehensive system of medicine, derived largely from ancient India, that places equal emphasis on the body, mind, and spirit, and strives to restore the body's innate harmony through diet, exercise, meditation, herbs, massage, exposure to sunlight, and controlled breathing.

background distressors Environmental stressors of which people are often unaware.

bacteria (singular: *bacterium*) Simple, single-celled microscopic organisms; about 100 known species of bacteria cause disease in humans.

barbiturates Drugs that depress the central nervous system and have sedating, hypnotic, and anesthetic effects.

barrier method Contraceptive methods that block the meeting of egg and sperm by means of a physical barrier (such as condom, diaphragm, or cervical cap), a chemical barrier (such as spermicide), or both.

basal body temperature The lowest temperature the body reaches, usually during sleep.

basal metabolic rate (BMR) The rate of energy expenditure by a body at complete rest in a neutral environment.

behavioral genetics The science that studies the role of inheritance in human behavior.

behavioral methods Temporary or permanent abstinence or planning intercourse in accordance with fertility patterns.

belief Appraisal of the relationship between some object, action, or idea and some attribute of that object, action, or idea.

benign Harmless; refers to a noncancerous tumor.

benzodiazepines A class of central nervous system depressant drugs with sedative, hypnotic, and muscle relaxant effects.

bereavement Loss or deprivation experienced by a survivor when a loved one dies.

bidis Hand-rolled flavored cigarettes.

binge drinking A pattern of drinking alcohol that brings BAC to 0.08% gram-percent or above; corresponds to consuming five or more drinks (adult male) or four or more drinks (adult female) in 2 hours.

binge-eating disorder A type of eating disorder characterized by gorging on food once a week or more, but not typically followed by a purge.

biofeedback A technique using a machine to self-monitor physical responses to stress.

biopsy Removal and examination of a tissue sample to determine if a cancer is present.

biopsychosocial model of addiction Theory of the relationship between an addict's biological (genetic) nature and psychological and environmental influences.

bipolar disorder Form of mood disorder characterized by alternating mania and depression; also called *manic depression.*

birth control (contraception) Methods of preventing conception.

bisexual Experiencing attraction to and preference for sexual activity with people of both sexes.

blood alcohol concentration (BAC) The ratio of alcohol to total blood volume; the factor used to measure the physiological and behavioral effects of alcohol.

body composition The relative proportions of fat and fat-free (muscle, bone, water, organs) tissues in the body.

body dysmorphic disorder (BDD) Psychological disorder characterized by an obsession with one's appearance and a distorted view of one's body or with a minor or imagined flaw in appearance.

body image How you see yourself in your mind, what you believe about your appearance, and how you feel about your body.

body mass index (BMI) A number calculated from a person's weight and height that is used to assess risk for possible present or future health problems.

brain death Irreversible cessation of all functions of the entire brainstem.

bronchitis An inflammation and eventual scarring of the lining of the bronchial tubes.

budget An estimate of spending and income over a set period of time.

budget deficit Spending more money than your income.

budget surplus Money left over for savings after expenses have been paid.

bulimia nervosa Eating disorder characterized by binge eating followed by inappropriate purging measures or compensatory behavior, such as vomiting or excessive exercise, to prevent weight gain.

caffeine A stimulant drug that is legal in the United States and found in many coffees, teas, chocolates, energy drinks, and certain medications.

calorie A unit of measure that indicates the amount of energy obtained from a particular food.

cancer A large group of diseases characterized by the uncontrolled growth and spread of abnormal cells.

cancer staging A classification system that describes how far a person's disease has advanced.

candidiasis Yeast-like fungal infection often transmitted sexually; also called *moniliasis* or *yeast infection.*

capillaries Minute blood vessels that branch out from the arterioles and venules; their thin walls permit exchange of oxygen, carbon dioxide, nutrients, and waste products among body cells.

capitation Prepayment of a fixed monthly amount for each patient without regard to the type or number of services provided.

carbapenem-resistant Enterobacteriaceae (CRE) A form of Enterobacteriaceae resistant to nearly all conventional antibiotics.

carbohydrates Basic nutrients that supply the body with glucose, the energy form most commonly used to sustain normal activity.

carbon footprint Amount of greenhouse gases produced, usually expressed in equivalent tons of carbon dioxide emissions.

carbon monoxide Gas found in cigarette smoke that reduces the ability of blood to carry oxygen.

carcinogens Cancer-causing agents.

cardiometabolic risks Physical and biochemical changes that are risk factors for the development of cardiovascular disease and type 2 diabetes.

cardiomyopathy Damage to heart muscle due to enlargement, atrophy, and/or rigidity that results in decreased heart function.

cardiopulmonary resuscitation (CPR) Emergency technique to provide lifesaving chest compression and mouth-to-mouth resuscitation when an individual has stopped breathing and has no pulse.

cardiorespiratory fitness The ability of the heart, lungs, and blood vessels to supply oxygen to skeletal muscles during sustained physical activity.

cardiovascular disease (CVD) Diseases of the heart and blood vessels.

cardiovascular system Organ system, consisting of the heart and blood vessels, that transports nutrients, oxygen, hormones, metabolic wastes, and enzymes throughout the body.

carpal tunnel syndrome A common occupational injury in which the median nerve in the wrist becomes irritated, causing numbness, tingling, and pain in the fingers and hands.

carrier Individual who has one copy of an autosome with a recessive allele for a particular trait, but is unaffected by it.

carrying capacity of the earth The largest population that can be supported indefinitely given the resources available in the environment.

cataracts Clouding of the lens that interrupts the focusing of light on the retina, resulting in blurred vision or eventual blindness.

celiac disease An inherited immune disorder causing malabsorption of nutrients from the small intestine and triggered by the consumption of gluten, a protein found in certain grains.

celibacy State of not engaging in sexual activity.

cell-mediated immunity Aspect of immunity that is mediated by specialized white blood cells that attack pathogens and antigens directly.

cervical cap Small cup made of silicone that is designed to fit snugly over the entire cervix; should always be used with spermicide.

cervix Lower end of the uterus that opens into the vagina.

cesarean section (C-section) Surgical birthing procedure in which a baby is removed through an incision made in the mother's abdominal wall and uterus.

chancre Sore often found at the site of syphilis infection.

chemotherapy The use of drugs to kill cancerous cells.

chewing tobacco Stringy form of tobacco that is placed in the mouth and then sucked or chewed.

chickenpox A highly infectious disease caused by the herpes varicella zoster virus.

child abuse Deliberate, intentional words or actions that cause harm, potential for harm, or threat of harm to a child.

child maltreatment Any act or series of acts of commission or omission by a parent or caregiver that results in harm, potential for harm, or threat of harm to a child.

chiropractic medicine Manipulation of the spine and neuromuscular structure to promote proper energy flow.

chlamydia Bacterially caused STI of the urogenital tract; most commonly reported STI in the United States.

chlorofluorocarbons (CFCs) Chemicals that contribute to the depletion of the atmospheric ozone layer.

cholesterol A lipid found in foods and synthesized by the body. Although essential to functioning, cholesterol circulating in the blood can accumulate on the inner walls of blood vessels.

chorionic villus sampling (CVS) Prenatal test that involves snipping tissue from the fetal sac to be analyzed for genetic defects.

chromosome Discrete bundle of DNA, 46 of which are present in the nucleus of almost all cells of the human body.

chromosome disorder A disorder arising from a damaged, missing, or extra chromosome or transfer of one portion of a chromosome to another.

chronic disease A disease that typically begins slowly, progresses, and persists, with a variety of signs and symptoms that can be treated but not cured by medication.

chronic lower respiratory disease (CLRD) Lung diseases such as emphysema, asthma, and some forms of bronchitis that are long-term in nature.

chronic mood disorder Experience of persistent emotional states, such as sadness, despair, hopelessness, or euphoria.

chronic obstructive pulmonary disease (COPD) A collection of chronic lung diseases, including emphysema and chronic bronchitis, where some form of obstruction interferes with a person's ability to breathe.

chronic stress An ongoing state of physiological arousal in response to ongoing or numerous perceived threats.

circadian rhythm The 24-hour cycle by which you are accustomed to going to sleep, waking up, and performing habitual behaviors.

cirrhosis The last stage of liver disease associated with chronic heavy alcohol use, during which liver cells die and damage becomes permanent.

climate change A shift in typical weather patterns that includes fluctuations in seasonal temperatures, rain or snowfall amounts, and the occurrence of catastrophic storms.

clitoris Pea-sized nodule of tissue located at the top of the labia minora; central to sexual arousal and pleasure in women.

Clostridium difficile (C. difficile) A highly resistant bacteria that affects the intestinal tract.

club drugs Synthetic analogs (drugs that produce similar effects) of existing illicit drugs.

Coccidioidomycosis (Valley Fever) An infection that occurs when humans or pets inhale soil-dwelling fungal spores.

codependence A self-defeating relationship pattern in which a person is controlled by an addict's addictive behavior.

cognitive restructuring The modification of thoughts, ideas, and beliefs that contribute to stress.

cohabitation Intimate partners living together without being married.

collateral circulation Adaptation of the heart to partial damage accomplished by rerouting needed blood through unused or underused blood vessels while the damaged heart muscle heals.

collective violence Violence perpetrated by groups against other groups.

colonization The process of bacteria or some other infectious organisms establishing themselves in a host without causing infection.

common-law marriage Cohabitation lasting a designated period of time (usually 7 years) that is considered legally binding in some states.

comorbidities The presence of one or more diseases at the same time.

complementary medicine Treatment used in conjunction with conventional medicine.

complete proteins Proteins that contain all nine of the essential amino acids.

complex carbohydrates A carbohydrate consisting of long chains of sugar molecules; also called a polysaccharide.

compulsion Preoccupation with a behavior and an overwhelming need to perform it.

compulsive buying disorder People who are preoccupied with shopping and spending.

compulsive exercise Disorder characterized by a compulsion to engage in excessive amounts of exercise and feelings of guilt and anxiety if the level of exercise is perceived as inadequate.

computerized axial tomography (CAT) scan A scan by a machine that uses radiation to view internal organs not normally visible in X-rays.

conception Fertilization of an ovum by a sperm.

conflict Emotional state that arises when opinions differ or the behavior of one person interferes with the behavior of another.

conflict resolution Concerted effort by all parties to constructively resolve differences or points of contention.

congeners Forms of alcohol that are metabolized more slowly than ethanol and produce toxic by-products.

congenital cardiovascular defect Cardiovascular problem that is present at birth.

consummate love A relationship that combines intimacy, compassion, and commitment.

contemplation Practice of concentrating the mind on a spiritual or ethical question or subject, a view of the natural world, or an icon or other image representative of divinity.

contraceptive sponge Contraceptive device made of polyurethane foam and containing nonoxynol-9 that fits over the cervix to create a barrier against sperm.

coping Managing events or conditions to lessen the physical or psychological effects of excess stress.

coronary artery disease (CAD) A narrowing or blockage of coronary arteries, usually caused by atherosclerotic plaque buildup.

coronary bypass surgery A surgical technique whereby a blood vessel taken from another part of the body is implanted to bypass a clogged coronary artery.

coronary calcium score A type of ultrafast CT used to diagnose levels of calcium in heart vessels or plaque formation and heart attack risk (involves radiation exposure).

coronary heart disease (CHD) A narrowing of the small blood vessels that supply blood to the heart.

coronary thrombosis A blood clot occurring in a coronary artery.

corpus luteum Cells that form from the remains of the graafian follicle following ovulation; it secretes estrogen and progesterone during the second half of the menstrual cycle.

cortisol Hormone released by the adrenal glands that makes stored nutrients more readily available to meet energy demands.

countering Substituting a desired behavior for an undesirable one.

Cowper's glands Glands that secrete a pre-ejaculate fluid that lubricates the urethra and neutralizes any acid remaining in the urethra after urination.

credit limit The maximum amount a person can charge on a credit card account.

credit The ability to buy goods and services in advance of paying for them.

Crohn's disease An autoimmune inflammatory bowel disease that can affect several parts of the gastrointestinal tract as well as other body organs and systems.

cross-tolerance Development of a physiological tolerance to one drug that reduces the effects of another, similar drug.

cunnilingus Oral stimulation of a woman's genitals.

death The permanent ending of all vital functions.

debt Money owed for goods and services that have been purchased.

defensive medicine The use of medical practices designed to avert the possibility of malpractice suits in the future.

dehydration Abnormal depletion of body fluids; a result of lack of water.

dehydration Loss of water from body tissues.

delayed ejaculation Persistent difficulty in reaching orgasm despite normal desire and stimulation.

delirium tremens (DTs) State of confusion, delusions, and agitation brought on by withdrawal from alcohol.

dementias Progressive brain impairments that interfere with memory and normal intellectual functioning.

denial Inability to perceive or accurately interpret the self-destructive effects of the addictive behavior.

dentist Specialist who diagnoses and treats diseases of the teeth, gums, and oral cavity.

Depo-Provera, Depo-subQ Provera Injectable method of birth control that lasts for 3 months.

depressants Drugs that slow down the activity of the central nervous and muscular systems and cause sleepiness or calmness.

determinants of health The range of personal, social, economic, and environmental factors that influence health status.

detoxification The early abstinence period during which an addict adjusts physically and cognitively to being free from the influences of the addiction.

diabetes mellitus A group of diseases characterized by elevated blood glucose levels.

diaphragm Latex, cup-shaped device designed to cover the cervix and block access to the uterus; should always be used with spermicide.

diastolic blood pressure The lower number in the fraction that measures blood pressure, indicating pressure on the walls of the arteries during the relaxation phase of heart activity.

Dietary Reference Intakes (DRIs) Set of recommended intakes for each nutrient published by the Institute of Medicine.

dietary supplement fraud A type of product fraud similar to food fraud but not controlled or monitored by the FDA as food or food additives would be.

dietary supplements Products taken by mouth and containing dietary ingredients such as vitamins and minerals that are intended to supplement existing diets.

digestive process The process by which the body breaks down foods and either absorbs or excretes them.

dilation and evacuation (D&E) Abortion technique that uses a combination of instruments and vacuum aspiration.

dioxins Highly toxic chlorinated hydrocarbons contained in herbicides and produced during certain industrial processes.

dipping Placing a small amount of chewing tobacco between the lower lip and teeth for rapid nicotine absorption.

disaccharides Combinations of two monosaccharides.

discretionary spending Goods and services that are not life essentials.

discrimination Actions that deny equal treatment or opportunities to a group, often based on prejudice.

disease prevention Actions or behaviors designed to keep people from getting sick.

disordered eating A pattern of atypical eating behaviors that is used to achieve or maintain a lower body weight.

distillation Process in which alcohol vapors are condensed and mixed with water to make hard liquor.

distress Stress that can have a detrimental effect on health; negative stress.

DNA (deoxyribonucleic acid) Compound residing in the nucleus of body cells that stores in its sequence of chemical subunits the instructions for assembling body proteins.

domestic violence The use of force to control and maintain power over another person in the home environment, including both actual harm and the threat of harm.

dominant Term describing an allele that is expressed even if there is only one copy in the pair.

Down syndrome A genetic disorder caused by the presence of an extra chromosome that results in mental disabilities and distinctive physical characteristics.

downshifting Taking a step back and simplifying a lifestyle that is hectic, packed with pressure and stress, and focused on trying to keep up; also known as *voluntary simplicity*.

drug abuse Excessive use of a drug.

drug misuse Use of a drug for a purpose for which it was not intended.

drug resistance That which occurs when microbes, such as bacteria, viruses, or other pathogens grow and proliferate in the presence of chemicals that would normally kill them or slow their growth.

drug-resistant *Neisseria gonorrhoeae* Drug-resistant form of *Neisseria gonorrhoeae.*

drunkorexia A colloquial term to describe the combination of disordered eating, excessive physical activity, and heavy alcohol consumption.

dying Process of decline in body functions that results in the death of an organism.

dysfunctional families Families in which there is violence; physical, emotional, or sexual abuse, significant parental discord; or other negative family interactions.

dysmenorrhea Condition of pain or discomfort in the lower abdomen just before or during menstruation.

dyspareunia Pain experienced by women during intercourse.

dyspnea Shortness of breath, usually associated with disease of the heart or lungs.

dysthymic disorder (dysthymia) Type of depression that is milder and harder to recognize than major depression; chronic; and often characterized by fatigue, pessimism, or a short temper.

eating disorder A psychiatric disorder characterized by severe disturbances in body image and eating behaviors.

ecological or public health model A view of health in which diseases and other negative health events are seen as a result of an individual's interaction with his or her social and physical environment.

ecosystem Collection of physical (nonliving) and biological (living) components of an environment and the relationships between them.

ectopic pregnancy Dangerous condition that results from the implantation of a fertilized egg outside the uterus, usually in a fallopian tube.

ejaculation Propulsion of semen from the penis.

ejaculatory duct Tube formed by the junction of the seminal vesicle and the vas deferens that carries semen to the urethra.

electrocardiogram (ECG) A record of the electrical activity of the heart; may be measured during a stress test.

embolus A blood clot that becomes dislodged from a blood vessel wall and moves through the circulatory system.

embryo Fertilized egg from conception through the eighth week of development.

emergency contraceptive pills (ECPs) Drugs taken within 3 to 5 days after unprotected intercourse to prevent pregnancy.

emotional health The feeling part of psychological health; includes your emotional reactions to life.

emotional intelligence (EI) A person's ability to identify, understand, use, and manage emotional states in positive and constructive ways.

emotions Intensified feelings or complex patterns of feelings.

emphysema A respiratory disease in which the alveoli become distended or ruptured and are no longer functional.

emphysema Chronic lung disease in which the tiny air sacs in the lungs are destroyed, making breathing difficult.

enablers People who knowingly or unknowingly protect addicts from the natural consequences of their behavior.

endemic Present at expected prevalence rates in a given population or area.

endometriosis Disorder in which endometrial tissue establishes itself outside the uterus.

endometrium Soft, spongy matter that makes up the uterine lining.

endorphins Opioid-like hormones that are manufactured in the human body and contribute to natural feelings of well-being.

energy medicine Therapies using energy fields, such as magnetic fields or biofields.

enhanced greenhouse effect Warming of the earth's surface due to increases in greenhouse gas concentration in the atmosphere, which traps more of the sun's radiation than is normal.

environmental stewardship Responsibility for environmental quality shared by all those whose actions affect the environment.

environmental tobacco smoke (ETS) Smoke from tobacco products, including secondhand and mainstream smoke.

epidemic Disease outbreak that affects many people in a community or region at the same time.

epididymis Duct system where sperm mature and are stored.

epigenome The sum total of chemical compounds that influence the activity of an individual's genes.

epilepsy A neurological disorder caused by abnormal electrical brain activity; can be accompanied by altered consciousness or convulsions.

epinephrine Also called *adrenaline,* a hormone that stimulates body systems in response to stress.

episodic acute stress The state of regularly reacting with wild, acute stress about one thing or another.

erectile dysfunction (ED) Difficulty in achieving or maintaining an erection sufficient for intercourse.

ergogenic drug Substance believed to enhance athletic performance.

erogenous zones Areas of the body that, when touched, lead to sexual arousal.

essential amino acids The nine basic nitrogen-containing building blocks of human proteins that must be obtained from foods.

estimated average glucose (eAG) A method for reporting A1C test results that gives the average blood glucose levels for the testing period using the same units (milligrams per deciliter, or mg/dL) that patients are used to seeing in self-administered glucose tests.

estrogens Hormones secreted by the ovaries that control the menstrual cycle and assist in the development of female secondary sex characteristics.

ethnoviolence Violence directed at persons affiliated with a particular ethnic group.

ethyl alcohol (ethanol) Addictive drug produced by fermentation that is the intoxicating substance in alcoholic beverages.

eustress Stress that presents opportunities for personal growth; positive stress.

evidence-based medicine Decisions regarding patient care based on clinical expertise, patient values, and current best scientific evidence.

excessive daytime sleepiness A disorder characterized by unusual patterns of falling asleep during normal waking hours.

exercise addicts People who exercise compulsively to try to meet needs of nurturance, intimacy, self-esteem, and self-competency.

exercise metabolic rate (EMR) The energy expenditure that occurs during exercise.

exercise Planned, structured, and repetitive bodily movement done to improve or maintain one or more component of physical fitness.

extensively drug-resistant TB (XDR-TB) Form of TB that is resistant to nearly all existing antibiotics.

fallopian tubes Tubes that extend from near the ovaries to the uterus; site of fertilization and passageway for fertilized eggs.

family of origin People present in the household during a child's first years of life—usually parents and siblings.

fats Essential nutrients needed for energy, cell function, insulation of body organs, maintenance of body temperature, and healthy skin and hair.

federal student loans Student financial aid loans that are financed by the government.

federal work study A type of financial aid in which part-time jobs for students are arranged to help them pay for school.

fellatio Oral stimulation of a man's genitals.

female athlete triad A syndrome of three interrelated health problems seen in some female athletes: disordered eating, amenorrhea, and poor bone density.

female condom (FC) Single-use nitrile sheath for internal use during vaginal intercourse to catch semen upon ejaculation.

female orgasmic disorder A woman's inability to achieve orgasm.

fermentation Process in which yeast organisms break down plant sugars to yield ethanol.

fertility A person's ability to reproduce.

fertility awareness methods (FAMs) Several types of birth control that require alteration of sexual behavior rather than chemical or physical intervention in the reproductive process.

fertility rate Average number of births a female in a certain population has during her reproductive years.

fetal alcohol syndrome (FAS) Birth defect involving physical and mental impairment that results from the mother's alcohol consumption during pregnancy.

fetal alcohol syndrome (FAS) Pattern of birth defects, learning, and behavioral problems in a child caused by the mother's alcohol consumption during pregnancy.

fetus Developing human from the ninth week until birth.

fiber The indigestible portion of plant foods that helps move food through the digestive system and softens stools by absorbing water.

fibrillation A sporadic, quivering pattern of heartbeat that results in extreme inefficiency in moving blood through the cardiovascular system.

fight-or-flight response Physiological arousal response in which the body prepares to combat or escape a real or perceived threat.

FITT Acronym for *frequency, intensity, time,* and *type,* the terms that describe the recommended levels of exercise to improve a health-related component of physical fitness.

flexibility The range of motion, or the amount of movement possible, at a particular joint or series of joints.

foams Spermicide packaged in aerosol cans and inserted into the vagina with an applicator.

food allergy An immune response against a specific food that the majority of people can eat without problem.

food fraud The deliberate and intentional substitution, addition, tampering or misrepresentation of food, food ingredients or food packing, or false or misleading statements about a product.

food intolerance Difficulty or inability to digest certain foods due to problems with the physical, hormonal, or biochemical systems in your digestive tract.

food irradiation Exposing foods to low doses of radiation to kill microorganisms or keep them from reproducing.

formaldehyde Colorless, strong-smelling gas released through outgassing; causes respiratory and other health problems.

fossil fuels Carbon-based material used for energy; includes oil, coal, and natural gas.

frequency As part of the FITT prescription, refers to how many days per week a person should exercise.

functional foods Foods believed to have specific health benefits beyond their basic nutrients.

fungi A group of multicellular and unicellular organisms that obtain their food by infiltrating the bodies of other organisms, both living and dead; several microscopic varieties are pathogenic.

gambling disorder Compulsive gambling that cannot be controlled.

gamma knife surgery *See* stereotactic radiosurgery.

gastroesophageal reflux disease (GERD) Chronic condition in which stomach acid backflows into the esophagus, causing heartburn and potential damage to the esophagus.

gay Sexual orientation involving primary attraction to people of the same sex.

gender Characteristics and actions associated with being feminine or masculine as defined by the society or culture in which one lives.

gender identity Personal sense or awareness of being masculine or feminine, a male or a female.

gender roles Expression of maleness or femaleness in everyday life that conforms to society's expectations.

gender-role stereotypes Generalizations concerning how men and women should express themselves and the characteristics each possess.

gene Discrete segment of DNA in a chromosome that stores the code for assembling one or more body proteins.

general adaptation syndrome (GAS) The pattern followed in the physiological response to stress, consisting of the alarm, resistance, and exhaustion phases.

generalized anxiety disorder (GAD) A constant sense of worry that may cause restlessness, difficulty in concentrating, tension, and other symptoms.

generic drugs Medications sold under chemical names rather than brand names.

genetically modified (GM) foods Foods derived from organisms whose DNA has been altered using genetic engineering techniques.

genital herpes STI caused by the herpes simplex virus.

genital warts Warts that appear in the genital area or the anus; caused by the human papillomavirus (HPV).

genome All of the genetic information an organism possesses.

gerontology The study of individual and collective aging processes.

gestational diabetes Form of diabetes mellitus in which women who have never had diabetes have high blood sugar (glucose) levels during pregnancy.

glaucoma Elevation of pressure within the eyeball, leading to hardening of the eyeball, impaired vision, and possible blindness.

global warming A type of climate change in which average temperatures increase.

globesity Global rates of obesity.

glycemic index (GI) Compares foods with the same amount of carbohydrates and determines how much each raises blood glucose levels.

glycemic load (GL) A means of assessing the likely rise in blood glucose based on dietary quality and quantity of food. Determined by consumption of carbohydrates in grams times glycemic index divided by 100.

glycogen The polysaccharide form in which glucose is stored in the liver and, to a lesser extent, in muscles.

gonads Reproductive organs that produce germ cells and sex hormones; in males, the testes, and in females, the ovaries.

gonorrhea Second most common bacterial STI in the United States; if untreated, may cause sterility.

graafian follicle Mature ovarian follicle that contains a fully developed egg (ovum).

grant Financial student aid that does not need to be repaid.

greenhouse gases Gases that accumulate in the atmosphere, where they contribute to global warming by trapping heat near the earth's surface.

grief An individual's reaction to significant loss, including one's own impending death, the death of a loved one, or a quasi-death experience; grief can involve mental, physical, social, or emotional responses.

grief work Process of accepting the reality of a person's death and coping with memories of the deceased.

hallucinogens Substances capable of creating auditory or visual distortions and unusual changes in mood, thoughts, and feelings.

hangover Physiological reaction to excessive drinking, including headache, upset stomach, anxiety, depression, diarrhea, and thirst.

hate crime Crime targeted against a particular societal group and motivated by bias against that group.

hay fever A chronic allergy-related respiratory disorder that is most prevalent when ragweed and flowers bloom, also known as *pollen allergy*.

hazardous waste Toxic waste that poses a hazard to humans or to the environment.

health The ever-changing process of achieving individual potential in the physical, social, emotional, mental, spiritual, and environmental dimensions.

health belief model (HBM) Model for explaining how beliefs may influence behaviors.

health disparities Differences in the incidence, prevalence, mortality, and burden of diseases and other health conditions among specific population groups.

health promotion The combined educational, organizational, procedural, environmental, social, and financial supports that help individuals and groups reduce negative health behaviors and promote positive change.

health-income gradient The relationship between the health of individuals or communities and income, where health outcomes increase as income increases.

health-related quality of life Assessment of impact of health status—including elements of physical, mental, emotional, and social function—on overall quality of life.

healthy life expectancy Expected number of years of full health remaining at a given age, such as at birth.

healthy weight Those with BMIs of 18.5 to 24.9, the range of lowest statistical health risk

heart failure (HF) or congestive heart failure (CHF) An abnormal cardiovascular condition that reflects impaired cardiac pumping and blood flow; pooling blood leads to congestion in body tissues.

heat cramps Involuntary and forcible muscle contractions that occur during or following exercise in hot and/or humid weather.

heat exhaustion A heat stress illness caused by significant dehydration resulting from exercise in hot and/or humid conditions.

heatstroke A deadly heat stress illness resulting from dehydration and overexertion in hot and/or humid conditions.

hepatitis A viral disease in which the liver becomes inflamed, producing symptoms such as fever, headache, and possibly jaundice.

herpes gladiatorum A skin infection caused by the herpes simplex type 1 virus and seen among athletes participating in contact sports.

heterosexual Experiencing primary attraction to and preference for sexual activity with people of the opposite sex.

high-density lipoproteins (HDLs) Compounds that facilitate the transport of cholesterol in the blood to the liver for metabolism and elimination from the body.

histamine Chemical substance that dilates blood vessels, increases mucous secretions, and produces other symptoms of allergies.

holistic Relating to or concerned with the whole body and the interactions of systems, rather than treatment of individual parts.

homeopathic medicine Unconventional Western system of medicine based on the principle that "like cures like."

homeostasis A balanced physiological state in which all the body's systems function smoothly.

homicide Death that results from intent to injure or kill.

homosexual Experiencing primary attraction to and preference for sexual activity with people of the same sex.

hormonal methods Contraceptive methods that introduce synthetic hormones into a woman's system to prevent ovulation, thicken cervical mucus, or prevent a fertilized egg from implanting.

hormone replacement therapy (menopausal hormone therapy) Use of synthetic estrogens and progesterone to compensate for hormonal changes in a woman's body during menopause.

hospice Type of end-of-life care designed to maximize quality of life and help dying people have peace, comfort, and dignity.

hostility The cognitive, affective, and behavioral tendencies toward anger and cynicism.

human chorionic gonadotropin (HCG) Hormone detectable in blood or urine samples of a mother within the first few weeks of pregnancy.

human immunodeficiency virus (HIV) The virus that causes AIDS by infecting helper T cells.

human papillomavirus (HPV) A group of viruses, many of which are transmitted sexually; some types of HPV can cause genital warts or cervical cancer.

humoral immunity Aspect of immunity that is mediated by antibodies secreted by white blood cells.

hunger The physiological impulse to seek food.

hymen In some women, a thin tissue covering the vaginal opening.

hyperglycemia Elevated blood glucose level.

hyperplasia A condition characterized by an excessive number of fat cells.

hypertension Sustained elevated blood pressure.

hypertrophy The act of swelling or increasing in size, as with cells.

hypnosis A trancelike state that allows people to become unusually responsive to suggestion.

hyponatremia or water intoxication Overconsumption of water, which leads to a dilution of sodium concentration in the blood, with potentially fatal results.

hypothalamus A structure in the brain located near the pituitary gland that controls the sympathetic nervous system and directs the stress response; works in conjunction with the pituitary gland to control reproductive functions.

hypothermia Potentially fatal condition caused by abnormally low body core temperature.

hysterectomy Surgical removal of the uterus.

ideal cardiovascular health (ICH) The absence of clinical indicators of CVD and the presence of certain behavioral and health factor metrics.

identity theft Stealing personal information and using it without permission.

idiopathic Of unknown cause.

imagined rehearsal Practicing, through mental imagery, to become better able to perform a task in actuality.

immunocompetence The ability of the immune system to respond to attack.

immunocompromised Having an immune system that is impaired.

immunotherapy Treatment strategies based on the concept of regulating the immune system by administering antibodies or desensitizing shots of allergens.

in vitro fertilization (IVF) Fertilization of an egg in a nutrient medium and subsequent transfer back to the mother's body.

income inequality The discrepancy in income between the wealthy and the poor.

incomplete proteins Proteins that lack one or more of the essential amino acids.

incubation period The time between exposure to a disease and the appearance of symptoms.

induction abortions Abortion technique in which chemicals are injected into the uterus through the uterine wall; labor begins, and the woman delivers a dead fetus.

infection The state of pathogens being established in or on a host and causing disease.

infertility Inability to conceive after a year or more of trying.

inflammatory bowel disease (IBD) A group of disorders in which the intestines become inflamed.

influenza A common viral disease of the respiratory tract.

informed consent Acknowledgment that you have been told of the potential risks and benefits of a recommended test or treatment, understand what you have been told, and agree to the care.

inhalants Chemical vapors that are sniffed or inhaled in order to produce highs.

inhalation The introduction of drugs through the respiratory tract via sniffing, smoking, or inhaling.

inheritance Process by which physical and biological characteristics—called traits—are transmitted from parents to their offspring.

Inhibited sexual desire Lack of sexual appetite or lack of interest and pleasure in sexual activity.

inhibition A drug interaction in which the effects of one drug are eliminated or reduced by the presence of another drug at the same receptor site.

injection The introduction of drugs into the body via a hypodermic needle.

insomnia A disorder characterized by difficulty in falling asleep quickly, frequent arousals during sleep, or early morning awakening.

insulin Hormone secreted by the pancreas and required by body cells for the uptake and storage of glucose.

insulin resistance State in which body cells fail to respond to the effects of insulin; obesity increases the risk that cells will become insulin resistant.

intact dilation and extraction (D&X) Late-term abortion procedure in which the body of the fetus is extracted up to the head and then the contents of the cranium are aspirated.

intensity As part of the FITT prescription, refers to how hard or how much effort is needed when a person exercises.

intentional injuries Injury, death, or psychological harm inflicted with the intent to harm.

interest A fee paid by the borrower of a loan.

Internet addiction Compulsive use of a computer, personal digital device, cell phone, or other forms of technology to access the Internet for activities such as e-mail, games, shopping, social networking, or blogging.

interpersonal violence Violence inflicted against one individual by another or by a small group of others.

intersexuality Not exhibiting exclusively male or female sex characteristics; also known as disorders of sexual development (DSD).

intervention A planned confrontation with an alcoholic/addict led by a professional counselor in which family members and/or friends try to get the alcoholic/addict to face the reality of his or her problem and to seek help.

intestate Dying without a will.

intimate partner violence (IPV) Describes physical, sexual, or psychological harm by a current or former partner or spouse.

intimate relationships Relationships with family members, friends, and romantic partners, characterized by behavioral interdependence, need fulfillment, emotional attachment, and emotional availability.

intolerance A drug interaction in which the combination of two or more drugs in the body produces extremely uncomfortable reactions.

intrauterine device (IUD) A device, often T-shaped, that is implanted in the uterus to prevent pregnancy.

ionizing radiation Electromagnetic waves and particles having short wavelengths and energy high enough to ionize atoms.

irritable bowel syndrome (IBS) A functional bowel disorder caused by certain foods or stress that is characterized by nausea, pain, gas, or diarrhea.

ischemia Reduced oxygen supply to a body part or organ.

jealousy Aversive reaction evoked by a real or imagined relationship involving a person's partner and a third person.

jellies and creams Spermicide packaged in tubes and inserted into the vagina with an applicator.

labia majora "Outer lips," or folds of tissue covering the female sexual organs.

labia minora "Inner lips," or folds of tissue just inside the labia majora.

leach To dissolve and filter through soil.

lead Highly toxic metal found in emissions from lead smelters and processing plants; also sometimes found in pipes or paint in older buildings.

learned behavioral tolerance The ability of heavy drinkers to modify behavior so they appear to be sober even when they have high BAC levels.

learned helplessness Pattern of responding to situations by giving up because of repeated failure in the past.

learned optimism Teaching oneself to think positively.

lesbian Sexual orientation involving attraction of women to other women.

leukoplakia Condition characterized by leathery white patches inside the mouth, which is produced by contact with irritants in tobacco juice.

libido Sexual drive or desire.

life expectancy Expected number of years of life remaining at a given age, such as at birth.

living will Type of advance directive.

loan Giving money to someone today with an agreement that it will be paid off under certain terms in the future.

locavore A person who primarily eats food grown or produced locally.

locus of control The location, *external* (outside oneself) or *internal* (within oneself), that an individual perceives as the source and underlying cause of events in his or her life.

loss of control Inability to reliably predict whether a particular instance of involvement with the addictive substance or behavior will be healthy or damaging.

low back pain (LBP) Pain or discomfort in the lumbosacral region (lowest vertebrae) of the back.

low sperm count Sperm count below 20 million sperm per milliliter of semen.

low-density lipoproteins (LDLs) Compounds that facilitate the transport of cholesterol in the blood to the body's cells and cause the cholesterol to build up on artery walls.

lymphocyte A type of white blood cell involved in the immune response.

macrophage A type of white blood cell that ingests foreign material.

macular degeneration Breakdown of the macula, the light-sensitive part of the retina responsible for sharp, direct vision.

magnetic resonance imaging (MRI) A device that uses magnetic fields, radio waves, and computers to generate an image of internal tissues of the body for diagnostic purposes without the use of radiation.

mainstream smoke Smoke that is drawn through tobacco while inhaling.

major depression Severe depressive disorder with physical effects such as sleep disturbance and exhaustion, and mental effects such as the inability to concentrate; also called *clinical depression.*

male condom Single-use sheath of thin latex or other material designed to fit over an erect penis and to catch semen upon ejaculation.

malignant Very dangerous or harmful; refers to a cancerous tumor.

malignant melanoma A virulent cancer of the melanocytes (pigment-producing cells) of the skin.

managed care Cost-control procedures used by health insurers to coordinate treatment.

manipulative and body-based practices Treatments involving manipulation or movement of one or more body parts.

marijuana Chopped leaves and flowers of *Cannabis indica* or *Cannabis sativa* plants (hemp); a psychoactive stimulant.

massage therapy Soft tissue manipulation by trained therapists for relaxation and healing.

masturbation Self-stimulation of genitals.

measles A viral disease that produces symptoms such as an itchy rash and a high fever.

Medicaid A federal-state matching funds program that provides health insurance to low-income people.

medical abortion Termination of a pregnancy during the first 9 weeks using hormonal medications that cause the embryo to be expelled from the uterus.

medical model A view of health in which health status focuses primarily on the individual and a biological or diseased organ perspective.

Medicare A federal health insurance program that covers people age 65 and older, the permanently disabled, and people with end-stage kidney disease.

meditation A relaxation technique that involves deep breathing and concentration.

melatonin A hormone that affects sleep cycles, increasing drowsiness.

menarche The first menstrual period.

meningitis An infection of the meninges, the membranes that surround the brain and spinal cord.

menopause Permanent cessation of menstruation; generally occurs between the ages of 45 and 55.

mental health The thinking part of psychological health; includes your values, attitudes, and beliefs.

mental illnesses Disorders that disrupt thinking, feeling, moods, and behaviors and that impair daily functioning.

metabolic syndrome (MetS) A group of metabolic conditions occurring together that increase a person's risk of heart disease, stroke, and 2 diabetes.

metabolic syndrome: Cluster of risks for CVD and diabetes; persons with more than three of these risks greatly increase their risks of CVD and type diabetes.

metastasize Process by which cancer spreads from one area to different areas of the body.

methicillin-resistant *Staphylococcus aureus* (MRSA) Highly resistant form of staph infection that is growing in international prevalence.

migraine A type of headache characterized by debilitating symptoms that possibly results from alternating dilation and constriction of blood vessels.

mind-body medicine Techniques designed to enhance the mind's ability to affect bodily functions and symptoms.

mindfulness Practice of purposeful, nonjudgmental observation in which we are fully present in the moment.

minerals Inorganic, indestructible elements that aid physiological processes.

miscarriage Loss of the fetus before it is viable; also called *spontaneous abortion.*

modeling Learning specific behaviors by watching others perform them.

monogamy Exclusive sexual involvement with one partner.

mononucleosis A viral disease that causes pervasive fatigue and other long-lasting symptoms.

monosaccharides Simple sugars that contain only one molecule of sugar.

mons pubis Fatty tissue covering the pubic bone in females; in physically mature women, the mons is covered with coarse hair.

morbidly obese Having a body weight 100 percent or more above healthy recommended levels; in an adult, having a BMI of 40 or more.

mortality The proportion of deaths to population.

motivation A social, cognitive, and emotional force that directs human behavior.

mourning Culturally prescribed behavior patterns for the expression of grief.

multidrug-resistant TB (MDR-TB) Form of TB that is resistant to at least two of the best antibiotics available.

multifactorial disease Disease caused by interactions of several factors.

multifactorial disorder A disorder attributable to more than one of a variety of factors.

mumps A once common viral disease that is controllable by vaccination.

municipal solid waste (MSW) Solid waste such as durable and nondurable goods, containers and packaging, food waste, yard waste, and miscellaneous waste from residential, commercial, institutional, and industrial sources.

muscle dysmorphia Body image disorder in which men believe that their bodies are insufficiently lean or muscular.

muscular endurance A muscle's ability to exert force repeatedly without fatiguing or the ability to sustain a muscular contraction for a length of time.

muscular strength The amount of force that a muscle is capable of exerting in one contraction.

mutant cells Cells that differ in form, quality, or function from normal cells.

myocardial infarction (MI) or heart attack A blockage of normal blood supply to an area in the heart.

narcolepsy A neurological disorder that causes people to fall asleep involuntarily during the day.

natural disaster Any extreme environmental event that causes widespread destruction of land and/or property, injuries, and sometimes deaths.

naturopathy (naturopathic medicine) System of medicine in which practitioners work with nature to restore people's health.

negative consequences Severe problems associated with addiction, such as physical damage, legal trouble, financial problems, academic failure, or family dissolution.

neglect Failure to provide a child's basic needs such as food, clothing, shelter, and medical care.

neoplasm A new growth of tissue that results from uncontrolled, abnormal cellular development and serves no physiological function.

neurotransmitter A chemical that relays messages between nerve cells or from nerve cells to other body cells.

neurotransmitters Chemicals that relay messages between nerve cells or from nerve cells to other body cells.

Nexplanon (Implanon) A plastic capsule inserted in a woman's upper arm that releases a low dose of progestin to prevent pregnancy.

nicotine Primary stimulant chemical in tobacco products that is highly addictive.

nicotine poisoning Symptoms often experienced by beginning smokers, including dizziness, diarrhea, lightheadedness, rapid and erratic pulse, clammy skin, nausea, and vomiting.

nicotine withdrawal Symptoms including nausea, headaches, irritability, and intense tobacco cravings suffered by nicotine-addicted individuals who stop using tobacco.

nocturia Frequent urination at night caused by an overactive bladder.

non-REM (NREM) sleep A period of restful sleep dominated by slow brain waves; during non-REM sleep, rapid eye movement is rare.

nonionizing radiation Electromagnetic waves having relatively long wavelengths and enough energy to move atoms around or cause them to vibrate.

nonpoint source pollutant Pollutant that runs off or seeps into waterways from broad areas of land.

nonverbal communication Unwritten and unspoken messages, both intentional and unintentional.

nuclear meltdown Accident that results when the temperature in the core of a nuclear reactor increases enough to melt the nuclear fuel and breach the containment vessel.

nurse Health professional who provides many services for patients and who may work in a variety of settings.

nurse practitioner (NP) Professional nurse with advanced training obtained through either a master's degree program or a specialized nurse practitioner program.

nutraceuticals Food or food-based supplements that have combined nutritional and pharmaceutical benefits; used interchangeably with the term *functional foods.*

nutrients The constituents of food that sustain humans physiologically: water, proteins, carbohydrates, fats, vitamins, and minerals.

nutrition The science that investigates the relationship between physiological function and the essential elements of foods eaten.

NuvaRing Soft, flexible ring inserted into the vagina that releases hormones, preventing pregnancy.

obesity A body weight more than 20 percent above healthy recommended levels; in an adult, a BMI of 30 or more.

obesogenic Characterized by environments that promote increased food intake, non healthful foods, and physical inactivity; refers to conditions that lead people to become excessively fat.

obsession Excessive preoccupation with an addictive object or behavior.

obsessive-compulsive disorder (OCD) Form of anxiety disorder characterized by recurrent, unwanted thoughts and repetitive behaviors.

oncogenes Suspected cancer-causing genes present on chromosomes.

one repetition maximum (1 RM) The amount of weight or resistance that can be lifted or moved only once.

open relationship A relationship in which partners agree that sexual involvement can occur outside the relationship.

ophthalmologist Physician who specializes in the medical and surgical care of the eyes, including prescriptions for glasses.

opioids Drugs that induce sleep, relieve pain, and produce euphoria, including derivatives of opium and synthetics with similar chemical properties; also called *narcotics.*

opium The parent drug of the opioids; made from the seedpod resin of the opium poppy.

opportunistic infections Infections that occur when the immune system is weakened or compromised.

optometrist Eye specialist whose practice is limited to prescribing and fitting lenses.

oral contraceptives Pills containing synthetic hormones that prevent ovulation by regulating hormones.

oral ingestion Intake of drugs through the mouth.

organic Grown without use of toxic and persistent pesticides, chemicals, or hormones.

Ortho Evra Patch that releases hormones similar to those in oral contraceptives; each patch is worn for 1 week.

osteoarthritis (OA) Progressive deterioration of bones and joints that has been associated with the wear-and-tear theory of aging; also called *degenerative joint disease.*

osteopath General practitioner who receives training similar to a medical doctor's but with an emphasis on the skeletal and muscular systems; often uses spinal manipulation as part of treatment.

osteoporosis Degenerative bone disorder characterized by increasingly porous bones.

other specified feeding or eating disorder (OSFED) Eating disorders that are a true psychiatric illness but that do not fit the strict diagnostic criteria for anorexia nervosa, bulimia nervosa, or binge-eating disorder.

ovarian follicles Areas within the ovary in which individual eggs develop.

ovaries Almond-sized organs that house developing eggs and produce hormones.

overload A condition in which a person feels overly pressured by demands.

overuse injuries Injuries that result from the cumulative effects of day-after-day stresses placed on tendons, muscles, and joints.

overweight Having a body weight more than 10 percent above healthy recommended levels; in an adult, having a BMI of 25 to 29.

ovulation The point of the menstrual cycle at which a mature egg ruptures through the ovarian wall.

ovum Single mature egg cell.

palliative care Any form of medical care focused on relieving the pain, symptoms, and stress of serious illness to improve the quality of life for patients and their families.

palliative treatment Those treatments designed to treat or ease symptoms but not cure the disease.

pancreas Organ that secretes digestive enzymes into the small intestine and hormones, including insulin, into the bloodstream.

pandemic Global epidemic of a disease that occurs in several countries at the same time.

panic attack Severe anxiety reaction in which a particular situation, often for unknown reasons, causes terror.

Pap test A procedure in which cells taken from the cervical region are examined for abnormal cellular activity.

parasitic worms The largest of the pathogens, most of which are more a nuisance than a threat.

parasympathetic nervous system Branch of the autonomic nervous system responsible for slowing systems stimulated by the stress response.

passive euthanasia Intentional withholding of treatment that would prolong life.

pathogen A disease-causing agent.

pelvic inflammatory disease (PID) Term used to describe various infections of the female reproductive tract; can be caused by chlamydia or gonorrhea.

pelvic inflammatory disease (PID) Inflammation of the female genital tract that may cause scarring or blockage of the fallopian tubes, resulting in infertility.

penis Male sexual organ that releases sperm into the vagina.

perceived exertion The subjective perception of effort during exercise that can be used to monitor exercise intensity

perfect-use failure rate The number of pregnancies (per 100 users) likely to occur in the first year of use of a particular birth control method if the method is used consistently and correctly.

perineum Tissue that forms the "floor" of the pelvic region, found between the vulva and the anus.

peripheral artery disease (PAD) Atherosclerosis occurring in the lower extremities, such as in the feet, calves, or legs, or in the arms.

personal flotation device A device worn to provide buoyancy and keep the wearer, conscious or unconscious, afloat with the nose and mouth out of the water; also known as a life jacket.

personality disorder Mental disorder characterized by inflexible patterns of thought and beliefs that lead to socially distressing behavior.

pesticides Chemicals that kill pests such as insects or rodents.

phobia Deep and persistent fear of a specific object, activity, or situation that results in a compelling desire to avoid the source of the fear.

physical activity Refers to all body movements produced by skeletal muscles resulting in substantial increases in energy expenditure, but generally refers to movement of the large muscle groups.

physical fitness A balance of health-related attributes that allows you to perform moderate to vigorous physical activities on a regular basis and complete daily physical tasks without undue fatigue.

physician assistant (PA) A midlevel practitioner trained to handle most standard cases of care under the supervision of a physician.

physiological dependence The adaptive state that occurs with regular addictive behavior and results in withdrawal syndrome.

phytochemicals Naturally occurring nonnutrient plant chemicals believed to have beneficial health effects.

pituitary gland Endocrine gland that controls the release of hormones from the gonads.

placenta Network of blood vessels connected to the umbilical cord that transports oxygen and nutrients to a developing fetus and carries away fetal wastes.

plant sterols Essential components of plant membranes that, when consumed in the diet, appear to help lower cholesterol levels.

plaque Buildup of deposits in the arteries.

platelet adhesiveness Stickiness of red blood cells associated with blood clots.

pneumonia Inflammatory disease of the lungs characterized by chronic cough, chest pain, chills, high fever, and fluid accumulation; may be caused by bacteria, viruses, fungi, chemicals, or other substances.

point source pollutant Pollutant that enters waterways at a specific location.

poison Any substance harmful to the body when ingested, inhaled, injected, or absorbed through the skin.

pollutant Substance that contaminates some aspect of the environment and causes potential harm to living organisms.

polychlorinated biphenyls (PCBs) Toxic chemicals that were once used as insulating materials in high-voltage electrical equipment.

polydrug use Taking several medications, vitamins, recreational drugs, or illegal drugs simultaneously.

pornography Visual or literary depictions of sexual activity intended to be sexually arousing.

positive reinforcement Presenting something positive following a behavior that is being reinforced.

post-traumatic stress disorder (PTSD) Collection of symptoms that may occur as a delayed response to a traumatic event or series of events.

postpartum depression Mood disorder experienced by women who have given birth; involves depression, fatigue, and other symptoms and may last for weeks or months.

power Ability to make and implement decisions.

prayer Communication with a transcendent Presence.

pre-gaming Drinking heavily at home before going out to an event or other location.

preconception care Medical care received prior to becoming pregnant that helps a woman assess and address potential health issues.

prediabetes Condition in which blood glucose levels are higher than normal, but not high enough to be classified as diabetes.

preeclampsia Pregnancy complication characterized by high blood pressure, protein in the urine, and edema.

prehypertensive Blood pressure is above normal, but not yet in the hypertensive range.

prejudice A negative evaluation of an entire group of people that is typically based on unfavorable and often wrong ideas about the group.

premature ejaculation Ejaculation that occurs prior to or almost immediately following penile penetration of the vagina; also known as *early ejaculation.*

premenstrual dysphoric disorder (PMDD) Group of symptoms similar to but more severe than PMS, including severe mood disturbances.

premenstrual syndrome (PMS) Mood changes and physical symptoms that occur in some women 1 to 2 weeks prior to menstruation.

premium Payment made to an insurance carrier, usually in monthly installments, that covers the cost of an insurance policy.

primary aggression Goal-directed, hostile self-assertion that is destructive in nature.

primary care practitioner (PCP) A medical practitioner who treats routine ailments, advises on preventive care, gives general medical advice, and makes appropriate referrals when necessary.

primary idiopathic hypersomnia Excessive daytime sleepiness without narcolepsy or the associated features of other sleep disorders.

principal Either the original loan amount or the amount left outstanding on a loan, excluding interest.

prion A recently identified self-replicating protein-based pathogen.

private student loans Student financial aid loans that are financed by private banks or other institutions.

process addictions Behaviors such as disordered gambling, compulsive buying, compulsive Internet or technology use, work addiction, compulsive exercise, and sexual addiction that are known to be addictive because they are mood altering.

procrastinate To intentionally put off doing something.

progesterone Hormone secreted by the ovaries; helps the endometrium develop and helps maintain pregnancy.

proof Measure of the percentage of alcohol in a beverage; the proof is double the percentage of alcohol in the drink.

prostaglandin Hormone-like substance associated with muscle contraction and inflammation.

prostate gland Gland that secretes chemicals that help sperm fertilize an ovum and secretes neutralizing fluids into the semen.

prostate-specific antigen (PSA) An antigen found in prostate cancer patients.

prostitution Practice of engaging in sexual acts for money.

proteins Large molecules made up of chains of amino acids; essential constituents of all body cells.

protozoans Microscopic single-celled organisms that can be pathogenic.

psychoactive drugs Drugs that affect brain chemistry and have the potential to alter mood or behavior.

psychological hardiness A personality trait characterized by control, commitment, and the embrace of challenge.

psychological health The mental, emotional, social, and spiritual dimensions of health.

psychological resilience The process of adapting well in the face of adversity, trauma, tragedy, threats, or significant sources of stress, such as family and relationship problems, serious health problems, or workplace and financial stressors.

psychoneuroimmunology (PNI) The study of the interactions of behavioral, neural, and endocrine functions and the functioning of the body's immune system.

puberty Period of sexual maturation.

pubic lice Parasitic insects that can inhabit various body areas, especially the genitals.

rabies A viral disease of the central nervous system; often transmitted through animal bites.

radiation absorbed dose (rad) Unit of measure of radiation exposure.

radiotherapy The use of radiation to kill cancerous cells.

radon Naturally occurring radioactive gas resulting from the decay of certain radioactive elements.

rape Sexual penetration without the victim's consent.

rational suicide The decision to kill oneself rather than endure constant pain and slow decay.

reactive aggression Hostile emotional reaction brought about by frustrating life experiences.

receptor sites Specialized areas of cells and organs where chemicals, enzymes, and other substances interact.

recessive Term describing an allele that is expressed only in the absence of a dominant allele; that is, if both alleles are recessive or if the recessive gene is on the X chromosome of the twenty-third pair.

relapse The tendency to return to the addictive behavior after a period of abstinence.

relative deprivation The inability of lower income groups to sustain the same lifestyle as higher income groups in their same community, often resulting in feelings of anxiety and inferiority.

religion System of beliefs, practices, rituals, and symbols designed to facilitate closeness to the sacred or transcendent.

REM sleep A period of sleep characterized by brain-wave activity similar to that seen in wakefulness; rapid eye movement and dreaming occur during REM sleep.

repetitive motion disorder (RMD) An injury to soft tissue, tendons, muscles, nerves, or joints due to the physical stress of repeated motions.

resiliency The ability to adapt to change and stressful events in healthy and flexible ways.

resting metabolic rate (RMR) The energy expenditure of the body under BMR conditions plus other daily sedentary activities.

restless legs syndrome (RLS) A neurological disorder characterized by an overwhelming urge to move the legs when they are at rest.

Rh factor Antigen present in the red blood cells of 85 percent of people; those with the Rh factor are known as Rh positive (Rh+); those without it are Rh negative (Rh−).

rheumatic heart disease A heart disease caused by untreated streptococcal infection of the throat.

rheumatoid arthritis An autoimmune inflammatory joint disease.

RICE Acronym for the standard first-aid treatment for virtually all traumatic and overuse injuries: rest, ice, compression, and elevation.

rickettsia A small form of bacteria that live inside other living cells.

risk behaviors Actions that increase susceptibility to negative health outcomes.

rubella (German measles) A milder form of measles that causes a rash and mild fever in children and may damage a fetus or a newborn baby.

satiety The feeling of fullness or satisfaction at the end of a meal.

saturated fats Fats that are unable to hold any more hydrogen in their chemical structure; derived mostly from animal sources; solid at room temperature.

schizophrenia Mental illness with biological origins characterized by irrational behavior, severe alterations of the senses, and often an inability to function in society.

scrotum External sac of tissue that encloses the testes.

seasonal affective disorder (SAD) Type of depression that occurs in the winter months, when sunlight levels are low.

secondary sex characteristics Characteristics associated with sex but not directly related to reproduction, such as vocal pitch, amount of body hair, breasts, and location of fat deposits.

self-disclosure Sharing feelings or personal information with others.

self-efficacy Describes a person's belief about whether he or she can successfully engage in and execute a specific behavior or task.

self-esteem One's realistic sense of self-respect or self-worth.

self-injury Intentionally causing injury to one's own body in an attempt to cope with overwhelming negative emotions; also called *self-mutilation, self-harm,* or *nonsuicidal self-injury* (NSSI).

self-nurturance Developing individual potential through a balanced and realistic appreciation of self-worth and ability.

self-talk The customary manner of thinking and talking to yourself, which can affect your self-image.

semen Fluid containing sperm and nutrients that increase sperm viability and neutralize vaginal acid.

seminal vesicles Glandular ducts that secrete nutrients for the semen.

serial monogamy Series of monogamous sexual relationships.

set point theory Theory that a form of internal thermostat controls our weight and fights to maintain this weight around a narrowly set range.

sexual addiction Compulsive involvement in sexual activity.

sexual assault Any act in which one person is sexually intimate with another without that person's consent.

sexual aversion disorder Desire dysfunction characterized by sexual phobias and anxiety about sexual contact.

sexual dysfunction Problems associated with achieving sexual satisfaction.

sexual fantasies Sexually arousing thoughts and dreams.

sexual harassment Any form of unwanted sexual attention related to any condition of employment, education, or performance evaluation.

sexual identity Recognition of oneself as a sexual being; a composite of biological sex characteristics, gender identity, gender roles, and sexual orientation.

sexual orientation A person's enduring emotional, romantic, or sexual attraction to other persons.

sexual performance anxiety Sexual difficulties caused by anticipating some sort of problem during a sex act.

sexual prejudice Negative attitudes and hostile actions directed at those with a different sexual orientation.

sexuality Thoughts, feelings, and behaviors associated with being male or female, experiencing attraction, being in love, and being in relationships that include sexual intimacy.

sexually transmitted infections (STIs) Infectious diseases caused by pathogens transmitted through some form of sexual contact.

shaping Using a series of small steps to gradually achieve a particular goal.

shift and persist A strategy of reframing appraisals of current stressors and focusing on a meaningful future that protects a person from the negative effects of too much stress.

shingles A disease characterized by a painful rash that occurs when the chickenpox virus is reactivated.

sick building syndrome (SBS) Describes a situation in which occupants of a building experience acute health effects linked to time spent in a building, but no specific illness or cause can be identified

sidestream smoke Smoke from the burning end of a cigarette, pipe, or cigar or exhaled by smokers, commonly called *secondhand smoke.*

simple carbohydrates A carbohydrate made up of only one sugar molecule, or of two sugar molecules bonded together; also called simple sugars.

simple rape Rape by one person, usually known to the victim, that does not involve physical beating or use of a weapon.

single-gene disorder A disorder characterized by structural and/or functional impairments resulting from a defect involving only one gene.

sinoatrial node (SA node) Cluster of electric pulse-generating cells that serves as a natural pacemaker for the heart.

situational inducement Attempts to influence a behavior through situations and occasions that are structured to exert control over that behavior.

sleep apnea A disorder in which breathing is briefly and repeatedly interrupted during sleep.

sleep debt The difference between the number of hours of sleep an individual needed in a given time period and the number of hours he or she actually slept.

sleep inertia A state characterized by cognitive impairment, grogginess, and disorientation that is experienced upon rising from short sleep or an overly long nap.

sleep study A clinical assessment of sleep in which the patient is monitored while spending the night in a sleep disorders center.

smog Brownish haze that is a form of pollution produced by the photochemical reaction of sunlight with hydrocarbons, nitrogen compounds, and other gases in vehicle exhaust.

snuff Powdered form of tobacco that is sniffed or absorbed through the mucous membranes in the nose or placed inside the cheek and sucked.

social anxiety disorder Phobia characterized by fear and avoidance of social situations; also called *social phobia.*

social bonds The level of closeness and attachment with other individuals.

social cognitive model (SCM) Model of behavior change emphasizing the role of social factors and thought processes (cognition) in behavior change.

social death A seemingly irreversible situation in which a person is not treated as an active member of society.

social health Aspect of psychological health that includes interactions with others, ability to use social supports, and ability to adapt to various situations.

social learning theory Theory that people learn behaviors by watching role models—parents, caregivers, and significant others.

social physique anxiety (SPA) A desire to look good that has a destructive effect on a person's ability to function well in social interactions and relationships.

social support Network of people and services with whom you share ties and from whom you get support.

socialization Process by which a society communicates behavioral expectations to its members.

socioeconomic status (SES) An individual or family's social and economic position in relation to others with regards to education, income, and occupation.

spermatogenesis The development of sperm.

spermicide Substance designed to kill sperm.

spiritual health Aspect of psychological health that relates to having a sense of meaning and purpose to one's life, as well as a feeling of connection with others and with nature.

spiritual intelligence (SI) The ability to access higher meanings, values, abiding purposes, and unconscious aspects of the self, a characteristic that helps us find a moral and ethical path to guide us through life.

spirituality An individual's sense of peace, purpose, and connection to others and beliefs about the meaning of life.

stalking Willful, repeated, and malicious following, harassing, or threatening of another person.

standard drink Amount of any beverage that contains about 14 grams of pure alcohol.

staphylococci A group of round bacteria, usually found in clusters, that cause a variety of diseases in humans and other animals.

starches Polysaccharides that are the storage forms of glucose in plants.

static stretching Stretching techniques that slowly and gradually lengthen a muscle or group of muscles and their tendons.

stent A stainless steel, mesh-like tube that is inserted to prop open the artery.

stereotactic radiosurgery A type of radiation therapy that can be used to zap tumors; also known as gamma knife surgery.

sterilization Permanent fertility control achieved through surgical procedures.

stigma Negative perception about a group of people or a certain situation or condition.

stillbirth Fetus that is dead at birth.

stimulants Drugs that increase activity of the central nervous system.

Streptococcus A round bacterium, usually found in chain formation.

stress A series of mental and physiological responses and adaptations to a real or perceived threat to one's well-being.

stress inoculation Stress-management technique in which a person consciously anticipates and prepares for potential stressors.

stressor A physical, social, or psychological event or condition that upsets homeostasis and produces a stress response.

stroke A condition occurring when the brain is damaged by disrupted blood supply; also called *cerebrovascular accident*.

student loans Financial student aid that must be repaid in the future.

subjective well-being An uplifting feeling of inner peace.

suction curettage Abortion technique that uses gentle suction to remove fetal tissue from the uterus.

sudden cardiac death Death that occurs as a result of abrupt, profound loss of heart function.

sudden infant death syndrome (SIDS) Sudden death of an infant under 1 year of age for no apparent reason.

suicidal ideation A desire to die and thoughts about suicide.

super obese Having a body weight higher than morbid obesity; in an adult, having a BMI of 50 or more.

Superfund Fund established under the Comprehensive Environmental Response, Compensation, and Liability Act to be used for cleaning up toxic waste dumps.

suppositories Mixtures of drugs and a waxy medium (designed to melt at body temperature) that are inserted into the anus or vagina.

surgical methods Surgically altering a man's or woman's reproductive system to permanently prevent pregnancy.

survivorship Physical, psychological, emotional, and economic issues of cancer from diagnosis until the end of life.

sustainable development Development that meets the needs of the present without compromising the ability of future generations to meet their own needs.

sympathetic nervous system Branch of the autonomic nervous system responsible for stress arousal.

sympathomimetics Food substances that can produce stresslike physiological responses.

synergism The interaction of two or more drugs that produces more profound effects than would be expected if the drugs were taken separately; also called *potentiation*.

syphilis One of the most widespread bacterial STIs; characterized by distinct phases and potentially serious results.

systolic blood pressure The upper number in the fraction that measures blood pressure, indicating pressure on the walls of the arteries when the heart contracts.

tar Thick, brownish sludge condensed from particulate matter in smoked tobacco.

target heart rate The heart rate range of aerobic exercise that leads to improved cardiorespiratory fitness (i.e., 64% to 96% of maximal heart rate).

temperature inversion Weather condition that occurs when a layer of cool air is trapped under a layer of warmer air, preventing the air from circulating.

teratogenic Causing birth defects; may refer to drugs, environmental chemicals, radiation, or diseases.

terrorism Unlawful use of force or violence against persons or property to intimidate or coerce a government, civilian population, or any segment thereof in furtherance of political or social objectives.

testes Male sex organs that manufacture sperm and produce hormones.

testosterone Male sex hormone manufactured in the testes.

tetrahydrocannabinol (THC) The chemical name for the active ingredient in marijuana.

thanatology The study of death and dying.

thrombolysis Injection of an agent to dissolve clots and restore some blood flow, thereby reducing the amount of tissue that dies from ischemia.

thrombus A blood clot attached to a blood vessel's wall.

time As part of the FITT prescription, refers to the duration of an exercise session.

tolerance Phenomenon in which progressively larger doses of a drug or more intense involvement in a behavior is needed to produce the desired effects.

toxic shock syndrome (TSS) Potentially life-threatening disease that occurs when specific bacterial toxins multiply and spread to the bloodstream, most commonly through improper use of tampons, diaphragms, or cervical caps.

toxoplasmosis Disease caused by an organism found in cat feces that, when contracted by a pregnant woman, may result in stillbirth or birth defects.

traditional Chinese medicine (TCM) Ancient comprehensive system of healing that uses herbs, acupuncture, and massage to bring vital energy, *qi*, into balance and to remove blockages of *qi* that lead to disease.

***trans* fats (*trans* fatty acids)** Fatty acids that are produced when polyunsaturated oils are hydrogenated to make them more solid.

transdermal The introduction of drugs through the skin.

transgender Having a gender identity that does not match one's biological sex.

transient ischemic attack (TIA) Brief interruption of the blood supply to the brain that causes only temporary impairment, often an indicator of impending major stroke.

transsexual Person who is psychologically of one sex but physically of the other.

transtheoretical model Model of behavior change that identifies six distinct stages people go through in altering behavior patterns; also called the *stages of change model*.

traumatic injuries Injuries that are accidental and occur suddenly and violently.

traumatic stress A physiological and mental response that occurs for a prolonged period of time after a major accident, war, assault, natural disaster, or an event in which one may be seriously hurt, or killed, or witness horrible things.

trichomoniasis Protozoan STI characterized by foamy, yellowish discharge and unpleasant odor.

triglycerides The most common form of fat in our food supply and in the body; made up of a molecule called glycerol and three fatty acid chains; excess calories are converted into triglycerides and stored as body fat.

trimester A 3-month segment of pregnancy.

triple marker screen (TMS) Common maternal blood test that can be used to identify fetuses with certain birth defects and genetic abnormalities.

tubal ligation Sterilization of a woman that involves cutting and tying off or cauterizing the fallopian tubes.

tuberculosis (TB) A disease caused by bacterial infiltration of the respiratory system.

tumor A neoplasmic mass that grows more rapidly than surrounding tissue.

type As part of the FITT prescription, refers to what kind of exercises a person should do.

type 1 diabetes Form of diabetes mellitus in which the pancreas is not able to make insulin, and therefore blood glucose cannot enter the cells to be used for energy.

type 2 diabetes Form of diabetes mellitus in which the pancreas does not make enough insulin or the body is unable to use insulin correctly.

typical-use failure rate The number of pregnancies (per 100 users) likely to occur in the first year of use of a particular birth control method if the method's use is not consistent or always correct.

ulcerative colitis An inflammatory bowel disease that affects the mucous membranes of the large intestine and can lead to ulcers, erosion of the outer lining of the colon, and serious bleeding.

ultrafast computed tomography (CT) A newer, faster form of heart X-ray used to evaluate bypass grafts, diagnose ventricular function, and identify other heart irregularities.

ultrasonography (ultrasound) Common prenatal test that uses sound waves to create a visual image of a developing fetus.

underweight Having a body weight more than 10 percent below healthy recommended levels; in an adult, having a BMI below 18.5.

unintentional injuries Injury, death, or psychological harm caused unintentionally or without premeditation.

unsaturated fats Fats with one or more chemical bonds that exclude hydrogen; derived mostly from plants; liquid at room temperature.

urethral opening Opening through which urine is expelled.

urinary incontinence Inability to control urination.

urinary tract infection (UTI) Infection, more common among women than men, of the urinary tract; causes include untreated STIs.

uterus (womb) Hollow, pear-shaped muscular organ whose function is to house a developing fetus.

vaccination Inoculation with killed or weakened pathogens or similar, less dangerous antigens to prevent or lessen the effects of some disease.

vagina Muscular, tube-shaped organ in females that serves as a passageway connecting the vulva to the uterus.

vaginal contraceptive film A thin film infused with spermicidal gel that is inserted into the vagina so that it covers the cervix.

vaginal intercourse Insertion of the penis into the vagina.

vaginismus State in which the vaginal muscles contract so forcefully that penetration cannot occur.

values Principles that influence our thoughts and emotions and guide the choices we make in our lives.

variant sexual behavior A sexual behavior that is not commonly practiced.

vas deferens Tube that transports sperm from the epididymis to the ejaculatory duct.

vasectomy Male sterilization procedure that involves cutting and tying off the vasa deferentia.

vasocongestion Engorgement of the genital organs with blood.

vegetarian A person who follows a diet that excludes some or all animal products.

veins Vessels that transport waste and carry blood back to the heart from other regions of the body.

ventricles The heart's two lower chambers, which pump blood through the blood vessels.

venules Branches of the veins.

very-low-calorie diets (VLCDs) Diets with a daily caloric value of 400 to 700 calories.

violence Aggressive behaviors that produce injuries and can result in death.

virulent Strong enough to overcome host resistance and cause disease.

viruses Pathogens that invade and inject their own DNA or RNA into a host cell, take it over, and force it to make copies of the pathogen.

visualization The creation of mental images to promote relaxation.

vitamins Essential organic compounds that promote metabolism, growth, and reproduction and help maintain life and health.

vulva External female genitalia.

waist circumference Simple measure of circumference around waist, measured one inch above naval in inches or centimeters.

waist circumference-to-height ratio Measure of a person's waist circumference, divided by their height; measures under .50 are desirable.

waist circumference-to-hip ratio Waist circumference divided by hip circumference; a high ratio indicates increased health risks due to unhealthy fat distribution.

wellness The achievement of the highest level of health possible in each of several dimensions.

whole grains Grains that are milled in their complete form and thus include the bran, germ, and endosperm, with only the husk removed.

withdrawal (1) A series of temporary physical and biopsychosocial symptoms that occurs when an addict abruptly abstains from an addictive chemical or behavior; (2) contraceptive method that involves withdrawing the penis from the vagina before ejaculation; also called *coitus interruptus*.

work addiction The compulsive use of work and the work persona to fulfill needs for intimacy, power, and success.

X-linked dominant disorder Single-gene disorder that occurs in individuals who have inherited at least one copy of an X chromosome with the affected dominant allele.

X-linked recessive disorder Single-gene disorder that occurs in males who have inherited one copy of an X chromosome with the affected recessive allele and in females who have inherited two copies.

yo-yo diets Cycles in which people diet and regain weight.

yoga System of physical and mental training involving controlled breathing, physical postures (*asanas*), meditation, chanting, and other practices believed to cultivate unity with the *Atman,* or spiritual life principle of the universe.

zoonotic diseases Diseases of animals that may be transmitted to humans.

REFERENCES

Chapter 1

1. Centers for Disease Control and Prevention, "Table A," *National Vital Statistics Report* 61, no. 6 (2012), www.cdc.gov/nchs/data/nvsr/nvsr61/nvsr61_06.pdf.
2. Centers for Disease Control and Prevention, "Achievements in Public Health, 1900–1999: Control of Infectious Diseases," *Morbidity and Mortality Weekly Report* 48, no. 29 (1999): 621–29, www.cdc.gov/mmwr/preview/mmwrhtml/mm4829a1.htm.
3. H. L. Walls et al., "Obesity and Trends in Life Expectancy," *Journal of Obesity*, 2012: 107989, doi:10.1155/2012/107989.
4. Organization for Economic Cooperation and Development, *Health at a Glance 2013: OECD Indicators*, 2013, doi:10.1787/health_glance-2013-en.
5. U.S. Department of Health and Human Services (DHHS), *Healthy People 2020* (Washington, DC: U.S. Government Printing Office, 2011), www.healthypeople.gov/2020/about/QoL.WBabout.aspx.
6. The Brookings Institution, "Obesity, Prevention, and Health Care Costs," May 2012, www.brookings.edu/research/papers/2012/05/04-health-care-hammond
7. S. Drenkard, "Overreaching on Obesity: Governments Consider New Taxes on Soda and Candy," *Tax Foundation Special Report* 196, October 31, 2011, Available at http://taxfoundation.org/article/overreaching-obesity-governments-consider-new-taxes-soda-and-candy; R. R. Friedman and K. D. Brownell, "Sugar-Sweetened Beverage Taxes: An Updated Policy Brief," Yale Rudd Center for Food Policy & Obesity, *Rudd Report*, October 2012, www.yaleruddcenter.org/resources/upload/docs/what/reports/Rudd_Policy_Brief_Sugar_Sweetened_Beverage_Taxes.pdf.
8. World Health Organization (WHO), "Constitution of the World Health Organization," *Chronicles of the World Health Organization* (Geneva: WHO, 1947), www.who.int/governance/eb/constitution/en/index.html.
9. R. Dubos, *So Human an Animal: How We Are Shaped by Surroundings and Events* (New York: Scribner, 1968), 15.
10. U.S. Department of Health and Human Services (DHHS), *Healthy People 2020* , 2011.
11. Centers for Disease Control and Prevention, "Chronic Disease Prevention and Health Promotion," August 2012, www.cdc.gov/chronicdisease/overview/index.htm#2.
12. U.S. Burden of Disease Collaborators, "The State of US Health, 1990–2010: Burden of Diseases, Injuries, and Risk Factors," *Journal of the American Medical Association* 310, no. 6 (2013): 591–606, doi:10.1001/jama.2013.13805; Centers for Disease Control and Prevention, "Alcohol Use and Health Fact Sheets," December 2013, www.cdc.gov/alcohol/fact-sheets/alcohol-use.htm; Centers for Disease Control and Prevention, "Smoking and Tobacco Use Fast Facts," February 2014, www.cdc.gov/tobacco/data_statistics/fact_sheets/fast_facts.
13. U.S. Burden of Disease Collaborators, "The State of US Health," 2013.
14. Ibid.
15. CDC, "Alcohol Use and Health Fact Sheets," 2013; CDC, "Smoking and Tobacco Use Fast Facts," 2014.
16. CDC, "Alcohol Use and Health Fact Sheets," 2013; CDC, "Smoking and Tobacco Use Fast Facts," 2014.
17. E. Kvaavik et al, "Influence of Individual and Combined Health Behaviors on Total and Cause-Specific Mortality in Men and Women: The United Kingdom Health and Lifestyle Survey," *Archives of Internal Medicine* 170, no. 8 (2010): 711–18.
18. U.S. DHHS, *Healthy People* 2020, 2011.
19. American College Health Association, *American College Health Association-National College Health Assessment II: Reference Group Executive Summary Spring* 2013 (Linthicum, MD: American College Health Association, 2013), www.acha.org.
20. D. Ding et al. "Neighborhood Environment and Physical Activity among Youth: A Review," *American Journal of Preventive Medicine* 41, no. 4 (2011): 442–55; J. Sallis et al., "Role of Built Environments in Physical Activity, Obesity, and Cardiovascular Disease," *Circulation* 125 (2012): 729–37, Available at https://circ.ahajournals.org/content/125/5/729.full.
21. M. J. Trowbridge and T. L. Schmid, "Built Environment and Physical Activity Promotion: Place-Based Obesity Prevention Strategies," *Journal of Law, Medicine & Ethics*, Weight of the Nation Supplement, (Winter, 2013): 46–51, Available at https://www.aslme.org/media/downloadable/files/links/j/l/jlme-41-4-supp_trowbridge.pdf.
22. S. Cummins, E. Flint, and S.A. Matthews, "New Neighborhood Grocery Store Increased Awareness of Food Access but Did Not Alter Dietary Habits or Obesity," *Health Affairs* 33, no. 2 (2014): 283–91.
23. Gallup, "U.S. Uninsured Rate Holds Steady at 13.4%," Accessed July 2014, http://www.gallup.com/poll/170882/uninsured-rate-holds-steady.aspx.
24. U.S. Department of Health & Human Services, "Enrollment in Health Insurance Marketplace Increases by 53% in January," February 2014, www.hhs.gov/news/press/2014pres/02/20140212a.html.
25. U.S. DHHS, *Healthy People 2020*, 2011.
26. I. Rosenstock, "Historical Origins of the Health Belief Model," *Health Education Monographs* 2, no. 4 (1974): 328–35.
27. Bandura, A. "Human Agency in Social Cognitive Theory." *Am Psychol.* 1989 Sep. 44(9): 1175–84.
28. P.J. Morgan et al. "The 'Healthy Dads, Healthy Kids' Community Randomized Controlled Trial: A Community-Based Healthy Lifestyle Program for Fathers and Their Children," *BMC Public Health,* no. 11 (2011): 876, doi:10.1186/1471-2458-11-876.
29. Centers for Disease Control and Prevention, "Understanding Youth Violence: Fact Sheet 2012," 2012, www.cdc.gov/violenceprevention/pdf/yv_factsheet2012-a.pdf; Centers for Disease Control and Prevention, "Striving to Reduce Youth Violence Everywhere," 2012, Available at http://vetoviolence.cdc.gov/STRYVE/docs/Stryve.pdf.
30. J. O. Prochaska and C. C. DiClemente, "Stages and Processes of Self-Change of Smoking: Toward an Integrative Model of Change," *Journal of Consulting and Clinical Psychology* 51 (1983): 390–95.
31. J. Huang, F. J. Chaloupka, and G. T. Fong, "Cigarette Graphic Warning Labels and Smoking Prevalence in Canada: A Critical Examination and Reformulation of the FDA Regulatory Impact Analysis." *Tobacco Control* (2013), doi: 10.1136/tobaccocontrol-2013-051170.
32. K. Simmen-Janevska, V. Brandstatter, and A. Maercker. "The Overlooked Relationship between Motivational Abilities and Posttraumatic Stress: A Review," *European Journal of Psychotraumatology* 10, no. 3 (2012), doi:10.3402/ejpt.v3i0.18560
33. A. Ellis and M. Benard, *Clinical Application of Rational Emotive Therapy* (New York: Plenum, 1985).

Pulled statistics:

p. 3, J. A. Salomon, et al., "Healthy life Expectancy for 187 Countries, 1990–2010: A Systematic Analysis for the Global Burden Disease Study 2010," *The Lancet* 380, no. 9859 (2012): 2144–2162, doi:10.1016/S0140-6736(12)61690-0.

p. 11, Centers for Disease Control and Prevention, "Health Insurance Coverage," August 2012, www.cdc.gov.

Chapter 1A

1. W. Evans, B. Wolfe, and N. Adler, "The Income-Health Gradient," *Institute for Research on Poverty: Focus* 30, no. 1 (2013), www.irp.wisc.edu/publications/focus/pdfs/foc301b.pdf; E. R. Cheng and D. A. Kindig, "Disparities in Premature Mortality Between High- and Low-Income US Counties," *Preventing Chronic Disease* 9 (2012): 110120, DOI: http://dx.doi.org/10.5888/pcd9.110120.
2. World Health Organization, "Social Determinants of Health: Key Concepts," *Commission on Social Determinants of Health, 2005–2008*, Accessed April 2014, www.who.int/social_determinants/thecommission/finalreport/key_concepts/en.
3. Centers for Disease Control and Prevention, "Obesity and Socioeconomic Status in Adults: United States, 2005–2008," *NCHS Data Brief*, no. 50 (2010), www.cdc.gov.
4. G. Georgiadis, F. R. Rodriguea, and J. Pineda, "Has the Preston Curve Broken Down?," United Nations Development Programme Human Development Reports, Research Paper 2010/32 (October 30, 2010), dx.doi.org/10.2139/ssrn.2031504.
5. M. O. Weeks, "Tobacco and Media Exposure in Poor Neighbourhoods: Implications for the Incidence of Smoking among Community Residents," *International Journal of Nursing Practice* 17, no. 5 (2011): 534–38.
6. A. Carlsson et al., "Financial Stress in Late Adulthood and Diverse Risks of Incident Cardiovascular Disease and All-Cause Mortality in Women and Men," *BMC Public Health* 14, no. 1 (2014): 17, DOI:10.1186/1471-2458-14-17.
7. Pruchno et al., "Neighborhood Food Environment and Obesity in Community-Dwelling Older Adults: Individual and Neighborhood Effects," *Journal of Public Health* 104, no. 5 (2014); D. Viola et al., "Overweight and Obesity: Can We Reconcile Evidence about Supermarkets and Fast Food Retailers for Public Health Policy?," *Journal of Public Health Policy* 34, no. 3 (2013): 424–38, DOI: 10.1057/jphp.2013.19.
8. Centers for Disease Control and Prevention, "A Look inside Food Deserts," September 2012, www.cdc.gov/Features/fooddeserts.
9. E. R. Cheng and D. A. Kindig, "Disparities in Premature Mortality," 2012.
10. N. Spencer, T. M. Thanh, S. Louise, "Low Income/Socio-Economic Status in Early Childhood and Physical Health in Later Childhood/Adolescence: A Systematic Review," *Maternal Child Health Journal* 17, no. 3 (2013): 424–31, DOI: 10.1007/s10995-012-1010-2.
11. E. R. Cheng and D. A. Kindig, "Disparities in Premature Mortality," 2012.
12. Ibid.
13. College Board, Trends in Higher Education, "Tuition and Fee and Room and Board Charges over Time, 1973–74 through 2013–14, Selected Years," Accessed May 2014, http://trends.collegeboard.org/college-pricing/figures-tables/tuition-and-fee-and-room-and-board-charges-over-time-1973-74-through 2013-14-selected-years.
14. National Survey of Student Engagement, *NSSE Annual Results 2012: Promoting Student Learning and Institutional Improvement: Lessons from NSSE at 13* (Bloomington, IN: Indiana University Center for Postsecondary Research, 2012).
15. American College Health Association, *American College Health Association-National College Health Assessment II (ACHA-NACHA II): Undergraduate Students, Reference Group Data Report, Spring 2013* (Hanover, MD: American College Health Association, 2013).
16. K. Eagan et al., *The American Freshman: National Norms for Fall 2013* (Los Angeles: Higher Education Research Institute, UCLA, 2013).
17. Sallie Mae and Ipsos, *How America Pays for College 2013: A National Study*, Accessed May 2014, http://news.salliemae.com/research-tools/america-pays-2013.
18. The White House, Office of the Press Secretary, "FACT SHEET on the President's Plan to Make College More Affordable: A Better Bargain for the Middle Class," August 22, 2013, www.whitehouse.gov/the-press-office/2013/08/22/fact-sheet-president-s-plan-make-college-more-affordable-better-bargain.
19. D. Lederman, M. Stratford, and S. Jaschik, "Rating (and Berating) the Ratings," *Inside Higher Ed*, February 7, 2014, www.insidehighered.com/news/2014/02/07/colleges-and-analysts-respond-obama-ratings-proposal#sthash.v0KEa9dC.dpbs.
20. Sallie Mae and Ipsos, *How America Pays for College 2013*, 2014.
21. OECD, *Education at a Glance 2013: OECD Indicators* (Paris: OECD Publishing, 2013), DOI: 10.1787/eag-2013-en.
22. State Higher Education Executive Officers Association, "The Economic Benefit of Post Secondary Degrees," December 2012, www.sheeo.org/resources/publications/economic-benefit-postsecondary-degrees.
23. M. Heron, "Deaths: Leading Causes for 2010, Table 1," *National Vital Statistics Reports* 62, no. 6 (2013): 17–18, www.cdc.gov/nchs/data/nvsr/nvsr62/nvsr62_06.pdf.
24. Healthcare.gov, "Why Should I Have Health Coverage?," Accessed April 2014, www.healthcare.gov/why-should-i-have-health-coverage.
25. Bankruptcy Abuse Prevention and Consumer Protection Act of 2005, Pub.L. 109–8, 109th Cong. (2005). Full text available at www.govtrack.us.
26. Federal Reserve Bank of New York, Research and Statistics Group, Microeconomic Studies, "Quarterly Report on Household Debt and Credit," November 2012, www.newyorkfed.org.
27. Credit Card Accountability Responsibility and Disclosure Act, The CARD Act of 2009, Pub.L. 111–24, 111th Cong. (2009). Full text available at www.gpo.gov.
28. Javelin Strategy & Research, "The 2014 Identity Fraud Report: Card Data Breaches and Inadequate Consumer Password Habits Fuel Disturbing Fraud Trends," February 2014, www.javelinstrategy.com/brochure/314.
29. Ibid.
30. Federal Trade Commission, Consumer Information, "Medical Identity Theft," August 2012, www.consumer.ftc.gov/articles/0171-medical-identity-theft.

Pulled statistics:

p. 28, Sallie Mae, "A Snapshot of How America Pays for College 2013," 2013, www1.salliemae.com.

p. 31, Nerd Wallet, "American Household Credit Card Debt Statistics: 2014," April 2014, http://www.nerdwallet.com/blog/credit-card-data/average-credit-card-debt-household.

p. 32, Javelin Strategy & Research, "The 2014 Identity Fraud Report: Card Data Breaches and Inadequate Consumer Password Habits Fuel Disturbing Fraud Trends," February 2014, www.javelinstrategy.com.

Chapter 2

1. A. H. Maslow, *Motivation and Personality*, 2nd ed. (New York: Harper and Row, 1970).
2. D. J. Anspaugh and G. Ezell, *Teaching Today's Health*, 10th ed. (Boston: Pearson, 2013).
3. D. Goleman, R. Boyatzis, and A. McKee, *Primal Leadership: Unleashing the Power of Emotional Intelligence* (Boston: Harvard Business Review Press, 2013); M. A. Brackett, S. E. Rivers, and P. Salovey, "Emotional Intelligence: Implications for Personal, Social, Academic, and Workplace Success," *Social and Personality Psychology Compass* 5, no. 1 (2011): 88–103.
4. J. Holt-Lunstad, T. B. Smith, and J. B. Layton, "Social Relationships and Mortality Risk: A Meta-Analytic Review," *PLoS Medicine* 7, no. 7 (2010): e1000316, DOI: 10.1371/journal.pmed.1000316; N. I. Eisenberger and S. W. Cole, "Social Neuroscience and Health: Neurophysiological Mechanisms Linking Social Ties with Physical Health," *Nature Neuroscience* 15 (2012): 669–74, DOI:10.1038/nn.3086; Y. Luo et al., "Loneliness, Health, and Mortality in Old Age: A National Longitudinal Study," *Social Science & Medicine* 74, no. 6 (2012): 907–14.
5. K. Karren et al., *Mind/Body Health: The Effects of Attitudes, Emotions, and Relationships*, 5th ed. (San Francisco: Benjamin Cummings, 2013).
6. National Cancer Institute, "Spirituality in Cancer Care," Revised 2012, www.cancer.gov/cancertopics/pdq/supportivecare/spirituality/patient.
7. C. Carter, *Raising Happiness: 10 Simple Steps for More Joyful Kids and Happier*

Parents (New York: Ballantine Publishing, 2010).

8. W. Cheng, W. Ickes, and L. Verhofstadt, "How is Family Support Related to Students' GPA Scores? A Longitudinal Study," *Higher Education* 64, no. 3 (2012): 399–420; L. Rice et al., "The Role of Social Support in Students' Perceived Abilities and Attitudes toward Math and Science," *Journal of Youth and Adolescence* 42, no. 7 (2013): 1028–40; J. Cullum et al., "Ignoring Norms with a Little Help from my Friends: Social Support Reduces Normative Influence on Drinking Behavior," *Journal of Social & Clinical Psychology* 32, no. 1 (2013): 17–33; J. Hirsch and A. Barton, "Positive Social Support, Negative Social Exchanges, and Suicidal Behavior in College Students," *Journal of American College Health* 59, no. 5 (2011): 393–98; I. Yalcin, "Social Support and Optimism as Predictors of Life Satisfaction of College Students," *International Journal for the Advancement of Counseling* 33, no. 2 (2011): 79–87.
9. M. Seligman, *Helplessness: On Depression, Development, and Death* (New York: W. H. Freeman, 1975).
10. K. Huffman and C. A. Sanderson, *Real World Psychology* (Hoboken, NJ: Wiley, 2014).
11. Ibid.
12. P. L. Hill et al., "Examining Concurrent and Longitudinal Relations Between Personality Traits and Social Well-Being in Adulthood," *Social Psychological and Personality Science* 3 (2012): 698–705.
13. Ibid.
14. S. Rimer, Harvard School of Public Health, "The Biology of Emotion—And What It May Teach Us about Helping People to Live Longer," 2012, www.hsph.harvard.edu/news/hphr/chronic-disease-prevention/happiness-stress-heart-disease.
15. Ibid; Steptoe, C. de Oliveira, P. Demakakos, and P. Zaninotto, "Enjoyment of Life and Declining Physical Function at Older Ages: A Longitudinal Cohort Study," *Canadian Medical Association Journal* 186, no. 4 (2014): e150–e156.
16. Ibid.; E. A. Wheeler, "Amusing Ourselves to Health: A Selected Review of Lab Findings" in *Positive Psychology: Advances in Understanding Adult Motivation*, ed. J. D. Sinnott (New York: Springer, 2013).
17. B. Fredrickson, et al., "A Functional Genomic Perspective on Human Well-Being," *Proceedings of the National Academy of Sciences* 110, no. 33 (2013): 13684-13689.
18. R. I. Dunbar et al., "Social Laughter Is Correlated with an Elevated Pain Threshold," *Proceedings of the Royal Society*, September 14, 2011, DOI: 10.1098/rspb.2011.1373.
19. J. DeNeve, "Functional Polymorphism (*5-HTTLPR*) in the Serotonin Transporter Gene Is Associated with Subjective Well Being: Evidence from a U.S. Nationally Representative Sample," *Journal of Human Genetics* 56 (2011): 456–59, DOI: 10.1038/jhg.2011.39.
20. M. Seligman, *Flourish: A Visionary New Understanding of Happiness and Well-Being* (New York: Free Press, 2011).
21. Mayo Clinic Staff, MayoClinic.com, "Mental Illness: Causes," September 2012, www.mayoclinic.org/diseases-conditions/mental-illness/basics/causes/con-20033813.
22. Ibid.
23. Substance Abuse and Mental Health Services Administration, "Results from the 2012 National Survey on Drug Use and Health: Mental Health Findings," NSDUH Series H-47, HHS Publication no. (SMA) 13-4805 (Rockville, MD: Substance Abuse and Mental Health Services Administration, 2013); R. C. Kessler et al., "Twelve-Month and Lifetime Prevalence and Lifetime Morbid Risk of Anxiety and Mood Disorders in the United States," *International Journal of Methods in Psychiatric Research* 21, no. 3 (2012): 169–84, DOI: 10.1002/mpr.1359.
24. H. A. Whiteford et al., "Global Burden of Disease Attributable to Mental and Substance Use Disorders: Findings from the Global Burden of Disease Study 2010," *The Lancet* 382, no. 9904 (2013): 1575–86; T. L. Mark et al., "Changes in U.S. Spending on Mental Health and Substance Abuse Treatment, 1986–2005, and Implications for Policy," *Health Affairs* 30, no. 2 (2011): 284–92.
25. R. P. Gallagher, *National Survey of College Counseling 2012* (Pittsburg, PA: The American College Counseling Association, 2012), Available at http://www.iacsinc.org/NSCCD%202012.pdf; D. Gruttadaro and D. Crudo, College Students Speak: A Survey Report on Mental Health, (Arlington, VA: National Alliance on Mental Health, 2012), Available at http://www.nami.org/Content/NavigationMenu/Find_Support/NAMI_on_Campus1/NAMI_Survey_on_College_Students/collegereport.pdf.
26. American College Health Association, *National College Health Assessment II: Reference Group Data Report, Spring 2013, 2013.*
27. Ibid.
28. R. C. Kessler et al., "Twelve-Month and Lifetime Prevalence and Lifetime Morbid Risk of Anxiety and Mood Disorders in the United States," 2012.
29. Ibid.
30. National Institute of Mental Health, "Depression," Revised 2011, http://www.nimh.nih.gov/health/publications/depression/index.shtml.
31. Ibid.
32. American College Health Association, *American College Health Association–National College Health Assessment II (ACHA–NCHA II): Reference Group Data Report Spring 2013* (Baltimore: American College Health Association, 2013), Available at www.acha-ncha.org/reports_ACHA-NCHAII.html.33.
33. C. Blanco et al., "The Epidemiology of Chronic Major Depressive Disorder and Dysthymic Disorder: Results from the National Epidemiologic Survey on Alcohol and Related Conditions," *Journal of Clinical Psychiatry* 71, no. 12 (2010): 1645–56, DOI: 10.4088/JCP.09m05663gry.
34. R. C. Kessler et al., "Twelve-Month and Lifetime Prevalence and Lifetime Morbid Risk of Anxiety and Mood Disorders in the United States," 2012.
35. WebMD, "Seasonal Depression (Seasonal Affective Disorder)," 2012, www.webmd.com/depression/guide/seasonal-affective-disorder.
36. Mayo Clinic Staff, MayoClinic.com, "Depression: Causes," 2013, www.mayoclinic.org/diseases-conditions/depression/basics/causes/con-20032977.
37. R. C. Kessler et al., "Twelve-Month and Lifetime Prevalence and Lifetime Morbid Risk of Anxiety and Mood Disorders in the United States," 2012.
38. Ibid.
39. American College Health Association, *ACHA–NCHA II: Reference Group Data Report Spring 2013,* 2013.
40. National Institute of Mental Health, "Generalized Anxiety Disorder, GAD," Accessed February 2014, www.nimh.nih.gov/health/publications/anxiety-disorders/generalized-anxiety-disorder-gad.shtml.
41. R. C. Kessler et al., "Twelve-Month and Lifetime Prevalence and Lifetime Morbid Risk of Anxiety and Mood Disorders in the United States," 2012.
42. Mayo Clinic Staff, MayoClinic.com, "Panic Attacks and Panic Disorder: Symptoms," May 2012, www.mayoclinic.org/diseases-conditions/panic-attacks/basics/symptoms/con-20020825.
43. R. C. Kessler et al., "Twelve-Month and Lifetime Prevalence and Lifetime Morbid Risk of Anxiety and Mood Disorders in the United States," 2012.
44. Ibid.
45. Ibid.
46. Mayo Clinic Staff, Mayo Clinic.com, "Generalized Anxiety Disorder: Causes," September 2011, www.mayoclinic.org/diseases-conditions/generalized-anxiety-disorder/basics/causes/con-20024562.
47. R. C. Kessler et al., "Twelve-Month and Lifetime Prevalence and Lifetime Morbid Risk of Anxiety and Mood Disorders in the United States," 2012.
48. National Institute of Mental Health, "Obsessive Compulsive Disorder," http://www.nimh.nih.gov/health/topics/obsessive-compulsive-disorder-ocd/index.shtml.
49. Ibid.; R. H. Pietrzak et al., "Prevalence and Axis I Comorbidity of Full and Partial PTSD in the U.S.: Results from Wave 2 of the National Epidemiologic Survey on Alcohol and Related Conditions," *Journal of Anxiety Disorders* 25, no. 3 (2011): 456–65.
50. R. H. Pietrzak et al., "Prevalence and Axis I Comorbidity of Full and Partial PTSD

in the U.S.," 2011; J. Gradus, United States Department of Veterans Affairs, National Center for PTSD, "Epidemiology of PTSD," January 2014, www.ptsd.va.gov/professional/PTSD-overview/epidemiological-facts-ptsd.asp; S. Staggs, PsychCentral. "Myths and Facts about PTSD," February 2014, http://psychcentral.com/lib/myths-and-facts-about-ptsd.

51. American Psychiatric Association, *Diagnostic and Statistical Manual of Mental Disorders (DSM-5)*, 5th ed. (Washington, DC: American Psychiatric Association, 2013).
52. R. A. Sansone and L. A. Sansone, "Personality Disorders: A Nation-Based Perspective on Prevalence," *Innovations in Clinical Neuroscience* 8, no. 4 (2011): 13–18.
53. A.D.A.M. Medical Encyclopedia, "Antisocial Personality Disorder," PubMed Health (Bethesda, MD: U.S. National Library of Medicine, 2012).
54. Mayo Clinic Staff, MayoClinic.com, "Borderline Personality Disorder," August 2012, www.mayoclinic.com/health/borderline-personality-disorder/DS00442.
55. M. C. Zanarini et al., "Reasons for Self-Mutilation Reported by Borderline Patients over 16 Years of Prospective Follow-Up," *Journal of Personality Disorders* 27, no. 6 (2013): 783–94, DOI: 10.1521/pedi_2013_27_115.
56. National Institute of Mental Health, "Schizophrenia," reviewed February 2013, www.nimh.nih.gov/health/topics/schizophrenia/index.shtml.
57. Ibid.
58. Ibid.
59. M. Heron, "Deaths: Leading Causes for 2010," National Vital Statistics Reports 62, no. 6 (2013), Available at http://www.cdc.gov/nchs/data/nvsr/nvsr62/nvsr62_06.pdf.
60. Ibid.; Centers for Disease Control and Prevention, "National Suicide Statistics at a Glance," January 2014, www.cdc.gov/violenceprevention/suicide/statistics/index.html.
61. D. L. Hoyert and J. Xu, "Deaths: Preliminary Data for 2011, Table 7," 2012.
62. Centers for Disease Control and Prevention, "National Suicide Statistics at a Glance," January 2014, www.cdc.gov/violenceprevention/suicide/statistics/mechanism02.html.
63. American Foundation for Suicide Prevention, "Warning Signs of Suicide," Accessed February 2014, www.afsp.org/preventing-suicide/risk-factors-and-warning-signs.
64. Ibid; Befrienders Worldwide, "The Warning Signs of Suicide," http://www.befrienders.org/warning-signs.
65. Ibid; Befrienders Worldwide, "Helping a Suidical Friend or Relative," http://www.befrienders.org/helping-a-friend and Befrienders Worldwide, "Suicidal Feelings," http://www.befrienders.org/suicidal-feelings.
66. Substance Abuse and Mental Health Services Administration, "Results from the 2012 National Survey on Drug Use and Health: Mental Health Findings," 2013.
67. A. Lasalvia et al., "Global Pattern of Experienced and Anticipated Discrimination Reported by People with Major Depressive Disorder: A Cross-Sectional Survey," *The Lancet* 381, no. 9860 (2013): 55–62. DOI:10.1016/S0140-6736(12)61379-8.
68. K. Huffman and C. A. Sanderson, *Real World Psychology* (Hoboken, NJ: Wiley, 2014).
69. Ibid.
70. Mayo Clinic, Cognitive Behavioral Therapy, February 2013, www.mayoclinic.com/health/cognitive-behavioral-therapy/MY00194.
71. U.S. Food and Drug Administration, "Antidepressant Use in Children, Adolescents, and Adults," August 2010, www.fda.gov/Drugs/DrugSafety/InformationbyDrugClass/UCM096273.
72. B. K. Hölzel et al., "Mindfulness Practice Leads to Increases in Regional Brain Gray Matter Density," *Psychiatry Research: Neuroimaging* 191, no. 1 (2011): 36–43; Mayo Clinic, "St. John's Wort (*Hypericum perforatum*)," November 2013, www.mayoclinic.org/drugs-supplements/st-johns-wort/background/HRB-20060053.

Pulled statistics:

p. 39, Bureau of Labor Statistics, "Economic News Release: Volunteering in the United States, 2012." U.S. Department of Labor, 2013.

p. 44, Substance Abuse and Mental Health Services Administration, Results from the 2012 National Survey on Drug Use and Health: Mental Health Findings, NSDUH Series H-47, HHS Publication no. (SMA) 13-4805 (Rockville, MD: Substance Abuse and Mental Health Services Administration, 2013).

p. 54, National Alliance on Mental Illness, "College Students Speak: A Survey Report on Mental Health", 2012, Available at: http://www.nami.org/Content/NavigationMenu/Find_Support/NAMI_on_Campus1/collegereport.pdf.

Chapter 2A

1. J. H Pryor et al., *The American Freshman: National Norms Fall 2012* (Los Angeles: Higher Education Research Institute, UCLA, 2013), Available at http://heri.ucla.edu/monographs/TheAmericanFreshman2013-Expanded.pdf.
2. Ibid.
3. Ibid.
4. H. G. Koenig, "Religion, Spirituality and Health: The Research and Clinical Implications," *ISRN Psychiatry* (2012), DOI: 10.5402/2012/27830.
5. Ibid.
6. Pew Research Center, "The Global Religious Landscape: A Report on the Size and Distribution of the World's Major Religious Groups as of 2010," December 2012, www.pewforum.org/files/2014/01/global-religion-full.pdf.
7. Ibid.
8. B. L. Seaward, *Managing Stress: Principles and Strategies for Health and Well Being*, 7th ed. (Sudbury, MA: Jones and Bartlett, 2012).
9. DanahZohar.com, "Learn the Qs," accessed January 2014, http://dzohar.com/?page_id=622.
10. C. Wigglesworth, "Spiritual Intelligence and Why It Matters," Deep Change, 2011, www.deepchange.com/SpiritualIntelligenceEmotionalIntelligence2011.pdf.
11. Cochraine Summaries: Complementary Medicine, March 2014, http://summaries.cochrane.org/search/site?f[0]=im_field_terms_archie_topics%3A948&f[1]=im_field_stage%3A3; NIH, NCCAM—Research Results, accessed March 2014, http://nccam.nih.gov/research/results.
12. Ibid.
13. Ibid.
14. B. C. Bock et al., "Yoga as a Complementary Treatment for Smoking Cessation in Women," *Journal of Women's Health* 21, no. 2 (2012): 240–48; L. Carim-Todd, S. H. Mitchell, B. S. Oken, "Mind-Body Practices: an Alternative, Drug-Free Treatment for Smoking Cessation? A Systematic Review of the Literature," *Drug and Alcohol Dependence* 132, no. 3 (2013): 399–410; V. Conn, "The Power of Being Present: The Value of Mindfulness Interventions in Improving Health and Well-Being," *Western Journal of Nursing Research* 33 (2011): 993–95; Y. Matchim, J. Armer, and B. Stewart, "Effects of Mindfulness-Based Stress Reduction on Health among Breast Cancer Survivors," *Western Journal of Nursing Research* 33, no. 8 (2011): 996–1016.
15. L. Carim-Todd, S. H. Mitchell, B. S. Oken, "Mind-Body Practices: an Alternative, Drug-Free Treatment for Smoking Cessation? A Systematic Review of the Literature," *Drug and Alcohol Dependence* 132, no. 3 (2013): 399–410.
16. Jean L. Kristeller and Ruth Q. Wolever, "Mindfulness-Based Eating Awareness Training for Treating Binge Eating Disorder: The Conceptual Foundation," *Eating Disorders* 19: 1, 49–61.
17. National Cancer Institute (NCI), "Spirituality in Cancer Care," September 20, 2012, www.cancer.gov/cancertopics/pdq/supportivecare/spirituality/HealthProfessional.
18. C. Lysne and A. Wachholtz, "Pain, Spirituality and Meaning Making: What Can We Learn from the Literature?" *Religions*, no. 2 (2011): 1–16, DOI:10.3390/rel2010001; H. Koenig and A. Bussing, "Spiritual Needs of Patients with Chronic Diseases." *Religions* 1, no. 1 (2010): 18–27.
19. ClinicalTrials.gov, "Mind–Body Interventions in Cardiac Patients," January 2011, http://clinicaltrials.gov/ct2/show/NCT01270568.
20. G. Lucchetti, A. Lucchetti, and H. Koenig, "Impact of Spirituality/Religiosity on Mortality: Comparison with Other Health Interventions," *The Journal of Science and Healing* 7, no. 4 (2011): 234–38.
21. NCI, "Spirituality in Cancer Care," 2012.

22. Ibid.; NCCAM, "Prayer and Spirituality in Health," 2005; NCI, "Spirituality in Cancer Care," 2009.
23. G. G. Ano and E. B. Vasconcelles, "Religious Coping and Psychological Adjustment to Stress: A Meta-Analysis," *Journal of Clinical Psychology* 61, no. 4 (2005): 461–80; U. Winter et al., "The Psychological Outcome of Religious Coping with Stressful Life Events in a Swiss Sample of Church Attendees," *Psychotherapy and Psychosomatics* 78, no. 4 (2009): 240–44; Lucchetti, "Impact of Spirituality/Religiosity," 2011; Matchim, "Breast Cancer Survivors Benefit," 2011.
24. A. Chiesa and A. Serretti, "Mindfulness-Based Stress Reduction for Stress Management in Healthy People: A Review and Meta-Analysis," *Journal of Alternative and Complementary Medicine* 15, no. (2009): 593–600; Lucchetti, "Impact of Spirituality/Religiosity," 2011; Matchim, "Breast Cancer Survivors Benefit," 2011.
25. D. R. Vago and D. A. Silbersweig, "Self-Awareness, Self-Regulation, and Self-Transcendence (S-ART): A Framework for Understanding the Neurobiological Mechanisms of Mindfulness," *Human Neuroscience* 6, no. 269 (2012), Available at http://www.ncbi.nlm.nih.gov/pmc/articles/PMC3480633.
26. G. Desbordes et al., "Effects of Mindful-Attention and Compassion Meditation Training on Amygdala Response to Emotional Stimuli in an Ordinary, Non-Meditative State," *Frontiers in Human Neuroscience* 6, no. 292 (2012). DOI: 10.3389/fnhum.2012.00292.
27. National Center for Complementary and Alternative Medicine (NCCAM), "Research Spotlight: Meditation May Increase Empathy," Modified January 2012, http://nccam.nih.gov/research/results/spotlight/060608.htm.
28. G. Desbordes et al., "Effects of Mindful-Attention and Compassion Meditation Training" 2012.
29. NCCAM, "Research Spotlight," 2013; A. Chiesa and A. Serretti, "Mindfulness-Based Stress Reduction for Stress Management in Healthy People," 2009; N. Y. Winbush, C. R. Gross, and M. J. Kreitzer, "The Effects of Mindfulness-Based Stress Reduction on Sleep Disturbance: A Systematic Review," *EXPLORE: The Journal of Science and Healing* 3, no. 6 (2007): 585–91; N. E. Morone et al., "'I Felt Like a New Person.' The Effects of Mindfulness Meditation on Older Adults with Chronic Pain: Qualitative Narrative Analysis of Diary Entries," *Journal of Pain*, no. 9 (2008): 841–48. Y. Matchim, "Breast Cancer Survivors Benefit," 2011.
30. Ibid.
31. American Cancer Society, "Spirituality and Prayer," December 2012, www.cancer.org/treatment/treatmentsandsideeffects/complementaryandalternativemedicine/mindbodyandspirit/spirituality-and-prayer; University of Minnesota Center for Spirituality and Healing, "What is Prayer?," August 2013, www.takingcharge.csh.umn.edu/explore-healing-practices/prayer.
32. R. Jahnke, et al. "A Comprehensive Review of Health Benefits of Qigong and Tai Chi," *American Journal of Health Promotion* 24, no. 6 (2010): e1–e25. www.ncbi.nlm.nih.gov/pubmed/20594090; American Tai Chi Association, "Psychiatric Expert: Tai Chi and Qigong Can Improve Mood in Older Adults, September 2013, www.americantaichi.net/TaiChiQigongForHealthArticle.asp?cID=2&sID=10&article=chi_201309_1&subject=Mental Health.
33. C. Carter, *Raising Happiness: 10 Simple Steps for More Joyful Kids and Happier Parents* (New York: Ballantine Publishing, 2010); R. I. Dunbar et al., "Social Laughter Is Correlated with an Elevated Pain Threshold," *Proceedings of the Royal Society*, September 14, 2011, DOI: 10.1098/rspb.2011.1373.39%.

Pulled statistics:

p. 62, B. Kosman and A. Keysar, "Religious, Spiritual and Secular: The Emergence of Three Distinct Worldviews among American College Students," September 2013, Available at http://www.trincoll.edu/Academics/centers/isssc/Documents/ARIS_2013_College%20Students_Sept_25_final_draft.pdf.

p. 64, Higher Education Research Institute, "Attending to Student's Inner Lives," April 2011, Available at http://spirituality.ucla.edu/docs/white%20paper/white%20paper%20final.pdf.

p. 69, Yoga Journal, "New Study Finds More Than 20 Million Yogis in U.S.," December 5, 2012, http://blogs.yogajournal.com/yogabuzz/2012/12/new-study-find-more-than-20-million-yogis-in-u-s.html.

Chapter 3

1. American Psychological Association (APA), "Stress in America: Missing the Health Care Connection," February 2013, www.apa.org/news/press/releases/stress/2012/full-report.pdf; S. Bethune, "Health-care Falls Short on Stress Management," *Monitor on Psychology* 44, no. 4 (2013): 22.
2. S. Cohen and D. Janicki-Deverts, "Who's Stressed? Distributions of Psychological Stress in the United States in Probability Samples from 1983, 2006, and 2009," *Journal of Applied Social Psychology* 42, no. 6 (2012): 1320–34, DOI: 10.1111/j.1559-1816.2012.00900.x.
3. B. Vanaelst et al. "The Association between Childhood Stress and Body Composition, and the Role of Stress-Related Lifestyle Factors—Cross-Sectional Findings from the Baseline ChiBS Survey," *International Journal of Behavioral Medicine* (2013), DOI: 10.1007/s12529-013-9294-1; S. M. Wilson and A. F. Sato, "Stress and Paediatric Obesity: What We Know and Where To Go," *Journal of the International Society for the Investigation of Stress*. 2013 DOI: 10.1002/smi.2501.
4. American Psychological Association, "Stress: The Different Kinds of Stress," Accessed February 2014, www.apa.org/helpcenter/stress-kinds.aspx.
5. B. L. Seaward, *Managing Stress: Principles and Strategies for Health and Well-Being*, 8th ed. (Sudbury, MA: Jones and Bartlett, 2013), 8; National Institute of Mental Health (NIMH), "Stress Fact Sheet," Accessed January 2014, www.nimh.nih.gov/health/publications/stress/stress_factsheet_ln.pdf.
6. H. Selye, *Stress without Distress* (New York: Lippincott, Williams & Wilkins, 1974), 28–29.
7. W. B. Cannon, *The Wisdom of the Body* (New York, NY: Norton, 1932).
8. M. P. Picard and D. M. Turnbull, "Linking the Metabolic State and Mitochondrial DNA in Chronic Disease, Health and Aging," *Diabetes* 62, no. 3 (2013), Available at http://diabetes.diabetesjournals.org/content/62/3/672.full; S. Cohen et al., "Chronic Stress, Glucocorticoid Receptor Resistance, Inflammation and Disease Risk," *Proceedings of the National Academy of Sciences of the United States of America* 109, no. 16 (2012): 5995–99, DOI: 10.1073/pnas.1118355109.
9. Shelly Taylor, "The Tending Instinct: Women, Men and the Biology of Our Relationships," Time Books (New York, NY: Henry Holt and Company, 2002).
10. J. Lee, V. R. Harley, "The Male Fight-Flight Response: A Result of SRY Regulation of Catecholamines?," *BioEssays* 34, no. 6 (2012): 454–57, DOI: 10.1002/bies.201100159.
11. A. Crum, P. Salovey, and S. Achor, "Rethinking Stress: The Role of Mindsets in Determining the Stress Response," *Journal of Personality and Social Psychology* 104, no. 4 (2013): 716–33.
12. P. Thoits, "Stress and Health: Major Findings and Policy Implications," *Journal of Health and Social Behavior*, no. 51 (2010): 554–55, DOI: 10.1177/0022146510383499; K. M. Scott et al., "Associations between Lifetime Traumatic Events and Subsequent Chronic Physical Conditions: A Cross-National, Cross-Sectional Study," *PLoS One* 8, no. 11 (2013), DOI: 10.1371/journal.pone.0080573.
13. K. M. Scott et al., "Associations between Lifetime Traumatic Events and Subsequent Chronic Physical Conditions: A Cross-National, Cross-Sectional Study," *PLoS One* 8, no. 11 (2013), DOI: 10.1371/journal.pone.0080573.
14. A. Steptoe and M. Kivimaki. "Stress and Cardiovascular Disease: An Update on Current Knowledge," *Annual Review of Public Health* 34 (2013): 337–54; E. Backe et al., "The Role of Psychosocial Stress at Work for the Development of Cardiovascular Disease: A Systematic Review," *International Archives of Occupational and Environmental Health* 85, no. 1 (2011): 67–79; A. Steptoe, A. Rosengren, and P. Hjemdahl,

"Introduction to Cardiovascular Disease, Stress, and Adaptation" in *Stress and Cardiovascular Disease,* eds. A. Steptoe, A. Rosengren, and P. Hjemdahl (New York, NY: Springer, 2012), 1–14.

15. A. Steptoe and Mike Kivimaki, "Stress and Cardiovascular Disease: An Update on Current Knowledge," *Annual Review of Public Health* 34 (2013): 337–54; S. Richardson et al., "Meta-Analysis of Perceived Stress and Its Association with Incident Coronary Heart Disease," *American Journal of Cardiology* 110, no. 12 (2012): 1711–17.
16. T. Lang et al, "Social Determinants of Cardiovascular Diseases," *Public Health Reviews* 33, no. 2 (2012): 601–22; M. Kivimaki et al., "Job Strain as a Risk Factor for Coronary Heart Disease: A Collaborative Meta-Analysis of Individual Participants," *The Lancet* 380, no. 9852 (2012): 1491–97; E. Mostofsky et al., "Risk of Acute Myocardial Infarction after the Death of a Significant Person on One's Life. The Determinants of Myocardial Infarction Onset Study," *Circulation* 125, no. 3 (2012): 491–96, DOI: 10.1161/CIRCULATIONAHA.111.061770.
17. K. Scott, S. Melhorn, and R. Sakai. "Effects of Chronic Social Stress on Obesity," *Current Obesity Reports Online First,* Accessed January 12, 2012, DOI: 10.1007/s13679-011-0006-3; F. Ippoliti, N. Canitano, and R. Businare, "Stress and Obesity as Risk Factors in Cardiovascular Diseases: A Neuroimmune Perspective, Journal of Neuroimmune Pharmacology 8, no. 1 (2013): 212–26; S. Pagota et al., "Association of Post-Traumatic Stress Disorder and Obesity in a Nationally Representative Sample," *Obesity* 20, no. 1 (2012): 200–205.
18. N. Ribertim et al., "Corticotropin Releasing Factor-Induced Amygdala Gamma Aminobutyric Acid Release Plays a Key Role in Alcohol Dependence," *Biological Psychiatry* 67, no. 9 (2010): 831–39, E. P Zorrilla et al., "Behavioral, Biological, and Chemical Perspectives on Targeting CRF(1) Receptor Antagonists to Treat Alcoholism," *Find all citations by this author (default). Or filter your current search Find all citations by this author (default). Or filter your current search Find all citations in this journal (default). Or filter your current search* Drug and *Alcohol Dependence* 128, no. 3 (2013): 175–86.
19. Mayo Clinic, "Stress and Hair Loss: Are They Related?," January 2014, www.mayoclinic.com/health/stress-and-hair-loss/AN01442.
20. American Diabetes Association, "How Stress Affects Diabetes," 2013, www.diabetes.org/living-with-diabetes/complications/mental-health/stress.html; A. Pandy et al, "Alternative Therapies Useful in the Management of Diabetes: A Systematic Review," *Journal of Bioallied Science* 3, no. 4 (2011): 504–12.
21. National Digestive Diseases Information Clearinghouse (NDDIC), "Irritable Bowel Syndrome: How Does Stress Affect IBS?," October 2013, http://digestive.niddk.nih.gov/ddiseases/pubs/ibs/#stress.
22. H. F. Herlong, "Digestive Disorders 2013," *The Johns Hopkins White Papers* (2013) www.johnshopkinshealthalerts.com.
23. G. Marshall, ed., "Stress and Immune-Based Diseases," *Immunology and Allergy Clinics of North America* 31, no. 1 (2011): 1–148; L. Christian, "Psychoneuroimmunology in Pregnancy: Immune Pathways Linking Stress with Maternal Health, Adverse Birth Outcomes and Fetal Development," *Neuroscience and Biobehavioral Reviews* 36, no. 1 (2012): 350–61, DOI: 10.1016/j.neubiorev.2011.07.005; A. Pedersen, R. Zachariae, and D. Bovbjerb, "Influence of Psychological Stress on Upper Respiratory Infection: A Meta-Analysis of Prospective Studies," *Psychosomatic Medicine* 7 (2010): 823–32.
24. American College Health Association (ACHA), *American College Health Association–National College Health Assessment II (ACHA-NCHA II): Reference Group Data Report Spring, 2013* (Baltimore, MD: American College Health Association, 2014).
25. M. Marin et al., "Chronic Stress, Cognitive Functioning and Mental Health," *Neurobiology of Learning and Memory* 96, no. 4 (2011): 583–95; R. M. Shansky and J. Lipps, "Stress-Induced Cognitive Dysfunction: Hormone-Neurotransmitter Interactions in the Prefrontal Cortex," *Neuroscience and Biobehavioral Reviews* 7 (2013): 123, Available at www.ncbi.nlm.nih.gov/pmc/articles/PMC3617365.
26. E. Dias-Ferreira et al., "Chronic Stress Causes Frontostriatal Reorganization and Affects Decision-Making," *Science* 325, no. 5940 (2009): 621–25; D. de Quervan et al., "Glucocorticoids and the Regulation of Memory in Health and Disease," *Frontiers in Neuroendocrinology* 30, no. 3 (2009): 358–70.
27. L. Johansson. "Can Stress Increase Alzheimer's Disease Risk in Women?," *Expert Review of Neurotherapeutics* 14, no. 2 (2014): 123–125, DOI: 10.1586/14737175.2014.878651.
28. T. Frodi and V. O'Keane, " How Does the Brain Deal with Cumulative Stress? A Review with Focus on Developmental Stress, HPA Axis Function and Hippocampal Structure in Humans," *Neurobiology of Disease* 52 (2013): 24–37; P .S. Nurius, E. Uehara, and D. F. Zatzick, "Intersection of Stress, Social Disadvantage, and Life Course Processes: Reframing Trauma and Mental Health," *American Journal of Psychiatric Rehabilitation* 16 (2013): 91–114; K. Scott et al., "Association of Childhood Adversities and Early-Onset Mental Disorders with Adult-Onset Chronic Physical Conditions," *Archives of General Psychiatry* 68, no. 8 (2011): 833–44.
29. J. Hunt and D. Eisenbe, "Mental Health Problems and Help Seeking Behaviors among College Students-Review Article," *Journal of Adolescent Health* 46, no. 1 (2010): 3–10; C. Segrin and S. Passalacqua, "Functions of Loneliness, Social Support, Health Behaviors, and Stress in Association with Poor Health," *Health Communication* 25, no. 4 (2010): 312; R. C. Chao, "Managing Perceived Stress among College Students: The Role of Social Support and Dysfunctional Coping," *Journal of College Counseling* 15, no. 1 (2012): 5–21.
30. APA, "Stress in America," 2013.
31. R. Lazarus, "The Trivialization of Distress," in *Preventing Health Risk Behaviors and Promoting Coping with Illness,* eds. J. Rosen and L. Solomon (Hanover, NH: University Press of New England, 1985), 279–98.
32. D. Hellhammer, A. Stone, J. Hellhammer, and J. Broderick, "Measuring Stress," *Encyclopedia of Behavioral Neurosciences* 2 (2010): 186–91.
33. A. Nixon et al., "Can Work Make You Sick? A Meta-Analysis of the Relationships between Job Stressors and Physical Symptoms," *Work and Stress,* no. 1 (2011): 1–22.
34. S. Schwartz et al., "Acculturation and Well-Being among College Students from Immigrant Families," *Journal of Clinical Psychology* (2012): 1–21, DOI: 10.1002/jclp21847; A. Pieterse, R. Carter, S. Evans, and R. Walter, "An Exploratory Examination of the Associations among Racial and Ethnic Discrimination, Racial Climate, and Trauma-Related Symptoms in a College Student Population," *Journal of Counseling Psychology* 57, no. 3 (2010): 255–63; A. McAleavey, L. Castonguay, and B. Locke, "Sexual Orientation Minorities in College Counseling: Prevalence, Distress, and Symptom Profiles," *Journal of College Counseling* 14, no. 2 (2011): 127–42.
35. K. Cokley et al., "An Examination of the Impact of Minority Status Stress and Imposter Feelings on the Mental Health of Diverse Ethnic Minority College Students," *Journal of Multicultural Counseling and Development* 41, no. 2 (2013): 82–95; D. Iwamoto, L, Kenji, and W. Ming, "The Impact of Racial Identity, Ethnic Identity, Asian Values and Race-Related Stress on Asian Americans and Asian International College Students' Psychological Well-Being," *Journal of Counseling Psychology* 57, no. 1 (2010): 79–91.
36. E. Brondolo et al., "Racism and Hypertension: A Review of the Empirical Evidence and Implications for Clinical Practice," *American Journal of Hypertension* 24, no. 5 (2011): 518–24; F. Fuchs, "Editorial: Why Do Black Americans Have Higher Prevalence of Hypertension?," *Hypertension* 57 (2011): 370–80.
37. K. Karren, L. Smith, B. Hafen, and K. Frandren, *Mind/Body Health: The Effects of Attitudes, Emotions, and Relationships,* 4th ed. (San Francisco, CA: Benjamin Cummings, 2010).
38. B. L. Seaward, *Managing Stress: Principles and Strategies for Health and Well-Being,*

8th ed. (New York: Barnes and Noble, 2013).

39. Brown, K., *Predictors of Suicide Ideation and the Moderating Effects of Suicide Attitudes,* masters thesis, University of Ohio, 2011, http://etd.ohiolink.edu/view.cgi?acc_num=tolego1301765761; J. Gomez, R. Miranda, and L. Polanco, "Acculturative Stress, Perceived Discrimination and Vulnerability to Suicide Attempts among Emerging Adults," *Journal of Youth and Adolescence* 40, no. 11 (2011): 1465–76.

40. K. Glanz, B. Rimer, and F. Levis, eds., *Health Behavior and Health Education: Theory, Research, and Practice,* 4th ed. (San Francisco, CA: Jossey-Bass, 2008).

41. S. Abraham, "Relationship between Stress and Perceived Self-Efficacy among Nurses in India," *International Conference on Technology and Business Management,* March 2012, www.icmis.net/ictbm/ictbm12/ICTBM12CD/pdf/D2144-done.pdf; B. L. Seaward, *Managing Stress,* 2013.

42. M. Friedman and R. H. Rosenman, *Type A Behavior and Your Heart* (New York, NY: Knopf, 1974).

43. M. Whooley and J. Wong, "Hostility and Cardiovascular Disease," *Journal of the American College of Cardiology* 58, no. 12 (2011): 1228–30; J. Newman et al. "Observed Hostility and the Risk of Incident Ischemic Heart Disease: A Perspective Population Study from the 1995 Canadian Nova Scotia Health Survey," *Journal of the American College of Cardiology* 58, no. 12 (2011): 1222–28; T. Smith., B. Uchino, B. Berg, and P. Florscheim, "Marital Discord and Coronary Artery Disease: A Comparison of Behaviorally Defined Discrete Groups," *Journal of Consulting and Clinical Psychology* 80, no. 1 (2012): 87–92.

44. G. Mate, *When the Body Says No: Understanding the Stress-Disease Connection,* (Hoboken, NJ: John Wiley and Sons, 2011).

45. H. Versteeg, V. Spek, and S. Pedersen, "Type D Personality and Health Status in Cardiovascular Disease Populations: A Meta-Analysis of Prospective Studies," *European Journal of Cardiovascular Prevention and Rehabilitation* (2011), DOI: 10.1177/1741826711425338; F. Mols and F. J. Denollet, "Type D Personality in the General Population: A Systematic Review of Health Status, Mechanisms of Disease and Work-Related Problems," *Health and Quality of Life Outcomes* 8, no. 9 (2010): 1–10, Available at www.hqlo.com/content/8/1/9.

46. S. Kobasa, "Stressful Life Events, Personality, and Health: An Inquiry into Hardiness," *Journal of Personality and Social Psychology* 37 (1979): 1–11.

47. C. D. Schetter and C. Dolbier, "Resilience in the Context of Chronic Stress and Health in Adults," *Social and Personality Psychology Compass* 5 (2011): 634–52, DOI: 10.1111/j.1751-9004.2011.00379.x.

48. C. Ryff et al., "Psychological Resilience in Adulthood and Later Life: Implications for Health," *Annual Review of Gerontology and Geriatrics* 32, no. 1 (2012): 73–92.

49. The American Psychological Association, "The Road to Resilience: What Is Resilience?," Accessed February 2014, www.apa.org/helpcenter/road-resilience.aspx.

50. E. Chen et al., "Protective Factors for Adults from Low-Childhood Socioeconomic Circumstances: The Benefits of Shift-and-Persist for Allostatic Load," *Psychosomatic Medicine* 74, no. 2 (2012): 178–186, DOI:10.1097/PSY.0B013e31824206fd.

51. J. H. Pryor et al., *The American Freshman: National Norms Fall 2012* (Los Angeles, CA: Higher Education Research Institute, 2013), Available at www.heri.ucla.edu/tfsPublications.php; J. Pryor, "The Changing First-Year Student: Challenges for 2011. Higher Education Research Institute of UCLA-Freshman Survey 2010," presented at AAC&U 2011 Annual Meeting (San Francisco, CA).

52. J. Pryor, "The Changing First-Year Student," 2011.

53. J. Boardman and K. Alexander, "Stress Trajectories, Health Behaviors and the Mental Health of Black and White Young Adults," *Social Science and Medicine* 72, no. 10 (2011): 1659–66; M. Cerda and V. Johnson-Lawrence, "Lifetime Income Patterns and Alcohol Consumption: Investigating the Association between Long and Short Term Income Trajectories and Drinking," *Social Science and Medicine* 73, no. 8 (2011): 1178–85; E. Avant, J. Davis, and C. Cranston, "Posttraumatic Stress Symptom Clusters, Trauma History, and Substance Use among College Students," *Journal of Aggression, Maltreatment and Trauma* 20, no. 5 (2011): 539–55; M. Terlecki, J. Buckner, M. Larimer, and A. Copeland, "The Role of Social Anxiety in a Brief Alcohol Intervention for Heavy-Drinking College Students," *Journal of Cognitive Psychotherapy* 25, no. 1 (2011): 7–21.

54. B. L. Seaward, *Managing Stress,* 2013.

55. J. Moskowitz et al., "A Positive Affect Intervention for People Experiencing Health-related Stress: Development and Non-randomized Pilot Test," *Journal of Health Psychology* 17, no. 5 (2012): 676–92, DOI: 10.1177/1359105311425275; P. Thoits, "Mechanisms Linking Social Ties and Support to Physical and Mental Health," *Journal of Health and Social Behavior* 52, no. 2 (2011): 145–61; B. Lake and E. Oreheck, "Relational Regulation Theory: A New Approach to Explain the Link between Perceived Social Support and Mental Health," *Psychological Review* 118, no. 3 (2011): 482–95.

56. B. L. Seaward, *Managing Stress,* 2012.

57. G. Colom, C. Alcover, C. Sanchez-Curto, and J. Zarate-Osuna, "Study of the Effect of Positive Humour as a Variable That Reduces Stress. Relationship of Humour with Personality and Performance Variables," *Psychology in Spain* 15, no. 1 (2011): 9–21.

58. L. Poole et al., "Associations of Objectively Measured Physical Activity with Daily Mood Ratings and Psychophysiological Stress Responses in Women," *Psychophysiology* 48 (2011): 1165–72, DOI: 10.1111/j.1469-8986.2011.01184.x; D. A. Girdano, D. E. Dusek, and G. S. Everly, *Controlling Stress and Tension,* 9th ed. (San Francisco, CA: Benjamin Cummings, 2012), 375.

59. M. A. Stults-Kolehmainen and R. Sinha, "The Effect of Stress on Physical Activity and Exercise," *Sports Medicine* 44, no. 1 (2014): 81–121; EM Jackson, "Stress Relief: The Role of Exercise in Stress Management," *ACSM Health and Fitness Journal* 17, no. 3 (2013), DOI, 10.1249/FIT.0b013e31828cb1c9.

60. P. M. Gollwitzer and G. Oettingen (2013). "Implementation Intentions." In M. Gellman and J. R. Turner (eds.), *Encyclopedia of Behavioral Medicine* (Part 9, pp. 1043–1048). New York: Springer-Verlag; C. Stern et al. "Effects of Implementation Intention on Anxiety, Perceived Proximity and Motor Performance," *Personality and Social Psychology Bulletin* 39, no. 5 (2013): 623–35; A. Dalton and S. Spiller, "Too Much of a Good Thing: The Benefits of Implementation Intentions Depend on the Number of Specific Goals," *Journal of Consumer Research* 39, no. 3 (2012): 600–14.

61. Yoga Journal, "Yoga in America," Accessed February 2014, www.yogajournal.com/press/yoga_in_america?print=1.

62. NIH Medline Plus, "What Yoga Can and Can't Do for You," December 2013, www.nlm.nih.gov/medlineplus/news/fullstory_143813.html; J. Kiecolt-Glaser et al., "Stress, Inflammation, and Yoga Practice," *Psychosomatic Medicine* 72, no. 2 (2010): 113–21.

63. V. Barnes and D. Orme-Johnson, "Prevention and Treatment of Cardiovascular Disease in Adolescents through the Transcendental Meditation Program," *Current Hypertension Reviews* 8, no. 3 (2012): 1573–1621.

64. M. Rapaport, P. Schettler, and C. Bresee, "A Preliminary Study of the Effects of a Single Session of Swedish Massage on Hypothalamic-Pituitary-Adrenal and Immune Function in Normal Individuals," *The Journal of Alternative and Complementary Medicine* 16, no. 10 (2010): 1–10.

65. NIH Medline Plus, "Avid Cellphone Use by College Kids Tied to Anxiety, Lower Grades," December 2013, www.nlm.nih.gov/;medlineplus/news/fullstory_143389.html.

Pulled statistics:

p. 73, American Psychological Association. "Stress in America—Making the Health Care Connection." 2013.

p. 77, American College Health Association, *American College Health Association National College Health Assessment II: Reference Group Executive Summary Spring,*

2013 (Hanover, MD: American College Health Association, 2014), www.acha.org.

p. 87, American Psychological Association. "Stress in America—Making the Health Care Connection." 2013.

Chapter 3A

1. National Heart, Lung, and Blood Institute, "Sleep Disorders & Insufficient Sleep: Improving Health through Research," Accessed February 2014, www.nhlbi.nih.gov/news/spotlight/fact-sheet/sleep-disorders-insufficient-sleep-improving-health-through-research.html.
2. National Sleep Foundation, "National Consumer Research Institute Predicts Top Five Health Trends for 2012," 2012, www.sleepfoundation.org/alert/national-consumer-research-institute-predicts-top-five-health-trends-2012; The Philips Center for Health and Well-Being, "Philips Index for Health and Well-Being: A Global Perspective Report 2010," October 2011, www.newscenter.philips.com/pwc_nc/main/standard/resources/corporate/press/2010/Global%20Index%20Results/20101111%20Global%20Index%20Report.pdf.
3. American College Health Association, *American College Health Association–National College Health Assessment II (ACHA-NCHA II): Reference Group Data Report Spring 2013* (Hanover, MD: American College Health Association, 2014), Available at www.achancha.org/reports_ACHA-NCHAII.html.
4. K. Ahrberg et al., "Interaction between Sleep Quality and Academic Performance," *Journal of Psychiatric Research* 46, no. 12 (2012): 1618–22; J. Gaultney, "The Prevalence of Sleep Disorders in College Students," 2010; H. Lund, B. Reider, A. Whiting, and J. Prichard, "Sleep Predictors of Disturbed Sleep in a Large Population of College Students," *Journal of Adolescent Health* 46, no. 2 (2010): 124–32; D. Taylor and A. Bramoweth, "Patterns and Consequences of Inadequate Sleep in College Students: Substance Abuse and Motor Vehicle Accidents," *Journal of Adolescent Health* 46, no. 6 (2010): 610–12.
5. J. Gaultney, "The Prevalence of Sleep Disorders in College Students," 2010; K. Ahrberg et al., "Interaction between Sleep Quality and Academic Performance," 2012.
6. National Sleep Foundation, "2011 Sleep in America Poll: Communications Technology and Sleep," March 2011, www.sleepfoundation.org/article/sleep-america-polls/2011-communications-technology-use-and-sleep.
7. American Academy of Sleep Medicine, *The International Classification of Sleep Disorders: Diagnostic—Coding Manual*, 2nd ed. (Westchester, IL: American Academy of Sleep Medicine; 2005).
8. Centers for Disease Control and Prevention, "Insufficient Sleep is a Public Health Epidemic," January 2014, www.cdc.gov/features/dssleep/; National Highway Traffic Safety Administration, "Drowsy Driving and Automobile Crashes," February 2014, www.nhtsa.gov/people/injury/drowsy_driving1/Drowsy.html#NCSDR/NHTSA; J. Gaultney, "The Prevalence of Sleep Disorders," 2010.
9. M. Meeker and L. Wu, "How Much Time Do We Really Spend on Our Smartphones Every Day?," *Business Insider*, June 6, 2013, www.businessinsider.com.au/how-much-time-do-we-spend-on-smartphones-2013-6; Marketing Charts, "College Students Own an Average of 7 Tech Devices," June 2013, www.marketingcharts.com/wp/topics/demographics/college-students-own-an-average-of-7-tech-devices-30430.
10. Ibid.
11. National Sleep Foundation, "Sleep in America Poll: Communications Technology in the Bedroom," 2011, http://www.sleepfoundation.org/sites/default/files/sleepinamericapoll/SIAP_2011_Summary_of_Findings.pdf.
12. National Highway Traffic Safety Administration, "Drowsy Driving and Automobile Crashes," 2014; Centers for Disease Control and Prevention, "Drowsy Driving: Asleep at the Wheel," 2014.
13. National Heart Lung and Blood Institute, "Why Is Sleep Important?," February 2012, www.nhlbi.nih.gov/health/health-topics/topics/sdd/why.html; F. P. Cappuccio et al., "Sleep Duration and All-Cause Mortality: A Systematic Review and Meta-Analysis of Prospective Studies," *Sleep* 33, no. 5 (2010): 585–92.
14. K. M. Orzech et al., "Sleep Patterns Are Associated with Common Illness in Adolescents," *Journal of Sleep Research* (2013), DOI: 10.1111/jsr.12096; J. M. Krueger and J. A. Majde, "Sleep and Host Defense," in *Principles and Practice of Sleep Medicine*, eds. M. H. Kryger, T. Roth, and W. C. Dement (St. Louis, MO: Saunders 2011), 261–90; M. Manzer and M. Hussein, "Sleep-Immune System Interaction: Advantages and Challenges of Human Sleep Loss Model," *Frontiers of Neurology* 3, no. 2 (2012), DOI: 10.3389/fneur.2012.00002.
15. X. Yu et al., "TH17 Cell Differentiation Is Regulated by Circadian Clock," *Science* 342, no. 6159 (2013): 727–30; A. Bollinger, A. Bollinger, H. Oster, and W. Scolbach, "Sleep, Immunity and Circadian Clocks: A Mechanistic Model," *Gerontology* 56, no. 6 (2010): 574–80, DOI: 10.1159/000281827.
16. R. Lanfranchi, F. Prince, D. Filipini, and J. Carrier, "Sleep Deprivation Increases Blood Pressure in Healthy Normotensive Elderly and Attenuates the Blood Pressure Response to Orthostatic Challenges," *Sleep* 34, no. 3 (2010): 335–39; F. Cappucio, D. Cooper, and D. Lanfranco, "Sleep Duration Predicts Cardiovascular Outcomes: A Systematic Review and Meta-Analysis of Prospective Studies," *European Heart Journal*, first published online February 7, 2011. DOI: 10.1093/eurheart.
17. M. A. Miller and F. P. Cappuccio. "Biomarkers of Cardiovascular Risk in Sleep Deprived People." *Journal of Human Hypertension* 27 (2013): 583–8; F. P. Cappuccio et al. "Sleep Duration Predicts Cardiovascular Outcomes," 2011; S. Agarwal, N. Bajaj, and C. Bae, "Association between Sleep Duration and Cardiovascular Disease: Results from the National Health and Nutrition Examination Survey (NHANES 2005–2008)," *Journal of the American College of Cardiology* 59, no. 13, Supplement 1 (2012): e1514; F. Sofi et al. "Insomnia and Risk of Cardiovascular Disease: A Meta-Analysis, *European Journal of Preventive Cardiology* 21, no. 1 (2014): 51–67.
18. M. A. Miller et al., "Sustained Short Sleep and Risk of Obesity. Evidence in Children and Adults," chap. 7 in *Handbook of Obesity*, vol. 1, 3rd ed., eds. G. A. Bray and C. Bouchard (Boca Raton, FL: CRC Press, Taylor & Francis Group, 2014), 397–41; Q. Xiao et al., "A Large Prospective Investigation of Sleep Duration, Weight Change and Obesity in the NIH-AARP Diet and Health Study," *American Journal of Epidemiology* 178, no. 11 (2013): 1600–1610.
19. M. A. Miller et al., "Sustained Short Sleep and Risk of Obesity," 2014; Q. Xiao et al., "A Large Prospective Investigation of Sleep Duration," 2013; L. Nielson, T. Danielson, and A. Serensen, "Short Sleep Duration as a Possible Cause of Obesity: Critical Analysis of the Epidemiological Evidence," *Obesity Reviews* 12, no. 2 (2011): 78–92; National Sleep Foundation, "Obesity and Sleep," Accessed January 2014, www.sleepfoundation.org/article/sleep-topics/obesity-and-sleep.
20. C. L. Jackson et al., "Association between Sleep Duration and Diabetes in Black and White Adults," *Diabetes Care* 36, no. 11 (2013): 3557–65; E. G. Holliday et al., "Short Sleep Duration Is Associated with Risk of Future Diabetes but Not Cardiovascular Disease: A Prospective Study and Meta-Analysis," *PLoS ONE* 8, no. 11 (2013): e82305, DOI:10.1371/journal.pone.0082305; American Diabetes Association, "Too Little Sleep Linked to Higher A1C," January 2014, www.diabetesforecast.org/2014/Jan/too-little-sleep-linked-to.html.
21. T. K. Jensen et al., "Association of Sleep Disturbances with Reduced Semen Quality: A Cross-Sectional Study among 953 Healthy Young Danish Men," *American Journal of Epidemiology* 177, no. 10 (2013): 1027–37.
22. National Institutes of Health, "Information about Sleep," Accessed 2014, http://science.education.nih.gov/supplements/nih3/sleep/guide/info-sleep.htm; C. Peri and M. Smith, "What Lack of Sleep Does to Your Mind," WebMD, Accessed January 20, 2012, www

.webmd.com/sleep-disorders/excessive-sleepiness-10/emotions-cognitive.

23. E. Fortier-Brochu, S. Beauliew-Bonneau, H. Ivers, and C. Morin, "Insomnia and Daytime Cognitive Performance: A Meta-Analysis," *Sleep Medicine Reviews* 16, no. 1, (2011), DOI: 10-1016/j.smrv.2011.03.008; W. Klemm, "How Sleep Helps Memory," *Psychology Today*, March 11, 2011, www.psychologytoday.com/blog/memory-medic/201103/how-sleep-helps-memory; M. A. Miller et al., "Sleep and Cognition," in *Sleep Disorders* (2014), in press.
24. A. Gomes, J. Tavares, and M. Azevedo, "Sleep and Academic Performance in Undergraduates: A Multi-Measure, Multi-Predictor Approach," *Chronobiology* 28, no. 9 (2011): 786–801, DOI:10.3109/07420528.2011.606518. Yu-Chih Chiang, "The effects of sleep on performance of undergraduate students working in the hospitality industry as compared to those who are not working in the industry," http://lib.dr.iastate.edu/cgi/viewcontent.cgi?article=4067&context=etd.
25. Z. Terpening et al., "The Contributors of Nocturnal Sleep to the Consolidation of Motor Skill Learning in Healthy Aging and Parkinson's Disease," *Journal of Sleep Research* 22, no. 4 (2013): 398–405; L. Genzel et al., "Complex Motor Sequence Skills Profit from Sleep," *Neuropsychobiology* 66, no. 4 (2012): 237–43, DOI: 10.1159/000341878
26. Centers for Disease Control and Prevention, "Drowsy Driving," 2014.
27. National Sleep Foundation, "Young People More Likely to Drive Drowsy," November 2012, www.sleepfoundation.org/alert/young-people-more-likely-drive-drowsy.
28. National Sleep Foundation, "Drowsy Driving Prevention Week, Sleep in America Poll–November, 2011, Facts about Drowsy Driving," 2012, http://drowsydriving.org/2010/11/drowsy-driving-prevention-week%C2%AE-highlights-prevalent-and-preventable-accidents/; Centers for Disease Control and Prevention, "Drowsy Driving—19 States and the District of Columba. 2009–2010," *Morbidity and Mortality Weekly Report* 61, no. 51 (2013): 1033–37, Available at www.cdc.gov/mmwr/preview/mmwrhtml/mm6151a1.htm.
29. National Institutes of Health (NIH), "Teacher's Guide–Information about Sleep," Accessed January, 2012, http://science.education.nih.gov/supplements/nih3/sleep/guide/info-sleep.htm.
30. H. Oster, "Does Late Sleep Promote Depression?" *Expert Reviews of Endocrinology and Metabolism* 7, no. 1 (2012): 27–29, www.expert-reviews.com/doi/abs/10.1586/eem.11.80; C. Baglioni et al., "Insomnia as a Predictor of Depression: A Meta-Analytic Evaluation of Longitudinal Epidemiological Studies," *Journal of Affective Disorders* 135, no. 1 (2011): 10–19.
31. National Institute of General Medical Sciences, "Circadian Rhythms Fact Sheet," November 2013, www.nigms.nih.gov/Education/Pages/Factsheet_CircadianRhythms.aspx.
32. E. Carlson et al., "Tick Tock: New Clues About Biological Clocks and Health," *Inside Life Science,* November 1, 2012, http://publications.nigms.nih.gov/insidelifescience/biological-clocks.html; M. Vitaterna, J. Takahashi, and F. Turek, "Overview of Circadian Rhythms," National Institute on Alcohol Abuse and Alcoholism, 2014, http://pubs.niaaa.nih.gov/publications/arh25-2/85-93.htm.
33. NIH, "Teacher's Guide–Information about Sleep," Accessed February 2014, http://science.education.nih.gov/supplements/nih3/sleep/guide/info-sleep.htm
34. B. Rasch and J. Born, "About Sleep's Role in Memory," *Physiological Reviews* 93, no. 2 (2013): 681–766.
35. Centers for Disease Control and Prevention, "Insufficient Sleep is a Public Health Epidemic," January 2014, www.cdc.gov/features/dssleep/; F. Cappuccio et al. "Sleep Duration and All Cause Mortality. Systematic Review," *Sleep* 33, no. 5 (2010): 585–92.
36. NIH, "Teacher's Guide–Information About Sleep," Accessed February 2014.
37. E. Carlson et al., "Tick Tock," 2012; CDC, "Insufficient Sleep Is a Public Health Epidemic," 2014, http://www.cdc.gov/features/dssleep.
38. Q. Xiao et al., "A Large Prospective Investigation of Sleep Duration," 2013; C .L. Jackson et al., "Association between Sleep Duration and Diabetes," 2013; F. Cappuccio et al., "Sleep Duration Predicts Cardiovascular Outcomes: A Systematic Review and Meta-Analysis of Prospective Studies," *European Heart Journal* 32, no. 12 (2011): 1484–92; A. Tamakoshi et al., "Multiple Roles and All-Cause Mortality: The Japan Collaborative Cohort Study," *European Journal of Public Health,* January, 2012, DOI: 10.1093/crpub/ckr194; E. Kronholm et al., "Self-Reported Sleep Duration, All-Cause Mortality, Cardiovascular Mortality and Morbidity in Finland," *Sleep Medicine* 12, no. 3 (2011): 215–21; F. Cappucino et al. "Sleep Duration and All-Cause Mortality," 2010.
39. National Sleep Foundation, "How Much Sleep Do We Really Need?," 2011, www.sleepfoundation.org/article/how-sleep-works/how-much-sleep-do-we-really-need.
40. National Sleep Foundation, "Napping," 2011, www.sleepfoundation.org/article/sleep-topics/napping; National Sleep Foundation, "Drowsy Driving—Is There a Perfect Time to Take a Nap?," Accessed January 19, 2012; B. Faraut et al., "Benefits of Napping and an Extended Duration of Recovery Sleep on Alertness and Immune Cells After Acute Sleep Restriction," *Brain, Behavior and Immunity* 25, no. 1 (2011): 18–24, DOI: 10.1016/j.bbi.2010.08.001.
41. National Sleep Foundation, "Exercise and Sleep," 2013, www.sleepfoundation.org/article/sleep-america-polls/2013/exercise-and-sleep.
42. National Sleep Foundation, "Caffeine and Sleep," Accessed February, 2014, www.sleepfoundation.org/article/sleep-topics/caffeine-and-sleep.
43. American College Health Association, *National College Health Assessment II: Reference Group Data Report Spring 2013*, 2014.
44. National Sleep Foundation, "Caffeine and Sleep," Accessed February 2014; American College Health Association, *National College Health Assessment II: Reference Group Data Report Spring 2013*, 2014.
45. National Sleep Foundation, "What Is Insomnia?," 2013, www.sleepfoundation.org/insomnia/what-is-insomnia/facts/; D. J. Buysse, "Insomnia," *Journal of the American Medical Association* 309, no. 7 (2013): 706–716; J. K. Walsh et al., "Nighttime Insomnia Symptoms and Perceived Health in the America Insomnia Survey (AIS)," *Sleep* 34, no. 8 (2011): 997–1011.
46. Ibid.
47. National Sleep Foundation, "Can't Sleep? What to Know About Insomnia,"Accessed February 2014, www.sleepfoundation.org/article/sleep-related-problems/insomnia-and-sleep.
48. American College Health Association, *National College Health Assessment II: Reference Group Data Report Spring 2013*, 2014.
49. Y. Chong, C. D. Fryar, and Q. Gu, "Prescription Sleep Aid Use among Adults: United States, 2005–2010," *NCHS Data Brief*, no. 127 (2013), Available at http://www.cdc.gov/nchs/data/databriefs/db127.htm.
50. National Sleep Foundation, "Sleep Apnea and Sleep," Accessed January 2014, www.sleepfoundation.org/article/sleep-related-problems/obstructive-sleep-apnea-and-sleep.
51. Sleep Disorders Guide, "Sleep Apnea Statistics," Accessed February 2014, www.sleepdisordersguide.com/sleepapnea/sleep-apnea-statistics.html.
52. National Sleep Foundation, "Sleep Apnea and Sleep," Accessed January 2014.
53. Ibid.
54. Ibid.
55. National Institute of Neurological Disorders and Stroke, "Restless Legs Syndrome Fact Sheet," updated December 13, 2013, www.ninds.nih.gov/disorders/restless_legs/detail_restless_legs.htm.
56. Ibid.
57. National Institute of Neurological Disorders and Stroke, "Narcolepsy Fact Sheet," updated July 18, 3013, www.ninds.nih.gov/disorders/narcolepsy/detail_narcolepsy.htm.
58. National Sleep Foundation, "Narcolepsy and Sleep," 2014, www.sleepfoundation.org/article/sleep-related-problems/narcolepsy-and-sleep.

Pulled statistics:

p. 99, American College Health Association, *American College Health Association—*

National College Health Assessment II: Reference Group Executive Summary, Spring 2013, Baltimore, MD: American College Health Association, 2014.

p. 100, Ibid.

Chapter 4

1. Y. Luo et al., "Loneliness, Health, and Mortality in Old Age: A National Longitudinal Study," *Social Science and Medicine* 74, no. 6 (2012): 907–14; N. I. Eisenberger and S. W. Cole, "Social Neuroscience and Health: Neurophysiological Mechanisms Linking Social Ties with Physical Health," *Nature Neuroscience* 15, no. 5 (2012): 669–74, DOI:10.1038/nn.3086.
2. M. T. Frías, A. Brassard, and P. R. Shaver, "Childhood Sexual Abuse and Attachment Insecurities as Predictors of Women's Own and Perceived-Partner Extradyadic Involvement," *Child Abuse & Neglect* (2014), http://dx.doi.org.proxy.lib.uni.edu/10.1016/j.chiabu.2014.02.009; A. Lowell, K. Renk, and A. H. Adgate, "The Role of Attachment in the Relationship between Child Maltreatment and Later Emotional and Behavioral Functioning," *Child Abuse & Neglect* (2014), http://dx.doi.org.proxy.lib.uni.edu/10.1016/j.chiabu.2014.02.006.
3. R. Sternberg, "A Triangular Theory of Love," *Psychological Review* 93 (1986): 119–35.
4. R. Sternberg, "Cupid's Arrow: The Course of Love through Time," (1998) Cambridge University Press.
5. H. Fisher, *Why We Love* (New York: Henry Holt, 2004); H. Fisher et al., "Defining the Brain System of Lust, Romantic Attraction, and Attachment," *Archives of Sexual Behavior* 31, no. 5 (2002): 413–19.
6. Ibid.
7. Ibid.
8. J. K. Rempel, J. G. Holmes, and M. P. Zanna, "Trust in Close Relationships," *Journal of Personality and Social Psychology*, 49 no. 1, (1985): 95–112.
9. S. Levay and J. Baldwin, *Human Sexuality*, 4th ed. (Sunderland, MA: Sinauer Associates, 2012).
10. C. R. Rogers, "Interpersonal Relationship: The Core of Guidance" in *Person to Person: The Problem of Being Human,* eds. C. R. Rogers and B. Stevens (Lafayette, CA: Real People Press, 1967).
11. L. A. Nadig, "Tips on Effective Listening," July 2010, www.drnadig.com/listening.htm.
12. S. A. Beebe, S. J. Beebe, and M. V. Redmond, *Interpersonal Communication: Relating to Others,* 6th ed. (Boston: Allyn & Bacon, 2011).
13. Ibid.
14. J. Wood, *Interpersonal Communication: Everyday Encounters,* 7th ed. (Belmont, CA: Cengage, 2012).
15. Ibid.
16. L. A. Nadig, "Relationship Conflict: Healthy or Unhealthy," http://www.drnadig.com/conflict.htm.
17. F. Newport and J. Wilke, "Most in U.S. Want Marriage, but Its Importance Has Dropped," Gallup, August 2, 2013, www.gallup.com/poll/163802/marriage-importance-dropped.aspx.
18. J. Wood, *Interpersonal Communication: Everyday Encounters, 7th ed.* (Belmont, CA: Cengage, 2012); F. Newport and J. Wilke, "Most in U.S. Want Marriage, but Its Importance Has Dropped," Gallup, August 2, 2013, www.gallup.com/poll/163802/marriage-importance-dropped.aspx.
19. U.S. Census Bureau, "Families and Living Arrangements: 2013, Table MS-2 Estimated Median Age at First Marriage, by Sex: 1890 to the Present," Accessed April 2014, www.census.gov/hhes/families/data/marital.html.
20. A. J. Cherlin, "Multiple Partners, but One at a Time," *New York Times* (Blog), May 21, 2013.
21. I. Siegler et al., "Consistency and Timing of Marital Transitions and Survival During Midlife: The Role of Personality and Health Risk Behaviors," *Annals of Behavioral Medicine* 45, no. 3 (2013): 338-47, DOI: 10.1007/s12160-012-9457-3; A. A. Aizer et al., "Marital Status and Survival in Patients with Cancer," *Journal of Clinical Oncology* 31, no. 31 (2013): 3869–76. DOI: 10.1200/JCO.2013.49.6489.
22. U.S. Department of Health and Human Services, Vital and Health Statistics, "Health Behaviors of Adults: United States, 2008–2010," *DHHS Pub* 10, No. 257 (2013):7–78, Available at www.cdc.gov/nchs/data/series/sr_10/sr10_257.pdf.
23. Ibid.
24. Ibid.
25. U.S. Department of Health and Human Services, Division of Vital Statistics, "First Premarital Cohabitation in the United States: 2006–2010 National Survey of Family Growth," *National Health Statistics Report* 64 (2013), Available at www.cdc.gov/nchs/data/nhsr/nhsr064.pdf.
26. Ibid.
27. A. Kuperberg, "Age at Co-Residence, Premarital Cohabitation and Marriage Dissolution: 1985–2009," *Journal of Marriage and Family*, 76 no. 2, (2014): 352–369.
28. U.S. Census Bureau, "Frequently Asked Questions about Same-Sex Couple Households," 2013, www.census.gov/hhes/samesex/files/SScplfactsheet_final.pdf.
29. National Gay and Lesbian Task Force, "Relationship Recognition Map for Same-Sex Couples in the U.S.," January 2014, www.thetaskforce.org/downloads/reports/issue_maps/rel_recog_1_6_14_color.pdf.
30. D. Masci et al., "Gay Marriage Around the World," *Pew Research Religion and Public Life Project*, February 5, 2014, www.pewforum.org/2013/12/19/gay-marriage-around-the-world-2013/#allow.
31. U.S. Census Bureau, "Marital Status: 2007–2011 American Community Survey, 5-Year Estimates, Table S1201," Accessed April 2014, http://factfinder2.census.gov/faces/tableservices/jsf/pages/productview.xhtml?src=bkmk.
32. R. M. Kreider and D. A. Loftquist, U.S. Census Bureau, "Adopted Children and Stepchildren: 2010," (April 2014), http://www.census.gov/content/dam/Census/library/publications/2014/demo/p20-572.pdf.
33. U.S. Census Bureau, "Table C2. Household Relationship and Living Arrangements of Children Under 18 Years, by Age and Sex: 2012," *America's Families and Living Arrangements: 2012*, November 2013, www.census.gov/hhes/families/data/cps2012.html.
34. M. Lino, *Expenditures on Children by Families, 2012* (Alexandria, VA: U.S. Department of Agriculture, Center for Nutrition Policy and Promotion, 2013), Available at www.cnpp.usda.gov/Publications/CRC/crc2012.pdf.
35. U.S. Bureau of Labor Statistics, "Women in the Labor Force: A Databook, 2012 Edition," March 2013, www.bls.gov/cps/wlf-databook-2012.pdf .
36. National Association of Child Care Resource and Referral Agencies, "Parents and the High Cost of Child Care, 2013 Report," *Child Care Aware of American,* 2013, http://usa.childcareaware.org/sites/default/files/cost_of_care_2013_103113_0.pdf.
37. L. Finer and M. R. Zoina, "Shifts in Intended and Unintended Pregnancies in the United States, 2001–2008," *American Journal of Public Health* 104, no. S1 (2014): S43–S48.
38. M. Gatzeva and A. Paik, "Emotional and Physical Satisfaction in Noncohabiting, Cohabiting, and Marital Relationships: The Importance of Jealous Conflict," *Journal of Sex Research* 48, no. 1 (2011): 29–42, DOI: 10.1080/00224490903370602; B. Sagarin et al., "Sex Differences in Jealousy: A Meta-Analytic Examination," *Evolution & Human Behavior* 33, no. 6 (2012): 595–614.
39. United States Department of Labor, Bureau of Labor Statistics, "American Time Use Survey Summary–2012 Results," January 2014, www.bls.gov/tus/datafiles_2012.htm.
40. K. Heller, "The Myth of the High Rate of Divorce," *Psych Central*, April 2, 2014, http://psychcentral.com/lib/2012/the-myth-of-the-high-rate-of-divorce.
41. Ibid.
42. R. M. Kreider and R. Ellis, "Number, Timing, and Duration of Marriages and Divorces: 2009," *Current Population Reports,* P70-125 (Washington, DC, U.S. Census Bureau, 2011), Available at www.census.gov/prod/2011pubs/p70-125.pdf.
43. Ibid.
44. The Gottman Institute, "Research FAQs," Accessed April, 2014, www.gottman.com/research/research-faqs.
45. G.F. Kelly, *Sexuality Today*, 10th ed. (New York, NY: McGraw-Hill, 2010).

Pulled statistics:

p. 122, W. Wang and P. Taylor, "For Millennials, Parenthood Trumps Marriage," Pew Research (2011), http://www.pewsocialtrends.org/2011/03/09/for-millennials-parenthood-trumps-marriage.

p. 123, A. Kuperberg, "Age at Co-Residence, Premarital Cohabitation and Marriage Dissolution: 1985–2009," Forthcoming at *Journal of Marriage and Family* (2014).

Chapter 5

1. I. A. Hughes et al., "Consensus Statement on Management of Intersex Disorders," *Archives of Disease in Childhood* 91, no. 7 (2006): 554–63.
2. J. S. Greenberg, C. E. Bruess, and S. B. Oswalt, *Exploring the Dimensions of Human Sexuality,* 5th ed. (Burlington, MA: Jones and Bartlett, 2014).
3. Ibid.
4. G. M. Herek and K. A. McLemore, "Sexual Prejudice," *Annual Review of Psychology* 64 (2013): 309–33.
5. Federal Bureau of Investigation, "Hate Crime Statistics, 2012," Fall 2013, www.fbi.gov/about-us/cjis/ucr/hate-crime/2012.
6. M. Rosario and E. Schrimshaw, "Theories and Etiologies of Sexual Orientation," *APA Handbook of Sexuality and Psychology* 1 (2014): 555–96.
7. S. M. Cabrera et al., "Age of Thelarche and Menarche in Contemporary U.S. Females: A Cross-Sectional Analysis," *Journal of Pediatric Endocrinology and Metabolism* 27, 1–2 (2014): 47–51.
8. S. Levay and J. Baldwin, *Human Sexuality,* 4th ed. (Sunderland, MA: Sinauer Associates, 2012).
9. F. M. Biro et al., "Onset of Breast Development in a Longitudinal Cohort," *Pediatrics* 132, no. 6 (2013): 1019–27.
10. E. Weil, "The Timing of Puberty: Is It Changing? Does It Matter?," *New York Times Magazine*, March 30, 2012, Available at: www.nytimes.com/2012/04/01/magazine/puberty-before-age-10-a-new-normal.html?pagewanted=all&_r=0.
11. Office of Women's Health, DHHS, "Premenstrual Symptoms Fact Sheet," 2012, Available at: www.womenshealth.gov/publications/our-publications/fact-sheet/premenstrual-syndrome.html.
12. Mayo Clinic Staff, "What's the Difference between Premenstrual Dysphoric Disorder and Premenstrual Syndrome?," December 2012, www.mayoclinic.org/diseases-conditions/premenstrual-syndrome/expert-answers/pmdd/faq-20058315.
13. Ibid.
14. Mayo Clinic Staff, "Menstrual Cramps," May 2011, www.mayoclinic.com/Health/Menstrual-Cramps/Ds00506.
15. "WHI Follow-Up Study Confirms Risk of Long-Term Combination Hormone Therapy Outweigh Benefits for Postmenopausal Women," news release, March 4, 2008, public.nhlbi.nih.gov/newsroom/home/GetPressRelease.aspx?id=2554; NHLBI, "WHI Study Data Confirm Short-Term Health Disease Risks of Combination Hormone Therapy for Postmenopausal Women," news release, February 15, 2010, www.nih.gov/news/health/feb2010/nhlbi 15.htm.
16. M. Beck, "Benefits of Hormone-Replacement Therapy Outweigh Risks, Reviews of Studies Show," Health Blog, *The Wall Street Journal*, May 22, 2012, http://blogs.wsj.com/health/2012/05/22/benefits-of-hormone-replacement-therapy-outweigh-risks-reviews-of-studies-show.
17. Z. Shi, A. B. Araujo, S. Martin, P. O'Loughlin, and G. A. Wittert, "Longitudinal Changes in Testosterone Over Five Years in Community-Dwelling Men," *The Journal of Clinical Endocrinology and Metabolism* 98, no. 8, (2013): 3289–3297.
18. Mayo Clinic Staff, "Male Menopause: Myth or Reality?," July 23, 2011, www.mayoclinic.org/healthy-living/mens-health/in-depth/male-menopause/art-20048056.
19. Ibid.
20. Ibid.
21. G. F. Kelly, "Sexual Individuality and Sexual Values," in *Sexuality Today: The Human Perspective*, 9th ed. (New York: McGraw-Hill, 2008).22.
22. Ibid.
23. American College Health Association, *American College Health Association–National College Health Assessment II (ACHA-NCHA II) Reference Group Data Report, Spring 2013* (Baltimore, MD: American College Health Association, 2013), Available at www.acha-ncha.org/reports_ACHA-NCHAII.html.
24. J. A. Higgins, J. Trussell, N. B. Moore, and J. K. Davidson, "Young Adult Sexual Health: Current and Prior Sexual Behaviours among Non-Hispanic White U.S. College Students," *Sexual Health* 7, no. 1 (2010): 35–43.
25. American College Health Association, *National College Health Assessment II: Reference Group Data Report, Spring 2013,* 2013.
26. Ibid.
27. Ibid.
28. Mayo Clinic Staff, "Antidepressants: Get Tips to Cope with Side Effects," July 2013, www.mayoclinic.org/diseases-conditions/depression/in-depth/antidepressants/art-20049305.
29. Mayo Clinic Staff, "Erectile Dysfunction," February 2012, www.mayoclinic.org/diseases-conditions/erectile-dysfunction/basics/definition/con-20034244.
30. National Kidney and Urological Diseases Information Clearinghouse, "Erectile Dysfunction," March 2012, http://kidney.niddk.nih.gov/KUDiseases/pubs/ED/index.aspx.
31. Medscape, "Premature Ejaculation," April 2014, http://emedicine.medscape.com/article/435884-overview.
32. Womenshealth.gov, "Men's Health: Sexual Problems," January 2011, http://womenshealth.gov/mens-health/sexual-health-for-men/sexual-problems.html; J. A. Simon, "Problems of Sexual Function in Menopausal Women," *Menopausal Medicine* 20, no. 4 (2012): S1–S6.
33. A. Mullens et al., "The Amyl Nitrite Expectancy Questionnaire for Men Who Have Sex with Men (AEQ-MSM): A Measure of Substance-Related Beliefs," *Substance Use & Misuse* 46, no. 13 (2011): 1642–50; D. J. Snipes and E. G. Benotsh, "High-Risk Cocktails and High-Risk Sex: Examining the Relation between Alcohol Mixed with Energy Drink Consumption, Sexual Behavior, and Drug Use in College Students," *Addictive Behaviors* 38, no. 1 (2013): 1418–23.
34. J. Bliss, "Police, Experts: Alcohol Most Common in Sexual Assaults," *USA Today*, October 28, 2103, www.usatoday.com/story/news/nation/2013/10/28/alcohol-most-common-drug-in-sexual-assaults/3285139.
35. M. Ward, "Web Porn: Just How Much Is There?," *BBC News*, June 30, 2013, www.bbc.com/news/technology-23030090.
36. C. Morris, "Is the Porn Industry Imperiled?," *CNBC News*, January 18, 2012, www.cnbc.com/id/45989346.
37. D. J. Ley, "Porn Is Not the Problem, You Are," *Psychology Today*, May 20, 2013, www.psychologytoday.com/blog/women-who-stray/201305/porn-is-not-the-problem-you-are.
38. D. M. Szymanski and D. N. Stewart-Richardson, "Psychological, Relational, and Sexual Correlates of Pornography Use on Young Adult Heterosexual Men in Romantic Relationships," *The Journal of Men's Studies* 22, no. 1 (2014): 64–82; T. L. Tylka, "No Harm in Looking, Right? Men's Pornography Consumption, Body Image, and Well-Being," *Psychology of Men & Masculinity* (2014), in press, DOI: 10.1037/a0035774; T. L. Tylka and A. M. Kroom Van Diest, "You Looking at Her 'Hot' Body May Not Be 'Cool' for Me: Integrating Male Partners' Use of Pornography into Objectification Theory for Women," *Psychology of Women Quarterly* (2014), in press, DOI:10.1177/0361684314521784.
39. M. Dank et al., *Estimating the Size and Structure of the Underground Commercial Sex Economy in Eight Major U.S. Cities* (Washington, D.C.: Urban Institute 2014), Available at: www.urban.org/UploadedPDF/413047-Underground-Commercial-Sex-Economy.pdf.
40. Ibid.

Pulled statistics:

p. 135, Data from American College Health Association, *American College Health Association—National College Health Assessment II (ACHA-NCHA II) Reference Group Data Report Spring 2013* (Baltimore: American College Health Association, 2013).

p. 143, Ibid.

Chapter 6

1. American College Health Association, *American College Health Association—National College Health Assessment III (ACHA-NCHA III): Reference Group Data Report, Spring 2013* (Baltimore, MD: American College Health Association, 2013), www.achancha.org/docs/ACHA-NCHA-II_ReferenceGroup_DataReport_Spring2013.pdf.
2. L. B. Finer and M. R. Zolna, "Shifts in Intended and Unintended Pregnancies in the United States, 2001–2008," *American Journal of Public Health* 104, S1 (2014): S43–S48.
3. Centers for Disease Control and Prevention, "Incidence, Prevalence and Cost of Sexually Transmitted Infections in the United States," February 2013, www.cdc.gov/std/stats/sti-estimates-fact-sheet-feb-2013.pdf.
4. J. Trussell, "Contraceptive Efficacy," in *Contraceptive Technology*, 20th rev. ed., eds. R. A. Hatcher et al., (New York, NY: Ardent Media, 2011).
5. Ibid.
6. Ibid.
7. Ibid.
8. Ibid.
9. Ibid.
10. World Health Organization, Media Centre, "Nonoxynol-9 Ineffective in Preventing HIV Infection," Accessed May 2014, www.who.int/mediacentre/news/notes/release55/en.
11. J. Trussell, "Contraceptive Efficacy," 2011.
12. Ibid.
13. Ibid.
14. Ibid.
15. Ibid.
16. American College Health Association, *National College Health Assessment III): Reference Group Data Report, Spring 2013*, 2013.
17. Drug Information Online, Drugs.com, "Seasonale," October 2013, www.drugs.com/seasonale.html..
18. J. Trussell, "Contraceptive Efficacy," 2011.
19. Ibid.
20. O. Lidegaard et al., "Thrombotic Stroke and Myocardial Infarction with Hormonal Contraception," *New England Journal of Medicine* 366, no. 24 (2012): 2257–66, DOI: 10.1056/NEJMoa1111840.
21. J. Trussell, "Contraceptive Efficacy," 2011.
22. E. G. Raymond, "Progestin-Only Pills," in *Contraceptive Technology*, 20th rev. ed., eds. R. A. Hatcher et al. (New York, NY: Ardent Media, 2011).
23. Janssen Pharmaceuticals, "OrthoEvra," October 2012, www.orthoevra.com.
24. J. Trussell, "Contraceptive Efficacy," 2011.
25. Janssen Pharmaceuticals, "Important Safety Update for U.S. Health Care Professionals ORTHO EVRA," March 2011, www.orthoevra.com/isi-hcp.html.
26. J. Trussell, "Contraceptive Efficacy," 2011.
27. Ibid.
28. Pfizer, "Depo-subQ Provera," September 2013, www.depo-subqprovera104.com.
29. J. Trussell, "Contraceptive Efficacy," 2011.
30. Merck & Co., Inc., "Nexplanon," March 2014, www.merck.com/product/usa/pi_circulars/n/nexplanon/nexplanon_pi.pdf.
31. J. Jones, W. Mosher, and K. Daniels, "Current Contraceptive Use in the United States, 2006–2010, and Changes in Pattern of Use Since 1995," *National Health Statistics Reports* 60 (2012)1–25.
32. The American Congress of Obstetricians and Gynecologists, "ACOG Committee Opinion-Adolescents and Long-Acting Reversible Contraception: Implants and Intrauterine Devices, Number 539," October 2012, www.acog.org/Resources_And_Publications/Committee_Opinions/Committee_on_Adolescent_Health_Care/Adolescents_and_Long-Acting_Reversible_Contraception.
33. J. Trussell, "Contraceptive Efficacy," 2011.
34. Office of Population Research & Association of Reproductive Health Professionals, The Emergency Contraception Website, "Answers to Frequently Asked Questions about Effectiveness," Updated April 2014, http://ec.princeton.edu/questions/eceffect.html.
35. J. Jacobson, "Court Orders FDA to Make Emergency Contraception Available Over-the-Counter for All Ages," *RH Reality Check,* April, 5 2013, http://rhrealitycheck.org/article/2013/04/05/court-orders-fda-to-make-emergency-contraception-available-over-the-counter-for-all-ages.
36. American College Health Association, *National College Health Assessment III: Reference Group Data Report Spring, 2013*, 2013.
37. J. Trussell, "Contraceptive Efficacy," 2011.
38. Ibid.
39. J. Jones, W. Mosher, and K. Daniels, "Current Contraceptive Use in the United States, 2006–2010, and Changes in Patterns of Use since 1995," *National Health Statistics Reports*, no. 60 (Hyattsville, MD: National Center for Health Statistics, 2012).
40. J. Trussell, "Contraceptive Efficacy," 2011.
41. Ibid.
42. Guttmacher Institute, "Fact Sheet: Induced Abortion in the United States," February 2014, www.guttmacher.org/pubs/fb_induced_abortion.html.
43. American Psychological Association (APA), Task Force on Mental Health and Abortion, *Report of the Task Force on Mental Health and Abortion* (Washington, DC: American Psychological Association, 2008), Available at www.apa.org/pi/wpo/mental-health-abortion-report.pdf.
44. *Roe v. Wade*, 410 U.S. 113 (1973).
45. L. Saad, "Abortion," *Gallup Politics*, Blog, January 22, 2013, www.gallup.com/poll/160058/majority-americans-support-roe-wade-decision.aspx.
46. H. D. Boonstra and E. Nash, "A Surge of State Abortion Restrictions Puts Providers and the Women They Serve in the Crosshairs," *Guttmacher Policy Review* 17, no. 1 (2014), www.guttmacher.org/pubs/gpr/17/1/gpr170109.pdf.
47. APA, *Report of the Task Force*, 2008; J. R. Steinberg, C. E. McCulloch, and N. E. Adler, "Abortion and Mental Health: Findings from the National Comorbidity Survey-Replication," *Obstetrics & Gynecology* 123, no. 2 (2014): 263–70.
48. Ibid.
49. Ibid.
50. Guttmacher Institute, "Fact Sheet: Induced Abortion in the United States," 2014.
51. Ibid.
52. Ibid.
53. Planned Parenthood, "The Abortion Pill (Medication Abortion)," Accessed May 2014, www.plannedparenthood.org/health-topics/abortion/abortion-pill-medication-abortion-4354.asp.
54. K. Cleland et al., "Significant Adverse Events and Outcomes After Medical Abortion," *Obstetrics and Gynecology* 121, no. 1 (2013): 166–71.
55. Ibid.
56. Centers for Disease Control and Prevention, "Preconception Care and Health Care: Women," July 2013, www.cdc.gov/preconception/women.html.
57. Centers for Disease Control and Prevention, "Preconception Care and Health Care: Women," July 2014, www.cdc.gov/preconception/women.html.
58. S. M. Schrader and K. L. Marlow, "Assessing the Reproductive Health of Men with Occupational Exposures," *Asian Journal of Andrology* 16, no. 1 (2014): 23–30; Centers for Disease Control and Prevention, "Preconception Health and Healthcare," December 2013, http://www.cdc.gov/preconception/careformen/exposures.html.
59. Centers for Disease Control and Prevention, "Preconception Health and Healthcare," December 2013, http://www.cdc.gov/preconception/careformen/exposures.html.
60. B. M. D'Onofrio, M. E. Rickert, E. Frans, R. Kuja-Halkola, C. Almqvist, A. Sjölander, H. Larsson, and P. Lichtenstein, "Paternal Age at Childbearing and Offspring Psychiatric and Academic Morbidity," *Journal of the American Medical Association Psychiatry,* 71 no. 4 (2014): 432–438; E. Calloway, "Fathers Bequeath More Mutations as They Age," *Nature,* 488 no. 7412 (2012): 439.
61. Truven Health Analytics, "The Cost of Having a Baby in the United States," January 2013, http://transform.childbirthconnection.org/wp-content/uploads/2013/01/Cost-of-Having-a-Baby1.pdf.
62. M. Lino, *Expenditures on Children by Families, 2012* (Alexandria, VA: U.S. Department of Agriculture, Center for Nutrition Policy and Promotion, 2013), www.cnpp.usda.gov/ExpendituresonChildrenbyFamilies.htm.
63. National Association of Child Care Resource and Referral Agencies, "Parents and the High Cost of Child Care, 2013 Report," August 2013, www.naccrra.org/

sites/default/files/child_care_aware_of_america_annual_report_0.pdf.

64. Planned Parenthood, "Pregnancy Tests," Accessed May 2014, www.plannedparenthood.org/health-topics/pregnancy/pregnancy-test-21227.asp.
65. Committee on Obstetric Practice, "Committee Opinion no. 548, American Congress of Obstetricians and Gynecologists: Weight Gain During Pregnancy," *Obstetrics and Gynecology* 121, no. 1, (2013): 210–12, DOI: 10.1097/01.AOG.0000425668.87506.4c.
66. The American Congress of Obstetricians and Gynecologists, "Tobacco, Alcohol, Drugs, and Pregnancy," December 2013, www.acog.org/~/media/For%20Patients/faq170.pdf?dmc=1&ts=20140516T2242271513.
67. National Center for Chronic Disease Prevention and Health Promotion, "Tobacco Use and Pregnancy," *Reproductive Health*, Updated January 2014, http://www.cdc.gov/Reproductivehealth/TobaccoUsePregnancy/index.htm; The American Congress of Obstetricians and Gynecologists, "Tobacco, Alcohol, Drugs, and Pregnancy," December 2013, www.acog.org/~/media/For%20Patients/faq170.pdf?dmc=1&ts=20140516T2242271513.
68. J. A. Martin et al., U.S. Department of Health and Human Services, National Center for Health Statistics, "Births: Final Data for 2012," *National Vital Statistics Reports* 62, no. 9 (2013), Available at www.cdc.gov/nchs/data/nvsr/nvsr62/nvsr62_09.pdf#table01.
69. American Pregnancy Association, "Miscarriage," Updated November 2011, http://americanpregnancy.org/pregnancycomplications/miscarriage.html.
70. J. A. Martin, et al., "Births: Final Data for 2012," 2013.
71. J. Christensen, CNN News, "Why So Many C-sections Have Medical Groups Concerned," May 8, 2014, www.cnn.com/2014/05/08/health/c-section-report.
72. E. Puscheck, "Early Pregnancy Loss," *Medscape Reference: Drugs, Diseases & Procedures*, Updated October 2014, http://reference.medscape.com/article/266317-overview.
73. V. P. Sepilian et al., "Ectopic Pregnancy," *Medscape Reference*, Updated May 2014, http://emedicine.medscape.com/article/2041923-overview.
74. What To Expect, "Stillbirth," Accessed May 2014, www.whattoexpect.com/pregnancy/pregnancy-health/complications/stillbirth.aspx.
75. K. L. Wisner et al., "Onset Timing, Thoughts of Self-harm, and Diagnoses in Postpartum Women with Screen-Positive Depression Findings," *JAMA Psychiatry* 70, no. 5 (2013): 1–9, DOI:10.1001/jamapsychiatry.2013.87.
76. American Academy of Pediatrics, "Benefits of Breastfeeding for Mom," Updated May 2013, www.healthychildren.org/English/ages-stages/baby/breastfeeding/pages/Benefits-of-Breastfeeding-for-Mom.aspx.
77. Centers for Disease Control and Prevention, "Sudden Unexpected Infant Death and Sudden Infant Death Syndrome," May 2014, www.cdc.gov/sids.
78. Ibid.
79. March of Dimes, "Low BirthWeight," March 2014, www.marchofdimes.com/baby/low-birthweight.aspx.
80. MayoClinic.com, "Infertility: Causes," July 2013, www.mayoclinic.com/health/infertility/DS00310/DSECTION=causes.
81. U.S. Department of Health and Human Services, "Polycystic Ovary Syndrome (PCOS) Fact Sheet," July 2012, www.womenshealth.gov/publications/our-publications/fact-sheet/polycystic-ovary-syndrome.html.
82. B. Kumbak, E. Oral, and O. Bukulmez, "Female Obesity and Assisted Reproductive Technologies," *Seminars in Reproductive Medicine* 30, no. 6, (2012): 507–16, DOI: 10.1055/s-0032-1328879.
83. Centers for Disease Control and Prevention (CDC), "Pelvic Inflammatory Disease CDC Fact Sheet," *Sexually Transmitted Diseases*, Updated March 2014, www.cdc.gov/std/PID/STDFact-PID.htm.
84. Centers for Disease Control and Prevention (CDC), "Assisted Reproductive Technology, (ART)," Updated June 2013, www.cdc.gov/reproductivehealth/infertility.
85. Centers for Disease Control and Prevention, "Infertility: FAQs," February 2013, www.cdc.gov/reproductivehealth/Infertility/index.htm#4; S. Cabler, A. Agarwal, and S. S. du Plessis, "Obesity and Male Fertility," *Male Infertility* 33 (2012): 349–60.
86. Ibid.
87. Ibid.
88. WebMD Medical Reference, "Fertility Drugs," July 2012, www.webmd.com/infertility-and-reproduction/guide/fertility-drugs.
89. American Society for Reproductive Medicine, "Fertility Drugs and the Risk for Multiple Births," Accessed May 2014, www.asrm.org/uploadedFiles/ASRM_Content/Resources/Patient_Resources/Fact_Sheets_and_Info_Booklets/fertilitydrugs_multiplebirths.pdf.
90. WebMD, "Using a Surrogate Mother, What You Need to Know," September 2013, www.webmd.com/infertility-and-reproduction/guide/using-surrogate-mother.
91. R. M. Kreider and D. A. Loftquist, "Adopted Children and Stepchildren: 2010," *U.S. Census Bureau*, April 2014, www.census.gov/content/dam/Census/library/publications/2014/demo/p20-572.pdf.
92. Intercountry Adoption, U.S. Department of State, "Statistics: Adoptions by Year," Accessed May 2014, http://adoption.state.gov/about_us/statistics.php.
93. Adoption.com, "Adoption Costs," Accessed May 2014, http://costs.adoption.com.

Pulled statistics:

p. 157, W. D. Mosher and J. Jones, "Use of Contraception in the United States: 1982–2008," *Vital and Health Statistics* 23, no. 29 (Hyattsville, MD: National Center for Health Statistics, 2010), www.cdc.gov.

p. 175, Gallup, "U.S. Still Split on Abortion: 47% Pro-Choice, 46% Pro-Life," (2014) http://www.gallup.com/poll/170249/split-abortion-pro-choice-pro-life.aspx.

p. 177, American College Health Association, *American College Health Association—National College Health Assessment III (ACHA-NCHA III). Reference Group Data Report Spring 2013* (Baltimore: American College Health Association, 2013), www.achancha.org/docs/ACHA-NCHA-II_ReferenceGroup_DataReport_Spring2013.pdf.

Chapter 7

1. L. L. Wilkinson et al., "Attachment Anxiety, Disinhibited Eating and Body Mass Index in Adulthood," *Appetite* 57, no. 2 (2011): 543.
2. S. C. Killer, A. K. Blannin, and A. E. Jeukendrup, "No Evidence of Dehydration with Moderate Daily Coffee Intake: A Counterbalanced Cross-Over Study in a Free-Living Population." *PLoS ONE* 9 no. 1 (2014): e84154. doi:10.1371/journal.pone.0084154.
3. American College of Sports Medicine (ACSM), "Selecting and Effectively Using Hydration for Fitness," 2011, www.acsm.org/docs/brochures/selecting-and-effectively-using-hydration-for-fitness.pdf.
4. U.S. Department of Agriculture, Agricultural Research Service, Beltsville Human Nutrition Research Center, Food Surveys Research Group (Beltsville, MD) and U.S. Department of Health and Human Services, Centers for Disease Control and Prevention, National Center for Health Statistics (Hyattsville, MD), *What We Eat in America, NHANES 2009–2010 Data: Table 1. Nutrient Intakes from Food: Mean Amounts Consumed per Individual by Gender and Age, in the United States, 2009–2010*, www.ars.usda.gov/SP2UserFiles/Place/12355000/pdf/0910/tables_1-40_2009-2010.pdf.
5. Food and Nutrition Board, Institute of Medicine, *Dietary Reference Intakes for Energy, Carbohydrate, Fiber, Fat, Fatty Acids, Cholesterol, Protein, and Amino Acids (Macronutrients)* (Washington, DC: National Academies Press, 2005), Available at www.nap.edu/openbook.php?isbn=0309085373.
6. S. M. Phillips and L. J. C. van Loon, "Dietary Protein for Athletes: From Requirements to Optimum Adaptation," *Journal of Sports Science* 29, no. S1 (2011): S29–S38.
7. Institute of Medicine of the National Academies, "Dietary, Functional, and Total Fiber," in *Dietary Reference Intakes for Energy, Carbohydrate, Fiber, Fat, Fatty Acids, Cholesterol, Protein, and Amino Acids* (Washington, DC: The National Academies Press, 2005), 339–421, Available at www.nap.edu/openbook.php?isbn=0309085373.
8. Ibid.

9. Ibid.
10. Ibid.
11. C. E. Ramsden et al., "Use of Dietary Linoleic Acid for Secondary Prevention of Coronary Heart Disease and Death: Evaluation of Recovered Data from the Sydney Diet Heart Study and Updated Meta-Analysis," *British Medical Journal* 346 (2013): e8707, DOI: http://dx.doi.org/10.1136/bmj.e8707; L. Gillingham, S. Harris-Janz, and P. Jones, "Dietary Monounsaturated Fatty Acids Are Protective against Metabolic Syndrome and Cardiovascular Disease Risk Factors," *Lipids* 46, no. 3 (2011): 209–228, DOI: 10.1007/s11745-010-3524-y.
12. W. Willet, "Dietary Fats and Coronary Heart Disease," *Journal of Internal Medicine*, no. 1 (2012): 13–24; N. Bendson et al., "Consumption of Industrial and Ruminant Trans Fatty Acids and Risk of CHD: A Systemic Review and Meta-Analysis of Cohort Studies," *European Journal of Clinical Nutrition* 65 (2011): 773–83.
13. U.S. Food and Drug Administration, "FDA Targets Trans Fats in Processed Foods," *FDA Consumer Updates*, December 2013, www.fda.gov/ForConsumers/Consumer Updates/ucm372915.htm.
14. Ibid.
15. H. J. Silver et al., "Consuming a Balanced High Fat Diet for 16 Weeks Improves Body Composition, Inflammation and Vascular Function Parameters in Obese Premenopausal Women," *Metabolism*, January 17, 2014. DOI: 10.1016/ j.metabol.2014.01.004; Z. Shadman, "Association of High Carbohydrate versus High Fat Diet with Glycated Hemoglobin in High Calorie Consuming Type 2 Diabetics," *Journal of Diabetes and Metabolic Disorders* 12, no. 1 (2013): 27.
16. Food and Nutrition Board, Institute of Medicine, *Dietary Reference Intakes for Energy, Carbohydrate, Fiber, Fat, Fatty Acids, Cholesterol, Protein, and Amino Acids (Macronutrients)* (Washington, DC: National Academies Press, 2005), Available at www.nap.edu/openbook.php?isbn=0309085373.
17. National Institutes of Health Office of Dietary Supplements, "Dietary Supplement Fact Sheet: Vitamin D," June 2011, http://ods.od.nih.gov/factsheets/VitaminD-HealthProfessional.
18. Institute of Medicine Committee to Review Dietary Reference Intakes for Vitamin D and Calcium, *Dietary Reference Intakes for Calcium and Vitamin D*, eds. A. Ross, C. Taylor, A. Yaktine, H. Del Valle (Washington, DC: National Academies Press, 2011), www.iom.edu/Reports/2010/Dietary-Reference-Intakes-for-Calcium-and-Vitamin-D.aspx.
19. Ibid.
20. U.S. Department of Agriculture, *What We Eat in America*, NHANES 2009-2010 Data: Table 1, 2010, www.ars.usda.gov/Services/docs.htm?docid=18349.
21. Ibid; C. Ayala et al., "Application of Lower Sodium Intake Recommendations to Adults—United States, 1999–2006," *Morbidity and Mortality Weekly* (*MMWR*) 58, no. 11 (2009): 281–83.
22. American Heart Association, "Sodium (Salt)," February 2014, www.heart.org/HEARTORG/GettingHealthy/Nutrition-Center/HealthyDietGoals/Sodium-Salt-or-Sodium-Chloride_UCM_303290_Article.jsp.
23. R. L. Bailey et al., "Estimation of Total Usual Calcium and Vitamin D Intakes in the United States," *Journal of Nutrition* 140, no. 4 (2010): 817–22, DOI: 10.3945/jn.109.118539.
24. D. C. Bauer, "Calcium Supplements and Fracture Prevention," *New England Journal of Medicine* 369, no. 16 (2013): 1537–43. DOI: 10.1056/NEJMcp1210380, Available at www.aahs.org/medstaff/wp-content/uploads/CalciumSuppNEJM2013.pdf.
25. Institute of Medicine Committee, "Dietary Reference Intakes for Calcium and Vitamin D," 2011
26. World Health Organization, "Miconutrient Deficiencies: Iron Deficiency Anemia," 2014, www.who.int/nutrition/topics/ida/en/index.html.
27. U.S. Centers for Disease Control and Prevention (CDC), "Iron and Iron Deficiency," *Nutrition for Everyone*, February 23, 2011, www.cdc.gov/nutrition/everyone/basics/vitamins/iron.html.
28. C. Geissler and M. Singh, "Iron, Meat, and Health," *Nutrients* 3, no. 3 (2011): 283–316, DOI: 10.3390/nu3030283.
29. Academy of Nutrition and Dietetics, "Position of the Academy of Nutrition and Dietetics: Functional Foods" *Journal of the Academy of Nutrition and Dietetics*, 113 (2013): 1096–1103.
30. Ibid.
31. Ibid.
32. M. E. Obrenovich, et al., "Antioxidants in Health, Disease, and Aging," *CNS & Neurological Disorders Drug Targets* 10, no. 2 (2011):192–207; V. Ergin, R. E. Hariry, and C. Karasu, "Carbonyl Stress in Aging Process: Role of Vitamins and Phytochemicals as Redox Regulators," *Aging and Disease* 4, no. 5 (2013): 276–94, DOI: 10.14336/AD.2013.0400276.
33. E. A. Klein et al., "Vitamin E and the Risk of Prostate Cancer: The Selenium and Vitamin E Cancer Prevention Trial (SELECT)," *Journal of the American Medical Association* 306, no. 14 (2011): 1549–56, DOI: 10.1001/jama.2011.1437.
34. U.S. Department of Agriculture, Economic Research Service, "U.S. Per Capita Loss-Adjusted Food Availability: Total Calories," April 2010, www.ers.usda.gov/Data/Food-Consumption/app/reports/displayCommodities.aspx?reportName=Total+Calories&id=36#startForm; U.S. Department of Agriculture, Economic Research Service, "Summary Findings," *Food Availability (Per Capita) Data System*, August 2012, www.ers.usda.gov/data-products/food-availability-%28per-capita%29-data-system/summary-findings.aspx#.UYLNPcphris.
35. D. Grotto and E. Zied, "The Standard American Diet and Its Relationship to the Health Status of Americans," *Nutrition in Clinical Practice* 25, no. 6 (2010): 603–12, DOI: 10.1177/0884533610386234.
36. U.S. Department of Agriculture and U.S. Department of Health and Human Services, *Dietary Guidelines for Americans, 2010*, 7th ed. (Washington, DC: U.S. Government Printing Office, 2010), www.cnpp.usda.gov/publications/dietaryguidelines/2010/policy-doc/policydoc.pdf.
37. U.S. Department of Agriculture, "Empty Calories: How Do I Count the Empty Calories I Eat?," June 4, 2011, www.choosemyplate.gov/foodgroups/emptycalories_count_table.html.
38. U.S. Food and Drug Administration, "Nutrition Facts Label: Proposed Changes Aim to Better Inform Food Choices," February 2014, www.fda.gov/ForConsumers/ConsumerUpdates/ucm387114.htm.
39. U.S. Food and Drug Administration, "Label Claims for Conventional Foods and Dietary Supplements," December 2013, www.fda.gov/Food/IngredientsPackagingLabeling/LabelingNutrition/ucm111447.htm.
40. The Vegetarian Resource Group, "How Often Do Americans Eat Vegetarian Meals? and How Many Adults in the U.S. Are Vegetarian?," *Vegetarian Resource Group Blog*, May 2012, www.vrg.org/blog/2012/05/18/how-often-do-americans-eat-vegetarian-meals-and-how-many-adults-in-the-u-s-are-vegetarian.
41. Y. Yokoyama et al., "Vegetarian Diets and Blood Pressure: A Meta-Analysis," *Journal of the American Medical Association Internal Medicine*, February 2014, DOI:10.1001/jamainternmed.2013.14547.
42. C. G. Lee et al., "Vegetarianism as a Protective Factor for Colorectal Adenoma and Advanced Adenoma in Asians," *Digestive Diseases and Science*, 2013, DOI: 10.1007/s10620-013-2974-5.
43. Office of Dietary Supplements, "Frequently Asked Questions," July 2013, http://ods.od.nih.gov/Health_Information/ODS_Frequently_Asked_Questions.aspx#; V. A. Moyer, "Vitamin, Mineral, and Multivitamin Supplements for the Primary Prevention of Cardiovascular Disease and Cancer: U.S. Preventive Services Task Force Recommendation Statement," *Annals of Internal Medicine*, 2014, DOI:10.7326/M14-0198.
44. R. Chowdhury et al., "Association between Fish Consumption, Long Chain Omega 3 Fatty Acids, and Risk of Cerebrovascular Disease: Systematic Review and Meta-Analysis," *British Medical Journal* 345 (2012): e6698, Available at www.ncbi.nlm.nih.gov/pmc/articles/PMC3484317.
45. Office of Dietary Supplements, "Vitamin A Fact Sheet for Consumers," June 2013,

http://ods.od.nih.gov/factsheets/VitaminA-QuickFacts/; Office of Dietary Supplements, "Vitamin E Fact Sheet for Consumers," June 2013, http://ods.od.nih.gov/factsheets/list-all/VitaminE-QuickFacts/; Office of Dietary Supplements, "Vitamin D Fact Sheet for Consumers," June 2013, http://ods.od.nih.gov/factsheets/VitaminD-QuickFacts.

46. Academy of Nutrition and Dietetics, "It's About Eating Right: Dietary Supplements," January 2013, www.eatright.org/public/content.aspx?id=7918.
47. The Organic Trade Association, "Eight in Ten U.S. Parents Report They Purchase Organic Products," April 2013, www.ota.com/organic-consumers/consumersurvey2013.html.
48. The Organic Trade Organization, "Consumer-Driven U.S. Organic Market Surpasses $31 Billion in 2011," 2012, www.organicnewsroom.com/2012/04/us_consumerdriven_organic_mark.html.
49. K. Brandt et al., "Agroecosystem Management and Nutritional Quality of Plant Foods: The Case of Organic Fruits and Vegetables," *Critical Reviews in Plant Sciences* 30, no. 1–2 (2011): 177–97; C. Smith-Spangler et al., "Are Organic Foods Safer or Healthier Than Conventional Alternatives? A Systematic Review," *Annals of Internal Medicine* 157, no. 5 (2012): 348–66, DOI:10.7326/0003-4819-157-5-201209040-00007.
50. U.S. Environmental Protection Agency, "Pesticides and Foods: Health Problems Pesticides May Pose," May 2012, www.epa.gov/pesticides/food/risks.htm.
51. U.S. Department of Agriculture, Pesticide Data Program: 21st Annual Summary, Calendar Year 2011, Agricultural Marketing Service, February 2013, www.ams.usda.gov/AMSv1.0/getfile?dDocName=stelprdc5102692.
52. U.S. Department of Health and Human Services, "Food Safety Modernization Act (FSMA)," November 2013, www.fda.gov/Food/GuidanceRegulation/FSMA/ucm304045.htm.
53. CDC, "Estimates of Food-Borne Illnesses in the United States," January 2014, www.cdc.gov/foodborneburden/index.html.
54. CDC, "Trends in Foodborne Illness in the United States, 2012," April 2013, www.cdc.gov/features/dsfoodnet2012.
55. R. Johnson, "The U.S. Trade Situation for Fruit and Vegetable Products," *Congressional Research Service*, January 2014, www.fas.org/sgp/crs/misc/RL34468.pdf.
56. S. Clark et al., "Frequency of US Emergency Department Visits for Food-related Acute Allergic Reactions," *Journal of Allergy Clinical Immunology* 127, no. 3, (2011): 682-683, doi: 10.1016/j.jaci.2010.10.040.
57. U.S. Food and Drug Administration, "Food Irradiation: What You Need to Know," March 2014, http://www.fda.gov/Food/ResourcesForYou/Consumers/ucm261680.htm.
58. National Institute of Allergy and Infectious Diseases, "Food Allergy," August 2013, www.niaid.nih.gov/topics/foodallergy/Pages/default.aspx.
59. R. S. Gupta et al., "The Prevalence, Severity, and Distribution of Childhood Food Allergy in the United States," *Journal of Pediatrics* 128, no. 1 (2011): e9–e17, DOI: 10.1542/peds.2011-0204.
60. National Institute of Allergy and Infectious Diseases, "Food Allergy," August 2013, www.niaid.nih.gov/topics/foodallergy/Pages/default.aspx.
61. U.S. Food and Drug Administration, "Food Allergies: What You Need to Know," April 2013, www.fda.gov/food/resourcesforyou/consumers/ucm079311.htm.
62. A. Rubio-Tapia et al., "The Prevalence of Celiac Disease in the United States," *American Journal of Gastroenterology* 107 (2012):1 538–44.
63. J. N. Keith et al., "The Prevalence of Self-Reported Lactose Intolerance and the Consumption of Dairy Foods among African American Adults Less than Expected," *Journal of the National Medical Association* 103 (2011): 36–45.
64. U.S. Department of Agriculture, Economic Research Service, "Adoption of Genetically Engineered Crops in the U.S.," July 2013, www.ers.usda.gov/data-products/adoption-of-genetically-engineered-crops-in-the-us.aspx.
65. Center for Food Safety, "About Genetically Engineered Foods," Accessed March 2014, www.centerforfoodsafety.org/issues/311/ge-foods/about-ge-foods.
66. Union of Concerned Scientists, "Genetic Engineering Risks and Impacts," November 2013, www.ucsusa.org/food_and_agriculture/our-failing-food-system/genetic-engineering/risks-of-genetic-engineering.html.
67. L. P Brower et al., "Decline of Monarch Butterflies Overwintering in Mexico: Is the Migratory Phenomenon at Risk?," *Insect Conservation and Diversity* 5, no. 2 (2012): 95–100.
68. Union of Concerned Scientists, "Genetic Engineering Risks and Impacts," November 2013, www.ucsusa.org/food_and_agriculture/our-failing-food-system/genetic-engineering/risks-of-genetic-engineering.html.
69. G. Pinholster, "AAAS Board of Directors: Legally Mandating GM Food Labels Could 'Mislead and Falsely Alarm Consumers,'" *American Association for the Advancement of Science News*, October 2012, www.aaas.org/news/aaas-board-directors-legally-mandating-gm-food-labels-could-mislead-and-falsely-alarm; World Health Organization, "20 Questions on Genetically Modified Foods," Accessed March 2014, www.who.int/foodsafety/publications/biotech/20questions/en.

Pulled statistics:

p. 198, D. King, A. Mainous, C. Lambourne, "Trends in Dietary Fiber Intake in the United States, 1999–2008," *Journal of the Academy of Nutrition and Dietetics* 112, no. 5, (2012): 642-648, DOI: 10.1016/j.jand.2012.01.019).

p. 211, C. Ogden, B. Kit, M. Carroll, S. Park, "Consumption of Sugar Drinks in the United States, 2005–2008," *NCHS data brief*, no 71. Hyattsville, MD: National Center for Health Statistics. 2011, http://www.cdc.gov/nchs/data/databriefs/db71.htm.

p. 212, D. Graham and M. Laska, "Nutrition Label Use Partially Mediates the Relationship between Attitude toward Healthy Eating and Overall Dietary Quality among College Students," *Journal of the Academy of Nutrition and Dietetics* 112, no. 3, (2012): 414–418, doi: 10.1016/j.jada.2011.08.047, http://www.ncbi.nlm.nih.gov/pmc/articles/PMC3561724.

p. 215, K. Heidal, S. Colby, G. Mirabella, et al., "Cost and Calorie Analysis of Fast Food Consumption in College Students," *Food and Nutrition Sciences* 3, no. 7, (2012): 942–946, doi:10.4236/fns.2012.37124.

Chapter 8

1. M. Ng et al., "Global, Regional, and National Prevalence of Overweight and Obesity in Children and Adults during 1980–2013: A Systematic Analysis for the Global Burden of Disease Study, 2013." *The Lancet*, Early Online Publication, May 29, 2014, doi:10.1016/S0140-6736(14)60460-8; C. L. Ogden et al., "Prevalence of Childhood and Adult Obesity in the United States, 2011–2012," *Journal of the American Medical Association* 311, no. 8 (2014): 806–814, DOI:10.1001/jama.2014.732; C. L. Ogden et al, "Prevalence of Obesity among Adults: United States, 2011-2012," *National Center for Health Statistics Data Brief* 131 (2013), www.cdc.gov/nchs/data/databriefs/db131.htm.
2. U.S. Department of Health and Human Services, *The Surgeon General's Vision for a Healthy and Fit Nation* (Rockville, MD: U.S. Department of Health and Human Services, Office of the Surgeon General, 2010).
3. C. L. Ogden et al., "Prevalence of Childhood and Adult Obesity," 2014.
4. A. Go et al., "AHA Statistical Update Heart Disease and Stroke Statistics—2014 Update: A Report from the American Heart Association," *Circulation* 129 (2014): 399–410.
5. C. L. Ogden et al., "Prevalence of Childhood and Adult Obesity," 2014.
6. K. M. Flegal et al., "Association of All-Cause Mortality with Overweight and Obesity Using Standard Body Mass Index Categories: A Systematic Review and Meta-Analysis," *Journal of the American Medical Association* 309, no. 1 (2013): 71–82.
7. American Heart Association, "With a Very Heavy Heart: Obesity and Cardiovascular disease," February 2014, www.heart.org/idc/groups/heart-public/@wcm/@adv/documents/downloadable/ucm_461353.pdf.

8. A. Go et al., "AHA Statistical Update Heart Disease and Stroke Statistics," (2014).
9. Ibid.
10. American Diabetes Association, "Statistics about Diabetes," January 2011, www.diabetes.org/diabetes-basics/statistics.
11. C. L. Himes and S. L. Reynolds. "Effect of Obesity on Falls, Injury, and Disability," *Journal of the American Geriatrics Society* 60, no. 1 (2012): 124–29; L. A. Schaap, A Koster, M. Visser, "Adiposity, Muscle Mass, and Muscle Strength in Relation to Functional Decline in Older Persons," *Epidemiologic Reviews* 35, no. 1 (2013): 1.
12. World Health Organization, "Obesity and Overweight Fact Sheet," March 2013, www.who.int/mediacentre/factsheets/fs311/en.
13. Ibid.; International Obesity Taskforce, "Obesity—The Global Epidemic," 2014, www.iaso.org/iotf/obesity/obesitytheglobal epidemic.
14. International Obesity Taskforce, "Obesity—The Global Epidemic," 2014, http://www.iaso.org/iotf/obesity/obesitytheglobalepidemic.
15. D. Spruijt-Metz, "Etiology, Treatment, and Prevention of Obesity in Childhood and Adolescence: A Decade in Review," *Journal of Research on Adolescence* 21 (2011): 129–52, DOI: 10.1111/j.1532-7795.2010.00719.x; S. A. Affenito et al., "Behavioral Determinants of Obesity: Research Findings and Policy Implications," *Journal of Obesity* 2012, (2012), www.hindawi.com/journals/jobes/2012/150732.
16. S. A. Affenito et al., "Behavioral Determinants of Obesity," 2012.
17. K. Silventoinen et al., "The Genetic and Environmental Influences on Childhood Obesity: A Systematic Review of Twin and Adoption Studies," *International Journal of Obesity* 34, no. 1 (2010): 29–40; D. Cummings and M. Schwartz, "Genetics and Pathophysiology of Human Obesity," *Annual Review of Medicine* 54 (2003): 453–71.
18. T. Tanaka, J. S. Ngwa, and F. J. van Rooij, "Genome-Wide Meta-Analysis of Observational Studies Shows Common Genetic Variants Associated with Macronutrient Intake," *American Journal of Clinical Nutrition* 97, no. 6 (2013): 1395–402; M. M. Hetherington and J. E. Cecil, "Gene-Environment Interactions in Obesity," *Forum Nutrition* 63 (2010): 195–203; "Genome-Wide Analysis of BMI in Adolescents and Young Adults Reveals Additional Insights into the Effects of the Genetic Loci over the Life Course," *Human Molecular Genetics* 22 no. 17 (2013): 3597–3607.
19. Ibid.
20. T. O. Kilpelainen et al., "Physical Activity Attenuates the Influence of *FTO* Variants on Obesity Risk: A Meta-Analysis of 218,166 Adults and 19,268 Children," 2012, *PLoS Medicine* 8, no.11 (2012), e1001116, DOI:10.1371/journal.pmed.1001116; A. S. Richardson et al., "Moderate to Vigorous Physical Activity Interactions with Genetic Variants and Body Mass Index in a Large US Ethnically Diverse Cohort," *Pediatric Obesity* 9, no. 2 (2013): e35–46, DOI: 10.1111/j.2047-6310.2013.00152.
21. J. C. Wells, "The Evolution of Human Adiposity and Obesity: Where Did It All Go Wrong?," *Disease Models and Mechanisms* 5, no. 5 (2012): 595–607, DOI:10.1242/dmm.009613; J. R. Speakman et al., "Evolutionary Perspectives on the Obesity Epidemic: Adaptive, Maladaptive, and Neutral Viewpoints," *Annual Review of Nutrition* 33 (2013): 289–317.
22. A. Tremblay et al., "Adaptive Thermogenesis Can Make a Difference in the Ability of Obese Individuals to Lose Body Weight," *International Journal of Obesity* 37 (2013): 759–64.
23. J. Buss et al., "Associations of Ghrelin with Eating Behaviors, Stress, Metabolic Factors, and Telomere Length Among Overweight and Obese Women: Preliminary Evidence of Attenuated Ghrelin Effects in Obesity," *Appetite* 76, no. 1 (2014): 84–94; B. Biondi, "Thyroid and Obesity: An Intriguing Relationship," *Journal of Clinical Endocrinology and Metabolism* 95, no. 8 (2010): 3614–17; T. Reinehr, "Obesity and Thyroid Function," *Molecular and Cellular Endocrinology* 316, no. 2 (2010): 165–71.
24. M. Rotondi, F. Magri, and L. Chiovato, "Thyroid and Obesity: Not a One Way Interaction," *The Journal of Clinical Endocrinology and Metabolism* 96, no. 2 (2011): 344–56.
25. D. E. Cummings et al., "Plasma Ghrelin Levels After Diet-Induced Weight Loss or Gastric Bypass Surgery," *New England Journal of Medicine* 346, no. 21 (2002): 1623–30.
26. M. Khatib et al., "Effect of Ghrelin on Regulation of Growth Hormone Release: A Review," *The Health Agenda* 2, no. 1 (2014), Available at www.healthagenda.net/wp-content/uploads/2013/11/Effect-of-ghrelin-on-regulation-of-growth-hormone-release-A-review.pdf; C. DeVriese et al., "Focus on the Short- and Long-Term Effects of Ghrelin on Energy Homeostasis," *Nutrition* 26, no. 6 (2010): 579–84; T. Castaneda et al., "Ghrelin in the Regulation of Body Weight and Metabolism," *Frontiers in Neuroendocrinology* 31, no. 1 (2010): 44–60.
27. P. Marzullo et al. "Investigations of Thyroid Hormones and Antibodies in Obesity: Leptin Levels Are Associated with Thyroid Autoimmunity Independent of Bioanthropometric, Hormonal and Weight-Related Determinants," *The Journal of Clinical Endocrinology and Metabolism* 95, no. 8 (2010): 3965–72; H. Feng et al., "Review: The Role of Leptin in Obesity and the Potential for Leptin Replacement Therapy," *Endocrine* 44 (2013): 33–39.
28. L. K. Mahan and S. Escott-Stump, *Krause's Food, Nutrition, and Diet Therapy*, 13th ed. (New York: W. B. Saunders, 2012).
29. USDA Economic Research Service, "Food Availability (per capita) Data System," March 2014, www.ers.usda.gov/data-products/food-availability.
30. E. Ford and W. Dietz, "Trends in Energy Intake among Adults in the United States: Findings from NHANES," *American Journal of Clinical Nutrition*, April 2013, http://bit.ly/XUJ7Dq
31. Centers for Disease Control and Prevention, "Overweight and Obesity—A Growing Problem," April 2013, www.cdc.gov/obesity/childhood/problem.html; Centers for Disease Control and Prevention, "Overweight and Obesity: Facts about Physical Activity," February 2014, www.cdc.gov/physicalactivity/data/facts.html.
32. L. Poston, L. F. Harthoorn, and E. M. Van Der Beek, "Obesity in Pregnancy: Implications for the Mother and Lifelong Health of the Child—A Consensus Statement." *Pediatr Res* 69, no. 2 (2011): 175–80; K. L. Connor et al., "Nature, Nurture or Nutrition? Impact of Maternal Nutrition on Maternal Care, Offspring Development and Reproductive Function," *Journal of Physiology* 590, no. 9 (2012): 2167–80.
33. M. A. Schuster et al., "Racial and Ethnic Health Disparities among Fifth-Graders in Three Cities," *The New England Journal of Medicine* 367, no. 8 (2012): 735–45; C. L. Odgen et al., "Prevalence of Obesity and Trends in Body Mass Index among U.S. Children and Adolescents. 1999–2010," *Journal of the American Medical Association* 307 (2012): 483–90.
34. R. M. Puhl and K. M. King, "Weight Discrimination and Bullying: A Review," *Best Practices and Research Clinical Endocrinology and Metabolism* 27, no. 2 (2013): 117–27, http://dx.doi.org/10.1016/j.beem.2012.12.002; M. H. Schafer and K.F. Ferraro, "The Stigma of Obesity: Does Perceived Weight Discrimination Affect Identity and Physical Health?" *Social Psychology Quarterly* 74, no. 1 (2011): 76–97.
35. T. Lehey, J. LaRose, J. Fave, and R. Wing. "Social Influences Are Associated with BMI and Weight Loss Intentions in Young Adults," *Obesity* 19, no. 6 (2011): 1157–62.
36. C. Gillespie et al., "The Growing Concern of Poverty in the United States: An Exploration of Food Prices and Poverty on Obesity Rates for Low-Income Citizens," *Undergraduate Economic Review* 8, no. 1 (2012): 1–38.
37. J. F. Sallis et al.,"Role of Built Environments in Physical Activity, Obesity and Cardiovascular Disease," *Circulation* 125, no. 5 (2012): 729–37.
38. U.S. Department of Health and Human Services, "Summary Health Statistics for U.S. Adults: National Health Interview Survey, 2012," *Vital and Health Statistics* 10, no. 260 (2014), Available at www.cdc.gov/nchs/data/series/sr_10/sr10_260.pdf.
39. Centers for Disease Control and Prevention, "Prevalence of Underweight among Adults Aged 20 Years and Over: United

States 1960–1962 and 2007–2010," September 2012, www.cdc.gov/nchs/data/hestat/underweight_adult_07_10/underweight_adult_07_10.htm; Centers for Disease Control and Prevention, "Prevalence of Underweight among Children and Adolescents aged 2–19 Years: United States, 1963–1965 through 2007–2010, www.cdc.gov/nchs/data/hestat/underweight_child_07_10/underweight_child_07_10.htm.

40. Centers for Disease Control and Prevention, "About BMI for Adults," September 2011, www.cdc.gov/healthyweight/assessing/bmi/adult_bmi/index.html.
41. J. I. Mechanick et al., "Clinical Practice Guidelines for the Perioperative Nutritional, Metabolic and Nonsurgical Support of the Bariatric Surgery Patient—2013 Update," *Endocrine Practice* 19, no. 2 (2013): e1–36, www.aace.com/files/publish-ahead-of-print-final-version.pdf.
42. K. M. Flegal et al., "Prevalence and Trends in Obesity among U.S. Adults, 1999–2010," *Journal of the American Medical Association* 307, no. 5 (2012): 491–97.
43. American Heart Association, "Body Composition Tests," April 2013, www.heart.org/HEARTORG/GettingHealthy/NutritionCenter/Body-Composition-Tests_UCM_305883_Article.jsp; S. J. Mooney, A. Baecker, and A. G. Rundel, "Comparison of Anthropometric and Body Composition Measures as Predictors of Components of the metabolic Syndrome in the Clinical Setting," *Obesity Research and Clinical Practice* 7, no. 1 (2013): e55–e66.
44. C. L. Ogden et al., "Prevalence of Childhood and Adult Obesity in the United States," 2014; National Center for Health Statistics, "Health, United States, 2011: With Special Features on Socioeconomic Status and Health," Hyattsville, MD; U.S. Department of Health and Human Services, 2012, Available at www.cdc.gov/nchs/data/hus/hus11.pdf.
45. R. Puhl, "Weight Stigmatization toward Youth: A Significant Problem in Need of Societal Solutions," *Childhood Obesity* 7, no. 5 (2011): 359–63; S. A. Mustillo, K. Budd, and K. Hendrix, "Obesity, Labeling, and Psychological Distress in Late-Childhood and Adolescent Black and White Girls: The Distal Effects of Stigma," *Social Psychology Quarterly* 76, no. 3 (2013): 268–89.
46. L. Goh et al., "Anthropometric Measurements of General and Central Obesity and the Prediction of Cardiovascular Disease Risk in Women: A Cross-Sectional Study," *BMJ Open*. 2014. 4:e004138 doi:10.1136/bmjopen-2013-004138. http://bmjopen.bmj.com/content/4/2/e004138.full; M. Bombelli et al., "Impact of Body Mass Index and Waist Circumference on the Long Term Risk of Diabetes Mellitus, Hypertension and Cardiac Organ Damage," *Hypertension* 58, no. 6 (2011): 1029–1035; S. Czernichow et al., "Body Mass Index, Waist Circumference and Waist-Hip Ratio: Which is the Better Discriminator of Cardiovascular Disease Mortality Risk? Evidence from an Individual-Participant Meta-Analysis of 82,864 Participants from Nine Cohort Studies," *Obesity Reviews* 12, no. 9 (2011): 1467–78
47. National Heart, Lung, and Blood Institute, "Classification of Overweight and Obesity by BMI, Waist Circumference and Associated Disease Risks," 2012, www.nhlbi.nih.gov/health/public/heart/obesity/lose_wt/bmi_dis.htm.
48. University of Maryland Medical Center, Rush University, "Waist to Hip Ratio Calculator," Accessed March 2014, www.health-calculators.org/calculators/waist_hip.asp.
49. P. Brambilla et al., "Waist Circumference-to-Height Ratio Predicts Adiposity Better than Body Mass Index in Children and Adolescents," *International Journal of Obesity* 37, no. 7 (2013): 943–46.
50. World Health Organization, "Waist Circumference and Waist-Hip Ratio: Report of WHO Expert Consultation," 2011, http://whqlibdoc.who.int/publications/2011/9789241501491_eng.pdf.
51. V. M. Wheatley and J. Spink, "Defining the Public Health Threat of Dietary Supplement Fraud," *Comprehensive Reviews in Food Science and Food Safety* 12, no. 6 (2013): 599–613.
52. K. M. Flegal et al., "Association of ALL-Cause Mortality and Overweight Using Standard Body Mass Index Categories," *Journal of the American Medical Association* 309, no. 1 (2013): 71–82.
53. L. Gray, N. Cooper, A. Dunkley et al., "A Systematic Review and Mixed Treatment Comparison of Pharmacological Interventions for the Treatment of Obesity," *Obesity Reviews* 13, no. 6 (2012): 483–98.
54. Federal Drug Administration, "FDA Consumer Updates: HCG Diet Products are Illegal," March 2014, www.fda.gov/forconsumers/consumerupdates/ucm281333.htm.
55. Federal Drug Administration, "Questions and Answers about FDA's Initiative Against Contaminated Weight Loss Products," September 2013, www.fda.gov/drugs/resourcesforyou/consumers/questionsanswers/ucm136187.htm; U.S. Food and Drug Administration, "Follow-Up to the November 2009 Early Communication about an Ongoing Safety Review of Sibutramine, Marketed as Meridia," January 2010, www.fda.gov/Drugs/DrugSafety/PostmarketDrugSafetyInformationforPatientsandProviders/DrugSafetyInformationforHeathcareProfessionals/ucm198206.htm.
56. ConsumerSearch, "Diet Pills: Reviews," 2012, www.consumersearch.com/diet-pills.
57. C. E. Weber et al., "Obesity and Trends in Malpractice Claims for Physicians and Surgeons," *Surgery* 154, no. 2 (2013): 299–304.
58. Mayo Clinic, "Gastric Bypass Surgery," www.mayoclinic.com/health/gastric-bypass/MY00825.
59. John's Hopkins Health Library, "BPD/DS Weight-Loss Surgery," Accessed March 2014, www.hopkinsmedicine.org/health-library/test_procedures/gastroenterology/bpdds_weight-loss_surgery_135,64.
60. F. Rubino et al., "Metabolic Surgery to Treat Type 2 Diabetes: Clinical Outcomes and Mechanisms of Action," *Annual Review of Medicine* 61 (2010): 393–411; S. Brethauer et al., "Can Diabetes Be Surgically Cured? Long-Term Metabolic Effects of Bariatric Surgery in Obese Patients with Type 2 Diabetes Mellitus," *Annals of Surgery* 258, no. 4 (2013): 628–37.
61. D. E. Arterburn et al., "A Multi-SIte Study of Long Term Remission and Relapse of Type 2 Diabetes Mellitis Following Gastric Bypass Obesity Surgery," *Obesity Surgery* 23, no. 1 (2013): 93–102; C. D. Still et al., "Preoperative Prediction of Type 2 Diabetes Remission after Roux-en-Y Gastric Bypass Surgery: A Retrospective Cohort Study," *The Lancet Diabetes & Endocrinology* 2, no. 1 (2014): 38–45.

Pulled statistics:

p. 227, C. L. Ogden et al., "Prevalence of Childhood and Adult Obesity in the United States, 2011–2012" *JAMA* 311, no. 8(2014):806_814, doi:10.1001/jama.2014.732.

p. 232, C. D. Fryar and R. B. Ervin, "Caloric Intake from Fast Food among Adults: United States, 2007–2010," NCHS DATA BRIEF No. 114 (2013), www.cdc.gov.

Chapter 8A

1. University of the West of England, "30% of Women Would Trade at Least One Year of Their Life to Achieve Their Ideal Body Weight and Shape," March 2011, http://info.uwe.ac.uk/news/UWENews/news.aspx?id=1949.
2. M. Bucchianeri et al., "Body Dissatisfaction from Adolescence to Young Adulthood: Findings from a 10-Year Longitudinal Study," *Body Image* 10, no. 1, (2013): 1–7.
3. National Eating Disorder Association, "What Is Body Image?," 2014, http://www.nationaleatingdisorders.org/what-body-image.
4. University of Minnesota Health Talk, "Social Media May Inspire Unhealthy Body Image," May 2013, www.healthtalk.umn.edu/2013/05/15/thigh-gap-and-social-media.
5. Ibid.
6. Centers for Disease Control and Prevention, "FASTSTATS: Obesity and Overweight," November 2013, www.cdc.gov/nchs/fastats/overwt.htm.
7. J. B. Webb et al., "Do You See What I See?: An Exploration of Inter-Ethnic Ideal Body Size Comparisons among College Women" in *Body Image* 10, no. 3 (2013): 369–79.
8. Ibid.
9. E. Batha, "Mauritania Must Ban Deadly Force Feeding of Child Brides—Activists,"

Thomson Reuters Foundation, January 18, 2014, www.trust.org/item/20140117185616-fl4hq.

10. Mayo Clinic Staff, "Body Dysmorphic Disorder," May 2013, www.mayoclinic.com/health/body-dysmorphic-disorder/DS00559.
11. J. D. Feusner et al., "Abnormalities of object visual processing in body dysmorphic disorder," *Psychological Medicine* 41, no. 11 (2011): 2385–97, 1 DOI: 10.1017/S0033291711000572.
12. Body Image Health, "The Model for Healthy Body Image and Weight," Accessed March 2014, http://bodyimagehealth.org/model-for-healthy-body-image.
13. I. Ahmed et al., "Body Dysmorphic Disorder," Medscape Reference, January 2014, http://emedicine.medscape.com/article/291182-overview.
14. Mayo Clinic Staff, "Body Dysmorphic Disorder," 2013; KidsHealth, "Body Dysmorphic Disorder," May 2013, http://kidshealth.org/parent/emotions/feelings/bdd.html.
15. I. Ahmed et al., "Body Dysmorphic Disorder," 2014.
16. J. Reel, *Eating Disorders: An Encyclopedia of Causes, Treatment and Prevention*, (New York, NY: Greenwood Publishing, 2013); A. Taheri et al., "The Relationship between Social Physique Anxiety and Anthropometric Characteristics of the Nonathletic Female Students," *Annals of Biological Research* 3, no. 6 (2012): 2727–29; A. Sicilia et al, "Exercise Motivation and Social Physique Anxiety in Adolescents," *Psychologica Belgica* 54, no. 1 (2014): 111–29, DOI: http://dx.doi.org/10.5334/pb.ai.
17. American Psychiatric Association, "Feeding and Eating Disorders," 2013, http://www.dsm5.org/documents/eating%20disorders%20fact%20sheet.pdf.
18. Academy for Eating Disorders, "Prevalence of Eating Disorders," 2014, www.aedweb.org/Prevalence_of_ED.htm.
19. Danielle A. Gagne et al., "Eating Disorder Symptoms and Weight and Shape Concerns in a Large Web-based Convenience Sample of Women Ages 50 and Above: Results of the Gender and Body Image (GABI) Study," *International Journal of Eating Disorders* 45, no. 7 (2012): 832–44, DOI: 10.1002/eat.22030.
20. American College Health Association, *National College Health Assessment II: Undergraduates Reference Group Executive Summary Spring 2013* (Linthicum, MD: American College Health Association, 2013), Available at www.acha-ncha.org/reports_ACHA-NCHAII.html.
21. L. M. Gottschlich, "Female Athlete Triad," Medscape Reference, Drugs, Diseases & Procedures, January 25, 2012, http://emedicine.medscape.com/article/89260-overview#a0156.
22. Alliance for Eating Disorder Awareness, "What Are Eating Disorders?," 2013, www.allianceforeatingdisorders.com/portal/what-are-eating-disorders#.Uycs4_Pn9lY.
23. Ibid.
24. S. A. Swanson et al., "Prevalence and Correlates of Eating Disorders in Adolescents: Results from the National Comorbidity Survey Replication Adolescent Supplement," *Archives of General Psychiatry* 68, no. 7 (2011): 714–23, DOI: 10.1001/archgenpsychiatry.2011.22.
25. The Alliance for Eating Disorders Awareness, "DSM-V Diagnostic Criteria," 2013, http://www.allianceforeatingdisorders.com/portal/dsm-anorexia#.U3QHd_Pn9lY.
26. National Eating Disorders Association, "Anorexia Nervosa," Accessed April 2014, www.nationaleatingdisorders.org/anorexia-nervosa.
27. P. Crocker et al., "Body-Related State Shame and Guilt in Women: Do Causal Attributions Mediate the Influence of Physical Self-concept and Shame and Guilt Proneness," *Body Image* 11, no. 1 (2013): 19–26; A. R. Smith, T. E. Joiner, and D. R. Dodd, "Examining Implicit Attitudes Toward Emaciation and Thinness in Anorexia Nervosa," *International Journal of Eating Disorders* 47, no. 2 (2013): 138–47; R. N. Carey, N. Donaghue, and P. Broderick, "Concern among Australian Adolescent Girls: The Role of Body Comparisons with Models and Peers," *Body Image* 11, no. 1 (2014): 81–84.
28. A.D.A.M. Medical Encyclopedia, U.S. National Library of Medicine, "Anorexia Nervosa," February 2013, www.ncbi.nlm.nih.gov/pubmedhealth/PMH0001401/; B. Suchan et al., "Reduced Connectivity between the Left Fusiform Body Area and the Extrastriate Body Area in Anorexia Nervosa Is Associated with Body Image Distortion," *Behavioural Brain Research* 241 (2013): 80–85, DOI: 10.1016/j.bbr.2012.12.002; G. Frank et al., "Altered Temporal Difference Learning in Bulimia Nervosa," *Biological Psychiatry* 70, no. 8 (2011): 728–35, DOI: 10.1016/j.biopsych.2011.05.011.
29. R. Kessler et al., "The Prevalence and Correlates of Binge Eating Disorder in the World Health Organization World Mental Health Surveys," *Biological Psychiatry* 73, no. 9 (2013): 904–14, DOI: 10.1016/j.biopsych.2012.11.020.
30. The Alliance for Eating Disorders Awareness, "DSM-5 Diagnostic Criteria," 2013, http://www.allianceforeatingdisorders.com/portal/dsm-bulimia#.U3QHofPn9lY.
31. National Institute of Mental Health, "Eating Disorders," January 2013, www.nimh.nih.gov/health/topics/eating-disorders/index.shtml.
32. T. A. Oberndorfer et al., "Altered Insula Response to Sweet Taste Processing After Recovery from Anorexia and Bulimia Nervosa," *American Journal of Psychiatry* 170, no. 10 (2013): 1143–51.
33. Mayo Clinic, "Binge-Eating Disorder," April 2012, www.mayoclinic.com/health/binge-eating-disorder/DS00608.
34. R. Kessler et al., "The Prevalence and Correlates of Binge Eating Disorder," 2013.
35. The Alliance for Eating Disorders Awareness, "DSM-5 Diagnostic Criteria," 2013, http://www.allianceforeatingdisorders.com/portal/dsm-bulimia#.U3QHofPn9lY.
36. National Eating Disorder Association, "Other Specified Feeding or Eating Disorder," Accessed March 2014, www.nationaleatingdisorders.org/other-specified-feeding-or-eating-disorder.
37. K. N. Franco, Cleveland Clinic Center for Continuing Education, "Eating Disorders," 2011, www.clevelandclinicmeded.com/medicalpubs/diseasemanagement/psychiatry-psychology/eating-disorders; Mirasol Eating Disorder Recovery Centers, "Eating Disorder Statistics," Accessed March 2014, www.mirasol.net/eating-disorders/information/eating-disorder-statistics.php.
38. M. Smith, L. Robinson, and J. Segal, "Helping Someone with an Eating Disorder," *Helpguide.org*, February 2014, www.helpguide.org/mental/eating_disorder_self_help.htm; C. Biggs, "On the Outside: Helping a Friend through an Eating Disorder," *Act: Every Action Counts*, February 28, 2013, http://act.mtv.com/posts/neda-week-helping-a-friend-through-an-eating-disorder.
39. National Eating Disorder Association, "Find Help and Support," Accessed March 2014, www.nationaleatingdisorders.org/find-help-support.
40. H. Goodwin, E. Haycraft, and C. Meyer, "The Relationship between Compulsive Exercise and Emotion Regulation in Adolescents," *British Journal of Health Psychology* 17, no. 4 (2012): 699–710.
41. J. J. Waldron, "When Building Muscle Turns into Muscle Dysmorphia," Association for Sport Applied Psychology, Accessed March 2014, www.appliedsportpsych.org/resource-center/health-fitness-resources/when-building-muscle-turns-into-muscle-dysmorphia.
42. M. Silverman, "What is Muscle Dysmorphia?" Massachusetts General Hospital, February 18, 2011, https://mghocd.org/what-is-muscle-dysmorphia; J. J. Waldron, "When Building Muscle Turns into Muscle Dysmorphia," 2014.
43. L. M. Gottschlich et al., "Female Athlete Triad," 2014.
44. Brown University Health Education, "The Female Athlete Triad," Accessed March 2014, www.brown.edu/Student_Services/Health_Services/Health_Education/nutrition_&_eating_concerns/eating_concerns/female_athlete_triad.php.

Pulled statistics:

p. 250, C. Ross, "Why Do Women Hate Their Bodies?" World of Psychology (blog), Psych Central, June 2, 2012, http://psychcentral.com/blog/archives/2012/06/02/why-do-women-hate-their-bodies.

p. 260, National Eating Disorders Association, "Factsheet on Eating Disorders," 2010, http://www.umassmed.edu/uploadedFiles/eap2/resources/Mental_Health/Eating_Disorders/NEDA%20Fact%20sheet.pdf; T. Pekar, "Eating Disorders: Do Men and Women Differ?" *Science of Eating Disorders: Making Sense of the Latest Findings in Eating Disorder Research* (blog), July 3, 2012.

Chapter 9

1. A. Rausrop and M. Lindwall, "Physical Self-Esteem—A Ten-Year Follow-Up Study from Early Adolescence to Early Adulthood," *International Journal of Adolescent Medicine and Health,* doi: 10.1515/ijamh-2014-0001 (e-pub ahead of print); T. Baghurst and B. C. Kelley, "An Examination of Stress in College Students Over the Course of a Semester," *Health Promotion Practice 15,* no. 3(2014):438–447; C. Huang et al., "Cardiovascular Reactivity, Stress, and Physical Activity," *Frontiers in Physiology* 4(2013): 1–13, doi:10.3389/fphys.201300314.
2. Centers for Disease Control and Prevention, "Behavioral Risk Factor Surveillance System Prevalence and Trends Data," Accessed March 2014, http://apps.nccd.cdc.gov/BRFSS/display.asp?yr=2012&state=US&qkey=8041&grp=0&SUBMIT3=Go.
3. C. E. Garber et al., "American College of Sports Medicine Position Stand: Quantity and Quality of Exercise for Developing and Maintaining Cardiorespiratory, Musculoskeletal and Neuromotor Fitness in Apparently Healthy Adults: Guidance for Prescribing Exercise," *Medicine and Science in Sports and Exercise* 33, no. 7 (2011): 1334–59, DOI: 10.1249/MSS.0b013e318213fefb.
4. American College Health Association, *American College Health Association-National College Health Assessment II (ACHA-NCHA II) Reference Group Executive Summary Spring 2013* (Hanover, MD: American College Health Association, 2013), http://www.acha-ncha.org.
5. National Heart, Lung, and Blood Institute, U.S. Department of Health and Human Services, National Institutes of Health, "What Is Physical Activity," Updated September 2011, www.nhlbi.nih.gov/health/health-topics/topics/phys/; Office of Disease Prevention and Health Promotion, *2008 Physical Activity Guidelines for Americans, 2008.*
6. P. Kokkinos, H. Sheriff, and R. Kheirbek, "Physical Inactivity and Mortality Risk," *Cardiology Research and Practice* 11 (2011): 924–49, Article ID 924945, www.hindawi.com/journals/crp/2011/924945; D. Lemanne, B. Cassileth, and J. Gubili, "The Role of Physical Activity in Cancer, Prevention, and Treatment," *Oncology 27,* no. 6(2013): 580–585; H. Silveira et al., "Physical Exercise and Clinically Depressed Patients: A Systematic Review and Meta-Analysis," *Neurospychology 67* (2013): 61–68; D. L. Swift et al., "The Role of Exercise and Physical Activity in Weight Loss and Maintenance," *Progress in Cardiovascular Diseases 56* (2014): 441–447.
7. I. Lee et al., "Impact of Physical Inactivity on the World's Major Non-communicable Diseases," *Lancet* 380, no. 9838 (2012): 219–29.
8. S. Plowman and D. Smith, *Exercise Physiology for Health, Fitness, and Performance,* 3rd ed. (Philadelphia: Lippincott Williams & Wilkins, 2011).
9. S. Grover et al., "Estimating the Benefits of Patient and Physician Adherence to Cardiovascular Prevention Guidelines: The MyHealthCheckup Survey," *Canadian Journal of Cardiology* 27, no. 2 (2011): 159–66.
10. American Heart Association, "About Cholesterol," Updated May 1 2013, www.heart.org/HEARTORG/Conditions/Cholesterol/AboutCholesterol/AboutCholesterol_UCM_001220_Article.jsp.
11. L. Montesi et al., "Physical Activity for the Prevention and Treatment of Metabolic Disorders," *Internal and Emergency Medicine* 8, no. 8 (2013): 655–66.
12. Ibid.
13. D. C. Lee, et al., "Changes in Fitness and Fatness on the Development of Cardiovascular Disease Risk Factors Hypertension, Metabolic Syndrome, and Hypercholesterolemia," *Journal of the American College of Cardiology* 59, no. 7 (2012): 665–72.
14. M. Uusitupa, J. Tuomilehto, and P. Puska, "Are We Really Active in the Prevention of Obesity and Type 2 Diabetes at the Community Level?," *Nutrition and Metabolism in Cardiovascular Diseases* 21, no. 5 (2011): 380–89, DOI: 10.1016/j.numecd.2010.12.007
15. National Diabetes Information Clearinghouse, U.S. Department of Health and Human Services, *Diabetes Prevention Program (DPP),* NIH Publication no. 09–5099 (Bethesda, MD: National Diabetes Information Clearinghouse, 2008), Available at http://diabetes.niddk.nih.gov/dm/pubs/preventionprogram.
16. N. Magné et al., "Recommendations for a Lifestyle Which Could Prevent Breast Cancer and Its Relapse: Physical Activity and Dietetic Aspects," *Critical Reviews in Oncology and Hematology* 80, no. 3 (2011): 450–59, DOI: 10.1016/j.critrevonc.2011.01.013
17. L. H. Kushi et al., "American Cancer Society Guidelines on Nutrition and Physical Activity for Cancer Prevention," *CA: A Cancer Journal for Clinicians* 62, no. 1 (2012): 30–67.
18. World Cancer Research Fund/American Institute for Cancer Research, Policy and Action for Cancer Prevention, "Food, Nutrition, and Physical Activity: A Global Perspective" (Washington DC: AICR, 2009); A. Shibata, K. Ishii, and K. Oka, "Psychological, Social, and Environmental Factors of Meeting Recommended Physical Activity Levels for Colon Cancer Prevention among Japanese Adults," *Journal of Science and Medicine in Sport* 12, no. 2 (2010): e155–6; K. Y. Wolin et al., "Physical Activity and Colon Cancer Prevention: A Meta-Analysis," *British Journal of Cancer* 100, no. 4 (2009): 611–16.
19. C. M. Friedenreich and A. E. Cust, "Physical Activity and Breast Cancer Risk: Impact of Timing, Type, and Dose of Activity and Population Subgroup Effects," *British Journal of Sports Medicine* 42, no. 8 (2008): 636–47).
20. V. Gremeaux et al., "Exercise and Longevity," *Maturitas 73*(2012): 312–317.
21. R. Rizzoli, C A. Abraham, and M. L. Brandi, "Nutrition and Bone Health: Turning Knowledge and Beliefs in Healthy Behavior," *Current Medical Research & Opinion* 30, no. 1 (2014): 131–41.
22. D. L. Swift et al., "The Role of Exercise and Physical Activity in Weight Loss and Maintenance," *Progress in Cardiovascular Diseases 56* (2014): 441–447.
23. T. L. Gillum et al., "A Review of Sex Differences in Immune Function after Aerobic Exercise," *Exercise Immunology Review* 17 (2011):104–20.
24. MedLine Plus, National Institutes of Health, "Exercise and Immunity," May 2012, www.nlm.nih.gov/medlineplus/ency/article/007165.htm.
25. N. P. Walsh et al., "Position Statement. Part Two: Maintaining Immune Health," *Exercise and Immunology Review* 17 (2011): 64–103.
26. T. L. Gillum et al., "A Review of Sex Differences in Immune Function after Aerobic Exercise," *Exercise Immuniology Review* 17 (2011): 104–120.
27. C. Huang et al., "Cardiovascular Reactivity, Stress, and Physical Activity," *Frontiers in Physiology* 4 (2013): 1–13 doi:10.3389/fphys.201300314.
28. T. M. Burkhalter and C. H. Hillman, "A Narrative Review of Physical Activity, Nutrition, and Obesity to Cognitive and Scholastic Performance across the Human Lifespan," *Advances in Nutrition: An International Review Journal* 2, no. 2 (2011): 201S –206S.
29. J. E. Ashlskog, Y. E. Geda, N. R. Graff-Radford, and R. C. Petersen, "Physical Exercise as a Preventive or Disease-Modifying Treatment of Dementia and Brain Aging," *Mayo Clinic Proceedings* 86, no. 9 (2011): 876–84.
30. J. Berry et al., "Lifetime Risks for Cardiovascular Disease Mortality by Cardiorespiratory Fitness Levels Measured at Ages 45, 55, and 65 Years in Men: The Cooper Center Longitudinal Study," *Journal of the American College of Cardiology* 57, no. 15 (2011): 1604–10; J. Woodcock et al., "Non-Vigorous Physical Activity and All-Cause Mortality: Systematic Review and Meta-Analysis of Cohort Studies," *International Journal of Epidemiology* 40, no. 1 (2011): 121–38.
31. A. F. Ambrose, G. Paul., and J. M. Hausdorff, "Risk Factors for Falls among Older

Adults: A Review of the Literature," *Maturitas 75* (2013): 51–61.

32. C. E. Garber et al., "American College of Sports Medicine Position Stand: Quantity and Quality of Exercise for Developing and Maintaining Cardiorespiratory, Musculoskeletal and Neuromotor Fitness in Apparently Healthy Adults: Guidance for Prescribing Exercise," *Medicine and Science in Sports and Exercise* 43, no. 7 (2011): 1334–59
33. Ibid.
34. Ibid.
35. American College of Sports Medicine, *ACSM's Resource Manual for Guidelines for Exercise Testing and Prescription* (Philadelphia, PA: Lippincott Williams & Wilkins, 2014).
36. W. Micheo, L. Baerga, and G. Miranda, "Basic Principles Regarding Strength, Flexibility, Flexibility, and Stability Exercises," *Physical Medicine & Rehabilitation* 4, no. 11 (2012): 805–11, DOI: 10.1016/j.pmrj.2012.09.583
37. Ibid.
38. M. Pahor et al., "Effect of structured physical activity on prevention of major mobility disability in older adults The LIFE Study randomized clinical trial," JAMA doi:10.1001/jama.2014.5616
39. American College of Sports Medicine, "Guidelines for Exercise Testing and Prescription," 9th edition, (Philadelphia, PA, Lippincot, Williams, & Wilkins, 2014).
40. Ibid.
41. D. G. Behm and A. Chaouachi, "A Review of the Acute Effects of Static and Dynamic Stretching on Performance," *European Journal of Applied Physiology* 111, no. 11 (2011): 2633–51.
42. K. C. Huxel Bliven and B. E. Anderson, "Core Stability Training for Injury Prevention," *Sports Health: A Multidisciplinary Approach* 5, no.6 (2013): 514–22.
43. Ibid.
44. D. G. Behm and J. C. Colao Sanchez, "Instability Resistance Training across the Exercise Continuum," *Sports Health: A Multidisciplinary Approach* 5, no.6 (2013): 500–503.
45. Ibid.
46. Ibid.
47. M. N. Sawka et al., "American College of Sports Medicine Position Stand: Exercise and Fluid Replacement," *Medicine and Science in Sports and Exercise* 39, no. 2 (2007): 377–90.
48. Ibid.
49. K. Pritchett and R. Pritchett, "Chocolate Milk: Post-Exercise Recovery Beverage for Endurance Sports," *Medicine and Sports Science* 59 (2011): 127–34.
50. S. Cutts, N. Obi, C. Pasapula, and W. Chan, "Plantar Fasciitis," *Annals of the Royal College of Surgeons of England* 94, no.8 (2012): 539–42.
51. P. Newman et al., "Risk Factors Associated with Medial Tibial Stress Syndrome in Runners: A Systematic Review and Meta-Analysis," *Open Access Journal of Sports Medicine* 4 (2013): 229–41.
52. J. A. Rixe et al., "A Review of the Management of Patellofemoral Pain Syndrome," *The Physician and Sportsmedicine* 41, no. 3 (2013): 19–28.
53. K. B. Fields et al., "Prevention of Running Injuries," *Current Sports Medicine Reports* 9, no. 3 (2010): 176–82.
54. American Academy of Ophthalmology, "Eye Health in Sports and Recreation," March 2014, www.aao.org/eyesmart/injuries/eyewear.cfm.
55. Ibid.
56. Bicycle Helmet Safety Institute, "Helmet-Related Statistics from Many Sources," January 2014, www.helmets.org/stats.htm.
57. American College Health Association, *National College Health Assessment II: Reference Group Data Report, Spring 2013*, 2013.
58. Bicycle Helmet Safety Institute, "Helmet-Related Statistics from Many Sources," January 2014, www.helmets.org/stats.htm.
59. N. G. Nelson et al., "Evectional Heat-Related Injuries Treated in Emergency Departments in the U.S., 1997–2006," *American Journal of Preventive Medicine* 40, no. 1 (2011): 54–60.

Pulled statistics:

p. 267, U.S. Department of Health and Human Services, "Physical Activity," *HealthyPeople.Gov: 2020 Topics & Objectives,* Updated April 10, 2013, www.healthypeople.gov.

p. 275, Centers for Disease Control and Prevention, "How Much Physical Activity Do Adults Need?" Physical Activity for Everyone, updated December 1, 2011, www.cdc.gov; Office of Disease Prevention and Health Promotion, "Making America Healthier 10 Minutes at a Time," Be Active Your Way, Blog, May 9, 2013, www.health.gov.

Chapter 9A

1. American Society of Addiction Medicine, "Definition of Addiction," April 2011, www.asam.org/research-treatment/definition-of-addiction.
2. S. S. Alavi et al., "Behavioral Addiction versus Substance Addiction: Correspondence of Psychiatric and Psychological Views," *International Journal of Preventive Medicine* 3, no. 4 (2012): 290–294.
3. J. Grant et al., "Introduction to Behavioral Addictions," *American Journal of Behavioral Addictions* 36, no. 5 (2010): 233–41.
4. National Institute on Drug Abuse, "Drugs, Brains, and Behavior: The Science of Addiction," August 2010, www.drugabuse.gov/publications/science-addiction.
5. American Society of Addiction Medicine, "Definition of Addiction," April 2011, www.asam.org/for-the-public/definition-of-addiction.
6. J. Burns et al., "Delirium Tremens (DTs)," *Medscape* 2013, http://emedicine.medscape.com/article/166032-overview#a0156.
7. J. Kinney, *Loosening the Grip: A Handbook of Alcohol Information,* 10th ed. (Boston: McGraw-Hill, 2012), 175.
8. Howard J. Edenberg, "Genes Contributing to the Development of Alcoholism," *Alcohol Research: Current Reviews* 34, no. 3 (2012): 336–38.
9. T. Foroud et al., "Genetic Research: Who Is at Risk for Alcoholism," *Alcohol Research & Health* 33, No. 1 and 2 (2010): 64–75; A. Agrawal et al., "Linkage Scan for Quantitative Traits Identifies New Regions of Interest," *Drug Alcohol Depend* 93, no. 1 and 2 (2008): 12–20; American Society of Addiction Medicine, "Definition of Addiction," 2011.
10. J. Kinney, *Loosening the Grip,* 2012, 106.
11. G. Hanson and P. Venturelli, *Drugs and Society,* 11th ed. (Sudbury, MA: Jones and Bartlett, 2011), 49.
12. Ibid, 4.
13. J. Grant et al., "Introduction to Behavioral Addictions," 2010; National Institute on Drug Abuse, National Institutes of Health, U.S. Department of Health and Human Services, *Drugs, Brains, and Behavior: The Science of Addiction,* NIH Publication no. 07-5605 (Bethesda, MD: National Institute on Drug Abuse, Revised 2010), Available at www.nida.nih.gov/scienceofaddiction.
14. National Council on Problem Gambling, "FAQs—Problem Gamblers," Accessed September 28, 2011, www.ncpgambling.org/i4a/pages/index.cfm?pageid=3390.
15. American Psychiatric Association, *Diagnostic and Statistical Manual of Mental Disorders,* 5th ed. (Arlington, VA: American Psychiatric Publishing, 2013), p. 585.
16. National Council on Problem Gambling, "FAQs—Problem Gamblers," Accessed September 28, 2011.
17. D. W. Black et al., "A Direct, Controlled, Blind Family Study of DSM-IV Pathological Gambling." *The Journal of Clinical Psychiatry* 75, no. 3 (2014): 215–221; K-L Chou and T Afifi, "Disordered (Pathologic or Problem) Gambling and Axis I Psychiatric Disorders: Results from the National Epidemiologic Survey on Alcohol and Related Conditions," *Am. J. Epidemiol.* 173, no. 11 (2011): 1289–1297, doi: 10.1093/aje/kwr017; American Psychiatric Association, *Diagnostic and Statistical Manual of Mental Disorders,* 5th ed. (Arlington, VA: American Psychiatric Publishing, 2013), p. 589.
18. National Center for Responsible Gambling, "College Students: Facts and Stats," Accessed March 2014, www.collegegambling.org/just-facts/gambling-college-campuses.
19. Ibid.
20. H. Hatfield, "Shopping Spree or Addiction?" *WebMD*, 2014, www.webmd.com/mental-health/features/shopping-spree-addiction; M. Lejoyeux and A. Weinstein, "Compulsive

Buying," *The American Journal of Drug and Alcohol Issues* 36, no. 5 (2010): 248–53.

21. Ibid.
22. A. Harvanko et al., "Prevalence and Characteristics of Compulsive Buying in College Students," *Psychiatry Research* 210 (2013):1079–85.
23. Ibid.
24. K. Deryshire et al., "Problematic Internet Use and Associated Risks in a College Sample," *Comprehensive Psychiatry* 54, no. 5 (2013): 415–22.
25. Ibid.
26. Pew Research Internet Project, "Health Fact Sheet," December 2013, www.pewinternet.org/fact-sheets/health-fact-sheet.
27. eMarketer, "Digital Set to Surpass TV in Time Spent with US Media," August 2013, www.emarketer.com/Article/Digital-Set-Surpass-TV-Time-Spent-with-US-Media/1010096.
28. M. Duggan et al., "The Demographics of Social Media," *Pew Internet & American Life Project*, 2013, http://pewinternet.org/Reports/2013/Social-media-users.aspx.
29. Ibid.
30. A. Alexander, "Internet Addiction Statistics 2012," April 24, 2012, http://ansonalex.com/infographics/internet-addiction-statistics-2012-infographic.
31. J. Anthony et al., "Problematic Internet Use and Other Risky Behaviors in College Students: An Application of Problem-Behavior Theory," *American Psychological Association* 27 no. 1 (2012): 133–41.
32. American College Health Association, *American College Health Association—National College Health Assessment II: Reference Group Data Report Spring 2013* (Baltimore. MD: American College Health Association, 2013).
33. EDUCAUSEreviewOnline, "Exploring Students' Mobile Learning Practices in Higher Education," October 7, 2013, www.educause.edu/ero/article/exploring-students-mobile-learning practices higher-education.
34. re:fuel, "Tech-Savvy College Students Are Gathering Gadgets, Saying Yes to Showrooming and Rejecting Second Screening," June 13,2013, www.globenewswire.com/news-release/2013/06/13/554002/10036312/en/Tech-Savvy-College-Students-Are-Gathering-Gadgets-Saying-Yes-to-Showrooming-and-Rejecting-Second-Screening.html.
35. Wordpress.com, "How Much Time Do College Students Spend with Technology?" June 2013, www.researchresults.wordpress.com/2013/06/28/how-much-time-do-college-students-spend-with-technology.
36. S. Sussman, "Workaholism: A Review," *Journal of Addiction Research and Therapy* 10, no. 6 (2012): 4120, www.ncbi.nlm.nih.gov/pmc/articles/PMC3835604.
37. Ibid.
38. Ibid.
39. M. Clark, et al., "All Work and No Play? A Meta-Analytic Examination of the Correlates and Outcomes of Workaholism," *Journal of Management*, February 28, 2014: 1–38, http://jom.sagepub.com/content/early/2014/02/28/0149206314522301.full.pdf+html.
40. L. Kravina et al., "Workalcoholism and Work Engagement in the Family: The Relationship Between Parents and Children as a Risk Factor," *European Journal of Work and Organizational Psychology* September 17, 2013.
41. M. Clark, et al., "All Work and No Play? A Meta-Analytic Examination of the Correlates and Outcomes of Workaholism," *Journal of Management*, February 28, 2014: 1–38, http://jom.sagepub.com/content/early/2014/02/28/0149206314522301.full.pdf+html.
42. K. Berczik et al., "Exercise Addiction: Symptoms, Diagnosis, Epidemiology and Etiology," *Substance Use and Misuse* 47 (2012): 403–17.
43. R. Weiss, "Hypersexuality: Symptoms of Sexual Addiction," *Psych Central*, March 2014, http://psychcentral.com/lib/hypersexuality-symptoms-of-sexual-addiction.
44. Ibid; Mayo Clinic, "Compulsive Sexual Behavior," September 2011, www.mayoclinic.org/diseases-conditions/compulsive-sexual-behavior/basics/risk-factors/con-20020126.
45. Substance Abuse and Mental Health Services Administration, Center for Behavioral Health Statistics and Quality, "Treatment Episode Data Set (TEDS): 2000–2010. National Admissions to Substance Abuse Treatment Services," 2012, DASIS Series S-61, HHS Publication No. (SMA) 12-4701 (Rockville, MD: Substance Abuse and Mental Health Services Administration), Available at www.samhsa.gov/data/2k12/TEDS2010N/TEDS2010NWeb.pdf.
46. National Center on Addiction and Substance Abuse, "Addiction Medicine: Closing the Gap Between Science and Practice," June, 2012

Pulled statistics:

p. 294, National Council on Problem Gambling, "College Gambling Facts and Statistics," 2014, http://www.ncpgambling.org/files/NPGAWcollegefactsheet.pdf.

p. 296, Center for Personal Finance Editors, "Tough Times Series: It Was Such a Bargain: Help for Compulsive Shoppers" 2014 http://hffo.cuna.org/12433/article/353/html.

p. 297, S. Li, "Our Addiction to Technology Trumps Caffeine, Chocolate and Alcohol," Technology: The Business and Culture of Our Digital Lives (blog), *Los Angeles Times*, August 11, 2011, http://latimesblogs.latimes.com/technology/2011/08/technology-addiction-chocolate-caffeine.html.

Chapter 10

1. G. Chiva-Blanch et al., "Effects of Wine, Alcohol and Polyphenols on Cardiovascular Disease Risk Factors: Evidences from Human Studies," *Alcohol and Alcoholism* 48, no.3 (2013): 270–277.
2. T. Naimi et al., "Confounding and Studies of 'Moderate' Alcohol Consumption: The Case of Drinking Frequency and Implications for Low Risk Drinking Guidelines," *Addiction*, 108, no. 9 (2013): 1534–43; J. Marrone et al., "Moderate Alcohol Intake Lowers Biochemical Markers of Bone Turnover in Postmenopausal Women," *Menopause* 19, no. 9 (2012): 974–79; C. Stockley, "Is It Merely a Myth That Alcoholic Beverages Such as Red Wine Can Be Cardioprotective?," *Journal of the Science of Food and Agriculture* 92, no. 9 (2012): 1815–21; A. Klatsky, "Alcohol and Cardiovascular Health," *Physiology and Behavior* 100, no. 1 (2010): 76–81.
3. National Center for Health Statistics, "Summary Health Statistics for U.S. Adults: National Health Interview Survey, 2012," *Vital and Health Statistics* 10, no. 260 (2014): 34.
4. Ibid.
5. Centers for Disease Control and Prevention, "Vital Signs: Binge Drinking," October 2013, www.cdc.gov/Vitalsigns/BingeDrinking.
6. M.Davalos et al., "Easing the Pain of An Economic Downturn: Macroeconomic Conditions and Excessive Alcohol Consumption," *Health Economics* 21, no. 11 (2012): 1318–35.
7. National Institute on Alcohol Abuse and Alcoholism, "Apparent Per Capita Alcohol Consumption: National, State and Regional Trends, 1977–2010," August 2012, http://pubs.niaaa.nih.gov/publications/Surveillance95/CONS10.htm.
8. D. J. Rohsenow et al., "Hangover Sensitivity after Controlled Alcohol Administration as Predictor of Post-College Drinking," *Journal of Abnormal Psychology* 121, no. 1 (2012): 270–75.
9. M. A.White et al., "Hospitalizations for Alcohol and Drug Overdoses in Young Adults Ages 18–24 in the United States, 1999–2008: Results from the Nationwide Inpatient Sample," *Journal of Studies on Alcohol and Drugs* 72, no. 5 (2011): 774–76.
10. National Institute on Alcohol Abuse and Alcoholism, "Drinking Can Put a Chill on Your Summer Fun," May 2012, http://pubs.niaaa.nih.gov/publications/SummerSafety/SummerSafety.htm; Centers for Disease Control and Prevention, "Unintentional Drowning: Get the Facts," November 2012, www.cdc.gov/HomeandRecreationalSafety/Water-Safety/waterinjuries-factsheet.html.
11. Centers for Disease Control and Prevention, "Injury Prevention and Control: Home and Recreational Safety: Fire Deaths and Injuries: Fact Sheet," October 2011, www.cdc.gov/HomeandRecreationalSafety/Fire-Prevention/fires-factsheet.html.
12. U.S. Department of Health and Human Services (HHS) Office of the Surgeon General and National Action Alliance for Suicide

Prevention, "2012 National Strategy for Suicide Prevention: Goals and Objectives for Action," September 2012, www.surgeongeneral.gov/library/reports/national-strategy-suicide-prevention/full-report.pdf.
13. American College Health Association, *American College Health Association—National College Health Assessment II: Reference Group Executive Summary Spring 2013* (Linthicum, MD: American College Health Association, 2014), Available at www.acha-ncha.org/reports_ACHA NCHAII.html.
14. Bureau of Justice Statistics, "Criminal Victimization in the United States, 2008 Table 32, Percent Distribution of Victimizations by Perceived Drug or Alcohol Use by Offender, 2008," May 2011, www.bjs.gov/content/pub/pdf/cvus0802.pdf
15. S. Lawyer et al., "Forcible, Drug-Facilitated, and Incapacitated Rape and Sexual Assault among Undergraduate Women," *Journal of American College Health* 58, no. 5 (2010): 453–60.
16. Ibid.
17. National Institute of Justice, "The Campus Sexual Assault Study," 2007, Available at www.ncjrs.gov/pdffiles1/nij/grants/221153.pdf.
18. M. J. Griffin et al., "Recent Sexual Victimization and Drinking Behavior in Newly Matriculated College Students: A Latent Growth Analysis," *Psychology of Addictive Behaviors* 27, no. 4 (2013): 966–73.
19. C. Stappenbeck, "A Longitudinal Investigation of Heavy Drinking and Physical Dating Violence in Men and Women," *Addictive Behaviors* 35, no. 5 (2010): 479–85.
20. S. J. Nielsen et al., "Calories Consumed from Alcoholic Beverages by U.S. Adults, 2007–2010," *NCHS Data Brief,* no. 110 (2012), Available at www.cdc.gov.
21. M. Silveri, "Adolescent Brain Development and Underage Drinking in the United States: Identifying Risks of Alcohol Use in College Populations," *Harvard Review of Psychiatry* 20, no. 4 (2012): 189–200.
22. Ibid.
23. L. Arriola et al., "Alcohol Intake and the Risk of Coronary Heart Disease in Spanish EPIC Cohort Study," *Heart* 96, no. 10 (2010): 124–30; T. Wilson et al., eds., "Should Moderate Alcohol Consumption be Promoted?" *Nutrition and Health: Nutrition Guide for Physicians* (New York: Humana Press, 2010); The American Heart Association, "Alcohol and Cardiovascular Disease," 2011, www.heart.org/HEARTORG/Conditions/Alcohol-and-Cardiovascular-Disease_UCM_305173_Article.jsp.
24. Ibid.
25. The American Heart Association, "Alcohol and Cardiovascular Disease," 2011.
26. H. K. Seitz and P. Becker, "Alcohol Metabolism and Cancer Risk," *Alcohol Research and Health* 30, no. 1 (2007): 38–47, Available at http://pubs.niaaa.nih.gov/publications/arh301/38-47.htm.
27. W. Y. Chen et al., "Moderate Alcohol Consumption during Adult Life, Drinking Patterns, and Breast Cancer Risk," *Journal of the American Medical Association* 306, no. 17 (2011): 1884–90.
28. H. K. Seitz, "Epidemiology and Pathophysiology of Alcohol and Breast Cancer: Update 2012" *Alcohol and Alcoholism* 47, no. 3 (2012): 204–212.
29. C. S. Berkey et al., "Prospective Study of Adolescent Alcohol Consumption and Risk of Benign Breast Disease in Young Women," *Pediatrics* 125, no. 5 (2010): e1081–87.
30. I. O. Ebrahim et al., "Alcohol and Sleep: Effects on Normal Sleep," *Alcoholism: Clinical and Experimental Research* 37, no. 4 (2013): 539–49; I. Popovici et al., "Binge Drinking and Sleep Problems among Young Adults," *Drug and Alcohol Dependence* 132, no. 1 (2013): 207–15.
31. Centers for Disease Control and Prevention, "Alcohol Use and Binge Drinking among Women of Childbearing Age-United States, 2006-2010," *Morbidity and Mortality Weekly* 61, no. 28 (2012): 534–38, Available at www.cdc.gov/mmwr/preview/mmwrhtml/mm6128a4.htm; Y. Liu et al., "Alcohol Intake between Menarche and First Pregnancy: Prospective Study of Breast Cancer Risk," *Journal of the National Cancer Institute* 105, no. 20 (2013): 1571–78, Available at http://jnci.oxfordjournals.org/content/early/2013/08/24/jnci.djt213.full.
32. Centers for Disease Control and Prevention, "Fetal Alcohol Spectrum Disorders (FASDs) Data and Statistics," Updated August 2012, www.cdc.gov/ncbddd/fasd/data.html.
33. Fetal Alcohol Spectrum Disorders (FASD) Center for Excellence, "What Is FASD?," March 2014, www.Fasdcenter.samhsa.gov.
34. American College Health Association, *National College Health Assessment II: Reference Group Data Report, Spring 2013,* 2013.
35. Substance Abuse and Mental Health Services Administration, *Results from the 2011 National Survey on Drug Use and Health: Volume I. Summary of National Findings,* NSDUH Series H-44, DHHS Publication no. (SMA) 12-4713. Findings (Rockville, MD: Office of Applied Studies, U.S. Department of Health and Human Services, 2012).
36. U.S. Department of Health and Human Services, National Institute on Alcohol Abuse and Alcoholism, "Moderate and Binge Drinking," 2012, www.niaaa.nih.gov/alcohol-health/overview-alcohol-consumption/moderate-binge-drinking.
37. American College Health Association, *National College Health Assessment II: Reference Group Data Report, Spring 2013,* 2013.
38. C. Foster et al., "National College Health Assessment Measuring Negative Alcohol-Related Consequences among College Students," *American Journal of Public Health Research* 2, no. 1 (2014): 1–5.
39. S. Onyper et al., "Class Start Times, Sleep and Academic Performance in College: A Path Analysis," *Chronobiology* 29, no. 3 (2012): 318–35; S. Kenney et al., "Global Sleep Quality as a Moderator of Alcohol Consumption and Consequences in College Students," *Addictive Behaviors* 37, no. 4 (2012): 507–12.
40. American College Health Association, *National College Health Assessment II: Reference Group Data Report, Spring 2013,* 2013.
41. R. Hingson et al., "Magnitude of Alcohol-Related Mortality and Morbidity among U.S. College Students Ages 18–24: Changes from 1998 to 2005," *Journal of Studies on Alcohol and Drugs* (2009): 12–20.
42. C. C. Abar, "Examining the Relationship between Parenting Types and Patterns of Student Alcohol-Related Behavior during Transition to College," *Psychology of Addictive Behaviors* 26, no. 1, (2012): 20; L. Varvil-Weld, "Parents' and Students' Reports of Parenting: Which Are More Reliably Associated with College Student Drinking?," *Addictive Behaviors* 38, no. 3 (2013): 1699–1703.
43. L. D. Johnston, *Monitoring the Future National Survey Results on Drug Use, 1975–2012: Volume II, College Students and Adults Ages 19–50* (Ann Arbor, MI: Institute for Social Research, The University of Michigan, 2013), Available at www.monitoringthefuture.org/pubs/monographs/mtf-vol2_2012.pdf.
44. Ibid.
45. J. W. LaBrie et al., "Are They All the Same? An Exploratory, Categorical Analysis of Drinking Game Types," *Addictive Behaviors* 38, no. 5 (2013): 2133–39; N. P. Barnett et al., "Predictors and Consequences of Pregaming Using Day and Week-Level Measures," *Psychology of Addictive Behaviors* 27, no. 4 (2013): 921.
46. C. Neighbors et al., "Event Specific Drinking among College Students," *Psychology of Addictive Behaviors* 25, no. 4 (2011), 702–707, DOI: 10.1037/a0024051.
47. M. A. Lewis et al., "Use of Protective Behavioral Strategies and Their Association to 21st Birthday Alcohol Consumption and Related Negative Consequences: A between and within Person Evaluation," *Psychology of Addictive Behaviors* 26, no. 2 (2012), 179–86, DOI: 10.1037/a0023797.
48. J. Alfonso et al., "Do Drinking Games Matter? An Examination by Game Type and Gender in a Mandated Student Sample," *The American Journal of Drug and Alcohol Abuse* 39, no. 5 (2013): 312–19.
49. N. P. Barnett et al., "Predictors; and Consequences of Pregaming Using Day and Week-Level Measures," *Psychology of Addictive Behaviors* 27, no. 4 (2013): 921.
50. Ibid.

51. National Center on Addiction and Substance Abuse at Columbia University, *Wasting the Best and the Brightest: Substance Abuse at America's Colleges and Universities,* March 2007, www.casacolumbia.org/addiction-research/reports/wasting-best-brightest-substance-abuse-americas-colleges-universitys.
52. A. Barry et al., "Drunkorexia: Understanding the Co-occurrence of Alcohol Consumption and Eating/Exercise Weight Management Behaviors," *Journal of American College Health Association* 60, no. 3 (2012): 236–43.
53. S. Burke, et al., "Drunkorexia: Calorie Restriction Prior to Alcohol Consumption among College Freshmen," *Journal of Alcohol Drug Education* 54, (2010): 17–34.
54. A. Barry et al., "Drunkorexia: Understanding the Co-occurrence of Alcohol Consumption and Eating/Exercise Weight Behaviors," Journal of *American College Health* 60, no. 3 (2012): 236–43.
55. R. Hingson et al., "Magnitude of Alcohol-Related Mortality and Morbidity among U.S. College Students Ages 18–24: Changes from 1998 to 2005," *Journal of Studies on Alcohol and Drugs* 16 (2009): 12–20.
56. Ibid.
57. G. DiFulvio, et al., "Effectiveness of the Brief Alcohol and Screening Intervention for College Students (BASICS) Program for Mandated Students," *Journal of American College Health* 60, no. 4 (2012): 269–80.
58. National Social Norms Institute, "Case Studies: Alcohol," Accessed 2014, www.socialnorms.org/CaseStudies/alcohol.php.
59. Centers for Disease Control and Prevention, "Ten Leading Causes of Death by Age Group," August 2013, www.cdc.gov/injury/wisqars/leadingcauses.html.
60. Centers for Disease Control and Prevention (CDC), "Vital Signs: Drinking and Driving, a Threat to Everyone—October 2011" October 2013, www.cdc.gov/vitalsigns/drinkinganddriving.
61. Ibid.
62. National Highway Traffic Safety Administration, "Traffic Safety Facts: 2010 Data Alcohol-Impaired Driving," April 2012, www-nrd.nhtsa.dot.gov/Pubs/811606.pdf.
63. Centers for Disease Control and Prevention (CDC), "Vital Signs: Drinking and Driving," 2013.
64. American College Health Association, *National College Health Assessment II: Reference Group Data Report, Spring 2013,* 2013.
65. Insurance Institute for Highway Safety, "Alcohol-Impaired Driving," 2013, www.iihs.org/iihs/topics/t/alcohol-impaired-driving/fatalityfacts/alcohol-impaired-driving/2012#When-alcohol-impaired-crashes-occur.
66. Ibid.
67. Ibid.
68. K. Keyes et al., "The Role of Race/Ethnicity in Alcohol-Attributable Injury in the United States," *Epidemiologic Reviews* 34, no. 1 (2012): 89–102.
69. K. Keyes et al., "The Role of Race/Ethnicity in Alcohol-Attributable Injury in the United States," *Epidemiologic Reviews* (2011): 1–14.
70. T. Zaploski et al., "Less Drinking, yet More Problems: Understanding African American Drinking and Related Problems," *Psychological Bulletin* 140, no. 1 (2013): 188–223.
71. National Institute on Alcohol Abuse and Alcoholism, "Alcohol and the Hispanic Community," July 2013, http://pubs.niaaa.nih.gov/publications/HispanicFact/hispanicFact.htm.
72. Substance Abuse and Mental Health Services Administration, *Results from the 2011 National Survey on Drug Use and Health: National Findings,* 2012, www.samhsa.gov/data/NSDUH/2k11Results/NSDUHresults2011.htm.
73. Substance Abuse and Mental Health Services Administration, *Results from the 2011 National Survey on Drug Use and Health: National Findings,* 2012, www.samhsa.gov/data/NSDUH/2k11Results/NSDUHresults2011.htm.
74. J. Otto et al., "Association of the ALDHA1*2 Promoter Polymorphism with Alcohol Phenotyptes in Young Adults with or without ALDH2*2," *Alcoholism Clinical and Experimental Research* 37, no. 1 (2013): 164–69.
75. Medline Plus, "Alcoholism and Alcohol Abuse," February 2014, www.nlm.nih.gov/medlineplus/ency/article/000944.htm.
76. Center of Behavioral Health Statistics and Quality, "Nearly Half of College Student Treatment Admissions Were for Primary Alcohol Abuse," *Data Spotlight* (2012), www.samhsa.gov/data/spotlight/Spotlight054College2012.pdf.
77. A. Arria, "College Student Success: The Impact of Health Concerns and Substance Abuse," lecture presented at NASPA Alcohol and Mental Health Conference (Fort Worth, TX: January 19, 2013).
78. M. Waldron et al., "Parental Separation and Early Substance Involvement: Results from Children of Alcoholic and Cannabis Twins," *Drug and Alcohol Dependence* 134 (2014): 78–84.
79. A. Levin, "Determining Alcoholism Proves Complicated Endeavor," *Psychiatric News* 47, no. 24 (2012): 20, DOI: 10.1176/appi.pn.2012.12b13.
80. D. Stacey, "RASGRF2 Regulates Alcohol-Induced Reinforcement by Influencing Mesolimbic Dopamine Neuron Activity and Dopamine Release," *Proceedings of the National Academy of Sciences* 109, no. 51 (2012): 21128–33, DOI: 10.1073/pnas.1211844110.
81. J. Niels Rosenquist et al., "The Spread of Alcohol Consumption Behavior in a Large Social Network," *Annals of Internal Medicine* 152, no. 7 (2010): 426–33.
82. Centers for Disease Control and Prevention, Fact Sheet, "Excessive Alcohol Use and Risks to Women's Health: 2010," www.cdc.gov/alcohol/fact-sheets/womens-health.htm.
83. Join Together Staff, "7.5 Million Children in the U.S. Live with Alcoholic Parent," February 16, 2012, www.drugfree.org/join-together/alcohol/7-5-million-children-in-u-s-live-with-alcoholic-parent.
84. Centers for Disease Control and Prevention, "The High Cost of Excessive Drinking to States," August 19, 2013, www.cdc.gov/features/CostsOfDrinking
85. Ibid.
86. Underage Drinking Enforcement Training Center, Underage Drinking Costs, "Underage Drinking," September 2011, www.udetc.org/UnderageDrinkingCosts.asp.
87. Ibid.
88. Substance Abuse and Mental Health Services Administration, "The NSDUH Report—Alcohol Treatment: Need, Utilization, and Barriers," April 2009, www.samhsa.gov/data/2k9/AlcTX/AlcTX.htm.
89. A. Laudet et al., "Collegiate Recovery Community Programs: What Do We Know and What Do We Need to Know?" *Journal of Social Work Practice in the Addictions* 14 (2014): 84–100.

Pulled statistics:

p. 308, National Institute on Alcohol Abuse and Alcoholism, "Drinking Statistics," 2012, http://www.niaaa.nih.gov/alcohol-health/overview-alcohol-consumption/drinking-statistics.

p. 314, California Department of Alcohol and Drug Programs, "Frequently Asked Questions: General," 2012, http://www.adp.ca.gov/Criminal_Justice/DUI/faqs.shtml.

Chapter 11

1. U.S. Department of Health and Human Services, *The Health Consequences of Smoking—50 Years of Progress: A Report of the Surgeon General* (Atlanta, GA: U.S. Department of Health and Human Services, Centers for Disease Control and Prevention, National Center for Chronic Disease Prevention and Health Promotion, Office on Smoking and Health, 2014), Available at: www.surgeongeneral.gov/library/reports/50-years-of-progress/exec-summary.pdf.
2. Ibid; Campaign for Tobacco Free Kids, "The Toll of Tobacco Use in the USA," July 2013, www.tobaccofreekids.org/research/factsheets/pdf/0072.pdf.
3. Substance Abuse and Mental Health Services Administration, "Results from the 2012 National Survey on Drug Use and Health: Summary of National Findings," U.S. Department of Health and Human Services Series H-46, No. (SMA) 13-4795 (Rockville, MD: Substance Abuse and Mental Health Services Administration, 2013), Available at www.samhsa.gov/data/NSDUH/2012SummNatFindDetTables/NationalFindings/NSDUHresults2012.pdf.

4. Centers for Disease Control and Prevention, "50th Anniversary of the First Surgeon General's Report on Smoking and Health," January 2014, www.cdc.gov/mmwr/preview/mmwr html/mm6302a1.htm?s_cid–mm6302a1_w.
5. Substance Abuse and Mental Health Services Administration, "Results from the 2012 National Survey on Drug Use and Health: Summary of National Findings," 2013.
6. Centers for Disease Control and Prevention, "Smoking and Tobacco Use: Fast Facts," April 2014, www.cdc.gov/tobacco/data_statistics/fact_sheets/fast_facts.
7. Centers for Disease Control and Prevention, "Adult Cigarette Smoking in the United States: Current Estimates," February 2014, www.cdc.gov/tobacco/data_statistics/fact_sheets/adult_data/cig_smoking/; American Cancer Society, "Smokeless Tobacco," December 2013, www.cancer.org/cancer/cancercauses/tobaccocancer/smokeless-tobacco; Centers for Disease Control and Prevention, "Smoking and Tobacco Use: Cigars," November 2013, www.cdc.gov/tobacco/data_statistics/fact_sheets/tobacco_industry/cigars.
8. Campaign for Tobacco-Free Kids, "Toll of Tobacco in the United States of America," February 2014, www.tobaccofreekids.org/research/factsheets/pdf/0072.pdf?utm_source=factsheets_finder&utm_medium=link&utm_campaign=analytics.
9. American Lung Association, "General Smoking Facts," June 2011, www.lung.org/stop-smoking/about-smoking/facts-figures/general-smoking-facts.html.
10. Tobacco Free Providence, "Sweet Deceit Survey Results," January 2012, www.tobaccofreeprovidence.org/2012-01-27-sweet-deceit-survey-results.
11. American Cancer Society, "Cancer Facts & Figures 2014," Accessed April 2014, www.cancer.org/research/cancerfactsstatistics/cancerfactsfigures2014.
12. CASA Columbia, "Time to Ban Menthol," February 2014, www.casacolumbia.org/addiction-research/reports/time-to-ban-menthol-report-2014.
13. U.S. Department of Health and Human Services, *The Health Consequences of Smoking—50 Years of Progress*, 2014.
14. Campaign for Tobacco-Free Kids, "Toll of Tobacco in the United States of America," 2014.
15. Campaign for Tobacco-Free Kids, "State Cigarette Excise Tax Rates & Rankings," December 2013, www.tobaccofreekids.org/research/factsheets/pdf/0097.pdf.
16. American College Health Association, *American College Health Association–National College Health Assessment II: Reference Group Data Report, Spring 2013* (Baltimore, MD: American College Health Association, 2013), Available from www.achancha.org/reports_ACHA-NCHAII.html.
17. Ibid.
18. Substance Abuse and Mental Health Services Administration, "Results from the 2012 National Survey on Drug Use and Health: Summary of National Findings," 2013.
19. Ibid.
20. Ibid.
21. B. Primack, et al., "Associations of Mental Health Problems with Waterpipe and Cigarette Smoking Among College Students," *Substance Use & Misuse* 48, no. 3 (2013): 211–219; C. Berg et al., "Depression and Substance Abuse and Dependency in Relation to Current Smoking Status and Frequency of Smoking among Nondaily and Daily Smokers," *The American Journal on Addictions* 22, no. 6, (2013): 581–589.
22. Y. Choi et al., 'I Smoke but I Am Not a Smoker': Phantom Smokers and the Discrepancy between Self-identity and Behavior," *Journal of American College Health* 59, no. 2 (2011): 117–25.
23. E. Sutfin et al., "Tobacco Use by College Students: A Comparison of Daily and Nondaily Smokers," *American Journal of Health Behavior* 36, no. 2 (2012): 218–29.
24. American Cancer Society, "Light Smoking as Risky as a Pack a Day?," January 2013, www.cancer.org/cancer/news/expertvoices/post/2013/01/02/light-smoking-as-risky-as-a-pack-a-day.aspx; L. Stoner et al., "Occasional Cigarette Smoking Chronically Affects Arterial Function," *Ultrasound in Medicine and Biology* 34, no. 12 (2008): 1885–92.
25. L. An et al., "Symptoms of Cough and Shortness of Breath among Occasional Young Adult Smokers," *Nicotine & Tobacco Research* 11, no. 2 (2009): 126–33.
26. Stop Smoking!, "Smoking and Birth Control Pills Are Not Made for Each Other," Retrieved March 6, 2012, www.stop-smoking-updates.com/quitsmoking/smoking-factsheet/facts/smoking-and-birth-control-pills-are-not-made-for-each-other.htm.
27. U.S. Department of Health and Human Services, *The Health Consequences of Smoking—50 Years of Progress,* 2014; U.S. Department of Health and Human Services, *How Tobacco Smoke Causes Disease: The Biology and Behavioral Basis for Smoking-Attributable Disease. A Report of the Surgeon General* (Atlanta, GA: CDC, 2010), www.surgeongeneral.gov.
28. American Cancer Society, "Child and Teen Tobacco Use," November 2013, www.cancer.org/acs/groups/cid/documents/webcontent/002963-pdf.pdf.
29. C. A. Wassenaar et al., "Relationship between CYP2A6 and CHRNA5-CHRNA3-CHRNB4 Variation and Smoking Behaviors and Lung Cancer Risk," *JNCI Journal of the National Cancer Institute* 103, no. 17 (2011): 1342–46, DOI: 10.1093/jnci/djr237; F. Ducci et al., "TTC12-ANKK1-DRD2 and CHRNA5-CHRNA3-CHRNB4 Influence Different Pathways Leading to Smoking Behavior from Adolescence to Mid-Adulthood," *Biological Psychiatry* 69, no. 7 (2011): 650–60; C. Amos, M. Spitz, and P. Cinciripini, "Chipping Away at the Genetics of Smoking Behavior," *Nature Genetics* 42, no. 5 (2010): 366–68.
30. F. Ducci et al., "TTC12-ANKK1-DRD2 and CHRNA5-CHRNA3-CHRNB4 Influence Different Pathways Leading to Smoking Behavior from Adolescence to Mid-Adulthood," *Biological Psychiatry* 69, no. 7 (2011): 650-660; T. Korhonen and J. Kaprio, "Genetic Epidemiology of Smoking Behaviour and Nicotine Dependence," 2011, eLS, www.els.net/WileyCDA/ElsArticle/refId-a0023476.html.
31. T. Korhonen and J. Kaprio, "Genetic Epidemiology of Smoking Behaviour and Nicotine Dependence," 2011
32. C. Amos, M. Spitz, and P. Cinciripini, "Chipping Away at the Genetics of Smoking Behavior," 2010.
33. H. J. Aubin et al., "Weight gain in smokers after quitting cigarettes: meta-analysis," *British Medical Journal* 345 (2012): e4439.
34. American Cancer Society, "Cancer Facts & Figures 2013," 2013, Available at www.cancer.org.
35. K. Sterling et al., "Factors Associated with Small Cigar Use among College Students," *American Journal of Health Behavior* 37, no. 3 (2013): 325–33.
36. American Cancer Society, "Questions about Smoking, Tobacco, and Health: What about More Exotic Forms of Smoking Tobacco, Such as Clove Cigarettes, Bidis, and Hookahs?," February 2014, www.cancer.org/cancer/cancercauses/tobaccocancer/questionsaboutsmokingtobaccoandhealth/questions-about-smoking-tobacco-and-health-other-forms-of-smoking.
37. Centers for Disease Control and Prevention, "Smoking and Tobacco Use: Bidis and Kreteks," Updated July 2013, www.cdc.gov/tobacco/data_statistics/fact_sheets/tobacco_industry/bidis_kreteks.
38. Ibid.
39. Centers for Disease Control and Prevention, "Youth and Tobacco Use," February 2014, www.cdc.gov/tobacco/data_statistics/fact_sheets/youth_data/tobacco_use.
40. Campaign for Tobacco Free Kids, "Toll of Tobacco in the United States of America," 2014.
41. National Cancer Institute, "Lung Cancer Prevention," February 2014, www.cancer.gov/cancertopics/pdq/prevention/lung/HealthProfessional/page2.
42. American Cancer Society, "Cancer Facts & Figures 2014," Accessed April 2014, www.cancer.org/research/cancerfactsstatistics/cancerfactsfigures2014.
43. Ibid.
44. American Cancer Society, "What Are Oral Cavity and Oropharyngeal Cancers?," February 2014, www.cancer.org/cancer/oralcavityandoropharyngealcancer/

detailedguide/oral-cavity-and-oropharyngeal-cancer-what-is-oral-cavity-cancer.
45. American Cancer Society, "Cancer Facts & Figures 2014," 2014.
46. Ibid.
47. American Heart Association, *Heart Disease and Stroke Statistics—2014 Update* (Dallas, TX: American Heart Association, 2014), Available at http://circ.ahajournals.org/content/129/3/e28.
48. Ibid.
49. Ibid.
50. Ibid.
51. American Heart Association, "Stroke Risk Factors," October 2012, www.strokeassociation.org/STROKEORG/AboutStroke/UnderstandingRisk/Understanding-Risk_UCM_308539_SubHomePage.jsp; CDC, "Health Effects of Cigarette Smoking," February 2014, www.cdc.gov/tobacco/data_statistics/fact_sheets/health_effects/effects_cig_smoking.
52. American Lung Association, "Benefits of Quitting," March 2012, www.lungusa.org/stop-smoking/how-to-quit/why-quit/benefits-of-quitting.
53. U.S. Department of Health and Human Services, *The Health Consequences of Smoking—50 Years of Progress: A Report of the Surgeon General*, 2014.
54. John Hopkins Health Alerts, "Emphysema: Symptoms and Remedies," Accessed March 2012, www.johnshopkinshealthalerts.com/symptoms_remedies/emphysema/96-1.html.
55. C. B. Harte et al., "Association between Cigarette Smoking and Erectile Tumescence: The Mediating Role of Heart Rate Variability," *International Journal of Impotence Research* 25, no. 4 (2013):155–59, DOI: 10.1038/ijir.2012.43.
56. Centers for Disease Control and Prevention, "Tobacco Use and Pregnancy," Modified January 2014, www.cdc.gov/reproductivehealth/TobaccoUsePregnancy.
57. Ibid.
58. American Academy of Periodontology, "Gum Disease Risk Factors," Accessed April 2014, www.perio.org/consumer/risk-factors.
59. I. Moreno-Gonzalez, et al., "Smoking Exacerbates Amyloid Pathology in a Mouse Model of Alzheimer's Disease," *Nature Communications* 4 (2013), www.nature.com/ncomms/journal/v4/n2/abs/ncomms2494.html; J. Cataldo et al., "Cigarette Smoking Is a Risk Factor of Alzheimer's Disease: An Analysis Controlling for Tobacco Industry Affiliation," *Journal of Alzheimer's Disease* 19, no. 2 (2010): 465–80.
60. Centers for Disease Control and Prevention, "Smoking and Tobacco Use Facts: Secondhand Smoke," April 2014, www.cdc.gov/tobacco/data_statistics/fact_sheets/secondhand_smoke/general_facts.
61. American Nonsmokers' Rights Foundation, "Overview List-How Many Smoke-Free Laws," January 2014, www.no-smoke.org/pdf/mediaordlist.pdf.
62. Ibid.
63. Ibid.
64. Ibid.
65. National Cancer Institute, "Secondhand Smoke and Cancer," January 2011, www.cancer.gov/cancertopics/factsheet/Tobacco/ETS.
66. U.S. Department of Health and Human Services, *The Health Consequences of Involuntary Exposure to Tobacco Smoke*, November 2011; Centers for Disease Control and Prevention, "Smoking and Tobacco Use Fact Sheet," February 2014, www.cancer.org/docroot/ped/content/ped_10_2x_secondhand_smoke-clean_indoor_air.asp.
67. U.S. Department of Health and Human Services, *The Health Consequences of Involuntary Exposure to Tobacco Smoke*, 2011.
68. Z. Kabir, G. Connolly, and H. Alpert, "Secondhand Smoke Exposure and Neurobehavioral Disorders among Children in the United States," *Pediatrics* 128, no. 2 (2011), DOI: 10.1542/peds.2011-0023.
69. Ibid.
70. O. Shafey, M. Eriksen, H. Ross, and J. Mackay, "Secondhand Smoking," in *The Tobacco Atlas*, 3d ed. (Atlanta, GA: American Cancer Society, 2009), Available at www.cancer.org/aboutus/GlobalHealth/Cancerand-TobaccoControlResources/the-tobacco-atlas-3rd-edition.
71. U.S. Department of Health and Human Services, *The Health Consequences of Smoking—50 Years of Progress*, 2014.
72. Tobacco-Free Kids, "1998 State Tobacco Settlement 15 Years Later," February 2014, www.tobaccofreekids.org/what_we_do/state_local/tobacco_settlement.
73. *Family Smoking Prevention and Tobacco Control Act of 2009*, HR 1256, 111th Congress of the United States of America, Available at www.govtrack.us/congress/billtext.xpd?bill=h111-1256.
74. Centers for Disease Control and Prevention, "Tobacco Use: Smoking Cessation," February 2014, www.cdc.gov/tobacco/data_statistics/fact_sheets/cessation/quitting/index.htm#quitting.
75. American Lung Association, "Benefits of Quitting," www.lung.org/stop-smoking/how-to-quit/why-quit/benefits-of-quitting/; Centers for Disease Control and Prevention, "Quitting Smoking," Smoking and Tobacco Use, February 7, 2014, www.cdc.gov/tobacco/data_statistics/fact_sheets/cessation/quitting/index.htm?utm_source=feedburner&utm_medium=feed&utm_campaign=Feed%3A+CdcSmokingAndTobaccoUseFactSheets+%28CDC+-+Smoking+and+Tobacco+Use+-+Fact+Sheets%29.
76. N. Hopper, "What a Pack of Cigarettes Costs Now, State by State," *The Awl*, July 12, 2013, www.theawl.com/2013/07/what-a-pack-of-cigarettes-costs-now-state-by-state.
77. American Cancer Society, "Guide to Quitting Smoking: A Word about Quitting Success Rates," February 2014, www.cancer.org/Healthy/StayAwayfromTobacco/Guideto-QuittingSmoking/guide-to-quitting-smoking-success-rates.
78. D. Thompson, "A Guide to Using the Nicotine Patch," *EveryDay Health*, May 2011, www.everydayhealth.com/stop-smoking/smoking-cessation-aids-nicotine-patch.aspx.
79. U.S. Food and Drug Administration, "Public Health Advisory: FDA Requires New Boxed Warnings for the Smoking Cessation Drugs Chantix and Zyban," July 1, 2009, www.fda.gov/Drugs/DrugSafety/DrugSafetyPodcasts/ucm170906.htm.

Pulled statistics:

p. 325, American Lung Association, "General Smoking Facts," June 2011, http://www.lung.org/stop-smoking/about-smoking/facts-figures/general-smoking-facts.html.

p. 328, Ibid.

Chapter 12

1. Substance Abuse and Mental Health Services Administration, *Results from the 2011 National Survey on Drug Use and Health: Summary of National Findings*, NSDUH Series H 44, HHS Publication No. (SMA) 12-4713 (Rockville, MD: Substance Abuse and Mental Health Services Administration, 2012).
2. J. Swendsen et al., "Use and Abuse of Alcohol and Illicit Drugs in the US Adolescents: Results of the National Comorbidity Survey-Adolescent Supplement," *Archives of General Psychiatry* 69, no. 4 (2012): 390–98.
3. L. D. Johnston et al., *Monitoring the Future National Results on Drug Use: 2012 Overview, Key Findings on Adolescent Drug Use* (Ann Arbor: Institute for Social Research, The University of Michigan, 2013).
4. National Institute of Drug Abuse, "Drug Facts: Nationwide Trends," NIDA, *January* 2014, www.drugabuse.gov/publications/drugfacts/nationwide-trends.
5. National Drug Intelligence Center, "National Drug Threat Assessment 2011," 2011, www.justice.gov/archive/ndic/pubs44/44849/44849p.pdf.
6. Centers for Disease Control and Prevention, National Center for Health Statistics, Office of Analysis and Epidemiology, "Table 99: Prescription Drug Use in the Past 30 Days, by Sex, Age, Race and Hispanic Origin: United States Selected Years 1988–1994 through 2007–2010," *Health*, United States, 2011, www.cdc.gov.
7. Consumer Health Care Products Association, "The Value of OTC Medicine to the United States," January 2012, www.chpa.org/ValueofOTCMeds2012.aspx.
8. Ibid.

9. L. D. Johnston et al., *Monitoring the Future National Results on Drug Use*, 2013.
10. Erowid, "The DXM Vault," 2012, www.erowid.org/chemicals/dxm/dxm.shtml.
11. U.S. Food and Drug Administration, "GAO Report Assesses State Approaches to Control Pseudoephedrine," The Law, Blog, February 26, 2013, www.fdalawblog.net/fda_law_blog_hyman_phelps/2013/02/gao-report-assesses-state-approaches-to-control-pseudoephedrine.html.
12. Substance Abuse and Mental Health Services Administration, "Results from the 2012 National Survey," October 2013, www.samhsa.gov/data/NSDUH/2012SummNatFindDetTables/Index.aspx.
13. J. L. McCauley et al., "Non-medical Use of Prescription Drugs in a National Sample of College Women," *Addictive Behaviors* 36, no. 7 (2011): 690–95.
14. Substance Abuse and Mental Health Services Administration, "Results from the 2012 National Survey," October 2013, www.samhsa.gov/data/NSDUH/2012SummNatFindDetTables/Index.aspx.
15. Ibid.
16. L. D. Johnston et al., *Monitoring the Future National Results on Drug Use*, 2013.
17. Centers for Disease Control and Prevention, "Prescription Pain Killer Overdoses at Epidemic Levels," November 2011, www.cdc.gov/media/releases/2011/p1101_flu_pain_killer_overdose.html.
18. American College Health Association, *American College Health Association–National College Health Assessment, Spring 2013* (Baltimore, MD: American College Health Association, 2013), Available at www.acha-ncha.org/docs/ACHA-NCHA-II_ReferenceGroup_ExecutiveSummary_Spring2013.pdf.
19. Ibid.
20. Ibid.
21. Ibid.
22. L. M. Garnier-Dykstra et al., "Nonmedical Use of Prescription Stimulants during College: Four-Year Trends in Exposure Opportunity, Use, Motives, and Sources," *Journal of American College Health* 60, no. 3 (2012): 226–34.
23. Substance Abuse and Mental Health Services Administration, "Results from the 2012 National Survey," 2013.
24. Ibid.
25. L. D. Johnston et al., *Monitoring the Future National Survey Results on Drug Use,* 2013.
26. A. Arria et al., "Drug Use Patterns and Continuous Enrollment in College: Results from a Longitudinal Study," *Journal of Studies on Alcohol and Drugs* 74, no. 1 (2013): 71–83.
27. Substance Abuse and Mental Health Services Administration, "Results from the 2012 National Survey," October 2013, www.samhsa.gov/data/NSDUH/2012SummNatFindDetTables/Index.aspx.
28. National Center on Addiction and Substance Abuse at Columbia University, *Wasting the Best and the Brightest: Substance Abuse at America's Colleges and Universities* (New York: National Center on Addiction and Substance Abuse at Columbia University, 2007), Available at www.casacolumbia.org/addiction-research/reports/wasting-best-brightest-substance-abuse-americas-colleges-universitys.
29. Substance Abuse and Mental Health Services Administration, "Results from the 2012 National Survey," 2013.
30. L. D. Johnston et al., *Monitoring the Future National Results on Drug Use,* 2013.
31. CPDD Community Website, "Methamphetamine Abuse and Parkinson's Disease," July 2011, www.cpddblog.com/2011/07/methamphetamine-abuse-and-parkinsons.html.
32. N. Volkow, "Bath Salts: Emerging and Dangerous Products," *National Institute on Drug Abuse*, February 2011, www.drugabuse.gov/about-nida/directors-page/messages-director/2011/02/bath-salts-emerging-dangerous-products.
33. S. Melton, "Bath Salts: An 'Ivory Wave' Epidemic?," *Medscape*, August 26, 2011, www.medscape.com/viewarticle/748344.
34. Ibid.
35. Food Manufacturing, "Consumer Trends: 83 Percent of Americans Drink Coffee," April 2013, www.foodmanufacturing.com/news/2013/04/consumer-trends-83-percent-americans-drink-coffee.
36. Harvard Health Letter, "What Is It About Coffee?" January 2012, www.health.harvard.edu/press_releases/what-is-it-about-coffee.
37. Substance Abuse and Mental Health Services Administration, Results from the 2012 National Survey on Drug Use and Health: Detailed Tables, NSDUH Series H-44, HHS Publication No. (SMA) 12-4713 (Rockville, MD: Substance Abuse and Mental Health Services Administration, 2013).
38. Ibid.
39. National Institute on Drug Abuse, " Drug Facts: Marijuana," January 2014, www.drugabuse.gov/publications/drugfacts/marijuana.
40. National Institute on Drug Abuse, *Research Report: Marijuana Abuse,* NIH Publication no. 05-3859, 2005, www.drugabuse.gov/ResearchReports/Marijuana; National Institute on Drug Abuse, "NIDA InfoFacts: Drugged Driving," 2009, www.nida.nih.gov/infofacts/driving.html.
41. M. Asbridge et al., "Acute Cannabis Consumption and Motor Vehicle Collision Risk: Systematic Review of Observational Studies and Meta-analysis," *British Medical Journal* 344 (2012): 1–9.
42. National Institute on Drug Abuse, "Drug Facts: Marijuana," January 2014, www.drugabuse.gov/publications/drugfacts/marijuana.
43. Ibid.
44. S. Lev-Ran et al., "The Association between Cannabis Use and Depression: A Systematic Review and Meta-Analysis of Longitudinal Studies," *Psychological Medicine* 24, (2013); L. R. Pacek et al., "The Bidirectional Relationships between Alcohol, Cannabis, Co-occurring Alcohol and Cannabis Use Disorders with Major Depressive Disorder: Results from a National Sample," *Journal of Affective Disorders* 148, no. 2 (2013):188–95, DOI: 10.1016/j.jad.2012.11.059.
45. L. R. Pacek et al., "The Bidirectional Relationships between Alcohol, Cannabis, Co-occurring Alcohol and Cannabis Use Disorders with Major Depressive Disorder," 2013.
46. L. Degenhardt et al., "The Persistence of the Association between Adolescent Cannabis Use and Common Mental Disorders into Young Adulthood," *Addiction* 108, no. 1 (2013): 124–33.
47. J. Copeland, "Changes in Cannabis Use among Young People: Impact on Mental Health," *Current Opinion in Psychiatry* 26, no. 4 (2013): 325–29.
48. A. Norton, "A Hidden Effect of Marijuana Use: Findings on Sleep Give Clinicians an Opportunity to Discuss Marijuana's Harms," *Addiction Professional* (2011), www.findarticles.com/p/articles/mi_m0QTQ/is_4_6/ai_n27947952.
49. National Institute on Drug Abuse, "Marijuana: Facts for Teens," October 2013, www.drugabuse.gov/publications/marijuana-facts-teens; Science Daily, "Marijuana Use Prior to Pregnancy Doubles Risk of Premature Birth," July 17, 2012, www.sciencedaily.com/releases/2012/07/120717182953.htm.
50. National Institute on Drug Abuse, "Drug Facts: Is Marijuana Medicine?" April 2014, www.drugabuse.gov/publications/drugfacts/marijuana-medicine.
51. DrugRehab.us, "Pros and Cons of Legalizing Recreational Marijuana," April 2014, www.drugrehab.us/news/pros-cons-legalizing-recreational-marijuana.
52. Ibid.
53. National Institutes of Health, National Institute on Drug Abuse, "Drug Facts: Spice," December 2012, www.drugabuse.gov/publications/drugfacts/spice-synthetic-marijuana.
54. Ibid.; L. D. Johnston et al., *Monitoring the Future National Survey Results on Drug Use, 1975–2012: Volume I, Secondary School Students,* 2013.
55. National Institutes of Health, National Institute on Drug Abuse, "Drug Facts: Spice," 2012.
56. The Partnership at Drugfree.org, "GHB," Accessed May 2014, www.drugfree.org/drug-guide/ghb.
57. Substance Abuse and Mental Health Services Administration, "Results from the 2012 National Survey," October 2013.
58. Ibid.
59. L. D. Johnston et al., *Monitoring the Future National Survey Results on Drug Use,* 2013.

60. National Institute on Drug Abuse, "NIDA InfoFacts: MDMA (Ecstasy)," September 2013, www.drugabuse.gov/infofacts/ecstasy.html.
61. The Partnership at DrugFree.org, "Experts: People Who Think They Are Taking 'Molly' Don't Know What They Are Getting," June 24, 2013, www.drugfree.org/join-together/drugs/experts-people-who-think-they-are-taking-molly-dont-know-what-theyre-getting.
62. The National Collegiate Athletic Association, "Substance Use: National Study of Substance Use Trends among NCAA College Student-Athletes," 2012, www.ncaapublications.com/productdownloads/SAHS09.pdf.
63. American College Health Association, *American College Health Association–National College Health Assessment, Spring 2012*, 2013.
64. H. G. Pope et al., "The Lifetime Prevalence of Anabolic-Androgenic Steroid Use and Dependence in Americans: Current Best Estimates," *American Journal on Addictions* (2013), DOI: 10.1111/j.1521-0391.2013.12118.x.
65. Ibid.
66. Substance Abuse and Mental Health Services Administration, "Results from the 2012 National Survey," October 2013, www.samhsa.gov/data/NSDUH/2012SummNatFindDetTables/Index.aspx.
67. A. Grasgreen, "Students in Recovery," *Inside Higher Education*, July 13, 2011, www.insidehighered.com/news/2011/07/13/student_addiction_recovery_centers_communities_form_higher_education_association#ixzz1oq13UApD.
68. Texas Tech University, "The Center for the Study of Addiction and Recovery," Accessed May 2014, www.depts.ttu.edu/hs/csa.
69. Office of National Drug Control Policy, "How Illicit Drug Use Affects Business and the Economy," *Executive Office of the President*, www.whitehouse.gov/ondcp/ondcp-fact-sheets/how-illicit-drug-use-affects-business-and-the-economy.
70. Ibid.
71. Substance Abuse and Mental Health Services Administration, "Results from the 2012 National Survey," 2013.

Pulled statistics:

p. 348, American College Health Association. *American College Health Association—National College Health Assessment II: Reference Group Executive Summary, Spring 2013* (Hanover, MD: American College Health Association, 2013).

p. 360, Substance Abuse and Mental Health Services Administration, Results from the 2012 National Survey on Drug Use and Health: Summary of National Findings, NSDUH Series H-44, HHS Publication No. (SMA) 12-4713. Rockville, MD: Substance Abuse and Mental Health Services Administration, 2013.

p. 362, Ibid

Chapter 13

1. Flu.gov, "Pandemic Flu History," Accessed April 2014, www.flu.gov/pandemic/history.
2. F. Dawood et al., "Estimated Global Mortality Associated with the First Months of 2009 Pandemic Influenza A *H1N1* Virus Circulation: A Modelling Study," *The Lancet Infectious Diseases* 12, no. 9 (2012): 687–95.
3. C. B. Field, et al. IPCC, 2014: Summary for policymakers. In: *Climate Change 2014: Impacts, Adaptation, and Vulnerability. Part A: Global and Sectoral Aspects. Contribution of Working Group II to the Fifth Assessment Report of the Intergovernmental Panel on Climate Change* (eds.), Cambridge University Press, Cambridge, United Kingdom and New York, NY, USA, pp. 1–32;. S. Altizer et al., "Climate Change and Infectious Diseases: From Evidence to a Predictive Framework," *Science* 341, no. 6145 (2013): 514–19; WHO, "Climate Change and Infectious Disease," Accessed March 2014, www.who.int/globalchange/climate/en/Chapter6.pdf.
4. S. Altizer et al., "Climate Change and Infectious Diseases," 2013; WHO, "Climate Change and Infectious Disease," 2014; J. Remais et al., "Convergence of Non-communicable and Infectious Diseases in Low- and Middle-Income Countries," *International Journal of Epidemiology* 42, no. 1 (2013): 221–27, DOI:10.1093/ije/dys135; Environmental Protection Agency, "Climate Impacts on Human Health," April 2013, www.epa.gov/climatechange/effects/health.html; E. Shuman, "Global Climate Change and Infectious Diseases," *New England Journal of Medicine* 362 (2010): 1061–63.
5. B. T. Kerridge et al., "Conflict and diarrheal and related diseases: A global analysis," *Journal of Epidemiology and Global Health* 3, no. 4 (2013): 269–77; K. F. Cann et al., "Extreme Water-Related Weather Events and Waterborne Disease," *Epidemiology and Infection* 141, no. 4 (2013): 671–86.
6. National Institute of Environmental Health Sciences, "NIH News—New Study Shows 32 Million Americans Have Autoantibodies That Target Their Own Tissues," 2012, www.nih.gov/news/health/jan2012/niehs-13.htm; National Institute of Arthritis and Musculoskeletal and Skin Diseases, "Understanding Autoimmune Diseases," October 2012, www.niams.nih.gov/Health_Info/Autoimmune/default.asp.
7. American Autoimmune Related Diseases Association, "Autoimmune Statistics," 2011, www.aarda.org/autoimmune_statistics.php; National Institute of Arthritis and Musculoskeletal and Skin Diseases, "Understanding Autoimmune Diseases," 2012.
8. Centers for Disease Control and Prevention, "Birth–18 Years and 'Catch-up' Immunization Schedules," January 2014, www.cdc.gov/vaccines/schedules/hcp/child-adolescent.html.
9. Centers for Disease Control and Prevention, "FastStats–Allergies and Hay Fever," February 2014, www.cdc.gov/nchs/fastats/allergies.htm.
10. National Institute of Allergy and Infectious Diseases, "Pollen Allergy," June 2012, www.niaid.nih.gov/topics/allergicdiseases/understanding/pollenallergy/Pages/default.aspx.
11. Centers for Disease Control and Prevention, "Antibiotic Resistance Threats in the United States, 2013," April 2013, www.cdc.gov/drugresistance/threat-report-2013/pdf/ar-threats-2013-508.pdf.
12. Ibid., Centers for Disease Control and Prevention, "Antibiotics: Will They Work When You Really Need Them?," November 2013, www.cdc.gov/getsmart/campaign-materials/week/downloads/gsw-factsheet-parents.pdf.
13. Centers for Disease Control and Prevention, "Antibiotic Resistance Threats in the United States, 2013," April 2013, www.cdc.gov/drugresistance/threat-report-2013/pdf/ar-threats-2013-508.pdf; S. Stefani et al., "Methicillin-Resistant *Staphylococcus Aureus* (MRSA): Global Epidemiology and Harmonization of Typing Methods," *International Journal of Antimicrobial Agents* 39, no. 4 (2012): 273–82, DOI: 10.1016/j.ijantimicag.2011.09.030; Centers for Disease Control and Prevention, "MRSA Fact Sheet," March 2014, www.cdc.gov/mrsa/pdf/MRSA_ConsumerFactSheet_F.pdf.
14. Centers for Disease Control and Prevention, "Antibiotic Resistance Threats in the United States, 2013," 2013.
15. Ibid.; W. Jarvis, "Prevention and Control of Methicillin-Resistant *Staphylococcus aureus:* Dealing with Reality, Resistance, and Resistance to Reality," *Clinical Infectious Diseases* 50, no. 2 (2010): 218–20.
16. Centers for Disease Control and Prevention, "Antibiotic Resistance Threats in the United States, 2013," 2013.
17. Ibid.
18. Ibid.
19. Centers for Disease Control and Prevention, "Scarlet Fever: A Group A Streptococcal Infection," January 2014, www.cdc.gov/features/scarletfever.
20. Ibid.
21. Centers for Disease Control and Prevention, "Meningitis," April 2014, www.cdc.gov/meningitis/index.html; Centers for Disease Control and Prevention, "Meningococcal Disease: Technical and Clinical Information," April 2014, www.cdc.gov/vaccines/vpd-vac/mening/vac-mening-fs.htm.

22. World Health Organization, "Tuberculosis Fact Sheet," February 2013, www.who.int/mediacentre/factsheets/fs104/en/index.html; Centers for Disease Control and Prevention, "Tuberculosis (TB): Data and Statistics," March 2014, www.cdc.gov/tb/statistics/default.htm.
23. Ibid.; Centers for Disease Control and Prevention, "Trends in Tuberculosis, 2012," September 2013, www.cdc.gov/tb/publications/factsheets/statistics/TBTrends.htm.
24. World Health Organization, "WHO Global Tuberculosis Report 2013: Executive Summary," Accessed April 2014, Available at www.who.int/tb/publications/global_report/gtbr13_executive_summary.pdf?ua=1.
25. Ibid.
26. Centers for Disease Control and Prevention, "Tuberculosis," March 2014, http://www.cdc.gov/tb.
27. Centers for Disease Control and Prevention, "Tuberculosis (TB): Treatment," August 2012, www.cdc.gov/tb/topic/treatment/default.htm.
28. World Health Organization, "WHO Global Tuberculosis Report 2013: Executive Summary," 2014.
29. National Institute of Allergy and Infectious Diseases, "Common Cold," May 2011, www.niaid.nih.gov/topics/commonCold/Pages/cause.aspx.
30. National Center for Complementary and Alternative Medicine, "Echinacea," April 2013, http://nccam.nih.gov/health/echinacea.
31. National Institute of Allergy and Infectious Diseases, "Common Cold: Prevention," April 2011, www.niaid.nih.gov/topics/commoncold/Pages/prevention.aspx.
32. Centers for Disease Control and Prevention, "Seasonal Influenza: Key Facts about Influenza (Flu) and Flu Vaccine," September 2013, www.cdc.gov/flu/keyfacts.htm.
33. Centers for Disease Control and Prevention, " Cold vs Flu?," September 2013, www.cdc.gov/flu/about/qa/coldflu.htm.
34. Centers for Disease Control and Prevention, "Types of Influenza Viruses," January 2014, www.cdc.gov/flu/about/viruses/types.htm.
35. Centers for Disease Control and Prevention, "Selecting the Viruses in the Seasonal Influenza (Flu) Vaccine," February 2014, www.cdc.gov/flu/about/season/vaccine-selection.htm.
36. S. Doerr, "Mononucleosis," 2012, www.emedicinehealth.com/script/main/art.asp?articlekey=58850&pf=3; Centers for Disease Control and Prevention, "Epstein-Barr Virus and Infectious Mononucleosis," 2012, www.cdc.gov/ncidod/diseases/ebv.htm.
37. Centers for Disease Control and Prevention, "Viral Hepatitis," March 2014, www.cdc.gov/hepatitis.
38. Centers for Disease Control and Prevention, "Reported Cases of Acute Hepatitis A, by State, United States, 2007–2011," August 2013, www.cdc.gov/hepatitis/Statistics/2011Surveillance/Table2.1.htm.
39. Centers for Disease Control and Prevention, "Viral Hepatitis Statistics and Surveillance—2011," August 2013, www.cdc.gov/hepatitis/Statistics/2011Surveillance/Commentary.htm#hepB; World Health Organization, "Global Report on Prevention and Control of Viral Hepatitis in WHO Member States," July 2013, www.who.int/csr/disease/hepatitis/global_report/en.
40. Ibid.
41. Centers for Disease Control and Prevention, "Hepatitis C FAQs for Health Professionals," Updated February 2014, www.cdc.gov/hepatitis/HCV/HCVfaq.htm.
42. Ibid.
43. Centers for Disease Control and Prevention, "Shingles Vaccination: What You Need to Know," November 2013, www.cdc.gov/vaccines/vpd-vac/shingles/vacc-need-know.htm#notGet-vaccine.
44. Ibid.
45. E. Cohen, "U.S. Measles Cases in 2013 May Be Most in 17 Years," *CNN Health*, September 13, 2013, www.cnn.com/2013/09/12/health/worst-measles-year.
46. Centers for Disease Control and Prevention, "Measles: Make Sure your Child is Fully Immunized," March 2014, www.cdc.gov/features/measles.
47. Ibid.
48. Centers for Disease Control and Prevention, "Valley Fever Increasing in Some Southwestern States," March 2013, www.cdc.gov/media/releases/2013/p0328_valley_fever.html.
49. Ibid.
50. Centers for Disease Control and Prevention, " vCJD Factsheet (Variant Creutzfeldt-Jakob Disease)," February 2013, www.cdc.gov/ncidod/dvrd/vcjd/factsheet_nvcjd.htm.
51. Ibid.
52. Ibid.
53. Centers for Disease Control and Prevention, "Antibiotic Resistance Threats in the United States, 2013," April 2013, www.cdc.gov/drugresistance/threat-report-2013/pdf/ar-threats-2013-508.pdf; Centers for Disease Control and Prevention, "Get Smart: Know When Antibiotics Work: Fast Facts," November 2014, www.cdc.gov/getsmart/antibiotic-use/fast-facts.html.
54. Centers for Disease Control and Prevention, "West Nile Virus (WNV): Preliminary Maps and Data for 2013," January 2014, www.cdc.gov/westnile/statsMaps/preliminaryMapsData/index.html.
55. Ibid.
56. Ibid.
57. Ibid.
58. World Health Organization, "Cumulative Number of Confirmed Human Cases of Avian Influenza A (H5N1) Reported to WHO," January 2014, www.who.int/influenza/human_animal_interface/H5N1_cumulative_table_archives/en/index.html.
59. Ibid.
60. World Health Organization, "Factsheet on the World Malaria Report 2013," December 2013, www.who.int/malaria/media/world_malaria_report_2013.
61. Ibid.
62. Ibid.

Pulled statistics:

p. 386, World Health Organization, "Tuberculosis," March 2014, http://www.who.int/mediacentre/factsheets/fs104/en.

p. 388, Centers for Disease Control and Prevention, "Estimating Seasonal Influenza-Associated Deaths in the United States: CDC Study Confirms Variability of Flu," September 2013, http://www.cdc.gov/flu/about/disease/us_flu-related_deaths.htm.

Chapter 14

1. Mayo Clinic, "Sexually Transmitted Diseases (STDs): Definition," Accessed April 20, 2014, www.mayoclinic.org/diseases-conditions/sexually-transmitted-diseases-stds/basics/definition/con-20034128.
2. Planned Parenthood, 2014, "Sexually Transmitted Diseases," www.plannedparenthood.org/health-topics/stds-hiv-safer-sex-101.htm.
3. Centers for Disease Control and Prevention, "Sexually Transmitted Disease Surveillance, 2012," March 2014, www.cdc.gov/std/stats12/default.htm.
4. American College Health Association, *American College Health Association—National College Health Assessment II (ACHA-NCHA II) Reference Group Executive Summary, Spring 2013* (Hanover, MD: American College Health Association, 2013), Available at www.acha-ncha.org.
5. Centers for Disease Control and Prevention, "Chlamydia—CDC Fact Sheet, Detailed Version," January 2014, www.cdc.gov/std/chlamydia/STDFact-chlamydia-detailed.htm
6. MedlinePlus, "Pelvic Inflammatory Disease (PID)," Updated February 2014, www.nlm.nih.gov/medlineplus/ency/article/000888.htm; Mayo Clinic Staff, "Urinary Tract Infection: Risk Factors," August 2012, www.mayoclinic.com/health/urinary-tract-infection/DS00286/DSECTION=risk-factors.
7. Centers for Disease Control and Prevention, "Conjunctivitis (Pink Eye) in Newborns," January 2014, www.cdc.gov/conjunctivitis/newborns.html.
8. Centers for Disease Control and Prevention, "Gonorrhea: CDC Fact Sheet," January 2014, www.cdc.gov/std/gonorrhea/stdfact-gonorrhea.htm.
9. Centers for Disease Control and Prevention, "Sexually Transmitted Disease Surveillance, 2012," 2014.
10. Centers for Disease Control and Prevention, "Gonorrhea: CDC Fact Sheet," 2014.
11. Ibid.
12. Centers for Disease Control and Prevention, "Syphilis—CDC Detailed Fact Sheet," January 2014, www.cdc.gov/std/syphilis/STDFact-Syphilis-detailed.htm.

13. Ibid.
14. Centers for Disease Control and Prevention, "Genital Herpes—CDC Fact Sheet, Detailed Fact Sheet," Modified February 2013, www.cdc.gov/std/herpes/stdfact-herpes-detailed.htm.
15. American Sexual Health Association, "Learn about Herpes: Fast Facts," 2014, www.ashastd.org/std-sti/Herpes/learn-about-herpes.html.
16. Ibid.
17. Centers for Disease Control and Prevention, "Genital HPV Infection—CDC Fact Sheet," March 2014, www.cdc.gov/std/HPV/STDFact-HPV.htm; American Sexual Health Association, "Overview and Fast Stats," Accessed April 2014, www.ashastd.org/std-sti/hpv/overview-and-fast-facts.html; Centers for Disease Control and Prevention, "What is HPV?," February 2013, www.cdc.gov/hpv/whatishpv.html.
18. National Institute of Cancer, "HPV and Cancer," March 2012, www.cancer.gov/cancertopics/factsheet/Risk/HPV.
19. Centers for Disease Control and Prevention, "What is HPV?," 2013; Centers for Disease Control and Prevention, March 2014, "What Should I Know About Screening?," www.cdc.gov/cancer/cervical/basic_info/screening.htm; Centers for Disease Control and Prevention, "Cervical Cancer," March 2014, www.cdc.gov/cancer/cervical.
20. Centers for Disease Control and Prevention, "Human Papillomavirus (HPV) and Oropharyngeal Cancer–Fact Sheet," November 2013, www.cdc.gov/std/hpv/stdFact-HPVandoralcancer.htm.
21. Ibid.
22. Centers for Disease Control and Prevention, "Genital/Vulvovaginal Candidiasis," February 2014, www.cdc.gov/fungal/diseases/candidiasis/genital/index.html.
23. Centers for Disease Control and Prevention, "Trichomoniasis: CDC Fact Sheet," August 2012, www.cdc.gov/std/trichomonas/STDFact-Trichomoniasis.htm.
24. Ibid.
25. Centers for Disease Control and Prevention, "Pubic Lice FAQs,"September 2013, www.cdc.gov/parasites/lice/pubic/gen_info/faqs.html.
26. Joint United Nations Programme on HIV/AIDS (UNAIDS) and World Health Organization (WHO), *2013 UNAIDS Report on the Global AIDS Epidemic* (Geneva: UNAIDS, 2013), Available at www.unaids.org/en/resources/publications/2013/name,85053,en.asp.
27. Centers for Disease Control and Prevention, "HIV in the United States: At a Glance," December 2013, www.cdc.gov/hiv/resources/factsheets/us.htm; Care.org, "HIV&AIDS: Facts," January 2014, www.care.org/work/health/hiv-aids/hiv-aids-facts; UNAIDS, *UNAIDS Report on the Global AIDS Epidemic*," 2013.
28. Centers for Disease Control and Prevention, "Today's HIV/AIDS Epidemic" December 2013, www.cdc.gov/nchhstp/newsroom/docs/hivfactsheets/todaysepidemic-508.pdf.
29. AVERT, "Can You Get HIV from . . .?," Updated 2012, www.avert.org/can-you-get-hiv-aids.htm.
30. Ibid.
31. World Health Organization, "Mother to Child Transmission of HIV," Accessed April 2014, www.who.int/hiv/topics/mtct/en.
32. AVERT, "HIV Testing," 2012, www.avert.org/hiv-testing.htm.
33. M. Smith, "Researchers Report Treatment Clears HIV In Second Baby," *MedPage Today*, March 6, 2014, www.medpagetoday.com/MeetingCoverage/CROI/44630.
34. U.S. Department of Health and Human Services, "FDA-Approved Anti-HIV Medications," September 2013, http://aidsinfo.nih.gov/contentfiles/ApprovedMedstoTreatHIV_FS_en.pdf.

Pulled statistics:

p. 399, Centers for Disease Control and Prevention, "Incidence, Prevalence and Cost of Sexually Transmitted Infections in the United States," 2013, http://www.cdc.gov/std/stats/sti-estimates-fact-sheet-feb-2013.pdf.

p. 405, UNAIDS, "UNAIDSGlobal Report 2013," http://www.unaids.org/en/resources/campaigns/globalreport2013/globalreport.

Chapter 14A

1. Genetics Home Reference, "What Advances Are Being Made in DNA Sequencing?," March 2014, http://ghr.nlm.nih.gov/handbook/genomicresearch/sequencing.
2. Genetics Home Reference, "Chromosomes," March 2014, http://ghr.nlm.nih.gov/chromosomes.
3. The ENCODE Project Consortium, "An Integrated Encyclopedia of DNA Elements in the Human Genome," *Nature* 489, no. 7414 (2012): 57–74.
4. J. L. Thompson, M. M. Manore, and L. A. Vaughan, *The Science of Nutrition*, 3rd ed. (San Francisco: Benjamin Cummings, 2014).
5. Genetics Home Reference, "MC1R," March 2014, http://ghr.nlm.nih.gov/gene/MC1R.
6. Genetics Home Reference, "Huntington Disease," March 2014, http://ghr.nlm.nih.gov/condition/huntington-disease.
7. Genetics Home Reference, "How Genes Work.: What Is the Epigenome?" March 2014, http://ghr.nlm.nih.gov/handbook/howgeneswork?show=all.
8. R. C. Laker, M. E. Wlodek, J. J. Connelly, and Z. Yan, "Epigenetic Origins of Metabolic Disease: The Impact of the Maternal Condition to the Offspring Epigenome and Later Health Consequences," *Food Science and Human Wellness*, March 2013; 2(1): 1–11. Available at www.sciencedirect.com/science/article/pii/S221345301300013X.
9. Genetic Science Learning Center, University of Utah, "Nutrition and the Epigenome," Accessed March 2014, http://learn.genetics.utah.edu/content/epigenetics/nutrition.
10. Genetics Home Reference, "Mutations and Health: What Are Complex or Multifactorial Disorders?," March 2014, http://ghr.nlm.nih.gov/handbook/mutationsanddisorders/complexdisorders.
11. S. Ripke et al., "Genome-Wide Association Analysis Identifies 13 New Risk Loci for Schizophrenia," *Nature Genetics* 45, no. 10 (2013): 1150–59.
12. B. Georgi et al., "Genomic View of Bipolar Disorder Revealed by Whole Genome Sequencing in a Genetic Isolate," *PLoS Genetics* 10, no. 3 (2014): e1004229.
13. J. Flint and K. S. Kendler, "The Genetics of Major Depression," *Neuron* 81, no. 3 (2014): 484–503., DOI: 10.1016/j.neuron.2014.01.027.
14. S. Kolgeci et al., "Cytogenetic Study in Children with Down Syndrome Among Kosova Albanian Population Between 2000 and 2010," *Materia Sociomedica* 25, no. 2 (2013): 131–35.
15. Ibid.
16. Genetics Home Reference, "Inheriting Genetic Conditions," March 2014, http://ghr.nlm.nih.gov/handbook/inheritance.
17. National Human Genome Research Institute, "Learning about Tay-Sachs Disease," 2011, www.genome.gov/page.cfm?pageID=10001220.
18. Genetics Home Reference, "Cystic Fibrosis," August 2012, http://ghr.nlm.nih.gov/condition/cystic-fibrosis; Genetics Home Reference, "Huntington Disease," March 2014, http://ghr.nlm.nih.gov/condition/huntington-disease.
19. American Cancer Society, "Cancer Facts and Figures 2014," (Atlanta: American Cancer Society, 2014), Available at www.cancer.org/acs/groups/content/@research/documents/webcontent/acspc-042151.pdf.
20. Ibid.
21. National Society of Genetic Counselors, "About Genetic Counselors," Accessed May 1, 2014, http://nsgc.org/p/cm/ld/fid=175.
22. V. Knopik, 2011, "Grand Challenge in Behavioral and Psychiatric Genetics: Quantitative Challenges to Keeping Up with Molecular Advances," *Frontiers in Genetics* 2 (2011): 9, DOI:10.3389/fgene.2011.00009, Available at http://www.ncbi.nlm.nih.gov/pmc/articles/PMC3268568/#__ffn_sectitle.
23. D. Archontaki, G. J. Lewis, and T. C. Bates, "Genetic Influences on Psychological Well-Being: A Nationally Representative Twin Study," *Journal of Personality* 81, no. 2 (2013): 221–30, DOI: 10.1111/j.1467-6494.2012.00787.x; L. Kalasuniene, A. Gostautas, and A. Sinkus, "Heredity of Cognitive Functions and Personality in Twins," *Medicina (Kaunas)* 49, no. 7 (2013): 321–8, Available at http://medicina.kmu.lt/1307/1307-04e.pdf.
24. W. D. Hill et al., " Human Cognitive Ability Is Influenced by Genetic Variation in Components of Postsynaptic Signaling Complexes Assembled by NMDA Receptors and MAGUK Proteins," *Translational Psychiatry* 4, no. 1 (2014): e341.

25. M. A. Schuckit, " A Brief History of Research on the Genetics of Alcohol and Other Drug Use Disorders," *Journal of Studies on Alcohol and Drugs* 17 (2014): 59–67.

Pulled statistics:

p. 413, Genetics Home Reference, "What Is DNA?," March 2014, http://ghr.nlm.nih.gov/handbook/basics/dna.

Chapter 15

1. A. S. Go et al., "Heart Disease and Stroke Statistics—2014 Update: A Report from the American Heart Association," *Circulation* 129 (2014): e28–e292.
2. Ibid.
3. Ibid.
4. Ibid.
5. Ibid.
6. Ibid.
7. D. M. Lloyd-Jones et al., "Defining and Setting National Goals for Cardiovascular Health Promotion and Disease Reduction: The AHA's Strategic Impact Goal through 2020 and Beyond," *Circulation* 121, no. 4 (2010): e14–e31; E. Ford, "Ideal Cardiovascular Health: Start Young, Finish Strong," *Circulation* 125, no. 16 (2012): 1955–57.
8. D. M. Lloyd-Jones et al., "Defining and Setting National Goals for Cardiovascular Health Promotion and Disease Reduction," 2010.
9. A. Folsom et al., "Community Prevalence of Ideal Cardiovascular Health, by the American Heart Association Definition, and Relationship with Cardiovascular Disease Incidence," *Journal of the American College of Cardiology* 57, no. 16 (2011): 1690–96.
10. Ibid.
11. Ibid.
12. A. S. Go et al., "Heart Disease and Stroke Statistics—2014 Update: A Report from the American Heart Association," *Circulation* 129 (2014): e28–e292.
13. Ibid.
14. Ibid.
15. Ibid.
16. Ibid.
17. Ibid.
18. Ibid.
19. Ibid.
20. Ibid.
21. Ibid.
22. Ibid.
23. Ibid.
24. Ibid.
25. Ibid.
26. World Health Organization, "Cardiovascular Diseases (CVDs)—Key Facts," Accessed April 2014, www.who.int/mediacentre/factsheets/fs317/en/#.
27. Ibid.
28. Ibid.
29. American Heart Association, "Why Blood Pressure Matters," April 2012, www.heart.org/HEARTORG/Conditions/HighBloodPressure/WhyBloodPressureMatters/Why-Blood-Pressure-Matters_UCM_002051_Article.jsp.
30. A. S. Go et al., "Heart Disease and Stroke Statistics—2014," 2014.
31. Centers for Disease Control and Prevention, Media Relations, "MMWR–Morbidity and Mortality Weekly Report, News Synopsis for April 4, 2013," April 2013, www.cdc.gov/media/mmwrnews/2013/0404.html.
32. A. S. Go et al., "Heart Disease and Stroke Statistics—2014 Update," 2014.
33. Centers for Disease Control and Prevention, "High Blood Pressure Facts," March 2014, www.cdc.gov/bloodpressure/facts.htm.
34. A. S. Go et al., "Heart Disease and Stroke Statistics—2014 Update," 2014.
35. Centers for Disease Control and Prevention, "High Blood Pressure Facts," March 2014, www.cdc.gov/bloodpressure/facts.htm.
36. P. A. James et al., "2014 Evidence-Based Guideline for the Management of High Blood Pressure in Adults: Report from the Panel Members Appointed to the Eighth Joint National Committee (JNC 8)." *Journal of the American Medical Association* 311, no. 5 (2014): 507–20; A. Navar-Boggan, "Proportion of US Adults Potentially Affected by the 2014 Hypertension Guidelines," *Journal of the American Medical Association* 311, no. 14 (2014): 1424–29, DOI:10.1001/jama.2014.2531.
37. A. S. Go et al., "Heart Disease and Stroke Statistics—2014 Update," 2014.
38. American Heart Association, "Peripheral Artery Disease: Undertreated and Understudied in Women," 2012, http://newsroom.heart.org/pr/aha/peripheral-artery-disease-undertreated-228645.aspx; A. S. Go et al., "Heart Disease and Stroke Statistics—2014 Update," 2014.
39. American Heart Association, "Peripheral Artery Disease: Undertreated and Understudied in Women," 2012, http://newsroom.heart.org/pr/aha/peripheral-artery-disease-undertreated-228645.aspx.
40. A. S. Go et al., "Heart Disease and Stroke Statistics—2014 Update," 2014.
41. Ibid.
42. B. M. Kissela et al., "Age at Stroke: Temporal Trends in Stroke Incidence in a Large, Biracial Population," *Neurology* 79, no. 17 (2012): 1781–87.
43. N. E. Synhaeve et al., "Poor Long-Term Functional Outcome After Stroke among Adults Aged 18 to 50 Years Follow-Up of Transient Ischemic Attack and Stroke Patients and Unelucidated Risk Factor Evaluation (FUTURE) Study," *Stroke* 45, no. 4 (2014): 1157–60.
44. A. S. Go et al., "Heart Disease and Stroke Statistics—2014 Update," 2014.
45. Ibid.
46. Ibid.
47. Ibid.
48. Ibid.
49. Ibid.
50. C. J. L. Murray et al., "The State of US Health, 1990–2010 Burden of Diseases, Injuries, and Risk Factors," *Journal of the American Medical Association* 310, no. 6 (2013): 591–608.
51. S. Gardener et al., "Dietary Patterns Associated with Alzheimer's Disease and Related Chronic Disease Risk: A Review," *Journal of Alzheimers Disease & Parkinsonism* 10 (2013); S. Sharp et al., "Hypertension Is a Potential Risk Factor for Vascular Dementia: Systematic Review," *International Journal of Geriatric Psychiatry* 26, no. 7 (2011): 661–69; F. Testai and P. Gorelick, "Vascular Cognitive Impairment and Alzheimer's Disease: Are These Disorders Linked to Hypertension and Other Cardiovascular Risk Factors?," *Clinical Hypertension and Vascular Diseases*, Part 4 (2011): 195–210.
52. A. S. Go et al., "Heart Disease and Stroke Statistics—2014 Update," 2014.
53. S. Grundy et al., "Definition of Metabolic Syndrome. Report of the National Heart, Lung, and Blood Institute/American Heart Association Conference on Scientific Issues Related to Definition," *Circulation* 109, no. 2 (2011): 433–39.
54. A. S. Go et al., "Heart Disease and Stroke Statistics—2014 Update," 2014.
55. Ibid.
56. Ibid.
57. Ibid.
58. National Cancer Institute, "Fact Sheet: Harms of Smoking and Benefits of Quitting," January 2011, www.cancer.gov/cancertopics/factsheet/tobacco/cessation.
59. G. Taylor et al., "Change in Mental Health After Smoking Cessation: Systematic Review and Meta-Analysis," *British Medical Journal* 348 (2014): 1151–53; A. Parsons, A. Daley, R. Begh, and P. Aveyard, "Influence of Smoking Cessation After Diagnosis of Early Stage Lung Cancer on Prognosis: Systematic Review of Observational Studies with Meta-analysis," *British Medical Journal* 340 (2010): b5569.
60. G. Taylor et al., "Change in Mental Health After Smoking Cessation," 2014.
61. R. Chowdhury et al., "Association of Dietary, Circulating, and Supplement Fatty Acids with Coronary Risk: A Systematic Review and Meta-Analysis," *Annals of Internal Medicine* 160, no. 6 (2014): 398–406.
62. Mayo Clinic, "High Cholesterol," September 2012, www.mayoclinic.org/diseases-conditions/high-blood-cholesterol/in-depth/cholesterol-levels/art-20048245; Mayo Clinic, "HDL Cholesterol: How to Boost Your 'Good' Cholesterol," November 2012, www.mayoclinic.org/diseases-conditions/high-blood-cholesterol/in-depth/hdl-cholesterol/art-20046388.
63. G. Schwarts et al., "Effects of Dalcetrapib in Patients with a Recent Acute Coronary Syndrome," *New England Journal of Medicine* 367, no. 22 (2012): 2089–2099; C. Zheng and M. Aikawa, "High Density Lipoproteins: From Function to Therapy," *American College of Cardiology* 60, no. 23 (2012): 2380–83.
64. N. J. Stone et al., "2013 ACC/AHA Guideline on the Treatment of Blood Cholesterol

to Reduce Atherosclerotic Cardiovascular Risk in Adults: A Report of the American College of Cardiology/American Heart Association Task Force on Practice Guidelines," *Journal of American Cardiology* 2013, DOI:10.1016/j.jacc.2013.11.002.

65. A. S. Go et al., "Heart Disease and Stroke Statistics—2014 Update," 2014.
66. Mayo Clinic, "Top 5 Lifestyle Changes to Reduce Cholesterol," September 2012, www.mayoclinic.org/diseases-conditions/high-blood-cholesterol/in-depth/reduce-cholesterol/art-20045935.
67. A. S. Go et al., "Heart Disease and Stroke Statistics—2014 Update," 2014.
68. Ibid.
69. A. Steptoe and M. Kivimaki, "Stress and Cardiovascular Disease: An Update on Current Knowledge," *Annual Review of Public Health* 34 (2013): 337–54, DOI: 10.1146/annurev-publhealth-031912-114452; C. Vlachopoulous, P. Xaplanteris, and C. Stefanadis, "Mental Stress, Arterial Stiffness, Central Pressures and Cardiovascular Risk," *Hypertension* 56, no. 3 (2010): e28–e30.
70. A. Steptoe and M. Kivimaki, "Stress and Cardiovascular Disease: An Update on Current Knowledge," *Annual Review of Public Health* 34 (2013): 337–54; R. C. Thurston, M. Rewak, and L.D. Kubzansky, "An Anxious Heart: Anxiety and the Onset of Cardiovascular Diseases," *Progress in Cardiovascular Diseases* 55 no. 6 (2013): 524–37.
71. A. S. Go et al., "Heart Disease and Stroke Statistics—2014 Update," 2014.
72. T. Ong and L. Perusse, "Impact of Nutritional Epigenomics on Disease Risk and Prevention: Introduction," *Journal of Nutrigenetics and Nutrigenomics* 4, no. 5 (2011): 245–47; A. Angelakopoulou et al. "Comparative Analysis of Genome-wide Association Studies Signals for Lipids, Diabetes, and Coronary Heart Disease: Cardiovascular Biomarker Genetics Collaboration," *European Heart Journal* 33, no. 3 (2012): 393–407; G. Thanassoulis et al., "A Genetic Risk Score Is Associated with Incident Cardiovascular Disease and Coronary Artery Calcium," *Circulation: Cardiovascular Genetics,* no. 5 (2012): 11321; C. Chow et al., "Parental History and Myocardial Infarction Risk Across the World: The Interheart Study," *Journal of the American College of Cardiology* 57 (2011): 619–27.
73. American Heart Association, "Understand Your Risk of Heart Attack," October 2012, www.heart.org/HEARTORG/Conditions/HeartAttack/UnderstandYourRiskof-HeartAttack/Understand-Your-Risk-of-Heart-Attack_UCM_002040_Article.jsp.
74. Ibid.
75. The Emerging Risk Factors Collaboration, "C-Reactive Protein, Fibrinogen and CVD Prediction," *New England Journal of Medicine* 367, no. 14 (2012): 1310–20.
76. J. Bosch et al., "n-3 Fatty Acids and Cardiovascular Outcomes in Patients with Dysglycemia," *New England Journal of Medicine* 367, no. 4 (2012): 309–318, DOI: 10.1056/NEJMoa1203859.
77. A. Begg et al., "Omega-3 Fatty Acids in Cardiovascular Disease: Re-Assessing the Evidence," *British Journal of Cardiology* 19, no. 2 (2012): 79–84.
78. S. Kaptoge et al. "Inflammatory Cytokines and risk of Coronary Heart Disease. New Prospective Study and Updated Meta-Analysis," *European Heart Journal* (2013): DOI.10.1093/eurheari/eht.367; D. Tehrani et al., "Impact of Inflammatory Biomarkers on Relation of High Density Lipoprotein-Cholesterol with Incident Coronary Heart Disease: Cardiovascular Health Study," *Atherosclerosis* 231, no. 2 (2013): 246–51.
79. D. Wald, J. Morris, and N. Wald, "Reconciling the Evidence on Serum Homocysteine and Ischemic Heart Disease: A Meta-Analysis," *PLoS ONE* 6, no. 2 (2011): e16473; J. Abraham and L. Cho, "The Homocysteine Hypothesis: Still Relevant to the Prevention and Treatment of Cardiovascular Disease?," *Cleveland Clinic Journal of Medicine* 77, no. 12 (2010): 911–18.
80. American Heart Association, "Homocysteine, Folic Acid, and Cardiovascular Disease," January 2012, www.heart.org/HEARTORG/GettingHealthy/Nutrition-Center/Homocysteine-Folic-Acid-and-Cardiovascular-Disease_UCM_305997_article.jsp.
81. Y. Ji et al., "Vitamin B Supplementation, Homocysteine Levels, and the Risk of Cerebrovascular Disease: A Meta-Analysis," *Neurology*, 2013, DOI: 10.1212/WNL.0b013e3182a823cc; A. H. Ford et al., "Homocysteine, Grey Matter and Cognitive Function in Adults with Cardiovascular Disease," *PLoS ONE* 7, no. 3 (2012): e33345; R. Clarke et al., "Homocysteine and Coronary Heart Disease: Meta-Analysis of *MTHFR* Case-Control Studies, Avoiding Publication Bias," *PLoS Med* 9, no. 2 (2012): e1001177.
82. K. M. Moon et al., "Lipoprotein-Associated Phospholipase A2 Is Associated with Atherosclerotic Stroke Risk: The Northern Manhattan Study," *PLoS ONE* 9, no. 1(2014): e83393, doi:10.1371/journal.pone.0083393; C. A. Garza et al., "The Association between Lipoprotein-Associated Phospholipse A2 and Cardiovascular Disease: A Systematic Review," *Mayo Clinic Proceedings* 82, no. 2 (2007): 159–65.
83. B. M. Sondermeijer et al., "Non-HDL Cholesterol vs. Apo B for Risk of Coronary Heart Disease in Healthy Individuals: The EPIC-Norfolk Prospective Population Study," *European Journal of Clinical Investigation* 43, no. 10 (2013): 1009–1015.
84. C. M. Rembold, "Review: Aspirin Does Not Reduce CHD or Cancer Mortality but Increases Bleeding," *Annals of Internal Medicine* 156, no. 12 (2012): JC6–3; C. Ling et al., "Aspirin to Prevent Incident Cardiovascular Disease: Is It Causing More Damage Than It Prevents?," *Clinical Practice* 9, no. 3 (2012): 223–25.
85. American Heart Association, "Prevention and Treatment of Heart Attack," January 2013, www.heart.org/HEARTORG/Conditions/HeartAttack/PreventionTreatmentofHeartAttack/Prevention-and-Treatment-of-Heart-Attack_UCM_002042_Article.jsp.
86. A. S. Go et al., "Heart Disease and Stroke Statistics—2014 Update," 2014.

Pulled statistics:

p. 423, A. S. Go et al., "Heart Disease and Stroke Statistics—2014 Update," 2014.
p. 425, Ibid.
p. 426, Ibid.

Chapter 15A

1. The International Diabetes Federation, *IDF Diabetes Atlas,* 6th ed. (Brussels, Belgium: The International Diabetes Federation, 2013), Available at www.idf.org/diabetesatlas.
2. Ibid.
3. E. Selvin et al., "Trends in Prevalence and Control of Diabetes in the United States, 1988-1994 and 1999-2010," *Annals of Internal Medicine* 160, no. 8 (2014): 517–525.
4. Centers for Disease Control and Prevention. "National Diabetes Statistics Report, 2014." June, 2014. http://www.cdc.gov/diabeteS/pubs/statsreport14.htm.
5. Ibid.
6. Centers for Disease Control and Prevention, "Summary Health Statistics for U.S. Adults: National Health Interview Survey, 2012," *Vital and Health Statistics* 10, no. 260 (2014), Available at www.cdc.gov/nchs/products/series/series10.htm.
7. Centers for Disease Control and Prevention, "National Diabetes Statistics Report, 2014."
8. Ibid.
9. American Diabetes Association, "Diabetes Basics: Type 1," Accessed May 2014, www.diabetes.org/diabetes-basics/type-1.
10. Ibid.
11. The National Diabetes Information Clearinghouse (NDIC), "National Diabetes Statistics: 2011," September 2013, http://diabetes.niddk.nih.gov/dm/pubs/statistics/#fast
12. Centers for Disease Control and Preven tion, "National Diabetes Statistics Report, 2014."
13. D. Dabelea et al., "Is Prevalence of Type 2 Diabetes Increasing in Youth? The SEARCH for Diabetes in Youth Study," *American Diabetes Association 72nd Scientific Sessions* (Philadelphia, PA: June 8–12, 2012.)
14. D. J. Pettitt et al., "Prevalence of Diabetes in U.S. Youth in 2009: The Search for Diabetes in Youth Study," *Diabetes Care* 37, no. 2 (2014): 402–408.
15. Ibid.
16. A. M. Kanaya et al., "Understanding the High Prevalence of Diabetes in U.S. South

Asians Compared with Four Racial/Ethnic Groups: The MASALA and MESA Studies," *Diabetes Care* (2014), DOI: 10.2337/dc13-2656; American Heart Association, "Statistical Fact Sheet, 2013 Update: Diabetes," 2013, Available at www.heart.org/idc/groups/heart-public/@wcm/@sop/@smd/documents/downloadable/ucm_319585.pdf.

17. R. Mihaescu et al., "Genetic Risk Profiling for Prediction of Type 2 Diabetes," *PLoS Currents* 3 (2011): DOI: 10.1371/currents.RRN1208, www.ncbi.nlm.nih.gov/pmc/articles/PMC3024707; E. Ntzani, K. Evangelia, and F. Kavvoura, "Genetic Risk Factors for Type 2 Diabetes: Insights from the Emerging Genomic Evidence," *Current Vascular Pharmacology* 10, no. 2 (2012): 147–155.
18. J. Logue et al., "Association between BMI Measured within a Year After Diagnosis of Type 2 Diabetes and Mortality," *Diabetes Care* 36, no. 4 (2013): 887–893; M. Ashwell, P. Gunn, and S. Gibson, "Waist-to-Height Ratio Is a Better Screening Tool than Waist Circumference and BMI for Adult Cardiometabolic Risk Factors: Systematic Review and Meta-Analysis," *Obesity Reviews* 13, no. 3 (2012): 275–286.
19. M. Schulze et al., "Body Adiposity Index, Body Fat Content and Incidence of Type 2 Diabetes," *Diabetologia* (2012), DOI. 10.1007/s00125-012-2499-z.
20. L. Bromley et al., "Sleep Restriction Decreases the Physical Activity of Adults at Risk for Type 2 Diabetes," *Sleep* 35, no. 7 (2012): 977–84, DOI:10.5665/sleep.1964
21. S. Reutrakul, and E. V. Cauter, "Interactions between Sleep, Circadian Function, and Glucose Metabolism: Implications for Risk and Severity of Diabetes," *Annals of the New York Academy of Sciences* 1311, no. 1 (2014): 151–73; A. Bonnefond et al., "Rare *MTNRIB* Variants Impairing Melatonin Receptor 1B Function Contribute to Type 2 Diabetes," *Nature Genetics* 44 (2012): 297–301; F. Cappuccio et al., "Quantity and Quality of Sleep and Incidence of Type 2 Diabetes: A Systematic Review and Meta-Analysis," *Diabetes Care* 33, no. 2 (2010): 414–420, 287–289; R. Hancox and C. Landlus, "Association between Sleep Duration and Haemoglobin A1c in Young Adults," *Journal of Epidemiology & Community Health* (November 7, 2011), DOI: 10.1136/jech-2011-200217. (Epub ahead of print.)
22. E. Donga et al., "A Single Night of Partial Sleep Deprivation Induces Insulin Resistance," 2010; J. P. Chaput, et al. "Short Sleep Duration as a Risk Factor for Development of the Metabolic Syndrome in Adults," *Preventive Medicine* 57, no. 6 (2013): 872–77; R. Hancox and C. Landlus, "Associations between Sleep Duration and Haemoglobin," 2011.
23. E. Feracioli-Oda, A. Qawasmi, and M. Bloch, "Meta-Analysis: Melatonin for the Treatment of Primary Sleep Disorders," *PLoS ONE* 8, no. 5 (2013): e63773; J. P. Chaput, et al., "Short Sleep Duration as a Risk Factor for Development of the Metabolic Syndrome in Adults," 2013; F. Cappuccio et al., "Quantity and Quality of Sleep and Incidence of Type 2 Diabetes," 2010.
24. E. Feracioli-Oda, A Qawasmi, and M. Bloch, "Meta-Analysis: Melatonin for the Treatment of Primary Sleep Disorders," 2013.
25. M. Cosgrove, L. Sargeant, R. Caleyachetty, and S. Griffin, "Work Related Stress and Type 2 Diabetes: A Systematic Review and Meta-Analysis," *Occupational Medicine* (2012), DOI: 10.1093/occmed/kqs002; T. Monk and D. J. Buysse, "Exposure to Shiftwork as a Risk Factor for Diabetes," *Journal of Biological Rhythms* 28, no. 5 (2013): 356–59; M. Novak et al., "Perceived Stress and Incidence of Type 2 Diabetes: A 35 Year Follow up Study of Middle Aged Swedish Men," *Diabetic Medicine* 30, no. 1 (2013): e8-3-16.
26. E. Puterman, N. Adler, K., Matthews, and E. Epel, "Financial Strain and Impaired Fasting Glucose: The Moderating Role of Physical Activity in the Coronary Artery Ris Development in Young Adults Study," *Psychosomatic Medicine* 74, no. 2 (2012): 187–192.
27. P. Puustinen et al., "Psychological Distress Predicts the Development of Metabolic Syndrome: A Prospective Population-Based Study," *Psychosomatic Medicine* 73 (2011): 158–165.
28. Centers for Disease Control and Prevention. "National Diabetes Statistics Report, 2014."
29. J. M. Schilter and L. C. Dalleck, "Fitness and Fatness: Indicators of Metabolic Syndrome and Cardiovascular Disease Risk Factors in College Students?" *Journal of Exercise Physiology Online* 13, no. 4 (2010): 29–39; Centers for Disease Control and www.cdc.gov/diabetes/pubs/factsheet11.htm.
30. American Heart Association, "Metabolic Syndrome," 2014, www.americanheart.org/presenter.jhtml?identifier=4756.
31. National Heart Lung and Blood Institute, "What Is Metabolic Syndrome?," November 2011, www.nhlbi.nih.gov/health/dci/Diseases/ms/ms_whatis.html.
32. National Heart, Lung, and Blood Institute, "Who Is at Risk for Metabolic Syndrome?," November 2011, www.nhlbi.nih.gov/health/health-topics/topics/ms/atrisk.html.
33. Ibid.
34. American Diabetes Association, "What Is Gestational Diabetes?," March 2014, www.diabetes.org/diabetes-basics/gestational/what-is-gestational-diabetes.html.
35. Ibid.; C. Kim et al., "Gestational Diabetes and the Incidence of Type 2 Diabetes: A Systematic Review," *Diabetes Care* 25, no. 10 (2002): 1862–68; G. Chodick et al., "The Risk of Overt Diabetes Mellitus among Women with Gestational Diabetes: A Population-Based Study," *Diabetic Medicine* 27, no. 7 (2010): 779–85.
36. S. D. Sullivan et al., "Genetic Risk of Progression to Type 2 Diabetes and Response to Intensive Lifestyle or Metformin in Prediabetic Women with and without a History of Gestational Diabetes," *Diabetes Care* (2013), DOI:10.2337/dc13-0700.
37. P. M. Catalano et al., "The Hyperglycemia and Adverse Pregnancy Outcome Study: Associations of GDM and Obesity with Pregnancy Outcomes," *Diabetes Care* 35, no. 4 (2012): 780, DOI: 10.2337/dc11-1790.
38. Y. Nomura et al., "Exposure to Gestational Diabetes Mellitus and Low Socioeconomic Status: Effects on Neurocognitive Development and Risk of Attention-Deficit/Hyperactivity Disorder in Offspring," *Archives of Pediatrics and Adolescent Medicine* 166, no. 4 (2012): 337–43.
39. Centers for Disease Control and Prevention. "National Diabetes Statistics Report, 2014"; American Diabetes Association, Living with Diabetes: Complications," Accessed May 2014, www.diabetes.org/living-with-diabetes/complications/; K. Weinspach et al., "Level of Information about the Relationship between Diabetes Mellitus and Periodontitis—Results from a Nationwide Diabetes Information Program," *European Journal of Medical Research* 18, no. 1 (2013): 6, DOI: 10.1186/2047-783X-18-6.
40. National Kidney Foundation, "Fast Facts," January 2014, www.kidney.org/news/newsroom/factsheets/FastFacts.cfm.
41. Centers for Disease Control and Prevention. "National Diabetes Statistics Report, 2014."
42. Prevent Blindness America, "Diabetic Retinopathy Prevalence by Age," Accessed May 2014, www.visionproblemsus.org/diabetic-retinopathy/diabetic-retinopathy-by-age.html.
43. K. Behan, "New ADA Guidelines for Diagnosis, Screening of Diabetes," *Advance Laboratory* 20, no. 1 (2011): 22, Available at http://laboratory-manager.advanceweb.com.
44. American Diabetes Association, "Diagnosing Diabetes and Learning about Prediabetes," March 2014, www.diabetes.org/diabetes-basics/diagnosis.
45. Diabetes Prevention Program Research Group, "Reduction in the Incidence of Type 2 Diabetes in the Incidence of Type 2 Diabetes with Lifestyle Intervention or Metformin," *New England Journal of Medicine* 345 (2002): 393–403.
46. S. Jonnalagadda et al., "Putting the Whole Grain Puzzle Together: Health Benefits Associated with Whole Grains—Summary of American Society for Nutrition 2010 Satellite Symposium," *Journal of Nutrition* 41, no. 5 (2011): 10115–25.
47. R. Post et al., "Dietary Fiber for the Treatment of Type 2 Diabetes Mellitus: A Meta Analysis," *Journal of the American Board of Family Medicine* 25, no. 1 (2012): 16–23; S. Bhupathiraju et al., "Glycemic Index, Glycemic Load and Risk of Type 2 Diabetes:

Results from 3 Large US Cohorts and an Updated Meta-Analysis," *Circulation* 129, Supplement 1 (2014): AP140–AP140; A. Olubukola, P. English, and J. Pinkney, "Systematic Review and Meta-Analysis of Different Dietary Approaches to the Management of Type 2 Diabetes," *The American Journal of Clinical Nutrition* 97, no. 3 (2013): 505–516.
48. A. Wallin et al. "Fish Consumption, Dietary Long-Chain N-3 Fatty Acids, and the Risk of Type 2 Diabetes: Systematic Review and Meta Analysis of Prospective Studies," *Diabetes Care* 35, no. 4 (2012): 918–29; L. Djousse et al., "Dietary Omega-3 Fatty Acids and Fish Consumption and Risk of Type 2 Diabetes," *American Journal of Clinical Nutrition* 93, no. 1 (2011): 113–50.
49. C. Jeppesen, K. Schiller, and M. Schultze, "Omega-3 and Omega-6 Fatty Acids and Type 2 Diabetes," *Current Diabetes Reports* 13, no. 2 (2013): 279–88.
50. Linus Pauling Institute, "Glycemic Index and Glycemic Load," Accessed April 2014, http://lpi.oregonstate.edu/infocenter/foods/grains/gigl.html.
51. American Diabetes Association, "What We Recommend," December 2013, www.diabetes.org/food-and-fitness/fitness/types-of-activity/what-we-recommend.html; National Diabetes Information Clearing House, "Diabetes Prevention Program," September 2013, http://diabetes.niddk.nih.gov/dm/pubs/preventionprogram/index.aspx.
52. S. R. Kashyap et al., "Metabolic Effects of Bariatric Surgery in Patients with Moderate Obesity and Type 2 Diabetes," *Diabetes Care* 36, no. 8 (2013): 2175–82.
53. P. R. Schauer et al., "Bariatric Surgery versus Intensive Medical Therapy for Diabetes-3 Year Outcomes," *New England Journal of Medicine* 370 (2014): 2002–13, DOI:10.1056/NEJMoa1401329.
54. P. Poirier et al., on Behalf of the American Heart Association Obesity Committee of the Council on Nutrition, Physical Activity, and Metabolism, "Bariatric Surgery and Cardiovascular Risk Factors: A Scientific Statement from the American Heart Association," *Circulation* 123, no. 15 (2011): 1683–701, DOI:10.1161/CIR.0b013e3182149099.
55. Medtronic, "Medtronic Gains Approval of First Artificial Pancreas Device System with Threshold Suspend Automation," September 2013, http://newsroom.medtronic.com/phoenix.zhtml?c=251324&p=irol-newsArticle&id=1859361.

Pulled statistics:

p. 445, American Diabetes Association, "Diabetes Fast Facts," 2013, http://www.diabetes.org/diabetes-basics/diabetes-statistics.

p. 452, Diabetes Prevention Program Research Group, "Reduction in the Incidence of Type 2 Diabetes in the Incidence of Type 2 Diabetes with Lifestyle Intervention or Metformin," *New England Journal of Medicine* 345 (2002): 393–403.

Chapter 16

1. A. S. Go et al., "Heart Disease and Stroke Statistics—2014 Update: A Report from the American Heart Association," *Circulation* 129, no. 3 (2014): e28–e296.
2. American Cancer Society, "Cancer Facts and Figures," Accessed May 2014, www.cancer.org/research/cancerfactsstatistics/cancerfactsfigures2014/index.
3. Ibid.
4. Ibid.
5. Ibid.
6. American Cancer Society, "Staging," June 2012, www.cancer.org/treatment/understandingyourdiagnosis/staging.
7. American Cancer Society, "Cancer Facts and Figures," May 2014.
8. Ibid.
9. Ibid.
10. Ibid.
11. U.S. Surgeon General, *The Health Consequences of Smoking—50 Years of Progress: A Report of the Surgeon General, 2014*, Accessed May 2014, Available at www.surgeongeneral.gov/library/reports/50-years-of-progress/index.html; American Cancer Society, "Cancer Facts and Figures," May 2014; Centers for Disease Control and Prevention, "*Tobacco Use: Targeting the Nation's Leading Killer—At-a-Glance 2011,*" Accessed May 2014, www.cdc.gov/chronicdisease/resources/publications/aag/pdf/2011/tobacco_aag_2011_508.pdf.
12. U.S. Surgeon General, "The Health Consequences of Smoking," May 2014.
13. American Cancer Society, "Cancer Facts and Figures," May 2014.
14. American Cancer Society, "Cancer Facts and Figures," May 2014; National Cancer Institute, "Harms of Smoking and Health Benefits of Quitting—Fact Sheet," 2014, www.cancer.gov/cancertopics/factsheet/Tobacco/cessation.
15. World Health Organization, "Report on the Global Tobacco Epidemic, 2013," Accessed May 2014, Available at www.who.int/tobacco/global_report/2013/en.
16. Cancer Research UK, "Worldwide Cancer," February 2014, http://publications.cancerresearchuk.org/downloads/Product/CS_KF_WORLDWIDE.pdf.
17. W. Chen et al., "Moderate Alcohol Consumption During the Adult Life, Drinking Patterns and Breast Cancer Risk," *Journal of the American Medical Association* 306, no. 17 (2011): 1884–90; S.Y. Park et al., "Alcohol Consumption and Breast Cancer Risk among Women from Five Ethnic Groups with Light to Moderate Intake: The Multiethnic Cohort Study," *International Journal of Cancer* 134, no. 6 (2014):1504–10.
18. American Cancer Society, "Cancer Facts and Figures," May 2014; D. Parkin, "Cancers Attributable to Consumption of Alcohol in the UK in 2010," *British Journal of Cancer* 105 (2011): S14–S18, DOI:10:10.1038/bjc.2011.476; National Cancer Institute, "Alcohol and Cancer Risk Sheet," Accessed May 2014, www.cancer.gov/cancertopics/factsheet/Risk/alcohol; I. Tramacere et al., "A Meta-Analysis on Alcohol Drinking and Gastric Cancer Risk." *Annals of Oncology* 23, no. 1 (2012): 28–36; S. Gupta et al., "Risk of Pancreatic Cancer by Alcohol Dose, Duration, and Pattern of Consumption, Including Binge Drinking: A Population-Based Study," *Cancer Causes & Control* 21, no. 7 (2010): 1047–59.
19. M. Jin et al., "Alcohol Drinking and All Cancer Mortality: A Meta-Analysis," *Annals of Oncology* 24, no. 3 (2013): 807–816.
20. American Cancer Society, "Cancer Facts and Figures," May 2014.
21. C. Eheman et al., "Annual Report to the Nation on the Status of Cancer, 1975–2008, Featuring Cancers Associated with Excess Weight and Lack of Sufficient Physical Activity," *Cancer* 118, no. 9 (2012): 2338–66, DOI: 10.1002/cncr.27514/full; American Cancer Society, "Cancer Facts and Figures," May 2014.
22. H. R. Harris et al., "Body Fat Distribution and Risk of Premenopausal Breast Cancer in the Nurses' Health Study II," *Journal of the National Cancer Institute* 103, no. 3 (2011): 373–78.
23. L. Teras et al., "Weight Loss and Postmenopausal Breast Cancer in a Prospective Cohort of Overweight and Obese U.S. Women," *Cancer Causes and Control* 22, no. 4 (2011): 573–79.
24. American Cancer Society, "The Obesity-Cancer Connection and What We Can Do About It," February 2013, www.cancer.org/cancer/news/expertvoices/post/2013/02/28/the-obesity-cancer-connection-and-what-we-can-do-about-it.aspx; C. Eheman et al., "Annual Report to the Nation on the Status of Cancer, 1975–2008, Featuring Cancers Associated with Excess Weight and Lack of Sufficient Physical Activity," *Cancer* 118, no. 9 (2012): 2338–66, DOI: 10.1002/cncr.27514/full.
25. American Cancer Society, "The Obesity-Cancer Connection," 2013.
26. K. Heikkila et al., "Work Stress and Risk of Cancer: Meta-Analysis of 5700 Incident Cancer Events in 116,000 European Men and Women," *British Medical Journal* 346, (2013): 1165, DOI: 10.1136/bmj.1165.
27. American Cancer Society, "Cancer Facts and Figures," May 2014.
28. American Cancer Society, "Breast Cancer Overview: What Causes Breast Cancer?," January 2014, www.cancer.org/Cancer/BreastCancer/DetailedGuide/breast-cancer-what-causes.
29. American Cancer Society, "Cancer Facts and Figures for Hispanic/Latinos, 2012–2014," Accessed May 2014, www.cancer.org/acs/groups/content/@epidemiologysurveilance/documents/document/acspc-034778.pdf; M. Banegas et al., "The Risk of Developing Invasive Breast Cancer in Hispanic Women," *Cancer* 119, no. 7 (2013): 1373–80.

30. American Cancer Society, "Menopausal Hormone Therapy and Cancer Risk," 2013, www.cancer.org/Cancer/CancerCauses/OtherCarcinogens/MedicalTreatments/menopausal-hormone-replacement-therapy-and-cancer-risk; J. Manson et al., "Menopausal Hormone Therapy and Health Outcomes During the Intervention and Extended Poststoping Phases of the Somen's Health Initiative Randomized Trials," *Journal of the American Medical Association* 310, no. 13 (2013): 1353–68; A. Pesatori et al., "Reproductive and Hormonal Factors and Risk of Lung Cancer: The EAGLE Study," *International Journal of Cancer* 132, no. 11 (2013): 2630–39.
31. Y. Guo et al., "Association between C-Reactive Protein and Risk of Cancer: A Meta-Analysis of Prospective Cohort Studies," *Asian Pacific Journal of Cancer Prevention* 14 (2013), DOI: http://dx.doi.org/10.7314/APJCP.2013.14.1.243.
32. S. Grivennikov, F. Gretan, and M. Karin, "Immunity, Inflammation, and Cancer," *Cell* 140, no. 6 (2010): 883–99, DOI: 10.1016/j.cell.2010.01.025; R. Francescone, V. Hou and S. Grivennikov, "Microbrome, Inflammation and Cancer," *The Cancer Journal* 20, no. 3 (2014): 181–189.
33. S. Sebastian et al., "Colorectal Cancer in Inflammatory Bowel Disease: Results of the 3rd ECCO Pathogenesis Scientific Workshop(I)," *Journal of Crohn's and Coilitis* 8, no. 1 (2014): 5–18.
34. National Cancer Institute, "Fact Sheet—Cell Phones and Cancer Risk," May 2014, www.cancer.gov/cancertopics/factsheet/Risk/cellphones.
35. American Cancer Society, "Infectious Agents and Cancer," March 2014, www.cancer.org/Cancer/CancerCauses/OtherCarcinogens/InfectiousAgents/InfectiousAgentsandCancer/infectious-agents-and-cancer-intro.
36. American Cancer Society, "Expert Voices: Viruses, Bacteria and Cancer, or It's not all Smoke and Sunlight," March 2012, www.cancer.org/cancer/news/expertvoices/post/2012/03/04/viruses-bacteria-and-cancer-or-ite28099s-not-all-smoke-and-sunlight.aspx; American Cancer Society, "Cancer Facts and Figures," Accessed May 2014, Available at http://www.cancer.org/research/cancerfactsstatistics/cancer factsfigures2014/index.
37. Centers for Disease Control and Prevention, "Human Papillomavirus Vaccination Coverage Among Adolescent Girls, 2007–2012, and Postlicensure Vaccine Safety Monitoring, 2006–2013—United States," July 2013, www.cdc.gov/mmwr/preview/mmwrhtml/mm6229a4.htm; American Cancer Society, "Cancer Facts and Figures," May 2014, www.cancer.org/research/cancerfactsstatistics/cancerfactsfigures2014/index; National Cancer Institute, "Fact Sheet–HPV and Cancer," 2012, www.cancer.gov/cancertopics/factsheet/Risk/HPV.
38. M. Gross, C. Tran, K Sutherland, et al. "Pilot Study: Can an Educational Intervention Increase Human Papillomavirus Vaccination in Female College Students?" *Obstetrics and Gynecology* 123 (2014): 114S–115S; N. T. Ratanasiripong, "A Review of Human Papillomaviurs HPV Infection and HPV Vaccine-Related Attitudes and Sexual Behaviors among College-Aged Women in the United States," *Journal of American College Health* 60, no. 6 (2012): 461–70.
39. Ibid.
40. American Cancer Society, "Cancer Facts and Figures," May 2014, www.cancer.org/research/cancerfactsstatistics/cancerfacts-figures2014/index.
41. American Cancer Society, "Infectious Agents and Cancer," May 2014, www.cancer.org/cancer/cancercauses/othercarcinogens/infectiousagents/infectiousagentsandcancer/infectious-agents-and-cancer-toc.
42. American Cancer Society, "Cancer Facts and Figures," May 2014, www.cancer.org/research/cancerfactsstatistics/cancerfacts-figures2014/index.
43. Ibid.
44. American Cancer Society, "Why Lung Cancer Strikes Non-Smokers," October 2013, www.cancer.org/cancer/news/why-lung-cancer-strikes-nonsmokers.
45. American Cancer Society, "Cancer Facts and Figures," May 2014, www.cancer.org/research/cancerfactsstatistics/cancerfacts-figures2014/index.
46. Centers for Disease Control and Prevention, "Smoking and Tobacco Use: Quitting Smoking," February 2014, www.cdc.gov/tobacco/data_statistics/fact_sheets/cessation/quitting/index.htm?utm_source=feedburner&utm_medium=feed&utm_campaign=Feed%3A+CdcSmokingAndTobaccoUseFactSheets+(CDC+-+Smoking+and+Tobacco+Use+-+Fact+Sheets).
47. Ibid.
48. American Cancer Society, "Cancer Facts and Figures," May 2014.
49. American Cancer Society, "Magnetic Resonance Imaging," January 2014, www.cancer.org/cancer/breastcancer/moreinformation/breastcancerearlydetection/breast-cancer-early-detection-a-c-s-recs-m-r-i.
50. American Cancer Society, "Cancer Facts and Figures," May 2014.
51. Ibid.
52. Ibid.
53. Ibid.
54. Breast Cancer.org, "Genetics," April 2014, www.breastcancer.org/risk/factors/genetics.
55. Y. Wu, D. Zhang, and S. Kang, "Physical Activity and Risk of Breast Cancer: A Meta-Analysis of Prospective Studies," *Breast Cancer Research and Treatment* 137, no. 3 (2013): 869–82.
56. J. Dong et al., "Dietary Fiber Intake and Risk of Breast Cancer: A Meta-Analysis of Prospective Cohort Studies," *American Journal of Clinical Nutrition* 94, no. 3 (2011): 900–905; D. Aune et al. "Dietary Fiber and Breast Cancer Risks: A Systematic Review and Meta Analysis of Prospective Studies," *Annals of Oncology* (2012), DOI:10.1093/annuls/mdr589.
57. American Cancer Society, "Colorectal Cancer Facts and Figures, 2014–2016," May 2014, www.cancer.org/acs/groups/content/documents/document/acspc-042280.pdf; American Cancer Society, Cancer Facts and Figures, May 2014.
58. American Cancer Society, "Cancer Facts and Figures," May 2014.
59. Ibid.
60. American Cancer Society, "Colorectal Cancer Facts and Figures, 2014–2016," May 2014.
61. Ibid.
62. Ibid.
63. Ibid.
64. Ibid.
65. Ibid.; American Cancer Society, "Cancer Facts and Figures," May 2014.
66. Ibid.
67. American Cancer Society, "Cancer Facts and Figures," May 2014; American Cancer Society, "Colorectal Cancer Facts and Figures, 2014–2016," May 2014.
68. American Cancer Society, "Cancer Facts and Figures," May 2014.
69. Ibid.
70. Ibid.
71. Skin Cancer Foundation, "Skin Cancer Facts," October 2013, www.skincancer.org/skin-cancer-information/skin-cancer-facts.
72. C. Heckman et al., "Psychiatric and Addictive Symptoms of Young Adult Female Indoor Tanners," *American Journal of Health Promotion* 28, no. 3 (2014): 168–74; C. Harrington et al., "Activation of the Mesostriatal Reward Pathway with Exposure to Ultraviolet Radiation (UVR) vs. Sham UVR in Frequent Tanners: A Pilot Study," *Addictive Biology* 17, no. 3 (2012): 680–86.
73. American Cancer Society, "Cancer Facts and Figures," May 2014.
74. Ibid.
75. Ibid.
76. Ibid.
77. K. Zu., et al. "Dietary Lycopene, Angiogenesis, and Prostate Cancer: A Prospective Study in the Prostate-Specific Antigen Era," *Journal of the National Cancer Institute* 106, no. 2 (2014): 1093–97 .
78. American Cancer Society, "Cancer Facts and Figures," May 2014.
79. Ibid.
80. Ibid.
81. Ibid.
82. Ibid.
83. Ibid.
84. Ibid.
85. Ibid.
86. National Cancer Institute, "Endometrial Cancer," 2012, www.cancer.gov/cancertopics/types/endometrial.
87. American Cancer Society, "Cancer Facts and Figures," May 2014.

88. Ibid.
89. American Cancer Society, "Testicular Cancer," February 2014, www.cancer.org/cancer/testicularcancer/detailedguide/testicular-cancer-risk-factors; National Cancer Institute, "General Information about Testicular Cancer," December 2013, www.cancer.gov/cancertopics/pdq/treatment/testicular/Patient/page1#Keypoint2.
90. American Cancer Society, "Cancer Facts and Figures," May 2014.
91. Ibid.
92. Ibid.
93. Ibid.
94. Centers for Disease Control and Prevention, "Cancer Survivors—United States, 2007," 2012, www.cdc.gov/cancer/survivorship/what_cdc_is_doing/research/survivors_article.htm; National Cancer Survivors Day Foundation, "Cancer Survivorship Issues," 2010, www.ncsdf.org/Pages/Issues.html.
95. National Cancer Institute, "Dictionary of Cancer Terms," 2014, www.cancer.gov/dictionary.

Pulled statistics:

p. 458, Centers for Disease Control and Prevention, "Lung Cancer Risk Factors," February 2013, www.cdc.gov.

p. 465, American Cancer Society, "Colorectal Cancer Facts and Figures—2012–2016." 2014, Available at http://www.cancer.org/acs/groups/content/documents/document/acspc-042280.pdf.

Chapter 17

1. American Lung Association, "How the Lungs Work," Accessed May 2014, www.lung.org/your-lungs/how-lungs-work.
2. American Lung Association, "Estimated Prevalence and Incidence of Lung Disease," May 2014, www.lung.org/finding-cures/our-research/trend-reports/estimated-prevalence.pdf; Centers for Disease Control and Prevention, "Leading Causes of Death," December 2013, www.cdc.gov/nchs/fastats/lcod.htm.
3. American Lung Association, "Chronic Obstructive Pulmonary Disease (COPD) Fact Sheet," May 2014, www.lung.org/lung-disease/copd/resources/facts-figures/COPD-Fact-Sheet.html.
4. Ibid.
5. American Lung Association, "Trends in COPD (Chronic Bronchitis and Emphysema): Morbidity and Mortality," March 2013, www.lung.org/finding-cures/our-research/trend-reports/copd-trend-report.pdf.
6. Ibid.
7. American Lung Association, "Estimated Prevalence and Incidence of Lung Disease," May 2014, www.lung.org/finding-cures/our-research/trend-reports/estimated-prevalence.pdf.
8. Ibid; Centers for Disease Control and Prevention, "FastStats: Asthma," February 2014, www.cdc.gov/nchs/fastats/asthma.htm.
9. American Lung Association, "Reduce Asthma Triggers," Accessed June 2014, www.lung.org/lung-disease/asthma/taking-control-of-asthma/reduce-asthma-triggers.html.
10. Ibid.
11. American Lung Association, "Asthma," Accessed June 2014, www.lung.org/lung-disease/asthma/; U. Gohil, A. Modan, and P. Gohil, "Aspirin-Induced Asthma–A Review," *Global Journal of Pharmacology* 4, no. 1 (2010): 19–30; WebMD, "Aspirin and Other Drugs That Trigger Asthma," April 2014, www.webmd.com/asthma/guide/medications-trigger-asthma.
12. Centers for Disease Control and Prevention, "FastStats: Asthma," February 2014, www.cdc.gov/nchs/fastats/asthma.htm.
13. American Lung Association, "The Burden of Asthma on Hispanics," Accessed June 2014, www.lung.org/lung-disease/disparities-reports/burden-of-asthma-on-hispanics/asthma-in-hispanics-english.pdf.
14. Ibid.
15. National Institute of Allergy and Infectious Diseases, "Allergic Diseases," June 2014, www.niaid.nih.gov/topics/allergicdiseases/Pages/default.aspx.
16. American Academy of Allergy, Asthma, and Immunology, "Allergy Statistics," Accessed June 2014, www.aaaai.org/about-the-aaaai/newsroom/allergy-statistics.aspx.
17. Ibid.
18. Ibid.
19. Ibid. Centers for Disease Control and Prevention, "Allergies and Hay Fever," February 2014, www.cdc.gov/nchs/fastats/allergies.htm.
20. National Institute of Allergy and Infectious diseases, "Pollen Allergy," June 2012, www.niaid.nih.gov/topics/allergicdiseases/understanding/pollenallergy/Pages/default.aspx.
21. National Institute of Allergy and Infectious Diseases, "Food Allergies," July 2013, http://jama.jamanetwork.com/article.aspx?articleid=1719742.
22. Ibid.
23. American Academy of Allergy, Asthma, and Immunology, "Allergy Statistics," 2014.
24. Alzheimer's Association, "Alzheimer's Facts and Figures," Accessed June 2014, www.alz.org/alzheimers_disease_facts_and_figures.asp#prevalence; Centers for Disease Control and Prevention, "Leading Cause of Death," December 2013, www.cdc.gov/nchs/fastats/lcod.htm.
25. Alzheimer's Association, "Alzheimer's Facts and Figures," 2014; Centers for Disease Control and Prevention, "Leading Cause of Death," 2013.
26. J. Lucado, K. Paez, and A. Elixhauser, "Headaches in U.S. Hospitals and Emergency Departments, 2008," *HCUP Statistical Brief* 111 (2011), Available at www.hcup-us.ahrq.gov/reports/statbriefs/sb111.jsp.
27. National Headache Foundation, "Press Kits: Categories of Headache," Accessed June 2014, www.headaches.org/press/NHF_Press_Kits/Press_Kits_-_Categories_Of_Headache.
28. Mayo Clinic, "Tension Headache: Basics and Symptoms," July 2013, www.mayoclinic.org/diseases-conditions/tension-headache/basics/definition/con-20014295.
29. Ibid.
30. National Headache Foundation, "Migraines," May 2014, www.headaches.org/education/Headache_Topic_Sheets/Migraine.
31. Ibid.
32. Ibid.
33. National Headache Foundation, "The Complete Guide to Headache-Migraine," Accessed June 2014, http://headaches.org/educational_modules/completeguide/migraine3.html.
34. Ibid.
35. National Headache Foundation, "Migraines," 2014.
36. National Headache Foundation, "Headache Topic Sheets: Cluster Headaches," 2013, www.headaches.org/education/Headache_Topic_Sheets/Cluster_Headaches.
37. Centers for Disease Control and Prevention, "Epilepsy Fast Facts," January 2013, www.cdc.gov/epilepsy/basics/fast_facts.htm; Lundbeck Foundation, "Epilepsy," March 2014, www.lundbeck.com/global/brain-disorders/disease-areas/epilepsy.
38. Centers for Disease Control and Prevention, "Epilepsy Fast Facts," January 2013, www.cdc.gov/epilepsy/basics/fast_facts.htm; Lundbeck Foundation, "Epilepsy," March 2014, www.lundbeck.com/global/brain-disorders/disease-areas/epilepsy.
39. Centers for Disease Control and Prevention, "Epilepsy Fast Facts," 2013; Lundbeck Foundation, "Epilepsy," March 2014, www.lundbeck.com/global/brain-disorders/disease-areas/epilepsy.
40. Centers for Disease Control and Prevention, "Epilepsy Fast Facts," January 2013, www.cdc.gov/epilepsy/basics/fast_facts.htm; Lundbeck Foundation, "Epilepsy," 2014.
41. R. Preidt, "Your Digestive Tract's Surface Is the Size of a Studio Apartment," *Medline Plus*, April 24, 2014, www.nlm.nih.gov/medlineplus/news/fullstory_145876.html.
42. National Digestive Diseases Information Clearinghouse, "Digestive Diseases Statistics for the United States," June 2014, http://digestive.niddk.nih.gov/statistics/statistics.aspx.
43. IBD Support Foundation, "IBDSF Cheat Sheet: Inflammatory Bowel Disease Defined," Accessed June 2014, www.ibdsf.com/images/cheat-sheets/3.pdf; M. Basson et al., "Ulcerative Colitis," *Medscape*, May 22, 2014, http://emedicine.medscape.com/article/183084-overview.
44. IBD Support Foundation, "IBDSF Cheat Sheet:," 2014. M. Basson et al., "Ulcerative Colitis," *Medscape*, May 22, 2014, http://emedicine.medscape.com/article/183084-overview.

45. IBD Support Foundation, "IBDSF Cheat Sheet," 2014; M. Basson et al., "Ulcerative Colitis," 2014.
46. Herlong, H. F. *Digestive Disorders. The Johns Hopkins White Papers.* Baltimore, MD: Johns Hopkins Medicine, 2013.
47. Ibid.
48. Centers for Disease Control and Prevention, "Inflammatory Bowel Disease (IBD)," 2014, www.cdc.gov/ibd.
49. Crohn's and Colitis Foundation of America, "IBS and IBD: Two Very Different Disorders," June 2012, www.ccfa.org/resources/ibs-and-ibd-two-very.html.
50. Herlong, H. F. *Digestive Disorders. The Johns Hopkins White Papers.* Baltimore, MD: Johns Hopkins Medicine, 2013.
51. Ibid.
52. Centers for Disease Control, "Data and Statistics, Arthritis," February 2014, www.cdc.gov/arthritis/data_statistics.
53. Ibid.
54. Arthritis Foundation, "The Heavy Burden of Arthritis in the U.S.," March 2012, www.arthritis.org/files/images/AF_Connect/Departments/Public_Relations/Arthritis-Prevalence-Fact-Sheet–3-7-12.pdf.
55. Ibid.
56. National Institute of Arthritis and Musculoskeletal and Skin Disease, "Handout on Health: Osteoporosis," August 2013, www.niams.nih.gov/Health_Info/Osteoarthritis/default.asp; Arthritis Foundation, "Who Gets Rheumatoid Arthritis?" Accessed June 2014, www.arthritis.org/who-gets-rheumatoid-arthritis.php.
57. National Institute of Arthritis and Musculoskeletal and Skin Disease, "Handout on Health: Osteoporosis," 2013; Arthritis Foundation, "Who Gets Rheumatoid Arthritis?" 2014.
58. National Institute of Arthritis and Musculoskeletal and Skin Disease, "Handout on Health: Osteoporosis," 2013; Arthritis Foundation, "Who Gets Rheumatoid Arthritis?" 2014.
59. National Institute of Arthritis and Musculoskeletal and Skin Disease, "Handout on Health: Osteoporosis," 2013; Arthritis Foundation, "Who Gets Rheumatoid Arthritis?" June 2014.
60. Arthritis Foundation, "Who Gets Rheumatoid Arthritis?" 2014.
61. International Osteoporosis Foundation, "Epidemiology," Accessed June 2014, www.iofbonehealth.org/epidemiology.
62. Ibid.
63. D. Hoy et al., "The Global Burden of Low Back Pain: Estimates from the Global Burden of Disease 2010 Study," *Annals of Rheumatic Disease* 73 (2014): 968–74.
64. F. Balague et al., "Non-specific Low Back Pain," *The Lancet* 379, no. 9814 (2012): 482–91, DOI:10.1016/S0140-6736(11)60610-7; National Information Institute of Neurological Disorders and Stroke, "NINDS Back Pain Information Page," April 2014, www.ninds.nih.gov/disorders/backpain/backpain.htm.
65. Ibid.
66. National Institute of Neurological Disorders and Stroke, "Low Back Pain Fact Sheet," NIH Publication no. 03-5161, Updated April 2014, www.ninds.nih.gov/disorders/backpain/detail_backpain.htm.
67. I. Calvo-Munos, A. Gomes-Conesa, and J. Sanches-Meca, "Prevalence of low Back Pain in Children and Adolescents: A Meta-Analysis," *Pediatrics* 13, no. 14 (2013), www.biomedcentral.com/1471-2431/13/14.
68. American Academy of Pain Medicine, "AAPM Facts and Figures on Pain," Accessed June 2014, www.painmed.org/patientcenter/facts_on_pain.aspx; National Institute of Neurological Disorders and Stroke, "Low Back Pain Fact Sheet," 2014.
69. National Institute of Neurological Disorders and Stroke, "Low Back Pain Fact Sheet," 2014.; M. Mehra et al., "The Burden of Chronic Low Back Pain with and without a Neuropathic Component: A Healthcare Resource Use and Cost Analysis," *Journal of Medical Economics* 15, no. 2 (2011): 245–52.
70. Centers for Disease Control and Prevention, National Institute of Neurological Disorders, "NINDS Repetitive Motion Disorders Information Page," Updated October 2011, www.ninds.nih.gov/disorders/repetitive_motion/repetitive_motion.htm.

Pulled statistics:

p. 485, American Academy of Allergy, Asthma and Immunology. "Allergy Statistics." 2014. http://www.aaaai.org/about-the-aaaai/newsroom/allergy-statistics.aspx.

p. 486, H. F. Herlong, *Digestive Disorders, The Johns Hopkins White Papers,* Baltimore, MD: Johns Hopkins Medicine, 2013.

Chapter 18

1. American College Health Association, *American College Health Association-National College Health Assessment II: Reference Group Executive Summary Spring, 2013* (Baltimore, MD: American College Health Association, 2013).
2. M. A. Hillen et al., "How Can Communication by Oncologists Enhance Patients' Trust? An Experimental Study," *Annals of Oncology* 25, no. 4 (2014): 896–901.
3. J. Commins, "Defensive Medicine," *Health Leaders Media,* April 13, 2012, www.healthleadersmedia.com/page-4/MAG-278899/Defensive-Medicine.
4. A. T. Chien and M. B. Rosenthal, "Waste Not, Want Not: Promoting Efficient Use of Health Care Resources," *Annals of Internal Medicine* 158, no. 1 (2013): 67–68.
5. Consumer Health, "Patient Rights: Informed Consent," March 2013, www.emedicinehealth.com/patient_rights/article_em.htm#patient_rights.
6. Centers for Disease Control and Prevention, "Therapeutic Drug Use," May 2014, www.cdc.gov/nchs/fastats/drugs.htm.
7. W. Zhong et al., "Age and Sex Patterns of Drug Prescribing in a Defined American Population," *Mayo Clinic Proceedings* 88, no. 7 (2013): 697–707.
8. L. Gallelli et al., "Safety and Efficacy of Generic Drugs with Respect to Brand Formulation," *Journal of Pharmacology and Pharmacotherapeutics* 4, Supplement 1 (2013): S110–S114.
9. U.S. Food and Drug Administration, "Know Your Online Pharmacy," February 2014, www.fda.gov/Drugs/ResourcesForYou/Consumers/BuyingUsingMedicineSafely/BuyingMedicinesOvertheInternet/BeSafeRxKnowYourOnlinePharmacy/ucm318487.htm.
10. National Center for Complementary and Alternative Medicine, "Complementary, Alternative, or Integrative Health: What's in a Name?" May 2013. http://nccam.nih.gov/health/whatiscam.
11. Ibid.
12. National Center for Complementary and Alternative Medicine, "Health Topics A to Z," 2014, http://nccam.nih.gov/health/atoz.htm.
13. National Center for Complementary and Alternative Medicine, "Traditional Chinese Medicine: An Introduction," October 2013, http://nccam.nih.gov/health/whatiscam/chinesemed.htm.
14. National Center for Complementary and Alternative Medicine, "Ayurvedic Medicine: An Introduction," NCCAM Publication no. D287, August 2013, http://nccam.nih.gov/health/ayurveda/introduction.htm.
15. Ibid.
16. National Center for Complementary and Alternative Medicine, "Homeopathy: An Introduction," May 2013, http://nccam.nih.gov/health/homeopathy.
17. Ibid.
18. American Association of Naturopathic Physicians, "Definition of Naturopathic Medicine," Amended 2011, www.naturopathic.org/content.asp?contentid=59.
19. National Center for Complementary and Alternative Medicine, "Chiropractic: An Introduction," NCCAM Publication no. D403, Modified February 2012, http://nccam.nih.gov/health/chiropractic/introduction.htm.
20. Bureau of Labor Statistics, U.S. Department of Labor, "Chiropractors," *Occupational Outlook Handbook, 2012–2013 Edition,* March 29, 2012, www.bls.gov/ooh/Healthcare/Chiropractors.htm.
21. National Center for Complementary and Alternative Medicine, "Massage Therapy: An Introduction," February 2014, http://nccam.nih.gov/health/massage/massageintroduction.htm.
22. Ibid.
23. Bureau of Labor Statistics, U.S. Department of Labor, "Massage Therapists," *Occupational Outlook Handbook, 2012–2013 Edition,* January 2014, www.bls.gov/ooh/Healthcare/Massage-therapists.htm.
24. National Center for Complementary and Alternative Medicine, "Complementary, Alternative, or Integrative Health: What's in

a Name?" May 2013, http://nccam.nih.gov/health/whatiscam.
25. National Center for Complementary and Alternative Medicine, "Acupuncture: An Introduction," September 2012, http://nccam.nih.gov/health/acupuncture/introduction.htm.
26. A. J. Vickers et al., "Acupuncture for Chronic Pain: Individual Patient Data Meta-Analysis," *Archives of Internal Medicine* 172, no. 19 (2012): 1444–53.
27. National Center for Complementary and Alternative Medicine, "Acupuncture," 2012.
28. R. Jahnke et al., "A Comprehensive Review of Health Benefits of Qigong and Tai Chi," *American Journal of Health Promotion 24,* no. 6 (2010): e1–e25.
29. D. L. Fazzino et al., "Energy Healing and Pain: A Review of the Literature," *Holistic Nursing Practice* 24, no. 2 (2010): 79–88; National Center for Complementary and Alternative Medicine, "Reiki: An Introduction," April 2013, http://nccam.nih.gov/health/reiki/introduction.htm.
30. Psychoneuroimmunology Research Society, "Mission Statement," November 17, 2010, www.pnirs.org/society/index.cfm.
31. E. Broadbent and H. E. Koschwanez, "The Psychology of Wound Healing," *Current Opinions in Psychiatry* 25, no 2 (2012): 135–40.
32. M. R. Irwin and R. Olmstead, "Mitigating Cellular Inflammation in Older Adults: A Randomized Controlled Trial of Tai Chi," *American Journal of Geriatric Psychiatry 20,* no. 9 (2012): 764–72.
33. J. J. Mao et al., "Complementary and Alternative Medicine Use among Cancer Survivors: A Population-Based Study," *Journal of Cancer Survivorship: Research and Practice* 5, no. 1 (2011): 8–17.
34. Academy of Nutrition and Dietetics, "Position of the Academy of Nutrition and Dietetics: Functional Foods," *Journal of the Academy of Nutrition and Dietetics* 113, no. 8 (2013): 1096–1103.
35. K. Ried et al., "Effect of Cocoa on Blood Pressure," *Cochrane Database of Systematic Reviews* 8, No. CD008893 (2012), DOI: 10.1002/14651858.CD008893.pub2.
36. National Center for Complementary and Alternative Medicine, "Oral Probiotics: An Introduction," December 2012, http://nccam.nih.gov/health/probiotics/introduction.htm.
37. Office of Dietary Supplements, National Institutes of Health, "Dietary Supplements: Background Information," Updated June 2011, http://ods.od.nih.gov/factsheets/dietarysupplements.asp.
38. National Center for Complementary and Alternative Medicine, "Kava," April 2012, http://nccam.nih.gov/health/kava.
39. Mayo Clinic Staff, "Herbal Supplements: What to Know before You Buy," November 2011, www.mayoclinic.com/health/herbal-supplements/SA00044.
40. U. S. Pharmacopeial Convention, "USP & Patients/Consumers," 2012, www.usp.org/usp-consumers.
41. Kaiser Family Foundation, "Total HMO Enrollment, July 2012," May 2014, http://kff.org/other/state-indicator/total-hmo-enrollment.
42. Centers for Medicare & Medicaid Services, "National Health Expenditure Projections 2012–2022: Forecast Summary," November 2013, www.cms.gov/Research-Statistics-Data-and-Systems/Statistics-Trends-and-Reports/NationalHealthExpendData/Downloads/proj2012.pdf.
43. Ibid.
44. U.S. Department of Health & Human Services, "2014 Poverty Guidelines," January 2014, http://aspe.hhs.gov/poverty/14poverty.cfm.
45. Centers for Medicare & Medicaid Services, "National Health Expenditure Projections 2012–2022," 2013.
46. Centers for Medicare and Medicaid Services, "Children's Health Insurance Program," Accessed May 2014, www.medicaid.gov/Medicaid-CHIP-Program-Information/By-Topics/Childrens-Health-Insurance-Program-CHIP/Childrens-Health-Insurance-Program-CHIP.html.
47. National Conference of State Legislators, "Health Insurance: Premiums and Increases," March 2014, www.ncsl.org/issues-research/health/health-insurance-premiums.aspx.
48. K. G. Carman and C. Eibner, "Survey Estimates Net Gain of 9.3 Million American Adults with Health Insurance," April 8, 2014, www.rand.org/blog/2014/04/survey-estimates-net-gain-of-9-3-million-american-adults.html.
49. American College Health Association, *National College Health Assessment II: Reference Group Executive Summary, Spring 2013,* 2014.
50. R. A. Cohen et. al., Division of Health Interview Statistics, National Center for Health Statistics, "Health Insurance Coverage: Early Release of Estimates from the National Health Interview Survey, January–March 2014," Table 8, September 2014, http://www.cdc.gov/nchs/data/nhis/earlyrelease/insur201409.pdf.
51. Bureau of Labor Statistics, U.S. Department of Labor, "Physicians and Surgeons," *Occupational Outlook Handbook, 2014–2015,* Modified January 2014, www.bls.gov/ooh/healthcare/physicians-and-surgeons.htm.
52. American Hospital Association, "Fast Facts on U.S. Hospitals," January 2014, www.aha.org/research/rc/stat-studies/fast-facts.shtml.
53. O. W. Brawley, *How We Do Harm: A Doctor Breaks Ranks about Being Sick in America* (New York: St. Martin's Press, 2011).
54. Centers for Medicare and Medicaid Services, "National Health Expenditure Projections 2012–2022," 2013.
55. Ibid.
56. America's Health Insurance Plans, "Fast Check: Administrative Costs," November 2012, www.ahip.org/ACA-Toolbox/Documents/Communications-Toolkit/FactCheck–Administrative-Costs.aspx.
57. Central Intelligence Agency, "Country Comparison: Life Expectancy at Birth. CIA World Factbook," Accessed May 2014, www.cia.gov/library/publications/the-world-factbook/rankorder/2102rank.html.
58. Central Intelligence Agency, "Country Comparison: Infant Mortality Rate. CIA Factbook," Accessed May 2014, www.cia.gov/library/publications/the-world-factbook/rankorder/2091rank.html.
59. Department of Health and Human Services, "Report to Congress: National Strategy for Quality Improvement in Health Care," 2011, www.ahrq.gov/workingforquality/nqs/nqs2011annlrpt.htm.

Pulled statistics:

p. 501, Centers for Disease Control and Prevention, "Hospital Utilization," 2014, http://www.cdc.gov/nchs/fastats/hospital.htm.

p. 502, Robert Wood Johnson Foundation, "Survey: Physicians Are Aware That Many Medical Tests and Procedures Are Unnecessary, See Themselves as Solution," May 2014, http://www.rwjf.org/en/about-rwjf/newsroom/newsroom-content/2014/04/survey--physicians-are-aware-that-many-medical-tests-and-procedu.html.

p. 509, P. M. Barnes, B. Bloom, and R. L. Nahin, "Complementary and Alternative Medicine Use among Adults and Children: United States, 2007," *National Health Statistics Reports,* no. 12 (Hyattsville, MD: National Center for Health Statistics, 2008), Available at www.cdc.gov.

Chapter 19

1. Voltaire, "Semiramis," V.1, trans. by J. K. Hoyt, in *The Cyclopaedia of Practical Quotations,* 1896. New York: Funk & Wagnalls Company.
2. World Health Organization, *World Report on Violence and Health* (Geneva: World Health Organization, 2002), Available at www.who.int/violence_injury_prevention/violence/world_report/en.
3. Ibid.
4. Centers for Disease Control and Prevention, Injury Prevention and Control, "Ten Leading Causes of Injury and Deaths—2010" and "10 Leading Causes of Injury Deaths by Age Highlighting Violence-Related Injury Deaths, United States-2010," October 2012, www.cdc.gov/injury/wisqars/pdf/10LCID_All_Deaths_By_Age_Group_2010-a.pdf.
5. World Health Organization, "Violence Prevention—The Evidence," 2010, http://apps.who.int/iris/bitstream/10665/77936/1/9789241500845_eng.pdf.
6. U.S. Department of Justice, Federal Bureau of Investigation, *Crime in the United States, Preliminary Semiannual Uniform Crime Report for January–June 2013,* May 2014, www.fbi.gov/about-us/cjis/ucr/crime-in-the-u.s/2013/preliminary-semi-annual-uniform-crime-report-january-june-2013.
7. Terry Frieden, "U.S. Violent Crime Down for Fifth Straight Year," CNN, October 29,

2012, www.cnn.com/2012/10/29/justice/us-violent-crime; J. Rudolph, "Violent Crime Up in the U.S. for the First Time in Nearly 2 Decades, Despite FBI Claims," *Huffington Post,* October 17, 2012, www.huffingtonpost.com/2012/10/17/violent-crime-bureau-justice-statistics_n_1974123.html.

8. Bureau of Justice Statistics, "The Nation's Two Crime Measures," March 2013, http://bjs.ojp.usdoj.gov.
9. Bureau of Justice Statistics, "For Second Consecutive Year Violent and Property Crime Rates Increased in 2012," October 2013, www.bjs.gov/content/pub/press/cv12pr.cfm 2013.
10. Ibid.
11. American College Health Association, *American College Health Association—National College Health Assessment II: Reference Group Data Report, Spring 2013* (Baltimore, MD: American College Health Association, 2014), www.acha-ncha.org/reports_ACHA-NCHAII.html.
12. National Criminal Justice Reference Service, "Section 6: Statistical Overviews," *NCVRW Resource Guide,* 2012, http://bjs.ojp.usdoj.gov.
13. Center for Public Integrity, "Sexual Assault on Campus: A Frustrating Search for Justice," Updated February 2013, www.publicintegrity.org/accountability/education/sexual-assault-campus.
14. World Health Organization Violence Prevention Alliance, "The Ecological Framework," Accessed June 2014, www.who.int/violenceprevention/approach/ecology/en/index.html; Centers for Disease Control and Prevention, National Center for Injury Prevention and Control, "Understanding School Violence: Fact Sheet—2012," Accessed June 2014, http://www.cdc.gov/violenceprevention/pdf/schoolviolence_factsheet-a.pdf.
15. R. Felner and M. DeVries, "Poverty in Childhood and Adolescence: A Transactional-Ecological Approach to Understanding and Enhancing Resilience in Contexts of Disadvantage and Developmental Risks," in *Handbook of Resilience in Children* (2013): 105–126, New York: Springer; American Psychological Association, "Violence and Socioeconomic Status," Accessed June 2014, www.apa.org/pi/ses/resources/publications/factsheet-violence.aspx.
16. World Health Organization Violence Prevention Alliance, "The Ecological Framework," Accessed June 2014, www.who.int/violenceprevention/approach/ecology/en/index.html; J. H. Derzon, "The Correspondence of Family Features with Problem, Aggressive, Criminal and Violent Behaviors: A Meta-Analysis," *Journal of Experimental Criminology* 6, no. 3 (2010): 263–292, DOI: 10.1007/s11292-010-9098-0; L. Kiss et al., "Gender-based Violence and Socioeconomic Inequalities: Does Living in More Deprived Neighborhoods Increase Women's Risk of Intimate Partner Violence?," *Social Science and Medicine* 74, no. 8 (2012): 1172–79.
17. M. L. Hunt, A. W. Hughey, and M. G. Burke, "Stress and Violence in the Workplace and on Campus: A Growing Problem for Business, Industry and Academia," *Industry and Higher Education* 26, no. 1 (2012): 43–51.
18. T. Dishion, "A Developmental Model of Aggression and Violence: Microsocial and Macrosocial Dynamic within an Ecological Framework," *Handbook of Developmental Psychology* (Springer US, 2014): 449–65. New York.
19. K. Makin-Byrd and K. L. Bierman, "Individual and Family Predictors of the Perpetration of Dating Violence and Victimization in Late Adolescence," *Journal of Youth Adolescence* 42, no. 4 (2013): 536–50, DOI: 10.1007/s10964-012-9810-7; J. H. Derzon, "The Correspondence of Family Features with Problem, Aggressive, Criminal and Violent Behaviors: A Meta-Analysis," *Journal of Experimental Criminology* 6, no. 3 (2010): 263–92, DOI: 10.1007/s11292-010-9098-0; C. Cook et al., "Predictors of Bullying and Victimization in Childhood and Adolescence: A Meta-Analytic Investigation," *School Psychology Quarterly* 25, no. 2 (2010): 65–83.
20. R. Puff and J. Segher, *The Everything Guide to Anger Management: Proven Techniques to Understand and Control Anger* (Adams Media, Inc. A Division of F. and W. Media, 2014). Avon, MA.
21. C. J. Ferguson, "Genetic Contributions to Antisocial Personality and Behavior: A Meta-Analytic Review from an Evolutionary Perspective," *The Journal of Social Psychology* 150, no. 2 (2010): 160–80; D. Boisvert and J. Vaske, "Genetic Theories of Criminal Behavior," *The Encyclopedia of Criminology and Criminal Justice* (2014): 1–6, Boston, MA: Wiley-Blackwell.
22. R. Kendra, K. Bell, and J. Guimond, "The Impact of Child Abuse History, PTSD and Anger Arousal on Dating Violence Perpetrators among College Women," *Journal of Family Violence* 27, no. 3 (2012): 165–75; C. Sousa et al., "Longitudinal Study on the Effects of Child Abuse and Children's Exposure to Domestic Violence, Parent-Child Attachments and Antisocial Behavior in Adolescence," *Journal of Interpersonal Violence* 26, no. 1 (2011): 111–36.
23. W. Gunter and B. Newby, "From Bullied to Deviant: The Victim-Offender-Overlap among Bullying Victims," *Youth Violence and Juvenile Justice* (2014), DOI: 10.1177/1541204014521250, (Epub ahead of print.); M. M. Ttofi, D. P. Farrington, and F. Lösel, "School Bullying as a Predictor of Violence Later in Life: A Systematic Review and Meta-Analysis of Prospective Longitudinal Studies," *Aggression and Violent Behavior* 17, no. 5 (2012): 405–18.
24. K. M Devries et al., "Intimate Partner Violence Victimization and Alcohol Consumption in Women: A Systematic Review and Meta-Analysis," *Addiction* 109 (2014): 379–91, DOI: 10.1111/add.12393; A. Abbey, "Alcohol's Role in Sexual Violence Perpetration: Theoretical Explanations, Existing Evidence and Future Directions," *Drugs and Alcohol Review* 30, no. 5 (2012): 481–85; J. M. Boden, D. M. Fergusen, and L. J. Horwood, "Alcohol Misuse and Violent Behavior: Findings from a 30-Year Longitudinal Study," *Drugs and Alcohol Dependence* 122, (2012): 135–41; United Nations Office on Drugs and Crime, "World Drug Report," 2013, http://www.unodc.org/unodc/secured/wdr/wdr2013/World_Drug_Report_2013.pdf; A. Sanderlund et al. "The Association between Sports Participation, Alcohol Use and Aggression and Violence: A Systematic Review," *Journal of Science and Medicine in Sport* 17, no. 1 (2014): 2–7.
25. P. H. Smith et al., "Intimate Partner Violence and Specific Substance Use Disorders: Findings from the National Epidemiologic Survey on Alcohol and Related Conditions," *Psychology of Addictive Behaviors* 26, no. 2 (2012): 236–45.
26. A. Abbey, "Alcohol's Role in Sexual Violence Perpetration: Theoretical Explanations, Existing Evidence and Future Directions," *Drug and Alcohol Review* 30, no. 5 (2011): 481–89.
27. A. Sanderlund et al., "The Association between Sports Participation, Alcohol Use and Aggression and Violence: A Systematic Review," *Journal of Science and Medicine in Sport* 17, no. 1 (2014) :2–7.
28. A. Abbey, "Alcohol's Role in Sexual Violence Perpetration," 2011.
29. Mary McMurran, ed., *Alcohol-Related Violence Prevention and Treatment* (West Sussex, UK: John Wiley and Sons, 2013); K. Graham et al., "Alcohol-Related Negative Consequences among Drinkers Around the World," *Addiction* 106, no. 8 (2011): 1391–1405; A. Abbey, "Alcohol's Role in Sexual Violence Perpetration," 2011; J. M. Boden, D. M. Fergusson, and L. J. Horwood, "Alcohol Misuse and Violent Behavior," 2012.
30. W. Gunter and K. Daley, "Causal or Spurious? Using Propensity Score Matching to Detangle the Relationship between Violent Video Games and Violent Behavior," *Computers in Human Behavior* 4, no. 28 (2012): 1348–55.
31. T. Greitemeyer and D. Mugge, "Video Games Do Affect Social Outcomes: A Meta-Analytic Review of the Effects of Violent and Prosocial Video Game Play," *Personality and Social Psychology Bulletin* 40, no. 5 (2014): 578–89.
32. C. J. Ferguson et al, "Not Worth the Fuss After All? Cross-Sectional and Prospective Data on Violent Video Game Influences on Aggression, Visuospatial Cognition and Mathematics Ability in a Sample of Youth," *Journal of Youth and Adolescence* 42, no. 1 (2013): 109–22.

33. T. Niederkrotenthaler et al., "Changes in Suicide Rates Following Media Reports of Celebrity Suicide: A Meta-Analysis," *Journal of Epidemiology and Community Health* 66, no. 11 (2012): 1037–42, DOI: 10.1136/jech-2011-200707.
34. R. A. Ramos et al., "Comfortably Numb or Just Yet Another Movie? Media Violence Exposure Does NOT Reduce Viewer Empathy for Victims of Real Violence Among Primarily Hispanic Viewers," *Psychology of Popular Media Culture* 2, no. 1 (2013): 2–10.
35. ChildStats.Gov, "America's Children in Brief: Key National Indicators of Well-Being, 2012," Accessed June 2014, http://childstats.gov/pdf/ac2012/ac_12.pdf.
36. Centers for Disease Control and Prevention, "Youth Violence: Definitions," December 2013, www.cdc.gov/violenceprevention/youthviolence/definitions.html; L. L. Dahlberg and E. G. Krug, "Violence: A Global Public Health Problem," in *World Report on Violence and Health* (Geneva: World Health Organization, 2002), 1–21.
37. Centers for Disease Control and Prevention, "Health, United States, 2013," May 2014, www.cdc.gov/nchs/data/hus/hus13.pdf.
38. Centers for Disease Control and Prevention, "Deaths: Preliminary Data for 2013," *National Vital Statistics Reports* 61, no. 6 (2012), Available at www.cdc.gov/nchs/data/nvsr/nvsr61/nvsr61_06.pdf; Centers for Disease Control and Prevention, "Faststats: Assault or Homicide," December 2013, www.cdc.gov/nchs/fastats/homicide.htm.
39. Centers for Disease Control and Prevention, National Center for Injury Prevention and Control, Web-Based Injury Statistics Query and Reporting System (WISQARS), 2011, www.cdc.gov; U. S. Department of Justice, Federal Bureau of Investigation, *Crime in the United States 2011*, 2012, www.fbi.gov.
40. Centers for Disease Control and Prevention, WISQARS, 2011; U. S. Department of Justice, Federal Bureau of Investigation, *Crime in the United States 2011*, 2012, www.fbi.gov.
41. Federal Bureau of Investigation, "Hate Crime Statistics, 2012," November 2013, www.fbi.gov/news/stories/2013/november/annual-hate-crime-statistics-show-slight-decease/annual hate crime statistics show slight-decrease.
42. Ibid.
43. Bureau of Justice Statistics, "Hate Crime Victimization-2004-2012-Statistical Tables," February 2014, www.bjs.gov/index.cfm?ty=pbdetail&iid=4883.
44. Ibid.
45. P. Lin and J. Gill, "Homicides of Pregnant Women," *Journal of Forensic Medicine and Pathology* (2010), DOI: 10-1097/PAF.0b013e3181d3dc3b.
46. Violence Policy Center, *American Roulette: Murder-Suicide in the United States*, 4th ed. (Washington, DC: Violence Policy Center, 2012), Available at www.vpc.org.
47. M. C. Black et al., *The National Intimate Partner and Sexual Violence Survey (NISVS): 2010 Summary Report* (Atlanta, GA: National Center for Injury Prevention and Control, Centers for Disease Control and Prevention, 2011), Available at www.cdc.gov.
48. L. Walker, *The Battered Woman* (New York: Harper and Row, 1979).
49. L. Walker, *The Battered Woman Syndrome*, 3rd ed. (New York: Springer, 2009).
50. Psychiatric Times, "Battered Woman Syndrome," July 2009, www.psychiatrictimes.com/trauma-and-violence/battered-woman-syndrome.
51. Bureau of Justice Statistics, "Intimate Partner Violence, 1993-2010," November 2012, www.bjs.gov/index.cfm?ty=pbdetail&iid=4536.
52. Centers for Disease Control and Prevention, National Center for Injury Prevention and Control, "Understanding Intimate Partner Violence Fact Sheet," 2009, www.cdc.gov/violenceprevention/pdf/IPV_factsheet-a.pdf; National Domestic Violence Hotline, "Abuse in America," www.ndvh.org/get-educated/abuse-in-america.
53. U. S. Department of Health and Human Services Administration for Children and Families, "Definitions of Child Abuse and Neglect," February 2011, www.childwelfare.gov/systemwide/laws_policies/statutes/define.cfm.
54. Childhelp, National Child Abuse Statistics, "Child Abuse in America—2012," 2012, www.childhelp.org/pages/statistics; National Children's Alliance, "National Statistics on Child Abuse," Accessed June 2014, www.nationalchildrensalliance.org/NCANationalStatistics.
55. Centers for Disease Control and Prevention, "Elder Abuse Prevention," June 2014, www.cdc.gov/Features/ElderAbuse/; National Institute on Aging, "Elder Abuse," March 2014, www.nia.nih.gov/health/publication/elder-abuse.
56. J. Grohol, "DSM-5 Changes: PTSD, Trauma and Stress-Related Disorders," *Psych Central-Professional*, May 28, 2013, http://pro.psychcentral.com/dsm-5-changes-ptsd-trauma-stress-related-disorders/004406.html.
57. M. L. Walters, J. Chen, and M. J. Breiding, *The National Intimate Partner and Sexual Violence Survey (NISVS): 2010 Findings on Victimization by Sexual Orientation* (Atlanta, GA: National Center for Injury Prevention and Control, Centers for Disease Control and Prevention, 2013).
58. D. G. Kilpatrick et al., "Drug-Facilitated, Incapacitated, and Forcible Rape: A National Study," July 2007, www.ncjrs.gov/pdffiles1/nij/grants/219181.pdf; White House Task Force to Protect Students from Sexual Assault, *Not Alone: First Report of White House Task Force to Protect Students from Sexual Assault*, April 2014, www.whitehouse.gov/sites/default/files/docs/report_0.pdf.
59. National Criminal Justice Reference Service, "School and Campus Crime," *Resource Guide*, Accessed June 2014, www.victimsofcrime.org/docs/ncvrw2013/2013ncvrw_stats_school.pdf?sfvrsn=0.
60. White House Task Force to Protect Students from Sexual Assault, "Not Alone," 2014.
61. R. Bergen and E. Barnhill, National Online Resource Center on Violence Against Women, "Marital Rape: New Research and Directions," National Resource Center on Domestic Violence, 2011.
62. Ibid.
63. M. Stoltenborgh et al., "The Current Prevalence of Child Sexual Abuse Worldwide: A Systematic Review and Meta-Analysis," *International Journal of Public Health* 58, no. 3 (2013): 469–83; L. P. Chen et al., "Sexual Abuse and Lifetime Diagnosis of Psychiatric Disorders: Systematic Review and Meta-Analysis," *Mayo Clinic Proceedings* 85, no. 7 (2010): 618–29; Childhelp, "Child Abuse in America—2012," 2014; U.S. Department of Health and Human Services, Children's Bureau, "Child Maltreatment," February 2013, www.acf.hhs.gov/sites/default/files/cb/cm2012.pdf.
64. M. Stoltenborgh et al., "The Current Prevalence of Child Sexual Abuse Worldwide," 2013.
65. Ibid.; Childhelp, "Child Abuse in America—2012," 2014.
66. Childhelp, "Child Abuse in America—2012," 2014; L. P. Chen et al., "Sexual Abuse and Lifetime Diagnosis of Psychiatric Disorders," 2010; M. Stoltenborgh et al., "The Current Prevalence of Child Sexual Abuse Worldwide, 2013; T. Hilberg, C. Hamilton-Giachrtsis, and L. Dixon, "Review of Meta-Analyses on the Association between Child Sexual Abuse and Adult Mental Health Difficulties: A Systematic Approach," *Trauma, Violence, Abuse* 12, no. 1 (2011): 38–49.
67. Childhelp, "Child Abuse in America—2012," 2014.
68. Oregon State University, Sexual Harassment and Sexual Violence, Accessed June 2014, http://oregonstate.edu/oei/sexual-harassment-and-violence-policy.
69. Centers for Disease Control, "Sexual Violence, Stalking, and Intimate Partner Violence Widespread in the US," NISVS 2010 Summary Report, Press Release, December 2011.
70. Centers for Disease Control and Prevention, "Sexual Violence, Stalking, and Intimate Partner Violence Widespread in the US," 2011; National Criminal Justice Reference Service (NCVRW), "Crime Victimization in the United States: Statistical Overviews," in *NCVRW Resource Guide—2012*, Accessed June 2014, Available at www.ncjrs.gov/ovc_archives/ncvrw/2012/pdf/Statistical-Overviews.pdf.
71. Centers for Disease Control and Prevention, "Sexual Violence, Stalking, and Intimate

Partner Violence Widespread in the US," 2011; NCVRW "Crime Victimization in the United States," 2014.
72. U.S. Department of Justice, "Juvenile Justice Fact Sheet—Highlights of the 2011 National Youth Gang Survey," September 2013, www.ojjdp.gov/pubs/242884.pdf; Federal Bureau of Investigation, "2011 National Gang Threat Assessment-Emerging Trends," Accessed June 2014, www.fbi.gov/stats services/publications/2011-national-gang-threat-assessment.
73. FBI, "2011 National Gang Threat Assessment," 2014.
74. D. McDaniel, "Risk and Protective Factors Associated with Gang Affiliation among High-Risk Youth: A Public Health Approach," *Injury Prevention*, January 11, 2012, Available at http://injuryprevention.bmj.com/content/early/2012/01/04/injury-prev-2011-040083.full.pdf+html.
75. U.S. Code of Federal Regulations, Title 28CFR0.85.

Pulled statistics:

p. 534, CDC. "The National Intimate Partner and Sexual Violence Survey (NISVS): 2010 Summary Report," February 26, 2014, Available at http://www.cdc.gov/violenceprevention/nisvs/2010_ipvreport.html.

p. 536, White House Task Force to Protect Students from Sexual Assault. "Not Alone: First Report of White House Task Force to Protect Students from Sexual Assault, "April 2014, http://www.whitehouse.gov/sites/default/files/docs/report_0.

p. 537, CDC. "The National Intimate Partner and Sexual Violence Survey (NISVS): 2010 Summary Report," February 26, 2014. http://www.cdc.gov/violenceprevention/nisvs/2010_ipvreport.html.

Chapter 19A

1. M. Heron, "Deaths: Leading Causes for 2010," *National Vital Statistics Reports* 62, no. 6 (2013), www.cdc.gov/nchs/data/nvsr/nvsr62/nvsr62_06.pdf.
2. Ibid.
3. Centers for Disease Control and Prevention, "Wide-Ranging OnLine Data for Epidemiologic Research (WONDER)," May 2013, Available from: http://wonder.cdc.gov/mortsql.html.
4. National Highway Traffic Safety Administration, "Traffic Safety Facts: 2012 Data," April 2014, www-nrd.nhtsa.dot.gov/Pubs/812016.pdf; Centers for Disease Control and Prevention, "Web-Based Injury Statistics Query and Reporting System (WISQARS)," January 2014, www.cdc.gov/injury/wisqars.
5. National Highway Traffic Safety Administration, "Traffic Safety Facts: 2012 Data," 2014.
6. National Safety Council, "Motor Vehicle Safety," Accessed May 2014, www.nsc.org/safety_home/MotorVehicleSafety/Pages/MotorVehicleSafety.aspx.
7. Governors Highway Safety Association, *Distracted Driving: What Research Shows and What States Can Do*, Executive Summary, 2011, www.ghsa.org/html/publications/pdf/sfdist11execsum.pdf.
8. National Highway Traffic Safety Administration, "What Is Distracted Driving? Key Facts and Statistics," Accessed May 2014, www.distraction.gov/content/get-the-facts/facts and statistics.html.
9. U.S. Centers for Disease Control and Prevention, "Distracted Driving," January 2014, www.cdc.gov/Motorvehiclesafety/Distracted_Driving.
10. National Highway Traffic Safety Administration, "Traffic Safety Facts: 2012 Data," 2014; CDC, "WISQARS," 2014.
11. National Highway Traffic Safety Administration, "What Is Distracted Driving?," 2014.
12. Governors Highway Safety Association, "Cell Phone and Texting Laws," Accessed May 2014, www.ghsa.org/html/stateinfo/laws/cellphone_laws.html.
13. National Highway Traffic Safety Administration, "What Is Distracted Driving?," 2014.
14. National Highway Traffic Safety Administration, "Traffic Safety Facts: 2012 Data," 2014.
15. Ibid.
16. National Institute on Drug Abuse, "NIDA InfoFacts: Drugged Driving," Revised October 2013, http://drugabuse.gov/infofacts/driving.html.
17. Ibid.
18. Centers for Disease Control and Prevention, "Drowsy Driving: Asleep at the Wheel," 2014, www.cdc.gov/features/dsDrowsyDriving/index.html.
19. National Highway Traffic Safety Administration, "Traffic Safety Facts: 2012 Data," 2014.
20. Centers for Disease Control and Prevention, "Policy Impact: Seat Belts," Updated January 2014, www.cdc.gov/Motorvehicle-safety/seatbeltbrief.
21. National Highway Traffic Safety Administration, "Traffic Safety Facts: 2012 Data," 2014.
22. Insurance Institute for Highway Safety, "Vehicle Size and Weight," February 2014, www.iihs.org/iihs/topics/t/vehicle-size-and-weight/qanda.
23. National Highway Traffic Safety Administration, "Traffic Safety Facts: 2012 Data," 2014.
24. Ibid.
25. Governors Highway Safety Association, "Helmet Laws," May 2014, www.ghsa.org/html/stateinfo/laws/helmet_laws.html.
26. National Highway Traffic Safety Administration, "Traffic Safety Facts 2011 Data: Bicyclists and Other Cyclists," April 2013, www-nrd.nhtsa.dot.gov/Pubs/811743.pdf.
27. Ibid.
28. American College Health Association, *American College Health Association—National College Health Assessment (ACHA-NCHA): Reference Group Executive Summary, Spring 2013* (Baltimore, MD: American College Health Association, 2013), www.acha-ncha.org/docs/ACHA-NCHA-II_ReferenceGroup_ExecutiveSummary_Spring2013.pdf.
29. Consumer Product Safety Commission, "CPSC Fact Sheet: Skateboarding Safety," *CPSC Publication* 93 (2012), Available at www.cpsc.gov//PageFiles/122356/093.pdf.
30. Ibid.
31. National Ski Areas Association, "Facts About Skiing/Snowboarding Safety," October 2013, www.nsaa.org/media/175091/Facts_on_Skiing_and_Snowboarding_10_4_13.pdf.
32. Ibid.
33. College of Optometrists, "Look After Your Eyes: Skiing," Accessed May 2014, http://lookafteryoureyes.org/eye-care/sun-and-sunshine/skiing.
34. Centers for Disease Control and Prevention, "Unintentional Drowning: Get the Facts," May 2014, www.cdc.gov/HomeandRecreationalSafety/Water-Safety/waterinjuries-factsheet.html.
35. American Red Cross, "Summer Water Safety Guide," March 2009, http://american.redcross.org/site/DocServer/watersafety0609.pdf?docID=735.
36. Centers for Disease Control and Prevention, "Unintentional Drowning," 2014.
37. U. S. Coast Guard, "Coast Guard News: U.S. Coast Guard Releases 2013 Recreational Boating Statistics Report," May 2014, http://coastguardnews.com/u-s-coast-guard-releases-2013-recreational-boating-statistics-report/2014/05/14/?utm_source=feedburner&utm_medium=feed&utm_campaign=Feed%3A+CoastGuardNews+(Coast+Guard+News).
38. Ibid.
39. Ibid.
40. Ibid.
41. U. S. Coast Guard, "Boating Safety Resource Center: Boating Under the Influence Initiatives," April 2014, www.uscgboating.org/safety/boating_under_the_influence_initiatives.aspx.
42. American Boating Association, "Boating Safety—It Could Mean Your Life," 2013, www.americanboating.org/safety.asp.
43. U.S. Consumer Product Safety Division, "2011 Fireworks Annual Report," June 2012, www.cpsc.gov//PageFiles/108534/2011fwreport.pdf.
44. National Council on Fireworks Safety, "Key Fireworks Safety Information," Accessed May 2014, www.fireworksafety.com.
45. Centers for Disease Control and Prevention, "Drug Overdose," December 2013, www.cdc.gov/homeandrecreationalsafety/overdose/index.html.
46. U.S. Food and Drug Administration, "Acetaminophen Prescription Combination Drug Products with More than 325 mg: FDA Statement-Recommendation to Discontinue Prescribing and Dispensing," January 2014, www.fda.gov/safety/

medwatch/safetyinformation/safetyalerts-forhumanmedicalproducts/ucm381650.htm.

47. J. B. Mowry et al., "2012 Annual Report of the American Association of Poison Control Centers' National Poison Data System (NPDS): 30th Annual Report," *Clinical Toxicology* 51, no. 10 (2013): 949–1229, DOI: 10.3109/15563650.2013.863906.
48. American Association of Poison Control Centers, "Prevention," Accessed May 2014, www.aapcc.org/prevention.
49. Centers for Disease Control and Prevention, "Falls among Older Adults: An Overview," September 2013, www.cdc.gov/HomeandRecreationalSafety/Falls/adultfalls.html.
50. Centers for Disease Control and Prevention, "Fire Deaths and Injuries: Fact Sheet," October 2011, www.cdc.gov/HomeandRecreationalSafety/Fire-Prevention/fires-factsheet.html.
51. U.S. Fire Administration, "Campus Fire Safety: Safety Tips for Students and Parents," March 2014, www.usfa.fema.gov/citizens/college.
52. Ibid.
53. Ibid.
54. American Heart Association, "Hands-Only CPR," Accessed May 2014, http://handsonlycpr.org.
55. F. R. Lin, J. K. Niparko, and L. Ferrucci, "Hearing Loss Prevlaence in the United States," *Archives of Internal Medicine* 171, no. 20 (2011): 1851–53.
56. C. G. LePrell et al., "Evidence of Hearing Loss in a 'Normally-Hearing' College Student Population," *International Journal of Audiology* 50, Supplement 1 (2011): S21–1.
57. K. Hannah et al., "Evaluation of the Olivocochlear Efferent Reflex Strength in the Susceptibility to Temporary Hearing Deterioration After Music Exposure in Young Adults," *Noise Health* 16, no. 69 (2014):108–15, DOI: 10.4103/1463-1741.132094.
58. U.S. Bureau of Labor Statistics, "Census of Fatal Occupational Injuries Summary, 2012," August 2013, www.bls.gov/news.release/cfoi.nr0.htm.
59. National Institute of Neurological Disorders and Stroke, "Low Back Pain Fact Sheet," April 2014, www.ninds.nih.gov/disorders/backpain/detail_backpain.htm.
60. American College Health Association, *American College Health Association—National College Health Assessment (ACHA-NCHA): Reference Group Executive Summary, Spring 2013*, (Baltimore, MD: American College Health Association, 2013), www.acha-ncha.org/docs/ACHA-NCHA-II_ReferenceGroup_ExecutiveSummary_Spring2013.pdf.

Pulled statistics:

p. 548, C. Jones, K. A. Mack, and L. J. Paulozzi. "Pharmaceutical Overdose Deaths, United States, 2010," *Journal of the American Medical Association* (JAMA). 2013, 309(7). 657–659.

p. 549, American College Health Association. *American College Health Association—National College Health Assessment II: Reference Group Executive Summary Spring 2013.* Hanover, MD: American College Health Association; 2013.

Chapter 20

1. Mead, M. *Male and Female: A Study of Sexes in a Changing World.* (1950). London: Gollancz.
2. Worldwatch Institute, "Fertility Surprises Portend More Populous Future," July 2013, www.worldwatch.org/fertility-surprises-portend-more-populous-future; Worldwatch Institute, "U.N. Raises 'Low' Population Projections for 2050," June 2014, www.worlwatch.org/node/6038.
3. United Nations, *World Population Prospects, The 2012 Revision: Highlights and Advance Tables,* http://esa.un.org/unpd/wpp/Documentation/pdf/WPP2012_HIGHLIGHTS.pdf.
4. United Nations, *Global Environment Outlook: Environment for Development* (GEO-5): Summary for Policy Makers, 2012, www.uncsd2012.org/rio20/content/documents/280GEO5_SPM_English.pdf.
5. Central Intelligence Agency, *The World Factbook: Country Comparison: Total Fertility Rate,* Accessed June 2014, www.cia.gov/library/publications/the world factbook/rankorder/2127rank.html.
6. U.S. Census Bureau, Population Division, "International Database Country Rankings," Accessed June 2014, http://sasweb.ssd.census.gov/idb/ranks.html.
7. United States Census Bureau, "U.S. and World Population Clock," June 2014, http://www.census.gov/popclock.
8. Ibis.; Global Footprint Network, "Key Findings of the National Footprint Accounts, 2012 Edition," March 2014, http://outsidemagazine.typepad.com/.a/6a00d83453140969e20168eba7a7cb970c-pi.
9. World Wildlife Report, *Living Planet Report 2012,* www.worldwildlife.org/science/2012%20Living%20Planet%20Report/index.html; United Nations, *Global Environmental Outlook,* 2012.
10. United Nations, *UNEP Yearbook: Emerging Issues in our Global Environment, 2013,* 2013, www.unep.org/pdf/uyb_2013.pdf.
11. The IUCN Red List of Threatened Species, "IUCN Red List Status: Mammals," Accessed June 2014, www.iucnredlist.org/initiatives/mammals/analysis/red-list-status; J. Croxall, et al. "Seabird Conservation Status, Threats and Priority Actions: A Global Assessment," *Bird Conservation International,* 2012, 22: 1–34, doi: 10.1017/S0959270912000020.
12. United Nations Environmental Program, "New Elephant Poaching and Ivory Smuggling Figures Released," June 2014, www.unep.org/newscentre/default.aspx?DocumentID=2791&ArticleID=10895.
13. The IUCN Red List of Threatened Species, "IUCN Red List Status: Amphibians," 2014.
14. United Nations, *Global Environment Outlook,* 2012.
15. United Nations Environmental Program, "Towards a Green Economy: Pathways to Sustainable Development and Poverty Eradication," Accessed June 2014, Available at www.unep.org/greeneconomy/greeneconomy-report/tabid/29846/default.aspx.
16. United Nations, "UNEP Yearbook: Emerging Issues in our Global Environment, 2013," 2013.
17. Ibid.
18. U.S. Energy Information Administration, "Independent Statistics and Analysis," 2013, www.eia.gov/oiaf/aeo/tablebrowser/#release=IEO2013&subject=1-IEO2013&table=9-IEO2013&region=0-0&cases=Reference-0504a_1630.
19. U.S. Environmental Protection Agency, "Air Enforcement," June 2014, www2.epa.gov/enforcement/air-enforcement.
20. U.S. Environmental Protection Agency, "Overview of Greenhouse Gases: Emissions and Trends: Carbon Dioxide," April 2014, www.epa.gov/climatechange/ghgemissions/gases/co2.html.
21. S. M. Platt et al., "Two-Stroke Scooters Are a Dominant Source of Air Pollution in Many Cities," *Nature Communications* 5 (2014), DOI:10.1038/ncomms4749. (Epub ahead of print.)
22. Environmental Protection Agency, "Our Nation's Air: Status and Trends through 2010," http://www.epa.gov/airtrends/2011/, Updated February 2012; American Lung Association, "Health Effects of Ozone and Particle Pollution," in *State of the Air 2013* (Washington, DC: American Lung Association, 2014), Available at www.stateoftheair.org/2013/health-risks.
23. A. Soos, "Acid Rain Change," Environmental News Network, 2012, www.enn.com/enn_news/article/43885.
24. Ibid.; American Lung Association, "Health Effects of Ozone and Particle Pollution," 2014.
25. U.S. Environmental Protection Agency, "Reducing Acid Rain," December 2012, www.epa.gov/acidrain/reducing.
26. U.S. Environmental Protection Agency, "Acid Rain: Effects of Acid Rain—Surface Waters and Aquatic Animals," December 2012, www.epa.gov/acidrain/effects/surface_water.html.
27. Ibid.; A. Soos, "Acid Rain Change," 2012.
28. U.S. Environmental Protection Agency, "Acid Rain: Effects of Acid Rain—Human Health," 2012.
29. U.S. Energy Information Administration, "Independent Statistics and Analysis," 2013.
30. S. McMahon et al., "Common Toxins in our Homes, Schools and Workplaces," Global Indoor Health Network, December 2012, Available at http://globalindoorhealth-network.com/files/GIHN_position_statement_Revised_12_17_2012.pdf.
31. U.S. Environmental Protection Agency, "An Introduction to Indoor Air Quality," Updated November 2013, www.epa.gov/iaq/ia-intro.html.

32. Ibid.
33. U.S. Environmental Protection Agency, "Health Effects of Exposure to Secondhand Smoke," November 2011, www.epa.gov/smokefree/healtheffects.html; American Cancer Society, "Health Effects of Secondhand Smoke," March 2014, www.cdc.gov/tobacco/data_statistics/fact_sheets/secondhand_smoke/health_effects.
34. American Nonsmoker's Rights Foundation, "States, Commonwealths and Municipalities with 100 Percent Smokefree Laws in Workplaces, Restaurants and Bars," April 2014, www.no-smoke.org/pdf/100ordlist.pdf.
35. Ibid.
36. U.S. Environmental Protection Agency, "Indoor Air Quality: Radon: Health Risks," Updated March 2013, www.epa.gov/radon/healthrisks.html.
37. U.S. Environmental Protection Agency, "Why Is Radon the Health Risk That It Is? Homes above EPA's Radon Action Level," January 2014, www.epa.gov/radon/aboutus.html.
38. Centers for Disease Control and Prevention, "Lead," June 2014, www.cdc.gov/nceh/lead/; Centers for Disease Control and Prevention, "Blood Lead Levels in Children Aged 1–5 Years—United States, 1999–2010," *Morbidity and Mortality Weekly Report* 62, no. 13 (2013): 245–48, Available at www.cdc.gov.
39. U.S. Department of Housing and Urban Development, "Making Homes Healthier for Families," Accessed June 2014, http://portal.hud.gov/hudportal/HUD?src=/program_offices/healthy_homes/healthyhomes.
40. National Center for Environmental Health, "Mold: Basic Facts," May 2014, www.cdc.gov/mold/faqs.htm#affect.
41. National Safety Council, "Sick Building Syndrome," April 2009, www.nsc.org/news_resources/Resources/Documents/Sick_Building_Syndrome.pdf.
42. T. Stafford, "Indoor Air Quality and Academic Performance," Accessed June 2014, http://research.economics.unsw.edu.au/RePEc/papers/2013-25.pdf; B. Biro et al., "Ventilation Rates in Schools and Pupil's Performance," *Building and Environment* 48, no. 1, (2012): 215–23.
43. U.S. Environmental Protection Agency, "IAQ Tools for Schools: Improved Academic Performance: Evidence from Scientific Literature," Updated January 2013, www.epa.gov/iaq/schools/student_performance/evidence.html; B. Biro et al., "Ventilation Rates in Schools and Pupil's Performance," 2012.
44. U.S. Environmental Protection Agency, "Overview of Greenhouse Gases: Emissions and Trends: Carbon Dioxide," 2014; U.S. Global Change Research Group, "Climate Change Impacts in the United States," May 2014, Available at http://nca2014.globalchange.gov/downloads/report; National Aeronautics and Space Administration, "Ozone Hole Watch," June 2014, http://ozonewatch.gsfc.nasa.gov.
45. White House, "Remarks by the President on Climate Change-Georgetown University," Press Release, June 2013, www.whitehouse.gov/the-press—office/2013/06/25/remarks-president-climate-change.
46. U.S. Global Change Research Group, "Climate Change Impacts in the United States," May 2014, Available at http://nca2014.globalchange.gov/downloads/report; NASA, "Global Climate Change. Evidence of Change: How Do We Know?," Accessed June 2014, http://climate.nasa.gov/evidence; Environmental Protection Agency, "Climate Change Facts: Answers to Common Questions," 2014; J. C. L. Olivier et al., "Trends in Global CO_2 Emissions—2013 Report," October 2013, Available at www.pbl.nl/en/publications/trends-in-global-co2-emissions-2013-report.
47. Environmental Protection Agency, "Climate Change Facts: Answers to Common Questions," 2014.
48. Environmental Protection Agency, "Climate Change: Overview of Greenhouse Gases," 2014.
49. NASA, "Global Climate Change," 2014; Environmental Protection Agency, "Climate Change Facts: Answers to Common Questions," 2014; J. C. L Olivier et al., "Trends in Global CO_2 Emissions—2013 Report," 2013.
50. NASA, "Global Climate Change," 2014.
51. Ibid; J. C. L. Olivier et al., "Trends in Global CO_2 Emissions—2013 Report," 2013.
52. J. C. L. Olivier et al., "Trends in Global CO_2 Emissions—2013 Report," 2013; Environmental Protection Agency, "National Greenhouse Gas Emissions Data," April 2014, www.epa.gov/climatechange/ghgemissions/usinventoryreport.html.
53. Ibid.
54. World Commission on Environment and Development, *Our Common Future* (Oxford: Oxford University Press, 1987): 27.
55. J. C. L. Olivier et al., "Trends in Global CO_2 Emissions—2013 Report," 2013.
56. Ibid.
57. U.S. Geological Survey, "Where Is Earth's Water?," Modified March 2014, http://ga.water.usgs.gov/edu/earthwherewater.html.
58. Ibid.
59. Ibid.
60. Ibid.
61. Department of National Intelligence, "Global Water Security," 2012, www.dni.gov/nic/ICA_Global%20Water%20Security.pdf.
62. World Economic Forum, "Global Agenda Council on Water Security 2012–2014," Accessed June 2014, www.weforum.org/content/global-agenda-council-water-security-2012-2014.
63. Department of National Intelligence, "Global Water Security," 2012; World Economic Forum, "Global Agenda Council on Water Security 2012–2014," 2014.
64. Environmental Protection Agency, "Drinking Water Contaminants," June 2013, http://water.epa.gov/drink/contaminants/; U.S. Geological Survey, "Emerging Contaminants in the Environment," 2011, http://toxics.usgs.gov/regional/emc/; U.S. Environmental Protection Agency, "Pharmaceuticals and Personal Care Products (PPCPs) in Water," May 2014, http://water.epa.gov/scitech/swguidance/ppcp.
65. M. Kostich, A. Batt, and J. Lazorcheck, "Concentrations of Prioritized Pharmaceuticals in Effluents from 50 Large Wastewater Treatment Plants in the U.S. and Implications for Risk Estimation," *Environmental Pollution* 184 (2014): 354–59.
66. Ibid.
67. Environmental Protection Agency, Office of Underground Storage Tanks, "FY 2011 Annual Report on the Underground Storage Tank Program," December 2012, www.epa.gov/oust.
68. Ibid.
69. Environmental Protection Agency, "Natural Gas Extraction: Hydraulic Fracturing," June 2014, www.epa.gov/hydraulicfracture.
70. Ibid.
71. Agency for Toxic Substances and Disease Registry (ATSDR), "Toxic Substances Portal: Polychlorinated Biphenyls (PCBs)," March 2011, www.atsdr.cdc.gov/substances/toxsubstance.asp?toxid=26.
72. U.S. Environmental Protection Agency, "The EPA and Food Security," May 2012, www.epa.gov/pesticides/factsheets/securty.htm.
73. U.S. Environmental Protection Agency, *Municipal Solid Waste Generation, Recycling, and Disposal in the United States: Facts and Figures for 2012*, EPA-530-F-14-001 (Washington, DC: U.S. Environmental Protection Agency, 2011), Available at www.epa.gov/osw/nonhaz/municipal/pubs/2012_msw_fs.pdf.
74. Ibid.
75. Ibid.
76. U.S. Environmental Protection Agency, "Superfund: Superfund National Accomplishments Summary, Fiscal Year 2013," Accessed June 2014, www.epa.gov/superfund/accomp/pdfs/FY_2013_SF_EOY_accomp_sum_FINAL.pdf.
77. U.S. Environmental Protection Agency, "Hazardous Waste," 2012, http://www.epa.gov/osw/basic-hazard.htm; U.S. Environmental Protection Agency, "Household Hazardous Waste," 2014, http://www.epa.gov/osw/conserve/materials/hhw.htm.
78. U.S. Nuclear Regulatory Commission, "Radiation Basics," 2011, http://nrc.gov/about-nrc/radiation/health-effects/radiation-basics.html.
79. National Council on Radiation Protection and Measurements, "NCRP Report No. 160 Section 1 Pie Chart," 2010, www.ncrponline.org/Publications/160_Pie_charts.html.
80. R. Balmforth, "Factbox: Key Facts on Chernobyl Nuclear Accident," Reuters, March 15, 2011, www.reuters.com/article/2011/03/15/uk-nuclear-chernobyl-facts-idUSTRE72E69R20110315.

81. U.S. Energy Information Administration, "Independent Statistics and Analysis," 2012.
82. M. Penny and M. Selden, "The Severity of the Fukushima Daiichi Nuclear Disaster: Comparing Chernobyl and Fukushima," *Global Research*, 2011, www.globalresearch.ca/PrintArticle.php?articleId=24949.

Pulled statistics:

p. 561, Population Reference Bureau, "2013 World Population Data Sheet," 2013, http://www.prb.org/pdf13/2013-population-data-sheet_eng.pdf.

p. 574, EPA. Municipal Solid Waste Generation, Recycling and Disposal in the United States: Facts and Figures, 2012. EPA-503-F-14-001. February, 2014. http://www.epa.gov/osw/nonhaz/municipal/pubs/2012_msw_fs._pdf.

Chapter 21

1. J. C. Cavanaugh and F. Blanchard-Fields, *Adult Development and Aging*, 6th ed. (Belmont, CA: Wadsworth, Cengage Learning, 2011); S. Hillier and G. Barrow, *Aging, the Individual, and Society*, 9th ed. (Belmont, CA: Wadsworth, Cengage Learning, 2011).
2. National Institute on Aging, "Biology of Aging," March 2014, Available at www.nia.nih.gov/health/publication/biology-aging/preface; S. Krauss, "Fulfillment at Any Age," *Psychology Today*, June 23, 2012, www.psychologytoday.com/blog/fulfillment-any-age/201206/what-s-your-true-age.
3. S. Krauss, "Fulfillment at Any Age," *Psychology Today*, June 23, 2012, www.psychologytoday.com/blog/fulfillment-any-age/201206/what-s-your-true-age.
4. Administration on Aging, U.S. Department of Health and Human Services, "A Profile of Older Americans: 2013, Education," 2013, http://www.aoa.gov/Aging_Statistics/Profile/2013/docs/2013_Profile.pdf; http://www.americangeriatrics.org/files/documents/Adv_Resources/Profile.of.Older.Americans.May.2013.pdf.
5. A. Paganini-Hill et al., "Activities and Mortality in the Elderly: The Leisure World Cohort Study," *Journal of Gerontology* 66A, no. 5 (2011): 559–67; National Institute on Aging, "Healthy Aging: Lessons from the Baltimore Longitudinal Study of Aging," 2010, www.nia.nih.gov/health/publication/healthy-aging-lessons-baltimore-longitudinal-study-aging.
6. Central Intelligence Agency, "The World Factbook. Country Comparisons: Life Expectancy at Birth," 2013, www.cia.gov/library/publications/the-world-factbook/rankorder/2103rank.html.
7. Administration on Aging, U.S. Department of Health and Human Services, "A Profile of Older Americans: 2013, Education," 2013, http://www.aoa.gov/Aging_Statistics/Profile/2013/docs/2013_Profile.pdf.
8. Federal Interagency Forum on Aging Related Statistics, "Older Americans 2012: Key Indicators of Well-Being," June 2012, Available at www.agingstats.gov/Main_Site/Data/2012_Documents/docs/EntireChartbook.pdf.
9. Administration on Aging, U.S. Department of Health and Human Services, "A Profile of Older Americans: 2013, Education," 2013, http://www.aoa.gov/Aging_Statistics/Profile/2013/docs/2013_Profile.pdf; http://www.americangeriatrics.org/files/documents/Adv_Resources/Profile.of.Older.Americans.May.2013.pdf.
10. Administration on Aging, "A Profile of Older Americans: 2013," 2013.
11. Ibid.
12. Ibid.
13. Ibid.
14. Genworth, "Arizona State-Specific Data from the Genworth 2013 Cost of Care Survey," March 2013, www.genworth.com/dam/Americas/US/PDFs/Consumer/corporate/Arizona_gnw.pdf.
15. Administration on Aging, "A Profile of Older Americans: 2013," 2013.
16. National Osteoporosis Foundation, "Debunking the Myths," Accessed June 2014, http://nof.org/articles/4.
17. Centers for Disease Control and Prevention, "Osteoarthritis," 2011, www.cdc.gov/arthritis/basics/osteoarthritis.htm.
18. National Association for Continence, "Statistics," Accessed June 2014, www.nafc.org/media/statistics.
19. Ibid.
20. J. Solheim et al., "Daily Life Consequences of Hearing Loss in the Elderly," *Disability Rehabilitation* 33, no. 23–24 (2011): 2179–85, DOI: 10.3109/09638288.2011.563815; F. Lin et al., "Hearing Loss and Cognitive Decline in the Elderly," *Journal of American Medical Association-Internal Medicine* 173, no. 4 (2013): 293–99, DOI: 10.1001/jamainternmed.2013.1868.
21. J. Solheim et al., "Daily Life Consequences of Hearing Loss," 2011; F. Lin et al., "Hearing Loss and Cognitive Decline," 2013.
22. T. E. Howe, et al., "Exercise for Improving Balance in Older People," *Cochrane Database of Systematic Reviews*, 2011, www.summaries.cochrane.org/CD004963/exercise-for-improving-balance-in-older-people.
23. Medline Plus, "Aging Changes in the Senses," 2012, www.nlm.nih.gov/medlineplus/ency/article/004013.html.
24. B. J. Cowart, "Smell and Taste in Aging," 2011, *Perfumer and Flavorist* 36, no. 1 (2011): 34–36.
22. R. von Simson et al., "Sexual Health and the Older Adult," February 2, 2012, *Student British Medical Journal* 20 (2012): e688.
25. R. von Simson et al., "Sexual Health and the Older Adult," 2012.
26. M. N. Lochlainne et al., "Sexual Activity and Aging," *Journal of American Medical Directors Association* 14, no. 8 (2013): 565–72; R. von Simson et al., "Sexual Health and the Older Adult," 2012.
27. M. N. Lochlainne et al., "Sexual Activity and Aging," 2013; R. von Simson et al., "Sexual Health and the Older Adult," 2012.
28. Alzheimer's Association, *2012 Alzheimer's Disease Facts and Figures* (Chicago: Alzheimer's Association, 2012).
29. Ibid.
30. L. Hebert et al., "Alzheimer Disease in the United States (2010–2050) Estimated Using the 2010 Census," *Neurology* 80, no. 19 (2013): 1778–83, DOI: 10.1212/WNL.0b013e31828726f5.
31. Alzheimer's Association, *2012 Alzheimer's Disease Facts and Figures*, 2012.
32. Ibid.
33. Alzheimer's Association, "What Is Alzheimer's?," 2011.
34. Centers for Disease Control and Prevention, "Health, United States, 2013," May 2014, Available at www.cdc.gov/nchs/hus.htm; National Institute on Aging, "AgePage: Alcohol Use in Older People," Updated April 2012, www.nia.nih.gov/HealthInformation/Publications/alcohol.htm.
35. Centers for Disease Control and Prevention, "Health, United States, 2013," 2014; National Institute on Aging, "AgePage: Alcohol Use in Older People," Updated April 2012, www.nia.nih.gov/HealthInformation/Publications/alcohol.htm. Centers for Disease Control and Prevention, "The State of Aging and Health in American 2013" Accessed June 2014, www.cdc.gov/features/agingandhealth/state_of_aging_and_health_in_america_2013.pdf.
36. Substance Abuse and Mental Health Services Administration, "Older Americans Behavioral Health Issue Brief 5: Prescription Medication Misuse and Abuse Among Older Adults," 2012, www.aoa.gov/AoARoot/AoA_Programs/HPW/Behavioral/docs2/Issue%20Brief%205%20Prescription%20Med%20Misuse%20Abuse.pdf.
37. D. S. Budnitz et al., "Emergency Hospitalizations for Adverse Drug Events in Older Americans," *The New England Journal of Medicine* 365 (2011): 2002–2012.
38. Centers for Disease Control and Prevention, "Making Physical Activity a Part of an Older Adult's Life," 2011, www.cdc.gov/physicalactivity/everyone/getactive/olderadults.html.
39. Merriam-Webster, "Death," *Merriam-Webster's Collegiate® Dictionary*, 11th ed. (Springfield, MA: Merriam-Webster, Inc., 2011), www.merriam-webster.com. Used by permission.
40. President's Commission on the Uniform Determination of Death, *Defining Death: Medical, Ethical and Legal Issues in the Determination of Death* (Washington, DC: U.S. Government Printing Office, 1981).
41. Ad Hoc Committee of the Harvard Medical School to Examine the Definition of Brain Death, "A Definition of Irreversible Coma," *Journal of the American Medical Association* 205 (1968): 377.
42. Elisabeth Kübler-Ross and David Kessler, "The Five Stages of Grief," 2011, www.grief.com/the-five-stages-of-grief.

43. C. Corr, C. Nabe, and D. Corr, *Death and Dying, Life and Living*, 6th ed. (Belmont, CA: Wadsworth, 2009).
44. Victorian Government Health Information, "Death and Dying," 2011, www.health.vic .gov.au/dementia/index.htm.
45. Behavioural Neuropathy Clinic, "Grief and the Grieving Process," 2012, www.adhd .com.au/grief.htm.
46. American Bar Association, Commission on Law and Aging, *Consumer's Tool Kit for Health Care Advance Planning*, 2nd ed. (Washington, DC: American Bar Association, 2012), Available at www.abanet.org/ aging/toolkit/home.html.
47. Aging with Dignity, "Five Wishes," 2012, www.agingwithdignity.org/five-wishes .php.
48. Public Agenda, "Right to Die," 2011, www .publicagenda.org/articles/right-die.
49. Oregon Department of Human Services, "FAQs about the Death with Dignity Act," Updated 2011, www.public.health.oregon. gov/ProviderPartner Resources/Evaluation-Research/DeathwithDignityAct/Pages/faqs .aspx#similar; International Task Force on Euthanasia and Assisted Suicide, "Assisted Suicide Laws," Updated February 2012, www.internationaltaskforce.org/assisted_ suicide_laws.htm.
50. National Hospice and Palliative Care Organization, "NHPCO Facts and Figures: Hospice Care in America, 2012 Ed.," 2012, www.nhpco.org/sites/default/files/public/ Statistics_Research/2012_Facts_Figures. pdf.
51. U.S. National Library of Medicine, "Organ Donation" 2012, www.nlm.nih.gov/medlin-eplus/organdonation.html.
52. U.S. Department of Health and Human Services, "The Need Is Real," 2012, www .organdonor.gov/about/data.html.
53. Mayo Clinic, "Organ Donation: Don't Let These Myths Confuse You," 2011, www .mayoclinic.com/health/organ-donation/ FL00077.

Pulled statistics:

p. 584, Administration on Aging, U.S. Dept. of Health and Human Services, "A Profile of Older Americans: 2013," 2014, www.aoa.gov/ Aging_Statistics/Profile/2013/docs/2013_ Profile.pdf.

p. 588, U.S. Bureau of Labor Statistics, "The 2012 Statistical Abstract," January 2013, http:// www.census.gov/compendia/statab.

p. 593, U.S. Census Bureau, "2010 Census Shows 65 and Older Population Growing Faster than Total U.S. Population," November 2011, http://www.census.gov/newsroom/ releases/archives/2010_census/cb11-cn192 .html.

PHOTO CREDITS

Chapter 1 1: Aldo Murillo/E+/Getty Images; 2: Photo Alto/Getty Images; 4: David Gregerson/Sport Studio Photos/Getty Images; 3: Chine Nouvelle/SIPA/Newscom; 5: Maridav/Fotolia; 6: AGE Fotostock; 7: Stockbroker/MBI/Alamy; 8: Cat London/E+/Getty images; 8: Grantly Lynch/UK Stock Images Ltd/Alamy; 8: Webphotographeer/E+/Getty Images; 8: Yeko Photo Studio/Shutterstock; 10: Karl Weatherly/Photodisc/Getty Images; 12: Ringo Chiu/ZUMA Press/Newscom; 13: MagicEyes77/Shutterstock; 14: Wavebreakmedia Ltd/Shutterstock; 15: Mitchel Gray/Getty Images; 16: iStockphoto/Thinkstock/Getty Images; 18: Manley099/E+/Getty Images; 19: Steve Lindridge/Alamy

Focus On: Improving Your Financial Health 24: Kate Kunz/Fancy/Corbis; 26: Jack Frog/Shutterstock; 26: Robert Nickelsberg/Getty Images; 27: Matthew Benoit/Fotolia; 28: Wavebreakmedia Ltd/Shutterstock; 29: Sturti/Getty Images; 30: Michael Jung/Shutterstock; 32: Blend Images/Alamy

Chapter 2 34: Michael Blann/Ocean/Corbis; 37: Getty Images; 37: Terry Vine/Blend Images/Getty Images; 38: Pascal Broze/AGE Fotostock; 41: Aldo Murillo/Getty Images; 41: ArtFamily/Shutterstock; 43: Dmitri Maruta/Shutterstock; 45: Donvictorio/Shutterstock; 46: Comstock Images/Getty Images; 47: Atanasija1/Shutterstock; 48: Pavel L Photo and Video/Shutterstock; 49: John Bell/Getty Images; 50: Science Source; 51: Chris Rout/Bubbles Photolibrary/Alamy; 52: Alamy; 54: Endostock/Fotolia; 57: David H.Seymour/Shutterstock

Focus On: Cultivating Your Spiritual Health 61: Jupiter Images/Stockbyte/Getty Images; 62: Jim West/Alamy; 64: Anne-Marie Palmer/Alamy; 65: Rick Gomez/Solus/Corbis; 66: Jiang Hongyan/Shutterstock; 67: PhotoAlto sas/Alamy; 68: Blend Images/Alamy; 68: Igor S. Srdanovic/shutterstock; 69: Blend Images/Alamy; 70: Xiaofoto/Fotolia; 71: Malerapaso/E+/Getty Images

Chapter 3 72: Ocean/Corbis; 74: Jupiterimages/Stockbyte/Getty Images; 76: Oliver Furrer/Alamy; 77: Michael Krinke/iStock/Getty Images; 78: Brenda Carson/Shutterstock; 79: Adam Borkowski/Getty Images; 80: Matthew Benoit/Shutterstock; 80: David De Lossy/Photodisc/Getty Images; 81: Radius Images/Corbis; 82: Marili Forastieri/Getty Images; 83: Alexandra Gl/Fotolia; 83: Shahrul Azman/Shutterstock; 84: Chad Baker/Jason Reed/Ryan McVay/Photodisc/Getty Images; 85: Kate Sept 2004/E+/Getty Images; 86: Dmitriy Shironosov/Shutterstock; 87: PhotoAlto/Alamy; 89: Asia Images Group Pvt Ltd/Alamy; 90: Dex Image/Getty Images; 91: David L. Moore/Alamy; 92: Richard Rodvold/Getty Images; 93: Andy Crawford/DK Images; 94: John Dowland/Getty Images

Focus On: Improving Your Sleep 98: Rubberball/Fotolia; 99: Rubberball/Getty Images; 100: Spauln/E+/Getty Images; 101: Newscom; 103: Superstock/Alamy; 104: RubberBall/Alamy; 106: Getty Images; 107: Amy Walters/fotolia; 108: Loretta Hostettler/Getty Images; 108: Radius Images/Getty Images

Chapter 4 110: Henglein and Steets/Age Fotostock; 111: Jetta Productions/Blend Images/Getty Images; 112: Photo Library/Getty Images; 114: Alamy; 116: Zero Creatives/Cultura/AGE Fotostock; 117: Michael Jung/Shutterstock; 118: Blue Jean Images/Getty Images; 119: Teens/Alamy; 121: Abfotolv/Fotolia; 122: Purestock/Getty Images; 123: Purestock/Getty Images; 124: Corbis/Superstock; 124: Ryan McVay/Photodisc/Getty Images; 125: Maria Dubova/Getty Images; 126: JGI/Jamie Grill/Blend Images/AGE Fotostock; 127: PhotoAlto/John Dowland/Getty Images

Chapter 5 131: Image Source/Corbis; 133: Hannibal Hanschke/Newscom; 134: Echo/Cultura/Getty Images; 134: FS2 Wenn Photos/Newscom; 139: David J. Green/Lifestyle Themes/Alamy; 141: Nam Fook Voon/AGE Fotostock; 144: Allison Michael Orenstein/Photodisc/Getty Images; 145: Ozgur Donmaz/Getty Images; 146: iStock/Getty Images; 147: J.B Nicholas/Splash News/Newscom; 148: Frederic Cirou/Photo Alto/Alamy; 150: Banana Stock/Getty Images; 151: Ron Nickel/AGE Fotostock

Chapter 6 155: Hero Images/Corbis; 159: Echo/Cultura/Getty Images; 160: Picture Net/Corbis; 161: Jules Selmes and Debi Treloar/DK Images; 161: Pearson Education; 162: Alfred Shihata and FemCap Inc.; 162: Siu Biomed/Newscom; 163: Sean Justice/AGE Fotostock; 164: Magdalena Zurawska/Fotolia; 166: Vario Images/Alamy; 167: Phanie/Science Source; 167: SPL/Science Source; 168: Pearson Education; 172: Image Source/Getty Images; 173: David L Green/Lifestyle Themes/Alamy; 173: Michael Keller/Corbis; 176: Plattform/Johner Images/AGE Fotostock; 179: Lisa Spindler Photography Inc./Getty Images; 180: Claude Edelman/Science Source; 180: Petit Format/Nestle/Science Source; 180: Petit Format/Science Source; 181: Leland Bobbe/Stone/Getty Images; 184: Kablonk/Golden Pixels/Alamy; 185: Plush Studios/Getty Images; 188: Donna Coleman/Getty Images

Chapter 7 193: Minerva Studio/Fotolia; 194: Webphotographer/iStock/Getty Images; 196: Pearson Learning Photo Studio; 197: China Foto Press US/Sipa/Newscom; 199: Brian Leatart/Photolibrary/Getty Images; 200: Steve Debenport/E+/Getty Images; 201: David R. Frazier Photolibrary, Inc./Alamy; 207: Image Source/Getty Images; 207: Suzannah Skelton/E+/Getty Images; 208: Al Freni/Contributor/The Life Images Collection/Getty Images; 208: Matka Wariatka/Getty Images; 209: Chris Bence/Shutterstock; 209: Edward Westmacott/iStock/360/Getty Images; 209: Hurst Photo/Shutterstock; 209: JR Trice/Shutterstock; 209: JRB/Fotolia; 209: Stargazer/Shutterstock; 214: Clarke Canfield/AP Images; 215: Barbara Ayrapetyan/Shutterstock; 215: Brian Hagiwara/Getty Images; 216: Rolf Bruderer/Blend Images/Getty Images; 218: Eric Gevaert/iStock/360/Getty Images; 220: More Pixels/Getty Images; 221: R. Tyree/Getty Images

Chapter 8 225: Corbis/Fotolia; 227: Big Cheese Photo LLC/Alamy; 230: Bikeriderlondon/Shutterstock; 231: Brian Kersey/UPI/Newscom; 232: Brand X Pictures/Getty Images; 233: Alamy; 233: Ariel Skelley/Blend RF/Glow Images; 234: Steve Stock/Alamy; 237: BSIP/Science Souce; 237: David Madison/Getty Images; 237: Julie Brown/Custom Medical Stock; 237: Phanie/Science Source; 237: PhotoEdit; 238: EPF/Alamy; 238: Image Source/Getty Images; 241: UpperCut Images/Alamy

Focus On: Enhancing Your Body Image 249: Dangubic/Fotolia; 250: Pictorial Press Ltd/Alamy; 250: Trinity Mirror/Mirrorpix/Alamy; 251: Custom Medical Stock Photo/Alamy; 251: Sakala/Shutterstock; 252: Brand X Pictures/Getty images; 253: Eric Wells/LatitudeStock/Alamy; 254: Brand X Pictures/Stockbyte/Getty Images; 254: Li Kim Goh/E+/Getty Images; 255: Angela Hampton Picture Library/Alamy; 256: Favakeh/Custom Medical Stock Photo/Newscom; 257: Moodboard/Corbis; 258: Loretta Hostettler/iStock/360/Getty Images; 258: Pascal Broze/Onoky/Getty Images; 259: Photodisc/Getty Images; 259: Shutterstock

Chapter 9 261: Hero Images/Corbis; 263: Miroslav Georgijevic/Vetta/Getty Images; 264: Dylan Ellis/Corbis; 264: John Fryer/Alamy; 266: Anton Gvozdikov/Getty Images; 266: Graham Mitchell/Superstock; 266: Pearson Education; 266: Photodisc/Getty Images; 266: Teo Lannie/PhotoAlto Agency/Getty Images; 267: Cultura/Mischa Keijser/StockImage/Getty Images; 268: Jupiter Images/Getty Images; 270: Ali Ender Birer/Getty Images; 270: Ali Ender Birer/Shutterstock; 270: Craig Veltri/Getty Images; 270: Dandanian/Getty Images; 270: Deymos/Shutterstock; 270: GVictoria/Shutterstock; 270: Kirsty Pargeter/Getty Images; 270: PaulMaguire/Getty Images; 270: Rod Ferris/Shutterstock; 270: Stephen VanHorn/Alamy; 270: Tatuasha/Shutterstock; 270: Walter Cruz/MCT/Newscom; 271: Wave Royalty Free/Design Pics Inc/Alamy; 272: Dan Dalton/Digital Vision/Getty Images; 272: Eric Audras/PhotoAlto sas/Alamy; 272: MIXA/Getty Images; 273: Karl Weatherly/Photodisc/Getty Images; 273: Pearson Education; 273: Rolf Adlercreutz/Alamy; 274: Kathy Willens/AP Images; 275: Ammentorp Photography/Alamy; 276: Pearson Education; 276: Radu Razvan/Shutterstock; 277: Pearson Education; 278: Wavebreakmedia Ltd/Getty Images; 279: Goodshoot/Getty Image; 280: Michael Jung/Shutterstock; 282: Thomas Smith Photography/Alamy; 283: Dennis Welsh/UpperCut Images/Age Fotostock; 284: Radius Images/Getty Images; 285: Daniel Hurst/Getty Images; 285: Ingram Publishing/Getty Images; 286: JP Images/Getty Images

Focus On: Recognizing and Avoiding Addiction 289: Ken Seet/Cardinal/Corbis; 290: Allstar Picture Library/Alamy; 291: Berekin/Getty Images; 293: Cassiede Alain/Shutterstock; 294: John Howard/Digital Vision/Getty Images; 295: Alamy; 296: Denis Pepin/Getty Images; 298: Clover/Alamy; 299: Image Source/AGE Fotostock

Chapter 10 301: CandyBox Images/Fotolia; 303: Goodshoot/Getty Images; 304: Insadco Photography/Alamy; 306: Photo Library/Getty Images; 307: Image Source/Stockbyte/Getty Images; 309: Martin M. Rotker/Science Source; 309: SPL/Science Source; 310: Bill Roth/AP Images; 312: Stockbyte/Getty Images; 313: Roy McMahon/Cardinal/Corbis; 316: Roger Allyn Lee/Superstock; 317: Thinkstock/Stockbyte/Getty Images; 318: Joerg Lange/Vario Images/Alamy; 319: Jiang Jin/Superstock

Chapter 11 324: Anuwat Donkiewpri/123RF; 326: Pearson Education; 327: Elizabeth Weinberg/Getty Images; 329: Helen H. Richardson/Denver Post/Getty Images; 329: James Stevenson/Science Source; 329: James Steveson/Science Source; 330: Alamy; 331: Oral Health America; 332: All Over Photography/Alamy; 332: Getty Images; 334: Handout/MCT/Newscom; 335: Image Source/Alamy; 336: U.S. Food and Drug Administration; 339: Comstock Images/Getty Images; 340: Diego

Cervo/Fotolia; 341: Fstop/Alamy; 342: Bloomberg/Contributor/Getty Images; 342: Dorling Kindersley; 342: E. Nelson/Custom Medical Stock Photo; 342: Gusto Images/Science Source; 342: In Camera Stock/Alamy; 342: Josh Sher/Science Source; 342: Pearson Education

Chapter 12 347: Tomas Rodriguez/Fancy/Corbis; 349: Craig Wactor/Shutterstock; 349: Image Source/Getty Images; 350: Ian Hooton/Science Photo Library/Alamy; 351: Lori Sparkia/Shutterstock; 352: AF archive/Alamy; 353: Thomas M Perkins/Shutterstock; 357: Getty Images; 358: Faces of Meth Program; 359: Karen Mower/E+/Getty Images; 360: Chris Rout/Bubbles Photolibrary/Alamy; 362: Gregor/Shutterstock; 363: Alibi Productions/Alamy; 364: Bob Cheung/Shutterstock; 364: Martyn Vickery/Alamy; 365: Janine Wiedel Photolibrary/Alamy; 366: European Press Photo Agency/Alamy; 367: David Hoffman Photo Library/Alamy; 367: Manchan/Photographer's Choice/Getty Images; 368: Jupiterimages/Getty Images; 370: Bonnie Kamin/PhotoEdit

Chapter 13 374: Henrik Larsson/Fotolia; 378: Photo Alto/Superstock; 379: Ocean/Corbis; 380: Xy/Fotolia; 383: Science Photo Library/Getty Images; 384: Dr. Linda M. Stannard/University of Cape Town/Science Source; 384: Dr. Gary Gaugler/Science Source; 384: Eye of Science/Science Source; 384: Mediscan/Medical-on-Line/Alamy; 384: Steve Gschmeissner/Science Source; 386: Eric Raptosh/Blend Images/Getty Images; 387: Lezh/E+/Getty Images; 388: Newscom; 389: Sidea Revuz/Science Source; 390: Alexei Zaycev/Getty Images

Chapter 14 395: Phase4Photography/Fotolia; 396: Peter Bernik/Shutterstock; 397: By Ian Miles-Flashpoint Pictures/Alamy; 399: Centers for Disease Control and Prevention; 399: Western Ophthalmic Hospital/Science Source; 400: SPL/Science Source; 400: Martin M. Rotker/Science Source; 400: Science Source; 401: Center for Disease Control Prevention; 401: Custom Medical Stock Photo; 402: Centers for Disease Control and Prevention; 402: Dr. P. Marazzi/Science Source; 403: Pixtal/Glow Images; 404: Eye of Science/Science Source; 406: Kevin Foy/Alamy; 407: Nick UT/AP Images; 407: Shashank Bengali/MCT/Newscom; 409: Brandon Brown/Getty Images

Focus On: Understanding Your Health Inheritance 411: Blend Images/Fotolia; 413: Getty images; 413: Science Source; 414: L. Willatt/Science Source; 414: Spotmatik/Alamy; 416: Friedrich Stark/Alamy; 416: Science Source; 417: Jack Hollingsworth/Superstock; 418: Christina Kennedy/Alamy; 418: Marcel Jancovic/Shutterstock; 420: Leila Cutler/Alamy

Chapter 15 422: Tyler Olson/Shutterstock; 432: Stockbroker/MBI/Alamy; 433: Radius Images/Alamy; 434: Moodboard/Alamy; 436: Julien Bastide/Shutterstock; 437: Ariusz Nawrocki/Getty Images; 438: Moodboard/Getty Images; 438: Thinkstock/Getty Images; 440: Levent Konuk/Shutterstock; 440: Red Images, LLC/Alamy; 441: Max Delson/Martins Santos/E+/Getty Images

Focus On: Minimizing Your Risk for Diabetes 444: Bikeriderlondon/Shutterstock; 445: Eugene Bochkarev/Getty Images; 445: Kamdyn R Switzer/Cal Sport Media/Newscom; 448: Ted Foxx/Alamy; 449: William Perugini/Shutterstock; 450: Elina Manninen/Getty Images; 451: Paul Parker/Science Source; 451: VCM/Alamy; 452: Brian Jackson/Getty Images; 453: Jerilee Bennett/KRT/Newscom

Chapter 16 455: T.Tulik/Fotolia; 457: Science Source; 459: Dawn Poland/Getty Images; 459: Getty Images; 461: Altrendo Images/Getty Images; 462: CHASSENET/BSIP/BSIP SA/Alamy; 463: Garo/Science Source; 466: Digital Vision/Thinkstock; 466: Dr P. Marazzi/Science Source; 466: James Stevenson/Science Source; 466: Science Source; 468: dotshock/Shutterstock; 469: David Sacks/Getty Images; 472: Martin Dohrn/Science Source; 473: W. G. Murray/Alamy; 474: ERproductions Ltd/Blend Images/Alamy; 475: Martin Shields/Alamy

Chapter 17 478: Wavebreak Media Ltd./Alloy/Corbis; 479: All Over Images/Alamy; 480: Alexander Tsiaras/Science Source; 481: Andrey Popov/Getty Images; 482: Custom Medical Stock Photo/Alamy; 483: Eric Audras/Photo Alto/Alamy; 484: Ian Hooton/Science Photo Library/Alamy; 486: Vanja Gavric/Alamy; 488: Alamy; 489: Gladskikh Tatiana/Shutterstock; 493: Jack Sullivan/Alamy; 494: Simarik/Getty Images; 495: Gautier Willaume/Shutterstock

Chapter 18 499: Brooklyn Production/Flame/Corbis; 500: Tom Merton/OJO Images/Alamy; 502: Jiang Jin/Superstock; 503: Tatiana Popova/Shutterstock; 505: Alamy; 508: Jo Unruh/Getty Images; 510: Thomas Boehm/Alamy; 510: Thomas Boehm/Alamy; 511: Monkey Business Images/Shutterstock; 513: Rayman/Getty Images; 514: PhotoEdit; 515: Alisa/Shutterstock; 515: Elena Elisseeva/Shutterstock; 515: Joanna Wnuk/Shutterstock; 515: Shapiso/Shutterstock; 515: WEK/iStockphoto/Getty images; 517: Jochen Tack/Alamy; 517: Tetra Images/Alamy; 520: Alamy; 522: Fotosearch/AGE Fotostock

Chapter 19 526: Ana Blazic Pavlovic/Fotolia; 528: Jochen Tack/Alamy; 530: Catherine Ursillo/Science Source; 531: D. Hurst/Alamy; 533: Africa Studio/Shutterstock; 534: deanmillar/Getty Images; 537: Bill Aron/PhotoEdit; 538: The Sentinel/Jason Malmont/AP Images; 539: Roy McMahon/Corbis/Glow Images; 540: Hemant Mehta/Getty Images; 541: Michael Dwyer/Alamy; 542: Tariq Zehawi/KRT/Newscom; 543: A. Ramey/PhotoEdit; 544: Daniel Deitschel/cosmonaut/Getty Images; 544: Eric Ferguson/Getty Images

Focus On: Reducing Your Risk of Unintentional Injury 547: vadymvdrobot/Fotolia; 548: Radius Images/Alamy; 549: Paul Conklin/PhotoEdit; 549: Presselect/Alamy; 551: Pearson Education; 551: Stephen Bonk/Shutterstock; 552: PNC/Getty Images; 554: Jeff Greenberg/PhotoEdit; 556: Hybrid Images/AGE Fotostock; 557: Ian Hooton/Science Photo Library/Alamy; 557: Science Photo Library/Alamy

Chapter 20 560: Frank and Helena/Cultura/Corbis; 563: Brianindia/Alamy; 564: Brent Winebrenner/Getty Images; 566: Science Source; 568: Steve Froebe/Getty Images; 571: Dave King/DK Images; 572: Qaphotos/Alamy; 575: Image Source/Corbis; 576: Patrick Lane/Somos Images/Corbis/Glow Images; 578: John Henley/Blend Images/Alamy; 579: Chine Nouvelle/SIPA/Newscom; 580: Getty Images; 580: Thinkstock/Getty Images

Chapter 21 583: Caroline Woodham/Digital Vision/Getty Images; 584: Ronnie Kaufman/Blend Images/Getty Images; 585: Lia Toby/Wenn/Newscom; 586: Markos Dolopikos/Alamy; 587: Moodboard/Corbis; 589: Elnur/Shutterstock; 590: Alamy; 592: Jupiterimages/Comstock Images/Getty Images; 593: Monkey Business Images/Shutterstock; 596: Image Source/Corbis; 597: Matthew Plexman/Masterfile; 599: PhotoEdit

INDEX

A

B

C

D

E

F

G

H

J

K

L

M

N

O

P

Q

R

S

T

U

V

W

X

Y

Z

BEHAVIOR CHANGE CONTRACT

Complete the Assess Yourself questionnaire. After reviewing your results and considering the various factors that influence your decisions, choose a health behavior that you would like to change, starting this quarter or semester. Sign the contract at the bottom to affirm your commitment to making a healthy change and ask a friend to witness it.

My behavior change will be:

____

My long-term goal for this behavior change is:

____

These are three obstacles to change (things that I am currently doing or situations that contribute this behavior to make it harder to change):

1. ____
2. ____
3. ____

The strategies I will use to overcome these obstacles are:

1. ____
2. ____
3. ____

Resources I will use to help me change this behavior include:

a friend/partner/relative: _______________________________

a school-based resource: _______________________________

a community-based resource: _______________________________

a book or reputable website: _______________________________

In order to make my goal more attainable, I have devised these short-term goals.

short-term goal	target date	reward

When I make the long-term behavior change described above, my reward will be:

____ target date _______________

I intend to make the behavior change described above. I will use the strategies and rewards to achieve the goals that will contribute to a healthy behavior change.

Signed: _______________________________ Witness: _______________________________